D1567665

CHRONIC CORONARY ARTERY DISEASE

A Companion to Braunwald's Heart Disease

CHRONIC CORONARY ARTERY DISEASE

A Companion to Braunwald's Heart Disease

James A. de Lemos, MD
Professor of Medicine
University of Texas Southwestern Medical Center
Dallas, Texas

Torbjørn Omland, MD, PhD, MPH
Professor of Medicine
University of Oslo
Oslo, Norway

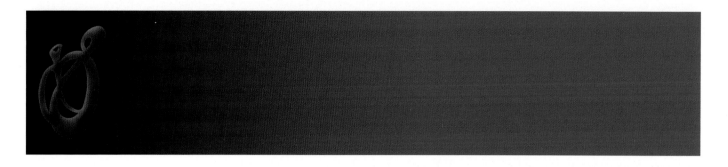

ELSEVIER

1600 John F. Kennedy Blvd.
Ste 1800
Philadelphia, PA 19103-2899

CHRONIC CORONARY ARTERY DISEASE:
A COMPANION TO BRAUNWALD'S HEART DISEASE ISBN: 978-0-323-42880-4

Copyright © 2018 by Elsevier, Inc. All rights reserved.

Cover images:
Optical coherence tomographic image from Tearney GJ, Regar E, Akasaka T, et al. Consensus standards for acquisition, measurement, and reporting of intravascular optical coherence tomography studies: a report from the International Working Group for Intravascular Optical Coherence Tomography Standardization and Validation. J Am Coll Cardiol 2012;59:1058-72.

Intravascular ultrasound study courtesy of sfam_photo, © Shutterstock; Stenosis of the left anterior descending coronary artery on angiography courtesy of Kalewa, © Shutterstock; Coronary Artery Bypass Graphs on Cardiac CT courtesy of wr588xlwnxj4cs, © 123RF.COM

No part of this publication may be reproduced or transmitted in any form or by any means, electronic or mechanical, including photocopying, recording, or any information storage and retrieval system, without permission in writing from the publisher. Details on how to seek permission, further information about the Publisher's permissions policies and our arrangements with organizations such as the Copyright Clearance Center and the Copyright Licensing Agency, can be found at our website: www.elsevier.com/permissions.

This book and the individual contributions contained in it are protected under copyright by the Publisher (other than as may be noted herein).

Notices

Knowledge and best practice in this field are constantly changing. As new research and experience broaden our understanding, changes in research methods, professional practices, or medical treatment may become necessary.

Practitioners and researchers must always rely on their own experience and knowledge in evaluating and using any information, methods, compounds, or experiments described herein. In using such information or methods they should be mindful of their own safety and the safety of others, including parties for whom they have a professional responsibility.

With respect to any drug or pharmaceutical products identified, readers are advised to check the most current information provided (i) on procedures featured or (ii) by the manufacturer of each product to be administered, to verify the recommended dose or formula, the method and duration of administration, and contraindications. It is the responsibility of practitioners, relying on their own experience and knowledge of their patients, to make diagnoses, to determine dosages and the best treatment for each individual patient, and to take all appropriate safety precautions.

To the fullest extent of the law, neither the Publisher nor the authors, contributors, or editors, assume any liability for any injury and/or damage to persons or property as a matter of products liability, negligence or otherwise, or from any use or operation of any methods, products, instructions, or ideas contained in the material herein.

Library of Congress Cataloging-in-Publication Data
Names: De Lemos, James A., editor. | Omland, Torbjørn, editor.
Title: Chronic coronary artery disease : a companion to Braunwald's heart disease / [edited by] James de Lemos, Torbjørn Omland.
Other titles: Complemented by (expression): Braunwald's heart disease. 10th edition.
Description: Philadelphia, PA : Elsevier, [2018] | Complemented by: Braunwald's heart disease / edited by Douglas L. Mann, Douglas P. Zipes, Peter Libby, Robert O. Bonow, Eugene Braunwald. 10th edition. [2015]. | Includes bibliographical references and index.
Identifiers: LCCN 2016036816 | ISBN 9780323428804 (hardcover : alk. paper)
Subjects: | MESH: Coronary Artery Disease
Classification: LCC RC685.C6 | NLM WG 300 | DDC 616.1/23–dc23 LC record available at https://lccn.loc.gov/2016036816

Executive Content Strategist: Dolores Meloni
Senior Content Development Specialist: Margaret Nelson
Publishing Services Manager: Patricia Tannian
Senior Project Manager: Cindy Thoms
Book Designer: Renee Duenow

Printed in China

Last digit is the print number: 9 8 7 6 5 4 3 2 1

Working together to grow libraries in developing countries

www.elsevier.com • www.bookaid.org

To my wife, Zena, and children, Nick, Mikaela, and Ben
Thank you for your constant support and love and for making sure I always stay focused on the things that really matter.

James A. de Lemos

To Anne Karin, and to my children, Dagne, Åsne, Tarjei, and Erlend
In memory of my father, Geirmund

Torbjørn Omland

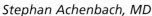

Contributors

Stephan Achenbach, MD
Professor of Medicine
Department of Cardiology
Friedrich-Alexander-Universitat Erlangen-Nurnberg
Erlangen, Germany

Krishna G. Aragam, MD
Fellow in Cardiovascular Medicine
Massachusetts General Hospital
Boston, Massachusetts, USA

Suzanne V. Arnold, MD, MHA
Associate Professor of Medicine
University of Missouri-Kansas City
Department of Cardiology
St. Luke's Mid America Heart Institute
Kansas City, Missouri, USA

Magnus Bäck, MD, PhD
Associate Professor of Cardiology
Department of Cardiology
Karolinska University Hospital
Center for Molecular Medicine
Karolinska Institutet
Stockholm, Sweden

Michael J. Blaha, MD, MPH
Assistant Professor of Medicine
Director of Clinical Research
Division of Cardiology
Johns Hopkins Ciccarone Center for the Prevention of Heart Disease
Baltimore, Maryland, USA

Stefan Blankenberg, MD
Professor of Internal Medicine
Director
Clinic for General and Interventional Cardiology
University Heart Center Hamburg
Hamburg, Germany

Roger S. Blumenthal, MD
The Kenneth Jay Pollin Professor of Cardiology
Johns Hopkins Professor of Medicine and Epidemiology
Director
Ciccarone Center for the Prevention of Heart Disease
Baltimore, Maryland, USA

Paolo G. Camici, MD
Professor of Cardiology
Vita Salute University and San Raffaele Hospital
Milan, Italy

Mina K. Chung, MD
Professor of Medicine
Cleveland Clinic Lerner College of Medicine
Case Western Reserve University
Staff, Cardiovascular Medicine
Cleveland Clinic
Cleveland, Ohio, USA

Joaquin E. Cigarroa, MD
Associate Professor of Medicine
Oregon Health and Science University
Knight Cardiovascular Institute
Portland, Oregon, USA

Filippo Crea, MD
Professor of Cardiology
Department of Cardiovascular Sciences
Catholic University of the Sacred Heart
Rome, Italy

Karina W. Davidson, PhD, MASc
Professor of Medicine and Psychiatry
Vice Dean, Organizational Effectiveness
Chief Academic Officer
New York Presbyterian Hospital-Columbia University College of Physicians and Surgeons
New York, New York, USA

Alban De Schutter, MD, MSc
Interventional Cardiology Fellow
New York University Langone Medical Center
New York, New York

Marcelo F. Di Carli, MD
Assistant Professor of Radiology and Medicine
Harvard Medical School
Chief of Nuclear Medicine
Brigham and Women's Hospital
Boston, Massachusetts, USA

Pamela S. Douglas, MD, MACC
Ursula Geller Professor of Research in Cardiovascular Disease
Department of Medicine (Cardiology)
Duke University School of Medicine
Durham, North Carolina, USA

Gregory Ducrocq, MD, PhD
Department of Cardiology
Bichat Hospital
Assistance Publique Hopitaux de Paris
Paris, France

Connor A. Emdin, HBSc
Broad Institute of Massachusetts Institute of Technology and Harvard
Cambridge, Massachusetts, USA

Obi Emeruwa, MD, MBA
Postdoctoral Resident
Department of Medicine
New York Presbyterian Hospital-Columbia University Medical Center
New York, New York, USA

Jonathan R. Enriquez, MD
Associate Professor of Medicine
Division of Cardiology
University of Missouri- Kansas City
Director, Coronary Care Unit
Truman Medical Center
Kansas City, Missouri, USA

William F. Fearon, MD
Professor of Medicine
Director of Interventional Cardiology
Stanford University Medical Center
Stanford, California, USA

Christopher B. Fordyce, MD, MSc
Clinical Assistant Professor
Division of Cardiology
University of British Columbia
Associate Director
Cardiac Intensive Care Unit
Vancouver General Hospital
Vancouver, British Columbia, Canada

Thomas A. Gaziano, MD, MHS, MSc
Assistant Professor
Harvard Medical School
Physician
Cardiovascular Medicine
Brigham and Women's Hospital
Boston, Massachusetts, USA

Bernard Gersh, MB, ChB, DPhil
Professor of Medicine
Mayo Clinic College of Medicine
Rochester, Minnesota, USA

Gitsios Gitsioudis, MD
Department of Cardiology
Friedrich-Alexander-Universitat Erlangen-Nurnberg
Erlangen, Germany

Yuanlin Guo, MD
Professor of Cardiology
David Geffen School of Medicine at UCLA
Los Angeles, California, USA
National Center for Cardiovascular Disease and FU WAI Hospital
Beijing, China

Rory Hachamovitch, MD
Staff Cardiologist
Department of Cardiovascular Medicine
Cardiovascular Imaging Section
Cleveland Clinic
Cleveland, Ohio, USA

Göran K. Hansson, MD, PhD
Professor of Cardiovascular Research
Department of Medicine and Center for Molecular Medicine
Karolinska University Hospital
Karolinska Institute
Stockholm, Sweden

Kristopher Heinzman, MD
Assistant Professor of Medicine
University of Texas Dell Medical School
Director of Clinical Electrophysiology
Seton Heart Institute
Austin, Texas, USA

Timothy D. Henry, MD
Director, Division of Cardiology
Lee and Harold Kapelovitz Chair in Research Cardiology
Cedars-Sinai Medical Center
Los Angeles, California, USA

Ayman A. Hussein, MD
Department of Cardiovascular Medicine
Heart and Vascular Institute
Section of Cardiac Electrophysiology and Pacing
Cleveland Clinic
Cleveland, Ohio, USA

Jesper K. Jensen, MD, PhD
Department of Cardiology
Aarhus University Hospital
Skejby, Denmark

E. Marc Jolicoeur, MD, MSc, MHS
Associate Professor of Medicine
Université de Montréal
Interventional Cardiologist
Montreal Heart Institute
Montréal, Quebec, Canada

Sekar Kathiresan, MD
Clinical Cardiologist and Human Geneticist
Director of Preventive Cardiology
Center for Human Genetic Research
Massachusetts General Hospital
Boston, Massachusetts, USA

Rajdeep S. Khattar, DM
Consultant Cardiologist and Head of Adult Echocardiography
Department of Cardiology and Echocardiography Laboratory
Royal Brompton and Harefield NHS Trust
Honorary Clinical Senior Lecturer
Cardiovascular Biomedical Research Unit
National Heart and Lung Institute, Imperial College
London, United Kingdom

Amit V. Khera, MD
Associate Professor of Internal Medicine
Director, Preventive Cardiology Program
University of Texas Southwestern Medical Center
Dallas, Texas

Mikhail Kosiborod, MD
Professor of Medicine
Department of Cardiology
Saint Luke's Mid America Heart Institute
University of Missouri-Kansas City
Kansas City, Missouri, USA

Lawrence Kwon, MD
Cardiology/Hypertension Research Fellow
Icahn School of Medicine at Mount Sinai and James J. Peters VA Medical Center
Bronx, New York, USA

Carl J. Lavie, MD
Professor of Medicine
Medical Director, Cardiac Rehabilitation
Department of Cardiovascular Disease
John Ochsner Heart and Vascular Institute
New Orleans, Louisiana, USA
Department of Preventive Medicine
Pennington Biomedical Research Center
Baton Rouge, Louisiana, USA

Matthew Lawlor, MD
Clinical Fellow in Medicine
Brigham and Women's Hospital
Boston, Massachusetts, USA

Steven P. Marso, MD
Chief Medical Officer of Cardiovascular Services
HCA Midwest Health Research Medical Center
Kansas City, Missouri, USA

Seth S. Martin, MD, MHS
Assistant Professor of Medicine (Cardiology)
Ciccarone Center for the Prevention of Heart Disease
Johns Hopkins Hospital
Baltimore, Maryland, USA

Nikolaus Marx, MD
Professor of Medicine/Cardiology
Head of the Department of Internal Medicine
University Hospital Aachen
Aachen, Germany

Puja K. Mehta, MD
Assistant Professor of Medicine
Director of Women's Translational Cardiovascular Research
Emory Women's Heart Center
Emory University
Atlanta, Georgia, USA

C. Noel Bairey Merz, MD
Professor of Medicine
Women's Guild Endowed Chair in Women's Health
Director, Barbra Streisand Women's Heart Center
Director, Linda Joy Pollin Women's Heart Health Program
Director, Preventive Cardiac Center
Barbra Streisand Women's Heart Center
Cedars-Sinai Medical Center
Los Angeles, California, USA

Erin D. Michos, MD, MHS
Associate Professor of Medicine (Cardiology) and Epidemiology
Johns Hopkins Ciccarone Center for Prevention of Heart Disease
Baltimore, Maryland, USA

Richard V. Milani, MD
Chief Clinical Transformation Officer
Vice-Chairman
Cardiovascular Diseases
Ochsner Health System
New Orleans, Louisiana, USA

Christopher J. O'Donnell, MD, MPH
Associate Clinical Professor
Harvard Medical School
Associate Director, Framingham Heart Study
Senior Advisor to the Director of NHLBI for Genome Research
Chief, Cardiovascular Epidemiology and Human Genomics Branch
NHLBI Division of Intramural Research
Boston, Massachusetts, USA

Lionel Opie, MD, DPhil (Oxon), DSc
Emeritus Professor and Scholar
Hatter Cardiovascular Institute for Research in Africa
University of Cape Town and Groote Schuur Hospital
Observatory, Cape Town
Western Cape, South Africa

Shailja V. Parikh, MD
Assistant Professor of Medicine
Division of Cardiology
University of Missouri- Kansas City
Director, Cardiac Rehab
Truman Medical Center
Kansas City, Missouri, USA

Eva Prescott, MD, DMSc
Clinical Professor
Department of Cardiology
Bispebjerg Hospital, University of Copenhagen
Copenhagen, Denmark

Sebastian Reith, MD
Department of Cardiology
University Hospital RWTH Aachen
Aachen, Germany

Ornella E. Rimoldi, MD
Senior Investigator
Institute of Molecular Bioimaging and Physiology
Consiglio Nazionale delle Ricerche
Segrate, Italy

Jennifer G. Robinson, MD, MPH
Professor of Epidemiology
Departments of Epidemiology and Medicine
University of Iowa
Director, Prevention Intervention Center
Department of Epidemiology
College of Public Health
Iowa City, Iowa, USA

George Rodgers, MD
Assistant Professor of Medicine
Seton Heart Institute
University of Texas Dell Medical School
Austin, Texas, USA

Anand Rohatgi, MD, MSCS
Associate Professor of Internal Medicine
Internal Medicine/Cardiology
University of Texas Southwestern Medical Center
Dallas, Texas, USA

Clive Rosendorff, MD, PhD, DScMed
Professor of Medicine
Icahn School of Medicine at Mount Sinai
New York, New York, USA
Physician and Director, Graduate Medical Education
Medicine
James J. Peters VA Medical Center
Bronx, New York, USA

Sheila Sahni, MD
Interventional Cardiology Fellow
David Geffen School of Medicine at UCLA
Los Angeles, California, USA

Daniel Sedehi, MD
Assistant Professor of Medicine
Knight Cardiovascular Institute
Oregon Health and Science University
Portland, Oregon, USA

Roxy Senior, MD
Professor of Clinical Cardiology
Consultant Cardiologist and Director of Echocardiography
Department of Cardiology and Echocardiography Laboratory
Royal Brompton Hospital and Harefield NHS Trust
Cardiovascular Biomedical Research Unit
National Heart and Lung Institute
Imperial College
London, United Kingdom

Philippe Gabriel Steg, MD
Professor of Cardiology
Universite Paris-Diderot
Professor, National Heart and Lung Institute
Imperial College
London, United Kingdom

Lauren Wasson, MD, MPH
Assistant Professor of Medicine
Division of Cardiology
Columbia University Medical Center
New York, New York, USA

Karol E. Watson, MD, PhD
Professor of Medicine/Cardiology
David Geffen School of Medicine at UCLA
Los Angeles, California, USA

Janet Wei, MD
Assistant Medical Director of the Biomedical Imaging Research Institute
Barbra Streisand Women's Heart Center
Cedars-Sinai Medical Center
Los Angeles, California, USA

Peter W. F. Wilson, MD
Professor of Medicine
Atlanta VA Medical Center and Clinical Cardiovascular Research Institute
Emory School of Medicine
Atlanta, Georgia, USA

Tanja Zeller, MD
Professor for Genomics and Systems Biology
Clinic for General and Interventional Cardiology
University Heart Center Hamburg
Hamburg, Germany

Preface

The past 50 years have witnessed remarkable achievements in the treatment and prevention of coronary artery disease, the most common cause of death in industrialized society. As the mortality rates from acute myocardial infarction have fallen by more than 50% since the 1970s; coronary artery disease has increasingly become a chronic disease. Outcomes among patients with chronic ischemic heart disease are heterogeneous, with excellent survival in many, while other high-risk subsets are at notably increased risk for death or major complications. Managing the growing population of patients with chronic coronary disease requires understanding of the full clinical spectrum of coronary disease, ranging from patients with advanced, but asymptomatic disease to those with ischemic cardiomyopathy at risk for heart failure and sudden cardiac death. Importantly, in this chronic condition understanding the impact of angina and other symptoms on *quality* of life and functional status is particularly important. Paralleling the growth in the chronic coronary disease population is the rapid pace of progress with regard to preventive strategies, diagnostic modalities, and new treatment options.

In this companion to ***Braunwald's Heart Disease*** we provide comprehensive coverage of chronic coronary artery disease. This text includes 30 chapters that are designed to provide the clinical practitioner and researcher with in depth understanding of factors responsible for disease development, as well as immediately actionable information regarding all available diagnostic and treatment modalities. We have assembled a superb team of international contributors who have provided authoritative coverage of their areas of expertise.

The text is divided into four sections, beginning with an introductory section reviewing the epidemiology of chronic coronary artery disease, and providing a global perspective on the disease spectrum. This is followed by sections covering pathogenesis, clinical evaluation, and management. As compared with broad-based cardiovascular textbooks, this focused companion "dives deep" into this important topic area. For example, we include individual chapters on each available testing modality for evaluating coronary disease. These chapters are followed by integrative chapters that provide algorithms to help clinicians select among the various testing options.

The chapters on management of chronic coronary artery disease first set the stage by identifying the unique goals of therapy for the patient with chronic coronary disease and how these are different from the acute coronary syndrome setting. Given the heterogeneity of disease phenotypes and outcomes, risk assessment tools are critically important for guiding therapy. We thus include several state-of-the-art chapters that cover existing and emerging risk assessment tools. Although the relationship of adverse lifestyle factors with atherosclerosis development is well established, obesity is a "special case." The relationship between obesity and outcomes among patients with existing coronary artery disease is complex, and the text includes a chapter focused on the obesity paradox. The chapter on medical therapy covers not only those agents that have established efficacy, but also a series of new and investigational agents to reduce symptoms and improve outcomes. The role of coronary revascularization, including selection between percutaneous coronary intervention and bypass surgery, is covered in depth, as are options for patients with refractory angina who do not have revascularization options. Finally, angina in the absence of epicardial coronary disease is increasingly recognized, and this text will outline the pathophysiological basis for ischemia in these patients, as well as emerging diagnostic and treatment algorithms for this challenging patient subset.

This text will be an invaluable resource for practitioners who care for patients across the full spectrum of coronary disease, including those with prior myocardial infarction, those with symptomatic angina, and those simply at risk for developing coronary disease in the future. We expect that readers will use the information provided in these chapters to improve the care of their many patients with chronic coronary artery disease.

James A. de Lemos, MD
Torbjørn Omland, MD, PhD

Acknowledgments

We offer our sincere gratitude to those who have supported this companion volume for *Braunwald's Heart Disease*. First, and most important, we thank Dr. Braunwald for inviting us to contribute to his illustrious series. Second, we would like to recognize Margaret Nelson, Cindy Thoms, and Dolores Meloni from Elsevier, for keeping us (and our authors) on task and providing expert advice and guidance at every step. Finally, we thank the authors who contributed so much of their busy time and expertise to make this textbook such an important contribution. We extend our gratitude to each of you.

Sincerely,
James A. de Lemos, MD
Torbjørn Omland, MD, PhD

Contents

Video Contents

Braunwald's Heart Disease Family of Books

BRAUNWALD'S HEART DISEASE COMPANIONS

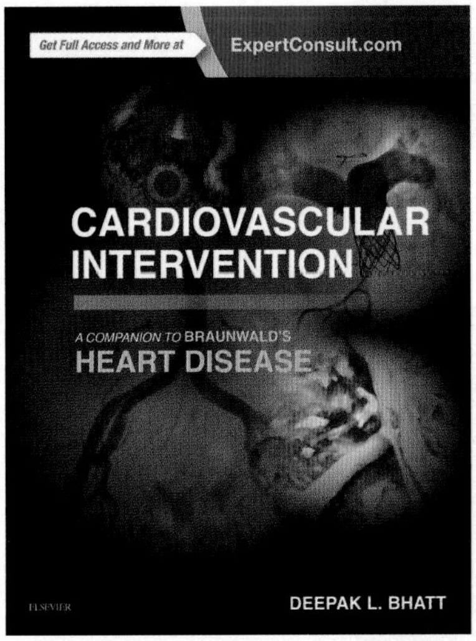

BHATT
Cardiovascular Intervention

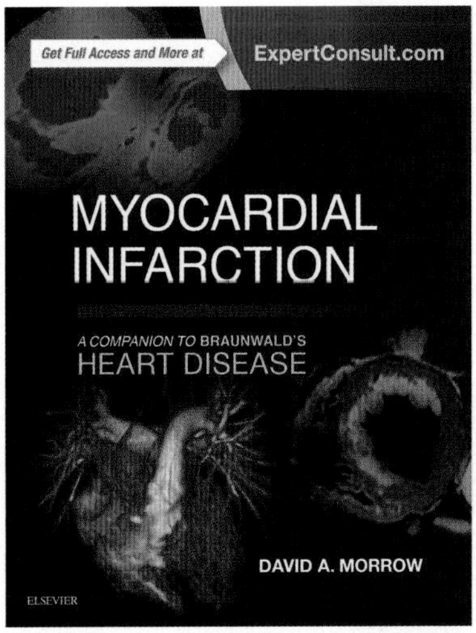

MORROW
Myocardial Infarction

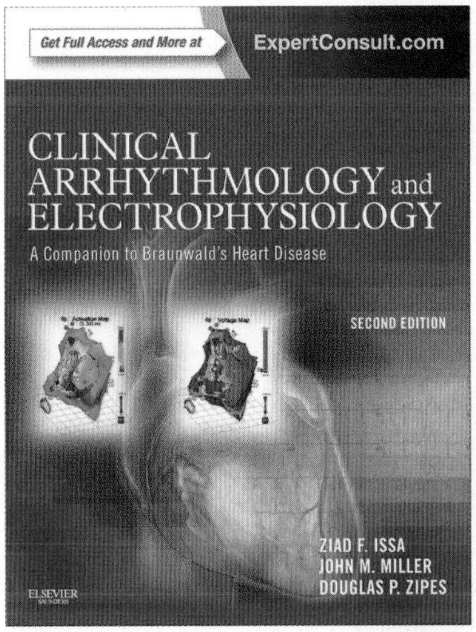

ISSA, MILLER, AND ZIPES
Clinical Arrhythmology and Electrophysiology

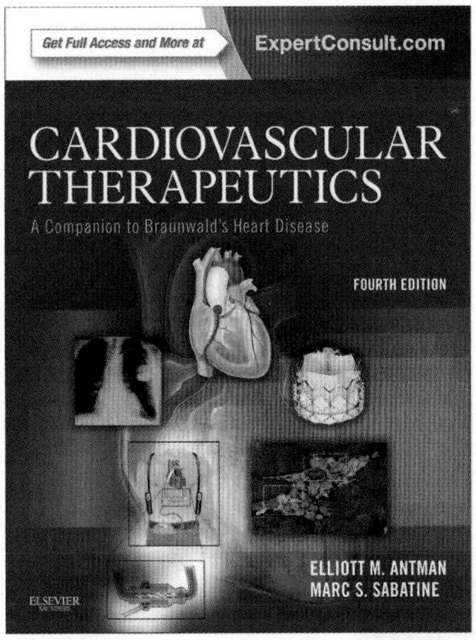

ANTMAN AND SABATINE
Cardiovascular Therapeutics

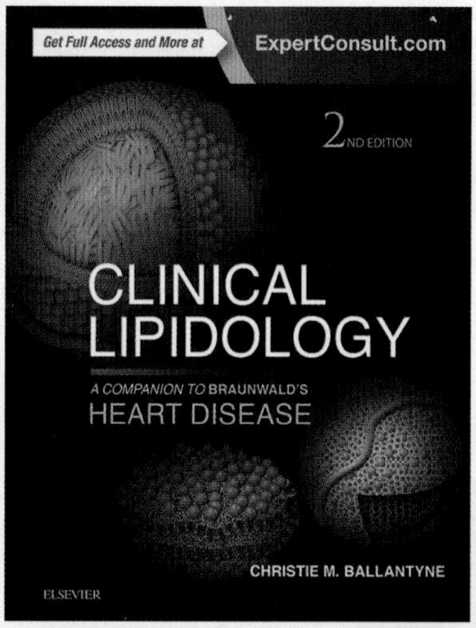

BALLANTYNE
Clinical Lipidology

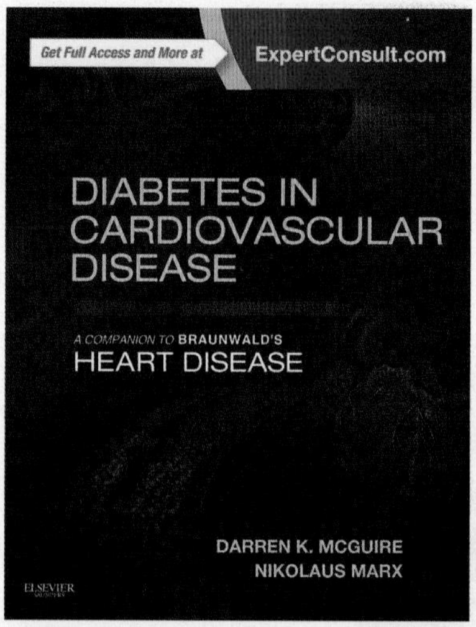

MCGUIRE AND MARX
Diabetes in Cardiovascular Disease

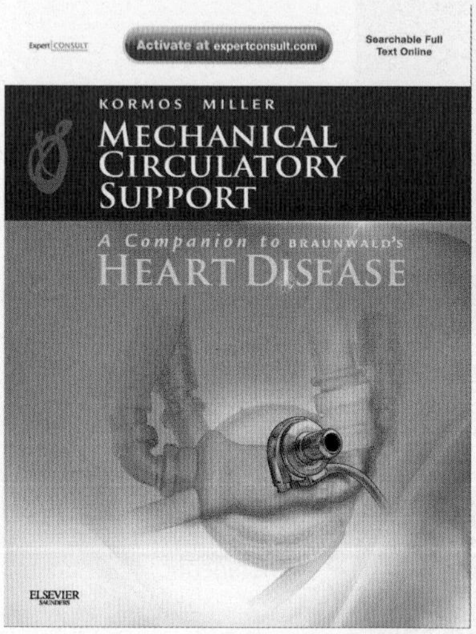

KORMOS AND MILLER
Mechanical Circulatory Support

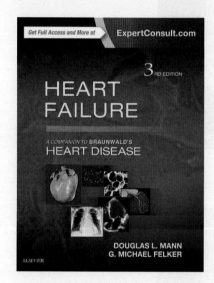

MANN AND FELKER
Heart Failure

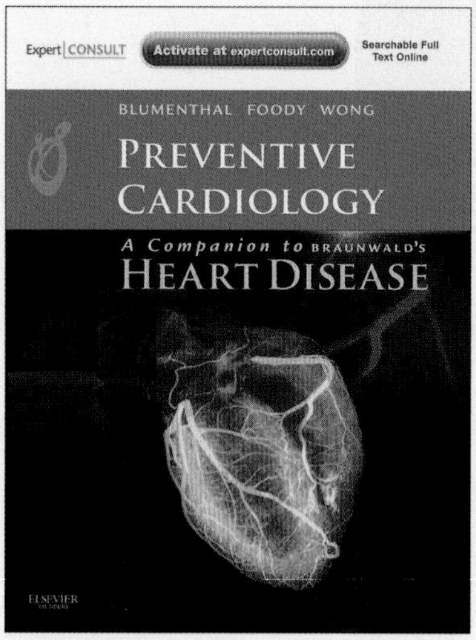

BLUMENTHAL, FOODY, AND WONG
Preventive Cardiology

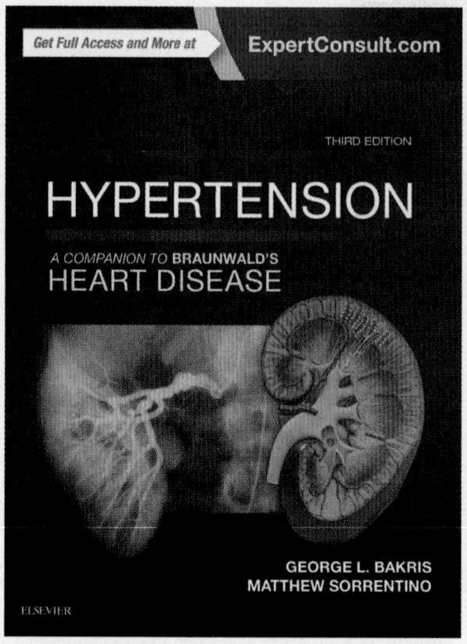

BAKRIS AND SORRENTINO
Hypertension

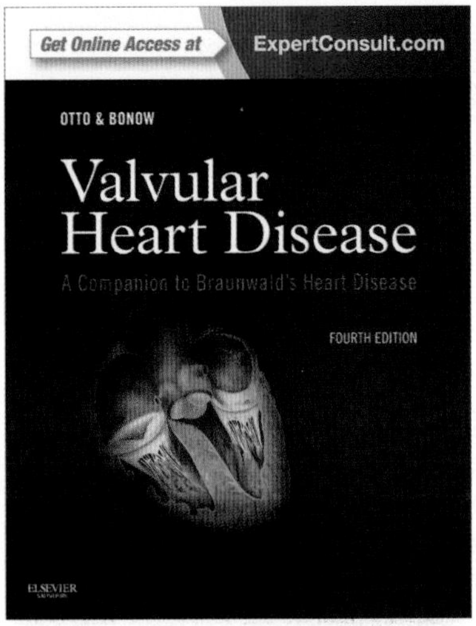

OTTO AND BONOW
Valvular Heart Disease

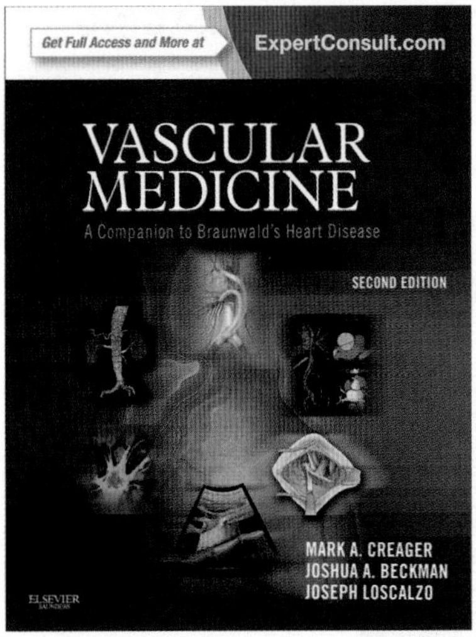

CREAGER, BECKMAN, AND LOSCALZO
Vascular Medicine

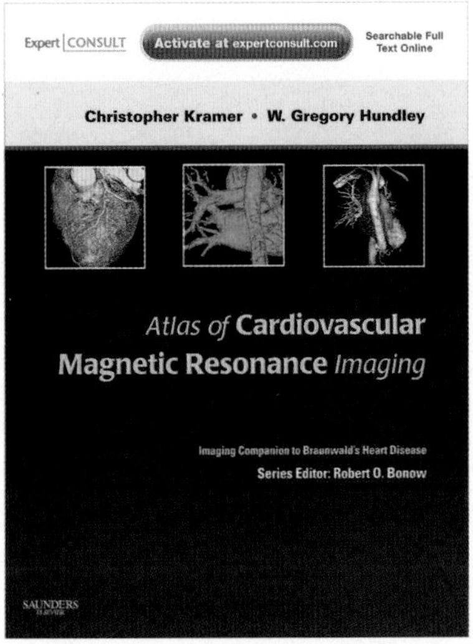

KRAMER AND HUNDLEY
Atlas of Cardiovascular Magnetic Resonance Imaging

BRAUNWALD'S HEART DISEASE REVIEW AND ASSESSMENT

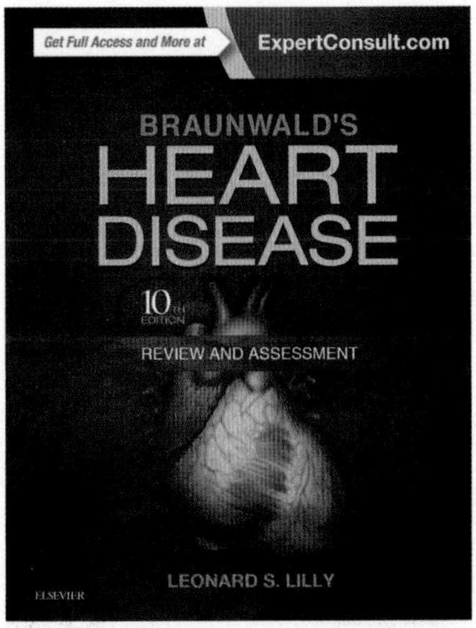

LILLY
Braunwald's Heart Disease Review and Assessment

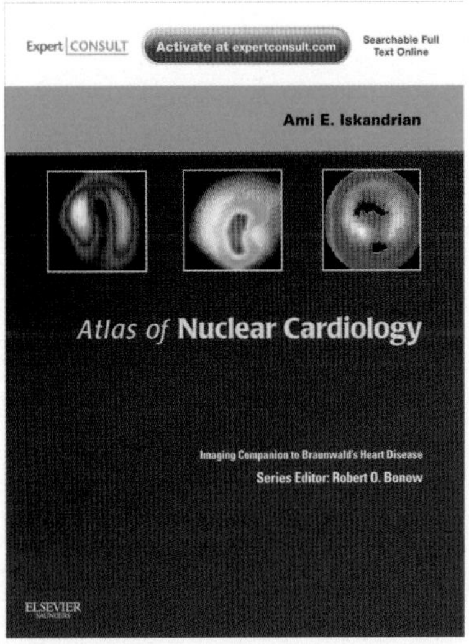

ISKANDRIAN AND GARCIA
Atlas of Nuclear Cardiology

BRAUNWALD'S HEART DISEASE IMAGING COMPANIONS

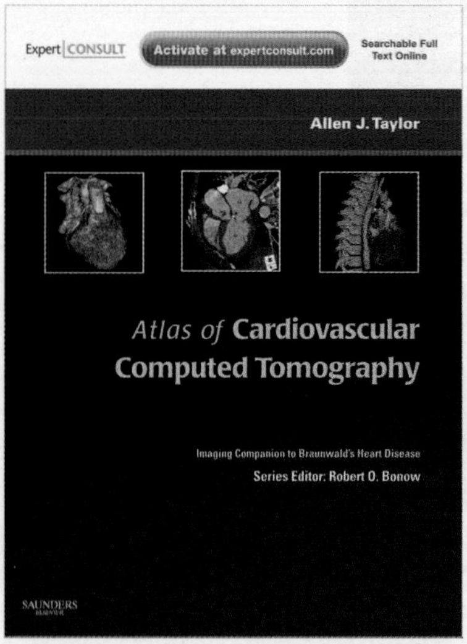

TAYLOR
Atlas of Cardiovascular Computer Tomography

COMING SOON!

SOLOMON
Essential Echocardiography

SECTION I

INTRODUCTION

1 Epidemiology of Chronic Coronary Artery Disease

Peter W.F. Wilson and Christopher J. O'Donnell

INTRODUCTION

Coronary artery disease (CAD) is a major cause of death and disability in developed countries. Although CAD mortality rates worldwide have declined over the past 4 decades, CAD remains responsible for approximately one-third or more of all deaths in individuals over age 35, and it has been estimated that nearly half of all middle-aged men and one-third of middle-aged women in the United States will develop clinical CAD.[1]

Population-based epidemiologic data and well-conducted surveys provide the best assessment of the CAD risk factors that contribute to the development of CAD outcomes. Such data are less encumbered by the unavoidable selection bias of clinical trials data. In addition, epidemiologic data provide critical information regarding targets for the primary and secondary prevention of CAD.

DEFINITIONS

The terms incidence, prevalence, coronary heart disease, CAD, and cardiovascular disease, as used in this chapter, are defined as follows:

Prevalence—The number of existing cases of a disease divided by the total population at a point in time.

Incidence—The number of new cases of a disease over a period of time divided by the population at risk. Incidence and prevalence are measures of disease burden in a population.

Coronary artery disease (CAD)—Often called coronary heart disease or CHD, is generally used to refer to the pathologic process affecting the coronary arteries (usually atherosclerosis). CAD includes the diagnoses of angina pectoris, myocardial infarction (MI), silent myocardial ischemia, and CAD mortality that result from CAD. Hard CAD endpoints generally include MI and CAD death. The term CHD is often used interchangeably with CAD.

CAD death—Includes sudden cardiac death (SCD) for circumstances when the death has occurred within 24 hours of the abrupt onset of symptoms, and the term non-SCD applies when the time course from the clinical presentation until the time of death exceeds 24 hours or has not been specifically identified.

Atherosclerotic cardiovascular disease (ASCVD, often shortened to CVD)—The pathologic process affecting the entire arterial circulation, not just the coronary arteries. Stroke, transient ischemic attacks, angina, MI, CAD death, claudication, and critical limb ischemia are manifestations of ASCVD.

Sources of Epidemiologic Data

Participants in observational studies are not necessarily under the care of clinicians, and generalizing research study or survey findings to clinical care should be undertaken with caution. For example, the observations in a report may be compiled over many years, the diagnosis may be self-reported or based on field survey methods, and it may be difficult to compare results across studies because of differences in methods. In addition, interpretation of the efficacy of treatments in observational studies can be difficult. Behavioral interventions and medications may be identified, but it can be difficult to be sure that the individual actually complied with what was prescribed or recommended.

Prevalence of Coronary Artery Disease

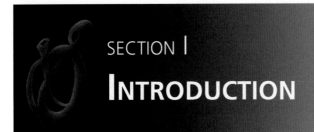

The 2016 Heart Disease and Stroke Statistics update of the American Heart Association (AHA) reports that 15.5 million adults (6.2% of the adult population) in the United States have CAD, including 7.6 million (2.8%) with MI and 8.2 million (3.3%) with angina pectoris. The self-reported National Health and Nutrition Examination Survey (NHANES) prevalence estimates for MI (Fig. 1.1) and angina pectoris (Fig. 1.2) increase with age for both women and men. Data from NHANES that rely on self-reported MI and angina from health interviews probably underestimate the actual prevalence of advanced CAD. Advanced occlusive CAD often exists with few symptoms or overt clinical manifestations.

Across the United States heart diseases head the list of direct health expenditures, costing approximately $100 billion per year. Approximately 60% of costs are attributable to hospitals, 16% to medications, 11% to physicians, 7% to nursing homes, 5% to home health care, and the remaining small percentage to other costs. Lost productivity due to heart diseases is estimated to cost society another $100 billion.[1]

There are 7 million healthcare discharges per year in the United States that have included cardiovascular procedures, and only obstetrical procedures are more common.[1] Approximately 7.5 million inpatient cardiovascular procedures are performed in the United States annually. Some of the inpatient cardiovascular procedures that are particularly relevant to ASCVD, listed in descending order from more common to less common along with the annual frequency, are cardiac catheterization (1,029,000 per year), percutaneous coronary intervention (500,000 per year), surgical cardiac revascularization (397,000 per year), and pacemaker implantation (370,000 per year).[1]

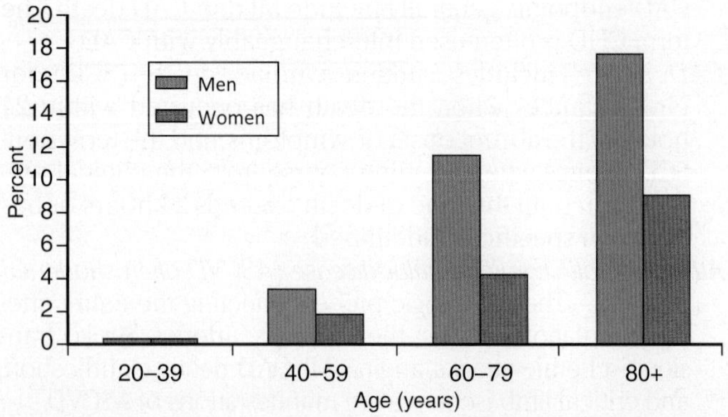

FIG. 1.1 Prevalence of myocardial infarction in US adults > 20 years of age. NHANES 2007–2012. *(From Mozaffarian D, Benjamin EJ, Go AS, et al. Heart Disease and Stroke Statistics—2016 update: a report from the American Heart Association.* Circulation. *2016;133(4):e38–e360; chart 19-1.)*

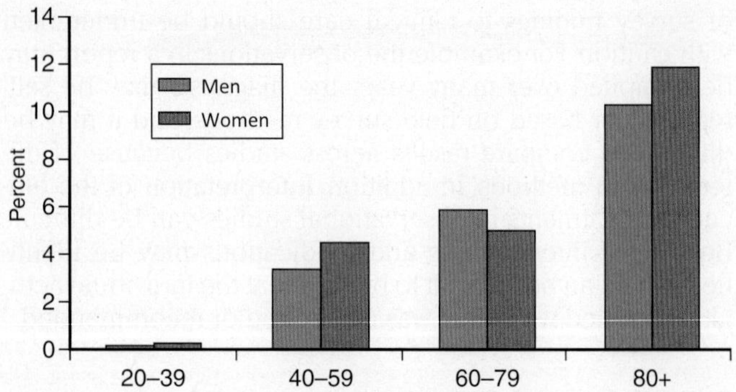

FIG. 1.2 Prevalence of self-reported angina pectoris in US adults >20 years of age. NHANES 2009–2012. *(From Mozaffarian D, Benjamin EJ, Go AS, et al. Heart Disease and Stroke Statistics—2016 update: a report from the American Heart Association.* Circulation. *2016;133(4):e38–e360; chart 19-9.)*

A Global Burden of Disease Study Group report from 2013 estimated that 17.3 million deaths worldwide in 2013 were related to ASCVD, a 41% increase since 1990.[2] Although the absolute numbers of ASCVD deaths had increased significantly since 1990, the age-standardized death rate decreased by 22% in the same period, primarily due to shifting age demographics and causes of death worldwide. In a 2009 report that used US NHANES data, MI prevalence was compared by sex in middle-aged individuals (35 to 54 years) during the 1988–1994 and 1999–2004 time periods.[3] Although MI prevalence was significantly greater in men than women in both time periods (2.5% vs 0.7% in 1988–1994 and 2.2% vs 1.0% in 1999–2004), the results suggested trends toward a decrease in prevalence for men and an increase in women.

Autopsy data have documented a reduced prevalence of anatomic CAD over time in both the general population and military personnel. In an analysis of 3832 autopsies performed on US military personnel (98% male, mean age 26 years) who died of combat or unintentional injuries between October 2001 and August 2011, the prevalence of CAD was 8.5%.[4] This represents a marked decline in the prevalence of autopsy-documented CAD compared with rates seen during the Korean War in the 1950s (77%) and the Vietnam War in the 1960s (45%).

Incidence

Historically, the incidence of ASCVD includes both morbid events (angina pectoris, MI) and death outcomes (cardiovascular disease death). Identification of morbid events can be challenging because assignment of an event requires review of hospital records and standardization of the adjudication process. This approach has been undertaken in cohort studies, registries, and occasionally in other groups such as adults followed in an insurance program. In addition, criteria for morbid events are in constant evolution. As an example, in the 1950s the diagnosis of an MI was largely based on electrocardiographic (ECG) information. Over time the diagnosis could be made on the basis of changes in blood tests such as troponin, as they have become increasingly more accurate, reliable, and capable of identifying smaller MIs than in the past.[5] Similarly, diagnosis of angina pectoris has evolved to be based on a composite of history and evaluation of ischemia with a variety of diagnostic modalities such as exercise and pharmacologic testing coupled with ECG and imaging—techniques that have led to greater accuracy.[6]

The following observations concerning lifetime incidence of CAD have been noted.

In Americans over 55 years of age, those with an optimal risk-factor profile (total cholesterol level < 180 mg/dL, blood pressure (BP) < 120/80 mm Hg, nonsmokers, no diabetes) had substantially lower risks of ASCVD death through the age of 80 years than participants with two or more major risk factors (4.7% vs 29.6% in men, 6.4% vs 20.5% in women). Those with an optimal risk-factor profile also had lower lifetime risks of fatal CHD or nonfatal MI (3.6% vs 37.5% among men, < 1% vs 18.3% among women) and fatal or nonfatal stroke (2.3% vs 8.3% among men, 5.3% vs 10.7% among women). Similar trends within risk-factor strata were observed among blacks and whites and across diverse birth cohorts (Table 1.1).[7] Berry et al. concluded that an individual's risk-factor burden translated into marked differences in the lifetime risk of cardiovascular disease, and these differences are consistent across race and birth cohorts.[7] For total coronary events, the incidence rises steeply with age, with women lagging behind men by 10 years.

Despite a lack of symptoms, the extent of nonobstructive CAD is associated with a worse prognosis compared to adults without CAD.[9,10] In a retrospective cohort study of American veterans without prior CAD who underwent coronary angiography and were followed for 1 year, the risk of MI over the ensuing year increased significantly and progressively in proportion to the extent of both nonobstructive (at least 1 stenosis ≥ 20% but < 70%) and obstructive (at least 1 stenosis ≥ 70%) CAD.[9]

Concerning the incidence of MI, the Atherosclerosis Risk in Communities (ARIC) Study in the United States has been a key source of information for the past 30 years, and recent results are shown in Fig. 1.3. Black men have the greatest incidence, followed by white men, black women, and white women. In general, women lag behind men in incidence by 20 years, but the sex ratio for incidence narrows with advancing age. The incidence at ages 65 to 94 versus ages 35 to 64 more than doubles in men and triples in women. In premenopausal women, serious manifestations of coronary disease, such as MI and SCD, are relatively rare.[1] Marked disparities in ASCVD health and treatment persist between the sexes, and more women die from ASCVD than men.[1] Despite a recent overall decline in ASCVD death rates, the burden of ASCVD death rates for women younger than 55 years has not changed over the last 2 decades.[11] ASCVD risk factors are more prevalent among women, as is mortality from acute MI.[12] It is unclear if these disparities persist due to pathophysiologic factors that affect ASCVD risk uniquely in women, or if they are related to differences in how detection and treatment algorithms are administered in women versus men.

TABLE 1.1 Lifetime Risk of Cardiovascular Disease (CVD) in Adults Without CVD at Age 55 Years

RISK FACTOR BURDEN	ATTAINED AGE 80 YEARS	ATTAINED AGE 90 YEARS
> 2 major risk factors	30%	42%
1 major risk factor	18%	32%
> 1 elevated risk factor	14%	28%
> 1 risk factor not optimal	9%	21%
All risk factors optimal	5%	18%

Data from Berry JD, Dyer A, Cai X, et al. Lifetime risks of cardiovascular disease. N Engl J Med. *2012;366(4):321–329.*

The incidence of CAD, especially CAD mortality, has decreased since the 1970s in developed countries.[13,14] Information on trends for total CAD that includes angina pectoris, MI, and coronary death is difficult to acquire. Only long-term cohort studies have such data, and the investigations have largely been concentrated in the United States. An analysis from the REasons for Geographic And Racial Differences in Stroke (REGARDS) study participants and Kaiser Permanente Southern California (KPSC) enrollees with baseline lipid measurements in 2003 to 2007 compared the recent experience to that for the ARIC study participants with baseline measurements in 1987 to 1989. The authors showed that CHD rates have declined in recent years and the association between lipids and CHD in contemporary studies may be attenuated by the preferential use of statins by high-risk individuals.[15]

Despite the declining incidence of CAD mortality in the United States, reductions in the incidence of MI have not been as large as might be expected.[16–18] In addition, the use of the more sensitive troponin assays, which began around 2000 and leads to the diagnosis of MI when less of the myocardium is infarcted, could potentially mask a reduction in MI incidence over time.

There has been a relative increase in non-ST elevation MI (NSTEMI) in relation to ST elevation MI (STEMI) in recent years.[17,19] For example, a report from the National Registry of Myocardial Infarction reviewed over 2.5 million MIs between 1990 and 2006 and found that the proportion of MIs due to NSTEMI increased from 19% in 1994 to 59% in 2006. This change in proportion was associated with an absolute decrease in the incidence of STEMI and either a rise (using MI defined by either CK-MB or troponin criteria)

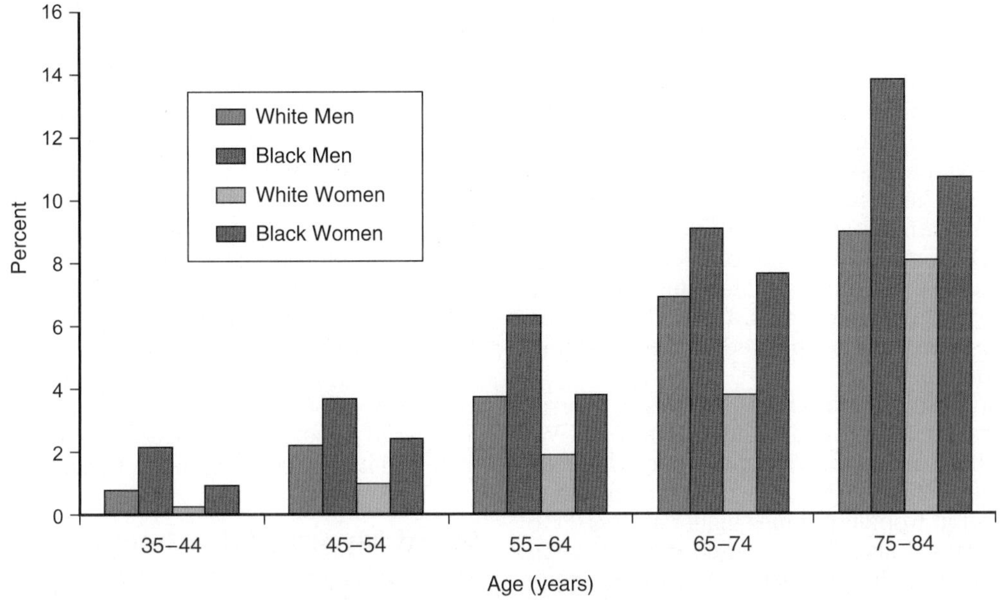

FIG. 1.3 Incidence of myocardial infarction in US adults > 35 years of age. ARIC Study 2007–2012. *(From Mozaffarian D, Benjamin EJ, Go AS, et al. Heart Disease and Stroke Statistics—2016 update: a report from the American Heart Association.* Circulation. *2016;133(4):e38–e360; chart 19-5.)*

TABLE 1.2 Worldwide Cardiovascular Disease (CVD) Death Rates

CVD DEATH RISK (PER 100,000/YEAR)	MEN	WOMEN
> 800	Belarus, Russian Federation, Ukraine	
600–800	Bulgaria	
400–600	Hungary	Ukraine, Russian Federation, Belarus
200–400	Croatia, Czechia, United States	Bulgaria, Romania, Hungary
100–200	United Kingdom, Austria, Taiwan, New Zealand, Belgium, Sweden, Italy, Portugal, Denmark, Spain, Japan, Netherlands, Australia, Norway, France, Switzerland, South Korea	Czechia, United States
0–100		Germany, New Zealand, United Kingdom, Austria, Belgium, Finland, Taiwan, Sweden, Portugal, Netherlands, Italy, Denmark, South Korea, Australia, Norway, Japan, Spain, Switzerland, Israel, France

Data from Mozaffarian D, Benjamin EJ, Go AS, et al. Heart Disease and Stroke Statistics—2016 update: a report from the American Heart Association. Circulation. *2016;133(4):e38–e360; Table 13-3.*

or no change (using MI defined by only CK-MB criteria) in the rate of NSTEMI.[20]

In summary, the incidence of ischemic CHD has declined in the United States over the past 40 years. Modern lab testing can identify smaller MIs than in the past, and the role of cholesterol levels has become more complex because of greater use of lipid-lowering medications.

Coronary Artery Disease Mortality

Heart disease mortality has declined since the 1970s in the United States and in regions where economies and healthcare systems are relatively advanced. Ischemic heart disease remains the number one cause of death in adults on a worldwide basis.[2] In a 2014 study using World Health Organization data from 49 countries in Europe and northern Asia, over 4 million annual deaths were attributable to ASCVD.[21] Current worldwide estimates for heart disease mortality show Eastern European countries have the highest ASCVD death rates (> 200 per 100,000/year), followed by an intermediate group that includes most countries with modern economies (100–200 per 100,000/year), and the lowest levels (0–100 per 100,000/year) are largely observed in European countries and a few non-European countries with advanced healthcare systems (Table 1.2). A detailed analysis of European country-specific data showed that CHD mortality rates dropped by more than 50% over the 1980–2009 interval, and the decline was observed across virtually all European countries for both sexes. The authors of the report concluded that the downward trends did not appear to show a plateau. Rather, CHD mortality was stable or continuing to decline across Europe.[22] Complementary analyses have been undertaken in the United States, and CHD mortality has been demonstrated to have peaked in the 1970s and declined since that date.[1]

The 2016 Heart Disease and Stroke Statistics update of the AHA shows that the 2013 overall death rate from ASCVD was 230 per 100,000/year and the CHD death rate is approximately 100 per 100,000/year (Fig. 1.4).[1] The death rate is higher in men than in women (3 times higher at ages 25 to 34, falling to 1.6 times at ages 75 to 84) and in blacks than in whites, an excess that disappears by age 75. Among the Hispanic population, coronary mortality is not as high as it is among blacks and whites.

The trends in mortality rates for ASCVD and CAD in men and women and in blacks and whites have fallen in most developed countries by 24% to 50% since 1975, although the decline has slowed since 1990. From 1996 to 2006 the ASCVD death rate declined by approximately 29%.[23] This trend has been associated with reductions in both total CAD and in the CAD case fatality rate.[14] The causes of the reduction in CAD mortality have been evaluated in adults between the ages of 25 and 84 in the United States from 1980 to 2000.[14] Approximately half of the decline was due to improvements in therapy, including secondary preventive measures after MI or revascularization, initial treatments for acute coronary syndromes, therapy for heart failure, and revascularization for chronic angina. The other half of this effect was due to changes in risk factors, including reductions in total cholesterol (24%), systolic BP (20%), smoking prevalence (12%), and physical inactivity (5%). These changes were partly offset by increases in body mass index (BMI) and the prevalence of diabetes, which together accounted for an 18% increase in the number of deaths.[13,14]

The international trends in CAD mortality are similar in many regions. Improvement in outcomes has been common in developed countries. Results have been variable in Eastern Europe, and some countries have shown an increase in CAD mortality in the early 1990s followed by a subsequent decline (Poland and the Czechia). The highest CAD mortality has been noted in the Russian Federation (330 and 154 per 100,000 in men and women, respectively, from 1995 to 1998). These values were similar to those in the period from 1985 to 1989. In Japan, CAD mortality has historically been much lower than in the United States and Europe. Mortality from CAD is expected to increase in developing countries (including China, India, sub-Saharan Africa, Latin America, and the Middle East), from an estimated 9 million in 1990 to a projected 19 million by 2020. This projected increase is thought to be a consequence of social and economic changes in non-Western countries, leading to decreased life expectancy, Westernized diets, physical inactivity, and increases in cigarette smoking.[2]

Silent Myocardial Ischemia and Infarction

Although many MIs appear to occur without warning, there is a large reservoir of detectable advanced silent CAD from which these apparently sudden events evolve. Such individuals may

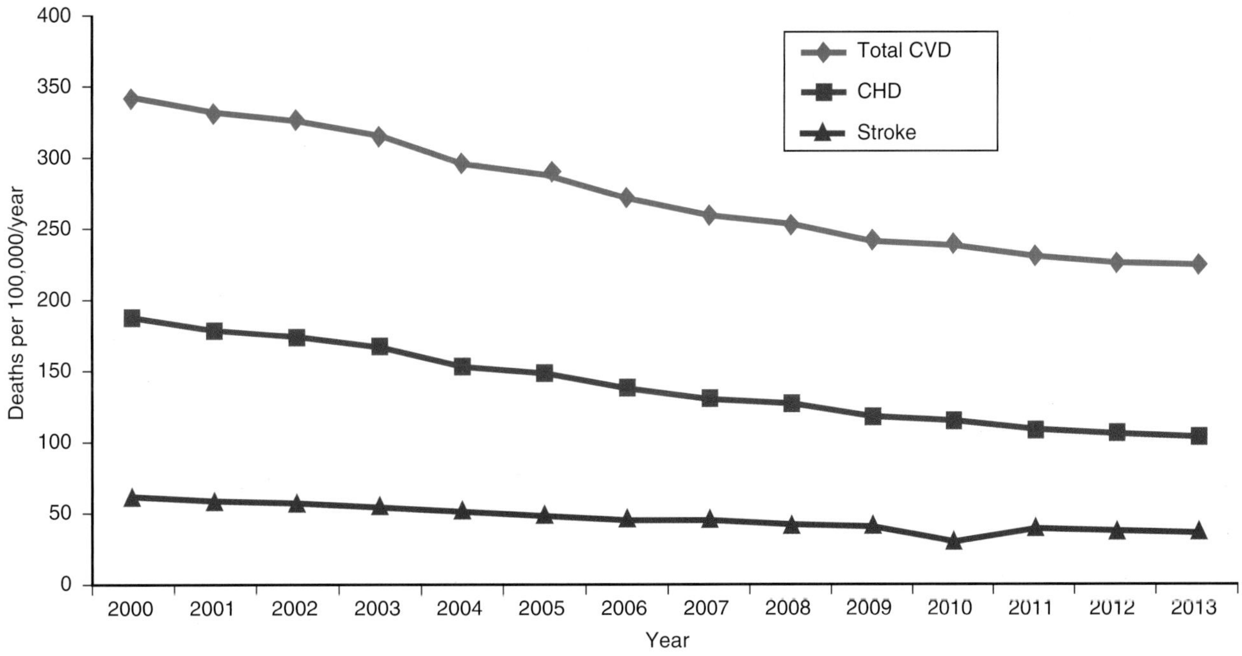

FIG. 1.4 US age-standardized death rates attributable to cardiovascular diseases 2000–2013. CVD, Cardiovascular disease; CHD, coronary heart disease. *(From Mozaffarian D, Benjamin EJ, Go AS, et al. Heart Disease and Stroke Statistics—2016 update: a report from the American Heart Association.* Circulation. *2016;133(4):e38–e360; chart 2-14.)*

have asymptomatic ischemic disease. The most specific ECG indication of silent myocardial ischemia is the development of a Q-wave MI in the absence of typical symptoms.[24,25] Diabetes mellitus is an established risk factor for unrecognized MI, and the Multiethnic Study of Atherosclerosis (MESA) investigators have described a higher prevalence of unrecognized MI in participants with impaired fasting glucose.[24] Researchers from Rotterdam have shown that the long-term prognosis for cardiovascular mortality and noncardiovascular mortality in men and women with unrecognized MI is worse than in those without MI.[25] Although the incidence of both unrecognized and recognized infarctions increases with the severity of hypertension, the fraction that goes undetected is substantially greater in hypertensive than in normotensive persons. This predisposition to hypertension persisted even when patients with diabetes, antihypertensive therapy, and left ventricular hypertrophy (LVH) were excluded.[26,27]

Sudden Cardiac Death

Survival after cardiac arrest is highly related to the type of treatment that is received immediately. The Resuscitation Outcomes Consortium has reported on the success of emergency therapy since 2006. Approximately 45% survival has been shown for bystander cardiopulmonary resuscitation, and in descending order lower survival rates have been observed for the following categories: first rhythm shockable, emergency medical services at the scene, and layperson use of automated external defibrillator.[1,28]

There is a clear relationship between SCD and CAD. Clinical and autopsy studies and data from death certificates have found that 62% to 85% of patients who experience out-of-hospital SCD have evidence of prior CAD, 10% have other structural cardiac abnormalities, and 5% have no structural cardiac abnormality.[29] A surveillance study of SCD from Ireland concluded that successful resuscitation of SCD was especially associated with ventricular fibrillation as the presenting rhythm.[30]

SCD is the initial clinical coronary event in 15% of patients with CAD. Most sudden deaths are cardiac. Arrhythmias and ischemic heart disease are the most common antecedents. Severe left ventricular systolic dysfunction is a key risk factor for sudden death in patients with ischemic or nonischemic cardiomyopathy.[31] In the Oregon Sudden Unexpected Death Study (Ore-SUDS), women were significantly less likely than men to have severe left ventricular dysfunction (odds ratio [OR] 0.51) or diagnosis of CAD (OR 0.34).[29,32]

Exertion may precipitate SCD during the time of the increased physical activity or after the activity has stopped. As an example, a recent Finnish study showed increased SCD risk with skiing, cycling, and snow shoveling.[29] The authors concluded that SCD during or immediately after exercise was related to male gender, ischemic heart disease, cardiac hypertrophy, and myocardial scarring.[29] For more information on this topic see Chapter 22 on SCD.

RISK FACTORS FOR CORONARY ARTERY DISEASE

Risk factors for CAD can be sorted into several different varieties. The traditional factors that are commonly available as part of a simple clinical evaluation or a screening program are the primary focus of this chapter and include age, sex, race/ethnicity and geography, heart rate, BP, total and low-density lipoprotein cholesterol (LDL-C), high-density lipoprotein cholesterol (HDL-C), diabetes mellitus, adiposity, smoking, and social class. The ECG has often been included in this traditional factor list because ECG information is typically available. An extension of these common factors are medical conditions and exposures such as environmental pollution and noise that may predispose individuals to greater risk from atherosclerosis. The second set of factors are biomarkers that are typically measured in the blood or potentially in other specimens such as urine. Examples of these factors are inflammatory markers such as C-reactive protein, uric acid, aldosterone, blood coagulation factors, and homocysteine. The list of candidate factors is long and constantly growing. The third set of factors includes information related to subclinical atherosclerotic disease, cardiovascular function, heart imaging findings, vascular calcification, intima-media thickness of major arteries, and vascular stiffness. These factors are discussed in the context of CAD risk factors in this section. More extensive coverage appears in Chapters 17 and 29. The fourth set of factors includes genetic information, and that will be mentioned only briefly because Chapter 3 provides full coverage of this topic.

Traditional Risk Factors

Many risk factors have been proposed for CAD. Greater age is an especially important determinant, and men experience greater risk for CAD than women throughout most of adulthood. In the worldwide INTERHEART study of patients from 52 countries, the authors identified nine potentially modifiable factors that accounted for over 90% of the population-attributable risk of a first MI: smoking, dyslipidemia, hypertension, diabetes, abdominal obesity, psychosocial factors, daily consumption of fruits and vegetables, regular alcohol consumption, and regular physical activity.[33] More information for each of these topics is provided in the following discussion.

Age

Atherosclerotic CAD is uncommon before age 40 in men and before menopause in women. The absolute risk of developing clinical CAD in women increases greatly after menopause, and by age 70 to 80 the incidence of CAD is roughly similar in both sexes.

Sex

Women tend to more commonly experience angina pectoris as the first evidence of CAD, and first CAD events in men are more commonly MI. Differences in CAD rates for men and women are discussed under the angina pectoris, MI, and coronary death headings.

Smoking

Current cigarette smoking typically doubles the risk of CAD events.[34] Relative risks may be much higher for heavy smokers. Older research has shown that filter and nonfilter cigarettes have similarly adverse effects on CAD risk.[35] Quitting smoking in persons with CAD is associated with improved long-term survival, and the benefit of smoking cessation is evident within a few years of stopping, as shown in the Multiple Risk Factor Intervention Trial.[36] The prevalence of current smoking in the United States has declined over the last 50 years and is now in the 15% to 25% range for men and 5% to 25% range for women (Fig. 1.5).[1]

Dyslipidemia

Higher levels of total cholesterol, LDL-C, or non-HDL-C are all associated with greater risk of CAD events. In recent times there is a more concentrated focus on LDL-C, non-HDL-C, apolipoprotein-B levels, and LDL particle number as important determinants of ASCVD risk.[37,38] Higher levels of HDL-C appear to be cardioprotective, and lifestyle factors such as lower BMI, greater alcohol intake, higher estrogen levels, avoidance of smoking, and greater physical activity are partially responsible for favorable HDL-C effects. Elevated triglyceride levels are a CAD risk factor when analyzed in tandem with cholesterol. However, when information from cholesterol, HDL-C, and triglycerides is available, the triglyceride effects appear to be modest. A large number of clinical trials have shown that lowering the concentration of atherogenic lipids such as LDL-C translates into reduced CAD risk.[39]

Hypertension

Elevated BP is a time-honored risk factor for CAD. Population studies have shown that the risk increases along a continuum and higher BP levels, even in the

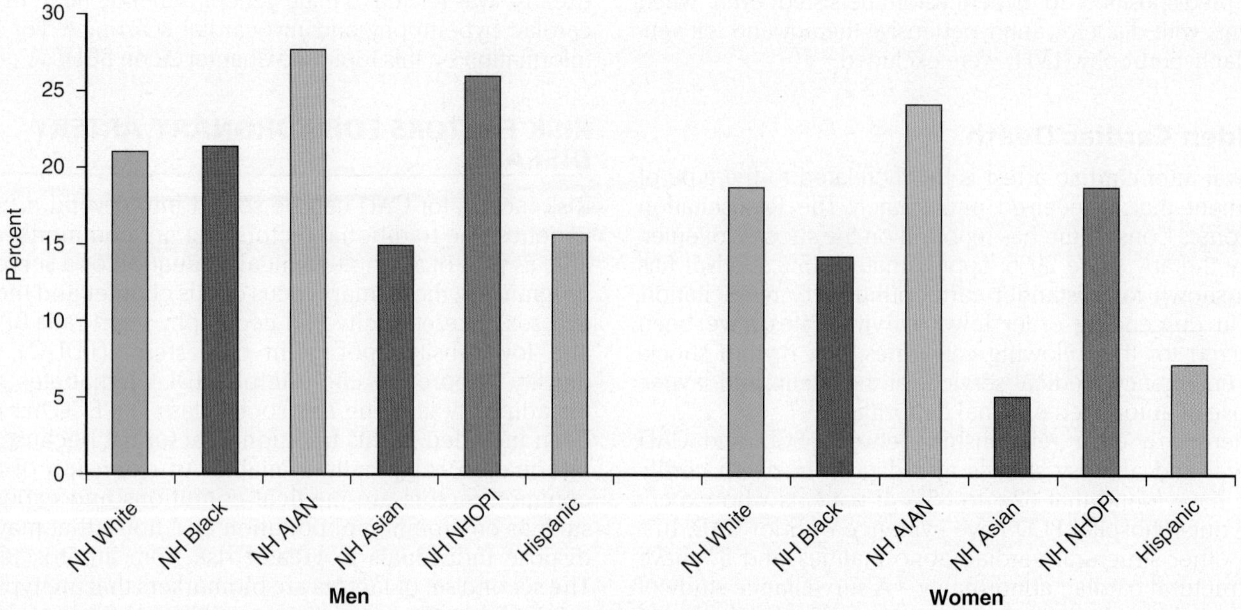

FIG. 1.5 Prevalence of current cigarette smoking in US adults > 18 years of age by age, race, and ethnicity. *AIAN*, American Indian/Alaska Native; *NH*, non-Hispanic; *NHOPI*, Native Hawaiian or Pacific Islander. *(From Mozaffarian D, Benjamin EJ, Go AS, et al. Heart Disease and Stroke Statistics—2016 update: a report from the American Heart Association.* Circulation. *2016;133(4):e38–e360; chart 3-4.)*

nonhypertensive range, are associated with greater CAD risk using 2007–2012 US NHANES data (Fig. 1.6).[1] The prevalence of hypertension (> 140/90 mm Hg or on BP medication) increases inexorably from an estimated 8% in young adults to 80% of the population aged over 75 years, and there is little difference in the prevalence estimates for men and women. In analyses across blacks, whites, and Hispanics, the awareness of hypertension is generally in the 70% to 90% range, BP treatment is in the 60% to 80% range, and BP control is in the 40% to 60% range. There is considerable heterogeneity in these estimates across the different ethnic/racial groups (Fig. 1.7).[1] The gradient of risk between CAD and BP is stronger for systolic pressure than for diastolic pressure, and systolic pressure is typically used as the BP measure to estimate risk for CAD events.[34] Lifestyle changes concerning dietary sodium intake and weight reduction if the person is obese are recommended for persons with BPs greater than 120 mm Hg systolic or 80 mm Hg diastolic. Pharmacotherapy is generally recommended for persons with greater than 140 mm Hg systolic or 90 mm Hg diastolic as recommended by expert guidelines.[40] The large National Institutes of Health (NIH)-funded Systolic Blood Pressure Intervention Trial (SPRINT) was stopped early because of benefit in the aggressive treatment arm. The investigators showed that targeting BP to less than 120/80 mm Hg for persons on BP-lowering therapy was more effective than the traditional goal of less than 140/90 mm Hg.[41]

Diabetes Mellitus

The presence of diabetes mellitus, typically type 2, doubles CAD risk for men and triples risk for women. The increased CAD risk in diabetic patients is attributable to higher BP levels, more dyslipidemia, elevated glucose levels, and increased levels of inflammatory markers.[42] The 2013 Action

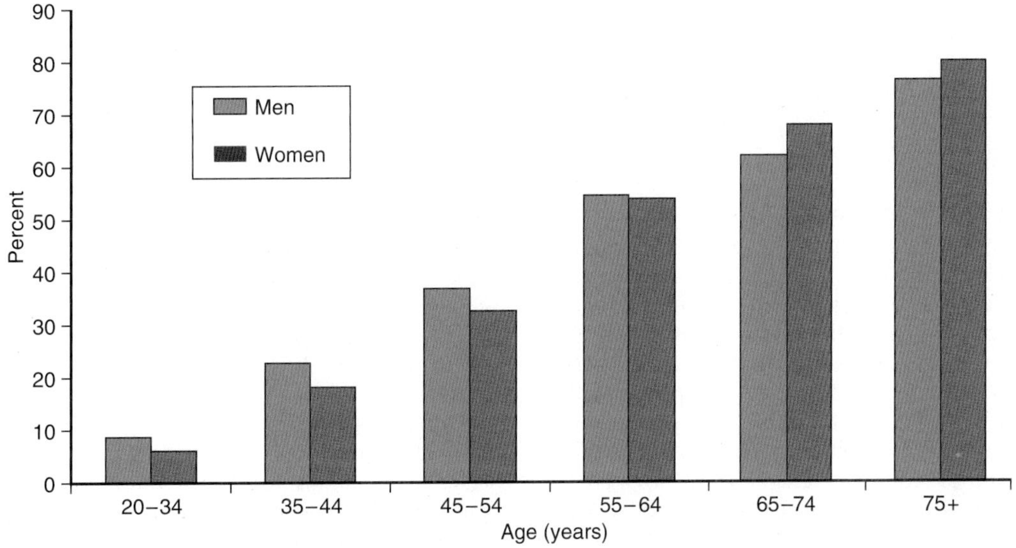

FIG. 1.6 Prevalence of high blood pressure (BP) in US adults > 20 years of age. NHANES (National Health and Nutrition Examination Survey) 2007–2012. Hypertension defined as systolic BP > 140 mm Hg, diastolic BP > 90 mm Hg, or taking hypertension medication. *(From Mozaffarian D, Benjamin EJ, Go AS, et al. Heart Disease and Stroke Statistics—2016 update: a report from the American Heart Association.* Circulation. *2016;133(4):e38–e360; chart 9-1.)*

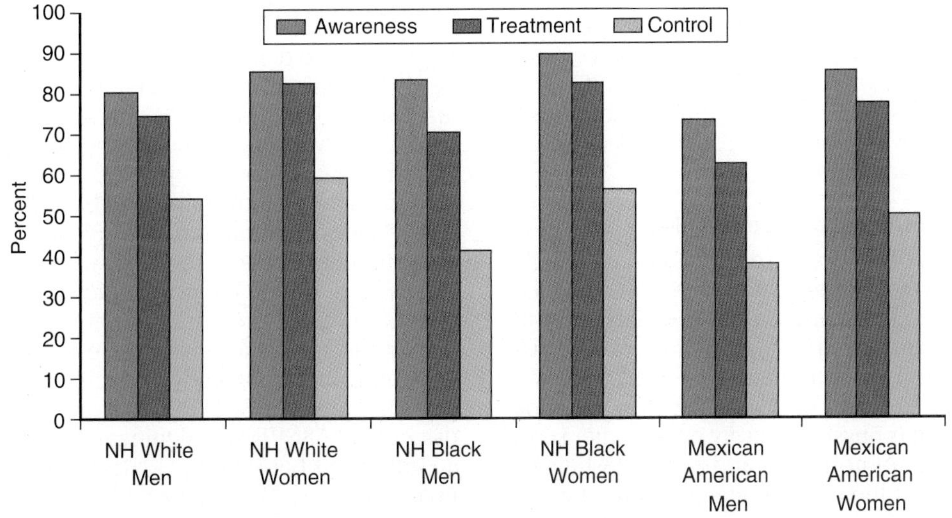

FIG. 1.7 Hypertension awareness, treatment, and control. NHANES (National Health and Nutrition Examination Survey) 2007–2012. Hypertension defined as systolic blood pressure (BP) > 140 mm Hg, diastolic BP > 90 mm Hg, or taking hypertension medication. *NH*, non-Hispanic. *(Modified from Mozaffarian D, Benjamin EJ, Go AS, et al. Heart Disease and Stroke Statistics—2016 update: a report from the American Heart Association.* Circulation. *2016;133(4):e38–e360; chart 9-5.)*

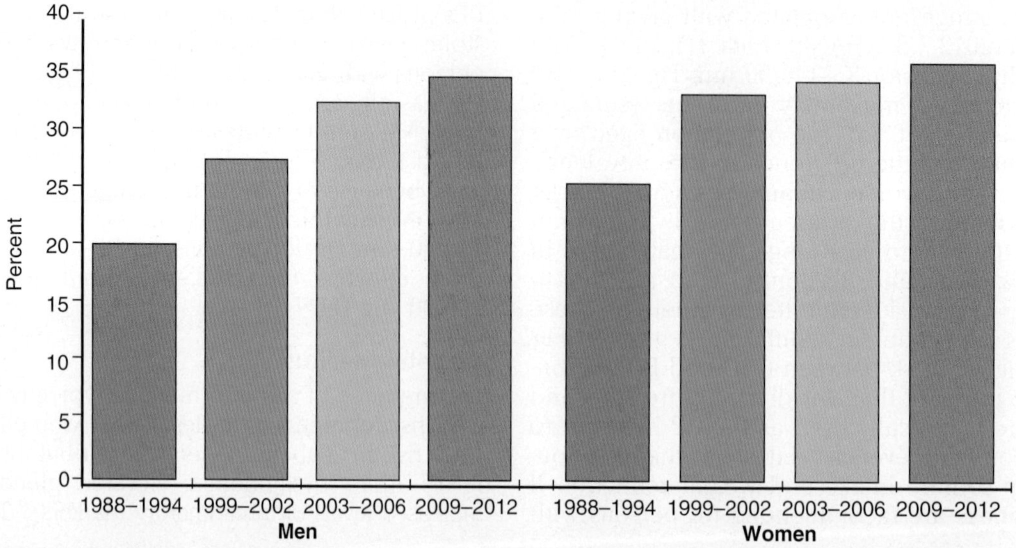

FIG. 1.8 Age-adjusted prevalence of obesity for US adults 20–74 years of age. NHANES (National Health and Nutrition Examination Survey) by sex and survey years. Obesity defined as body mass index > 30 kg/m^2. *(From Mozaffarian D, Benjamin EJ, Go AS, et al. Heart Disease and Stroke Statistics—2016 update: a report from the American Heart Association.* Circulation. *2016;133(4):e38–e360; chart 6-2.)*

for Health in Diabetes (LOOK AHEAD) trial investigated whether weight loss would affect risk of ASCVD outcomes in diabetic patients and the overall result was null.[43]

Excess Adiposity and the Metabolic Syndrome

Greater adiposity in the abdominal region is associated with increased CAD risk, and this risk is largely evident through the effects on BP, lipids, and diabetes mellitus. The prevalence of obesity in the United States has risen greatly over the past few decades (Fig. 1.8), and NHANES estimates that 35% of men and women are obese with a BMI greater than 30 kg/m^2.[1] Metabolic syndrome has been defined as present if an individual has at least three of the following: abdominal adiposity, elevated BP, low HDL-C, elevated triglycerides, and impaired fasting glucose. Each factor increases ASCVD risk approximately 1.5 times, and persons with metabolic syndrome have an elevated risk of developing CAD and a very elevated risk of developing type 2 diabetes mellitus.[44]

Psychosocial Factors

Personality type, educational status, income level, employment status, health insurance status, and other factors have been investigated as CAD risk factors. It can be difficult to generalize results across cultures on psychosocial measures. British investigators have incorporated such measures into CAD risk estimation formulations.[45]

Daily Consumption of Fruits and Vegetables

Greater consumption of fruits and vegetables and a healthy diet in general are typically associated with lower concentrations of atherogenic lipids and favorable effects on other blood factors that translates into a reduction in CAD risk. The AHA has developed a program called *Life's Simple Seven* that emphasizes seven lifestyle attributes: no smoking, normal BMI, regular physical activity, healthy diet score, normal blood cholesterol, normal BP, and normal fasting glucose. Surveys show that the healthy diet component is one of the least likely measures to be achieved and that 50% of US adults 20 to 49 years old and 31% of those over 50 years had poor scores related to healthy diet.[1]

Regular Physical Activity

Physical activity and physical fitness itself are associated with lower risk of CAD in a very large number of settings. The 2008 Physical Activity Guidelines for Americans recommend more than 150 minutes/week of moderate physical activity or 75 minutes of vigorous aerobic activity or an equivalent combination. In calendar year 2008, 43.5% of US adults were aerobically active, 28.4% were highly active, 21.9% met the muscle-strengthening guideline, and 18.2% both met the muscle-strengthening guideline and were aerobically active. Meeting the guidelines was associated with being male, being younger, being non-Hispanic white, having higher levels of education, and having a lower BMI (Fig. 1.9).[46] National Health Interview Survey data across the United States for 2014 showed that approximately 30% of adults did not undertake leisure-time physical activity. Inactivity was generally greater in women, more common with increasing age, and more prevalent in Hispanic and non-Hispanic blacks than in whites (Table 1.3).[1]

Electrocardiographic Abnormalities

Asymptomatic persons with resting ECG abnormalities such as ST depression, T-wave inversion, LVH or strain, and premature ventricular contractions have a 2- to 10-fold increased risk of CHD versus those with a normal ECG.[47] As examples, both minor (13%) and major (23%) ECG abnormalities were present in the Health, Aging, and Body Composition (Health ABC) Cohort participants over 65 years at baseline. These abnormalities were associated with an increased risk of CHD. When the ECG abnormalities were added to a model containing traditional risk factors alone, they improved the overall discrimination to a modest degree. Similarly, in the Copenhagen Heart Study participants who were over 65 years, the prevalence of ECG abnormalities was 30% and the risk of fatal ASCVD was significantly greater in persons with an abnormal baseline ECG (hazard ratio [HR] 1.33 vs normal baseline ECG, 95% confidence interval [CI] 1.29–1.36). Among 2192 adults aged 70 to 79 without known ASCVD who were followed for 8 years, persons with minor (defined as minor ST-T abnormalities) and major (defined as Q

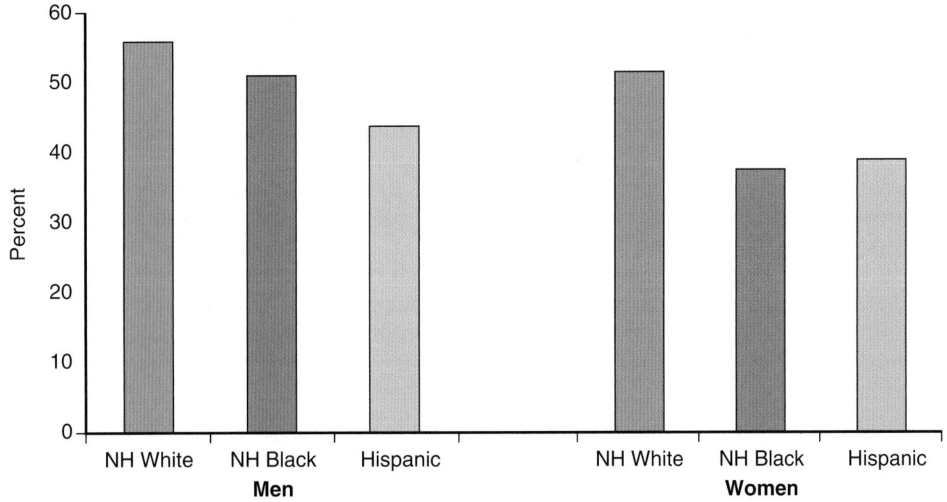

FIG. 1.9 Prevalence of meeting 2008 Aerobic Guidelines in US Adults > 18 years of age. NHANES (National Health Interview Survey) by age, race, and ethnicity. *(From Mozaffarian D, Benjamin EJ, Go AS, et al. Heart Disease and Stroke Statistics—2016 update: a report from the American Heart Association.* Circulation. *2016;133(4):e38–e360; chart 4-4.)*

TABLE 1.3 US Adults Meeting Federal Aerobic and Strengthening Physical Activity Guideline

POPULATION GROUP	2014 PREVALENCE (AGE > 18 YEARS, %)
Both sexes	21.4
Men	25.4
Women	17.6
Non-Hispanic white only	23.6
Non-Hispanic black only	20.0
Hispanic or Latino	15.3
Asian only	17.0
American Indian/Alaska Native only	24.0

Data from Mozaffarian D, Benjamin EJ, Go AS, et al. Heart Disease and Stroke Statistics—2016 update: a report from the American Heart Association. Circulation. *2016;133(4):e38–e360; Table 4-1.*

waves, LVH, bundle branch block, atrial fibrillation or flutter, Wolff–Parkinson–White syndrome, or major ST-T changes) ECG abnormalities were more likely to develop ASCVD than those with normal baseline ECGs (HR 1.35, 95% CI 1.02–1.81 and HR 1.51, 95% CI 1.20–1.90, respectively).[48]

The usual transition zone, where the R wave and S wave are equal in amplitude in the precordial leads, usually occurs between V_3 and V_4. In a cohort of 9067 persons (44% male) followed for 24 years, clockwise rotation (also called *late transition*) was associated with increased risk of ASCVD (HR 1.49, 95% CI 1.12–1.98), whereas counterclockwise rotation (also called *early transition*) was inversely associated with ASCVD (HR 0.74, 95% CI 0.59–0.94). Whereas these patterns are easily identified from the surface ECG, the exact mechanism by which cardiac rotation on ECG alters the risk of ASCVD remains undetermined.[49]

LVH is associated with hypertension, older age, and obesity. Among more than 15,000 patients in the ARIC study who were followed for 15 years, both women and men with baseline ECG-identified LVH were significantly more likely to die from ASCVD than from non-ASCVD causes (HR in women 8.4, 95% CI 4.5–15.6; HR in men 4.9, 95% CI 3.0–7.8).[50]

Resting heart rate and peak exercise heart rate are associated with greater CHD and ASCVD mortality.[51–53] Resting heart rate has been studied in several population-based cohorts, and it is associated with modest increases in ASCVD events. In a recent Framingham analysis, a positive difference of 11 beats/min was associated with higher all-cause (HR 1.17, 95% CI 1.11–1.24, $p < 0.0001$) and cardiovascular mortality (HR 1.18, 95% CI 1.04–1.33, $p = 0.01$).[52] Compared with persons with a resting heart rate of less than 60 beats/min, those with a resting heart rate of 80 beats/min or more had significantly higher all-cause (HR 1.66, 95% CI 1.45–1.89) and cardiovascular (HR 1.87, 95% CI 1.52–2.30) mortality. Change in resting heart rate over time also correlates with an increased risk of CHD death. In a prospective cohort study of 29,325 Norwegians (46% men) without known CHD, resting heart rate was measured on two occasions approximately 10 years apart, after which the group was followed for an average of 12 years. Persons with a resting heart rate of less than 70 beats/min at the initial visit but greater than 85 beats/min at the second visit had a significantly higher risk of CHD death compared with persons with resting heart rate of 70 beats/min at both visits, (adjusted hazard ratio [AHR] 1.9, 95% CI 1.0–3.6). Similar results were noted for persons with a resting heart rate of 70 to 85 beats/min at the initial visit but greater than 85 beats/min at second visit (AHR 1.8, 95% CI 1.2–2.8).[54]

Medical Diagnoses and Systemic Conditions That May Increase Risk for Coronary Artery Disease

Androgen Deficiency

Androgen deficiency in men with reduced serum testosterone concentrations is associated with the subsequent development of metabolic syndrome, diabetes mellitus, and elevated C-reactive protein levels in addition to higher overall mortality.[55] Among a cohort of 930 British men with angiographically documented CHD who were observed for a mean of 7 years, those with low testosterone levels (bioavailable testosterone < 2.6 nmol/L, 21% of the group) had significantly greater mortality than men with normal testosterone levels.[56] Additionally, several observational studies and retrospective analyses of randomized trials have shown an association between therapeutically reduced androgen levels (i.e., as treatment for prostate cancer) and higher rates of ASCVD and mortality. On the other hand, a systematic review and meta-analysis of randomized trials of exogenous testosterone replacement therapy (TRT) reported that TRT was not associated with increased risk of cardiovascular death.[57] Other reports suggest that normalization of testosterone levels with TRT may alter the risk of ASCVD. In a retrospective cohort analysis of 83,010 male veterans with low total testosterone levels, patients were separated into three groups: those taking TRT with normalized testosterone levels (n = 43,931), those taking TRT with persistently low testosterone levels (n = 25,701), and those not on TRT (n = 13,378).[58] Using propensity analysis, patients receiving TRT who had normalization of testosterone levels had significantly lower risk of total mortality, MI, and stroke over an average follow-up of up to 6 years. Two separate studies on the effects of TRT in veterans produced discordant results. Basaria[59] et al. showed an increase for CAD risk, while Sharma et al.[58] showed a decrease. The NIH-funded Testosterone Trial is underway to address this issue.

Estrogen Status

In the 1980s a large number of studies reported decreased CAD risk in women who took postmenopausal estrogen products. Subsequently, the Women's Health Initiative was developed by the NIH, and several clinical trials were undertaken to rigorously test the benefit and safety of postmenopausal estrogens. None of the trials demonstrated a reduction in CAD risk.[60,61]

Collagen Vascular Disease

Patients with collagen vascular disease, especially those with rheumatoid arthritis (RA) and systemic lupus erythematosus (SLE), have a significantly increased incidence of ASCVD.[62] High CAD risk has been demonstrated for young women with SLE.[63] Immunotherapeutic agents are being evaluated to potentially reduce inflammation and clinical CHD events in clinical trials.[64]

Acute Infectious Illnesses

Acute infectious illnesses may be associated with a transient increase in the risk of ASCVD events, and influenza vaccination reduces the risk of a clinical CAD event.[65,66] It has been proposed that certain types of infections may play a role in the pathogenesis of atherosclerosis by establishing a low-grade persistent inflammatory process. Acute or chronic inflammation may result in endothelial dysfunction and may be responsible for a cardiac event. The major organisms that have been studied with respect to chronic inflammation and ASCVD include *Chlamydia pneumoniae*, cytomegalovirus, and *Helicobacter pylori*. Enterovirus (Coxsackie viral infection), hepatitis A virus, and herpes simplex virus type 1 and type 2 have also been implicated. A large meta-analysis has shown that large randomized trials do not support benefit from antibiotic therapy against *C. pneumoniae* to reduce CAD risk.[67]

Nonalcoholic Fatty Liver Disease

Nonalcoholic fatty liver disease (NAFLD), also referred to as *nonalcoholic steatohepatitis*, is a clinico-histopathologic entity with features that resemble alcohol-induced liver injury. Although its etiology is unknown, NAFLD is frequently associated with obesity, type 2 diabetes mellitus, and hyperlipidemia. Patients with NAFLD often meet the diagnostic criteria for metabolic syndrome, and there is evidence for an increased risk of incident cardiovascular disease that is independent of the risk conferred by traditional risk factors and components of metabolic syndrome.[68,69]

Obstructive Sleep Apnea

Obstructive sleep apnea is associated with an increased risk for CAD, cardiac arrhythmias, and systemic hypertension.[70] It is difficult to disentangle the effects of obesity versus the effects of disordered breathing on the risk of CAD in such patients.[71]

Small for Gestational Age Infants

Adults who were small for gestational age infants experience an increased risk for ischemic heart disease and related disorders including hypertension, stroke, diabetes, and hypercholesterolemia.[72] Reports suggest that the mother of the small for gestational age infant may be at higher risk to develop CAD as well.[73]

Environmental Factors

Air Pollution

Air pollution has emerged as a potentially modifiable risk factor for the development of ASCVD. Multiple observational studies have demonstrated an association between fine particulate air pollution (primarily from the use of fossil fuels in automobiles, power plants, and heating purposes) and cardiovascular and cardiopulmonary mortality, as well as an increased risk for the development of acute coronary syndromes. More recent studies are controlling the analyses for usual CAD risk factors. Larger concentrations of particles in the air have been associated with a 25% increase in the risk of ASCVD death. In 2010 the AHA and in 2015 the European Society of Cardiology issued official statements discussing the association between long-term exposure to fine particulate air pollution and increased risk of developing cardiovascular disease.[74,75] Exposure to particulate matter less than 2.5 μm in diameter over a few hours to weeks can trigger cardiovascular disease-related mortality and nonfatal events; longer exposure over years increases the risk for cardiovascular mortality to an even greater extent than exposures over a few days and reduces life expectancy within more highly exposed segments of the population by several months to a few years. From the prevention vantage point, reductions in particulate matter levels are associated with decreases in cardiovascular mortality within a time frame as short as a few years. Possible mechanisms by which fine particulate air pollution may increase the risk of ASCVD include raising mean resting arterial BP, prothrombotic effects through transient increases in plasma viscosity and impaired endothelial dysfunction, and promoting the initiation of atherosclerosis.[75–77]

Environmental Noise

Environmental noise has been implicated in observational studies as a CAD risk factor. Chronic exposure to increased environmental noise levels from roadways, airplanes, and other sources has been linked to an increased risk of developing ASCVD. This effect is hypothesized to be caused by stress-related dysregulation of the autonomic nervous system, leading to increases in hypertension and subsequent ASCVD.[78]

Socioeconomic Factors

Socioeconomic factors, including where a person lives, his or her education, occupation, and income, or combinations of these, have been associated with risk for ASCVD, especially CHD and ASCVD mortality. Disadvantaged socioeconomic status is consistently associated with higher ASCVD risk in these studies.[79–81]

Elevated Blood Homocysteine

Elevated blood homocysteine levels in cross-sectional and prospective studies have been linked to increased risk for CHD. Higher serum homocysteine concentrations are frequently accompanied by reduced levels and intake of folate and vitamin B_{12}. On the other hand, numerous prospective randomized trials of folate and vitamin B_{12} supplementation to lower serum homocysteine have demonstrated no reduction in ASCVD outcomes.[82] The addition of a serum homocysteine measurement to the Framingham risk score has been shown to improve risk prediction, with net reclassification of between 13% and 20% of patients from two cohorts.[83] The majority of those affected were reclassified to a higher risk level.

Subclinical Atherosclerotic Disease

Carotid artery intima-media thickness (IMT) is linked to the atherosclerotic process because of its association with known cardiovascular risk factors. Thicker IMT of the common carotid artery is highly associated with greater risk for CAD events. Far wall common carotid artery IMT has been shown to have the strongest association with incident CHD, whereas mean IMT had the strongest associations with risk factors.[84–87] Arterial stiffness, measured as the aortic pulse wave velocity (PWV) between the carotid and femoral arteries, also predicts ASCVD events. This was demonstrated in a meta-analysis of 17 studies that included more than 15,000 patients in whom aortic PWV had been correlated to clinical outcome.[88] The pooled relative risks for total ASCVD events, ASCVD mortality, and all-cause mortality were significantly increased in comparisons of high versus low aortic PWV groups: 2.26 (95% CI 1.89–2.70), 2.02 (95% CI 1.68–2.42), and 1.90 (95% CI 1.61–2.24), respectively.

Calcium deposits in large arteries, particularly the aortic arch and abdominal aorta, may be an indicator for an increased risk for clinical ASCVD and overall mortality.[89] Calcification of the abdominal aorta has also been associated with an increased risk of ASCVD, and a meta-analysis showed calcification of the abdominal aorta was associated with significantly higher risk for CHD across five studies with a total of 11,250 patients (RR 1.81, 95% CI 1.54–2.14).[90]

Coronary artery calcification (CAC) detected by electron beam computed tomography or multidetector computed tomography can be used to quantify the amount of calcium present in the coronary arteries. After age 40 coronary calcium is frequently seen in the coronary arteries, an aggregate coronary calcium score can be developed from the images, and CAD risk is greater in persons in proportion to the quantity of calcium.[91] Coronary plaque volume, calcium density, and progression of the calcification are all related to greater risk for CAD events.[92,93]

Inherited Risk and Genetic Factors

First-Degree Relatives with a History of ASCVD

Parental history of CAD is associated with greater risk for CAD in the offspring. Risk is approximately double if one parent has a history of a heart attack and much higher if both parents have a history of a heart attack, especially if both parents had a heart attack before age 50, as shown in Table 1.4.[1] Additionally, a positive history of ASCVD in siblings has been reported to be associated with an increased risk for CAD.[94]

TABLE 1.4 Cardiovascular Disease Risk and Parental Heart Attack History

GROUP	ODDS RATIO (95% CONFIDENCE LIMIT)
No family history	1.00
One parent with heart attack > 50 years of age	1.67 (1.55–1.81)
One parent with heart attack < 50 years of age	2.36 (1.89–2.95)
Both parents with heart attack > 50 years of age	2.90 (2.30–3.66)
Both parents with heart attack, one < 50 years of age	3.26 (1.72–6.18)
Both parents with heart attack, both < 50 years of age	6.56 (1.39–30.95)

From Mozaffarian D, Benjamin EJ, Go AS, et al. Heart Disease and Stroke Statistics—2016 update: a report from the American Heart Association. Circulation. *2016;133(4):e38–e360; Table 7-1.*

TABLE 1.5 Heritability of Traits Estimated in the Framingham Heart Study

HERITABILITY	TRAITS
High (> 0.50)	Subcutaneous abdominal fat HDL cholesterol Total cholesterol LDL cholesterol
High intermediate (0.40–0.50)	Systolic blood pressure Waist circumference Triglycerides
Low intermediate (0.30–0.40)	Diastolic blood pressure Visceral abdominal fat Fasting glucose C-reactive protein Estimated glomerular filtration rate
Low (< 0.30)	Left ventricular mass Hemoglobin A_{1c} Ankle brachial index

HDL, High-density lipoprotein; *LDL*, low-density lipoprotein.
Data from Mozaffarian D, Benjamin EJ, Go AS, et al. Heart Disease and Stroke Statistics—2016 update: a report from the American Heart Association. Circulation. *2016;133(4):e38–e360; Table 7-3.*

Heritability of Risk Factors

Heritability of risk factors is an important contribution to inherited CAD risk. Studies like Framingham, which measured risk factors comprehensively across more than one generation and at similar ages for the generations being compared, provide reliable estimates for the risk factor heritability. Table 1.5 shows the heritability of several common risk factors according to several heritability strata. Of particular note is that most of the commonly measured lipids that are used to help estimate CAD risk are very heritable.

Genetic Variants

Genetic variants have been associated with greater CAD risk in multiple studies.[95,96] Among the various implicated single-nucleotide polymorphisms (SNPs), those appearing on locus 9p21 have shown the strongest association with CHD risk. In a 2010 systematic review that evaluated

47 distinct datasets, including 35,872 cases and 95,837 controls, persons with two abnormal alleles at this locus were more likely to have CHD when compared with persons with one at-risk allele (OR 1.25, 95% CI 1.21–1.29).[97] The association with 9p21 SNPs and an increased risk of developing CHD has also been shown in patients greater than 70 years of age without known prior CHD.[96] A 2014 systemic review and meta-analysis of 31 cohorts including 193,372 persons confirmed the association between 9p21 variants and the likelihood of a first CHD event (HR 1.19 per risk allele, 95% CI 1.17–1.22).[95] However, 9p21 variants were not associated with an increased likelihood of subsequent CHD events among persons with known CHD (HR 1.01 per risk allele, 95% CI 0.97–1.06). Despite an apparently clear association between variants and incident CHD, locus 9p21 SNPs have not been definitively shown to significantly improve on the discrimination or classification of predicted CHD risk compared with traditional risk factors.[95–101] Among 950 nondiabetic patients with early-onset CHD (mean age 56 years) displaying at least one angiographic epicardial stenosis greater than 50% on coronary angiography, the 9p21 genotype was associated with a risk of left main CHD (OR 2.38 per copy of risk allele, 95% CI 1.48–3.85), 3-vessel CHD (OR 1.45 per copy of risk allele, 95% CI 1.18–1.79), and need for bypass surgery (OR 1.37 per copy of risk allele, 95% CI 1.04–1.79). These data suggest more aggressive CHD occurring at a younger age in patients with 9p21 variants.

Different genetic variants have been associated with a variety of CHD diagnoses. Some increase the risk of coronary atherosclerosis and others increase the risk of plaque rupture and acute MI, suggesting different biologic effects.[101,102] The pathophysiologic impact of genetic variants likely varies depending on comorbidities. In a study that pooled CHD cases and controls from five large cohorts, the same SNP on chromosome 1q25 was associated with a significantly higher risk of CHD among patients with diabetes (OR 1.36 vs diabetic patients without this SNP, 95% CI 1.22–1.51) but no change in risk of CHD among patients without diabetes (OR 0.99, 95% CI 0.87–1.13).[103] These findings point toward the importance of other biologic factors in the development of CHD, including different mechanisms in patients with diabetes.

Many genetic variants have been reported to be associated with the risk of ASCVD. In a study of 180 genetic variants associated with height among 193,449 persons (including 65,066 cases with CAD and 128,383 control subjects without CAD), there was a significant increase in CAD risk with shorter stature (13.5% for each standard deviation [6 cm] decrease in height, 95% CI 5.4–22.1), with a significant decrease in CAD risk with increasing numbers of height-raising genetic variants.[104]

Although individual genetic markers are associated with ASCVD, their aggregate effect on risk beyond traditional factors has not been established. A genetic risk score created from 101 SNPs associated with ASCVD did not improve discrimination or reclassification of risk after adjustment for traditional factors in a cohort of over 19,000 white women.[105] Peripheral blood cell gene expression has also been investigated as a means of estimating the risk of ASCVD, specifically obstructive CAD, and based on limited data the technique may be comparable to stress testing with myocardial perfusion imaging in terms of accuracy of diagnosing CHD.[106–108]

Prediction of First ASCVD Event

Multivariable risk models have been developed in an attempt to estimate both 10-year and 30-year ASCVD risk in patients without clinical vascular disease at baseline. In the 1990s the Framingham Heart Study developed multivariable models using the traditional variables—age, sex, systolic BP level, BP treatment, total cholesterol (or LDL-C), HDL-C, diabetes mellitus status, and current smoking habit—to estimate risk of developing a first CAD event.

Since the late 1990s varieties of the multivariable-based CAD prediction models have been developed around the world. The Systematic COronary Risk Evaluation (SCORE) risk tool was developed in Europe to predict CAD death.[109] British investigators developed a QRISK tool that was updated to QRISK2 and in its most recent version became the Joint British Societies (JBS3) estimator. The British model included a region of the United Kingdom that was linked to socioeconomic status, family history of ASCVD, atrial fibrillation, rheumatoid arthritis, and BMI variables as predictive factors.[45] In the United States the expert committees developing guidelines for the prevention of vascular disease elected to focus on hard ASCVD as the vascular endpoint of interest, and this algorithm was published in a 2013 American College of Cardiology (ACC)/AHA report.[34] The 2013 estimator was based on the experience of the Framingham, ARIC, Cardiovascular Health Study (CHS), and Coronary Artery Risk Development in Young Adults (CARDIA) cohorts and was externally validated in REasons for Geographic and Racial Differences in Stroke (REGARDS). Follow-up validations undertaken by Reynolds and MESA investigators using Reynolds risk scores and MESA cohorts suggest that the 2013 ACC/AHA may overestimate ASCVD risk.[110,111]

Estimating lifetime risk of having CAD and other vascular events has been possible since the turn of century using methods that censored for competing causes of death and had follow-ups of long duration. A 2012 report that included information from 18 cohorts and more than 200,000 adults showed that the lifetime risk of ASCVD was 15% for persons without risk factors at age 55 years, and absolute risk rose to approximately 40% for those with two or more of the traditional risk factors.[7]

An example of hard ASCVD 10-year risk estimation using the 2013 ACC/AHA Risk Estimator is illustrated in Fig. 1.10 for hypothetical 55-year-old adults with different combinations of risk factors—cholesterol, HDL-C, systolic BP, BP treatment, smoking status, and diabetes status.

Prediction of Recurrent ASCVD

Persons with symptomatic ischemia experience greater risk for subsequent ischemia-related events, including hospitalizations for acute coronary syndrome (ACS), stroke, and ASCVD death.[112] Research into identifying the predictors of these events has focused on survivors of ACS or MI. Historically most risk scores have been based on inpatient or emergency department information, such as Thrombolysis in Myocardial Infarction (TIMI), Global Registry of Acute Coronary Events (GRACE), the emergency department History, ECG, Age, Risk factors, Troponin (HEART) algorithm, and the Dual Antiplatelet Therapy (DAPT) investigators.[113–116] In the outpatient setting and in observational studies the Reduction of Atherothrombosis for Continued Health (REACH) and the Secondary Manifestations of ARTerial disease (SMART) investigators developed prediction algorithms.[117,118] We will focus on the outpatient prediction of recurrent ASCVD events using outpatient information.

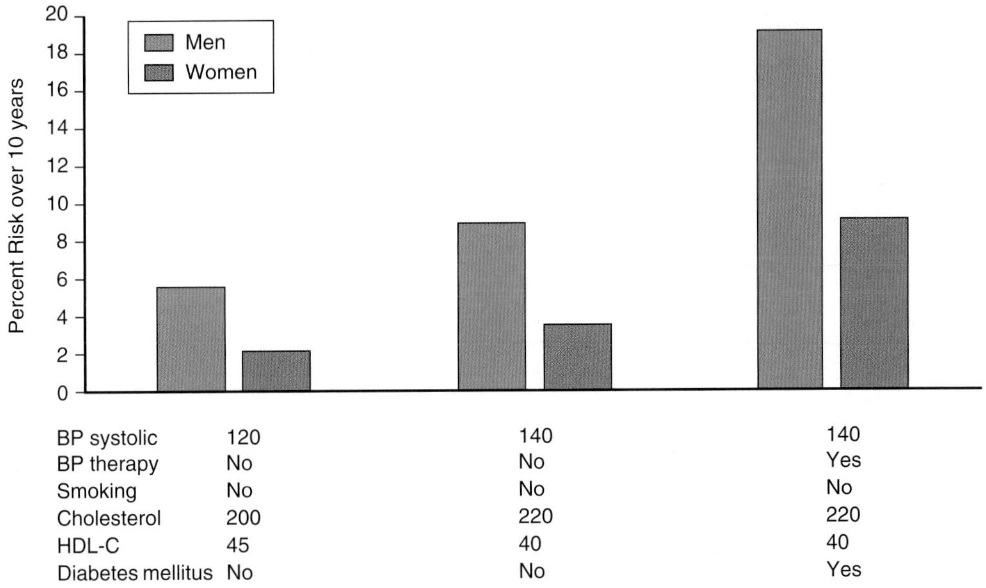

FIG. 1.10 Estimated 10-year hard cardiovascular disease risk based on 2013 ACC/AHA risk estimator. *BP*, Blood pressure; *HDL-C*, HDL cholesterol. *(Data from algorithm by Stone NJ, Robinson JG, Lichtenstein AH, et al. 2013 ACC/AHA guideline on the treatment of blood cholesterol to reduce atherosclerotic cardiovascular risk in adults: a report of the American College of Cardiology/American Heart Association Task Force on Practice Guidelines.* Circulation. *2014;129(25 suppl 2):S1–45.)*

TABLE 1.6 Recurrent Heart Disease Outpatient Prediction Algorithms

STUDY GROUP	REACH	SMART
Entry	Outpatient Post MI	Outpatient History of Arterial Disease
Sex	x	x
Age	x	x
Current smoking	x	x
Diabetes mellitus	x	x
Parental history of MI before age 60 years		x
Blood pressure level		x
Cholesterol level		x
eGFR		x
BMI > 20 kg/m^2	x	
Recent cardiac arrest		x
Cerebrovascular disease, peripheral arterial disease, or abdominal aortic aneurysm	x	x
Time since first vascular event	x	x
Heart failure	x	x
Carotid intima-media thickness	x	
Carotid stenosis		
Atrial fibrillation	x	
Antiplatelet therapy	x	x
Statin or lipid therapy	x	x
Blood pressure therapy		x
Geographic region	x	

Reduction of Atherothrombosis for Continued Health (REACH), Secondary Manifestations of Arterial Disease (SMART)

BMI, Body mass index; *eGFR*, estimated glomerular filtration rate; *MI*, myocardial infarction.

x indicates that the variable is included in the algorithm.

Table 1.6 shows the variables used in the REACH and SMART risk model. In REACH the investigators developed ASCVD prediction models from the 2-year follow-up data of 49,689 participants (2394 CV events and 1029 CV deaths).[117] Age, sex, number of vascular beds with clinical disease, diabetes, smoking, low BMI, history of atrial fibrillation, cardiac failure, region of the world, and history of CV event(s) within 1 year of the baseline examination increased risk of a subsequent CV event. The investigators in SMART had European data and found that age, sex, carotid findings, smoking, systolic BP, and lab biomarkers were significantly associated with recurrent vascular disease in a population of 5788 patients at risk and 788 recurrent events.

CONCLUSIONS

The epidemiology of ASCVD has evolved to the point where angina pectoris, MI, and CHD death are extremely common on a worldwide basis. The key traditional factors such as age, male sex, smoking, diabetes mellitus, hypertension, and lipid measures are important determinants of risk. Newer biomarkers continue to be studied and are complemented by research findings concerning genetic variants that augment ASCVD risk. In addition, a variety of other situations, conditions, and diagnoses such as use of testosterone or estrogen products, inhalation of pollutants, and obesity may affect risk of developing clinical ischemic heart disease. Finally, use of subclinical heart disease assessments using coronary artery calcium scoring and other modalities holds promise to refine the assessment of ASCVD risk in some individuals.

References

1. Mozaffarian D, Benjamin EJ, Go AS, et al.: Heart Disease and Stroke Statistics—2016 update: a report from the American Heart Association, *Circulation* 133(4):e38–e360, 2016.
2. GBD: 2013 Mortality and Causes of Death Collaborators. Global, regional, and national age-sex specific all-cause and cause-specific mortality for 240 causes of death, 1990–2013: a systematic analysis for the Global Burden of Disease Study 2013, *Lancet* 385(9963):117–171, 2015.
3. Towfighi A, Zheng L, Ovbiagele B: Sex-specific trends in midlife coronary heart disease risk and prevalence, *Arch Intern Med* 169(19):1762–1766, 2009.
4. Webber BJ, Seguin PG, Burnett DG, et al.: Prevalence of and risk factors for autopsy-determined atherosclerosis among US service members, 2001–2011, *JAMA* 308(24):2577–2583, 2012.
5. Roe MT, Messenger JC, Weintraub WS, et al.: Treatments, trends, and outcomes of acute myocardial infarction and percutaneous coronary intervention, *J Am Coll Cardiol* 56(4):254–263, 2010.

6. Fihn SD, Gardin JM, Abrams J, et al.: 2012 ACCF/AHA/ACP/AATS/PCNA/SCAI/STS guideline for the diagnosis and management of patients with stable ischemic heart disease: a report of the American College of Cardiology Foundation/American Heart Association Task Force on Practice Guidelines, and the American College of Physicians, American Association for Thoracic Surgery, Preventive Cardiovascular Nurses Association, Society for Cardiovascular Angiography and Interventions, and Society of Thoracic Surgeons, *Circulation* 126(25):e354–e471, 2012.
7. Berry JD, Dyer A, Cai X, et al.: Lifetime risks of cardiovascular disease, *N Engl J Med* 366(4): 321–329, 2012.
8. Reference deleted in proofs.
9. Chow BJ, Small G, Yam Y, et al.: Incremental prognostic value of cardiac computed tomography in coronary artery disease using CONFIRM: COroNary computed tomography angiography evaluation for clinical outcomes: an InteRnational Multicenter registry, *Circ Cardiovasc Imaging* 4(5):463–472, 2011.
10. Maddox TM, Stanislawski MA, Grunwald GK, et al.: Nonobstructive coronary artery disease and risk of myocardial infarction, *JAMA* 312(17):1754–1763, 2014.
11. Wilmot KA, O'Flaherty M, Capewell S, et al.: Coronary heart disease mortality declines in the United States from 1979 through 2011: evidence for stagnation in young adults, especially women, *Circulation* 132(11):997–1002, 2015.
12. Gupta A, Wang Y, Spertus JA, et al.: Trends in acute myocardial infarction in young patients and differences by sex and race, 2001 to 2010, *J Am Coll Cardiol* 64(4):337–345, 2014.
13. Capewell S, Ford ES, Croft JB, et al.: Cardiovascular risk factor trends and potential for reducing coronary heart disease mortality in the United States of America, *Bull World Health Organ* 88(2):120–130, 2010.
14. Young F, Capewell S, Ford ES, et al.: Coronary mortality declines in the U.S. between 1980 and 2000 quantifying the contributions from primary and secondary prevention, *Am J Prev Med* 39(3):228–234, 2010.
15. Colantonio LD, Bittner V, Reynolds K, et al.: Association of serum lipids and coronary heart disease in contemporary observational studies, *Circulation* 133(3):256–264, 2016.
16. Chen J, Normand SL, Wang Y, et al.: Recent declines in hospitalizations for acute myocardial infarction in Medicare fee-for-service beneficiaries: progress and continuing challenges, *Circulation* 121(11):1322–1328, 2010.
17. Roger VL, Weston SA, Gerber Y, et al.: Trends in incidence, severity, and outcome of hospitalized myocardial infarction, *Circulation* 121(7):863–869, 2010.
18. Parikh NI, Gona P, Larson MG, et al.: Long-term trends in myocardial infarction incidence and case fatality in the National Heart, Lung, and Blood Institute's Framingham Heart study, *Circulation* 119(9):1203–1210, 2009.
19. Kontos MC, Rennyson SL, Chen AY, et al.: The association of myocardial infarction process of care measures and in-hospital mortality: a report from the NCDR(R), *Am Heart J* 168(5):766–775, 2014.
20. Rogers WJ, Frederick PD, Stoehr E, et al.: Trends in presenting characteristics and hospital mortality among patients with ST elevation and non-ST elevation myocardial infarction in the National Registry of Myocardial Infarction from 1990 to 2006, *Am Heart J* 156(6):1026–1034, 2008.
21. Nichols M, Townsend N, Scarborough P, et al.: Cardiovascular disease in Europe 2014: epidemiological update, *Eur Heart J* 35(42):2929, 2014.
22. Nichols M, Townsend N, Scarborough P, Rayner M: Trends in age-specific coronary heart disease mortality in the European Union over three decades: 1980–2009, *Eur Heart J* 34(39):3017–3027, 2013.
23. Lloyd-Jones D, Adams RJ, Brown TM, et al.: Executive summary: heart disease and stroke statistics—2010 update: a report from the American Heart Association, *Circulation* 121(7):948–954, 2010.
24. Brandon Stacey R, Leaverton PE, Schocken DD, et al.: Prediabetes and the association with unrecognized myocardial infarction in the multi-ethnic study of atherosclerosis, *Am Heart J* 170(5):923–928, 2015.
25. Dehghan A, Leening MJ, Solouki AM, et al.: Comparison of prognosis in unrecognized versus recognized myocardial infarction in men versus women >55 years of age (from the Rotterdam Study), *Am J Cardiol* 113(1):1–6, 2014.
26. Valensi P, Lorgis L, Cottin Y: Prevalence, incidence, predictive factors and prognosis of silent myocardial infarction: a review of the literature, *Arch Cardiovasc Dis* 104(3):178–188, 2011.
27. Arenja N, Mueller C, Ehl NF, et al.: Prevalence, extent, and independent predictors of silent myocardial infarction, *Am J Med* 126(6):515–522, 2013.
28. Sasson C, Meischke H, Abella BS, et al.: Increasing cardiopulmonary resuscitation provision in communities with low bystander cardiopulmonary resuscitation rates: a science advisory from the American Heart Association for healthcare providers, policymakers, public health departments, and community leaders, *Circulation* 127(12):1342–1350, 2013.
29. Toukola T, Hookana E, Junttila J, et al.: Sudden cardiac death during physical exercise: characteristics of victims and autopsy findings, *Ann Med* 47(3):263–268, 2015.
30. Byrne R, Constant O, Smyth Y, et al.: Multiple source surveillance incidence and aetiology of out-of-hospital sudden cardiac death in a rural population in the West of Ireland, *Eur Heart J* 29(11):1418–1423, 2008.
31. Kuriachan VP, Sumner GL, Mitchell LB: Sudden cardiac death, *Curr Prob Cardiol* 40(4):133–200, 2015.
32. Chugh SS, Uy-Evanado A, Teodorescu C, et al.: Women have a lower prevalence of structural heart disease as a precursor to sudden cardiac arrest: the Ore-SUDS (Oregon Sudden Unexpected Death Study), *J Am Coll Cardiol* 54(22):2006–2011, 2009.
33. Yusuf S, Hawken S, Ounpuu S, et al.: Effect of potentially modifiable risk factors associated with myocardial infarction in 52 countries (the INTERHEART study): case-control study, *Lancet* 364(9438):937–952, 2004.
34. Goff Jr DC, Lloyd-Jones DM, Bennett G, et al.: 2013 ACC/AHA guideline on the assessment of cardiovascular risk: a report of the American College of Cardiology/American Heart Association Task Force on Practice Guidelines, *Circulation* 129(25 suppl 2):S49–S73, 2014.
35. Castelli WP, Garrison RJ, Dawber TR, et al.: The filter cigarette and coronary heart disease: the Framingham study, *Lancet* 2(8238):109–113, 1981.
36. Hammal F, Ezekowitz JA, Norris CM, et al.: Smoking status and survival: impact on mortality of continuing to smoke one year after the angiographic diagnosis of coronary artery disease, a prospective cohort study, *BMC Cardiovasc Dis* 14:133, 2014.
37. Sniderman AD, Lamarche B, Contois JH, et al.: Discordance analysis and the Gordian knot of LDL and non-HDL cholesterol versus apoB, *Curr Opin Lipidol* 25(6):461–467, 2014.
38. Sniderman AD, Williams K, Contois JH, et al.: A meta-analysis of low-density lipoprotein cholesterol, non-high-density lipoprotein cholesterol, and apolipoprotein B as markers of cardiovascular risk, *Circ Cardiovasc Qual Outcomes* 4(3):337–345, 2011.
39. Cholesterol Treatment Trialists' (CTT) Collaboration, Baigent C, Blackwell L, et al.: Efficacy and safety of more intensive lowering of LDL cholesterol: a meta-analysis of data from 170,000 participants in 26 randomised trials, *Lancet* 376(9753):1670–1681, 2010.
40. James PA, Oparil S, Carter BL, et al.: 2014 evidence-based guideline for the management of high blood pressure in adults: report from the panel members appointed to the Eighth Joint National Committee (JNC 8), *JAMA* 311(5):507–520, 2014.
41. Group SR, Wright Jr JT, Williamson JD, et al.: A randomized trial of intensive versus standard blood-pressure control, *N Engl J Med* 373(22):2103–2116, 2015.
42. Regensteiner JG, Golden S, Huebschmann AG, et al.: Sex differences in the cardiovascular consequences of diabetes mellitus: a scientific statement from the American Heart Association, *Circulation* 132(25):2424–2447, 2015.
43. Look ARG, Wing RR, Bolin P, et al.: Cardiovascular effects of intensive lifestyle intervention in type 2 diabetes, *N Engl J Med* 369(2):145–154, 2013.
44. Wilson PW, D'Agostino RB, Parise H, et al.: Metabolic syndrome as a precursor of cardiovascular disease and type 2 diabetes mellitus, *Circulation* 112(20):3066–3072, 2005.
45. JBS3 Board: Joint British Societies' consensus recommendations for the prevention of cardiovascular disease (JBS3), *Heart* 100(Suppl 2):ii1–ii67, 2014.
46. Carlson SA, Fulton JE, Schoenborn CA, et al.: Trend and prevalence estimates based on the 2008 physical activity guidelines for Americans, *Am J Prev Med* 39(4):305–313, 2010.
47. Auer R, Bauer DC, Marques-Vidal P, et al.: Association of major and minor ECG abnormalities with coronary heart disease events, *JAMA* 307(14):1497–1505, 2012.
48. Jorgensen PG, Jensen JS, Marott JL, et al.: Electrocardiographic changes improve risk prediction in asymptomatic persons age 65 years or above without cardiovascular disease, *J Am Coll Cardiol* 64(9):898–906, 2014.
49. Nakamura Y, Okamura T, Higashiyama A, et al.: Prognostic values of clockwise and counterclockwise rotation for cardiovascular mortality in Japanese subjects: a 24-year follow-up of the National Integrated Project for Prospective Observation of Noncommunicable Disease and Its Trends in the Aged, 1980–2004 (NIPPON DATA80), *Circulation* 125(10):1226–1233, 2012.
50. Desai CS, Ning H, Lloyd-Jones DM: Competing cardiovascular outcomes associated with electrocardiographic left ventricular hypertrophy: the Atherosclerosis Risk in Communities Study, *Heart* 98(4):330–334, 2012.
51. Saxena A, Minton D, Lee DC, et al.: Protective role of resting heart rate on all-cause and cardiovascular disease mortality, *Mayo Clin Proc* 88(12):1420–1426, 2013.
52. Ho JE, Larson MG, Ghorbani A, et al.: Long-term cardiovascular risks associated with an elevated heart rate: the Framingham Heart Study, *J Am Heart Assoc* 3(3):e000668, 2014.
53. Bohm M, Reil JC, Deedwania P, et al.: Resting heart rate: risk indicator and emerging risk factor in cardiovascular disease, *Am J Med* 128(3):219–228, 2015.
54. Nauman J, Janszky I, Vatten LJ, et al.: Temporal changes in resting heart rate and deaths from ischemic heart disease, *JAMA* 306(23):2579–2587, 2011.
55. Ohlsson C, Barrett-Connor E, Bhasin S, et al.: High serum testosterone is associated with reduced risk of cardiovascular events in elderly men. The MrOS (Osteoporotic Fractures in Men) study in Sweden, *J Am Coll Cardiol* 58(16):1674–1681, 2011.
56. Malkin CJ, Pugh PJ, Morris PD, et al.: Low serum testosterone and increased mortality in men with coronary heart disease, *Heart* 96(22):1821–1825, 2010.
57. Nguyen PL, Je Y, Schutz FA, et al.: Association of androgen deprivation therapy with cardiovascular death in patients with prostate cancer: a meta-analysis of randomized trials, *JAMA* 306(21):2359–2366, 2011.
58. Sharma R, Oni OA, Gupta K, et al.: Normalization of testosterone level is associated with reduced incidence of myocardial infarction and mortality in men, *Eur Heart J* 36(40):2706–2715, 2015.
59. Basaria S, Coviello AD, Travison TG, et al.: Adverse events associated with testosterone administration, *N Engl J Med* 363(2):109–122, 2010.
60. Clarkson TB, Melendez GC, Appt SE: Timing hypothesis for postmenopausal hormone therapy: its origin, current status, and future, *Menopause* 20(3):342–353, 2013.
61. Dous GV, Grodman R, Mornan A, et al.: Menopausal hormone treatment in postmenopausal women: risks and benefits, *South Med J* 107(11):689–695, 2014.
62. Mason JC, Libby P: Cardiovascular disease in patients with chronic inflammation: mechanisms underlying premature cardiovascular events in rheumatologic conditions, *Eur Heart J* 36(8):482–489c, 2015.
63. Kahlenberg JM, Kaplan MJ: Mechanisms of premature atherosclerosis in rheumatoid arthritis and lupus, *Annu Rev Med* 64:249–263, 2013.
64. Ridker PM, Howard CP, Walter V, et al.: Effects of interleukin-1beta inhibition with canakinumab on hemoglobin A1c, lipids, C-reactive protein, interleukin-6, and fibrinogen: a phase IIb randomized, placebo-controlled trial, *Circulation* 126(23):2739–2748, 2012.
65. Madjid M, Alfred A, Sahai A, et al.: Factors contributing to suboptimal vaccination against influenza: results of a nationwide telephone survey of persons with cardiovascular disease, *Tex Heart Inst J* 36(6):546–552, 2009.
66. Madjid M, Miller CC, Zarubaev VV, et al.: Influenza epidemics and acute respiratory disease activity are associated with a surge in autopsy-confirmed coronary heart disease death: results from 8 years of autopsies in 34,892 subjects, *Eur Heart J* 28(10):1205–1210, 2007.
67. Baker WL, Couch KA: Azithromycin for the secondary prevention of coronary artery disease: a meta-analysis, *Am J Health-System Pharm* 64(8):830–836, 2007.
68. Targher G, Day CP, Bonora E: Risk of cardiovascular disease in patients with nonalcoholic fatty liver disease, *N Engl J Med* 363(14):1341–1350, 2010.
69. Lonardo A, Ballestri S, Targher G, Loria P: Diagnosis and management of cardiovascular risk in nonalcoholic fatty liver disease, *Exp Rev Gastroenterol Hepatol* 9(5):629–650, 2015.
70. Weinreich G, Wessendorf TE, Erdmann T, et al.: Association of obstructive sleep apnoea with subclinical coronary atherosclerosis, *Atherosclerosis* 231(2):191–197, 2013.
71. Kim SH, Cho GY, Baik I, et al.: Association of coronary artery calcification with obstructive sleep apnea and obesity in middle-aged men, *Nutr Metab Cardiovasc Dis* 20(8):575–582, 2010.
72. Banci M, Saccucci P, Dofcaci A, et al.: Birth weight and coronary artery disease. The effect of gender and diabetes, *Int J Biol Sci* 5(3):244–248, 2009.
73. Bukowski R, Davis KE, Wilson PW: Delivery of a small for gestational age infant and greater maternal risk of ischemic heart disease, *PloS One* 7(3):e33047, 2012.
74. Brook RD, Rajagopalan S, Pope III CA, et al.: Particulate matter air pollution and cardiovascular disease: an update to the scientific statement from the American Heart Association, *Circulation* 121(21):2331–2378, 2010.
75. Newby DE, Mannucci PM, Tell GS, et al.: Expert position paper on air pollution and cardiovascular disease, *Eur Heart J* 36(2):83–93b, 2015.
76. Sun Q, Hong X, Wold LE: Cardiovascular effects of ambient particulate air pollution exposure, *Circulation* 121(25):2755–2765, 2010.
77. Bauer M, Moebus S, Mohlenkamp S, et al.: Urban particulate matter air pollution is associated with subclinical atherosclerosis: results from the HNR (Heinz Nixdorf Recall) study, *J Am Coll Cardiol* 56(22):1803–1808, 2010.
78. Munzel T, Gori T, Babisch W, Basner M: Cardiovascular effects of environmental noise exposure, *Eur Heart J* 35(13):829–836, 2014.
79. Virtanen M, Nyberg ST, Batty GD, et al.: Perceived job insecurity as a risk factor for incident coronary heart disease: systematic review and meta-analysis, *BMJ* 347:f4746, 2013.
80. Kivimaki M, Nyberg ST, Batty GD, et al.: Job strain as a risk factor for coronary heart disease: a collaborative meta-analysis of individual participant data, *Lancet* 380(9852):1491–1497, 2012.
81. Kivimaki M, Jokela M, Nyberg ST, et al.: Long working hours and risk of coronary heart disease and stroke: a systematic review and meta-analysis of published and unpublished data for 603,838 individuals, *Lancet* 386(10005):1739–1746, 2015.
82. Rafnsson SB, Saravanan P, Bhopal RS, I, et al.: Is a low blood level of vitamin B12 a cardiovascular and diabetes risk factor? A systematic review of cohort studies, *Eur J Nutr* 50(2):97–106, 2011.
83. Veeranna V, Zalawadiya SK, Niraj A, et al.: Homocysteine and reclassification of cardiovascular disease risk, *J Am Coll Cardiol* 58(10):1025–1033, 2011.

84. Polak JF, O'Leary DH: Edge-detected common carotid artery intima-media thickness and incident coronary heart disease in the multi-ethnic study of atherosclerosis, *J Am Heart Assoc* 4(6):e001492, 2015.
85. Polak JF, Szklo M, O'Leary DH: Associations of coronary heart disease with common carotid artery near and far wall intima-media thickness: the multi-ethnic study of atherosclerosis, *J Am Soc Echocardiogr* 28(9):1114–1121, 2015.
86. Berry JD, Liu K, Folsom AR, et al.: Prevalence and progression of subclinical atherosclerosis in younger adults with low short-term but high lifetime estimated risk for cardiovascular disease: the coronary artery risk development in young adults study and multi-ethnic study of atherosclerosis, *Circulation* 119(3):382–389, 2009.
87. Polak JF: Carotid intima-media thickness: an early marker of cardiovascular disease, *Ultrasound Q* 25(2):55–61, 2009.
88. Vlachopoulos C, Aznaouridis K, Stefanadis C: Prediction of cardiovascular events and all-cause mortality with arterial stiffness: a systematic review and meta-analysis, *J Am Coll Cardiol* 55(13):1318–1327, 2010.
89. Ong KL, McClelland RL, Rye KA, et al.: The relationship between insulin resistance and vascular calcification in coronary arteries, and the thoracic and abdominal aorta: the Multi-Ethnic Study of Atherosclerosis, *Atherosclerosis* 236(2):257–262, 2014.
90. Bastos Goncalves F, Voute MT, Hoeks SE, et al.: Calcification of the abdominal aorta as an independent predictor of cardiovascular events: a meta-analysis, *Heart* 98(13):988–994, 2012.
91. Detrano R, Guerci AD, Carr JJ, et al.: Coronary calcium as a predictor of coronary events in four racial or ethnic groups, *N Engl J Med* 358(13):1336–1345, 2008.
92. Budoff MJ, Young R, Lopez VA, et al.: Progression of coronary calcium and incident coronary heart disease events: MESA (Multi-Ethnic Study of Atherosclerosis), *J Am Coll Cardiol* 61(12):1231–1239, 2013.
93. Criqui MH, Denenberg JO, Ix JH, et al.: Calcium density of coronary artery plaque and risk of incident cardiovascular events, *JAMA* 311(3):271–278, 2014.
94. Murabito JM, Pencina MJ, Nam BH, et al.: Sibling cardiovascular disease as a risk factor for cardiovascular disease in middle-aged adults, *JAMA* 294(24):3117–3123, 2005.
95. Patel RS, Asselbergs FW, Quyyumi AA, et al.: Genetic variants at chromosome 9p21 and risk of first versus subsequent coronary heart disease events: a systematic review and meta-analysis, *J Am Coll Cardiol* 63(21):2234–2245, 2014.
96. Dutta A, Henley W, Lang IA, et al.: The coronary artery disease-associated 9p21 variant and later life 20-year survival to cohort extinction, *Circ Cardiovasc Genet* 4(5):542–548, 2011.
97. Palomaki GE, Melillo S, Bradley LA: Association between 9p21 genomic markers and heart disease: a meta-analysis, *JAMA* 303(7):648–656, 2010.
98. Paynter NP, Chasman DI, Buring JE, et al.: Cardiovascular disease risk prediction with and without knowledge of genetic variation at chromosome 9p21.3, *Ann Intern Med* 150(2):65–72, 2009.
99. Dandona S, Stewart AF, Chen L, et al.: Gene dosage of the common variant 9p21 predicts severity of coronary artery disease, *J Am Coll Cardiol* 56(6):479–486, 2010.
100. Palomaki GE, Melillo S, Neveux L, et al.: Use of genomic profiling to assess risk for cardiovascular disease and identify individualized prevention strategies—a targeted evidence-based review, *Genet Med* 12(12):772–784, 2010.
101. Fan M, Dandona S, McPherson R, et al.: Two chromosome 9p21 haplotype blocks distinguish between coronary artery disease and myocardial infarction risk, *Circ Cardiovasc Genet* 6(4):372–380, 2013.
102. Hernesniemi JA, Lyytikainen LP, Oksala N, et al.: Predicting sudden cardiac death using common genetic risk variants for coronary artery disease, *Eur Heart J* 36(26):1669–1675, 2015.
103. Qi L, Qi Q, Prudente S, et al.: Association between a genetic variant related to glutamic acid metabolism and coronary heart disease in individuals with type 2 diabetes, *JAMA* 310(8):821–828, 2013.
104. Nelson CP, Hamby SE, Saleheen D, et al.: Genetically determined height and coronary artery disease, *N Engl J Med* 372(17):1608–1618, 2015.
105. Paynter NP, Chasman DI, Pare G, et al.: Association between a literature-based genetic risk score and cardiovascular events in women, *JAMA* 303(7):631–637, 2010.
106. Elashoff MR, Wingrove JA, Beineke P, et al.: Development of a blood-based gene expression algorithm for assessment of obstructive coronary artery disease in non-diabetic patients, *BMC Med Genom* 4:26, 2011.
107. Rosenberg S, Elashoff MR, Beineke P, et al.: Multicenter validation of the diagnostic accuracy of a blood-based gene expression test for assessing obstructive coronary artery disease in nondiabetic patients, *Ann Intern Med* 153(7):425–434, 2010.
108. Thomas GS, Voros S, McPherson JA, et al.: A blood-based gene expression test for obstructive coronary artery disease tested in symptomatic nondiabetic patients referred for myocardial perfusion imaging the COMPASS study, *Circ Cardiovasc Genet* 6(2):154–162, 2013.
109. Conroy RM, Pyorala K, Fitzgerald AP, et al.: Estimation of ten-year risk of fatal cardiovascular disease in Europe: the SCORE project, *Eur Heart J* 24(11):987–1003, 2003.
110. Ridker PM, Cook NR: Statins: new American guidelines for prevention of cardiovascular disease, *Lancet* 382(9907):1762–1765, 2013.
111. DeFilippis AP, Young R, Carrubba CJ, et al.: An analysis of calibration and discrimination among multiple cardiovascular risk scores in a modern multiethnic cohort, *Ann Intern Med* 162(4):266–275, 2015.
112. Fihn SD, Gardin JM, Abrams J, et al.: 2012 ACCF/AHA/ACP/AATS/PCNA/SCAI/STS Guideline for the diagnosis and management of patients with stable ischemic heart disease: a report of the American College of Cardiology Foundation/American Heart Association Task Force on Practice Guidelines, and the American College of Physicians, American Association for Thoracic Surgery, Preventive Cardiovascular Nurses Association, Society for Cardiovascular Angiography and Interventions, and Society of Thoracic Surgeons, *J Am Coll Cardiol* 60(24):e44–e164, 2012.
113. Antman EM, Cohen M, Bernink PJ, et al.: The TIMI risk score for unstable angina/non-ST elevation MI: a method for prognostication and therapeutic decision making, *JAMA* 284(7):835–842, 2000.
114. Eagle KA, Lim MJ, Dabbous OH, et al.: A validated prediction model for all forms of acute coronary syndrome: estimating the risk of 6-month postdischarge death in an international registry, *JAMA* 291(22):2727–2733, 2004.
115. Brieger D, Fox KA, Fitzgerald G, et al.: Predicting freedom from clinical events in non-ST-elevation acute coronary syndromes: the Global Registry of Acute Coronary Events, *Heart* 95(11):888–894, 2009.
116. Yeh RW, Secemsky EA, Kereiakes DJ, et al.: Development and validation of a prediction rule for benefit and harm of dual antiplatelet therapy beyond 1 year after percutaneous coronary intervention, *JAMA* 315(16):1735–1749, 2016.
117. Wilson PW, D'Agostino Sr R, Bhatt DL, et al.: An international model to predict recurrent cardiovascular disease, *Am J Med* 125(7):695–703, 2012.
118. Dorresteijn JA, Visseren FL, Wassink AM, et al.: Development and validation of a prediction rule for recurrent vascular events based on a cohort study of patients with arterial disease: the SMART risk score, *Heart* 99(12):866–872, 2013.

2 The Global Perspective of Ischemic Heart Disease

Matthew Lawlor, Bernard Gersh, Lionel Opie, and Thomas A. Gaziano

INTRODUCTION

Cardiovascular disease (CVD) and specifically ischemic heart disease (IHD) have long been the leading cause of death in high-income countries (HICs); indeed, "disease of the heart," in all its manifestations, has topped the Centers for Disease Control and Prevention cause of death list since 1921.[1] Coronary artery disease accounts for the majority of this disease burden.

With the progression of global development, the burden of CVD has increasingly been borne by low- and middle-income countries (LMICs), with up to 80% of CVD deaths worldwide occurring in LMICs.[2] The shifting burden of CVD, first encountered in HICs and increasingly affecting the developing world, is the result of the epidemiologic transition and represents the contribution of sanitation, public health, industrialization, urbanization, and economic advances, leading to a reduction in the burden of infectious disease on the one hand and an increase in CVD risk factors on the other hand.

Epidemiologic Trends

The epidemiologic transition consists of four basic stages (Fig. 2.1): pestilence and famine, receding pandemics, degenerative and man-made disease, and delayed degenerative diseases.[3] The current trend in CVD burden is being driven by the transition of LMICs to stage 3 of this transition, namely the phase of degenerative and man-made disease.[4,5] In this stage, improvement in economic circumstances, as well as increased urbanization with its attendant sociopsychologic stresses, results in altered dietary patterns, decreased activity levels, and an increase in behaviors associated with CVD, including smoking. These changes lead to an increase in atherosclerosis and resultant CVD; between 35% and 65% of all deaths in this stage are attributable to CVD, with IHD the predominant cause. The majority of CVD deaths in this stage are seen among individuals of higher socioeconomic status, as they are the first to benefit from these improvements in circumstance.[4]

High-income countries currently occupy the fourth stage of the transition: delayed degenerative diseases. In this stage, primary and secondary prevention measures, as well as new therapeutic approaches, lead to significant decreases in age-adjusted mortality rates. CVD still accounts for between 40% and 50% of all deaths in this stage, though largely affecting older individuals. Importantly, the burden of premature CVD in HICs shifts to lower levels of socioeconomic status, as those of higher status are first to benefit from improvements in the measures noted previously.[3,4]

Importantly, there is mounting evidence of a possible fifth stage: the age of obesity and inactivity. In some HICs, declines in age-adjusted mortality rates of CVD have leveled off, with improvements in rates of smoking and hypertension plateauing and with increasing rates of obesity and its associated consequences, including diabetes and dyslipidemia. Although the trends are for continued age-adjusted declines in mortality, some increases in risk factors particularly evident in children have the potential to reverse gains in age-adjusted CVD mortality in the coming years.[3,4]

Burden of Disease

With the global advancement through the epidemiologic transition, the primary drivers of global mortality have shifted from malnutrition, infectious disease, and infant and child mortality to more chronic, noncommunicable diseases. In the most recent survey of the Global Burden of Disease (GBD) in 2010, noncommunicable diseases comprised 65.5% of all deaths worldwide and approximately 43% of years of life lost (YLL), a measurement of amount of life lost due to premature mortality. Chief among this advanced class of maladies stands CVD, and within this category, IHD, as the primary cause of mortality worldwide. Indeed, IHD has remained the top-ranked cause of mortality worldwide from 1990 to 2010, and in 2010 overtook lower respiratory tract infections as the top-ranked cause of both YLL and disability-adjusted life years (DALYs).[2,6] In 2010, IHD was the cause of 13.3% of all deaths globally.[6]

IHD manifests in three clinical presentations: chronic stable angina, ischemic heart failure, and acute myocardial infarction (AMI). Whereas YLL secondary to AMI make up the largest portion of DALYs lost to IHD (94% in men, 92% in women)[7] (Fig. 2.2), IHD drives a growing number of years lived with disability (YLDs) as a result of chronic stable angina, ischemic cardiomyopathy, and nonfatal AMI. The largest proportion of YLD due to IHD is secondary to chronic stable angina, which in 2010 was prevalent in 20.3 per 100,000 males and 15.9 per 100,000 females. Ischemic heart failure, an increasingly important outcome in chronic IHD, was prevalent in 2.7 males and 1.9 females per 100,000. Disability due to nonfatal AMI, consisting of the period up to 28 days post-AMI, was responsible for a small fraction of YLDs due to IHD (Fig. 2.3).

Importantly, the epidemiologic transition underlies the trends in the incidence and prevalence of IHD and

Description	Life expectancy	Proportion of death due to CVD (%)	Dominant form of CVD death
Stage 1 Pestilence and famine			
• Malnutrition • Infectious diseases	35 years	<10	Infectious (RHD) Nutritional
Stage 2 Receding pandemics			
• Improved nutrition and public health • Chronic disease • Hypertension	50 years	10–35	Infectious (RHD) Stroke–hemorrhagic
Stage 3 Degenerative and man-made diseases			
• ↑ fat and caloric intake • Tobacco use • Chronic disease deaths > infections, malnutrition	>60 years	35–65 Stroke	IHD* — Hemorrhagic — Ischemic
Stage 4 Delayed degenerative diseases			
• Leading causes of mortality CV and cancer deaths • Prevention and Tx delays onset • Age-adjusted CV death reduced	>70 years	40–50	• IHD** • Stroke–ischemic • CHF

* Greater in high socioeconomic groups
** Younger patient—lower socioeconmic status
Elderly—higher socioecnomic status

FIG. 2.1 Stages of epidemiologic transition. *CVD,* Cardiovascular disease; *CHF,* congestive heart failure; *IHD,* ischemic heart disease; *RHD,* rheumatic heart disease; *Tx,* therapy.

its growing burden of disease worldwide. Globally, the number of deaths due to IHD increased from 5.2 million to 7 million from 1990 to 2010, though in the same time period age-adjusted death rates decreased from 131.3 to 105.7 per 100,000, an almost 20% improvement.[2] Similarly, YLDs secondary to all chronic sequelae of IHD increased from 1990 to 2010: chronic angina from 5 million to 7.2 million (44% increase), ischemic cardiomyopathy from 890,000 to 1.5 million (70% increase), and nonfatal AMI from 29,000 to 42,000 (45% increase).[7] As with mortality secondary to fatal AMI, age-standardized prevalence of chronic stable angina and nonfatal AMI fell from 1990 to 2010, though there was a slight increase in the age-standardized prevalence of ischemic cardiomyopathy. Despite the almost universal improvement in age-standardized incidence and prevalence of IHD, the absolute global burden of IHD measured in DALYs increased by 29% from 1990 to 2010. This increase was driven primarily by the aging of the world's population and increasing size of the population, accountable for 32.4% and 22.1% of the growth of DALYs, respectively. These changes were attenuated by an overall decrease of 25.3% in the age-adjusted IHD DALY rate. Notably, in LMICs, the increase in IHD DALYs was driven primarily by the increasing size of the population, whereas in HICs, the increase was largely due to the increasing age of the population.[7]

Data on incident AMI and prevalent IHD are well documented; however there is a significant body of evidence that suggests that coronary atherosclerosis, the etiology of IHD, has a long detectable preclinical phase.[8] The biologic onset of disease occurs long before the manifestation of symptoms, resulting in a lengthy asymptomatic disease state. Efforts to characterize patients as low-, intermediate-, and high-risk for the development of IHD have been established through the use of risk scores. However, diagnosis prior to clinical onset of disease is largely prohibitive due to the invasive nature of the gold standard for IHD diagnosis, coronary angiography. Recent technical advances have resulted in the introduction of coronary computed tomography (CT) angiography to assess coronary artery calcification and stenosis. The modality has been shown to be highly sensitive and specific for the detection of greater than 50% stenosis versus coronary angiography.[9] In multiple large-scale trials, CT screening of middle-aged patients between 45 and 74 years old with no history of IHD was revealing for *any* degree of coronary artery calcification in one-half to two-thirds of people screened.[10,11] These numbers may be reflective only of asymptomatic IHD in HICs, though with the continued advancement of LMICs through the epidemiologic transition, this may soon be representative of larger swaths of the global population. Indeed, in a postmortem study of coronary artery atherosclerosis in

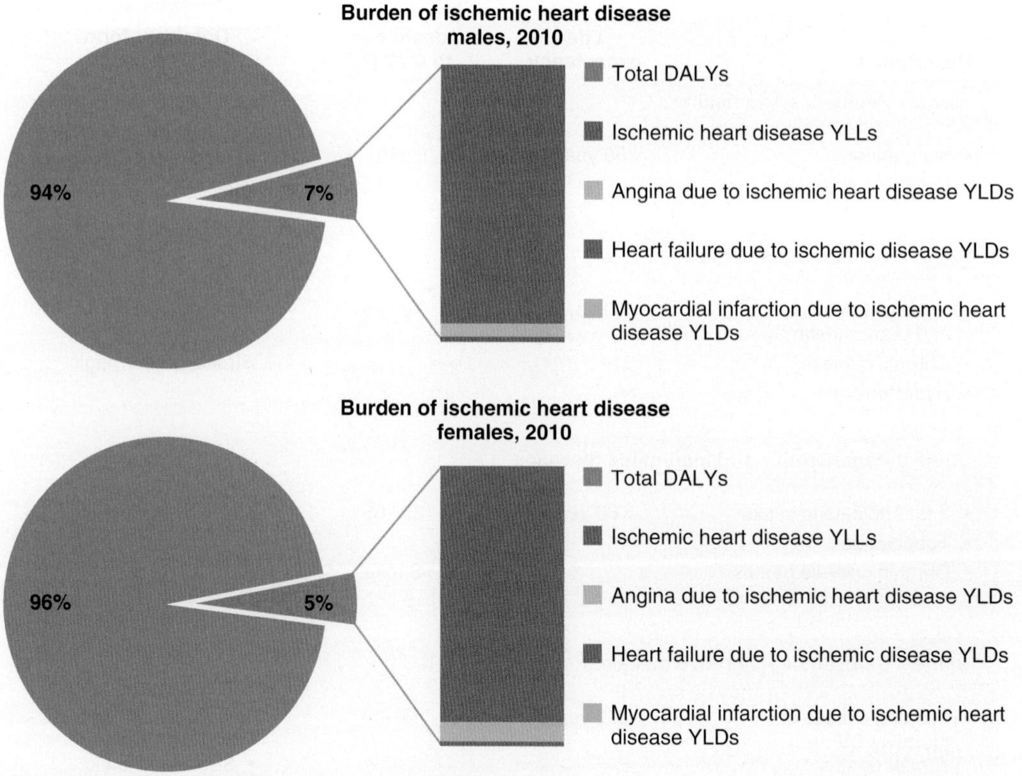

FIG. 2.2 Disability-adjusted life years (DALYs) secondary to ischemic heart disease. *YLL*, Years of life lost; *YLD*, years lived with disability. *(From Moran AE, Forouzanfar MH, Roth GA, et al. The global burden of ischemic heart disease in 1990 and 2010: the Global Burden of Disease 2010 study.* Circulation. *2014;129(14):1493–1501.)*

northern India, stenosis was found in approximately 30% of cases (mean age 35 years); of these, approximately two-thirds of cases were nonobstructive, with narrowing of less than 50% of the coronary lumen.[12] These results are consistent with the growing disease burden of IHD in LMICs.

Disease Burden by Region

With the progression of societies through the epidemiologic transition, larger proportions of IHD morbidity and mortality are borne by LMICs as previously discussed. In this section, we will detail incidence, prevalence, and trends in IHD in distinct regions as defined by the GBD study.[2,6,7,13,14] Figs. 2.4 and 2.5 depict regional variation in YLD and total DALYs lost to IHD, respectively. Figs. 2.6 and 2.7 graphically display temporal trends in IHD DALYs and proportion of DALYs driven by YLDs by GBD region, respectively. Data in this section on social and demographic indices in these regions are derived by World Bank World Development Indicators.

High-Income Countries

Social and Demographic Indices

Over 1 billion people live in HICs as defined by the GBD, including the regions of southern Latin America, Western Europe, high-income North America, Australasia, and high-income Asia Pacific. Of these countries, the largest is the United States, with approximately 318 million inhabitants. People in these countries enjoy relatively long life expectancies, with men born in this region in 2013 expected to live approximately 80 years and women 83 years. The median percentage of the population over 65 in these countries is 17%, though there is a significant range, from 10% in southern Latin America to greater than 18% in Western Europe. Notably, greater than 25% of the population of Japan is over the age of 65. The median gross national income (GNI) per capita and health expenditure per capita in this region are $46,550 and $3965, respectively. Median public spending on health expenditures as a percent of total spending is approximately 75%.

Disease Burden and Trends

There is great heterogeneity in the epidemiology of IHD throughout this region. HICs as a group enjoyed the lowest number of DALYs lost to IHD per population in 2010, from a low of 654 per 100,000 persons in high-income Asia Pacific, to 1636 in high-income North America. As a share of total morbidity and mortality, IHD was responsible for 4.7% of DALYs in this region in 2010. By comparison, this number was 7.88% in 1990. High-income Asia Pacific again bears the lowest percent of DALYs attributed to IHD at 2.7%, compared to 6.1% in high-income North America. It is worth noting that the high-income Asia Pacific region bears an aberrantly high stroke burden, with ischemic stroke driving almost half of the CVD burden in this region. This is compared to a greater than 2:1 global ratio in favor of IHD over stroke in CVD mortality.

As previously mentioned, the primary driver of DALYs lost secondary to IHD is YLL due to AMI. Of over 21 million DALYs lost to IHD in HICs in 2010, just over 10% were due to morbidity associated with IHD, including nonfatal AMI, angina, and ischemic cardiomyopathy. In 1990, this number was less than 7%, which belies the shifting

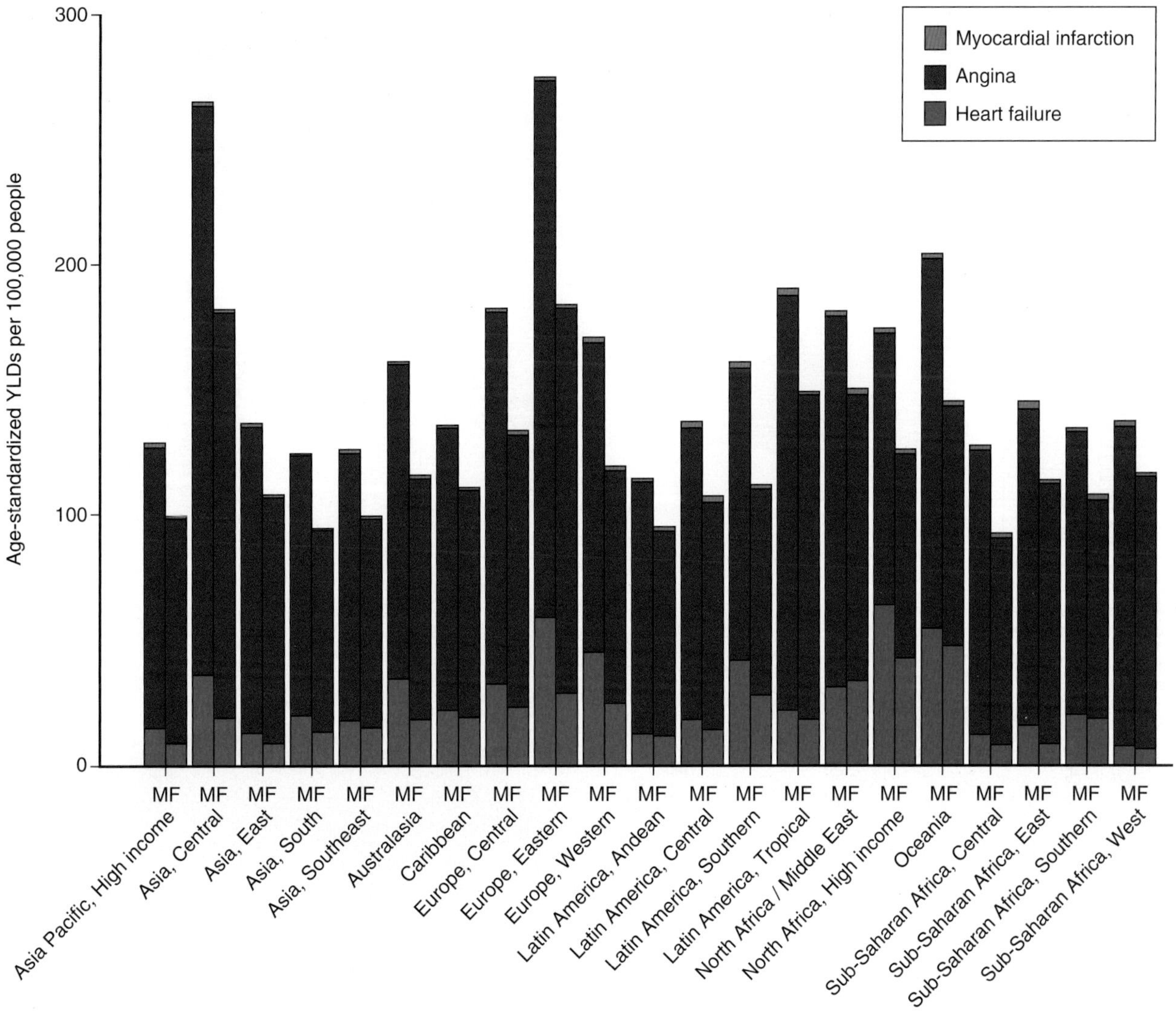

FIG. 2.3 Cause-specific years lived with disability (YLDs) secondary to chronic ischemic heart disease. *(From Moran AE, Forouzanfar MH, Roth GA, et al. The global burden of ischemic heart disease in 1990 and 2010: the Global Burden of Disease 2010 study.* Circulation. *2014;129(14):1493–1501.)*

burden of IHD from acute events to a chronic condition. YLDs in the high-income Asia Pacific region drove more than 15% of DALYs in 2010, as compared to less than 9% in high-income North America and southern Latin America. The mean age of onset of angina rose from 60.2 to 62.2 from 1990 to 2010, and its mean duration of 14 years did not change in the interceding decades. Mean age of first AMI rose from 69.9 to 71.4.

With advancement through the stages of epidemiologic transition, much of the improvement in IHD morbidity and mortality can be attributed to better preventive and therapeutic measures resulting in the decrease in age-standardized incidence and prevalence of IHD. The age-standardized incidence rates of AMI fell from 245 to 173 males per 100,000 and 119 to 85 females per 100,000 from 1990 to 2010. Incidence rates of angina similarly fell from 24 to 18 in males and 17 to 13 in females per 100,000. Notably, though, prevalence rates of ischemic cardiomyopathy increased during this same time frame, albeit as a less common outcome than either AMI or angina: 3.2 to 3.7 males and 2 to 2.3 females per 1000 persons.

Despite the improvement in age-standardized rates of morbidity and mortality secondary to IHD described, the global burden of IHD continues to rise. The exception to this phenomenon is in HICs, where not only age-adjusted rates of IHD but absolute IHD DALYs have fallen from 1990 to 2010 in three—Western Europe, high-income North America, and Australasia—of five regions in this grouping, with total burden remaining relatively stable in high-income Asia Pacific and southern Latin America. Total burden of DALYs due to IHD has fallen more than 30% in Western Europe, 28% in Australasia, and 17% in high-income North America due to large improvements in age-adjusted incidence; in Australasia, the age-adjusted incidence rate of IHD has been nearly halved in 20 years. High-income Asia Pacific additionally has seen dramatic reductions in age-adjusted incidence rates—approximately a 75% decrease. However, total burden of IHD DALYs has risen 10% due to a sharp increase in aging of the population.

Eastern Europe/Central Asia

Social Indices

There are 400 million inhabitants of the Central and Eastern Europe and Central Asia regions. The population is evenly divided among these three regions, with Russia being the

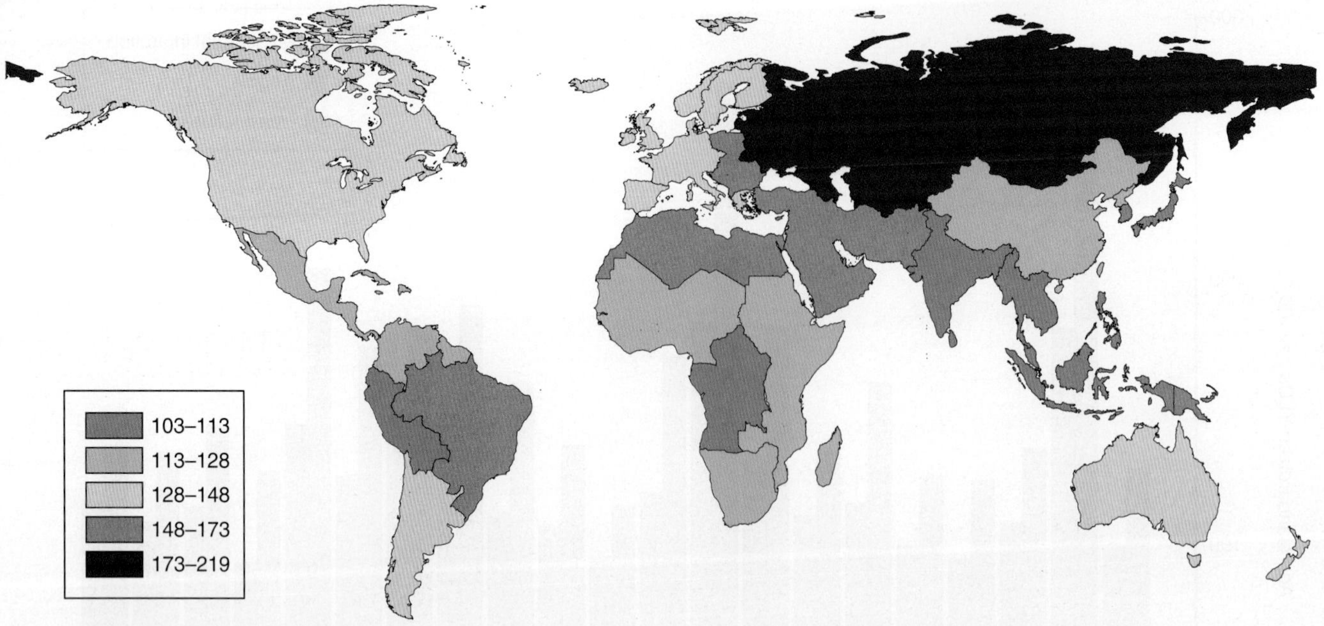

FIG. 2.4 Years lived with disability secondary to chronic ischemic heart disease per 100,000 population by region. *(From Moran AE, Forouzanfar MH, Roth GA, et al. The global burden of ischemic heart disease in 1990 and 2010: the Global Burden of Disease 2010 study.* Circulation. *2014;129(14):1493–1501.)*

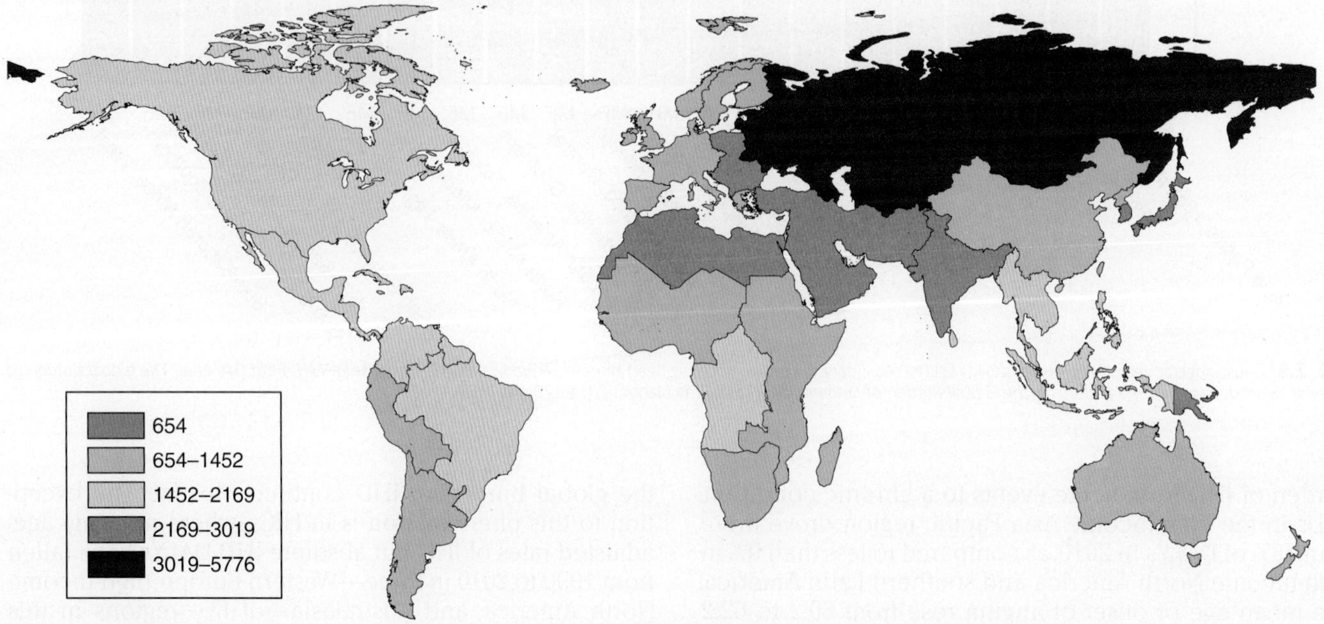

FIG. 2.5 Disability-adjusted life years secondary to chronic ischemic heart disease per 100,000 population by region. *(From Moran AE, Forouzanfar MH, Roth GA, et al. The global burden of ischemic heart disease in 1990 and 2010: the Global Burden of Disease 2010 study.* Circulation. *2014;129(14):1493–1501.)*

largest individual nation by population with 140 million people. This region has a high median percentage of the population over 65 at approximately 14%; however, this number masks vast differences in the population makeup between regions. Whereas Eastern and Central Europe have greater than 15% and 16% of persons over the age of 65, respectively, this number is only 4.6% in Central Asia. Median life expectancy across the region is approximately 71 years in men and 78 years in women, though men in Central Asia and Eastern Europe have life expectancies of 66 years and 67 years, respectively. Median GNI per capita is $7590, ranging from $13,220 in Eastern Europe to $4020 in Central Asia. Median health expenditure in the region is $462, which represents 6.5% of gross domestic product (GDP). Public spending makes up 60% of total health expenditures in the region.

Disease Burden and Trends

The Eastern Europe/Central Asia region holds the highest burden of DALYs secondary to IHD globally. Age-adjusted DALYs per 100,000 persons numbered 4614 in 2010, a figure that has not seen much change in two decades (4741 per 100,000 persons in 1990). The majority of disease in this region is driven by Eastern Europe and Central Asia, both of which have seen increases in IHD DALY rates from 1990 to 2010 and currently rank first and second in IHD DALY rates by region at 5776 and 5459 IHD DALYs per 100,000, respectively. These numbers represent 12.8% and 15.3% of total DALYs in

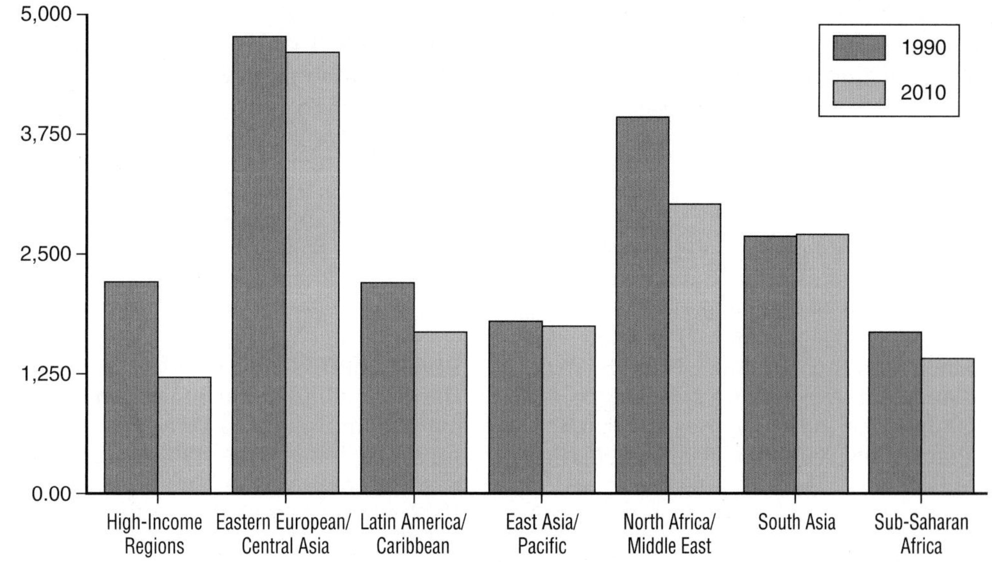

FIG. 2.6 Ischemic heart disease disability-adjusted life years per 100,000 persons.

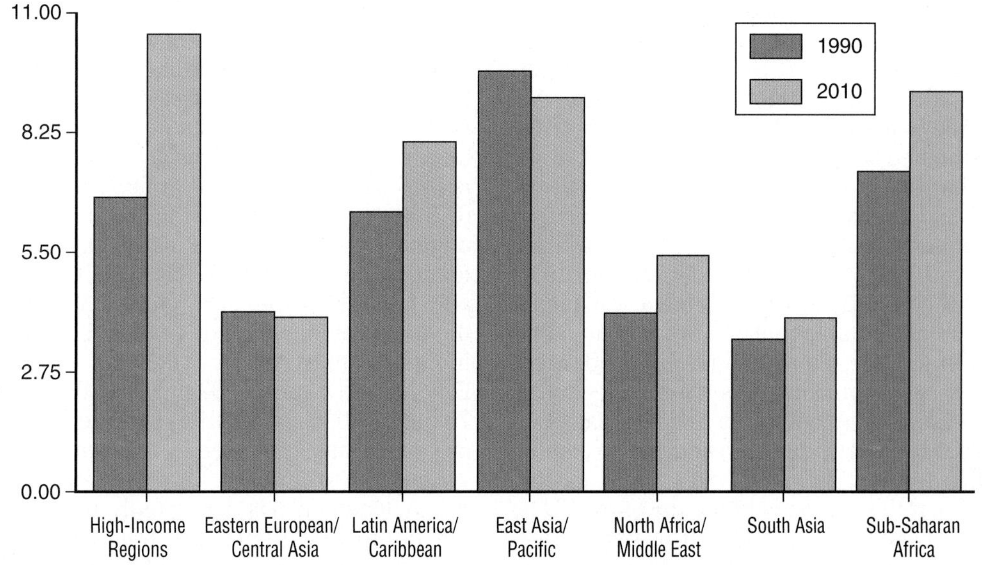

FIG. 2.7 Percent ischemic heart disease disability-adjusted life years secondary to years lived with disability.

these regions. Indeed, these are the only two regions globally where the rate of rise of YLLs outpaced increases in YLDs as they contribute to total IHD DALYs. YLDs secondary to IHD account for 3.65% in Eastern Europe and 4.08% in Central Asia. Central Europe, by contrast, has not only seen improvement in its age-adjusted rate of IHD DALYs per 100,000 persons from 3936 to 2608, but also a decrease in total burden of IHD DALYs from 1990 to 2010, the only non-HIC region to earn such a distinction. IHD DALYs account for less than 8% of total DALYs in this region, and an increasing proportion of DALYs is due to YLDs, from 4.11% in 1990 to 5.54% in 2010.

The mean age of onset of angina in this region is 60 years, ranging from 56 years in Central Asia to 62.3 years in Central Europe. The incidence of angina has remained stable overall in the region as a whole, at 30.5 and 22 per 100,000 men and women, respectively, in 2010. The mean age of incident AMI is 69.5, distributed from young (66.6) in Central Asia, to old (71.9) in Central Europe. The incidence of AMI has fallen for the region as a whole from 1990 to 2010 in both men and women from 343 to 338 and 186 to 175 per 100,000 persons, though it has risen for men in both Eastern Europe and Central Asia, as well as for women in Eastern Europe; these trends have been offset by greater improvement in AMI incidence in Central Europe. The prevalence of ischemic cardiomyopathy has increased for both men and women in all regions, and averages 4 per 1000 persons in men (5.5 in Eastern Europe, 3.0 in Central Europe) and 2 per 1000 persons in women.

The gains noted in Central Europe have been made by a decrease in age-adjusted rates of IHD DALYs of greater than 40%, resulting in an actual 12% improvement in IHD DALYs from 1990 to 2010. In contrast, age-adjusted rates in Central Asia have remained flat, and have increased in Eastern Europe by greater than 15%. Increases in actual IHD burden in these two regions total greater than 37% and 31%, respectively. Population growth and aging of the population have combined to result in the increase in actual IHD DALYs in Central Asia, whereas the aforementioned increase in age-adjusted rates of disease and aging of the population has driven the increase in Eastern Europe; notably, this region has seen a net decrease in the population of greater than 6% from 1990 to 2010. Central Europe, too, has seen a net negative decline in total population, with aging of the population offsetting some of the gains made in age-adjusted mortality rates.

Latin America/Caribbean

Social Indices

There are over 550 million people living in the Latin America/Caribbean region, which includes the Caribbean, central, tropical, and Andean regions of Latin America. Median life expectancy in the region is 70 in men and 77 in women, and 6.8% of the population is over 65. Median GNI in the region is $6770, and median health expenditure per capita is $431 annually; this ranges from $76 in Haiti to over $1000 in Brazil, Costa Rica, the Bahamas, and Barbados. Health expenditure represents 6.5% of GDP, and 57% of that figure stems from public spending.

Disease Burden and Trends

The Latin America/Caribbean grouping bears a relatively low rate of IHD DALYs as a region, ranging from 1144 in Andean Latin America to 2169 in the Caribbean. There has been improvement in the age-standardized IHD DALYs as a whole over two decades, from 2216 in 1990 to 1699 per 100,000 persons in 2010, representing 5.25% of total DALYs lost in the region. The percent that IHD DALYs contribute to total DALYs has remained stable over this time period; however this masks changes in disease proportions in subregions. Central and Andean Latin America have seen relative increases in the proportion of DALYs lost secondary to IHD, from 6.1% to 6.7% and 3.5% to 4.2%, respectively, from 1990 to 2010. In contrast, the Caribbean saw a dramatic decline in the percent of DALYs attributable to IHD, from 6.3% to 5.3%; although this region did see improvement in age-adjusted rates of IHD DALYs per population, this likely reflects the large increase in DALYs lost secondary to natural disaster in the setting of the 2010 Haiti earthquake. In addition to overall improvement in age-adjusted IHD DALY rates, an increasing proportion of DALYs in this region is being driven by YLDs, from 6.5% to 8.1% between 1990 and 2010. This percentage is highest in tropical Latin America at 9.3% and lowest in the Caribbean at 5.6%.

The mean age at onset of angina in this region is 57 years, and mean duration is 16 years. Mean age at incident AMI is 67 years. There has been a stable to mildly decreased incidence rate of angina, from 20.9 to 19.2 per 100,000 in men and 17 to 15.3 in women from 1990 to 2010. The AMI incidence rate has similarly trended down, from 219 to 191 in men and 144 to 121 in women per 100,000 over the same time period. Rates of ischemic cardiomyopathy have increased in this region as they have globally, from 1.47 to 1.77 per 1000 in men and 1.32 to 1.51 per 1000 in women.

The region as a whole has seen an increase in absolute DALYs lost to IHD primarily due to an increase in population growth and aging of the population. For instance, despite an improvement by over 30% in the age-adjusted rate of IHD morbidity and mortality in Central Latin America, actual IHD DALYs have jumped 62.2%, with over 50% change due to aging of the population and approximately 40% due to population growth. This story is similar in other parts of the region, with the exception of the Caribbean, which has seen little population growth at 3.4% and thus has had the lowest increase in actual rates of IHD DALYs at 22%.

East Asia/Pacific

Social Indices

Over 2 billion people live in the East Asia, Southeast Asia, and Oceania regions, including 1.36 billion in China alone. Median life expectancy in men is 67 years and in women 73 years. The median percentage of the population over 65 in the region as a whole is 5.18, but it is notably 9.18 in China. Median GNI per capita is $3460, and median health expenditure per capita is $123. Health expenditures represent a median 4.57% of GDP in the region, of which 67% is public spending.

Disease Burden and Trends

The East Asia/Pacific region, including populous China, has a combined IHD DALY rate of 1759 per 100,000 persons, which has been stable for the past two decades. The East Asia region, which includes China, has a lower rate at 1242, whereas Oceania has the highest rate in the region at 2324. IHD DALYs represent 5.2% of total DALYs lost in the superregion, and of them, 9% are due to YLD secondary to IHD. Notably, YLDs in East Asia contribute over 10% to total IHD DALYs, and in total number nearly 1.9 million YLD due to IHD; South Asia and Western Europe also contribute over 1 million YLDs to the global total.

The mean age at incidence of angina in the East Asia/Pacific region is 55.3 years, and mean age at incident AMI is 63.7 years. Oceania has notably earlier onset of disease than other regions in this grouping, with onset of angina at 52.6 and incident AMI at 60.7, compared with 57.5 and 67.5 years, respectively, in East Asia. The incidence rate of angina per 100,000 persons is 19.4 in males and 13.3 in females, and for AMI 179.5 and 103.3 per 100,000 males and females, respectively, both small improvements from the two previous decades. Oceania has nearly double the incident rate of AMI in males and females compared with East Asia: 212 versus 132 per 100,000 males and 130 versus 78 per 100,000 females. The prevalence of ischemic cardiomyopathy has increased in this region as well, from 2.3 to 2.7 and 2.1 to 2.3 per 1000 males and females, respectively. Again, Oceania has a markedly worse burden of disease per population than other regions in this grouping, with 5.22 per 1000 males and 4.53 per 1000 females affected by ischemic cardiomyopathy, compared with 1.19 and 0.83, respectively, in East Asia.

As a superregion, East Asia/Pacific has experienced a 70.9% increase in total DALYs secondary to IHD, which is second only to the South Asia superregion. Despite increases in actual DALYs across the board as a superregion, each region has been affected by different dynamics to arrive at a similar point. East Asia, including China, has seen an increase in actual DALYs by 75.5%, of which 47.1% can be attributed to aging of the population and 11.4% to an increase in age-adjusted DALY rates. Only 17% of this increase is the result of population growth, which coupled with a large effect due to aging can likely be linked to the one-child policy pursued in China over the past three decades. In contrast, Southeast Asia, which has seen a reduction in age-adjusted DALY rates by 16%, nevertheless saw actual disease burden increase by 61.5% due to both aging (44.4%) and population growth (33.2%). Oceania has unfortunately seen a 72.3% increase in actual disease burden due to population growth (31.6%), population aging (29.9%), and an increased age-adjusted DALY rate (10.9%).

North Africa/Middle East

Social Indices

483 million people live in the North Africa/Middle East region. Median life expectancy in this region is 72 in males and 76 in females, with 3.7% of the population over 65 years of age. Median GNI per capita in the region is $6500, and per capita health expenditures are $432; the latter figure ranges from $42 in Syria to $1507 in Kuwait. Health expenditures represent a median of 5.1% of GDP, of which 65% is public spending.

Disease Burden and Trends

The North Africa/Middle East region has a relatively high rate of IHD DALYs at 3019 per 100,000 in 2010; nevertheless, this has improved significantly from approximately 4000 per 100,000 in 1990. A high proportion of total DALYs is attributable to IHD in this region, at 10.8%, and it is increasing in share (from 9.7% in 1990). Of these, only 5.5% can be attributed to YLDs.

The mean age at onset of angina in this region is 54.7 years, and of AMI 63.8 years. Both angina and AMI incidence per 100,000 persons have improved from 1990 to 2010: angina from 25.3 to 23.2 in males and 20.5 to 18.0 in females per 100,000, and AMI from 290 to 257.5 in males and 178.1 to 152.6 in females per 100,000. Ischemic cardiomyopathy prevalence rates have remained stable through time, numbering 3 males per 1000 and 3.2 females per 1000 in 2010.

The North Africa/Middle East region experienced an actual increase in IHD DALYs of 37.2% from 1990 to 2010. Despite improvement in age-adjusted DALY rates by 47.2%, actual rates were driven by population growth (45.4%) and aging (39%).

South Asia

Social Indices

Approximately 1.7 billion people reside in South Asia, of whom 1.3 billion live in India. Median life expectancy in the region is 67 in men and 69 in women; this ranges from 58 to 70 for men and 61 to 72 for women in Afghanistan and Bangladesh, respectively. A median of 4.9% of the population is older than 65. Median GNI per capita is $1240, and median health expenditures per capita total $47. Health expenditures represent 3.85% of GDP, of which 36% is public spending.

Disease Burden and Trends

South Asia, including India, has seen a small increase in IHD DALYs per 100,000, from 2685 in 1990 to 2728 in 2010. Notably, by 2010 South Asia IHD contributed more than 30 million DALYs to the global total, more than any other superregion. In 2010, DALYs lost to IHD contributed 6.46% of total DALYs lost. Of these, only 4% were secondary to YLDs, up from 3.5% in 1990.

Age at onset of angina in South Asia was 54.7 in 2010, with average duration of 16 years. Average age at onset of incident AMI was 63.8. Incident angina increased in males from 1990 to 2010, from 13.7 to 16.3 per 100,000, and was stable in females, from 12.3 to 12.5 per 100,000. Incident AMI decreased for both males and females, from 254 to 245 in males and 169 to 155 in females per 100,000. Rates of ischemic cardiomyopathy were relatively low in both males and females, at 1.87 males per 1000 and 1.32 females per 1000 in 2010.

From 1990 to 2010, the South Asia superregion saw the single largest increase in actual DALYs lost to IHD: 75.5%. This change was driven primarily by aging of the population (47.1%), as well as by population growth (17%) and increase in age-adjusted rates of disease (11.4%).

Sub-Saharan Africa

Social Indices

Approximately 1 billion people live in sub-Saharan Africa, the great majority of whom are in Eastern and Western sub-Saharan Africa. The median life expectancy for men is 58 and for women is 61, ranging from 54 to 60 for men and 58 to 64 for women. Median GNI per capita is $975; in Eastern sub-Saharan Africa, where a plurality resides (> 400 million), this number is $790. Southern sub-Saharan Africa is relatively wealthy by comparison, with median GNI of $4590. Health expenditure per capita in the region is $54, ranging from $48 and $49 in Western and Eastern sub-Saharan Africa, respectively, to $397 in Southern sub-Saharan Africa. Health expenditures represent a median of 5.4% of GDP in the region, with public spending accounting for 50% of these expenditures.

Disease Burden and Trends

With the exception of the high-income superregion, sub-Saharan Africa had the lowest age-adjusted rate of IHD DALYs in 2010 at 1425 per 100,000 persons, down from 1693 in 1990. This rate represented the lowest proportion of IHD DALYs as contributing to total DALYs of any region, at 2%. Within this region, there was little significant variation in this trend. YLDs represented 9.26% of total IHD DALYs, from 5.5% in Central sub-Saharan Africa to 11% in Eastern sub-Saharan Africa.

The average age of onset of angina in this grouping was 52.75 years, and average age of incident AMI was 61.4 years. These represent the youngest average ages of onset of disease of any superregion. From 1990 to 2010, there was little change in incidence of angina in both men and women, at 19 per 100,000 males and 15 per 100,000 females in 2010. There were small improvements in the rates of incident AMI in both males and females in this time frame, from 199 to 188 per 100,000 males and 147 to 142 per 100,000 females. AMI rates for the grouping as a whole mask discrepancies between regions: whereas AMI incidence rates in males improved or were stable in Southern (210 to 174 per 100,000), Eastern (191 to 173 per 100,000), and Central sub-Saharan Africa (226 to 223 per 100,000), Western sub-Saharan Africa saw a slight increase in AMI incidence in males in this timeline, from 168 to 181 per 100,000. Ischemic cardiomyopathy prevalence rates for the grouping as a whole were lower than any other superregion, at 1.31 per 1000 males and 0.98 per 1000 females.

All regions in the sub-Saharan African superregion saw increases in their IHD DALY burden from 1990 to 2010, from 20.8% in Southern sub-Saharan Africa to 58.8% in Central sub-Saharan Africa. All of these regions additionally saw improvements in their age-adjusted IHD DALY rates, from a 57% improvement in Southern sub-Saharan Africa to a 10.5% improvement in Central sub-Saharan Africa. The offsetting factor in all four of the regions in this grouping was population growth, which was accountable for nearly all of the gain in actual IHD DALYs with the exception of Southern sub-Saharan Africa, for which aging of the population increased actual burden of IHD DALYs by 42.5%. Population aging was actually reversed in Central sub-Saharan Africa, with 9%

improvement in actual IHD DALYs due to a younger population in 2010 than in 1990.

Risk Factors

Risk factors for IHD, including smoking, hypertension, and dyslipidemia, were first identified in population-based cohort studies, including the Framingham Heart Study. Whereas these studies helped determine the etiology of IHD, the relationship of these risk factors to IHD was established in populations of largely European descent in HICs. In order to explore the applicability of these findings to other ethnic groups and other settings, including LMICs, the INTERHEART study published data in 2004 on risk factors associated with first AMI in 52 countries on every inhabited continent. The results of this case-control study reinforced the importance of traditional risk factors for IHD and MI across ethnic and geographic divides.[15] Using the results of this study, the INTERHEART score was devised, similar to Framingham and other studies, to predict incident CVD.

In a follow-up study, the Prospective Urban Rural Epidemiology (PURE) cohort investigated the prevalence of these risk factors and their relationship to incident CVD.[16] Notably, there was a higher burden of risk factors as determined by INTERHEART risk score in HICs as opposed to LMICs (Fig. 2.8). Despite this, there was a higher incidence of major cardiovascular events, including death from CVD, MI, stroke, and heart failure, in low-income versus middle-income and middle-income versus high-income countries. These findings likely belie more robust efforts at risk factor control, as well as appropriate management of incident and prevalent CVD, in urban and high-income areas.

Next, we will explore the global prevalence of the main risk factors for CVD, as well as the evidence for their etiologic relationship to development of CVD, including IHD. The population-attributable risk (PAR) for individual risk factors by geographic regions is summarized in Table 2.1.

Smoking

Smoking is the most important lifestyle risk factor associated with IHD and the second most important risk factor in IHD, as well as overall morbidity and mortality, worldwide; total DALYs attributable to smoking worldwide numbered greater than 115 million in men and approximately 41 million in women in 2010.[2] As reported in the GBD study, 31% of DALYs lost secondary to IHD can be attributed to smoking[17] (Table 2.2). Indeed, the odds ratio (OR) for AMI in current smokers versus nonsmokers is 2.95 and increases with the amount of smoking; in individuals smoking more than 40 cigarettes per day (equivalent of 2 packs), the OR for AMI is 9.16.[15]

As referenced previously, as the burden of morbidity and mortality secondary to IHD shifts from HICs to LMICs, risk factors for disease continue to comingle in HICs, with the notable exception of smoking. Whereas tobacco use, and specifically smoking, is still one of the most important causes of morbidity and mortality in HICs the prevalence of current smokers is higher in LMICs than HICs. The exception to this trend is in female smokers, although they are more prevalent in HICs, they make up a much smaller proportion of total smokers worldwide. In the PURE study previously referenced, approximately 16% of men and 11% of women in HICs were current smokers, as opposed to approximately 40% of men and less than 10% of women in LMICs. Furthermore, the inverse relationship between level of educational attainment and CVD risk factors does not appear to exist in LMICs.[18]

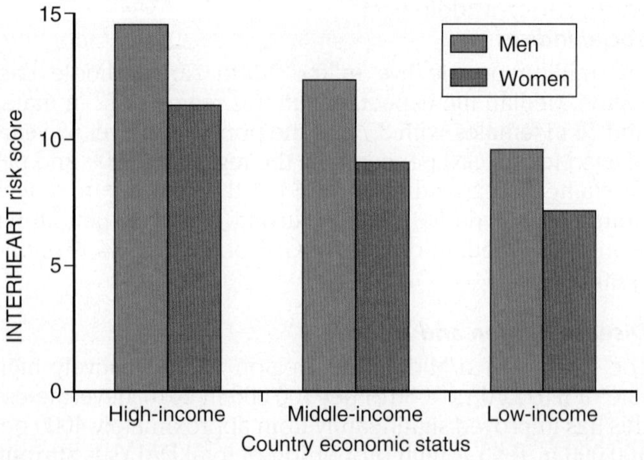

FIG. 2.8 Risk factor burden in high-, middle- and low-income countries, as measured by INTERHEART risk score. *(Data from Yusuf S, Rangarajan S, Teo K, et al. Cardiovascular risk and events in 17 low-, middle-, and high-income countries.* N Engl J Med. *2014;371(9):818–827.)*

Hypertension

Hypertension is the risk factor accounting for the most DALYs lost secondary to IHD; over 50% of PAR can be ascribed to it.[17] It is also, importantly, the major risk factor for global DALYs lost due to any cause. As shown in Table 2.2, the OR of AMI in hypertensive versus nonhypertensive individuals is 2.48.[15]

In the PURE study on global CVD risks and events, 49% of males and 37% of females in HICs had a self-reported history of hypertension, compared with 45% and 44% in middle-income countries and 32% and 34% in low-income countries, respectively. The PAR of hypertension for development of AMI varies geographically, but notably is highest in Southeast Asia and Japan (up to 38%), South America (32.7%), and Africa (29.6%).

In a large systematic review of systolic blood pressure (SBP) prevalent levels and trends, Danaei et al. found that global SBP fell by 0.8 mm Hg in men and 1.0 mm Hg in women per decade between 1980 and 2008.[19] Male SBP fell the most in high-income North America (2.8 mm Hg per decade), as well as in Australasia and Western Europe, which saw declines of greater than 2.0 mm Hg per decade. Female SBP fell by greater than 3.5 mm Hg in Australasia and Western Europe per decade. In contrast, SBP rose for both sexes in Oceania, Eastern sub-Saharan Africa, Southeast Asia, and South Asia. Rate of rise was between 0.8 mm Hg and 1.6 mm Hg per decade in men and 1.0 mm Hg and 2.7 mm Hg per decade in women. Highest SBP levels in men were seen in Eastern Europe and Eastern and Western sub-Saharan Africa, with a mean SBP of 138 mm Hg or greater. Highest SBP in women was noted in Eastern and Western sub-Saharan Africa, where mean SBP levels were as high as 135 mm Hg.

Dyslipidemia

Though hypertension has been noted to be the largest contributor to DALYs secondary to IHD worldwide, dyslipidemia, which contributes 29% of PAR to IHD DALYs, likely has a stronger relationship to development of disease. In Yusuf's study on the risk factors associated with AMI, the highest quintile of dyslipidemia, measured in apolipoprotein

TABLE 2.1 Regional Differences in Risk Factor Burden by Population-Attributable Risk

	SMOKING	DIET	EXERCISE	HYPERTENSION	DIABETES	OBESITY	DYSLIPIDEMIA
Western Europe	39	13.3	37.7	20.5	12.8	68.6	36.7
Central and Eastern Europe	40.4	7.6	−0.4	15.9	5.8	31.7	38.7
Middle East	51.4	5.8	1.9	5.8	13.1	23.9	72.7
Africa	45.2	−4.4	15.9	26.8	11.6	60.4	73.7
South Asia	42.0	16.0	25.5	17.8	10.5	36	60.2
China	45.3	15.1	16.6	19.9	7.9	4.9	41.3
Southeast Asia and Japan	39.2	8.5	31.4	34.3	19.1	57.9	68.7
Australia and New Zealand	46.1	8.0	20.6	18.3	5.6	49.5	48.7
South America	42.4	7.1	27.6	28.1	9.7	35.2	41.6
North America	30.9	22.4	24.7	13.9	6.1	64.7	60

From Yusuf S, Hawken S, Ounpuu S, et al. Effect of potentially modifiable risk factors associated with myocardial infarction in 52 countries (the INTERHEART study): case-control study. Lancet. *2004;364(9438):937–952.*

TABLE 2.2 Proportion of Ischemic Heart Disease Disability-Adjusted Life Years (DALYs) Attributable to Individual Risk Factors Worldwide in 2010

	DALYS (%)
Physiologic risk factors	
High blood pressure	53
High total cholesterol	29
High body mass index	23
High fasting plasma glucose	16
Alcohol use	5
Tobacco smoking, including second-hand smoke	31
Dietary risk factors and physical inactivity	
Diet low in nuts and seeds	40
Physical inactivity and low physical activity	31
Diet low in fruits	30
Diet low in seafood omega-3 fatty acids	22
Diet low in whole grains	17
Diet high in sodium	17
Diet high in processed meat	13
Diet low in vegetables	12
Diet low in fiber	11
Diet low in polyunsaturated fatty acids	9
Diet high in trans fatty acids	9
Diet high in sugar-sweetened beverages	2
Air pollution	
Ambient particulate matter pollution	22
Household air pollution from solid fuels	18
Other environmental risks	
Lead exposure	4

From Lim SS, Vos T, Flaxman AD, et al. A comparative risk assessment of burden of disease and injury attributable to 67 risk factors and risk factor clusters in 21 regions, 1990–2010: a systematic analysis for the Global Burden of Disease Study 2010. Lancet. *2012;380(9859):2224–2260.*

B/apolipoprotein A1 ratios, was associated with an OR of incident AMI of 3.87; indeed, this study found a graded relationship between severity of dyslipidemia and incident disease, with no effect plateau identified.[15] As reported by the GBD, the PAR of dyslipidemia was 29% for all IHD DALYs, including YLDs.[17,20]

IHD risk factors increase as populations urbanize and societies move through the epidemiologic transition. Whereas hypertension, diabetes, and obesity, as we will review later, increasingly affects people in LMICs, hypercholesterolemia remains largely a risk factor of HICs. In the PURE study, 48% of men and 53% of women in HICs had elevated cholesterol levels. This was in comparison to 32% and 37% in middle-income and 17% and 23% in low-income countries, respectively. These studies were notably conducted on total cholesterol levels, rather than low-density lipoprotein (LDL) or apolipoprotein B.

Farzadfar et al. conducted a systematic analysis of geographic and temporal trends in cholesterol levels that supports these findings.[21] They similarly surveyed total cholesterol and found that the highest levels were found in HICs, specifically Australasia, high-income North America, and Western Europe. Total cholesterol levels in these regions averaged 5.24 mmol/L in men and 5.23 mmol/L in women. In contrast, the lowest levels of total cholesterol were found in sub-Saharan Africa, where the average level was 4.08 mmol/L in men and 4.27 mmol/L in women. The study did note the temporal trend of gradual decline in high-income regions, including those with the highest concentrations mentioned previously, as well as in central and eastern Europe, where rates of decline averaged 0.2 mmol/L per decade in both men and women. In contrast, total cholesterol levels increased in some LMICs, including East Asia and Southeast Asia at a rate of 0.08 mmol/L in men and 0.09 mmol/L in women; these trends, however, were not enough to offset the difference in total cholesterol between HICs and LMICs.

Diabetes

Although not a traditional risk factor, diabetes has increasingly been identified as a major predisposition for the development of IHD. In the INTERHEART study, this risk was noted to be outsized in women: the OR for development of AMI in men with diabetes compared with controls was 2.67, though in women the OR was 4.26, and it represented a PAR of greater than 19% versus 10% in men.[15] In the PURE study, diabetes prevalence was fairly even among high-, middle-, and low-income countries, ranging from 7.6% to 10.9% in men and 7.2% to 8.3% in women.[16]

Danaei et al. carried out a large-scale study on the prevalence and temporal trends in diabetes from 1980 to 2008.[22] Their findings suggest more nuance than the homogeneity found in diabetes prevalence across income strata in the PURE study. The highest prevalence found in this study was in the Oceania region at 15.5% of men and 15.9% of women, followed by South Asia, Latin America and the Caribbean, and Central Asia, North Africa, and the Middle East. Of high-income regions, high-income North America and Australasia also had a high prevalence of diabetes. This was in comparison to a lower prevalence of diabetes found in both HIC and LMIC regions, including high-income Asia Pacific, Western Europe, East and Southeast Asia, and sub-Saharan Africa. Globally, age-standardized prevalence of diabetes increased from 1990 to 2008, from 8.3% to 9.8% in men and 7.5% to 9.2% in women. Increases were seen in virtually every country in all regions.

Obesity

Obesity, a risk factor for hypertension, dyslipidemia, and diabetes, has also been noted to be an independent predictor of IHD. Indeed, as will be expanded upon hereafter, obesity has been substituted for dyslipidemia in risk scoring for primary prevention in IHD with good correlation. In the INTERHEART study, abdominal obesity (as measured by waist/hip ratio > 0.95 in men and > 0.90 in women) was associated with an OR of 2.24 for AMI and a PAR of greater than 33% for incident AMI when controlling for age, sex, and smoking.[15] When controlling for other risk factors that confound effects of obesity, these measurements were less profound but still significant: OR of 1.62 and PAR of 20.1%. In the PURE study, obesity as measured by body mass index (BMI) rather than waist/hip ratio showed marked variation in distribution among HICs and LMICs: in HICs, BMI greater than 30 was prevalent in more than 25% of both men and women. In middle-income countries, the percent of obese men and women was 14% and 21%, and in low-income countries 5% and 11%, respectively.[16]

In a study on global geographic and temporal trends in obesity, Finucane et al. found a worldwide increase in BMI by 0.4 kg/m^2 in men and 0.5 kg/m^2 in women from 1980 to 2008.[23] These global trends were consistent in all regions with the exception of Central sub-Saharan Africa and South Asia in men, which saw small decreases in average BMI. Increases in BMI were largest in Oceania in both men (1.3 kg/m^2) and women (1.8 kg/m^2). In 2008, the highest mean BMI levels in men were in high-income North America at 28.4 kg/m^2 and Australasia 27.6 kg/m^2; the correlating regions for women were high-income North America, North Africa and Middle East, and Southern sub-Saharan Africa, all with BMIs greater than 28 kg/m^2. The lowest BMI in men was seen in Central, East, and West sub-Saharan Africa and East, Southeast, and South Asia, all at less than 23 kg/m^2. In women, lowest BMI values were found in Central and East sub-Saharan Africa, South Asia, East Asia and high-income Asia Pacific, also at less than 23 kg/m^2. As a whole, men had higher BMIs than women in high-income subregions and lower BMIs in most low- and middle-income regions. Globally, obesity (BMI > 30) was prevalent in 9.8% of men and 13.8% of women, numbers that nearly doubled in the interim from 1980.

Diet and Physical Activity

Apart from their effects on risk factors for IHD, diet, particularly consumption of fruits and vegetables, and lack of physical activity play a significant role in the development of IHD, as well as overall morbidity and mortality globally. In a GBD report on burden of disease and risk factors, low dietary fruit was listed as the fourth largest cause of lost DALYs globally, physical inactivity was tenth, and low dietary vegetables was seventeenth. Diets low in fruit and vegetables were associated with over 100 million DALYs and approximately 40 million DALYs lost, respectively, worldwide in 2010. Along with lack of physical activity and other dietary risk factors, including diets low in whole grains, nuts, seeds, and milk and high in red meat and processed meats, these risk factors altogether accounted for over 250 million DALYs lost in 2010.[17]

In the INTERHEART study, regular intake of fruits and vegetables and regular physical activity were individually associated with an OR of 0.70 of incident AMI. PAR for these lifestyle risk factors was 12.9% for dietary fruit and vegetable intake and greater than 25% for regular exercise.[15] The prevalence of these risk factors in the PURE study was divergent, with less people in HICs endorsing low physical activity (10.8% males, 11.7% females) compared with LMICs (20.1–22.5% males and 13.8–17.1% females). Interestingly, men in HICs were more likely to ascribe to unhealthful diet compared with LMICs (40.4% vs 30.1–32.5%), though the same was not true of women, with a relatively similar number of women endorsing unhealthy diet across the economic spectrum (28.4–33.1%).[16] In addition to the traditional risk factors, other nontraditional risk factors such as air pollution, stress due to migration, and HIV may apply additional roles in CVD risk in LMICs.[24,25]

Management by Region

The increasing incidence and prevalence of IHD have prompted need for response both in primary and secondary prevention of disease. Here we will review global trends in individual treatment, population management, and policy measures to combat IHD.

Prevention

In the early 20th century, the growing epidemic of CVD in HICs prompted the creation of population-based studies in Europe and the United States to examine the risk factors associated with incidence of disease. These studies, including the Framingham Heart Study, have generated much of the foundational understanding of the natural history of CVD. Using data gathered on risk factors for disease, prediction models were published to help guide clinicians in the identification of individuals at high risk of development of IHD. These models have been updated over the years, though they still largely rely on several foundational risk factors, including smoking, hypertension, and dyslipidemia, to inform clinical decision-making in individual patients. These risk scores have been formally incorporated into guidelines on the treatment of cholesterol for the express purpose of prevention of CVD.[26]

More recently, the American College of Cardiology/ American Heart Foundation Blood Cholesterol Guidelines have set a standard for primary and secondary prevention of arteriosclerotic CVD (ASCVD). The Guidelines' recommendations include the use of statin therapy in all patients with clinically apparent ASCVD (secondary prevention), as well as in all patients at high risk of ASCVD as determined by a new sum risk score (primary prevention). The latter of these two aims breaks from previous guidelines, which encouraged treatment thresholds and goals based on cholesterol levels and informed by overall IHD risk.[20,27] The Heart Outcomes Prevention Evaluation-3 (HOPE-3) trial also supports the notion that overall risk including age as a risk factor is perhaps more important than LDL cholesterol level, at least for those with intermediate levels. Other guidelines[28] have suggested that treatment decisions should rely on lifetime risk, which diminishes the importance of age as a risk factor, but there are limited data on lifetime treatment of lipids from a young age to confirm if this strategy is more cost-effective.

The delineation of IHD risk factors and creation of risk scores for prediction of incident IHD have allowed for the implementation of previously mentioned screening and treatment guidelines for primary prevention of IHD. With these treatment guidelines in mind, one can examine the success of primary and secondary prevention efforts at both a public health and an economic level. We will start with the evidence found in HICs.

High-Income Countries

Primary Prevention

Screening efforts for IHD have been directed at two related but distinct populations: patients with risk factors for disease, for example, dyslipidemia, hypertension, etc., and patients with high risk of development of IHD based on sum risk scores as described previously. Whereas current screening efforts have shifted to favor more the sum risk score approach, previous guidelines included treatment thresholds and goals based on lipid profiling, that is, treating the risk factor rather than the sum risk. These guidelines included recommendations on individual lipid components, including LDL and triglycerides. Similar guidelines exist on the treatment of hypertension based on treatment thresholds and blood pressure goals.

In light of dynamic recommendations on who and how to screen, metrics for success of screening programs have shifted in accord. The outcomes of screening programs can be measured in the number of patients treated according to guidelines, as well as by the adequacy of control obtained by these treatments, whether it be improvement in risk factor profile or in composite cardiovascular outcomes.

In the mid-1990s, Steinberg et al. reviewed achievement of risk factor goals, including blood pressure and cholesterol levels, in outpatients with clinically evident CVD or risk factors for disease (including dyslipidemia, hypertension, diabetes mellitus, and the metabolic syndrome). This study took place in the United States and Europe over a 9-year period between 1998 and 2006. Among the primary prevention group, 58% of patients in the United States at high risk of development of CVD had LDL levels at or below target level in 2006 based on treatment goals at the time. In Europe, this number was 35%, with a large minority of patients at risk for CVD undergoing no testing for LDL cholesterol levels. The group found that 65% of all subjects in the United States met the blood pressure goal of less than 140/90 mm Hg in 2006; this number was only 49% in Europe.[29] A similar level of poor risk factor control was seen in the Future Revascularization Evaluation in patients with Diabetes mellitus: optimal management of Multivessel disease (FREEDOM) trial.[30]

In a similar study on treatment goals in primary (as well as secondary) prevention, Bhatt et al. published the baseline characteristics of the REduction of Atherothrombosis for Continued Health (REACH) registry in 2006, a large global registry of patients with CVD and risk factors for CVD.[31] They defined subjects at risk of disease as having three or more risk factors for CVD, among which were hypertension, hypercholesterolemia, diabetes, and smoking. Of all patients with hypertension in high-income regions (North America, Western Europe, Australia, and Japan), including those with risk factors and with clinical CVD, 96% were on at least one antihypertensive agent. In this same cluster of regions, 66% of all patients were prescribed an aspirin, and 72% were prescribed a statin. Despite these efforts, between 40% and 60% of subjects in HICs had inadequately controlled blood pressure, and between 25% and 50% of subjects in these same regions had elevated cholesterol levels.[31]

In 2010, follow-up data on the REACH registry were released. After a 4-year interval, 9.1% of patients who were at risk of CVD but without clinically overt disease on presentation experienced an ischemic event, including either MI or stroke. Hazard ratio (HR) for development of cardiovascular death in this group was 4.34, and HR was 2.26 for nonfatal MI. These data were inclusive of patients in both HIC and LMIC regions. Importantly, both aspirin and statin therapy were associated with a lower risk of CV death, MI, or stroke.[32]

Secondary Prevention

The strongest evidence for medical management of IHD is in secondary prevention in patients with known IHD. In this population, four classes of medications have been associated with improvement in survival: antiplatelet agents, statins, β-blockers, and in a subset of individuals, angiotensin-converting enzyme (ACE) inhibitors. Unlike the dynamic therapeutic targets in primary prevention, there is agreement that the secondary prevention population benefits from optimal medical therapy with these four classes of medications if tolerated.

As previously mentioned, the PURE study was a multinational epidemiologic survey on CVD first published in 2011 that enrolled over 150,000 thousand subjects in 17 countries on five continents. Among subjects with a history of IHD in HICs, statins were prescribed to 70.9%, antiplatelet agents (including aspirin) to 64.1%, β-blockers to 46.5%, and ACE inhibitors to 51.7%. Among patients with IHD in HICs, almost 50% reported use of at least three out of four proven effective medications for CVD, with only 12% reporting no medication usage.[33]

Data on the REACH registry convey that a significant proportion of patients in HICs, both with overt CVD and risk factors for disease, were on antihypertensive therapy, antiplatelet agents, and statins. In all participants with IHD in this registry, including both high-income and low- and middle-income regions, 86% of subjects were on an antiplatelet agent, 76% were on a statin, 63% were on a β-blocker, and 51% were on ACE inhibitors. In the follow-up data published in 2010, 12.2% of subjects with stable CVD at baseline had experienced a CV event. In subjects with a history of an ischemic event, this number was 18.3%. Both aspirin and statins had protective effects on the development of CV events in follow-up.[31,32] The Synergy Between Percutaneous Coronary Intervention with Taxus and Cardiac Surgery (SYNTAX) trial also showed poor use of optimal medical therapy in those with IHD.[34]

Low- and Middle-Income Countries

LMICs are increasingly bearing the burden of IHD as the population ages and continues to expand; as discussed previously, approximately 80% of the burden of IHD is now born by LMICs. Whereas guidelines for treatment in the primary

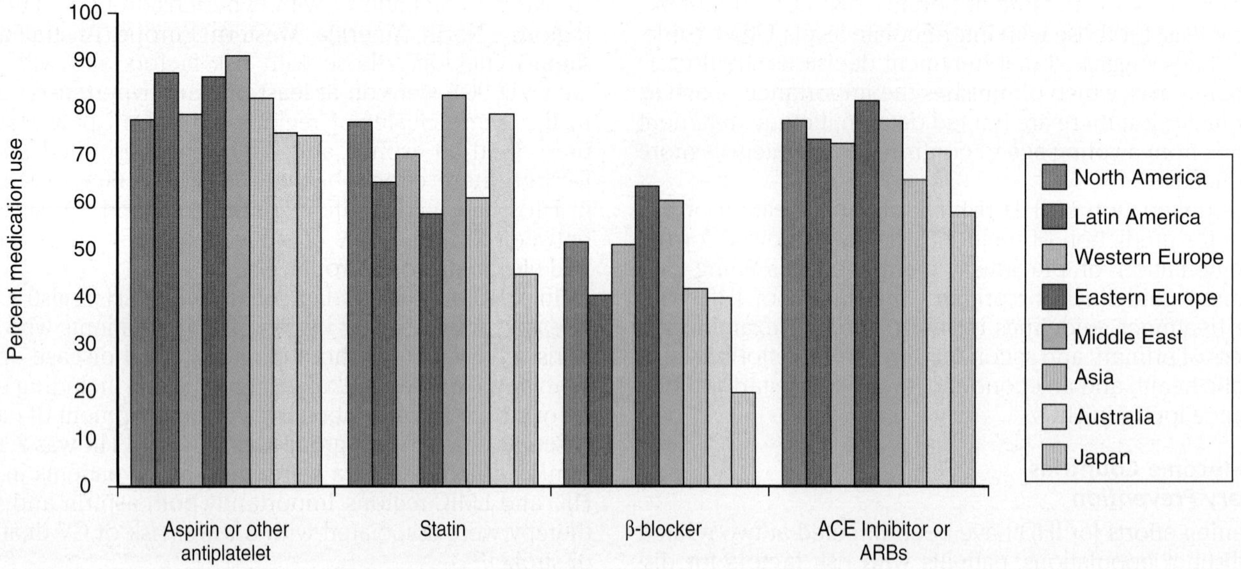

FIG. 2.9 Medication use among patients in the REACH registry, percentage of population. *(Data from Bhatt DL, Steg PG, Ohman EM, et al. International prevalence, recognition, and treatment of cardiovascular risk factors in outpatients with atherothrombosis.* JAMA. *2006;11;295(2):180–189.)*

and secondary prevention of CVDs have been developed in HICs based on evidence of improvement in CVD outcomes, many of the diagnostics and therapeutics discussed are not readily available in LMICs. Accordingly, there have been calls for investigation into the appropriateness of these guidelines in resource-poor settings. Here we present data on the use of alternative risk scores to guide treatment and use of effective medications for primary and secondary prevention of IHD, as well as an economic analysis of treatment costs in LMICs.

Primary Prevention

In patients at high risk of developing disease, complex risk scores as described previously have been used to help guide clinicians in selecting an appropriate treatment for primary prevention. A key component of these various risk scores is laboratory data, including cholesterol levels, to help determine risk. In LMICs, such routine data are often unavailable, rendering these risk scores largely unhelpful in identifying high-risk patient populations. As a result, the World Health Organization (WHO) has designed and implemented the use of nonlaboratory-based risk prediction tools to guide treatment in primary prevention[35] in resource-poor settings. In 2008, Gaziano et al. presented data supporting the accuracy of these substituted risk prediction tools. Their results demonstrated that scores incorporating BMI rather than laboratory cholesterol data could predict future cardiovascular events with accuracy similar to more traditional laboratory-based models.[36] These tools allow for focused treatment of high-risk individuals in resource-poor settings without sacrificing accurate risk prediction.

In LMICs, primary and secondary prevention of IHD is underutilized to a greater extent than in HICs. In the PURE study, use of proven effective medications in primary prevention was 15% to 65% as common in middle-income countries compared with HICs, with ACE inhibitors the most commonly prescribed medication and statins the least. This same pattern holds true for low-income countries, with proven effective medications used as little as 3% as often as in HICs for statins for primary prevention purposes.[16]

In subjects in LMICs treated for both primary and secondary prevention of CVD in the REACH registry, 96.3% with hypertension were on at least one antihypertensive, 75.6% were on aspirin, and 63.5% were on a statin. Regional differences in medication use are displayed in Fig. 2.9. Between 55% and 65% of subjects in LMICs had uncontrolled blood pressure, and between 35% and 65% of subjects had cholesterol levels above target.[31] Of note, at 4-year follow-up, two distinct LMIC regions, Eastern Europe and the Middle East, had significantly increased risk of CV death, MI, or stroke compared with the other regions studied.[32]

Secondary Prevention

As in HICs, there is little dispute regarding the indication for secondary prevention of IHD with proven effective medications in LMICs. Despite this, significant proportions of these individuals are untreated or undertreated in these regions.

In the PURE study, uptake of proven effective medications for the secondary prevention of CVD in LMICs was notably lower than that seen in HICs. In subjects with IHD, those taking statin therapy were 21.1%, 4.9%, and 4.5% in upper middle-, lower middle-, and low-income countries, respectively. Similar trends were seen for antihypertensives (51.0%, 36.1%, and 21.8%) and antiplatelet agents (27.1%, 20.1%, and 11.0%). Additional differences were seen between urban and rural areas, with higher percentage of subjects receiving treatment in urban centers; the trend toward disparity between urban and rural subjects was inverse to the wealth of a given country: HICs saw little difference in prescription rates between urban and rural subjects. Patients in LMICs were also more likely to be on no treatment at all, with 48.4%, 67.5%, and 82.8% of subjects in upper middle-, lower middle-, and low-income countries taking none of the four proven effective drugs[33] (Fig. 2.10).

One way to address drug availability and affordability is a combination of generic CVD medications or "polypill" given to all adults with significant risk for CVD.[37] It has been estimated that this single intervention could reduce IHD events by as much as 50%. The potential advantages of a polypill for primary prevention include[38] reduced need for dose titrations, improved adherence, and use of cheap generics in single formulation.

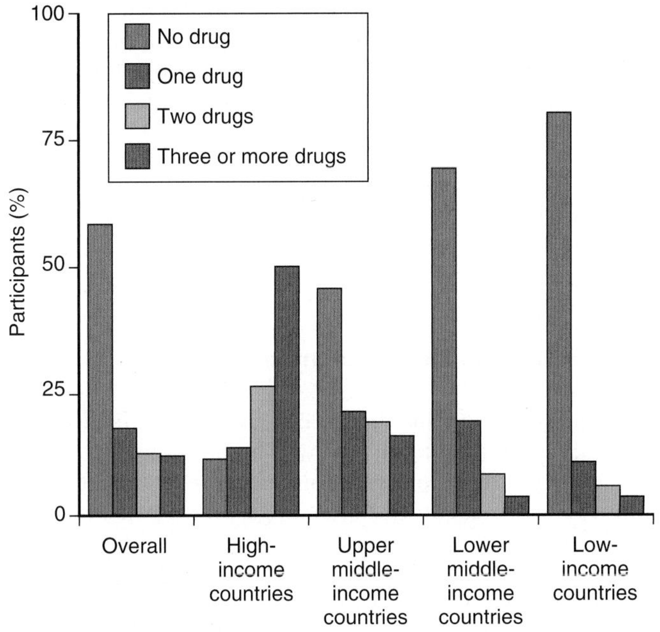

FIG. 2.10 Number of drugs taken by individuals by country economic status. Drugs counted were aspirin, β-blockers, angiotensin-converting enzyme inhibitors or angiotensin-receptor blockers, or statins. *(From Yusuf S, Islam S, Chow CK, et al. Use of secondary prevention drugs for cardiovascular disease in the community in high-income, middle-income, and low-income countries (the PURE Study): a prospective epidemiological survey.* Lancet. *2011;378(9798):1231–1243.*

TABLE 2.3 Cost-Effectiveness for a Selection of Ischemic Heart Disease Interventions in Developing Regions

	COST-EFFECTIVENESS RATIO ($US/DALY)
Drug treatments	
Primary prevention	
Cholesterol lowering (Brazil)	441/LY
Multidrug regimen (AR > 20–25%) (global)	771–1195
Secondary prevention	
Multidrug regimen (ASA, BB, ACEI, statin)	306–388
Policy interventions	
Tobacco	
Price increase of 33%	2–85
Nonprice interventions	33–1432
Salt reduction	
2 to 8 mm Hg reduction	Cost saving –250
Fat-related interventions	
Reduced saturated fat intake	Cost saving –2900
Trans fat replacement –7% reduction in CHD	50–1500

ACEI, Angiotensin-converting enzyme inhibitor; *ASA,* aspirin; *BB,* β-blocker; *AR,* absolute risk; *DALY,* disability-adjusted life years.

Whereas several studies have shown reductions in risk factors such as blood pressure and cholesterol[39] and improvement in adherence, no such study with reductions in IHD or stroke endpoints has been published, though several are currently under way.[38–40]

The use of a polypill in secondary prevention is less controversial because, even though there has been no trial proving its efficacy in this setting, there are multiple trials showing that the individual component drugs (aspirin, statins, β-blockers, and blockers of the renin-angiotensin system) improve outcomes in patients with known CVD or high risk factor levels.[38] In addition, a large case-control analysis of 13,029 patients with IHD in the United Kingdom indicated that combinations of drugs (statin, aspirin, and β-blockers) rather than single agents decreased mortality in patients with known CVD.[41] Finally, the use of combination therapy was shown to be cost-effective for LMICs for both primary and secondary prevention, with the best cost-effectiveness ratio for secondary prevention.[42,43]

Cost-Effectiveness

In resource-constrained settings, the question of cost-effectiveness must often be addressed before large-scale investment in treatment options can be scaled up. The WHO has established guidelines on the cost-effectiveness of treatments based on national resources and has set the standard to be incremental cost-effectiveness ratios of 3 × the GNI per head. Incremental cost-effectiveness ratios allow comparison between strategies, and they are calculated as the difference in costs divided by the difference in quality-adjusted life years (QALYs) gained. Notwithstanding criticism of the premise, these guidelines offer at least a barometer for a discussion on best use of limited resources.

In another study, modeling of primary and secondary prevention strategies in LMICs yielded a gain of 2 years of life expectancy in regions studied, at costs of less than $400/QALY in secondary prevention and less than $900/QALY in primary prevention in patients identified to be at high risk (10-year absolute CVD risk score > 25%).[44] The regimens studied were proven effective medications as previously discussed, with the exchange of calcium-channel blockers for β-blockers in primary prevention. Primary prevention strategies were more expensive per QALY gained due to the increased number needed to treat in order to prevent an event. However, in all areas studied, these treatment regimens were shown to be cost-effective per WHO guidelines when treating to absolute CVD risk of 5% in primary prevention. Notably, if the model were half as effective as predicted in prevention of CVD, treating to an absolute risk of 25% would remain cost-effective in these regions[44] (Table 2.3).

A similar study of cost-effectiveness of scaling up primary and secondary prevention of CVD by Lim et al.[45] found that over 17.9 million deaths could be averted in a 10-year period over 23 LMICs studied. This was at an average cost of $1.08 per head per year saved, ranging from less than $1 per year in low-income countries to less than $3 per year in middle-income countries. This study evaluated the use of proven effective medications in secondary prevention and substituted an alternate antihypertensive for β-blockers in primary prevention. The primary prevention analysis was limited to individuals with 15% or greater 10-year absolute risk of CVD, which was calculated using country-specific risk charts incorporating easy-to-measure variables, including the substitution of BMI for cholesterol as noted above.

Policy and Community Interventions

Whereas efforts at expanding IHD prevention and management at the individual level have been crucial to improving outcomes in HICs and remain a focal point of development for LMICs, risk factor modification through policy and community intervention also holds the potential to substantially blunt the rise in IHD incidence. Here we will explore the effectiveness of various population-level interventions in both HICs and LMICs, as well as remark on the cost-effectiveness of these programs.

High-Income Countries

Policy

Investigational models into public policy maneuvers to improve the population risk factor profile have resulted in effective and cost-effective mechanisms to combat the rising epidemic of IHD. One such study from the GBD project focused on decreasing salt intake, both through voluntary agreements and legislative action directed at producers of processed foods, as well as on cholesterol and BMI education through mass media. These investigators conducted an analysis on effect size, health outcomes, and costs of these interventions in three world regions, including high-income Western Europe. Their evaluation of these interventions in a high-income region found between 700,000 and 2.4 million DALYs saved per year through the use of either reduction in salt intake through processed food interventions, reduction in cholesterol levels and BMI through mass media campaigns, or both. These population-based measures were compared with personal interventions for blood pressure and dyslipidemia. Policy-based interventions were far more cost-effective in preventing morbidity and mortality, though the number of DALYs averted using a strategy based on personal interventions was greater.[46] A combination of both personal and nonpersonal measures was found to prevent the largest number of DALYs lost to CVD. Notably, both policy and personal measures, as well as their combination, were found the be cost-effective in this high-income region.

A similar study on policy measures to decrease salt intake in the United States was completed using health outcomes estimates derived from the Coronary Heart Disease Policy Model, a computer-based model of the incidence, prevalence, mortality, and costs related to IHD in the United States. This model predicted a decrease in incident cases of IHD by 60 to 120,000 cases per year based on a decrease of 3 g of dietary salt per day; this represented a 6% to 10% reduction in incidence rates of IHD. These outcomes were found to be cost-saving, with conservative estimates of dollars saved approximating $10 billion dollars per year.[47]

Community

Complementary to policy efforts in controlling population risk for IHD, community efforts centered on education, screening, and prevention have additionally been variably shown to be effective at reducing incidence of IHD. The most well-known example of successful community intervention to prevent IHD was carried out in North Karelia, Finland, starting in the 1970s. Combined mass media communication, educational efforts, and outreach by both medical professionals and "lay" personnel, including journalists and community leaders, spearheaded a campaign that saw risk factor rates, including cholesterol levels, diastolic blood pressure, and smoking prevalence, decrease at a faster rate over the first 5 years of study versus other parts of the country over the same time period[48] Importantly, this series of interventions decreased cardiovascular mortality in the communities of interest compared to other regions in the country.[49] A similar study carried out in the United States, called the Stanford Five City Project, studied differences in IHD risk factors and mortality in communities randomized to education campaigns through both media and direct education versus control communities. Those communities randomized to intensive education had lower rates of important risk factors including smoking, cholesterol levels, and blood pressure at 5 years compared with controls; however there was not a significant difference in cardiovascular mortality between the two groups in the same time period.[50,51]

Low- and Middle-Income Countries

Policy

Policy efforts at management of disease at a population level serve the foundation of any well-functioning health system; however, these interventions have been of significant importance in resource-poor settings, where personal intervention in noncommunicable diseases, including IHD, has often been seen as a luxury of more developed nations. In the previously mentioned GBD study, both policy and nonpolicy interventions were found to be effective at preventing DALYs lost to CVD in a high-income region, as well as cost-effective. While these findings are not surprising, further exploration of these same methods in LMICs came to the same conclusion. Specifically, policy interventions, including reducing salt intake through voluntary agreements and legislative action directed at producers of processed foods, as well as mass media campaigns on cholesterol and BMI, were found to be both effective and cost-effective at averting lost DALYs in low-income regions (with high rates of adult and child mortality) and in middle-income regions (with low adult and child mortality). These measures, if applied, could avert between 300,000 and 1.2 million DALYs in Latin America (the middle-income region of interest in this study), and nearly double that number in Southeast Asia (the low-income region of interest). These interventions were found to be cost-effective for each region studied.[46] Similar data by Gaziano et al. have supported the cost-effectiveness of salt reduction and fat-related interventions in developing regions as shown in Table 2.1.

Further studies have since claimed similar findings of both effectiveness and cost-effectiveness of policy level interventions in LMICs for reducing cardiovascular morbidity and mortality. A single study on tobacco control through taxation, bans on smoking in the workplace, packaging warnings regarding the dangers of cigarette smoking, and bans on advertisement, combined with similar salt-reduction campaigns, including reduction of salt in processed food and mass media education on the health effects of a salt-heavy diet, found combined reduction of over 10 million deaths attributable to CVDs in a 23-nation representative sample of LMICs over a 10-year period.[52] Across all countries in this study, the per person per year implementation cost of these plans was $0.36; this ranged from $0.14 to $0.38 in low-income and lower middle-incomes countries and from $0.52 to $1.04 in upper middle-income countries. Similar results were found in modeling cost-effectiveness of a price increase on tobacco and nonprice interventions in a separate study as shown in Table 2.1. Where they are available, data on experience with these measures as they have been carried out have been promising; for instance, in South Africa, smoking rates have shown an inverse relationship with taxation rates on cigarettes.[53]

Community

Studies on community intervention in LMICs are sparse, and where data exist, results have been variable. One study of mass media education, including mass media education plus interpersonal education for high-risk individuals, versus control in communities in South Africa showed an improvement in blood pressure, smoking rates, and overall risk profile in intervention groups compared to control groups, with no difference between interventions. This same study did not reveal a difference in lipid profile or BMI, though statistical significance was not able to be determined due to sampling patterns. Whereas this study represents a single experience, it expands on the premise that community-level interventions, both in HICs and LMICs, hold some promise for the improvement in risk factors and potentially for prevention of morbidity and mortality secondary to IHD.[54]

CONCLUSIONS

IHD continues to be the most common cause of mortality worldwide, as well as an increasingly important contributor to global morbidity. The burden of IHD is shifting from high-income to LMICs as societal advancement results in advancing age, growing populations, and increasing prevalence of risk factors for disease. Proven effective therapies for IHD have resulted in improved outcomes in HICs where their use is most prevalent; however, these medications have been shown to be cost-effective in all settings in which they have been studied. Improved uptake of medical therapy and policy and community interventions have the potential to improve outcomes for IHD in low- and middle-income regions as they continue to progress in the epidemiologic transition.

References

1. Historical Data, 1900–1998. Centers for Disease Control and Prevention, *Centers for Disease Control and Prevention* 12, Nov. 2009. Web. 27 Mar. 2016. http://www.cdc.gov.
2. Murray CJL, Vos T, Lozano R, et al.: Disability-adjusted life years (DALYs) for 291 diseases and injuries in 21 regions, 1990–2010: a systematic analysis for the Global Burden of Disease Study 2010, *Lancet* 380:2197–2223, 2012.
3. Gaziano T, et al.: Fundamentals of cardiovascular disease. In Libby P, Bonow RO, Mann DL, Zipes DP, editors: *Braunwald's Heart Disease: A Textbook of Cardiovascular Medicine*, ed 8, Philadelphia, 2008, Saunders, pp 1–21.
4. Ruff CT, Braunwald E: The evolving epidemiology of acute coronary syndromes, *Nat Rev Cardiol* 8(3):140–147, 2011.
5. Gaziano TA, Bitton A, Anand S, et al.: Growing epidemic of coronary heart disease in low- and middle-income countries, *Curr Probl Cardiol* 35(2):72–115, 2010.
6. Lozano R, Naghavi M, Foreman K, et al.: Global and regional mortality from 235 causes of death for 20 age groups in 1990 and 2010: a systematic analysis for the Global Burden of Disease Study 2010, *Lancet* 380(9859):2095–2128, 2012.
7. Moran AE, Forouzanfar MH, Roth GA, et al.: The global burden of ischemic heart disease in 1990 and 2010: the Global Burden of Disease 2010 study, *Circulation* 129(14):1493–1501, 2014.
8. Joseph A, Ackerman D, Talley JD, et al.: Manifestations of coronary atherosclerosis in young trauma victims—an autopsy study, *J Am Coll Cardiol* 22(2):459–467, 1993.
9. Janjua SA, Hoffmann U: New insights from major prospective cohort studies with cardiac CT, *Curr Cardiol Rep* 17(4):19, 2015.
10. Detrano R, Guerci AD, Carr JJ, et al.: Coronary calcium as a predictor of coronary events in four racial or ethnic groups, *N Engl J Med* 358(13):1336–1345, 2008.
11. Arad Y, Goodman KJ, Roth M, et al.: Coronary calcification, coronary disease risk factors, C-reactive protein, and atherosclerotic cardiovascular disease events: the St. Francis Heart Study, *J Am Coll Cardiol* 46(1):158–165, 2005.
12. Bansal YS, Mandal SP, Kumar S, et al.: Prevalence of atherosclerotic coronary stenosis in asymptomatic north Indian population: a post-mortem coronary angiography study, *J Clin Diagn Res* 9(9): HC01–4, 2015.
13. Roth GA, Forouzanfar MH, Moran AE, et al.: Demographic and epidemiologic drivers of global cardiovascular mortality, *N Engl J Med* 372(14):1333–1341, 2015.
14. Roth GA, Huffman MD, Moran AE, et al.: Global and regional patterns in cardiovascular mortality from 1990 to 2013, *Circulation* 132(17):1667–1678, 2015.
15. Yusuf S, Hawken S, Ounpuu S, et al.: Effect of potentially modifiable risk factors associated with myocardial infarction in 52 countries (the INTERHEART study): case-control study, *Lancet* 364(9438):937–952, 2004.
16. Yusuf S, Rangarajan S, Teo K, et al.: Cardiovascular risk and events in 17 low-, middle-, and high-income countries, *N Engl J Med* 371(9):818–827, 2014.
17. Lim SS, Vos T, Flaxman AD, et al.: A comparative risk assessment of burden of disease and injury attributable to 67 risk factors and risk factor clusters in 21 regions, 1990–2010: a systematic analysis for the Global Burden of Disease Study 2010, *Lancet* 380(9859):2224–2260, 2012.
18. Goyal A, Bhatt DL, Steg PG, et al.: Attained educational level and incident atherothrombotic events in low- and middle-income compared with high-income countries, *Circulation* 122:1167–1175, 2010.
19. Danaei G, Finucane MM, Lin JK, et al.: Global Burden of Metabolic Risk Factors of Chronic Diseases Collaborating Group (Blood Pressure). National, regional, and global trends in systolic blood pressure since 1980: systematic analysis of health examination surveys and epidemiological studies with 786 country-years and 5.4 million participants, *Lancet* 377(9765):568–577, 2011.
20. Yusuf S, Bosch J, Dagenais G, et al.: Cholesterol lowering in intermediate-risk persons without cardiovascular disease, *N Engl J Med* 374(21):2021–2031, 2016.
21. Farzadfar F, Finucane MM, Danaei G, et al.: Global Burden of Metabolic Risk Factors of Chronic Diseases Collaborating Group (Cholesterol). National, regional, and global trends in serum total cholesterol since 1980: systematic analysis of health examination surveys and epidemiological studies with 321 country-years and 3.0 million participants, *Lancet* 377(9765):578–586, 2011.
22. Danaei G, Finucane MM, Lu Y, et al.: Global Burden of Metabolic Risk Factors of Chronic Diseases Collaborating Group (Blood Glucose). National, regional, and global trends in fasting plasma glucose and diabetes prevalence since 1980: systematic analysis of health examination surveys and epidemiological studies with 370 country-years and 2.7 million participants, *Lancet* 378(9785):31–40, 2011.
23. Finucane MM, Stevens GA, Cowan MJ, et al.: Global Burden of Metabolic Risk Factors of Chronic Diseases Collaborating Group (Body Mass Index). National, regional, and global trends in body-mass index since 1980: systematic analysis of health examination surveys and epidemiological studies with 960 country-years and 9.1 million participants, *Lancet* 377(9765):557–567, 2011.
24. Gersh BJ, Sliwa K, Mayosi BM, et al.: Novel therapeutic concepts: the epidemic of cardiovascular disease in the developing world: global implications, *Eur Heart J* 31:642–648, 2010.
25. Sliwa K, Acquah L, Gersh BJ, et al.: Impact of socioeconomic status, ethnicity, and urbanization on risk factor profiles of cardiovascular disease in Africa, *Circulation* 133:1199–1208, 2016.
26. Tsao CW, Vasan RS: Cohort profile: The Framingham Heart Study (FHS): overview of milestones in cardiovascular epidemiology, *Int J Epidemiol* 44(6):1800–1813, 2015.
27. Stone NJ, Robinson JG, Lichtenstein AH, et al.: 2013 ACC/AHA guideline on the treatment of blood cholesterol to reduce atherosclerotic cardiovascular risk in adults: a report of the American College of Cardiology/American Heart Association Task Force on Practice Guidelines, *J Am Coll Cardiol* 63(25 Pt B):2889–2934, 2014.
28. Board J: Joint British Societies' consensus recommendations for the prevention of cardiovascular disease (JBS3), *Heart* 100:ii1–ii67, 2014.
29. Steinberg BA, Bhatt DL, Mehta S, et al.: Nine-year trends in achievement of risk factor goals in the US and European outpatients with cardiovascular disease, *Am Heart J* 156(4):719–727, 2008.
30. Bansilal S, Farkouh ME, Hueb W, et al.: The Future REvascularization Evaluation in patients with Diabetes mellitus: optimal management of Multivessel disease (FREEDOM) trial: clinical and angiographic profile at study entry, *Am Heart J* 164:591–599, 2012.
31. Bhatt DL, Steg PG, Ohman EM, et al.: International prevalence, recognition, and treatment of cardiovascular risk factors in outpatients with atherothrombosis, *JAMA* 295(2):180–189, Jan 11, 2006.
32. Bhatt DL, Eagle KA, Ohman EM, et al.: Comparative determinants of 4-year cardiovascular event rates in stable outpatients at risk of or with atherothrombosis, *JAMA* 304(12):1350–1357, 2010.
33. Yusuf S, Islam S, Chow CK, et al.: Use of secondary prevention drugs for cardiovascular disease in the community in high-income, middle-income, and low-income countries (the PURE Study): a prospective epidemiological survey, *Lancet* 378(9798):1231–1243, 2011.
34. Iqbal J, Zhang YJ, Holmes DR, et al.: Optimal medical therapy improves clinical outcomes in patients undergoing revascularization with percutaneous coronary intervention or coronary artery bypass grafting: insights from the Synergy Between Percutaneous Coronary Intervention with TAXUS and Cardiac Surgery (SYNTAX) trial at the 5-year follow-up, *Circulation* 131:1269–1277, 2015.
35. Mendis S, Lindholm LH, Mancia G, et al.: World Health Organization (WHO) and International Society of Hypertension (ISH) risk prediction charts: assessment of cardiovascular risk for prevention and control of cardiovascular disease in low and middle-income countries, *J Hypertens* 25(8):1578–1582, 2007.
36. Gaziano TA, Young CR, Fitzmaurice G, et al.: Laboratory-based versus non-laboratory-based method for assessment of cardiovascular disease risk: the NHANES I Follow-up Study cohort, *Lancet* 371(9616):923–931, 2008.
37. Wald NJ, Law MR: A strategy to reduce cardiovascular disease by more than 80%, *BMJ* 326:1419, 2003.
38. Lonn E, Bosch J, Teo KK, et al.: The polypill in the prevention of cardiovascular diseases: key concepts, current status, challenges, and future directions, *Circulation* 122:2078–2088, 2010.
39. Yusuf S, Pais P, Afzal R, et al.: Effects of a polypill (Polycap) on risk factors in middle-aged individuals without cardiovascular disease (TIPS): a phase II, double-blind, randomised trial, *Lancet* 373:1341–1351, 2009.
40. Heart Outcomes Prevention Evaluation-3 (HOPE-3).
41. Hippisley-Cox J, Coupland C: Effect of combinations of drugs on all cause mortality in patients with ischaemic heart disease: nested case-control analysis, *BMJ* 330:1059–1063, 2005.
42. Gaziano TA, Steyn K, Cohen DJ, et al.: Cost-effectiveness analysis of hypertension guidelines in South Africa: absolute risk versus blood pressure level, *Circulation* 112:3569–3576, 2005.
43. Lim SS, Gaziano TA, Gakidou E, et al.: Chronic disease 4—prevention of cardiovascular disease in high-risk individuals in low-income and middle-income countries: health effects and costs, *Lancet* 370:2054–2062, 2007.
44. Gaziano TA, Opie LH, Weinstein MC: Cardiovascular disease prevention with a multidrug regimen in the developing world: a cost-effectiveness analysis, *Lancet* 368(9536):679–686, 2006.
45. Lim SS, Gaziano TA, Gakidou E, et al.: Prevention of cardiovascular disease in high-risk individuals in low-income and middle-income countries: health effects and costs, *Lancet* 370(9604):2054–2062, 2007.
46. Murray CJ, Lauer JA, Hutubessy RC, et al.: Effectiveness and costs of interventions to lower systolic blood pressure and cholesterol: a global and regional analysis on reduction of cardiovascular-disease risk, *Lancet* 361(9359):717–725, 2003. Erratum in Lancet 366(9481):204, 2005.
47. Bibbins-Domingo K, Chertow GM, Coxson PG, et al.: Projected effect of dietary salt reductions on future cardiovascular disease, *N Engl J Med* 362(7):590–599, 2010.
48. Vartiainen E, Puska P, Jousilahti P, et al.: Cardiovascular diseases and risk factors in Finland, *Prev Med* 29(6 Pt 2):S124–129, 1999.
49. Tuomilehto J, Geboers J, Salonen JT, et al.: Decline in cardiovascular mortality in North Karelia and other parts of Finland, *BMJ (Clin Res Ed)* 293(6554):1068–1071, 1986.
50. Farquhar JW, Fortmann SP, Flora JA, et al.: Effects of communitywide education on cardiovascular disease risk factors. The Stanford Five-City Project, *JAMA* 264(3):359–365, 1990.
51. Fortmann SP, Varady AN: Effects of a community-wide health education program on cardiovascular disease morbidity and mortality: the Stanford Five-City Project, *Am J Epidemiol* 152(4):316–323, 2000.
52. Asaria P, Chisholm D, Mathers C, et al.: Chronic disease prevention: health effects and financial costs of strategies to reduce salt intake and control tobacco use, *Lancet* 370(9604):2044–2053, 2007.
53. Gaziano TA, Pagidipati N: Scaling up chronic disease prevention interventions in lower- and middle-income countries, *Annu Rev Public Health* 34:317–335, 2013.
54. Gaziano TA, Galea G, Reddy KS: Scaling up interventions for chronic disease prevention: the evidence, *Lancet* 370(9603):1939–1946, 2007.

SECTION II

PATHOGENESIS

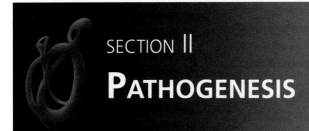

3 Genetics of Coronary Atherosclerosis

Krishna G. Aragam and Sekar Kathiresan

INTRODUCTION

This chapter reviews current understanding of the genetic architecture of coronary atherosclerosis as gleaned from Mendelian and common, complex forms of the disease. Newly identified pathways and biologic mechanisms are highlighted before discussing the present and future role of genetic testing for the diagnosis, prognosis, and treatment of patients with coronary artery disease (CAD).

HERITABILITY OF CORONARY ARTERY DISEASE

Familial clustering of CAD has long been observed and suggests an inherited basis for CAD and its downstream complication of myocardial infarction (MI).[1–3] In the offspring cohort of the Framingham Heart Study, a parental history of premature CAD conferred a two- to three-fold increase in the age-specific incidence of cardiovascular events after adjustment for conventional CAD risk factors—implying a genetic basis for the observed susceptibility to CAD.[4] Twin and family studies have estimated that the heritability of CAD is approximately 40% to 60%.[5] Heritable effects appear most pronounced for early-onset CAD, denoting the importance of inherited over acquired risk factors for the development of premature disease.[6] Furthermore, several risk factors for CAD, including plasma lipid concentrations, blood pressure, and type II diabetes mellitus, are themselves heritable and as such contribute to the overall heritability of the CAD/MI phenotype.[7–11]

Varying patterns of inheritance have provided insights into the genetic underpinnings of CAD. Some forms of CAD demonstrate a simple, Mendelian inheritance pattern, manifest at a young age without the influence of environmental risk factors, and are typified by a single causal gene with a large effect size.[12] Candidate gene studies and linkage analyses have elucidated these monogenic disorders through the study of patients and families with extreme phenotypes to identify causal genes contributing to the disease of interest.

However, the majority of CAD in the population exhibits a more complex and multifactorial inheritance pattern inconsistent with the ratios of Mendel. Such polygenic forms of CAD involve the interplay of many common DNA variants of small to moderate effect sizes, together with nongenetic factors, including both lifestyle and environment.[13] Advancements in high-throughput DNA microarray technologies have permitted the identification of nearly 60 common DNA variants associated with CAD/MI through large-scale genetic association studies, accounting for approximately 13% of the cumulative genetic variance of CAD.[14] Next-generation sequencing technologies and additional studies interrogating potential gene-environment interactions have begun to bridge the gap on the missing heritability of CAD and its risk factors.[15–17]

MENDELIAN CAUSES OF CORONARY ARTERY DISEASE

Examples of Mendelian forms of CAD largely involve gene defects that lead to extremely high plasma concentrations of low-density lipoprotein cholesterol (LDL-C). One such disease is familial hypercholesterolemia (FH) where defects in the LDL receptor mediate disordered uptake of cellular LDL particles from the bloodstream (Table 3.1).[18] Investigations of homozygous FH patients led to the sequencing and identification of mutations in the LDL receptor (*LDLR*) gene, resulting in defective cellular uptake of LDL-C.[19,20] *LDLR* mutations are associated with elevated plasma concentrations of LDL-C, typical physical stigmata of severe hypercholesterolemia—ie, tendon xanthomas and corneal arcus (see Chapter 7, Figs. 7.4 and 7.5)—and premature coronary atherosclerosis. FH is inherited in a codominant pattern where the number of abnormal allelic copies (1 or 2) correlates directly with the severity of the FH phenotype.[18]

Subsequent studies in FH patients without *LDLR* mutations led to the discovery of additional causal mutations in the *APOB* and *PCSK9* genes, which encode for apolipoprotein B (ApoB) and proprotein convertase subtilisin/kexin type 9 (PCSK9), respectively. ApoB is a key protein on the LDL particle that facilitates its binding to the LDL receptor for cellular uptake and degradation. *APOB* mutations associating with FH were found to interrupt the binding of the ApoB protein to LDL receptor on the cell surface, leading to reduced LDL uptake and higher plasma LDL concentrations.[21]

PCSK9 is highly expressed in the liver and regulates cholesterol homeostasis by binding to the LDL receptor and inducing its degradation. Gain-of-function mutations in the *PCSK9* gene are associated with FH presumably due to reduced LDL receptor availability and a resultant decrease in LDL particle uptake.[22] Similar to *LDLR* and *APOB*, mutations in *PCSK9* demonstrate an autosomal dominant inheritance pattern, with one copy of the mutant allele leading to an FH phenotype. Notably, loss-of-function mutations in *PCSK9* are associated with upregulation of LDL receptors, a marked reduction in LDL-C concentrations, and an 88% reduction in CAD risk.[23]

Other Mendelian disorders of hypercholesterolemia mediate CAD but through an autosomal recessive pattern of inheritance. Two aberrant copies of the *LDLRAP1* gene are causative for autosomal recessive hypercholesterolemia (ARH), the mechanism of which remains uncertain but appears to involve a defect in an adapter protein that disrupts the interaction between the LDL receptor and clathrin-coated pits. Individuals with ARH manifest an intermediate form of hypercholesterolemia somewhere between that of *LDLR* heterozygotes and *LDLR* homozygotes.[24] Sitosterolemia is a rare autosomal recessive disorder of plant sterol metabolism caused by a defect in the genes encoding ATP-binding cassette (ABC) transporter proteins involved in the excretion of dietary plant sterols. The disease shares several clinical features with FH, such as tendon xanthomas and premature development of CAD. However, unlike FH, the disease is characterized by elevated plant sterol levels, whereas total cholesterol levels may be normal.[25–27]

Attempts to uncover Mendelian forms of CAD/MI independent of the aforementioned lipoprotein pathways have been unsuccessful. A 21-kb deletion within the *MEF2A* gene (which encodes the myocyte enhancer factor [MEF] 2A transcription factor strongly expressed in the coronary endothelium) was initially identified as a putative autosomal dominant form of CAD/MI in a 21-member family with 13 affected individuals.[28] However, the noted deletion and others in the *MEF2A* gene failed to segregate with the disease in a subsequent cohort analysis, casting doubt on whether the gene leads to CAD/MI.[29,30]

COMMON, COMPLEX FORMS OF CORONARY ARTERY DISEASE

Genome-Wide Association Studies

Beyond rare variants of Mendelian disorders that confer exceptional disease risk, common DNA variants (minor allele frequency [MAF] > 0.05) with more modest effect sizes have also been shown to impact CAD risk. Population-based association studies—ie, genome-wide association studies (GWAS)—compare the DNA profiles of CAD cases and control participants free of CAD to detect statistically significant differences. GWAS have been enabled by the systematic classification of millions of single-nucleotide polymorphisms (SNPs) in the human genome and the advent of high-throughput technologies permitting the interrogation of 1 million or more SNPs on a single microarray chip.[31] Due to linkage disequilibrium—the nonrandom association of alleles at different loci—it is possible to cover the entire human genome of certain populations with approximately 500,000 marker SNPs for the detection of common DNA variants.[32]

In GWAS, large populations are genotyped and allele frequencies of each SNP are compared in cases and controls to test for associations between common variants and a particular phenotype in a relatively unbiased manner. For GWAS of quantitative traits (ie, blood lipid concentrations), analysis is focused on whether SNPs associate with increases or decreases in the specific trait. Given the simultaneous interrogation of up to a million SNPs for association with the disease or quantitative trait, a stringent *p*-value criterion of 5×10^{-8} or less is required to achieve genome-wide significance. Accordingly, these studies have relied upon worldwide collaborations to recruit thousands of carefully phenotyped individuals with and without the disease of interest.

Genome-Wide Association Studies of Coronary Artery Disease/Myocardial Infarction

The first locus associated with CAD at a level of genome-wide significance was reported concurrently in 2007 by three independent groups employing distinct cohorts and genotype arrays. All three studies demonstrated a 58-kb interval on chromosome 9p21 containing multiple index SNPs strongly associated with CAD with high allele frequency and robust effect size.[33–35] Approximately 20% to 25% of the population were found to be homozygous for the variant, with homozygosity conferring a greater than 60% increase in risk of CAD. The locus has also been associated with the extent and severity of CAD, as increased allele frequency has been reported among patients with premature, as well as multivessel, disease.[36] Of note, it has been repeatedly demonstrated

TABLE 3.1 Major Mendelian Disorders That Cause Severe Hypercholesterolemia

DISEASE	CAUSAL GENE(S)	INHERITANCE PATTERN	PREVALENCE	METABOLIC DEFECT
Familial hypercholesterolemia	*LDLR* *APOB* *PCSK9*	Autosomal dominant	HeFH – 1: 500 HoFH – 1: 1×10^6	Reduced LDL clearance
Autosomal recessive hypercholesterolemia	*LDLRAP1*	Autosomal recessive	< 1: 5×10^6	Reduced LDL clearance
Sitosterolemia	*ABCG5* *ABCG8*	Autosomal recessive	< 1: 5×10^6	Reduced plant sterol clearance

ABC, ATP-binding cassette; *APOB*, apoliporotein B; *HeFH,* heterozygous familial hypercholesterolemia; *HoFH,* homozygous familial hypercholesterolemia; *LDL,* low-density lipoprotein; *LDLR,* LDL receptor; *PCSK9,* proprotein convertase subtilisin/kexin type 9. *(Adapted from Rader DJ, Cohen J, Hobbs HH. Monogenic hypercholesterolemia: new insights in pathogenesis and treatment.* J Clin Invest. *2003;111:1795–1803.)*

that the 9p21 locus is not associated with traditional CAD risk factors such as plasma lipids, blood pressure, diabetes, older age, or obesity. Furthermore, the 58-kb block does not harbor any annotated genes, which renders unclear the exact mechanism by which the locus confers an elevated risk of CAD. However, studies have associated the 9p21 locus with other vascular phenotypes including carotid atherosclerosis, abdominal aortic aneurysm, peripheral artery disease, and intracranial aneurysm, suggesting a pathogenic process related to vessel wall integrity.[37–41]

Subsequent meta-analyses of GWAS have involved international collaborations such as the Myocardial Infarction Genetics Consortium (MIGen), the Coronary ARtery DIsease Genome-Wide Replication and Meta-Analysis (CARDIoGRAM) consortium, the Coronary Artery Disease Genetics Consortium (C4D), and the combined CARDIoGRAMplusC4D consortium.[42–45] Together, these large cohorts identified 48 common variants attaining genome-wide significance for association with CAD. Whereas several of these CAD risk loci include genes linked to lipoprotein metabolism, hypertension, and other related pathways, a large proportion lie in gene regions not previously implicated in CAD pathogenesis. As expected for a complex phenotype with a multifactorial origin, most of these common variants have relatively small effect sizes, with only two of the susceptibility loci—the 9p21 locus and the *LPA* gene (which codes lipoprotein (a))—conferring a greater than 15% risk of CAD.[46]

The previous analyses were restricted to common SNPs (MAF > 0.05) derived from the International HapMap project. A GWAS published in 2015 leveraged more extensive human genetic data from the 1000 Genomes Project including lower frequency and insertion/deletion variants (indels). This GWAS meta-analysis comprised over 185,000 CAD cases and controls and interrogated 6.7 million common variants, as well as 2.7 million low-frequency (MAF = 0.005–0.05) variants. The study confirmed the majority of known CAD susceptibility loci and identified eight novel loci associated with CAD at a genome-wide level of significance, bringing the total number of replicated CAD susceptibility loci to 56 and accounting for approximately 13% of the overall heritability of CAD (Table 3.2). Of note, the eight novel CAD risk loci and all but one of the previously identified loci were represented by risk alleles

TABLE 3.2 Gene Regions Identified for CAD Using the Genome-Wide Association Approach

CHR	LOCUS NAME	LEAD SNP	EAF	RISK OF CAD (OR)	ASSOCIATION OF GENE VARIANT WITH TRADITIONAL RISK FACTORS
1p32	*PPAP2B*	rs17114036	0.92	1.13	
1p32	*PCSK9*	rs11206510	0.85	1.08	LDL
1p13	*SORT1*	rs7528419	0.79	1.12	LDL, HDL
1q21	*IL6R*	rs4845625	0.45	1.06	
1q41	*MIA3*	rs17465637	0.66	1.08	
2p24	*APOB*	rs515135	0.75	1.07	LDL
2p21	*ABCG5-ABCG8*	rs6544713	0.32	1.05	LDL
2p11	*VAMP5-VAMP8-GGCX*	rs1561198	0.46	1.06	
2q22	*ZEB2*	rs2252641	0.44	1.03	
2q33	*WDR12*	rs6725887	0.11	1.14	LDL
3q22	*MRAS*	rs9818870	0.14	1.07	
4q31	*EDNRA*	rs1878406	0.16	1.06	
4q32	*GUCY1A3*	rs7692387	0.81	1.07	BP
4q12	*REST-NOA1*	rs17087335	0.21	1.06	
5q31	*SLC22A4-SLC22A5*	rs273909	0.12	1.06	LDL
6p21	*ANKS1A*	rs17609940	0.82	1.03	
6p24	*PHACTR1*	rs9369640	0.43	1.14	
6p21	*KCNK5*	rs10947789	0.78	1.05	
6q23	*TCF21*	rs12190287	0.62	1.06	
6q25	*SLC22A3-LPAL2-LPA*	rs2048327 rs3789220	0.35 0.02	1.06 1.42	LDL
6q26	*PLG*	rs4252120	0.74	1.03	
7p21	*HDAC9*	rs2023938	0.10	1.06	
7q22	7q22	rs10953541	0.78	1.05	
7q32	*ZC3HC1*	rs11556924	0.69	1.08	HDL, BP
7q36	*NOS3*	rs3918226	0.06	1.14	BP
8p21	*LPL*	rs264	0.85	1.06	HDL, TG
8q24	*TRIB1*	rs2954029	0.55	1.04	LDL, HDL, TG

Continued

TABLE 3.2 Gene Regions Identified for CAD Using the Genome-Wide Association Approach—cont'd

CHR	LOCUS NAME	LEAD SNP	EAF	RISK OF CAD (OR)	ASSOCIATION OF GENE VARIANT WITH TRADITIONAL RISK FACTORS
9p21	*CDKN2BAS1*	rs4977574 rs3217992	0.49 0.39	1.21 1.14	
9q34	*ABO*	rs579459	0.21	1.08	LDL
10p11	*KIAA1462*	rs2505083	0.40	1.06	
10p11	*CXCL12*	rs501120 rs2047009	0.81 0.48	1.08 1.06	
10q23	*LIPA*	rs11203042 rs1412444	0.45 0.37	1.04 1.07	
10q24	*CYP17A1-CNNM2-NT5C2*	rs12413409	0.89	1.08	BP, BMI
11p15	*SWAP70*	rs10840293	0.55	1.06	
11q22	*PDGFD*	rs974819	0.33	1.07	
11q23	*ZNF259-APOA5-APOA1*	rs964184	0.18	1.05	LDL, HDL, TG
12q24	*SH2B3*	rs3184504	0.42	1.07	LDL, HDL, BP, BMI
12q21	*ATP2B1*	rs7136259	0.43	1.04	
12q24	*KSR2*	rs11830157	0.36	1.12	
13q12	*FLT1*	rs9319428	0.31	1.04	
13q34	*COL4A1-COL4A2*	rs4773144 rs9515203	0.43 0.76	1.05 1.07	
14q32	*HHIPL1*	rs2895811	0.41	1.04	
15q25	*ADAMTS7*	rs7173743	0.56	1.08	
15q22	*SMAD3*	rs56062135	0.79	1.07	
15q26	*MFGE8-ABHD2*	rs8042271	0.90	1.10	
15q26	*FURIN-FES*	rs17514846	0.44	1.05	BP
17q23	*BCAS3*	rs7212798	0.15	1.08	
17p11	*RAI1-PEMT-RASD1*	rs12936587	0.61	1.03	
17p13	*SMG6*	rs2281727	0.35	1.05	BMI
17q21	*UBE2Z*	rs15563	0.51	1.04	
18q21	*PMAIP1-MC4R*	rs663129	0.26	1.06	HDL, BMI
19p13	*LDLR*	rs1122608	0.77	1.08	LDL
19q13	*APOE-APOC1*	rs2075650 rs445925	0.13 0.09	1.07 1.09	LDL, HDL, TG, BMI
19q13	*ZNF507-LOC400684*	rs12976411	0.09	0.67	
21q22	*KCNE2*	rs9982601	0.13	1.12	
22q11	*POM121L9P-ADORA2A*	rs180803	0.97	1.20	

BMI, Body mass index; *BP,* blood pressure; *CAD,* coronary artery disease; *CHR,* chromosome; *EAF,* effect allele frequency in those of European ancestry; *HDL,* high-density lipoprotein; *LDL,* low-density lipoprotein; *OR,* odds ratio; *TG,* triglycerides.

with MAF greater than 0.5.[14] This suggests that low-frequency variants and insertion/deletion polymorphisms do not contribute significantly to the missing heritability of this complex disease, further supporting the common disease-common variant hypothesis for CAD.[47]

Genome-Wide Association Studies of Coronary Artery Disease Risk Factors

Common DNA variants impact several prominent CAD risk factors in a similar, polygenic manner, with GWAS over the past decade identifying numerous genetic loci associated with traits such as blood lipid levels, blood pressure (BP), type 2 diabetes, and some nontraditional CAD risk factors such as C-reactive protein (CRP).

The first reported GWAS of blood lipid concentrations assessed 2800 individuals genotyped at approximately 400,000 SNPs from the Diabetes Genetics Initiative and identified three loci reaching genome-wide significance, one associated with each of the three lipid traits: LDL-C, HDL-C, and triglyceride levels.[48] Two of these common variants were mapped to known lipid regulators, thereby validating the GWAS approach. Specifically, the index SNP for LDL-C was mapped to a region near *APOE* (encoding the apolipoprotein that mediates cellular uptake of chylomicrons and very-low-density lipoprotein [VLDL]), and the index SNP for HDL-C was found near *CETP* (encoding cholesteryl ester transfer protein [CETP], a component that facilitates transfer of cholesteryl esters from HDL to other lipoproteins). In addition, the GWAS identified an index SNP associated with triglyceride levels within *GCKR*, which encodes glucokinase regulatory protein.[49,50]

Additional GWAS have expanded the number of known lipid-related loci. In 2010, a large-scale GWAS of approximately 100,000 individuals identified 95 loci contributing to plasma LDL-C, HDL-C, and triglyceride levels, and a subsequent study of approximately 190,000 persons increased the loci count to 157.[51,52] Of these loci, 9 demonstrated the strongest associations with LDL-C, 46 with HDL-C, 16 with triglycerides, 18 with total cholesterol, and numerous loci affected multiple lipid fractions. Among the discovered loci are those containing other well-characterized lipid regulators, including *APOB*, *PCSK9*, *LDLR*, *LPL* (lipoprotein lipase—involved in triglyceride metabolism), and *HMGCR* (encoding for 3-hydroxy-3-methylglutaryl-coenzyme A reductase—the pharmacologic target of statins). Several loci are known to harbor rare mutations involved in monogenic lipid disorders such as FH. Notably, many of these causal genes for Mendelian disorders also have common variants that induce subtle effects on gene function resulting in more modest changes in plasma lipid levels.

Large genetic association studies of BP have identified 29 independent genetic variants associated with continuous BP and dichotomous hypertension at genome-wide levels of significance.[53–55] The majority of these variants affect systolic blood pressure (SBP) and diastolic blood pressure (DBP) in a concordant direction, although variants at three loci are reported to have discordant effects.[56] In most cases, the potential mechanistic links between each gene and the BP phenotype remain unclear. As compared to genetic variants for other CAD risk factors, variants identified for BP appear to exert less influence on the overall phenotype, as the 29 identified variants account for less than 1% of the variation in SBP and DBP. Notably, in a GWAS of 200,000 individuals, an aggregate genetic risk score comprised of the aforementioned genetic variants positively correlated with phenotypes such as CAD and stroke but were not associated with chronic kidney disease or measures of kidney function, suggesting a strong causal relationship between elevated BP and cardiovascular disease but not between elevated BP and renal dysfunction.[55]

Type 2 diabetes mellitus has been studied extensively through several GWAS, including early discovery of an association with *TCF7L2* (encoding a transcription factor that regulates proglucagon gene expression in the gastrointestinal tract) through a relatively small GWAS of 2000 cases and 3000 controls.[57] Subsequent larger meta-analyses have increased the total number of type 2 diabetes loci to 63, accounting for approximately 6% of the variation in disease risk.[58] Several of these risk loci harbor genes that alter the processing and secretion of insulin by the pancreatic beta cell, whereas a smaller proportion of genes appear to mediate insulin resistance. SNPs at these loci have therefore been associated with fasting glucose and insulin levels as well as other metabolic traits, such as lipids and adiposity. Of note, variants in the risk loci for type 2 diabetes have little overlap with those for type 1 diabetes and are poor predictors of the latter disease process.[59,60]

Several other risk biomarkers—including CRP—have also been studied via GWAS with identification of many associated risk loci. CRP is a well-described inflammatory biomarker predictive of CAD/MI in epidemiologic cohorts. GWAS have identified at least 18 loci associated with circulating levels of CRP, including SNPs in the *CRP* gene encoding for the protein of interest.[61–63] Other annotated genes at the identified risk loci directly or indirectly involve immune response pathways, as well as various metabolic regulatory pathways implicated in diabetes mellitus.

Studies of Causal Inference—Mendelian Randomization

Since the initial association of total plasma cholesterol and CAD risk, observational epidemiologic studies have identified numerous additional soluble biomarkers associated with CAD.[64] However, due to confounding and reverse causation, observational epidemiology as an approach is inherently limited in ability to draw causal inference. Distinguishing causal from noncausal biomarkers is particularly relevant for therapy, as only causal biomarkers have potential as therapeutic targets.

A study design termed *Mendelian randomization* affords the ability to assess causality by leveraging Mendel's law of allele segregation—the random assortment of genetic variants to offspring at the time of conception. This principle results in a natural randomization process akin to that of randomized clinical trials and lessens concerns of confounding and reverse causation. DNA variants associated with the biomarker are utilized as instruments to assess whether an established epidemiologic association between a biomarker and disease reflects a causal relationship. The methodology relies on the premise that if a biomarker is causal for a disease, then the genetic determinants of that biomarker should also be associated with the disease. Furthermore, the magnitude of association should be commensurate with the known effect sizes of the DNA variant on the biomarker and the biomarker on the disease.[65] Presuming adequate study power, lack of an association between a biomarker-related DNA variant (or set of variants) and the disease suggests that the given biomarker is not causal for disease pathogenesis.

The Mendelian randomization approach has several limitations. Importantly, these studies rely on the effect size estimates used for the variant-biomarker and biomarker-disease associations, placing great emphasis on the studies from which these estimates are derived. Furthermore, it is imperative that the variants included in the genetic instrument affect the disease only through the biomarker of interest. The existence of pleiotropy—where a single gene affects a number of unrelated phenotypic traits—undermines the determination of causality, as a proposed causal biomarker may serve as proxy for a separate pathologic mechanism influenced by the genetic variants used.

Over the past decade, Mendelian randomization studies have systematically evaluated which plasma biomarkers causally relate to CAD risk. These studies have provided supportive evidence for LDL-C, triglycerides, and Lp(a) as causal CAD risk factors. In contrast, these studies have cast doubt on HDL and CRP as causal factors for CAD.

Low-Density Lipoprotein

Initial insights into the causal relationship between LDL-C and CAD were derived from studies of patients with FH. As described previously, pathogenic FH mutations in *LDLR*, *APOB*, and *PCSK-9* mediate increased plasma LDL-C concentrations and are associated with premature CAD, providing strong evidence for a causal link between LDL-C and CAD risk. A formal Mendelian randomization experiment was performed in 50,000 cases and controls employing a genetic score for LDL-C comprised of 13 SNPs exclusively associated with LDL-C. Notably, genetically-elevated LDL-C (a 1-standard deviation increase, ~35 mg/dL) was associated with a 113% increase in risk of MI, exceeding the 54% increase in MI risk per 1-standard deviation increase in LDL expected from epidemiologic estimates (Fig. 3.1).[66] These results affirmed the

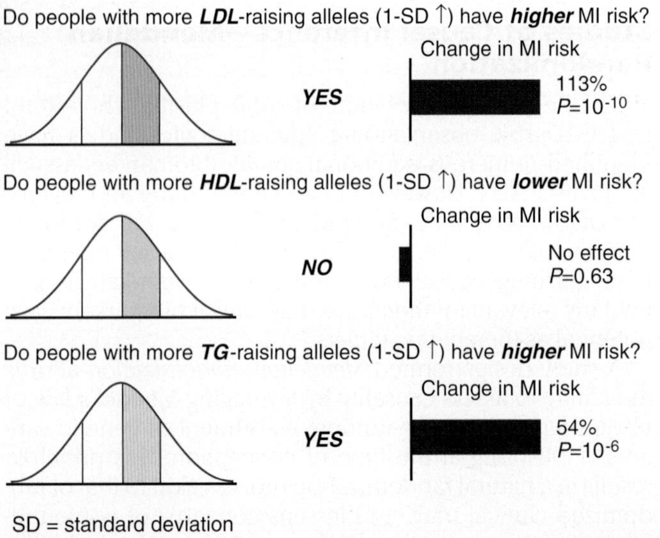
Do people with more LDL-raising alleles (1-SD ↑) have higher MI risk?
Change in MI risk
YES
113%
P=10-10
Do people with more HDL-raising alleles (1-SD ↑) have lower MI risk?
Change in MI risk
NO
No effect
P=0.63
Do people with more TG-raising alleles (1-SD ↑) have higher MI risk?
Change in MI risk
YES
54%
P=10-6
SD = standard deviation

FIG. 3.1 The cumulative effects of genetic variants that raise plasma low-density lipoprotein (LDL) cholesterol, high-density lipoprotein (HDL) cholesterol, and triglyceride (TG) levels on the risk of myocardial infarction (MI). *(From Musunuru K, Kathiresan S. Surprises from genetic analyses of lipid risk factors for atherosclerosis.* Circ Res. *2016;118:579–585.)*

causal nature of the association between LDL and CAD/MI. In addition, these data suggest the concept of cumulative, lifelong exposure to LDL-C (measured by genetic risk score) being particularly harmful.

A separate line of support for the causal link between LDL and CAD/MI has emerged from studies of genetic variants involved in the mechanisms of action of lipid-lowering therapies such as ezetimibe and statins. Ezetimibe reduces LDL-C through inhibition of the Niemann-Pick C1-like protein 1 (NPC1L1), a transporter responsible for the uptake of dietary and biliary cholesterol in the gastrointestinal tract. Despite an early randomized clinical trial showing no significant benefit with ezetimibe therapy on carotid intima-media thickness, other Mendelian randomization studies using genetic variants within or near the *NPC1L1* gene have demonstrated both lower plasma LDL-C levels and reduced risk of CAD. One such study of 7364 CAD cases and 14,728 controls in the MIGen consortium identified 34 loss-of-function mutations in *NPC1L1*, and in a larger replication cohort, one of these inactivating mutations (p.Arg406X) was associated with a 12 mg/dL decrease in LDL-C, as well as a 50% reduction in CAD risk.[67] In a separate 2 × 2 factorial study design of over 100,000 subjects from 14 clinical trials, patients harboring common genetic variants inactivating *NPC1L1*, *HMGCR*, or both demonstrated LDL-C reductions of 2.4, 2.9, and 5.8 mg/dL, respectively, with corresponding reductions in CAD risk of 4.8%, 5.3%, and 10.8%.[68] These studies have bolstered the causal relationship between LDL-C and CAD risk and lent credence to the pharmacologic lowering of LDL through statins, ezetimibe, or combination therapy by showing the independent and additive effects of NPC1L1 and HMGCR inhibition on LDL-C and CAD risk reduction. Indeed, the previously mentioned genetic data were corroborated by the Improved Reduction of Outcomes: Vytorin Efficacy International Trial (IMPROVE-IT) that demonstrated the additive benefit of ezetimibe on baseline statin therapy for reducing mean LDL-C concentrations and the composite endpoint of cardiovascular death, nonfatal MI, and nonfatal stroke in patients hospitalized following an acute coronary syndrome (ACS).[69]

Triglycerides

Epidemiologic studies have yielded, at best, modest associations between plasma triglyceride levels and CAD risk.[70] Even randomized clinical trials of triglyceride-lowering therapies—ie, gemfibrozil, fenofibrate, and omega-3 fatty acids—have offered mixed results regarding their efficacy for reducing cardiovascular events.[71–74] However, genetic data have supported a causal role for triglyceride-rich lipoproteins (TRLs) and their remnants in coronary atherosclerosis. Plasma triglyceride metabolism is primarily mediated by lipoprotein lipase (LPL), and genetic variants that decrease LPL function have been associated with increased cardiovascular risk.[75–77] LPL function is enhanced by apolipoprotein A5 and inhibited by apolipoprotein C3 and the angiopoietin-like proteins 3 and 4 (ANGPTL-3,-4). Accordingly, genetic determinants of these factors have been associated with plasma triglyceride levels and CAD risk in the expected directions.[78–82]

However, many of these Mendelian randomization approaches have been confounded by the pleiotropic relationships between triglyceride-associated SNPs and other lipid markers, as nearly all SNPs identified for plasma triglycerides have additional effects on LDL-C or HDL-C. A methodology termed *multivariable Mendelian randomization* has been developed to dissect the triglyceride-mediated effects of genetic variants on CAD risk from those mediated by other lipid traits. Employing the multivariable analytical approach on all triglyceride-associated SNPs to control for pleiotropic effects on secondary lipid fractions, genetic determinants of triglyceride levels were strongly associated with CAD after adjusting for their effects on LDL-C and HDL-C, with a magnitude of association comparable to that of LDL-C.[83] The data indicate that plasma triglycerides—likely through triglyceride-rich lipoproteins and remnant cholesterol—causally mediate CAD independent of other lipid traits. The inconsistent benefit of triglyceride-lowering therapies for lowering cardiovascular events in the previously mentioned trials may reflect particular characteristics of the trial populations and the variable degrees of triglyceride lowering attained in each study.

Lipoprotein (a)

Lp(a) is a lipoprotein comprised of an LDL-like particle attached to the glycoprotein apolipoprotein(a). Cohort studies have observed an association between elevated plasma levels of Lp(a) and increased risk of CAD (see Chapter 8).[84] Apolipoprotein(a) is encoded for by *LPA*, which largely controls plasma levels of Lp(a). Mendelian randomization studies utilizing common copy number variants and SNPs in or near the *LPA* gene have associated genetically elevated Lp(a) with increased CAD risk, providing sound evidence for a causal link between Lp(a) and CAD.[85,86]

Blood Pressure

As in the previous sections, nearly 30 SNPs have been uncovered that associate with SBP and DBP.[55] In an analysis of 22,500 CAD cases and 65,000 controls from the CARDIoGRAM consortium, 88% of these SNPs were positively associated with CAD risk. The average per-allele increase in CAD risk was 3.0% for SBP-related SNPs and 2.9% for DBP-related SNPs. Employing a genetic risk score comprised of BP-associated SNPs, patients in the highest versus lowest quintiles of genetic score distribution demonstrated 70% higher odds of CAD. Similar to genetic variants for LDL-C, SNPs associated with BP were found to have stronger effects on CAD risk than would have been expected from epidemiologic estimates.[87]

The finding that most SNPs associated with blood pressure also confer a higher risk for CAD supports a causal relationship between increased BP and CAD.

High-Density Lipoprotein

Observational data attest to a strong inverse association between HDL and CAD/MI, spurring decades-long efforts to reduce CAD risk through raising HDL-C pharmacologically (see Chapter 8).[88] However, genetic analyses do not support a causal relationship between HDL and CAD.[89] A recent Mendelian randomization study in approximately 20,000 MI cases and 95,000 controls investigated a loss-of-function coding SNP (Asn396Ser) in the *LIPG* gene encoding for endothelial lipase, an enzyme that mediates HDL metabolism with little effect on other lipid fractions. Carriers of the *LIPG* 396Ser allele had approximately 5.5 mg/dL higher average levels of HDL-C than noncarriers, which would correspond to an expected 13% decrease in MI risk per epidemiologic estimates. However, the *LIPG* 396Ser variant was not associated with risk of MI (odds ratio [OR] 0.99, 95% confidence interval [CI] 0.88–1.11, $p = 0.85$).[66]

In the same study, a genetic risk score was constructed utilizing 14 common variants associated with plasma HDL-C without pleiotropic effects on LDL-C or triglycerides. The genetic score for HDL was applied to over 50,000 MI cases and controls from the CARDIoGRAM consortium. Whereas a 1-standard deviation increase in HDL-C (~15 mg/dL) was expected to confer a 38% decrease in MI risk based on epidemiologic estimates, genetically elevated HDL-C (1-standard deviation increase) was not associated with a statistically significant change in MI risk (OR 0.93, 95% CI 0.68–1.26, $p = 0.63$) (see Fig. 3.1).[66]

Genetic evidence does not support a causal relationship between HDL-C and CAD, challenging the long-held notion that pharmacologic raising of HDL-C will consistently lead to reductions in CAD risk. Multiple randomized controlled trials of HDL-C raising therapies have failed to reduce risk for atherosclerotic CVD. Three separate CETP inhibitors—torcetrapib, dalcetrapib, and evacetrapib—did not significantly reduce the risk of CAD despite achieving anywhere between 30% and 90% increases in HDL-C.[90–92] Similarly, two randomized clinical trials assessing the efficacy of niacin in patients with established atherosclerotic vascular disease showed no significant reduction in the risk of major vascular events despite significant increases in HDL-C.[93,94]

C-Reactive Protein

Epidemiologic data have consistently associated higher plasma concentrations of CRP—an acute-phase, circulating biomarker of inflammation—with an increased risk of CAD.[95,96] However, Mendelian randomization studies of common genetic variants within the *CRP* locus associated with elevated plasma levels of CRP have not found an association with CAD risk.[62,97,98] Similarly, more recent studies of rare exonic variants linked with CRP levels have demonstrated no significant association with CAD, providing further evidence that CRP is more likely a marker than a causal mediator of coronary atherosclerosis.[99]

Nontraditional CAD Pathways and Implications for Novel Biology

Genetic association studies and studies of causal inference attest to the importance of ApoB-containing lipoproteins (LDL, TRL, and Lp(a)) as causal mediators of atherosclerosis. In fact, approximately 14 of the 58 GWAS-identified CAD risk loci are linked to ApoB-containing lipoproteins. Of the remaining CAD risk loci, a few have been associated with hypertension, although curiously, none have been specifically linked to diabetes mellitus or related pathways (see Table 3.2). However, the majority of known CAD susceptibility loci are not related to traditional CAD risk factors and appear to increase risk of coronary atherosclerosis by yet unidentified mechanisms, highlighting the potential of the GWAS approach to uncover novel biology. Whereas a few risk loci involve inflammatory pathways, several candidate genes implicate protein products with well-known roles in vessel wall biology, such as cellular adhesion, leukocyte and vascular smooth muscle cell (vSMC) migration, angiogenesis, and nitric oxide signaling.[14]

Of particular interest is ADAMTS7, an extracellular protease with disintegrin and metalloproteinase activity that regulates the migration of vSMCs. ADAMTS7 has been found to colocalize with vascular smooth muscle cells (VsMC) in human atherosclerotic plaques, with a particular predilection for the intima-media border and fibrous cap. SNPs within the *ADAMTS7* gene are among the CAD susceptibility loci identified via GWAS.[45,100] Certain genotypes within the *ADAMTS7* locus have been associated with lower atherosclerosis prevalence and severity. An in vitro mechanistic study of vSMCs harboring CAD-protective SNPs in *ADAMTS7* demonstrated normal expression but reduced maturation and activity of the ADAMTS7 protein, resulting in decreased substrate cleavage and attenuated vSMC migration.[101] In 2015, a study of atherosclerosis-prone mice (*APOE-/-* and *LDLR -/-*) found that deletion of *ADAMTS7* resulted in marked reduction of atherosclerosis formation despite comparable levels of plasma lipid content. *ADAMTS7*-deficient mice also demonstrated reduced neointimal formation after arterial injury, as well as reduced in vitro vSMC migration in response to tumor necrosis factor-α.[102]

Studies of ADAMTS7 have established a clear candidate gene with plausible biology for promoting the atherosclerotic phenotype. In addition, the data suggest that inhibition of ADAMTS7, which has narrow substrate specificity, provides a novel therapeutic strategy for CAD. Further investigations are required to establish similar mechanistic links for other CAD risk loci and may offer new insights into CAD pathogenesis and new therapeutic targets for disease management.

GENETIC TESTING FOR CORONARY ARTERY DISEASE IN THE CLINICAL SETTING

Significant advancements in the procurement of human genetic data coupled with the decreased cost and increased availability of point-of-care genetic testing have prompted considerable efforts to incorporate genetic information into the diagnosis, prognosis, and management of patients with CAD. At present, efforts are largely focused on the identification of monogenic disorders such as FH, the use of multilocus genetic models for assessing cardiovascular risk, and the application of pharmacogenomics to guide appropriate therapeutic strategies for CAD.

Familial Hypercholesterolemia

As discussed previously, FH classically results from single-gene mutations—usually in *LDLR*, *APOB*, or *PCSK9*—that negatively affect the LDL receptor and induce marked elevations in plasma LDL-C. The disease follows an autosomal dominant pattern of inheritance and, if untreated, confers a greater than 8-fold increase in lifetime risk of CAD.[103]

There are three different sets of diagnostic criteria for FH, and each relies variably on genetic testing, clinical history, family history, typical physical stigmata (ie, tendon xanthomas), and plasma LDL-C levels.[104–106] This variability has led to a wide range of prevalence estimates for FH. A 2012 analysis of approximately 70,000 participants from the Copenhagen General Population Study employing a score-based diagnostic tool yielded an FH prevalence estimate of 0.73%.[107] However, family history is often underreported, physical stigmata can be absent, LDL-C is not routinely assessed (particularly at a young age), and genetic testing is seldom employed. Therefore, FH has been presumed to be underdiagnosed at a population level, with detection usually occurring in adulthood after years of exposure to elevated LDL-C and development of subclinical or clinical CAD.[108]

Prevalence estimates of FH have also been variable in patients with known hyperlipidemia. Prior studies of patients with severe hypercholesterolemia (defined as LDL > 190 mg/dL) have estimated an FH mutation prevalence anywhere between 20% and 80% largely due to differing ascertainment schemes all enriching for a monogenic origin of disease, ie, positive family history or prominent features on physical examination.[109–112] However, in a 2016 analysis of 20,485 CAD-free multiethnic participants, 1386 were found to have severe hypercholesterolemia, of which only 1.7% carried a mutation for FH in *LDLR, APOB*, or *PCSK9*. The same study demonstrated that for any given LDL-C level, the risk of CAD was markedly higher in FH mutation carriers than in noncarriers. For example, in the subset of patients with LDL between 190 and 200 mg/dL, those with an FH mutation had 17-fold increased odds for CAD, whereas those without an FH mutation had fivefold increased odds for CAD (Fig. 3.2). Among participants with longitudinal data on serial lipid measurements, mutation carriers were shown to have a higher lifelong exposure to

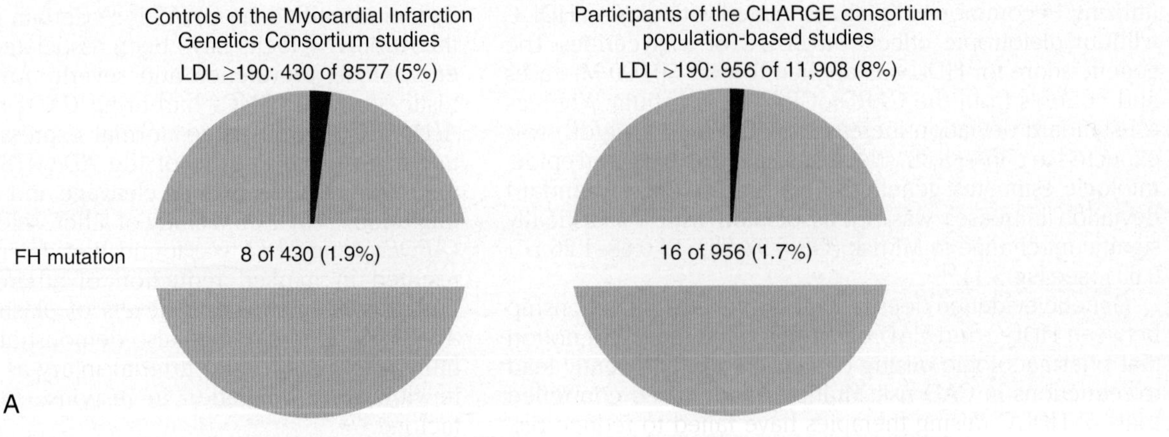

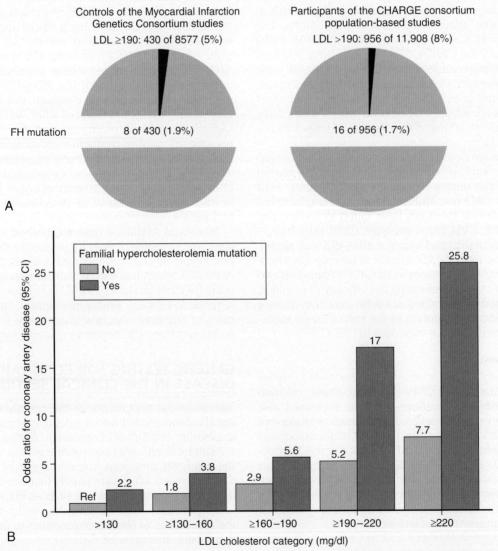

FIG. 3.2 Sequencing familial hypercholesterolemia genes in severe hypercholesterolemia: prevalence and impact. **(A)** Prevalence of a familial hypercholesterolemia (FH) mutation among severely hypercholesterolemic participants. **(B)** Risk of coronary artery disease (CAD) across low-density lipoprotein (LDL) cholesterol and FH mutations status categories. Odds ratios for CAD were calculated via logistic regression with adjustment for sex, cohort, and principal components of ancestry relative to a reference category of LDL cholesterol < 130 mg/dL without an FH mutation. The *p*-value for mutation carriers versus noncarriers across strata of LDL cholesterol was < 0.0001. The *p* interaction between LDL cholesterol category and mutation status was 0.51. *(From Khera AV, Son HH, Peloso GM, et al. Diagnostic yield and clinical utility of sequencing familial hypercholesterolemia genes in patients with severe hypercholesterolemia.* J Am Coll Cardiol. *2016;67:2578–2589.)*

LDL cholesterol than noncarriers, likely accounting for the elevated risk of CAD in this subgroup of patients.[113] The study suggests that FH may explain fewer cases of severe hypercholesterolemia than previously estimated. However, it also affirms that FH mutation status confers a substantial increase in CAD risk, thereby raising the possibility that routine genetic testing will be useful to decrease the population-level burden of CAD.

Genetic Risk Scores for Coronary Artery Disease Risk Prediction

Each of the nearly 60 identified CAD susceptibility variants confers a small but independent risk of CAD. Variants have therefore been aggregated to create weighted genetic risk scores based on their individual effect sizes, and risk scores have subsequently been validated in both case-control and prospective CAD cohorts. In all validation assessments, a higher genetic risk score has correlated with an increased risk of CAD. Furthermore, the predictive abilities of the genetic risk scores have improved over time with the discovery and incorporation of additional CAD-associated genetic variants.[114–116] The 2013 prospective evaluation of 24,124 participants from four cohorts demonstrated a positive association between a genetic risk score for CAD—comprised of 28 genetic variants—and incident cardiovascular events over a 12-year follow-up. Addition of the 28-SNP genetic risk score to conventional CAD risk factors and family history modestly improved risk discrimination of CAD (C-statistic 0.856 versus 0.851; $p = 0.0002$) and reclassified 12% of intermediate-risk patients into a high-risk category warranting statin therapy.[117]

In a separate retrospective study, a 27-SNP genetic risk score for CAD was applied to a community-based cohort and four randomized clinical trial populations of statin therapy for primary and secondary cardiovascular prevention. Higher genetic risk scores were associated with increased risk of CAD across the primary and secondary prevention populations. Furthermore, patients with the highest genetic risk derived the greatest benefit from statin therapy. Specifically, a 48% relative risk reduction was observed with statin therapy in the highest tertile of genetic risk versus a 13% relative risk reduction in the lowest tertile; absolute risk reductions were also more than threefold greater in the highest versus lowest subgroups of genetic risk for CAD.[118]

A recent study (2016) also analyzed the impact of disclosing a patient's genetic risk for CAD on health-related behaviors and outcomes. In the Myocardial Infarction Genes (MI-GENES) trial, 203 participants at intermediate risk for CAD were randomized to receive a 10-year estimate of CAD risk via a conventional risk score or a conventional plus a multilocus genetic risk score. Participants informed of their genetic risk for CAD were more likely to be initiated on and remain adherent to statin therapy (39% vs 22%, $p < 0.01$) and had lower LDL-C levels (~9.4 mg/dL) after 6 months. Of note, there was no discernible difference between the two groups in lifestyle changes such as diet or exercise. In addition, disclosure of genetic risk for CAD was not associated with an increase in patient anxiety.[119]

At present, guidelines do not endorse the inclusion of multilocus genetic risk scores into algorithms for longitudinal CAD risk prediction. The data suggest that genetic risk scores provide modest incremental benefit over conventional risk factors for the prognostication of CAD risk, although the incorporation of newer CAD risk loci into these multivariable models may improve discriminative capacity. However, there is apparent value in genetic risk stratification to identify patients most likely to benefit from statin therapy. In addition, trial results indicate that insight into genetic risk for CAD may motivate short-term statin use. Accordingly, further prospective studies and clinical trials are required over longer time horizons to determine the ultimate utility of multilocus genetic tools for assessing CAD risk, guiding appropriate therapies, and improving patient-specific behaviors and outcomes.

Pharmacogenomics

Pharmacogenomics involves the study of genetically determined variability in drug responses and the application of relevant genetic data to facilitate the study of efficacy and safety of pharmacologic treatments. Inherited differences in pharmacologic responses may reflect variability in the amount of drug delivered to its target receptor (pharmacokinetics) or variability within a drug target that results in differing responses to equivalent drug concentrations (pharmacodynamics). Whereas many pharmacogenomic interactions with cardiovascular agents have been interrogated, the most robust interactions with potential for clinical translation have been seen for statins, clopidogrel, and warfarin.

Genetic influences on statin efficacy have been well-studied through candidate gene analyses and larger meta-analyses achieving genome-wide significance, with the identification of numerous genes—ie, *HMGCR, LDLR, APOE, LPA, SORT1*, and genes encoding for statin transporters—associated with statin-induced LDL-C lowering.[120–123] However, polymorphisms at these genes have accounted for a minor fraction of the total variability in LDL-C lowering by statins and therefore have not been incorporated into mainstream clinical use.

Instead, there has been greater emphasis on pharmacogenomic interactions pertaining to adverse reactions from statin therapy. Variants in the *SLCO1B1* gene have been associated with simvastatin-related myopathy in patients taking 80 mg/day of simvastatin. As *SLCO1B1* encodes a statin transporter, the presumed mechanism of toxicity is reduced simvastatin metabolism resulting in elevated levels of circulating simvastatin. A nearly 17-fold increase in the risk of myopathy has been observed among homozygous carriers of the risk allele receiving high-dose simvastatin.[124] However, the risk of toxicity appears to be mitigated by reduced doses of simvastatin and has been inconsistently observed for other more potent statins such as atorvastatin and rosuvastatin that provide robust cardiovascular benefits, thereby diminishing the need to test for genetic variation in *SLCO1B1*.

Long-term dual antiplatelet therapy with aspirin and a P2Y12-receptor antagonist is recommended per consensus guidelines for patients with acute coronary syndromes and patients with stable ischemic heart disease after coronary stenting.[125] Clopidogrel, the prototypical P2Y12-receptor antagonist, is a prodrug that requires activation by cytochrome P-450 2C19 (CYP2C19). However, polymorphisms in the *CYP2C19* gene have been associated with variable clopidogrel activity due to differing levels of the resultant active metabolite of the drug. The loss-of-function variants *CYP2C19*2* and *CYP2C19*3* give rise to decreased clopidogrel activity and reduced platelet inhibition.[126,127] In an analysis of acute coronary syndrome patients on clopidogrel in the Trial to Assess Improvement in Therapeutic Outcomes by Optimizing Platelet Inhibition with Prasugrel-Thrombolysis in Myocardial Infarction (TRITON-TIMI) 38, carriers of at least one loss-of-function *CYP2C19* allele harbored a 53% relative increase in the composite endpoint of cardiovascular death, MI, or stroke and a threefold increase in the risk of stent thrombosis than noncarriers.[128] A meta-analysis of approximately 10,000 patients on clopidogrel after PCI and/or ACS confirmed this association and showed a direct correlation between the number of loss-of-function alleles and the risk of adverse cardiovascular outcomes.[129] Polymorphisms at another gene, *ABCB1*, which encodes an efflux transporter of clopidogrel, have also been associated with reduced clopidogrel activity, albeit to a lesser degree than *CYP2C19* variants.[130] Conversely, a gain-of-function *CYP2C19*17* allele has been associated with increased clopidogrel activity and an increase in hemorrhagic complications.[131]

Point-of-care systems for genetic testing are available and retrospective data suggest improved platelet inhibition and better clinical outcomes employing a therapeutic strategy guided by knowledge of the *CYP2C19* genotype.[132–134] However, the development of newer and more potent P2Y12-inhibitors—ie, prasugrel and ticagrelor—unaffected by *CYP2C19* variation calls into question the current and future need for genetic testing in this clinical context.[135,136] The ongoing Tailored Antiplatelet Initiation to Lessen Outcomes due to Decreased Clopidogrel Response after Percutaneous Coronary Intervention (TAILOR-PCI) and Patient Outcomes after primary PCI (POPular) genetics trials will prospectively assess the benefit of *CYP2C19* genotyping for selecting appropriate P2Y12 inhibitor therapy.[137,138]

The growing burden of concomitant CAD and atrial fibrillation merits combination antiplatelet and anticoagulant therapy to mitigate the risks of coronary thrombosis and venous thromboembolism, respectively. Consensus guidelines now promote situation-dependent combinations and durations of aspirin, P2Y12-inhibitor, and oral anticoagulant therapy to balance the net antithrombotic benefit of these agents with their inherent risks for inducing bleeding complications.[139] Warfarin is a vitamin K antagonist that acts through inhibition of the vitamin K epoxide reductase complex (VKORC1) and has remained the cornerstone of oral anticoagulation therapy for over 50 years. Warfarin has a narrow therapeutic window that requires close monitoring of the international normalized ratio (INR) to balance anticoagulant efficacy and safety. Variations in the gene encoding for the target of warfarin (*VKORC1*) and in the gene encoding for a warfarin metabolizer (*CYP2C9*) have been associated with increased warfarin sensitivity and a predisposition to bleeding complications.[140] Three separate clinical trials have evaluated the efficacy of genotype-guided warfarin dosing to reduce the time needed to achieve a therapeutic INR and to optimize the proportion of time spent in the therapeutic range. Whereas two trials showed minimal to no benefit of a genotype-guided approach over an optimized clinical algorithm employing more frequent INR checks, a third trial yielded superior results with a genotype-guided approach over standard of care for reducing time to therapeutic INR and maximizing time spent in the therapeutic range.[141–143] The trials suggest that genetic testing may assist with optimal warfarin dosing, although the marginal benefits of genotype guidance may be mitigated by more frequent INR testing.

Novel oral anticoagulants like the direct thrombin and Factor Xa inhibitors are alternatives to Vitamin K antagonists and provide the potential to circumvent the aforementioned genetic variation predisposing to inconsistent warfarin response. Compared with warfarin, these agents have demonstrated noninferior efficacy in randomized clinical trials of atrial fibrillation patients and even a favorable overall safety profile, albeit with a slight increase in the risk of gastrointestinal bleeding.[144] A prespecified genetic subgroup analysis of the Effective Anticoagulation with Factor Xa Next Generation in Atrial Fibrillation-Thrombolysis in Myocardial Infarction (ENGAGE AF-TIMI) 48 trial assessed the differential safety profile of warfarin and edoxaban-treated patients as stratified by warfarin-sensitivity genotype. Notably, patients classified as "sensitive" and "highly-sensitive" warfarin responders—based on *VKORC1* and *CYP2C9* genotyping—had less bleeding complications on edoxaban than on warfarin during the first 90 days of the study. These findings suggest the utility of genetic testing for identifying patients at increased risk of bleeding with warfarin and the early safety benefit of edoxaban therapy over warfarin in this subgroup.[145]

The previous examples point to the potential for genetic testing to facilitate the optimal medical management of CAD by maximizing the efficacy and safety of key pharmacologic agents with robust data for preventing the progression of coronary atherosclerosis. Whereas alternative, higher-potency pharmacologic agents in each class may obviate the need for routine genetic testing, current and future studies will continue to determine the net utility of genotype guidance for selecting and dosing appropriate CAD pharmacotherapies.

CONCLUSIONS

The advent of large-scale genetic association studies and Mendelian randomization experiments has enabled the recognition of numerous CAD susceptibility loci, discernment between causal and noncausal risk factors, and identification of novel biologic mechanisms involved in the pathogenesis of coronary atherosclerosis. Next-generation sequencing technologies, which permit interrogation of the whole genome, are now available at reasonable cost and may facilitate additional gene discovery. Moreover, studies of gene-environment interactions may further elucidate the as yet unexplained heritability of CAD. Future studies will continue the transition in focus from gene discovery to clinical translation in an effort to refine risk stratification schemes and provide more tailored therapeutic strategies for primary and secondary prevention of CAD.

References

1. Gertler MM, Garn SM, White PD: Young candidates for coronary heart disease, *JAMA* 147:621–625, 1951.
2. Thomas CB, Cohen BH: The familial occurrence of hypertension and coronary artery disease, with observations concerning obesity and diabetes, *Ann Intern Med* 42:90–127, 1955.
3. White PD: Genes, the heart and destiny, *N Engl J Med* 256:965–969, 1957.
4. Lloyd-Jones DM, et al.: Parental cardiovascular disease as a risk factor for cardiovascular disease in middle-aged adults: a prospective study of parents and offspring, *JAMA* 291:2204–2211, 2004.
5. Zdravkovic S, Wienke A, Pederson NL, et al.: Heritability of death from coronary heart disease: a 36-year follow-up of 20 966 Swedish twins, *J Intern Med* 252:247–254, 2002.
6. Nora JJ, Lortscher RH, Spangler RD, et al.: Genetic—epidemiologic study of early-onset ischemic heart disease, *Circulation* 61:503–508, 1980.
7. Namboodiri KK, Kaplan EB, Heuch I, et al.: The Collaborative Lipid Research Clinics Family Study: biological and cultural determinants of familial resemblance for plasma lipids and lipoproteins, *Genet pidemiol* 2:227–254, 1985.
8. Heller DA, de Faire U, Pedersen NL, et al.: Genetic and environmental influences on serum lipid levels in twins, *N Engl J Med* 328:1150–1156, 1993.
9. Havlik RJ, Garrison RJ, Feinleib M, et al.: Blood pressure aggregation in families, *Am J Epidemiol* 110:304–312, 1979.

10. Levy D, DeStefano AL, Levy MG, et al.: Evidence for a gene influencing blood pressure on chromosome 17. Genome scan linkage results for longitudinal blood pressure phenotypes in subjects from the framingham heart study, *Hypertension* 36:477–483, 2000.
11. Barroso I: Genetics of type 2 diabetes, *Diabet Med* 22:517–535, 2005.
12. Stitziel NO, MacRae CA: A clinical approach to inherited premature coronary artery disease, *Circ Cardiovasc Genet* 7:558–564, 2014.
13. Altshuler D, Daly MJ, Lander ES: Genetic mapping in human disease, *Science* 322:881–888, 2008.
14. Nikpay M, Goel A, Won HH, et al.: A comprehensive 1,000 genomes-based genome-wide association meta-analysis of coronary artery disease, *Nat Genet* 47:1121–1130, 2015.
15. Peloso GM, et al.: Association of low-frequency and rare coding-sequence variants with blood lipids and coronary heart disease in 56,000 whites and blacks, *Am J Hum Genet* 94:223–232, 2014.
16. Lange LA, Hu Y, Zhang H, et al.: Whole-exome sequencing identifies rare and low-frequency coding variants associated with LDL cholesterol, *Am J Hum Genet* 94:233–245, 2014.
17. Cole CB, Nikpay M, McPherson R: Gene-environment interaction in dyslipidemia, *Curr Opin Lipidol* 26:133–138, 2015.
18. Rader DJ, Cohen J, Hobbs HH: Monogenic hypercholesterolemia: new insights in pathogenesis and treatment, *J Clin Invest* 111:1795–1803, 2003.
19. Lehrman MA, Schneider WJ, Sudhof TC, et al.: Mutation in LDL receptor: Alu-Alu recombination deletes exons encoding transmembrane and cytoplasmic domains, *Science* 227:140–146, 1985.
20. Brown MS, Goldstein JL: A receptor-mediated pathway for cholesterol homeostasis, *Science* 232:34–47, 1986.
21. Soria LF, Ludwig EH, Clarke HR, et al.: Association between a specific apolipoprotein B mutation and familial defective apolipoprotein B-100, *Proc Natl Acad Sci U S A* 86:587–591, 1989.
22. Abifadel M, Varret M, Rabes JP, et al.: Mutations in PCSK9 cause autosomal dominant hypercholesterolemia, *Nat Genet* 34:154–156, 2003.
23. Cohen JC, Boerwinkle E, Mosley Jr TH, et al.: Sequence variations in PCSK9, low LDL, and protection against coronary heart disease, *N Engl J Med* 354:1264–1272, 2006.
24. Soutar AK, Naoumova RP: Autosomal recessive hypercholesterolemia, *Semin Vasc Med* 4:241–248, 2004.
25. Salen G, Shefer S, Nguyen L, et al.: Sitosterolemia, *J Lipid Res* 33:945–955, 1992.
26. Berge KE, Tian H, Graf GA, et al.: Accumulation of dietary cholesterol in sitosterolemia caused by mutations in adjacent ABC transporters, *Science* 290:1771–1775, 2000.
27. Lee MH, Lu K, Hazard S, et al.: Identification of a gene, ABCG5, important in the regulation of dietary cholesterol absorption, *Nat Genet* 27:79–83, 2001.
28. Wang L, Fan C, Topol SE, et al.: Mutation of MEF2A in an inherited disorder with features of coronary artery disease, *Science* 302:1578–1581, 2003.
29. Weng L, Rao S, Topol EJ, et al.: Lack of MEF2A mutations in coronary artery disease, *J Clin Invest* 115:1016–1020, 2005.
30. Altshuler D, Hirschhorn JN: MEF2A sequence variants and coronary artery disease: a change of heart? *J Clin Invest* 115:831–833, 2005.
31. International HapMap Consortium, Frazer KA, Ballinger DG, et al.: A second generation human haplotype map of over 3.1 million SNPs, *Nature* 449:851–861, 2007.
32. Dudbridge F, Gusnanto A: Estimation of significance thresholds for genomewide association scans, *Genet Epidemiol* 32:227–234, 2008.
33. McPherson R, Pertsemlidis A, Kavaslar N, et al.: A common allele on chromosome 9 associated with coronary heart disease, *Science* 316:1488–1491, 2007.
34. Helgadottir A, Thorleifsson G, Manolescu A, et al.: A common variant on chromosome 9p21 affects the risk of myocardial infarction, *Science* 316:1491–1493, 2007.
35. Samani NJ, Erdmann J, Hall AS, et al.: Genomewide association analysis of coronary artery disease, *N Engl J Med* 357:443–453, 2007.
36. Chan K, Patel RS, Newcombe P, et al.: Association between the chromosome 9p21 locus and angiographic coronary artery disease burden: a collaborative meta-analysis, *J Am Coll Cardiol* 61:957–970, 2013.
37. Smith JG, Melander O, Lovkvist H, et al.: Common genetic variants on chromosome 9p21 confers risk of ischemic stroke: a large-scale genetic association study, *Circ Cardiovasc Genet* 2:159–164, 2009.
38. Anderson CD, Biffi A, Rost NS, et al.: Chromosome 9p21 in ischemic stroke: population structure and meta-analysis, *Stroke* 41:1123–1131, 2010.
39. Bown MJ, Braund PS, Thompson J, et al.: Association between the coronary artery disease risk locus on chromosome 9p21.3 and abdominal aortic aneurysm, *Circ Cardiovasc Genet* 1:39–42, 2008.
40. Helgadottir A, Thorleifsson G, Magnusson KP, et al.: The same sequence variant on 9p21 associates with myocardial infarction, abdominal aortic aneurysm and intracranial aneurysm, *Nat Genet* 40:217–224, 2008.
41. Cluett C, McDermott MM, Guralnik J, et al.: The 9p21 myocardial infarction risk allele increases risk of peripheral artery disease in older people, *Circ Cardiovasc Genet* 2:347–353, 2009.
42. Myocardial Infarction Genetics Consortium, Kathiresan S, Voight BF, et al.: Genome-wide association of early-onset myocardial infarction with single nucleotide polymorphisms and copy number variants, *Nat Genet* 41:334–341, 2009.
43. Schunkert H, Konig IR, Kathiresan S, et al.: Large-scale association analysis identifies 13 new susceptibility loci for coronary artery disease, *Nat Genet* 43:333–338, 2011.
44. Coronary Artery Disease (C4D) Genetics Consortium: A genome-wide association study in Europeans and South Asians identifies five new loci for coronary artery disease, *Nat Genet* 43:339–344, 2011.
45. CARDIoGRAMplusC4D Consortium, Deloukas P, Kanoni S, et al.: Large-scale association analysis identifies new risk loci for coronary artery disease, *Nat Genet* 45:25–33, 2013.
46. Tregouet DA, Konig IR, Erdmann J, et al.: Genome-wide haplotype association study identifies the SLC22A3-LPAL2-LPA gene cluster as a risk locus for coronary artery disease, *Nat Genet* 41:283–285, 2009.
47. Schork NJ, Murray SS, Frazer KA, et al.: Common vs. rare allele hypotheses for complex diseases, *Curr Opin Genet Dev* 19:212–219, 2009.
48. Diabetes Genetics Initiative of Broad Institute of Harvard and MIT, Lund University, and Novartis Institutes of BioMedical Research, et al.: Genome-wide association analysis identifies loci for type 2 diabetes and triglyceride levels, *Science* 316:1331–1336, 2007.
49. Orho-Melander M, Melander O, Guiducci C, et al.: Common missense variant in the glucokinase regulatory protein gene is associated with increased plasma triglyceride and C-reactive protein but lower fasting glucose concentrations, *Diabetes* 57:3112–3121, 2008.
50. Raimondo A, Rees MG, Gloyn AL: Glucokinase regulatory protein: complexity at the crossroads of triglyceride and glucose metabolism, *Curr Opin Lipidol* 26:88–95, 2015.
51. Teslovich TM, et al.: Biological, clinical and population relevance of 95 loci for blood lipids, *Nature* 466:707–713, 2010.
52. Global Lipids Genetics Consortium, Willer CJ, Schmidt EM, et al.: Discovery and refinement of loci associated with lipid levels, *Nat Genet* 45:1274–1283, 2013.
53. Newton-Cheh C, Johnson T, Gateva V, et al.: Genome-wide association study identifies eight loci associated with blood pressure, *Nat Genet* 41:666–676, 2009.
54. Levy D, Ehret GB, Rice K, et al.: Genome-wide association study of blood pressure and hypertension, *Nat Genet* 41:677–687, 2009.
55. International Consortium for Blood Pressure Genome-Wide Association Studies, Ehret GB, Munroe PB, et al.: Genetic variants in novel pathways influence blood pressure and cardiovascular disease risk, *Nature* 478:103–109, 2011.
56. Wain LV, Verwoert GC, O'Reilly PF, et al.: Genome-wide association study identifies six new loci influencing pulse pressure and mean arterial pressure, *Nat Genet* 43:1005–1011, 2011.
57. Wellcome Trust Case Control Consortium, et al.: Genome-wide association study of 14,000 cases of seven common diseases and 3,000 shared controls, *Nature* 447:661–678, 2007.
58. Morris AP, Voight BF, Teslovich TM, et al.: Large-scale association analysis provides insights into the genetic architecture and pathophysiology of type 2 diabetes, *Nat Genet* 44:981–990, 2012.
59. Raj SM, Howson JM, Walker NM, et al.: No association of multiple type 2 diabetes loci with type 1 diabetes, *Diabetologia* 52:2109–2116, 2009.
60. Winkler C, Raab J, Grallert H, et al.: Lack of association of type 2 diabetes susceptibility genotypes and body weight on the development of islet autoimmunity and type 1 diabetes, *PLoS One* 7:e35410, 2012.
61. Ridker PM, Pare G, Parker A, et al.: Loci related to metabolic-syndrome pathways including LEPR, HNF1A, IL6R, and GCKR associate with plasma C-reactive protein: the Women's Genome Health Study, *Am J Hum Genet* 82:1185–1192, 2008.
62. Elliott P, Chambers JC, Zhang W, et al.: Genetic loci associated with C-reactive protein levels and risk of coronary heart disease, *JAMA* 302:37–48, 2008.
63. Dehghan A, Dupuis J, Barbalic M, et al.: Meta-analysis of genome-wide association studies in >80 000 subjects identifies multiple loci for C-reactive protein levels, *Circulation* 123:731–738, 2011.
64. Kannel WB, Dawber TR, Kagan A, et al.: Factors of risk in the development of coronary heart disease–six year follow-up experience. The Framingham Study, *Ann Intern Med* 55:33–50, 1961.
65. Evans DM, Davey Smith G: Mendelian randomization: new applications in the coming age of hypothesis-free causality, *Annu Rev Genomics Hum Genet* 16:327–350, 2015.
66. Voight BF, Peloso GM, Orho-Melander M, et al.: Plasma HDL cholesterol and risk of myocardial infarction: a mendelian randomisation study, *Lancet* 380:572–580, 2012.
67. Myocardial Infarction Genetics Consortium, I: Inactivating mutations in NPC1L1 and protection from coronary heart disease, *N Engl J Med* 371:2072–2082, 2014.
68. Ference BA, Majeed F, Penumetcha R, et al.: Effect of naturally random allocation to lower low-density lipoprotein cholesterol on the risk of coronary heart disease mediated by polymorphisms in NPC1L1, HMGCR, or both: a 2 x 2 factorial Mendelian randomization study, *J Am Coll Cardiol* 65:1552–1561, 2015.
69. Cannon CP, Blazing MA, Giugliano RP, et al.: Ezetimibe added to statin therapy after acute coronary syndromes, *N Engl J Med* 372:2387–2397, 2015.
70. Sarwar N, Danesh J, Eiriksdottir G, et al.: Triglycerides and the risk of coronary heart disease: 10,158 incident cases among 262,525 participants in 29 Western prospective studies, *Circulation* 115:450–458, 2007.
71. Rubins HB, Robins SJ, Collins D, et al.: Gemfibrozil for the secondary prevention of coronary heart disease in men with low levels of high-density lipoprotein cholesterol. Veterans Affairs High-Density Lipoprotein Cholesterol Intervention Trial Study Group, *N Engl J Med* 341:410–418, 1999.
72. Keech A, Simes RJ, Barter P, et al.: Effects of long-term fenofibrate therapy on cardiovascular events in 9795 people with type 2 diabetes mellitus (the FIELD study): randomised controlled trial, *Lancet* 366:1849–1861, 2005.
73. ACCORD Study Group, Ginsberg HN, Elam MB, et al.: Effects of combination lipid therapy in type 2 diabetes mellitus, *N Engl J Med* 362:1563–1574, 2010.
74. ORIGIN Trial Investigators, Bosch J, Gerstein HC, et al.: n-3 fatty acids and cardiovascular outcomes in patients with dysglycemia, *N Engl J Med* 367:309–318, 2012.
75. Nordestgaard BG, Abildgaard S, Wittrup HH, et al.: Heterozygous lipoprotein lipase deficiency: frequency in the general population, effect on plasma lipid levels, and risk of ischemic heart disease, *Circulation* 96:1737–1744, 1997.
76. Wittrup HH, Tybjaerg-Hansen A, Abildgaard S, et al.: A common substitution (Asn291Ser) in lipoprotein lipase is associated with increased risk of ischemic heart disease, *J Clin Invest* 99:1606–1613, 1997.
77. Wittrup HH, Tybjaerg-Hansen A, Nordestgaard BG: Lipoprotein lipase mutations, plasma lipids and lipoproteins, and risk of ischemic heart disease. A meta-analysis, *Circulation* 99:2901–2907, 1999.
78. Do R, Stitziel NO, Won HH, et al.: Exome sequencing identifies rare LDLR and APOA5 alleles conferring risk for myocardial infarction, *Nature* 518:102–106, 2015.
79. Pollin TI, Damcott CM, Shen H, et al.: A null mutation in human APOC3 confers a favorable plasma lipid profile and apparent cardioprotection, *Science* 322:1702–1705, 2008.
80. TG and HDL Working Group of the Exome Sequencing Project, National Heart, Lung, and Blood Institute, Crosby J, Peloso GM, et al.: Loss-of-function mutations in APOC3, triglycerides, and coronary disease, *N Engl J Med* 371:22–31, 2014.
81. Jorgensen AB, Frikke-Schmidt R, Nordestgaard BG, et al.: Loss-of-function mutations in APOC3 and risk of ischemic vascular disease, *N Engl J Med* 371:32–41, 2014.
82. Folsom AR, Peacock JM, Demerath E, et al.: Variation in ANGPTL4 and risk of coronary heart disease: the Atherosclerosis Risk in Communities Study, *Metabolism* 57:1591–1596, 2008.
83. Do R, Willer CJ, Schmidt EM, et al.: Common variants associated with plasma triglycerides and risk for coronary artery disease, *Nat Genet* 45:1345–1352, 2013.
84. Emerging Risk Factors Collaboration, Erqou S, Kaptoge S, et al.: Lipoprotein(a) concentration and the risk of coronary heart disease, stroke, and nonvascular mortality, *JAMA* 302:412–423, 2009.
85. Clarke R, Peden JF, Hopewell JC, et al.: Genetic variants associated with Lp(a) lipoprotein level and coronary disease, *N Engl J Med* 361:2518–2528, 2009.
86. Kamstrup PR, Tybjaerg-Hansen A, Steffensen R, et al.: Genetically elevated lipoprotein(a) and increased risk of myocardial infarction, *JAMA* 301:2331–2339, 2009.
87. Lieb W, Jansen H, Loley C, et al.: Genetic predisposition to higher blood pressure increases coronary artery disease risk, *Hypertension* 61:995–1001, 2013.
88. Emerging Risk Factors Collaboration, Di Angelantonio E, Sarwar N, et al.: Major lipids, apolipoproteins, and risk of vascular disease, *JAMA* 302:1993–2000, 2009.
89. Frikke-Schmidt R, Nordestgaard BG, Stene MC, et al.: Association of loss-of-function mutations in the ABCA1 gene with high-density lipoprotein cholesterol levels and risk of ischemic heart disease, *JAMA* 299:2524–2532, 2008.
90. Barter PJ, Caulfield M, Eriksson M, et al.: Effects of torcetrapib in patients at high risk for coronary events, *N Engl J Med* 357:2109–2122, 2007.
91. Schwartz GG, Olsson AG, Abt M, et al.: Effects of dalcetrapib in patients with a recent acute coronary syndrome, *N Engl J Med* 367:2089–2099, 2012.
92. Eli Lilly and Company: Lilly to Discontinue Development of Evacetrapib for High-risk Atherosclerotic Cardiovascular disease. https://investor.lilly.com/releasedetail.cfm?releaseid = 936130. Accessed 2016.
93. AIM-HIGH Investigators, Boden WE, Probstfield JL, et al.: Niacin in patients with low HDL cholesterol levels receiving intensive statin therapy, *N Engl J Med* 365:2255–2267, 2011.
94. HPS2-THRIVE Collaborative Group, Landray MJ, Haynes R, et al.: Effects of extended-release niacin with laropiprant in high-risk patients, *N Engl J Med* 371:203–212, 2014.
95. Danesh J, Wheeler JG, Hirschfield GM, et al.: C-reactive protein and other circulating markers of inflammation in the prediction of coronary heart disease, *N Engl J Med* 350:1387–1397, 2004.
96. Shah T, Casas JP, Cooper JA, et al.: Critical appraisal of CRP measurement for the prediction of coronary heart disease events: new data and systematic review of 31 prospective cohorts, *Int J Epidemiol* 38:217–231, 2009.
97. Zacho J, Tybjaerg-Hansen A, Jensen JS, et al.: Genetically elevated C-reactive protein and ischemic vascular disease, *N Engl J Med* 359:1897–1908, 2008.
98. C Reactive Protein Coronary Heart Disease Genetics Collaboration (CCGC), Wensley F, Gao P, et al.: Association between C reactive protein and coronary heart disease: mendelian randomisation analysis based on individual participant data, *BMJ* 342:d548, 2011.

99. Schick UM, Auer PL, Bis JC, et al.: Association of exome sequences with plasma C-reactive protein levels in >9000 participants, *Hum Mol Genet* 24:559–571, 2015.
100. Reilly MP, Li M, He J, et al.: Identification of ADAMTS7 as a novel locus for coronary atherosclerosis and association of ABO with myocardial infarction in the presence of coronary atherosclerosis: two genome-wide association studies, *Lancet* 377:383–392, 2011.
101. Pu X, Xiao Q, Kiechl S, et al.: ADAMTS7 cleavage and vascular smooth muscle cell migration is affected by a coronary-artery-disease-associated variant, *Am J Hum Genet* 92:366–374, 2013.
102. Bauer RC, Tohyama J, Cui J, et al.: Knockout of Adamts7, a novel coronary artery disease locus in humans, reduces atherosclerosis in mice, *Circulation* 131:1202–1213, 2015.
103. Umans-Eckenhausen MA, Sijbrands EJ, Kastelein JJ, et al.: Low-density lipoprotein receptor gene mutations and cardiovascular risk in a large genetic cascade screening population, *Circulation* 106:3031–3036, 2002.
104. Williams RR, Hunt SC, Schumacher MC, et al.: Diagnosing heterozygous familial hypercholesterolemia using new practical criteria validated by molecular genetics, *Am J Cardiol* 72:171–176, 1993.
105. Risk of fatal coronary heart disease in familial hypercholesterolaemia. Scientific Steering Committee on behalf of the Simon Broome Register Group, *BMJ* 303:893–896, 1991.
106. Nordestgaard BG, Chapman MJ, Humphries SE, et al.: Familial hypercholesterolaemia is underdiagnosed and undertreated in the general population: guidance for clinicians to prevent coronary heart disease: consensus statement of the European Atherosclerosis Society, *Eur Heart J* 34:3478–3490a, 2013.
107. Benn M, Watts GF, Tybjaerg-Hansen A, et al.: Familial hypercholesterolemia in the Danish general population: prevalence, coronary artery disease, and cholesterol-lowering medication, *J Clin Endocrinol Metab* 97:3956–3964, 2012.
108. Schmidt HH, Hill S, Makariou EV, et al.: Relation of cholesterol-year score to severity of calcific atherosclerosis and tissue deposition in homozygous familial hypercholesterolemia, *Am J Cardiol* 77:575–580, 1996.
109. Graham CA, McIlhatton BP, Kirk CW, et al.: Genetic screening protocol for familial hypercholesterolemia which includes splicing defects gives an improved mutation detection rate, *Atherosclerosis* 182:331–340, 2005.
110. Civeira F, Ros E, Jarauta E, et al.: Comparison of genetic versus clinical diagnosis in familial hypercholesterolemia, *Am J Cardiol* 102:1187–1193, 2008.
111. Taylor A, Wang D, Patel K, et al.: Mutation detection rate and spectrum in familial hypercholesterolaemia patients in the UK pilot cascade project, *Clin Genet* 77:572–580, 2010.
112. Ahmad Z, Adams-Huet B, Chen C, et al.: Low prevalence of mutations in known loci for autosomal dominant hypercholesterolemia in a multiethnic patient cohort, *Circ Cardiovasc Genet* 5:666–675, 2012.
113. Khera AV, Won HH, Peloso GM, et al.: Diagnostic yield and clinical utility of sequencing familial hypercholesterolemia genes in patients with severe hypercholesterolemia, *J Am Coll Cardiol* 67:2578–2589, 2016.
114. Davies RW, Dandona S, Stewart AF, et al.: Improved prediction of cardiovascular disease based on a panel of single nucleotide polymorphisms identified through genome-wide association studies, *Circ Cardiovasc Genet* 3:468–474, 2010.
115. Ripatti S, Tikkanen E, Orho-Melander M, et al.: A multilocus genetic risk score for coronary heart disease: case-control and prospective cohort analyses, *Lancet* 376:1393–1400, 2010.
116. Ganna A, Magnusson PK, Pedersen NL, et al.: Multilocus genetic risk scores for coronary heart disease prediction, *Arterioscler Thromb Vasc Biol* 33:2267–2272, 2013.
117. Tikkanen E, Havulinna AS, Palotie A, et al.: Genetic risk prediction and a 2-stage risk screening strategy for coronary heart disease, *Arterioscler Thromb Vasc Biol* 33:2261–2266, 2013.
118. Mega JL, Stitziel NO, Smith JG, et al.: Genetic risk, coronary heart disease events, and the clinical benefit of statin therapy: an analysis of primary and secondary prevention trials, *Lancet* 385:2264–2271, 2015.
119. Kullo IJ, Jouni H, Austin EE, et al.: Incorporating a genetic risk score into coronary heart disease risk estimates: effect on low-density lipoprotein cholesterol levels (the MI-GENES Clinical Trial), *Circulation* 133:1181–1188, 2016.
120. Medina MW, Gao F, Ruan W, et al.: Alternative splicing of 3-hydroxy-3-methylglutaryl coenzyme A reductase is associated with plasma low-density lipoprotein cholesterol response to simvastatin, *Circulation* 118:355–362, 2008.
121. Polisecki E, Muallem H, Maeda N, et al.: Genetic variation at the LDL receptor and HMG-CoA reductase gene loci, lipid levels, statin response, and cardiovascular disease incidence in PROSPER, *Atherosclerosis* 200:109–114, 2008.
122. Kajinami K, Brousseau ME, Ordovas JM, et al.: Interactions between common genetic polymorphisms in ABCG5/G8 and CYP7A1 on LDL cholesterol-lowering response to atorvastatin, *Atherosclerosis* 175:287–293, 2004.
123. Postmus I, Trompet S, Deshmukh HA, et al.: Pharmacogenetic meta-analysis of genome-wide association studies of LDL cholesterol response to statins, *Nat Commun* 5:5068, 2014.
124. SEARCH Collaborative Group, Link E, Parish S, et al.: SLCO1B1 variants and statin-induced myopathy–a genomewide study, *N Engl J Med* 359:789–799, 2008.
125. Levine GN, Bates ER, Bittl JA, et al.: 2016 ACC/AHA Guideline Focused Update on Duration of Dual Antiplatelet Therapy in Patients With Coronary Artery Disease: a report of the American College of Cardiology/American Heart Association Task Force on Clinical Practice Guidelines, *J Am Coll Cardiol* 68:1082–1115, 2016.
126. Shuldiner AR, O'Connell JR, Bliden KP, et al.: Association of cytochrome P450 2C19 genotype with the antiplatelet effect and clinical efficacy of clopidogrel therapy, *JAMA* 302:849–857, 2009.
127. Mega JL, Hochholzer W, Frelinger AL, et al.: Dosing clopidogrel based on CYP2C19 genotype and the effect on platelet reactivity in patients with stable cardiovascular disease, *JAMA* 306:2221–2228, 2011.
128. Mega JL, Close SL, Wiviott SD, et al.: Cytochrome p-450 polymorphisms and response to clopidogrel, *N Engl J Med* 360:354–362, 2009.
129. Mega JL, Simon T, Collet JP, et al.: Reduced-function CYP2C19 genotype and risk of adverse clinical outcomes among patients treated with clopidogrel predominantly for PCI: a meta-analysis, *JAMA* 304:1821–1830, 2010.
130. Mega JL, Close SL, Wivott SD, et al.: Genetic variants in ABCB1 and CYP2C19 and cardiovascular outcomes after treatment with clopidogrel and prasugrel in the TRITON-TIMI 38 trial: a pharmacogenetic analysis, *Lancet* 376:1312–1319, 2010.
131. Sibbing D, Koch W, Gebhard D, et al.: Cytochrome 2C19*17 allelic variant, platelet aggregation, bleeding events, and stent thrombosis in clopidogrel-treated patients with coronary stent placement, *Circulation* 121:512–518, 2010.
132. Sorich MJ, Vitry A, Ward MB, et al.: Prasugrel vs. clopidogrel for cytochrome P450 2C19-genotyped subgroups: integration of the TRITON-TIMI 38 trial data, *J Thromb Haemost* 8:1678–1684, 2010.
133. Roberts JD, Wells GA, Le May MR, et al.: Point-of-care genetic testing for personalisation of antiplatelet treatment (RAPID GENE): a prospective, randomised, proof-of-concept trial, *Lancet* 379:1705–1711, 2012.
134. Xie X, Ma YT, Yang YN, et al.: Personalized antiplatelet therapy according to CYP2C19 genotype after percutaneous coronary intervention: a randomized control trial, *Int J Cardiol* 168:3736–3740, 2013.
135. Wiviott SD, Braunwald E, McCabe CH, et al.: Prasugrel versus clopidogrel in patients with acute coronary syndromes, *N Engl J Med* 357:2001–2015, 2007.
136. Wallentin L, Becker RC, Budaj A, et al.: Ticagrelor versus clopidogrel in patients with acute coronary syndromes, *N Engl J Med* 361:1045–1057, 2009.
137. Mayo Clinic. Tailored Antiplatelet Therapy Following PCI (TAILOR-PCI). https://ClinicalTrials.gov NCT01742117. Accessed 2016.
138. Bergmeijer TO, Janssen PW, Schipper JC, et al.: CYP2C19 genotype-guided antiplatelet therapy in ST-segment elevation myocardial infarction patients-rationale and design of the Patient Outcome after primary PCI (POPular) genetics study, *Am Heart J* 168:16–22, 2014. e11.
139. Lip GY, Windecker S, Huber K, et al.: Management of antithrombotic therapy in atrial fibrillation patients presenting with acute coronary syndrome and/or undergoing percutaneous coronary or valve interventions: a joint consensus document of the European Society of Cardiology Working Group on Thrombosis, European Heart Rhythm Association (EHRA), European Association of Percutaneous Cardiovascular Interventions (EAPCI) and European Association of Acute Cardiac Care (ACCA) endorsed by the Heart Rhythm Society (HRS) and Asia-Pacific Heart Rhythm Society (APHRS), *Eur Heart J* 35:3155–3179, 2014.
140. International Warfarin Pharmacogenetics Consortium, Klein TE, Altman RB, Eriksson N, et al.: Estimation of the warfarin dose with clinical and pharmacogenetic data, *N Engl J Med* 360:753–764, 2009.
141. Kimmel SE, French B, Kasner SE, et al.: A pharmacogenetic versus a clinical algorithm for warfarin dosing, *N Engl J Med* 369:2283–2293, 2013.
142. Verhoef TI, Ragia G, de Boer A, et al.: A randomized trial of genotype-guided dosing of acenocoumarol and phenprocoumon, *N Engl J Med* 369:2304–2312, 2013.
143. Pirmohamed M, et al.: A randomized trial of genotype-guided dosing of warfarin, *N Engl J Med* 369:2294–2303, 2013.
144. Ruff CT, Giugliano RP, Braunwald E, et al.: Comparison of the efficacy and safety of new oral anticoagulants with warfarin in patients with atrial fibrillation: a meta-analysis of randomised trials, *Lancet* 383:955–962, 2014.
145. Mega JL, Walker JR, Ruff CT, et al.: Genetics and the clinical response to warfarin and edoxaban: findings from the randomised, double-blind ENGAGE AF-TIMI 48 trial, *Lancet* 385:2280–2287, 2015.

4 Basic Mechanisms of Atherosclerosis

Magnus Bäck and Goran K. Hansson

INTRODUCTION

Atherosclerosis is a chronic inflammatory process triggered by accumulation of cholesterol-containing low-density lipoprotein (LDL) particles in the arterial wall.[1,2] Major etiologic factors include hyperlipidemia, hypertension, diabetes, and cigarette smoking, all of which are thought to initiate and promote vascular inflammation. The notion of atherosclerosis as an inflammatory disease has emerged based on observations of immune activation and inflammatory signaling in human atherosclerotic lesions, inflammatory biomarkers as independent risk factors for cardiovascular events, and an LDL-induced immune activation.

The use of animal models of atherosclerosis, such as hyperlipidemic rabbits and mice lacking either apolipoprotein E ($ApoE^{-/-}$) or the LDL receptor ($LDLr^{-/-}$), has provided major mechanistic insight into the basic mechanisms of atherosclerosis.

INITIATION OF ATHEROSCLEROSIS

Atherosclerosis is initiated by the infiltration of apolipoprotein B (apoB)-containing LDL in the arterial wall (Fig. 4.1). Atherosclerotic lesions preferentially occur in arterial bifurcations and when the caliber of the arterial tree changes. The switch from a laminar longitudinal to a turbulent flow at those sites will lead to a local recirculation and consequently increased concentrations of plasma LDL adjacent to the luminal surface.[3] As a result, an increased radial LDL transport will occur into the arterial wall, where LDL can be retained by proteoglycans. Endothelial cells are sensitive to shear stress and the frictional force generated by blood flow. Whereas the normal laminar shear stress may be atheroprotective, a disturbed flow activates proinflammatory transcriptional programs in endothelial cells,[4] which participate in the initiation of the inflammatory reaction at sites prone to develop atherosclerotic lesions. In addition, endothelial dysfunction hampers the barrier function of this cell layer, leading to increased influx of cholesterol-containing lipoproteins into the arterial intima.

Modification of the retained LDL by, for example, oxidation, may serve as an initiating stimulus for inflammatory reactions, by being recognized as a so-called danger-associated-molecular-pattern (DAMP). Specific pattern recognition, such as toll-like receptor (TLR) activation by oxidized LDL, subsequently stimulates endothelial cells to express adhesion molecules. Oxidatively modified LDL particles induce endothelial cell surface expression of leukocyte adhesion molecules such as E-selectin, intercellular adhesion molecule (ICAM)-1, and vascular cell adhesion molecule (VCAM)-1, which bind to their ligands sialyl-Lewis^{X}, integrins CD11/18, and VLA-4, expressed on leukocytes. The combinatorial expression of endothelial adhesion molecules and leukocyte integrins and selectins provides a sophisticated regulation of the inflammatory process and determines the type and place for recruitment of a certain type of myeloid or lymphoid cell during atherosclerosis development as depicted in Fig. 4.1.

ATHEROSCLEROTIC INFLAMMATION AND IMMUNE ACTIVATION

The leukocytes recruited to the developing atherosclerotic lesion produce a number of inflammatory mediators (Fig. 4.2) that will amplify the inflammatory reaction through a continued activation of both leukocytes and endothelial cells and by recruiting further immune cells to the forming lesion. These mediators are further discussed hereafter.

Monocytes represent the most numerous white blood cells recruited into atherosclerotic plaques. Once resident in the arterial wall, they differentiate into tissue macrophages under the influence of monocyte-colony stimulating factor (M-CSF) present in forming lesions. Activated macrophages in the atherosclerotic lesion further enrich the proinflammatory milieu, by means of inflammatory proteins and lipid mediators, such as cytokines and leukotrienes. This subtype, which is referred to as *classically activated* or *M1 macrophages*, will hence sustain inflammatory responses and result in tissue damage. In contrast, the alternatively activated, or M2, macrophages secrete antiinflammatory mediators such as lipoxin (LX) A_4, interleukin (IL)-10, and transforming growth factor (TGF)-β and may promote the resolution of inflammation by means of clearance of apoptotic cells (efferocytosis) and dampening of immune responses, hence promoting tissue repair and healing.[5] Both M1 and M2 macrophages are present at different stages of human atherosclerotic plaque development, and data suggest that the atherosclerotic lesion macrophages constitute a unique subset. This may necessitate further subclass characterization depending on their specific functions and signaling pathways,[5] although it should be kept in mind that the macrophage is a highly plastic cell that can modulate its phenotype depending on its local environment.

The number of mast cells is low in the normal vessel. However, mast cell numbers increase with lipid

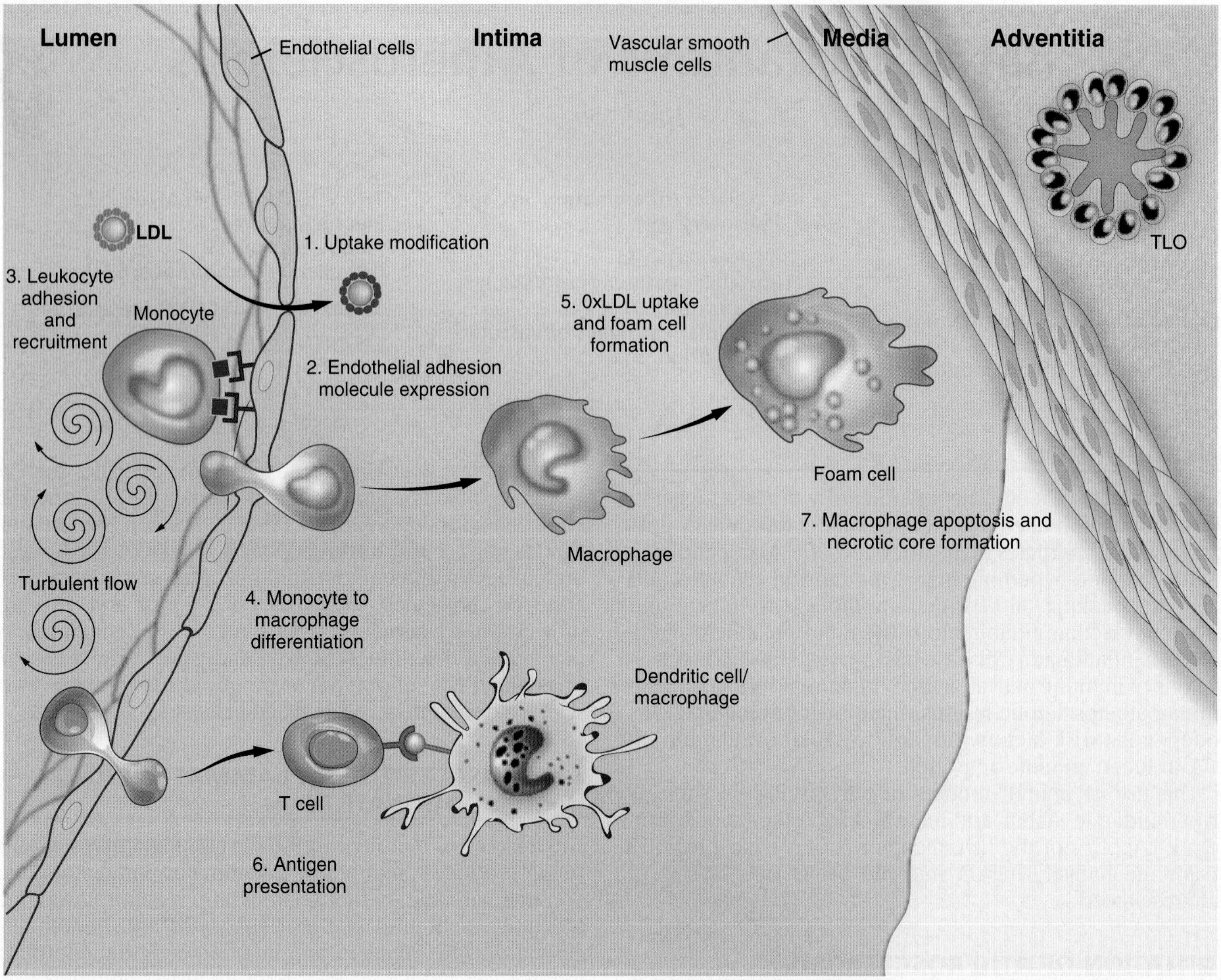

FIG. 4.1 Cellular mechanisms of atherosclerosis. *(1)* Low-density lipoprotein (LDL) is retained in the vascular wall, where it is modified by oxidation. *(2)* Oxidized LDL (oxLDL) stimulates endothelial cells to express adhesion molecules, which *(3)* induces leukocyte adhesion and recruitment. *(4)* Infiltrating monocytes differentiate into macrophages that *(5)* take up oxLDL and become foam cells. *(6)* Dendritic cells and macrophages present antigens to T cells. *(7)* Macrophage death, for example by apoptosis, creates a lipid-filled necrotic core. Note also the presence of mast cells within the lesion. Tertiary lymphoid organs (TLOs) in the adventitia are also depicted (see text for details).

accumulation in the vascular wall in early atherosclerosis, implying that mast cell progenitors are recruited from the arterial lumen.[6]

At this stage, with the presence of both retained naïve and modified LDL, together with activated leukocytes, the atherosclerotic lesion is emerging. Oxidized and otherwise modified forms of LDL particles can bind to scavenger receptors, such as SRA-1, CD36, and LOX-1, all of which are expressed on resident macrophages.[7] The resulting uptake of lipoprotein particles will induce the conversion of macrophages into foam cells, a pathogenic process that results in the microscopic appearance of lipid-laden macrophages, which is a characteristic of the atherosclerotic lesion.

The internalization of oxidized LDL (oxLDL) by macrophages and dendritic cells will lead not only to foam cell formation, but also antigen presentation. The processing of modified lipoproteins and other antigens followed by a subsequent presentation to T cells will hence activate the adaptive immune system within the atherosclerotic lesion. Although oxidation of LDL has been thought to be the source of neoantigens, this hypothesis has been challenged by results showing that T cells in atherosclerotic mice recognize peptide motifs of native LDL particles and its ApoB100 moiety. This suggests that cellular immunity toward LDL as an autoantigen might drive atherosclerosis.[7]

Effector CD4+ T cells are recruited to the atherosclerotic lesion by leukocyte adhesion molecules and chemotactic factors produced as a consequence of innate immune activation. In addition to Th1 cells, effector T cells of the Treg subtype are present in atherosclerotic lesions and act by inhibiting immune responses and inflammation; hence they are considered as atheroprotective.[8] The Th17 cell subtype, finally, promotes fibrosis through action of its signature cytokine, IL-17. Therefore, Th17 activity enhances formation of the lesion's fibrous cap and, hence, presumably, plaque stability.[9]

Several factors in the atherosclerotic lesions induce macrophage apoptosis.[10] Under normal conditions, apoptotic cells are cleared by a specific phagocytosis process, termed *efferocytosis,* from the Greek word "to bury." Efferocytosis is an immune response essential for normal steady state of a tissue and a critical phenomenon in the resolution of inflammation.[11] Defective clearance of lipid-laden apoptotic macrophages in the atherosclerotic lesion will create a lipid necrotic core, as depicted in Fig. 4.1.

In addition to the previously mentioned inflammatory circuits, which take place in the intima, complex adaptive

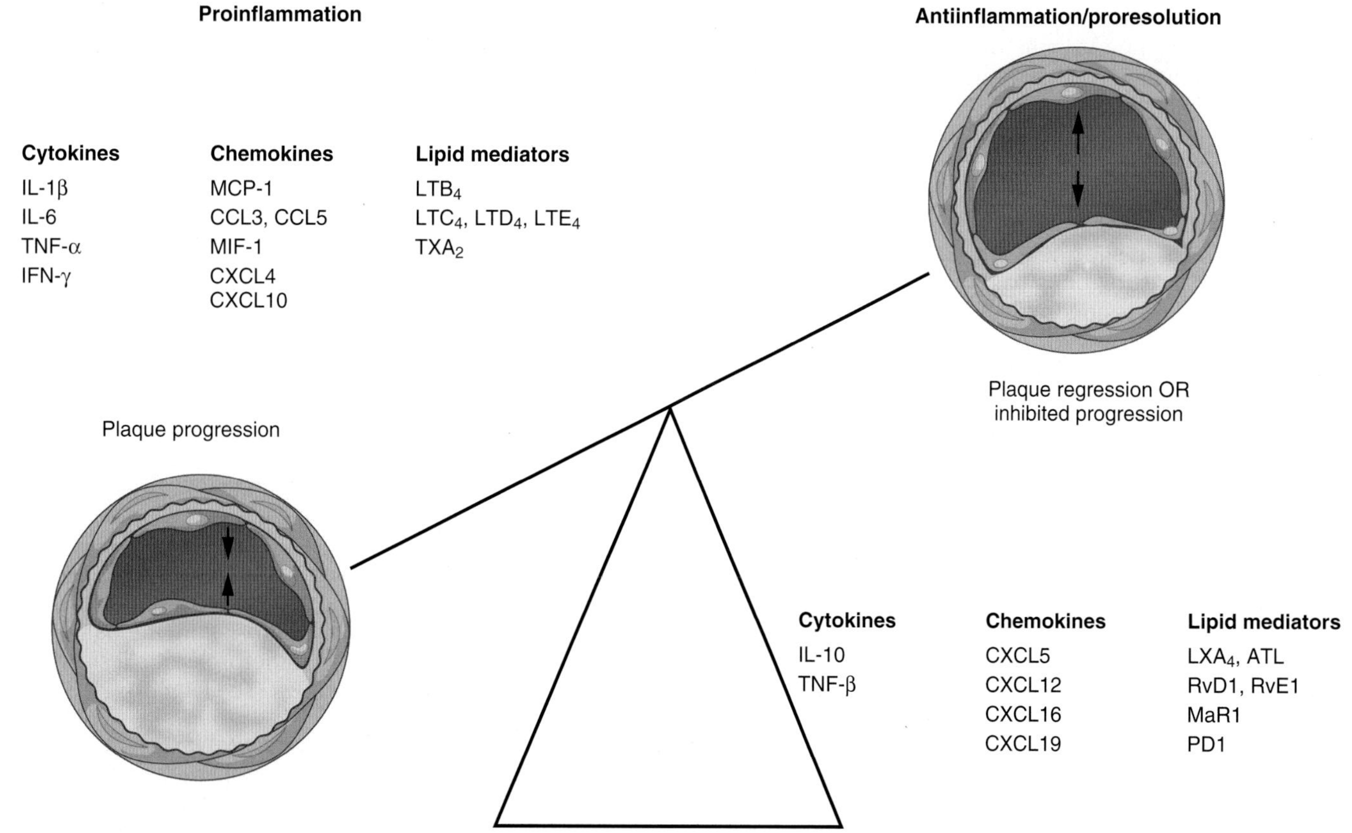

FIG. 4.2 Mediators transducing proinflammation, antiinflammation, and proresolution in atherosclerosis. *ATL,* Aspirin-triggered lipoxin; *CCL,* C-C chemokine ligand; *CXCL,* C-X-C chemokine ligand; *IL,* interleukin; *LT,* leukotriene; *LX,* lipoxin; *MaR1,* maresin 1; *MCP-1,* macrophage chemoattractant protein 1; *MIF-1,* migration inhibitory factor; *PD1,* protectin 1; *Rv,* resolvin; *TGF,* transforming growth factor; *TNF,* tumor necrosis factor; *TXA_2,* thromboxane A_2.

immune responses also develop in the adventitia and the periadventitial connective tissues. Antigens reach the adventitia via the vasa vasorum and also through convection of macromolecules from the arterial lumen.[12] Inflammatory cells observed in the adventitia of atherosclerotic lesions include dendritic cells, macrophages, mast cells, and lymphocytes. T and B cell activation is present in the adventitia of atherosclerotic vessels, and in advanced stages of atherosclerosis, large lymphoid structures may develop, referred to as *adventitial tertiary lymphoid organs*[13] (see Fig. 4.1). The latter contain germinal centers with B cells going through differentiation to centrocytes and plasma cells. Surrounding them, dendritic cells, T cells, and macrophages form organized structures of interacting cells. These adventitial tertiary lymphoid organs are sites of antibody production, including antibodies to plasma lipoproteins. Interestingly, deposits of ceroid-containing oxidized lipids are also found here, suggesting that they may serve as antigenic stimuli for antibody production.[13]

Inflammatory and Antiinflammatory Proteins

Cytokines

In the 1980s, IL-1 was identified as a cytokine of the vasculature, regulating hemostatic properties and leukocyte adhesion. The discovery that macrophages initiate IL-1β production as a response to cholesterol accumulation by means of a multiprotein oligomer called the inflammasome[14,15] and the development of IL-1β-neutralizing antibodies for clinical use have renewed the interest in this cytokine in the context of atherosclerosis, as discussed later. Other cytokines that have been studied for their proatherogenic role include tumor necrosis factor (TNF), interferon (IFN)-γ, and IL-6, as well as others listed in Fig. 4.2. Retrospective analysis of studies of rheumatoid arthritis patients receiving TNF blockade has strengthened the importance of cytokine signaling in atherosclerosis, because these patients exhibit a decreased cardiovascular risk compared with those given alternative treatment.[16] These observations reinforce the notion of TNF being an important proinflammatory signaling factor in atherosclerosis and have suggested that TNF blockade may be useful for cardiovascular prevention.[16]

Several lines of experimental evidence implicate IFN-γ, the signature cytokine of Th1 cells, as a powerful proatherosclerotic cytokine. IFN-γ increases lesion development, modulates lipoprotein metabolism, and inhibits fibrous cap formation. Its presence in culprit lesions of human atherosclerosis supports the notion that Th1/IFN-γ activity may be deleterious in atherosclerosis.

IL-6 is produced in large amounts by IL-1-stimulated cells, including vascular and blood-derived ones. As large amounts of IL-6 are produced by IL-1-stimulated cells, this cytokine acts as an amplifier of vascular inflammation, and circulating IL-6 levels have been reported to predict clinical events. When IL-6 reaches the liver, it induces an acute-phase response that involves increased production of C-reactive protein and fibrinogen and subsequent higher circulating levels of these acute-phase reactants. Therefore, C-reactive protein measurement has become an attractive way of estimating atherosclerosis-associated inflammation.[17,18]

In contrast to these proinflammatory cytokines, TGF-β and IL-10, produced by M2 macrophages and Tregs, activate suppressive pathways and have antiatherosclerotic effects (see Fig. 4.2). Finally, IL-17 produced by Th17 cells may both increase atherosclerosis formation and promote collagen synthesis, which stabilizes the atherosclerotic lesion.[8]

Chemokines

Chemokines are a specific family of chemotactic proteins, classified in subgroups based on the position of the N-terminal cysteine residues (CC, CXC, CX3C, XC).[19] Several studies have supported a key role of chemokines in atherosclerosis by means of mediating immune cell recruitment and regulating the activation of different immune cell types and subsets.[19] Endothelium-derived CXCL1 and monocyte chemoattractant protein 1 (MCP-1, also referred to as CCL2) are involved in early atherosclerosis by means of specific chemokine receptors. In addition, the chemokine-like protein migration inhibitory factor (MIF) also binds to chemokine receptors (CXCR2 and CXCR4) to mediate monocyte and T lymphocyte recruitment to atherosclerotic lesions. Inhibiting MCP-1 binding to CCR2 reduces inflammatory biomarkers in subjects with cardiovascular risk factors, supporting the importance of chemokine signaling as a regulator of inflammation in atherosclerosis[16] (see Fig. 4.2).

In contrast to the previously mentioned proinflammatory chemokine-induced effects, other chemokines, such as CCL19/CCL21, CXCL5, and CXCL12, mediate macrophage regression from atherosclerotic lesions, block foam cell formation, improve endothelial repair, and increase plaque stability under certain conditions,[5] illustrating that changes in chemokine profiles may drive the atherosclerotic lesion to either progression or regression (see Fig. 4.2).

Lipid Mediators of Inflammation and Resolution

In addition to the aforementioned proteins, bioactive lipids (see Fig. 4.2) provide important signaling in atherosclerosis. Their generation may derive from either extracellular metabolism of phospholipids from circulating lipoproteins or intracellular enzymatic pathways using membrane phospholipids as substrate.

Phospholipases

The hydrolysis of phospholipids into fatty acids by the phospholipase A_2 (PLA_2) family of enzymes releases arachidonic acid and lysophospholipids.[20] The secreted $sPLA_2$ has been detected in human atherosclerotic lesions and participates in LDL modification by hydrolysis of phosphatidylcholine, hence rendering the LDL molecule more atherogenic[21] (Fig. 4.3). Another PLA_2 isoenzyme, LpPLA2, which hydrolyzes oxidized phospholipids in LDL particles to proinflammatory lysophosphatidylcholine and oxidized nonesterified fatty acids (oxNEFAs), has also been identified as a risk marker for atherosclerosis[22] (see Fig. 4.3). However, although apparently reducing atherosclerosis in animal models of atherosclerosis and surrogate markers in early clinical trials, large randomized clinical trials (RCTs) have not demonstrated any beneficial effects for PLA_2 inhibitors in terms of cardiovascular prevention.[16]

The Cyclooxygenase Pathway

The two cyclooxygenase (COX) enzymes, COX-1 and COX-2, catalyze the formation of prostaglandins (PGs) and thromboxane (TX). The COX isoenzymes are the targets for nonsteroidal antiinflammatory drugs (NSAIDs). The use of low-dose aspirin in secondary prevention relies on its irreversible inhibition of COX-1 in platelets, which lack the ability to resynthesize COX enzymes, leading to a selective inhibition of platelet proaggregatory TXA_2 formation.[23] In contrast to the constitutively expressed COX-1, the COX-2 isoform is induced by proinflammatory stimuli at sites of inflammation, such as atherosclerotic lesions. The use of NSAIDs being either selective or preferential for the COX-2 isoform (COX-2 inhibitors or coxibs) has however been associated with an increased cardiovascular risk in several RCTs and observational studies and has led to withdrawal and precautions in their prescription to subjects with an increased cardiovascular risk (see Bäck et al.[24] and references therein). Despite potential antiinflammatory effects, the detrimental outcome of COX-2 inhibition in atherosclerosis may be due to a disturbed balance between TXA_2 and prostacyclin, which exert opposing effects in terms of platelet aggregation, pro- and antiatherogenic signaling, and alterations of vascular reactivity.[23] However, other prostaglandins also affect several responses in the vascular wall and inflammatory cells with potential importance for atherosclerosis, and the balance of the COX pathway, both locally in atherosclerotic lesions and systemically, may be more complex (see Fig. 4.3).

The Lipoxygenase/Leukotriene Pathways

Arachidonic acid also serves as a substrate for the 5-lipoxygenase (5-LO) enzyme and leukotriene (LT) biosynthesis (see Fig. 4.3). Arachidonic acid metabolism by the 5-LO enzyme together with the 5-LO activating protein (FLAP) leads to the formation of the unstable LTA_4, which subsequently is either hydrolyzed into the dihydroxy LTB_4 or conjugated with glutathione to yield the cysteinyl-LTs (LTC_4, LTD_4, and LTE_4). These LTs act on specific receptors, BLT and CysLT receptors,[25] respectively, to transduce several proinflammatory effects with implications for atherosclerosis development, such as leukocyte recruitment and activation, smooth muscle cell (SMC) proliferation, and endothelial dysfunction.[26] Local LT biosynthesis and expression of LT forming enzymes are detected in human atherosclerotic lesions, and biomarker studies have associated LTs with acute coronary syndromes and subclinical atherosclerosis.[27] Genetic or pharmacologic targeting of 5-LO and FLAP has, however, generated contradictory results in terms of atherosclerosis development in hyperlipidemic mouse models.[27] Nevertheless, antileukotrienes that are in clinical use for the treatment of asthma and allergic rhinitis have been associated with a reduced risk of recurrent cardiovascular events in retrospective analysis.[28]

Specialized Proresolving Mediators

In addition to the formation of proinflammatory leukotrienes, lipoxygenases also participate in the formation of antiinflammatory lipid mediators, which participate in the resolution of inflammation.[11] For example, arachidonic acid metabolism by means of dual lipoxygenation leads to the formation of lipoxin A_4 (LXA_4) (see Fig. 4.3), whereas the metabolite resulting from the consecutive action of LO and COX-2 acetylated by aspirin[11] is an LXA_4 analogue termed *aspirin-triggered lipoxin* (ATL). These lipoxins are produced locally in coronary atherosclerotic lesions, and their levels increase after aspirin treatment.[29]

In addition to arachidonic acid, omega-3 fatty acids can serve as the substrate for lipoxygenase metabolism, yielding a number of bioactive lipids, such as resolvins, maresins, and protectins, which also promote the resolution of

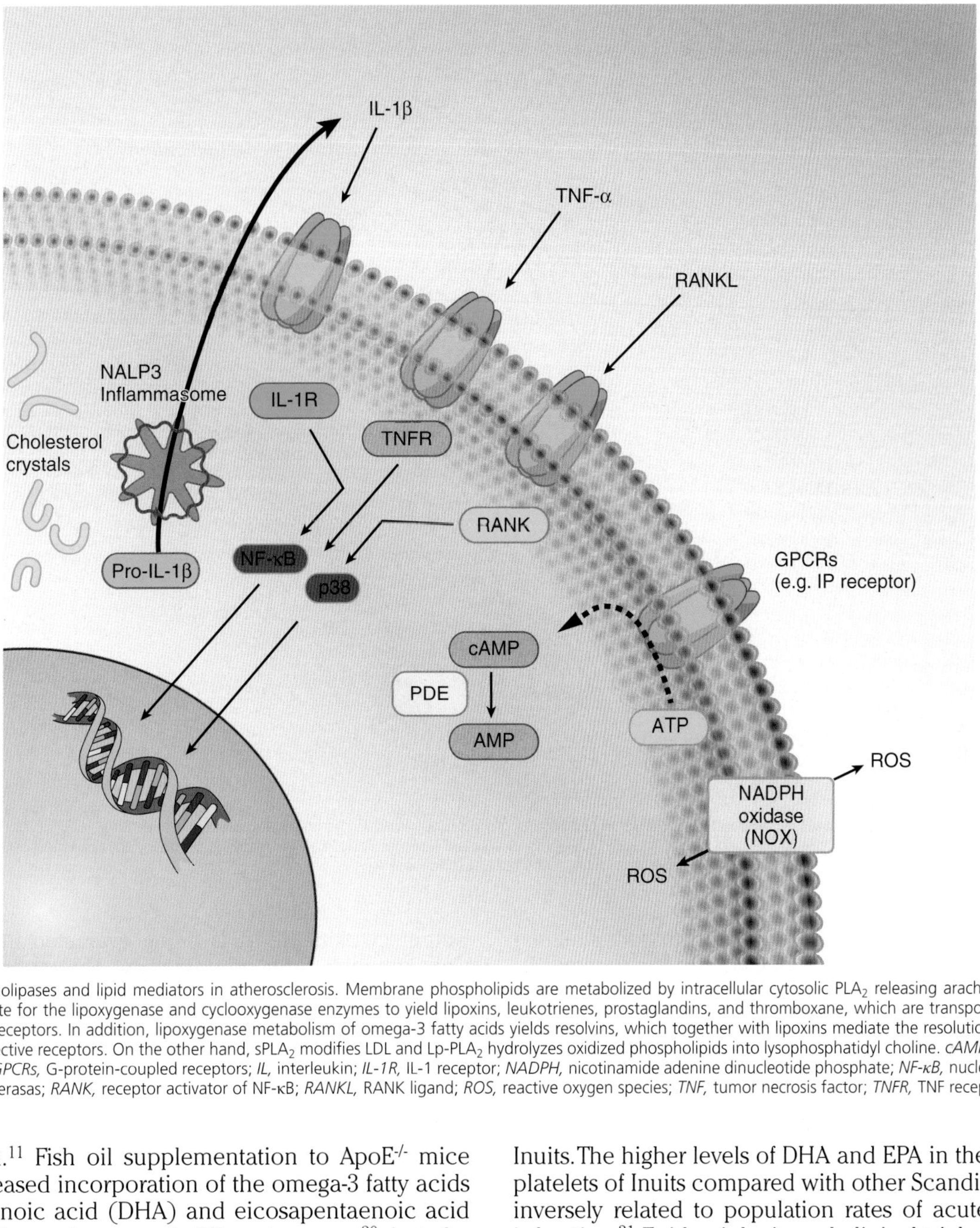

FIG. 4.3 Phospholipases and lipid mediators in atherosclerosis. Membrane phospholipids are metabolized by intracellular cytosolic PLA_2 releasing arachidonic acid, which serves as a substrate for the lipoxygenase and cyclooxygenase enzymes to yield lipoxins, leukotrienes, prostaglandins, and thromboxane, which are transported extracellularly to act on specific receptors. In addition, lipoxygenase metabolism of omega-3 fatty acids yields resolvins, which together with lipoxins mediate the resolution of inflammation through their respective receptors. On the other hand, $sPLA_2$ modifies LDL and Lp-PLA_2 hydrolyzes oxidized phospholipids into lysophosphatidyl choline. *cAMP,* Cyclic adenosine monophosphate; *GPCRs,* G-protein-coupled receptors; *IL,* interleukin; *IL-1R,* IL-1 receptor; *NADPH,* nicotinamide adenine dinucleotide phosphate; *NF-κB,* nuclear factor-kappa B; *PDE,* phosphodiesterasas; *RANK,* receptor activator of NF-κB; *RANKL,* RANK ligand; *ROS,* reactive oxygen species; *TNF,* tumor necrosis factor; *TNFR,* TNF receptor.

inflammation.[11] Fish oil supplementation to $ApoE^{-/-}$ mice leads to increased incorporation of the omega-3 fatty acids docosahexeanoic acid (DHA) and eicosapentaenoic acid (EPA) in cell membranes of different organs,[30] but the effects on atherosclerosis have been somewhat varying between different studies, time points, and models.[31]

Lipoxins and resolvins stimulate efferocytosis,[11,32] which is an important mechanism of the resolution of inflammation and may serve to decrease the necrotic core formation in atherosclerosis (see previous section and Fig. 4.1). LXA_4, ATL, and RvD1 exert their proresolving actions by means of the receptor FPR2/ALX (formyl peptide receptor 2 and A type lipoxin receptor), which is also activated by a number of proinflammatory agonists in the atherosclerotic lesion.[32,33] Studies in human carotid atherosclerotic plaques and animal models have implicated this receptor in atherosclerosis progression and plaque stability.[32,34,35] In addition to macrophages, the FPR2/ALX receptor is also expressed on vascular SMCs, and ATL inhibits vascular SMC migration and proliferation,[36] suggesting additional benefits of aspirin in the treatment of coronary atherosclerosis.

A link between omega-3 fatty acids and decreased cardiovascular inflammation was first observed in Greenland Inuits. The higher levels of DHA and EPA in the plasma and platelets of Inuits compared with other Scandinavians were inversely related to population rates of acute myocardial infarction.[31] Epidemiologic and clinical trial evidence subsequently accumulated in further support of antiinflammatory effects for omega-3 fatty acids.[31] However, the effects of omega-3 supplementation in secondary prevention of coronary artery disease have not been consistently replicated,[37] and further studies are ongoing. The structural elucidation of the active proresolution omega-3-derived mediators as resolvins, maresins, and protectins[11] (see Figs. 4.2 and 4.3) suggests specific stimulations of these pathways as putative therapeutic options in atherosclerosis.

Intracellular Inflammatory Signaling Pathways

p38 Mitogen-Activated Protein Kinase

Among the intracellular pathways that transduce the cellular responses to the extracellular proinflammatory stimuli discussed previously, phosphorylation cascades play a key role in regulating cellular activity (Fig. 4.4). The p38 serine kinase is one of the mitogen-activated protein kinase

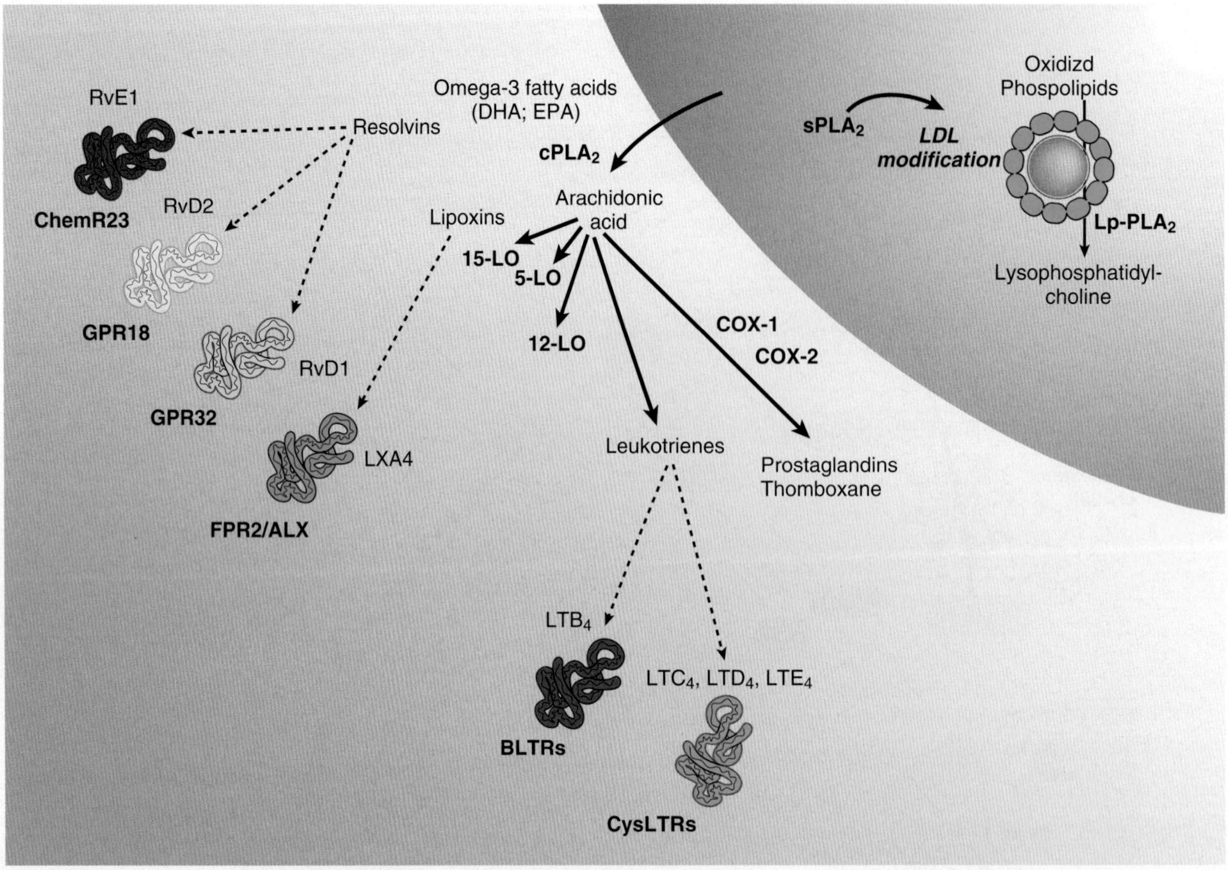

FIG. 4.4 Intracellular signalling pathways in atherosclerosis. *BLTRs,* B leukotriene receptors; *ChemR23,* chermerin and resolvin E1 receptor; *COX,* cyclooxygenase; *CysLTRs,* cysteinyl-leukotriene receptors; *cPLA₂,* cytosolic phospholipase A_2; *GPR18,* G-protein coupled receptor 18; *LDL,* low-density lipoprotein; *LO,* lipoxygenase; *LT,* leukotriene; *Lp-PLA₂,* lipoprotein associated-phospholipase A_2; *LX,* lipoxin, *Rv,* resolvin, *sPLA₂,* secreted phospholipase A_2.

(MAPK) pathways transducing and amplifying intracellular inflammatory responses, such as cytokine production (IL-1β, TNF, and IL-6) and enzyme activity (COX-2-derived PGE_2 formation).[16] Furthermore, p38 phosphorylation may be inhibited by specialized proresolving mediators as part of their role in the resolution of inflammation. Recent clinical evaluations have suggested a potential antiinflammatory and therefore beneficial effect of p38 inhibitors in the treatment of atherosclerosis.[16]

Inflammasome

In classic crystal-induced inflammation, monosodium urate and calcium pyrophosphate dehydrate crystals taken up by macrophages activate the caspase-1-activating NALP3 inflammasome, resulting in cleavage of pro-IL-1β and secretion of active IL-1β.[38] In atherosclerosis, cholesterol crystallization in macrophages may trigger activation of the NLRP3 inflammasome and stimulate IL-1β production as a direct inflammatory response to cholesterol accumulation[14] (see Fig. 4.3).

A possible strategy for the inhibition of crystal-induced inflammasome activation and IL-1β secretion is offered by the microtubule inhibitor colchicine,[38] which reduces atherosclerosis in hypercholesterolemic mice and is associated with decreased cardiovascular risk in observational studies and a prospective randomized trial.[16] However, the perspectives of inhibiting inflammasome activation in secondary prevention by means of colchinine may be limited by its side effects. An alternative approach to targeting inflammasome-dependent activation, by neutralizing its output cytokine, IL-1β, is being evaluated in the ongoing Canakinumab Anti-inflammatory Thrombosis Outcomes Study (CANTOS) for effects in secondary prevention after myocardial infarction.[39]

Nuclear Factor-Kappa B

Nuclear factor-kappa B (NF-κB) is a redox-sensitive transcription factor that is activated in human atherosclerotic plaques, downstream of the IL-1β receptor. In addition, TLR signal transduction is linked to the NF-κB pathway through a chain of transducing proteins, including MyD88 and IRAK. The TNF receptor-associated factor (TRAF) then conveys the signal to either the MAP kinase/AP-1 pathway or activation of Iκ-kinase, leading to nuclear NF-κB translocation to regulate a large number of inflammatory genes. Another NF-κB activator, which will be discussed later in the context of calcification pathways in atherosclerosis, is the receptor activator of NF-κB (RANK), which is a member of the TNF receptor family. Subsequent to its activation by RANK ligand (RANKL), the cytoplasmic domain of RANK signals through TRAFs to activate NF-κB (see Fig. 4.3).

The Jak/STAT Pathway

The Janus kinase (Jak) family is activated by several receptors ligating cytokines, including IFN-γ and IL-6. Jak receptors signal through the signal transducer and activator of transcription (STAT) family of intracellular proteins. Targeting the Jak/STAT pathway downstream of IFN receptors has profound effects on inflammation, foam cell formation, and atherosclerosis.

NADPH Oxidase

The generation of reactive oxygen species (ROS) may be a key driver of atherosclerosis. Increased levels of ROS provoke nitric oxide (NO) dysregulation leading to endothelial dysfunction and induce mitogenic effects of SMCs in the development of intimal hyperplasia. In addition, ROS formation may be directly involved in regulation of inflammatory circuits within the vascular wall. In this context, the nicotinamide adenine dinucleotide phosphate (NADPH) oxidase family of enzymes catalyze 1-electron transfer of oxygen to generate superoxide or hydrogen peroxide (see Fig. 4.3). In human atherosclerotic coronary arteries, the NADPH subunit Nox2 is expressed in macrophages, whereas Nox4 expression prevails in the vascular wall.

Phosphodiesterases

Cyclic nucleotides are important second messengers, with implications for inflammation. The adenylyl cyclase and guanylyl cyclase enzymes catalyze the formation of cyclic adenosine monophosphate (cAMP) and cyclic guanosine monophosphate (cGMP), respectively. Several endogenous antiinflammatory mediators, such as prostacyclin, may negatively regulate inflammatory cells through increased intracellular cAMP levels as a second messenger. In addition, cGMP is typically stimulated by NO through activation of soluble guanylyl cyclase. The intracellular increase in cyclic nucleotides is transient, because cAMP and cGMP are degraded by phosphodiesterases (PDEs), a group of enzymes consisting of multiple isoforms with particular tissue expression and substrate affinities. Blocking cAMP and cGMP hydrolysis by means of PDE inhibitors (see Fig. 4.3) therefore could serve to enhance the effects of endogenous antiinflammatory mediators and SPMs.

CALCIFICATION

In addition to lipid accumulation and inflammation, vascular calcification plays an important role in atherosclerosis. Scoring the amount of calcium in the coronary arteries by means of computed tomography provides a noninvasive measure of the total atherosclerosis burden. Increased coronary artery calcification (CAC) has been associated with increased cardiovascular risk and shown to provide further prognostic information in addition to traditional cardiovascular risk factors. Novel concepts in vascular calcification imaging also include using positron emission tomography to detect vascular uptake of 18F-fluoride, which is a radiotracer of active calcification.[40]

Arterial calcification increases the stiffness of the vascular wall, which can be measured, for example, as an increased arterial pulse wave velocity (PWV).[41] In addition, a pattern of punctate vascular calcification has been described in atherosclerotic lesions. Such microcalcifications are of particular importance, as they may be a site of plaque destabilization and drive plaque rupture, as will be further discussed hereafter. Accordingly, coronary atherosclerotic lesions derived from subjects with acute coronary syndromes exhibit multiple small calcium deposits, whereas those derived from subjects with stable coronary disease have few and larger calcium deposits.[42] Hence regardless if it is on a systemic level as part of a general arteriosclerosis or localized in atherosclerotic lesions, vascular calcification has a major impact on vascular biomechanics.[3]

Although initially considered purely degenerative, atherosclerotic calcification is in fact an active process, which involves calcium deposits, procalcifying particles, and a phenotypic transdifferentiation of vascular SMCs toward an osteoblastic phenotype. Importantly, calcification is also linked to inflammation.[43]

Intracellular Pathways of Vascular Calcification

Wnt Signaling

Agonists of the canonical wingless (Wnt) pathway, also referred to as *the Wnt/β-catenin pathway*, bind LDL-receptor related proteins (LRP) 5 and 6 with Frizzled proteins as coreceptors. This will lead to the cytoplasmatic accumulation of β-catenin and subsequent translocation to the nucleus and the induction of gene expression (Fig. 4.5), such as, for example, bone morphogenic protein (BMP)-2.[44]

SMAD Signaling

BMPs are members of the TGF-β ligand superfamily, which regulate osteoblastic differentiation and calcification of vascular SMCs. The canonical BMP signaling pathway is coupled to phosphorylation of SMAD-1/5/8.[45] The TGF-β and BMP pathways converge when their respective phosphorylated SMADs bind to co-SMAD-4 and translocate into the nucleus to induce gene expression (see Fig. 4.5). In contrast, SMAD-6 acts as an inhibitor of BMP signaling by preventing the formation of the SMAD-1–SMAD-4 complex.[45]

Notch1 Signaling

Finally, another important signaling pathway in arterial calcification is the transmembrane protein Notch1, which upon binding to delta-like or jagged ligands on neighboring cells is cleaved, after which the liberated intracellular domain translocates into the nucleus to regulate gene expression (see Fig. 4.5).

Extracellular Pathways of Vascular Calcification

Matrix Gla Protein

The use of vitamin K antagonists, such as warfarin, as anticoagulant therapy has been associated with increased vascular calcification. The mechanism involves an inhibition of extrahepatic vitamin K-dependent carboxylation of glutamate residues in the matrix Gla protein (MGP), which is an inhibitor of calcification. The γ-carboxylated form of MGP sequesters BMP-2 to protect nonosseous tissues from calcification. Consequently, mice lacking MGP exhibit extensive cardiovascular calcifications.[43]

Likewise, coadministration of warfarin and vitamin K (to specifically inhibit extrahepatic carboxylation) to rodents induces arterial medial calcification and increases vascular stiffness. Importantly, when administered to $ApoE^{-/-}$ mice, warfarin also increases the intimal atherosclerotic plaque microcalcifications.[46] Taken together, these findings suggest that novel anticoagulants (NOACs), such as direct thrombin inhibitors (dabigatran) and factor X inhibitors (rivaroxaban, apixaban), would offer an advantage compared with vitamin K antagonists in terms of vascular calcification and atherosclerotic plaque stability. RCTs are ongoing to test this hypothesis, comparing NOAC with AVK treatment using CAC and PWV as study endpoints.[47]

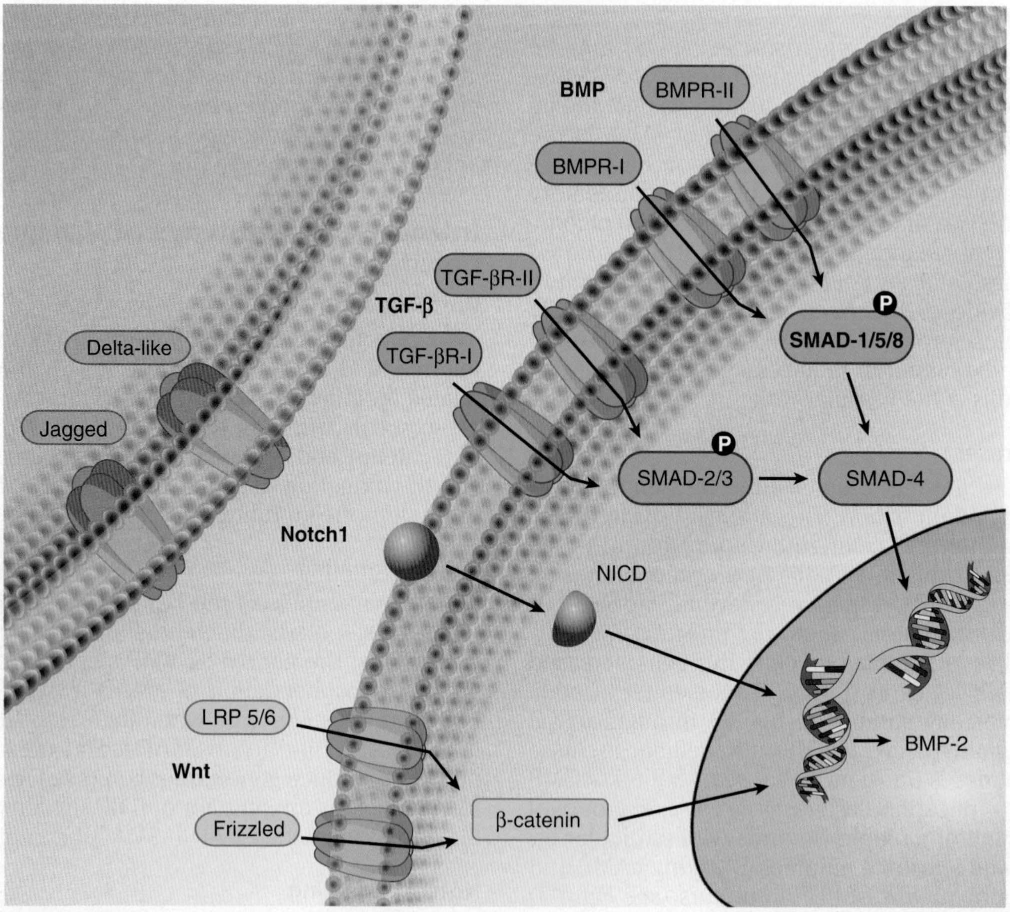

FIG. 4.5 Calcification pathways in atherosclerosis. Notch-1 binding to delta-like or jagged ligands on neighboring cells liberates its intracellular domain (NICD), which translocates into the nucleus and negatively regulates gene expression. The canonical wingless (Wnt) pathway is initiated when Wnt agonists bind LRP 5 and 6, with Frizzled proteins as coreceptors, which will lead to accumulation of β-catenin, which translocates to the nucleus and regulates expression of target genes, including BMP-2. TGF-β and BMPs activate canonical pathways by phosphorylation of the receptor-regulated SMAD-2/3 and SMAD-1/5/8, respectively. *BMP,* Bone morphogenic protein; *LRP,* LDL receptor-related protein; *NICD,* notch intracellular domain; *TGF,* transforming growth factor.

OPG/RANKL/RANK Pathway

Activation of RANK (discussed previously), which is expressed on the surface of osteoclasts by RANKL, is critical for osteoclast differentiation. In contrast, osteoprotegerin (OPG), a soluble receptor that is part of the TNF receptor superfamily, binds to RANKL and hence blocks its interaction with RANK to prevent bone destruction.

Systemic OPG levels and gene expression of OPG, RANKL, and RANK in leukocytes have been detected in subjects with coronary artery disease.[48] One study identified increased expression of RANKL in T lymphocytes derived from patients with acute coronary syndrome compared with those derived from patients with stable coronary disease—thus illustrating the link between the OPG/RANKL/RANK pathway and inflammation in atherosclerosis. In $ApoE^{-/-}$ mice, OPG, RANK, and RANKL are expressed in both immune cells and vascular SMCs,[48] and OPG treatment promotes fibrous cap formation.[49] Furthermore, older mice lacking both ApoE and OPG exhibit increased calcification of atherosclerotic lesions of the innominate artery and increased MMP activity in macrophages and SMCs.[50]

In contrast to its effects in osseous tissue, RANKL induces calcification of vascular SMCs by means of RANK and NF-κB pathway activation.[51] Furthermore, OPG decreases the in vitro calcification of vascular SMCs, both by inhibiting RANKL-induced effects[51] and by direct effects on Notch1 signaling.[52]

THE VULNERABLE PLAQUE

Plaque Rupture

As the atherosclerotic plaque develops, SMCs and collagen form a cap to protect the lipid and inflammatory content from contact with blood. Degradation of this fibrous cap surrounding the core of a coronary atherosclerotic lesion induces plaque rupture and provokes acute thrombosis[53] (Fig. 4.6). If complete coronary artery occlusion occurs in this setting, the myocardium distal to the coronary occlusion will become ischemic, and the patient develops an ST elevation myocardial infarction.

Atherosclerotic plaque rupture results from a loss of mechanical stability of the fibrous cap surrounding the plaque. Therefore, control of cap formation and renewal is critical for plaque stability. Cytokines that stimulate smooth muscle differentiation and collagen production tend to stabilize plaques, whereas cytokines that inhibit these processes destabilize them. TGF-β and IL-17A are powerful fibrogenic cytokines and therefore promote plaque stability. The latter is secreted by Th17 cells; TGF-β is produced by several different cell types including Treg, certain macrophages, SMCs, and platelets. Counteracting these cytokines, the proinflammatory Th1 cytokine, IFN-γ, strongly inhibits smooth muscle differentiation and collagen production. It has, therefore, been implicated as a plaque-destabilizing cytokine.

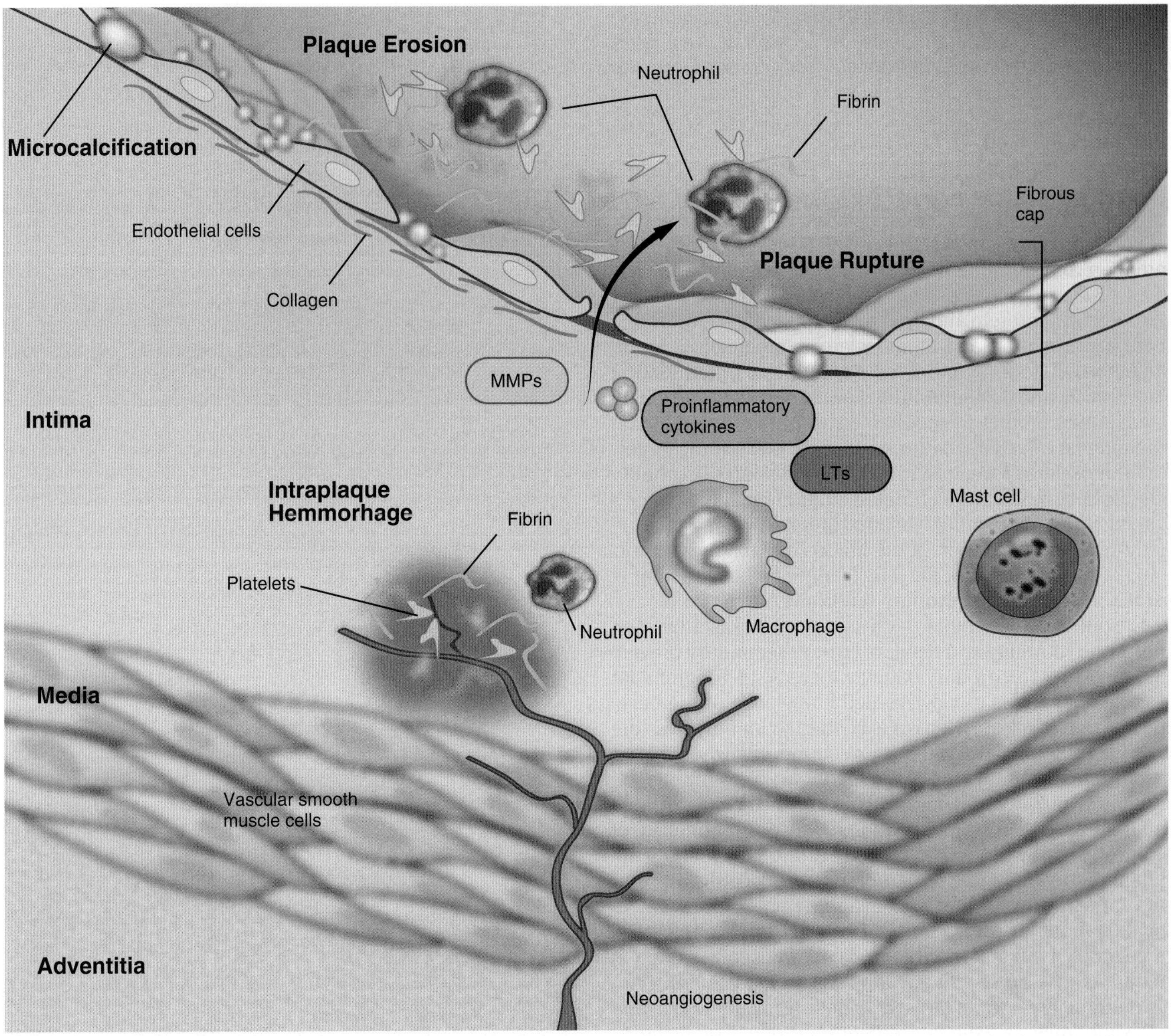

FIG. 4.6 The vulnerable plaque. The fibrous cap, containing mainly smooth muscle cells and collagen, protects the lipid and inflammatory content of the atherosclerotic lesion from contact with blood. In plaque erosion, endothelial cells detach and the exposure of the subendothelial matrix will lead to neutrophil activation and thrombus formation. Degradation of this fibrous cap surrounding the core of a coronary atherosclerotic lesion induces plaque rupture—provoking acute thrombosis and vessel occlusion. Hypoxia and growth factors contribute to neoangiogenesis within the atherosclerotic lesions, which is the source of intraplaque hemorrhage, another important characteristic of vulnerable plaques. *LTs,* Leukotrienes; *MMPs,* matrix metalloproteinases.

Plaque-destabilization can be caused by a number of proteinases released by, for example, macrophages,[53] mast cells,[6] lymphocytes,[53] and neutrophil granulocytes[54] (see Fig. 4.5). Examples of such proteinases are the matrix metalloproteinase (MMP)[55] or cathepsin families. The MMPs are zinc-containing endopeptidases involved in the metabolism of extracellular matrix, as well as in the cleavage of other proteins. Several of the MMPs are locally expressed within human atherosclerotic lesions, and biomarker, genetic, and experimental studies have supported their involvement in plaque rupture and an increased risk for acute coronary events.[55] Microcalcifications in the fibrous cap may also be part of plaque destabilization and drive plaque rupture (see Fig. 4.6).

Plaque Erosion

Atherosclerotic lesions generally remain covered by an intact endothelium until the late stages of the disease.[53] However, in the vulnerable plaque, endothelial cells may detach and, as a result, the exposure of the subendothelial matrix will lead to neutrophil activation and thrombus formation.[53] The latter process, depicted in Fig. 4.5, is referred to as plaque erosion.[53] Pathology studies suggest that the proportion of myocardial infarctions caused by plaque rupture versus erosion is changing, with more cases due to plaque erosion and fewer due to plaque rupture.[53,56]

Intraplaque Hemorrhage

Hypoxia and growth factors contribute to neoangiogenesis within the atherosclerotic lesions. This neovascularization is however considered to be immature and highly susceptible to leakage.[54] The resulting intraplaque hemorrhage (see Fig. 4.5) is an important characteristic of vulnerable plaques and a possible predictor of plaque rupture.[54] Magnetic resonance imaging (MRI) allows the detection of iron deposition in atherosclerotic plaques and thus may detect intraplaque hemorrhages.[57] Although such MRI imaging has been reported to distinguish symptomatic from nonsymptomatic carotid artery atherosclerotic lesions,[57] the possibilities of imaging intraplaque hemorrhage in coronary atherosclerosis are today limited.

SUMMARY AND CONCLUSIONS

The basic mechanisms of atherosclerosis involve lipid accumulation and immune activation in the vascular wall (see Fig. 4.1). These processes are highly regulated by a number of specialized protein and lipid mediators, which either stimulate inflammation and atherosclerosis progression or are antiatherosclerotic by inducing resolution of inflammation (see Figs. 4.2 and 4.3). Inhibiting proinflammatory and stimulating antiinflammatory mediators and/or their intracellular signaling (see Fig. 4.4) may present novel therapeutic targets for atherosclerosis treatment.[16] The progression of coronary atherosclerosis toward a vulnerable plaque includes microcalcifications, extracellular matrix breakdown, intraplaque hemorrhage, degradation of the fibrous cap, plaque erosion, and plaque rupture (see Fig. 4.5), leading to the clinical presentation of an acute coronary syndrome.

Despite a considerable decrease in cardiovascular morbidity and mortality as a result of current secondary prevention measures in coronary patients, there is still a significant residual risk in this group. Detailed knowledge of the basic mechanism of atherosclerosis is needed to identify possible novel therapeutic targets that show superiority when added to currently used strategies for secondary prevention. The results of ongoing and future RCTs on the effects of antiinflammatory agents in preventing the consequences of atherosclerosis will shed light on the future prospect of antiinflammatory treatment as part of secondary cardiovascular prevention. To reach this goal, experimental studies providing the rationale and the proof of concept for the respective targets, observational and biomarker studies in the context of human disease, and finally the design of large clinical trials defining the correct target population, treatment periods, and outcomes, as well as predicting potential side effects, will be crucial for the future development of therapies for atherosclerosis.

References

1. Hansson GK: Inflammation, atherosclerosis, and coronary artery disease, *N Engl J Med* 352:1685–1695, 2005.
2. Libby P, Ridker PM, Hansson GK: Progress and challenges in translating the biology of atherosclerosis, *Nature* 473:317–325, 2011.
3. Bäck M, Gasser TC, Michel JB, et al.: Biomechanical factors in the biology of aortic wall and aortic valve diseases, *Cardiovasc Res* 99:232–241, 2013.
4. Kwak BR, Bäck M, Bochaton-Piallat ML, et al.: Biomechanical factors in atherosclerosis: mechanisms and clinical implications, *Eur Heart J* 35:3013–3020, 2014. 3020a–3020d.
5. Bäck M, Weber C, Lutgens E: Regulation of atherosclerotic plaque inflammation, *J Intern Med* 278:462–482, 2015.
6. Shi GP, Bot I, Kovanen PT: Mast cells in human and experimental cardiometabolic diseases, *Nat Rev Cardiol* 12:643–658, 2015.
7. Hansson GK, Hermansson A: The immune system in atherosclerosis, *Nat Immunol* 12:204–212, 2011.
8. Spitz C, Winkels H, Burger C, et al.: Regulatory T cells in atherosclerosis: critical immune regulatory function and therapeutic potential, *Cell Mol Life Sci* 73:901–922, 2016.
9. Gisterå A, Robertson AK, Andersson J, et al.: Transforming growth factor-beta signaling in T cells promotes stabilization of atherosclerotic plaques through an interleukin-17-dependent pathway, *Sci Transl Med* 5:196ra100, 2013.
10. Seimon T, Tabas I: Mechanisms and consequences of macrophage apoptosis in atherosclerosis, *J Lipid Res* 50(Suppl):S382–S387, 2009.
11. Serhan CN: Pro-resolving lipid mediators are leads for resolution physiology, *Nature* 510:92–101, 2014.
12. Michel JB, Thaunat O, Houard X, et al.: Topological determinants and consequences of adventitial responses to arterial wall injury, *Arterioscler Thromb Vasc Biol* 27:1259–1268, 2007.
13. Weih F, Grabner R, Hu D, et al.: Control of dichotomic innate and adaptive immune responses by artery tertiary lymphoid organs in atherosclerosis, *Front Physiol* 3:226, 2012.
14. Duewell P, Kono H, Rayner KJ, et al.: NLRP3 inflammasomes are required for atherogenesis and activated by cholesterol crystals, *Nature* 464:1357–1361, 2010.
15. Rajamaki K, Lappalainen J, Oömi K, et al.: Cholesterol crystals activate the NLRP3 inflammasome in human macrophages: a novel link between cholesterol metabolism and inflammation, *PLoS One* 5:e11765, 2010.
16. Bäck M, Hansson GK: Anti-inflammatory therapies for atherosclerosis, *Nat Rev Cardiol* 12:199–211, 2015.
17. Ridker PM: From C-reactive protein to interleukin-6 to interleukin-1: moving upstream to identify novel targets for atheroprotection, *Circ Res* 118:145–156, 2016.
18. Libby P, Ridker PM: Inflammation and atherosclerosis: role of C-reactive protein in risk assessment, *Am J Med* 116(Suppl 6A):9S–16S, 2004.
19. van der Vorst EP, Doring Y, Weber C: Chemokines, *Arterioscler Thromb Vasc Biol* 35:e52–e56, 2015.
20. Burke JE, Dennis EA: Phospholipase A2 structure/function, mechanism, and signaling, *J Lipid Res* 50(Suppl):S237–S242, 2009.
21. Suckling KE: Phospholipase A2 inhibitors in the treatment of atherosclerosis: a new approach moves forward in the clinic, *Expert Opin Investig Drugs* 18:1425–1430, 2009.
22. Rosenson RS, Hurt-Camejo E: Phospholipase A2 enzymes and the risk of atherosclerosis, *Eur Heart J* 33:2899–2909, 2012.
23. Capra V, Bäck M, Angiolillo DJ, et al.: Impact of vascular thromboxane prostanoid receptor activation on hemostasis, thrombosis, oxidative stress, and inflammation, *J Thromb Haemost* 12:126–137, 2014.
24. Bäck M, Yin L, Ingelsson E: Cyclooxygenase-2 inhibitors and cardiovascular risk in a nation-wide cohort study after the withdrawal of rofecoxib, *Eur Heart J* 33:1928–1933, 2012.
25. Bäck M, Dahlen SE, Drazen JM, et al.: International Union of Basic and Clinical Pharmacology. LXXXIV: leukotriene receptor nomenclature, distribution, and pathophysiological functions, *Pharmacol Rev* 63:539–584, 2011.
26. Bäck M, Hansson GK: Leukotriene receptors in atherosclerosis, *Ann Med* 38:493–502, 2006.
27. Bäck M: Inhibitors of the 5-lipoxygenase pathway in atherosclerosis, *Curr Pharm Des* 15:3116–3132, 2009.
28. Ingelsson E, Yin L, Bäck M: Nationwide cohort study of the leukotriene receptor antagonist montelukast and incident or recurrent cardiovascular disease, *J Allergy Clin Immunol* 129:702–707, 2012. e2.
29. Brezinski DA, Nesto RW, Serhan CN: Angioplasty triggers intracoronary leukotrienes and lipoxin A4. Impact of aspirin therapy, *Circulation* 86:56–63, 1992.
30. Van Noolen L, Bäck M, Arnaud C, et al.: Docosahexaenoic acid supplementation modifies fatty acid incorporation in tissues and prevents hypoxia induced-atherosclerosis progression in apolipoprotein-E deficient mice, *Prostaglandins Leukot Essent Fatty Acids* 91:111–117, 2014.
31. Laguna-Fernandez A, Petri M, Thul S, et al.: In Steinhilber D, editor: *Lipoxygenases in Inflammation*, Springer, Switzerland, 2016, http://dx.doi.org/10.1007/978-3-319-27766-0_6.
32. Petri MH, Laguna-Fernandez A, Gonzalez-Diez M, et al.: The role of the FPR2/ALX receptor in atherosclerosis development and plaque stability, *Cardiovasc Res* 105:65–74, 2015.
33. Bäck M, Powell WS, Dahlen SE, et al.: Update on leukotriene, lipoxin and oxoeicosanoid receptors: IUPHAR Review 7, *Br J Pharmacol* 171:3551–3574, 2014.
34. Drechsler M, de Jong R, Rossaint J, et al.: Annexin A1 counteracts chemokine-induced arterial myeloid cell recruitment, *Circ Res* 116:827–835, 2015.
35. Fredman G, Kamaly N, Spolitu S, et al.: Targeted nanoparticles containing the proresolving peptide Ac2-26 protect against advanced atherosclerosis in hypercholesterolemic mice, *Sci Transl Med* 7, 2015. 275ra20.
36. Petri MH, Laguna-Fernandez A, Tseng CN, et al.: Aspirin-triggered 15-epi-lipoxin A(4) signals through FPR2/ALX in vascular smooth muscle cells and protects against intimal hyperplasia after carotid ligation, *Int J Cardiol* 179:370–372, 2015.
37. ORIGIN Trial Investigators, Bosch J, Gerstein H, et al.: n-3 fatty acids and cardiovascular outcomes in patients with dysglycemia, *N Engl J Med* 367:309–318, 2012.
38. Martinon F, Petrilli V, Mayor A, et al.: Gout-associated uric acid crystals activate the NALP3 inflammasome, *Nature* 440:237–241, 2006.
39. Ridker PM, Thuren T, Zalewski A, et al.: Interleukin-1beta inhibition and the prevention of recurrent cardiovascular events: rationale and design of the Canakinumab Anti-inflammatory Thrombosis Outcomes Study (CANTOS), *Am Heart J* 162:597–605, 2011.
40. Adamson PD, Newby DE, Dweck MR: Translational coronary atherosclerosis imaging with PET, *Cardiol Clin* 34:179–186, 2016.
41. Reference Values for Arterial Stiffness Collaboration: Determinants of pulse wave velocity in healthy people and in the presence of cardiovascular risk factors: "establishing normal and reference values," *Eur Heart J* 31:2338–2350, 2010.
42. Demer LL, Tintut Y: Vascular calcification: pathobiology of a multifaceted disease, *Circulation* 117:2938–2948, 2008.
43. Krohn JB, Hutcheson JD, Martinez-Martinez E, et al.: Extracellular vesicles in cardiovascular calcification: expanding current paradigms, *J Physiol* 594(11):2895–2903, 2016.
44. Miller JD, Weiss RM, Heistad DD: Calcific aortic valve stenosis: methods, models, and mechanisms, *Circ Res* 108:1392–1412, 2011.
45. Massague J, Wotton D: Transcriptional control by the TGF-beta/Smad signaling system, *EMBO J* 19:1745–1754, 2000.
46. Schurgers LJ, Uitto J, Reutelingsperger CP: Vitamin K-dependent carboxylation of matrix Gla-protein: a crucial switch to control ectopic mineralization, *Trends Mol Med* 19:217–226, 2013.
47. Brandenburg VM, Schurgers LJ, Kaesler N, et al.: Prevention of vasculopathy by vitamin K supplementation: can we turn fiction into fact? *Atherosclerosis* 240:10–16, 2015.
48. Sandberg WJ, Yndestad A, Øie E, et al.: Enhanced T-cell expression of RANK ligand in acute coronary syndrome: possible role in plaque destabilization, *Arterioscler Thromb Vasc Biol* 26:857–863, 2006.
49. Ovchinnikova O, Gylfe A, Bailey L, et al.: Osteoprotegerin promotes fibrous cap formation in atherosclerotic lesions of ApoE-deficient mice—brief report, *Arterioscler Thromb Vasc Biol* 29:1478–1480, 2009.
50. Bennett BJ, Scatena M, Kirk EA, et al.: Osteoprotegerin inactivation accelerates advanced atherosclerotic lesion progression and calcification in older $ApoE^{-/-}$ mice, *Arterioscler Thromb Vasc Biol* 26:2117–2124, 2006.
51. Panizo S, Cardus A, Encinas M, et al.: RANKL increases vascular smooth muscle cell calcification through a RANK-BMP4-dependent pathway, *Circ Res* 104:1041–1048, 2009.
52. Zhou S, Fang X, Xin H, et al.: Osteoprotegerin inhibits calcification of vascular smooth muscle cell via down regulation of the Notch1-RBP-Jkappa/Msx2 signaling pathway, *PLoS One* 8:e68987, 2013.
53. Hansson GK, Libby P, Tabas I: Inflammation and plaque vulnerability, *J Intern Med* 278:483–493, 2015.
54. Michel JB, Martin-Ventura JL, Nicoletti A, et al.: Pathology of human plaque vulnerability: mechanisms and consequences of intraplaque haemorrhages, *Atherosclerosis* 234:311–319, 2014.
55. Bäck M, Ketelhuth DF, Agewall S: Matrix metalloproteinases in atherothrombosis, *Prog Cardiovasc Dis* 52:410–428, 2010.
56. Falk E, Nakano M, Bentzon JF, et al.: Update on acute coronary syndromes: the pathologists' view, *Eur Heart J* 34:719–728, 2013.
57. Raman SV, Winner MW 3rd, Tran T, et al.: In vivo atherosclerotic plaque characterization using magnetic susceptibility distinguishes symptom-producing plaques, *JACC Cardiovasc Imaging* 1:49–57, 2008.

5 Coronary Microvascular Dysfunction

Paolo G. Camici, Ornella E. Rimoldi, and Filippo Crea

INTRODUCTION

Atherosclerotic disease of the epicardial coronary arteries has been recognized as the cause of angina pectoris for more than 2 centuries, and sudden thrombotic occlusion of an epicardial coronary artery has been well established as the cause of acute myocardial infarction (AMI) for more than 100 years. The introduction of coronary arteriography in the late 1950s has made it possible to visualize the contour of the epicardial coronary arterial tree in vivo. This was followed in the 1970s by the development of coronary artery bypass grafting and of percutaneous coronary intervention (PCI). These three techniques have been refined progressively over the years and successfully applied to millions of patients worldwide.

However, the epicardial arteries are only one segment of the arterial coronary circulation. They give rise to smaller arteries and arterioles that in turn feed the capillaries and constitute the coronary microcirculation, which is the main site of regulation of myocardial blood flow. During the past 2 decades several studies have demonstrated that abnormalities in the function and structure of the coronary microcirculation occur in different clinical conditions. In some instances, these abnormalities represent epiphenomena, whereas in others they represent important markers of risk or may even contribute to the pathogenesis of myocardial ischemia, thus becoming therapeutic targets.[1–3]

FUNCTIONAL ANATOMY OF THE CORONARY CIRCULATION

The coronary arterial system is composed of three compartments with different functions, although the borders of each compartment cannot be clearly defined anatomically (Fig. 5.1). The proximal compartment is represented by the large epicardial coronary arteries, known also as *conductance vessels*. They are surrounded largely by adipose tissue, have a thick wall with three, well-represented layers (adventitia, media, and intima), possess vasa vasorum, and have diameters ranging from approximately 500 μm up to 2–5 mm. These arteries have a capacitance function and offer little resistance to coronary blood flow (CBF) (Fig. 5.1A). Their distribution has been divided into three patterns.[4] The type I branching pattern is characterized by numerous branches reducing their diameter as they approach the endocardium. The type II pattern is characterized by fewer proximal branches that channel transmurally toward the subendocardium of the trabeculae and papillary muscles, an arrangement that favors blood flow to the subendocardium. The type III pattern is characterized by epicardial vessels with small proximal branches that vascularize the subepicardial layer. During systole, the epicardial arteries accumulate elastic energy as they increase their blood content up to approximately 25%. This elastic energy is converted into blood kinetic energy at the beginning of diastole and contributes to the prompt reopening of intramyocardial vessels that are squeezed closed by systole. The latter function is of particular relevance if one considers that 90% of CBF occurs in diastole. The more distal branches of the coronary arteries have an intramyocardial path (intramural arteries) and thinner walls than the epicardial branches, and they do not possess vasa vasorum (see Fig. 5.1A).

The intermediate compartment is represented by the prearteriolar vessels (Fig. 5.1B). These small arteries have diameters ranging from approximately 100 to 500 μm, are characterized by a measurable pressure drop along their length, and are not under direct vasomotor control by diffusible myocardial metabolites. Their specific function is to maintain pressure at the origin of arterioles within a narrow range when coronary perfusion pressure or flow changes. The more proximal (500 to 150 μm) are predominantly responsive to changes in flow, whereas the more distal (150 to 100 μm) are more responsive to changes in pressure. The distal compartment is represented by the arterioles, which have diameters of less than 100 μm and are characterized by a considerable drop in pressure along their path. Arterioles are the site of metabolic regulation of blood flow, as their tone is influenced by substances produced by surrounding cardiac myocytes during their metabolic activity.[2,5,6]

REGULATION OF MYOCARDIAL BLOOD FLOW

Myocardial blood flow (MBF) is used to indicate tissue perfusion, ie, the volume of blood per unit of time per unit of cardiac mass (mL/min per g). MBF should be kept distinct from CBF, which is used to indicate the volume of blood that flows along a vascular bed over a time unit (mL/min).

The cardiac pump is an aerobic organ that requires continuous perfusion with oxygenated blood to generate the adenosine triphosphate (ATP) that is necessary for contraction. The role of the coronary circulation is to provide an adequate matching between myocardial oxygen demand and supply. Under resting conditions, the tone of the coronary microvasculature is high. This intrinsically high resting tone allows the coronary circulation to increase flow when myocardial oxygen consumption increases (as oxygen extraction from arterial blood is already close to 60–70% under baseline conditions) through rapid changes in arteriolar diameter, a mechanism known as *functional hyperemia*. The fall in arteriolar resistance drives a number of subsequent vascular adaptations that involve all upstream coronary vessels. The initial arteriolar response is driven by the strict cross-talk that exists between these vessels and contracting cardiomyocytes, which is the basis of metabolic vasodilatation.[7]

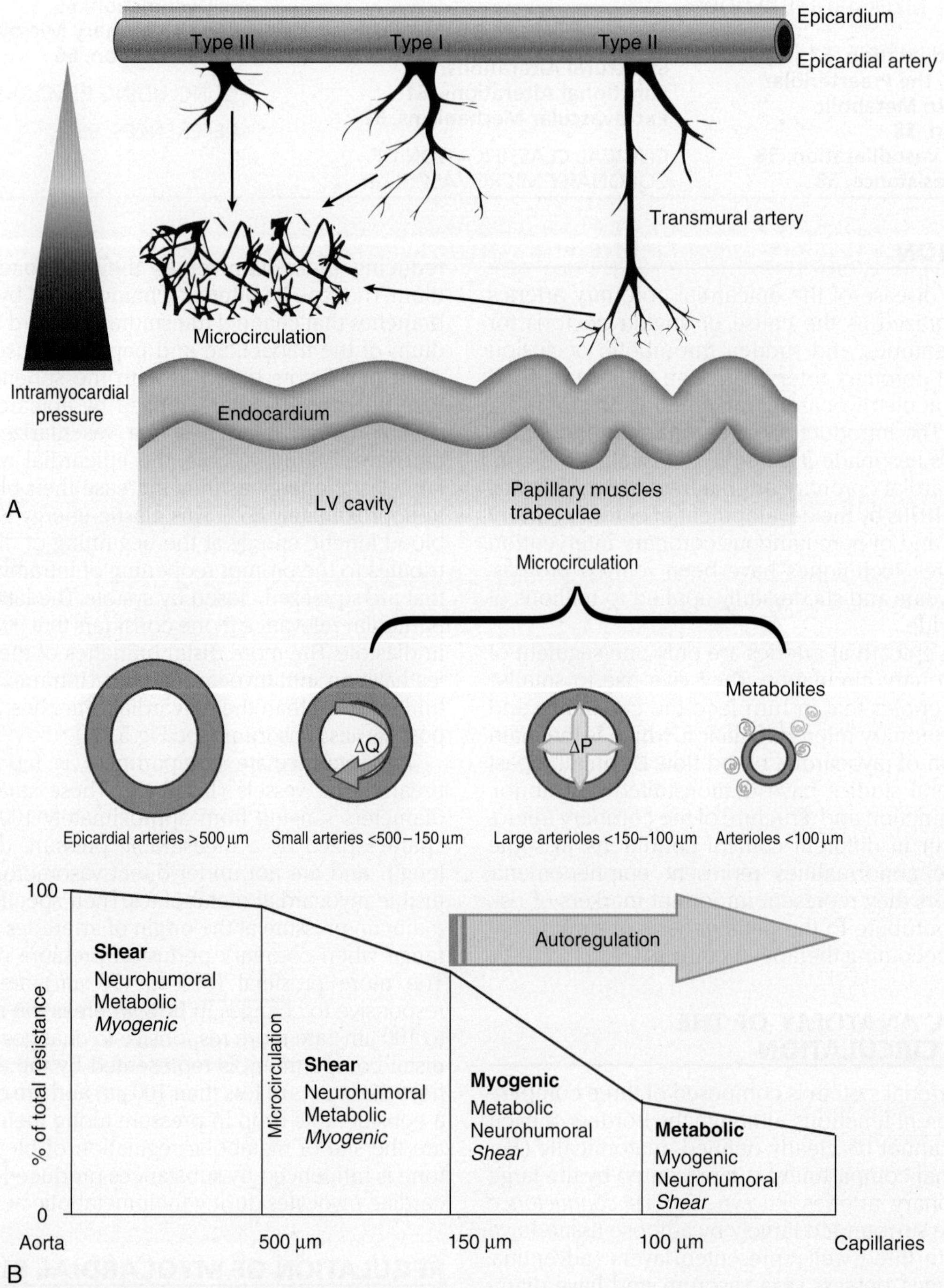

FIG. 5.1 **(A)** Coronary artery branching patterns. Type I pattern is characterized by multiple early intramural branches; type II distribution is directed to the subendocardial myocardium and papillary muscles with less initial branching. Type III consists of short branches that supply mainly the subepicardial myocardium. Transition to microcirculation corresponds to a diameter of <500 μm. Intramyocardial pressure progressively increases from the epicardium to the subendocardium. **(B)** Small arteries are more responsive to flow-dependent dilatation. Large arterioles are more responsive to changes in intravascular pressure and are mainly responsible for autoregulation of coronary blood flow (CBF). Arterioles are more responsive to changes in the intramyocardial concentration of metabolites and are mainly responsible for the metabolic regulation of CBF. The proportion of total resistance in epicardial arteries is negligible; small arteries account for 20% and arterioles are the largest accounting for 40%. Control mechanisms are listed by their importance in the global control of the segment of microcirculation. *P*, coronary pressure; *Q*, coronary blood flow. *(Panel B modified from Toyota E, Koshida R, Hattan N, et al. Regulation of the coronary vasomotor tone: what we know and where we need to go.* J Nucl Cardiol. *2001;8(5):599–605.)*

The integrated coronary response to changes in myocardial oxygen consumption involves (1) metabolic vasodilation, (2) prearteriolar autoregulation, (3) flow-mediated (endothelium-dependent) vasodilation, (4) extravascular tissue pressure, and (5) neurohumoral control.

Metabolic Vasodilatation

During Normoxic Conditions

Metabolites that control blood flow in a feed-forward manner are produced at a rate directly proportional to oxidative metabolism (Fig. 5.2). Examples of such metabolites are carbon dioxide (CO_2), which is generated in decarboxylation reactions of the citric acid cycle, and reactive oxygen species (ROS), which are formed in the respiratory chain in proportion to oxygen consumption.[3] CO_2 is produced in proportion to oxygen consumption and results from the pyruvate dehydrogenase reaction and further decarboxylation reactions in the citric acid cycle. Increased concentrations of CO_2 result in an increase of proton (H^+) concentration, which likely constitutes the direct stimulus for coronary vasodilatation.[3] Similar to the production of CO_2, the production of hydrogen peroxide (H_2O_2) is a feed-forward response, in that the production of this ROS is directly linked to myocardial oxygen consumption.[8] H_2O_2 is generated by two-electron reduction of oxygen. This can occur in one enzymatic step, or more typically it involves generation of the intermediate ROS, superoxide anion ($^{\bullet}O_2^-$).[3,9] With regard to the origin of H_2O_2 associated with metabolic vasodilatation, there is evidence supporting its endothelial mitochondrial generation.[10,11] The vasodilator properties of H_2O_2 have been recognized for a number of years. H_2O_2-induced dilatation is principally mediated by 4-aminopyridine sensitive ion channels, presumably Kv channels. The coronary dilator effect of H_2O_2 might also be mediated by the large conductance Maxi-K channel or by prostanoids.[11,12]

During Hypoxic Conditions

Hypoxia is the most powerful physiologic stimulus for coronary vasodilatation, and adenosine has been proposed as a regulator of CBF in response to hypoxia.[3] Adenosine is formed by degradation of adenine nucleotides under conditions in which ATP utilization exceeds the capacity of myocardial cells to resynthesize high-energy compounds. This results in the formation of adenosine monophosphate, which in turn is converted to adenosine by the enzyme 5′-nucleotidase. Adenosine then diffuses from the myocytes into the interstitial fluid, where it exerts powerful arteriolar dilator effects through the direct stimulation of A_2 adenosine receptors on vascular smooth muscle cells. Several findings support the critical role of adenosine in the metabolic regulation of blood flow.[5,13] Indeed, its production increases in cases of imbalance in the supply/demand ratio of myocardial oxygen, with the rise in interstitial concentration of adenosine paralleling the increase in CBF.[14]

Vasodilatation ensues when Ca^{2+} concentration in the cytosol of the vascular smooth muscle decreases or sensitivity to Ca^{2+} of contractile elements is impaired. Ca^{2+} entry is prevented by vascular smooth muscle membrane hyperpolarization in response to K_{ATP} channels activation[3,15] (see Fig. 5.2).

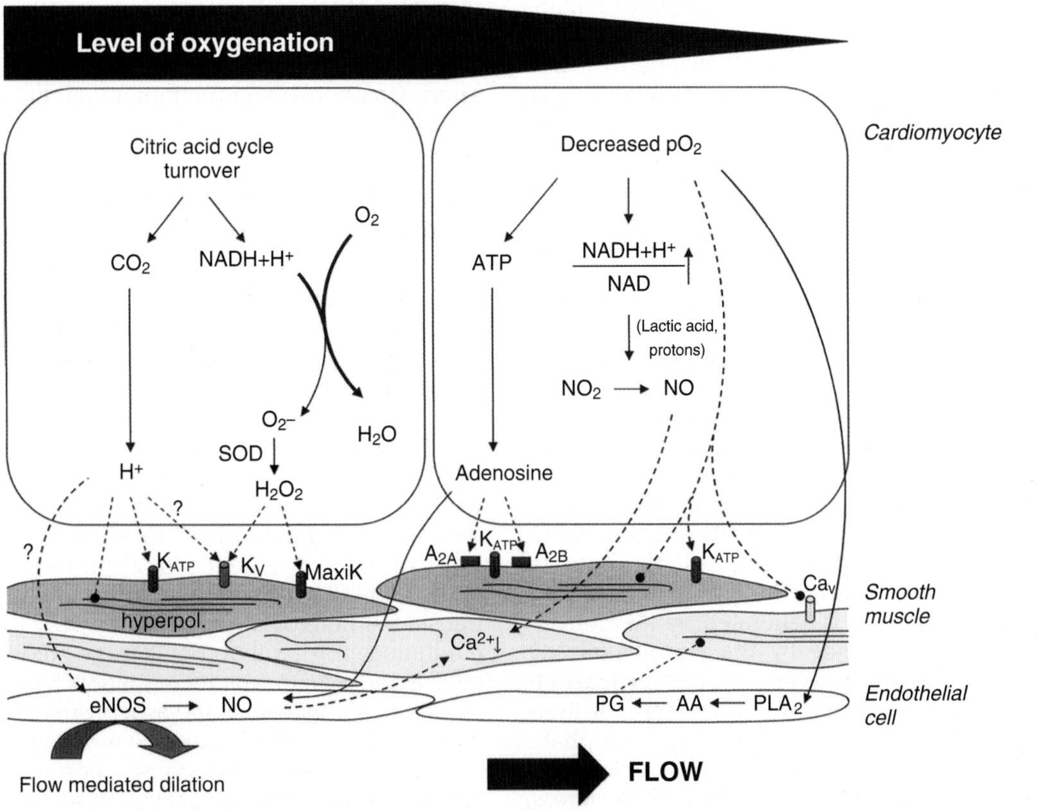

FIG. 5.2 Metabolic coronary flow regulation. The concepts are separated for physiologic conditions (unchanged level of myocardial oxygenation) and pathologic conditions (decreased oxygenation). Biochemical reactions and metabolic interaction are indicated by *solid arrows*, links to effectors are indicated by *broken arrows*. *Blue* and *yellow colors* indicate the primary response on the level of smooth muscle cells, membrane hyperpolarization, and decreased cytosolic calcium concentration, respectively. *Arrows* indicate activation; *closed pointed ends* indicate inhibition. See text for more details. *AA*, arachidonic acid; *PG*, prostaglandins; *PLA₂*, phospholipase A2. *(From Deussen A, Ohanyan, V, Jannasch , et al. Mechanisms of metabolic coronary flow regulation.* J Mol Cell Cardiol. *2012;52(4):794.)*

Autoregulation, the Prearteriolar Adaptations to Metabolic Vasodilatation

Arteriolar dilatation decreases both resistance in overall network and pressure in distal prearteriolar vessels, which in turn induce the dilatation of these vessels. It is worth noting that the coronary circulation exhibits an intrinsic tendency to maintain blood flow at a constant rate despite changes in perfusion pressure, a mechanism known as *autoregulation*. The mechanism responsible for autoregulation is a myogenic response to transmural distending pressure eliciting wall tension, which involves primarily distal prearteriolar vessels: they dilate in response to a reduction of perfusion pressure and constrict in response to an increase of perfusion pressure.[14,16] In vitro, active smooth muscle tone increases almost linearly with transmural pressure, leading to a substantial diameter reduction.[2] A key mechanism of this myogenic response is membrane depolarization of vascular smooth muscle in response to stretch detected by a sensor (extracellular matrix-integrin interactions) that then initiates signaling mechanisms that lead to the opening of nonspecific cation channels promoting an inward Na^+ and/or Ca^{2+} current, although other mechanisms also contribute to this phenomenon[2,17] (Fig. 5.3). Myogenic contraction is ultimately caused by activation of smooth muscle contractile proteins by myosin light chain kinase.[18,19]

Flow-Mediated Vasodilatation

Shear stress, the tractive force that acts on the vascular wall, is proportional to blood shear rate, or velocity, and to viscosity. When flow changes, epicardial coronary arteries and proximal prearterioles have an intrinsic tendency to maintain a given level of shear stress by endothelial-dependent dilatation, ie, the production of endothelial-derived factors such as nitric oxide (NO) and prostacyclin (PGI_2), and endothelial-derived hyperpolarizing factors (EDHFs) stimulated by the activation of specific receptors (muscarinic, bradykinin, histamine) or mechanical deformation sensed by cytoskeletal elements and glycocalix[5,6,15,17] (see Fig. 5.3). In fact, both very high and very low shear stress may jeopardize the interaction between blood elements and the vascular endothelium. In the absence of changes in perfusion pressure, variations of flow in epicardial coronary arteries can be achieved by intracoronary injection of arteriolar vasodilators such as adenosine. Human angiographic studies have shown that epicardial coronary arteries dilate in response to an increase in blood flow, and that the increase in coronary diameter is proportional to the increase in flow, thus maintaining shear stress constant.[1] Vasodilators released by endothelial cells in response to an increase in shear stress, NO, EDHFs, and PGI_2 operate through different mechanisms on the underlying smooth muscle[14,17] (see Fig. 5.3). NO is generated by the conversion of L-arginine to L-citrulline by the endothelial NO synthase (eNOS) in the presence of cofactors such as tetrahydrobiopterin (BH4).[12] NO induces hyperpolarization primarily by activating cyclic guanosine monophosphate (cGMP) signaling and K_{Ca} channels. In the human heart more than one EDHF is produced during shear stress, and it appears that the common pathway is the opening of K^+ channels causing hyperpolarization and relaxation of smooth muscle cells. PGI_2 causes relaxation by activating adenylyl cyclase/cyclic adenosine monophosphate (cAMP)-dependent hyperpolarization; the latter are released into the coronary circulation mainly during episodes of hypoxia/ischemia[12,15] (see Fig. 5.3).

Endothelial-derived vasoconstrictors under normal conditions exert a relatively weak effect on the coronary microcirculation (see Fig. 5.3). There is some evidence supporting a more significant role of endothelin-1 in atherosclerotic disease or for angiotensin-II in obesity, hypertension, or coronary artery disease.[5,6,20–22]

Extravascular Resistance

In addition to vascular resistance there is an extravascular component of resistance due to the compressive forces produced during cardiac contraction that impinge upon the walls of intramyocardial vessels.[23] These extravascular systolic compressive forces have two components: the first is related to the pressure developed within the left ventricular (LV) cavity, which is directly transmitted to the subendocardium, but falls off to almost zero at the epicardial surface. The second is vascular narrowing caused by compression and bending of vessels coursing through the ventricular wall (see Fig. 5.1A). Because of this cyclic extravascular pressure, both vascular resistance and flow vary considerably during the cardiac cycle. Extravascular pressure can exceed coronary perfusion pressure during systole, particularly in the inner subendocardial layers. As a consequence, during systole, subendocardial microvessels become more narrowed, or even occluded, in comparison to those in the subepicardium, and, at the onset of diastole, they present a higher resistance to flow, needing a longer time to resume their full diastolic caliber. This is the reason why most of the blood flow to the left ventricle occurs during diastole when perfusion pressure exceeds the value of extravascular pressure. At peak systole there is even backflow in the coronary arteries, particularly in the intramural and small epicardial vessels.[6,23]

Neural and Biohumoral Regulation of the Microcirculation

Small arteries and arterioles are richly innervated by both sympathetic and parasympathetic nerve terminals that play an important role in the regulation of CBF. Under normal circumstances, in addition to its well-known β_1 adrenoceptor-mediated chronotropic, inotropic, and dromotropic effects, the net effect of sympathetic activation is to increase CBF through β_2 adrenoceptor-mediated vasodilatation of small coronary arterioles,[24] thus contributing to the feed-forward control that does not require an error signal such as decreased oxygen tension.[5] In isolated subepicardial arterioles of swine, β_2 adrenoceptor mRNA is expressed nearly 3-fold more than in subendocardial arterioles,[25] indicating transmural heterogeneity. Coronary vessels are also rich in α adrenoceptors, with α_1 being more predominant in larger vessels and α_2 in the microcirculation. Activation of vascular α-adrenoceptors results in vasoconstriction that competes with metabolic vasodilatation. Sympathetic α adrenoceptor-mediated coronary vasoconstriction has been demonstrated during adrenergic activation, such as during exercise or during a cold pressor reflex in humans.[26]

Based on experimental evidence, Feigl hypothesized that there was a beneficial effect of this paradoxic vasoconstrictor influence in that it helps preserve flow to the vulnerable

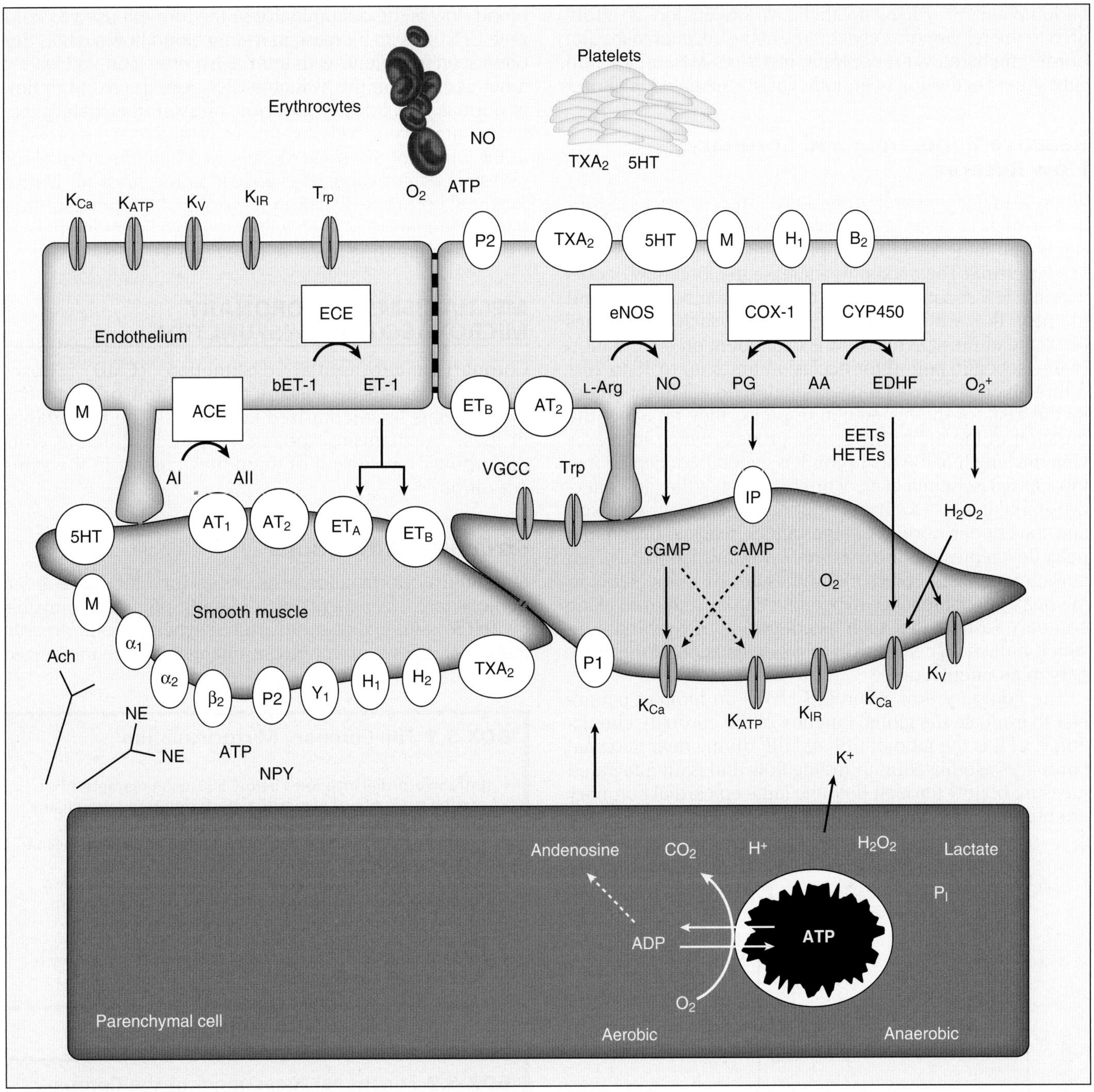

FIG. 5.3 Schematic drawing of endothelium, vascular smooth muscle, and cardiomyocyte. Illustrating neurohumoral, endothelial, and metabolic influences. α_1, α_1-adrenergic receptor; α_2, α_2-adrenergic receptor; *ACh,* acetylcholine; *AA,* arachidonic acid; *ACE,* angiotensin-converting enzyme; *AI,* angiotensin I; *AII,* angiotensin II; AT_1, angiotensin type 1 receptor; AT_2, angiotensin type 2 receptor; *ATP,* adenosine triphosphate; β_2, β_2-adrenergic receptor; B_2, bradykinin type 2 receptor; *bET-1,* big endothelin-1; *COX-1,* cyclooxygenase 1; *CYP450,* cytochrome P450; *ECE,* endothelin-converting enzyme; *EDHF,* endothelium-derived hyperpolarizing factor; *EETs,* epoxyeicosatrienoic acids; *eNOS,* endothelial nitric oxide synthase; ET_A, endothelin type A receptor; ET_B, endothelin type B receptor; *ET-1,* endothelin-1; *5HT,* 5-hydroxytryptamine and receptor; H_1 and H_2, histamine type 1 and 2 receptors; *HETEs,* hydroxyeicosatetraenoic acids; H_2O_2, hydrogen peroxide; *IP,* prostacyclin receptor; K_{ATP}, ATP-sensitive K^+ channel; K_{Ca}, calcium-activated K^+ channel; K_{IR}, inward rectifying K^+ channel; K_V, voltage-gated K^+ channel; *L-arg,* L-arginine; *M,* muscarinic receptor; *NE,* norepinephrine; *NO,* nitric oxide; *NPY,* neuropeptide Y; O_2, oxygen; $\bullet O_2^-$, superoxide anion; *P1,* purinergic type 1 receptor; *P2,* purinergic type 2 receptor; *PG,* prostaglandins; *Trp,* transient receptor potential channels; TXA_2, thromboxaneA$_2$ and receptor; *VGCC,* voltage-gated calcium channels; Y_1, neuropeptide Y receptor. *(Modified from Duncker DJ, Koller A, Merkus D, et al. Regulation of coronary blood flow in health and ischemic heart disease.* Prog Cardiovasc Dis. *2015;57(5):409.)*

inner layer of the left ventricle, but only when heart rate, contractility, and coronary flow are high.[27] However, this hypothesis was not confirmed by subsequent studies that failed to demonstrate a favorable effect of α-adrenergic coronary vasoconstriction on the transmural blood flow distribution under physiologic conditions. On the other hand, α-adrenergic coronary vasoconstriction is operative in ischemic myocardium, and several studies have demonstrated improved subendocardial blood flow following administration of α-adrenergic blockers.[28]

Parasympathetic control of CBF has been extensively studied in dogs. Vagal stimulation produces uniform vasodilation across the LV wall independent of changes in myocardial metabolism. The vagal response, which is activated during carotid baroreceptor and/or chemoreceptor stimulation, depends on the species and the integrity of the endothelium.[5,29] Parasympathetic vasodilatation is attributed to the release of acetylcholine at the adventitial-medial border mediated via muscarinic receptors M1 and M2 and subsequent activation of endothelial NO mediated dilation.[5]

Reactive Hyperemia and Coronary Flow Reserve

When a major epicardial coronary artery is occluded for a short period of time, occlusion release is followed by a significant increase in CBF, a phenomenon known as *reactive hyperemia*. The maximum increase in blood flow occurs within a few seconds after the release of the occlusion, and the peak flow, which has been shown to reach 4 or 5 times the value of preischemic flow, is dependent on the duration of the ischemic period for occlusion times up to 15 to 20 s. Although occlusions of longer duration do not further modify the peak of the hyperemic response, they do affect the duration of the entire hyperemic process, which increases with the length of the occlusion. It is generally accepted that myocardial ischemia, even of brief duration, is the most effective stimulus for vasodilatation of coronary resistive vessels and that, under normal circumstances, reactive hyperemic peak flow represents the maximum flow available at a given coronary perfusion pressure.[6] Values of CBF comparable to the peak flow of reactive hyperemia can be achieved using coronary vasodilators such as adenosine or dipyridamole, which induce a "near maximal" vasodilatation of the coronary microcirculation.[30]

The coronary flow reserve (CFR) is an indirect parameter to evaluate the global function of the coronary circulation.[31] CFR is the ratio of CBF or MBF during near maximal coronary vasodilatation to resting flow and is an integrated measure of flow through both the large epicardial coronary arteries and the microcirculation[6,30,31] (Fig. 5.4). Resting blood flow is the denominator in the formula used to compute CFR; thus an increase in resting blood flow, such as that often seen in patients with arterial hypertension, will lead to a net decrease in the available CFR even if maximum flow is normal. The driving perfusion pressure that determines flow at any given level of vascular resistance is the pressure at the origin of arteriolar vessels, which, under normal circumstances, corresponds closely to aortic pressure. During maximal coronary dilatation, the slope of the pressure/flow curve becomes very steep with a sizeable linear increase of CBF with increasing pressure (see Fig. 5.4).

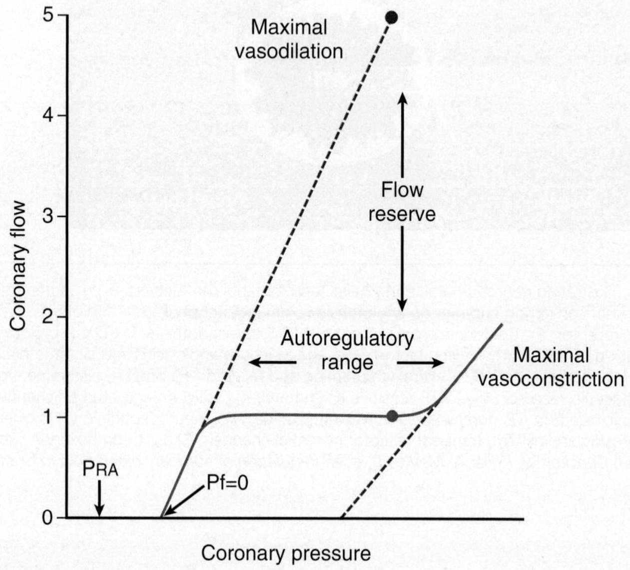

FIG. 5.4 Relationship between coronary blood flow (CBF) and coronary perfusion pressure in the left ventricle. At a constant level of myocardial oxygen consumption, CBF is maintained constant over a wide range of coronary perfusion pressures *(solid line)*, included within the boundaries of maximal resistive coronary vessel dilatation or constriction *(dashed lines)*. In the presence of maximal resistive vessels dilatation, CBF and coronary perfusion pressure are linearly related *(dashed line on the left)*. The blue dot represents the baseline CBF and the red dot maximal CBF for that given perfusion pressure, resulting in a CFR of around 5. *Pf = 0*, pressure at zero flow; *PRA*, right atrial pressure. *(From Crea F, Lanza GA, Camici PG.* Coronary Microvascular Dysfunction. *Milan: Springer Verlag Italia; 2014.)*

MECHANISMS OF CORONARY MICROVASCULAR DYSFUNCTION

Coronary microvascular dysfunction (CMD) (Boxes 5.1 and 5.2) can be sustained by several pathogenetic mechanisms, as summarized in Table 5.1. The importance of these mechanisms appears to vary in different clinical settings, but several of them may coexist in the same condition.[1,6]

Structural Alterations

Structural abnormalities responsible for CMD have been demonstrated in patients with hypertrophic cardiomyopathy (HCM) and in those with arterial hypertension.[32] In both these conditions morphologic changes are characterized

BOX 5.1 The Coronary Microcirculation

- Intramyocardial arterioles below 500 μm in diameter that are the main site of myocardial perfusion regulation make up the coronary microcirculation.
- Coronary microvascular dysfunction is an additional mechanism of myocardial ischemia.
- Dysfunction of the coronary microcirculation is caused by functional and/or structural alterations of the intramyocardial arterioles as well as by increased extravascular compression.
- No technique allows direct visualization of the anatomy of the coronary microcirculation in vivo in humans.

BOX 5.2 Functional Assessment of the Coronary Microcirculation

- Microvascular function is assessed indirectly, by measuring coronary (CBF) or myocardial blood flow (MBF) and coronary flow reserve (CFR) or by calculating the index of microvascular resistance (IMR).
- CBF is the volume of blood that flows along a vascular bed over a time unit (mL/min).
- MBF is the volume of blood per unit of time per unit of cardiac mass (mL/min per g).
- CFR is the ratio of CBF or MBF during near maximal vasodilation achieved by means of drugs such as adenosine or dipyridamole to baseline CBF or MBF.
- IMR is calculated as the product of distal coronary pressure and mean transit time using a combined pressure/temperature wire.
- Invasive and noninvasive techniques can be used to assess CBF/MBF and CFR including intracoronary Doppler flow wires, transthoracic Doppler, positron emission tomography, and cardiac magnetic resonance imaging.

TABLE 5.1 Pathogenetic Mechanisms and Clinical Classification of Coronary Microvascular Dysfunction

	CLINICAL SETTING	MAIN PATHOGENETIC MECHANISMS
Type 1: In the absence of myocardial diseases and obstructive CAD	Risk factors Microvascular angina	Endothelial dysfunction SMC dysfunction Vascular remodelling
Type 2: In myocardial diseases	Hypertrophic cardiomyopathy Dilated cardiomyopathy Anderson-Fabry disease Amyloidosis Myocarditis Aortic stenosis	Vascular remodelling SMC dysfunction Extramural compression Luminal obstruction
Type 3: In obstructive CAD	Stable angina Acute coronary syndrome	Endothelial dysfunction SMC dysfunction Luminal obstruction
Type 4: Iatrogenic	PCI Coronary artery grafting	Luminal obstruction Autonomic dysfunction

CAD, coronary artery diseases; *PCI*, percutaneous coronary intervention; *SMC*, smooth muscle cells.

(From Crea F, Camici PG, Bairey Merz CN. Coronary microvascular dysfunction: an update. Eur Heart J. *2014;35(17):1101.)*

by an adverse remodeling of intramural coronary arterioles responsible for vessel wall thickening, mainly due to hypertrophy of smooth muscle cells and increased collagen deposition in the tunica media, with variable degrees of intimal thickening.[32,33] The remodeled, hypertrophied vascular wall leads to an increase in medial wall area, with a relative reduction of the vessel lumen. Although qualitatively similar in the two conditions, these anatomic changes are usually more severe in patients with HCM. An important feature, common to patients with arterial hypertension and those with HCM, is the diffuse nature of the microvascular remodeling, which is extended to the entire left ventricle independently of the distribution of ventricular hypertrophy (ie, symmetric vs asymmetric) and may also involve portions of the right ventricle.[30,32,34] The functional counterpart of these structural changes of the vessel wall is the demonstration that, in most of these patients, maximum MBF and CFR are blunted in the whole left ventricle.[32] Structural abnormalities of coronary microcirculation have also been described in other clinical conditions characterized by CMD, including primary microvascular angina (MVA). This condition is defined as the occurrence of anginal symptoms in the absence of significant coronary artery disease (CAD) or cardiomyopathies.[35,36] Analysis of endomyocardial biopsies obtained from these patients, however, has given discordant results, showing no alterations in some and heterogeneous findings in others, including medial hyperplasia and hypertrophy, intimal proliferation and degeneration, proliferation of endothelial cells, and capillary rarefaction.[6] Finally, structural alterations of intramural coronary arterioles have been demonstrated in other myocardial diseases including amyloidosis and Fabry disease.[37]

Functional Alterations

Functional CMD may be caused by a variable combination of mechanisms leading to impaired coronary microvascular dilatation and mechanisms resulting in increased coronary microvascular constriction[1,5,6,11,13] (see Fig. 5.3).

Alterations of Endothelium-Dependent Vasodilatation

Alterations in endothelial function may impair CBF both at rest, favoring susceptibility to constrictor stimuli, and during increased myocardial workload, as typically occurs during exercise.[2,14] NO production and release are the primary mechanisms of endothelium-mediated vasodilatation, and also the most vulnerable in the case of endothelial dysfunction. Unfortunately, NO is a volatile molecule, with a very short half-life (56 s); thus its direct measurement in vivo is difficult.

The detection of abnormalities in endothelium-dependent coronary microvascular dilatation in the clinical setting is mainly based on the blunting or even decrease of CBF in response to stimuli known to exert their vasodilator effect by inducing release of NO from endothelial cells. Stimulation of muscarinic receptors by intracoronary acetylcholine, in association with intracoronary Doppler flow recording, has been the most widespread stimulus used in clinical research, although it is limited to invasive procedures.[38,39] A valid alternative to assess endothelium-dependent CMD is represented by cold pressure testing (CPT), which can be applied noninvasively in association with imaging techniques (eg, positron emission tomography [PET]) to measure MBF.[40] If the endothelium is dysfunctional, the vasodilator response to these stimuli is blunted and can even turn into vasoconstriction in case of severe impairment of endothelial function, due to the complex vasoconstrictor effects elicited by CPT.[6]

Impaired NO generation as a cause of endothelial dysfunction has been shown in several experimental studies.[41,42] The most common cause is reduced activity of endothelial eNOS, the enzyme that catalyzes NO synthesis from the amino acid L-arginine, which can be caused by noxious stimuli activating acetylcholine/muscarinic, bradykinin, histamine receptors, or increasing frictional forces (ie, shear stress).[42] In some cases, the administration of the NO synthase cofactor BH4 can improve and even normalize endothelial dysfunction,[43] thus suggesting that a reduction of this cofactor can be involved in the impairment of endothelium-mediated dilatation, at least in some cases. Impairment of endothelium-dependent vasodilatation can be caused not only by impaired NO generation, but also by increased degradation. NO can be inactivated by several factors, with superoxide anion $^{\cdot}O_2^-$ playing a major role. Excess generation of ROS reduces NO bioavailability by reacting directly with NO to form peroxynitrite ($^{\cdot}ONOO^-$) and altering eNOS coupling. When uncoupled, instead of releasing NO, eNOS produces ROS, and ROS-mediated oxidation of the eNOS cofactor BH4 is the main mechanism responsible for eNOS uncoupling.[15,43] This chain of events has been demonstrated in several conditions that are associated with impaired endothelium-dependent coronary microvascular dilatation, including diabetes, obesity,[44] smoking, and other cardiovascular risk factors.[1,41] Accordingly, antioxidant administration, which prevents superoxide anion formation including glutathione and antioxidant vitamins,[43] has been shown to improve or even normalize endothelium-dependent coronary microvascular dilatation in both experimental and clinical conditions.[1,45]

NO exerts its vasodilator effects by diffusing into smooth muscle cell cytoplasm and activating the guanylyl cyclase (GC) pathway by binding to the heme groups of the enzyme.[46] Under certain circumstances, NO-dependent vasodilatation can be impaired despite normal levels of

NO production. This might be due to oxidation of the heme groups of GC that renders the enzyme unresponsive to NO.[46]

Endothelial dysfunction is also likely to reduce the activity of the EDHF and prostacyclin PGI_2.[47] Peroxynitrite can inhibit prostacyclin synthase, thus reducing PGI_2 release. This induces a shift in the PGI_2 precursor PGH_2 toward the synthesis of thromboxane A_2 (TXA_2), a powerful vasoconstrictor. How much and in which cases perturbation of these factors significantly contributes to CMD in the clinical setting remains substantially unknown, largely due to the lack of specific tests to assess these pathways in vivo.

Alterations of Endothelium-Independent Vasodilatation

An impaired endothelium-independent dilatation as a cause of CMD has been demonstrated in several experimental and clinical conditions, in which CBF increases and/or microvascular resistance decreases in response to direct arteriolar/prearteriolar vasodilators (eg, adenosine, dipyridamole, papaverine) were clearly abnormal.[13]

Despite the large amount of data documenting the role of endothelium-independent dilatation of the coronary microcirculation, the cellular mechanisms involved remain incompletely understood. There are two main known intracellular pathways leading to smooth muscle cell relaxation.[15,17] One pathway is based on activation of the enzyme adenylyl cyclase that results in the production of cAMP, which acts by opening K_{ATP} channels and inhibiting calcium influx into smooth muscle cells (see Fig. 5.3). This pathway is mainly activated by stimulation of purinergic A_2 receptors and β_2 adrenoceptors.[14,48] The second intracellular pathway, mentioned previously, relies on the activation of GC, which results in the production of cGMP. This latter pathway is mainly activated by NO released by the endothelium, as discussed previously.[17,46,49,50]

Thus the mechanisms responsible for an impaired smooth muscle cell response to vasodilator stimuli are likely to be different in different clinical settings, as they may be related to abnormalities in specific receptors or in one or both of the main intracellular signaling pathways regulating smooth muscle cell relaxation. A reduced response to the vasodilator effect of prolonged nitrate administration (nitrate resistance), for instance, has been shown to occur because of a reduced production of cGMP, which might also be involved in a reduced response to NO (as shown previously).[6]

Abnormalities in endothelium-independent coronary microvascular dilatation can also involve impaired opening of K_{ATP} channels.[11,51] Indeed, activation of intracellular cAMP and cGMP leads to the opening of K_{ATP} channels, eventually resulting in cell hyperpolarization and closure of voltage-dependent calcium channels (see Fig. 5.3). Finally, alterations in other K^+ channels, such as K_{Ca} and K_v channels, may also be responsible for impairment of endothelium-independent coronary microvascular dilatation.[52]

In summary, alterations in endothelium-independent smooth muscle cell relaxation in the coronary microcirculation may result in impaired vasodilator response to factors that mediate the metabolic regulation of CBF, autoregulation, and reactive hyperemia, as well as flow-mediated dilatation.

Vasoconstriction

Enhanced vasoconstriction of coronary microcirculation can result from either an increased release of vasoconstrictor agonists (systemically or locally) (see Fig. 5.3) and/or an increased susceptibility of smooth muscle cells to vasoconstrictor stimuli.

The notion that coronary microvascular constriction may cause myocardial ischemia has been demonstrated in both experimental models and humans. Some vasoconstrictors cause intense, selective microvascular constriction with minimal effects on the epicardial coronary arteries.[5,6,20,21,26]

Experimental studies in dogs have provided evidence that administration of endothelin-1 in the left anterior descending coronary artery can cause a dose-dependent reduction of CBF leading to myocardial ischemia in the absence of any significant effect on epicardial arteries.[53] Similar effects were observed with intracoronary injection of angiotensin II or phenylephrine,[54] and, in rabbits, with the intracoronary injection of the tripeptide *N*-formyl-L-methionin-L-leucil-L-phenylamine, which acts through release of leukotrienes from activated neutrophils.[55] These substances act on both subendocardial and subepicardial small coronary arteries and induce transmural myocardial ischemia.

In humans, evidence of myocardial ischemia due to coronary microvascular constriction comes from studies showing that intracoronary injections of neuropeptide Y[56] or high doses of acetylcholine[38] can cause chest pain and objective evidence of myocardial ischemia in patients with normal coronary angiograms, in the absence of significant changes in epicardial coronary arteries. In patients with flow-limiting stenoses, the intracoronary infusion of serotonin has been shown to cause myocardial ischemia with evidence of diffuse constriction of distal branches and reduced filling of collateral vessels, but with only minimal changes in stenosis severity.[57] This response to serotonin is known to be due to stimulation of both endothelial and vascular smooth muscle 5HT receptors.

Abnormal microvascular constriction has been demonstrated in patients with chest pain and normal coronary arteries and in those with chronic stable angina.[39,57] Intense coronary microvascular constriction is an important pathogenetic component of microvascular obstruction (MVO) observed in a substantial proportion of patients with ST elevation myocardial infarction (STEMI) after primary PCI.[30,58]

Intravascular Plugging

Intravascular plugging caused by atherosclerotic debris and thrombus material typically occurs during PCI and is related to intracoronary manipulation of friable plaques, in particular in degenerated saphenous vein grafts.[59] In these cases, microvascular plugging often causes "infarctlets," characterized by a modest raise of biomarkers of myocardial injury, and it is associated with a worse prognosis compared with procedures that are not followed by any raise in these biomarkers.[58,60] Intravascular plugging caused by microemboli and leukocyte-platelet aggregates is an additional mechanism of MVO in STEMI patients.[58,61]

MVO is compounded by a complex interplay of ischemia/reperfusion-related events, including endothelial dysfunction with loss of vasodilator mechanisms, enhancement of vasoconstriction mediated by platelet activation, release of TXA_2 and 5HT, and inflammatory reaction.[61]

Extravascular Mechanisms

Extramural Compression

During the cardiac cycle the pulsatile pattern of CBF follows typical physiologic variations, which are influenced by the variations in intramyocardial and intracavitary pressures occurring during systole and diastole (see Fig. 5.1).[14,23] Approximately 90% of CBF occurs in diastole, and therefore diastolic abnormalities have a more significant impact on myocardial perfusion. Nevertheless, an increase in systolic intramyocardial and intracavitary pressures, for example in conditions of increased pressure overload, may negatively impact on myocardial perfusion. An increased microvascular compression during systole hinders subendocardial vessels' tone restoration in diastole, thus impairing diastolic microvascular CBF in the subendocardial layers.[62]

Diastolic CBF is impaired whenever intracavitary diastolic pressure is increased. This is the case in the presence of either primary or secondary LV hypertrophy (LVH)[32] and also in the presence of diastolic dysfunction consequent to increased interstitial and perivascular fibrosis.[63] Diastolic impairment of CBF is enhanced when arteriolar driving pressure during diastole is significantly lower than intracavitary pressure, as in patients with severe aortic stenosis, critical coronary stenoses, prearteriolar constriction, or merely hypotension.

Tissue Edema

Abnormalities of capillary permeability, which favor migration of intravascular fluid into the interstitium, cause myocardial edema and CMD. Experimental studies suggest that edema per se does not reduce CFR.[64] Nevertheless, edema can worsen the impairment of CBF in the setting of MVO in STEMI.[65,66] Edema results from a combination of several mechanisms,[64] including (1) increased osmolality, caused by ischemic myocardial catabolites diffusing to the interstitial space during the ischemic phase, which recalls fluid from the intravascular compartment during reperfusion; (2) increased vascular permeability to water and protein, as well as abnormal ionic transport, consequent to endothelial damage occurring during ischemia/reperfusion; and (3) inflammation associated with reperfusion.[67] Coronary microvascular compression is another component that favors intravascular cell plugging by neutrophil-platelet aggregates. Finally, myocardial edema can occur during open heart surgery.[64] Increased venous pressure, mainly in the right chambers, may contribute to interstitial edema due to increased hydrostatic capillary pressure. Clinically, noninvasive assessment of myocardial edema and MVO is now possible using T2-based and inversion recovery cardiac magnetic resonance imaging.[30,68]

Diastolic Time

Because CBF occurs predominantly during diastole, the duration of diastole plays a central role in preserving myocardial perfusion. In the normal heart both subendocardial and subepicardial perfusion is maintained at very short diastolic time, as during intense physical exercise. In contrast, a reduction of diastolic time can contribute to determine a critical reduction of myocardial perfusion at a time when coronary-driving pressure is significantly lower than intracavitary pressure, as in patients with aortic stenosis.[62]

CLINICAL CLASSIFICATION OF CORONARY MICROVASCULAR DYSFUNCTION

In 2007, Camici and Crea proposed a clinical classification of CMD involving four types: type 1: CMD occurring in the absence of CAD and myocardial diseases; type 2: CMD in patients with evidence of myocardial diseases; type 3: CMD in patients with obstructive CAD; and type 4: CMD consequent to interventions such as bypass surgery, percutaneous revascularization, etc., also defined as iatrogenic.[1] As discussed in the previous section, these types of CMD can be sustained by changes inherent to the microvasculature (both structural and/or functional), as well by factors that originate from the environment surrounding the microvasculature (eg, increased extravascular pressure). The importance of these mechanisms appears to vary in different clinical settings, although several of them may coexist in the same patient. Clinically, CMD can be severe enough to cause myocardial ischemia in isolation or in conjunction with the traditional "epicardial" mechanisms[35] (Fig. 5.5). It would be beyond the scope of this chapter to discuss type 2 CMD[32,34] as we will focus on the other three types.

Type 1 Coronary Microvascular Dysfunction

This type represents the functional counterpart of traditional coronary risk factors and is the cause of MVA. Type 1 CMD may not be associated with symptoms or signs of myocardial ischemia, but it can be unveiled by demonstrating a reduced CFR. The impairment of CFR can be significant, but most often it is not severe enough to limit the heart's functional capacity during normal daily life activities. The severity of CFR reduction has been demonstrated to correlate with the severity of underlying risk factors. Furthermore, correction of the risk factor is often paralleled by an improvement in CFR.[30]

Cigarette Smoking

Cigarette smoking is unquestionably a well-established risk factor for cardiovascular disease.[69] CMD has been demonstrated in asymptomatic smokers with no evidence of CAD, in whom CFR was reduced by more than 20% compared with the value in nonsmoking controls.[70] Further evidence linking smoking and CMD was derived from a study of twins demonstrating that CFR was lower in smoking twins compared to nonsmoking cotwins.[71] The gas phase of cigarette smoke contains large amounts of free radicals and prooxidant lipophilic quinones, which can form the highly reactive hydroxyperoxide radical.[72] The latter increases the amount of oxidized low-density lipoprotein, which in turn will impair eNOS and contribute to endothelial dysfunction.[3] This is consistent with the results of the study by Kaufmann et al. demonstrating that intravenous administration of the antioxidant vitamin C normalized CFR in smokers with no significant effects in nonsmoking control subjects.[70]

Hypercholesterolemia

Reduced CFR has been demonstrated in asymptomatic subjects with hypercholesterolemia and angiographically normal coronary arteries using PET. A significant inverse correlation between CFR and low-density lipoprotein cholesterol has been shown in subjects with elevated total cholesterol, although no relation between total cholesterol and CFR could be demonstrated. This supports a direct pathogenic role of this subfraction in the development of CMD.[73] There is evidence that the CFR reduction in dyslipidemic patients can be improved, at least in part, by cholesterol-lowering strategies.[1] Furthermore, in patients with familial combined hyperlipidemia, treatment with the peroxisome proliferator-activated receptor (PPAR)-γ

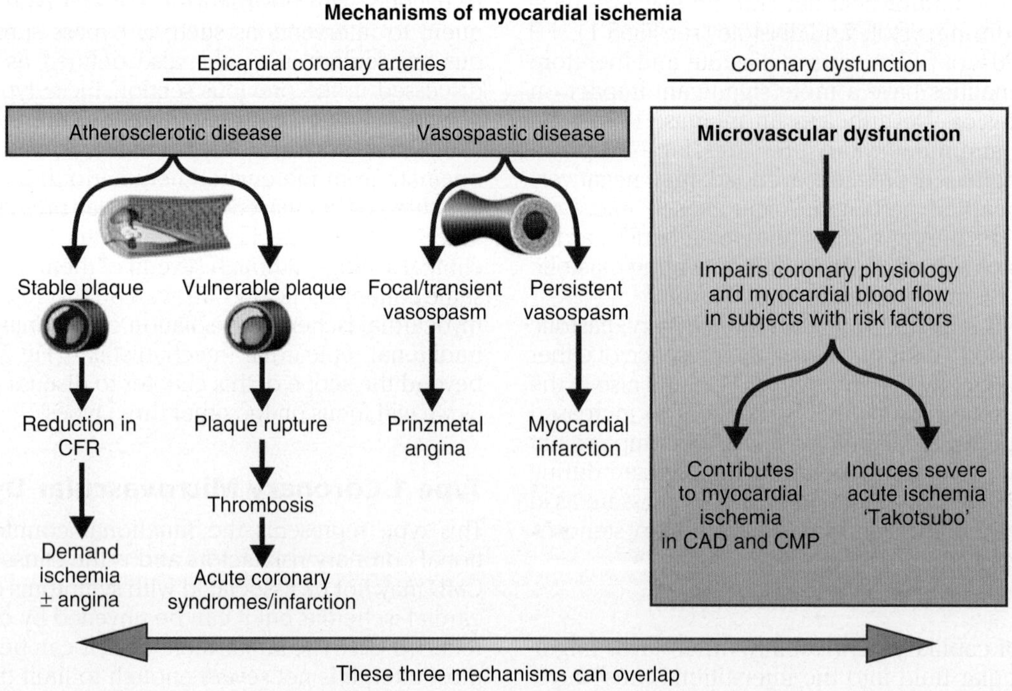

FIG. 5.5 In addition to the "classic" mechanisms (ie, atherosclerotic disease and vasospastic disease) that lead to myocardial ischemia, coronary microvascular dysfunction (CMD) has emerged as a third potential mechanism. As with the other two mechanisms, CMD (alone or in combination with the other two) can lead to transient myocardial ischemia, as in patients with coronary artery disease (CAD) or cardiomyopathy (CMP), or to severe acute ischemia, as observed in Takotsubo syndrome. *CFR*, coronary flow reserve. *(From Crea F, Camici PG, Bairey Merz CN. Coronary microvascular dysfunction: an update.* Eur Heart J. *2014;35(17):1101.)*

agonist pioglitazone, in addition to conventional lipid-lowering therapy, led to significant improvement in myocardial glucose utilization that was paralleled by an increase in hyperemic MBF.[74]

Hypertension

Arterial hypertension is a major independent risk factor for adverse cardiovascular events. Patients with hypertension have evidence of CMD and may present signs and symptoms suggestive of myocardial ischemia even in the absence of obstructive CAD.[75] The blunting of CFR in hypertension is severe, particularly if there is concomitant LVH. In patients with stage 1–2 hypertension and LVH, CFR was shown to be transmurally blunted due to a reduced hyperemic response to stress inversely related to systolic blood pressure.[76] This finding may be explained by the increased extravascular compressive forces, with elevated systolic/diastolic wall stress and impaired relaxation, which contribute to impaired microvascular function. However, the impairment of CFR in hypertension is not necessarily related to the degree of cardiomyocyte hypertrophy. It is strictly linked to the degree of arteriolar remodeling and capillary rarefaction due, at least in part, to excessive activation of the renin-angiotensin-aldosterone system.[32,77] Treatment with angiotensin-converting enzyme inhibitors can improve CFR in patients with arterial hypertension. These drugs have also been shown to improve coronary flow and revert arteriolar remodeling in the spontaneously hypertensive rat model.[78]

Diabetes and Insulin Resistance

A direct deleterious effect of diabetes on vascular and, in particular, endothelial function has been suggested, thereby increasing the potential for vasoconstriction and thrombosis. There is, indeed, consistent evidence that patients with diabetes exhibit CMD and that this may be an early marker of atherosclerosis that precedes clinically overt CAD.[1] The worsening of glucose intolerance and insulin resistance in patients with the metabolic syndrome is paralleled by progressive impairment of coronary microvascular function.[79,80] Furthermore, in patients with diabetes mellitus, coronary vasodilator dysfunction is a powerful, independent correlate of cardiac mortality and all-cause mortality.[81] The impairment in stress perfusion in patients with type 2 diabetes can be normalized acutely by means of insulin infusion and glycemic control with glyburide and metformin or insulin-sensitizing thiazolidinediones.[82–84]

Inflammation

Chronic inflammatory diseases such as rheumatoid arthritis, systemic lupus erythematosus, and systemic sclerosis are important risk factors for the development of ischemic heart disease and a source of high cardiovascular morbidity and mortality. In these patients inflammation can impair coronary microvascular function and contribute to the development of myocardial ischemia in the absence of obstructive CAD and even in the absence of other risk factors.[2,30] Increased levels of markers of inflammation, including C-reactive protein (CRP) and interleukin-1 receptor antagonist, have been reported in patients with MVA.[85] High CRP levels were associated with increased frequency of ischemic electrocardiographic changes.[86] More recently, objective evidence linking CMD with inflammation in patients with chest pain and angiographically normal coronary arteries without conventional risk factors for CAD has been provided by Recio-Mayoral et al.[87] They demonstrated that patients with elevated CRP levels have a severely reduced CFR compared with control subjects, a finding indicative of CMD.

Stable Microvascular Angina

MVA is the prototypical clinical manifestation of type 1 CMD. Primary stable MVA is defined as the occurrence of anginal attacks in relation to effort, in the absence of obstructive CAD, myocardial diseases, and any other significant cardiovascular disease. In these patients CMD is the cause of myocardial ischemia and chest pain. MVA is caused by a variable combination of (1) structural abnormalities, (2) alterations of endothelium-dependent and independent vasodilatation, (3) alterations of endothelium-independent vasodilatation, and (4) enhanced pain perception. MVA will be discussed in detail in Chapter 25.

Type 3 Coronary Microvascular Dysfunction

CMD plays an important role in both stable CAD and acute coronary syndromes. This section will focus only on the role of CMD in stable CAD. In acute coronary syndromes, CMD is involved in the pathogenesis of MVO, also known as *no reflow phenomenon*, which occurs in a sizeable proportion of patients with STEMI, who, despite successful recanalization of the culprit artery, have evidence of angiographic slow flow or of MVO and are at higher risk of adverse cardiovascular events at follow-up.

Pathophysiology of Coronary Microvascular Dysfunction in Stable Coronary Artery Disease

The role played by CMD in determining symptom severity in patients with chronic CAD was initially highlighted in the early 1990s in patients with angina, total occlusion of a single coronary artery, and no previous MI.[6] These patients showed remarkable variability in their anginal and ischemic threshold. Angina and electrocardiographic signs of ischemia on Holter monitoring were present at a relatively low heart rate; in contrast, at other times during the same day, both symptoms and signs of ischemia were absent despite much higher heart rates. As these patients did not have evidence of "dynamic" stenosis—ie, vasoconstriction at the site of a stenosis that further reduces a vessel's lumen and thus increases stenosis severity—in large epicardial arteries, the variability of anginal and ischemic threshold could only be explained by profound dynamic changes of coronary microvascular resistance.[88] In line with this finding, subsequent studies in patients with single-vessel CAD have documented an abnormal CFR, measured with PET, in regions subtended by angiographically normal coronary arteries.[89]

In patients with obstructive CAD, the development of myocardial ischemia during increased oxygen demand is generally attributed to an inadequate flow increase due to the exhaustion of the CFR.[89] However, it is worth noting that the correlation between stenosis severity and CFR measured in vivo is widely scattered and thus other factors might contribute to the development of myocardial ischemia.[31] Among patients with stable angina, the invasive measurement of resistance in the stenotic segment and the microvasculature in response to atrial pacing showed an increased resistance in both districts. The intracoronary infusion of adenosine during pacing reduced microvascular resistance, suggesting that CFR was not totally exhausted.[90] In patients with CAD, the physiologic arteriolar vasodilatation during increased oxygen demand is limited by the presence of the stenosis, which causes a consistent pressure drop. The intrinsic control mechanisms of the coronary circulation maintain driving pressure in a range of values high enough to perfuse vessels, but low enough to prevent capillary damage. Such a control could be as powerful as the metabolic control, although the two may go in opposite directions in the presence of CAD. The response of the microcirculation to an excessively low perfusion pressure could be a heterogeneous vasoconstriction aimed at maintaining pressure at the cost of excluding some vascular units.[6]

There is evidence that, on a background of optimal medical therapy, revascularization by PCI improves anginal symptoms compared with medical therapy, although it does not reduce the risk of mortality, cardiovascular death, nonfatal MI, or further revascularization.[91] However, in a substantial proportion of patients, the prevalence of angina at follow-up remains high despite successful revascularization. For instance, in the Clinical Outcomes Utilizing Revascularization and Aggressive Drug Evaluation (COURAGE) trial more than 30% of patients were still experiencing angina 1 year after PCI, and at 5-year follow-up, the incidence of angina was not significantly different from that in patients who did not undergo a revascularization procedure.[92] These findings suggest that, although revascularization is effective in removing coronary stenosis and its hemodynamic consequences, other mechanisms, including CMD, contribute to the pathogenesis of ischemia and angina in these patients.

In over 1000 patients who underwent elective measurement of both fractional flow reserve (FFR) and index of microvascular resistance (IMR),[93] Lee et al[94] found no correlation between IMR and either FFR or angiographic lesion severity. Furthermore, the predictors of high IMR were different from those for an ischemic FFR. It is foreseeable that integration of IMR into FFR measurement may provide additional insights regarding the relative contribution of macro- and microvascular disease in patients with ischemic heart disease.

The noninvasive quantification of MBF using PET has provided clear evidence that the inclusion of CFR in risk prediction models resulted in the correct reclassification of risk in a substantial proportion of patients, including a sizeable proportion of those at intermediate risk.[81,95–98] CFR is an integrated measurement of the function of both large vessels and the microvasculature.[30] An abnormal CFR gives incremental risk stratification over and above that obtained by the conventional semiquantitative evaluation of myocardial perfusion studies (ie, summed rest and stress scores). The measurement of absolute MBF and CFR provides information on both regional and diffuse perfusion abnormalities, the latter being a typical manifestation of CMD.

Support to this hypothesis is provided by data reported by Milo et al.[99] They found that patients with evidence of ST-segment depression during exercise stress testing had lower CBF response to adenosine following the procedure, although no significant clinical or procedural differences were observed between patients with positive and negative exercise stress test results.

In stable CAD, CMD is not only a likely explanation of symptoms persisting after successful recanalization, but also a predictor of an adverse outcome. Invasive measurement of coronary flow velocity reserve (CFVR) has shown that an abnormal CFVR in reference vessels was associated with a significant increase of mortality at long-term follow-up.[100] Another study from the same group has demonstrated that a normal FFR with an abnormal CFVR was associated with a significantly increased major adverse cardiac events rate throughout 10 years of follow-up, regardless of the FFR cut-off applied.[101] These findings strongly suggest that the outcome in these patients was determined by CMD rather than by functional stenosis severity.

These findings are further confirmed by Taqueti et al, who measured CFR noninvasively with PET and the extent and severity of coronary disease at angiography in a cohort of patients with chronic CAD. Although these two factors were weakly correlated, their severity was independently associated with cardiovascular death and heart failure admission at 3-year follow-up after adjustment for clinical risk score, ejection fraction, global ischemia, and early revascularization. Interestingly, global CFR had an impact on the effect of revascularization, so that only patients with low CFR appeared to benefit from revascularization, and only if the revascularization included coronary artery bypass grafting (CABG), and their event rate was comparable to patients with preserved CFR. These data raise the paradoxic hypothesis that invasive revascularization in patients with preserved CFR may contribute to increased events.[102]

Clinical Implications

A microvascular origin of angina in patients with obstructive CAD can be suspected in patients who have prolonged angina or angina poorly responsive to sublingual nitrates (clinical features frequently observed in patients with MVA). It can also be suspected in patients in whom angina is more severe than predicted by the severity of coronary stenoses. Finally, it may be suspected in patients in whom the angina threshold is remarkably variable, although this variability can also be accounted for by the presence of "dynamic" stenoses. In the individual patient, however, it is often very difficult to establish the role played by CMD in causing angina.

It is predictable, however, that up to 30% of patients will have persistence of angina and/or evidence of stress-induced ischemia due to persistent CMD, despite successful coronary revascularization. Thus, when the goal of revascularization is symptom control rather than outcome improvement, it is always worth testing optimal antianginal treatment, including drugs targeting CMD, before proposing a new or repeat revascularization procedure.

After myocardial revascularization, it would be highly desirable to identify those patients who have angina and inducible ischemia caused by CMD as opposed to that caused by restenosis. In this context, noninvasive assessment of CFR can provide useful, incremental information for the diagnosis of CMD and for further risk stratification.

The observation that the reduction of CFR is mainly due to progressive reductions in peak stress MBF indicates a primary abnormality in coronary vasodilator function and strongly supports the presence of CMD.[97]

Type 4 Coronary Microvascular Dysfunction

In addition to the CMD observed in patients with chronic CAD (ie, type 3), coronary revascularization by PCI or CABG can induce a further transient impairment of CFR in the territory subtended by a successfully recanalized artery. This is most likely triggered by an intracoronary reflex resulting in a reversible α-adrenergic receptor-mediated constriction of coronary microvessels that limits hyperemic blood flow and can be prevented by α-adrenergic receptor antagonists given before the procedure. This phenomenon may contribute to the delayed improvement of exercise-induced myocardial ischemia that can be observed after successful PCI.[1]

In addition to vasoconstriction, embolization of the coronary microcirculation can contribute to CMD in patients undergoing PCI and CABG. The material that is washed out of the plaques is dislodged distally in the microcirculation and may cause infarctlets as demonstrated by increased necrosis biomarkers. In a meta-analysis including over 7500 patients, troponin elevations after PCI were found in 29% of the patients, and in 15% the elevation reached the criterion for MI. Patients with PCI-related MI had an increased risk of death and re-PCI. At follow-up, any troponin elevation was associated with a 50% increased risk of major cardiovascular events.[103]

In the setting of PCI for obstructed saphenous vein grafts, mechanical prevention of distal embolization by filters or proximal protection devices has been demonstrated to reduce the occurrence of periprocedural MI and major cardiac events.[104] With regard to pharmacologic treatment, administration of statins was shown to halve periprocedural infarction both during elective and urgent PCI.[105] Similarly to PCI, substantial biomarker elevations measured 2 and 24 hours after CABG have been shown to have significant independent prognostic implications.[106] Surgical trauma and cardiopulmonary bypass contribute to a systemic inflammatory response, measurable by circulating cytokines, which promotes CMD. This can be compounded by many factors, including contact of blood with the bypass circuit, myocardial ischemia during bypass, aortic cross-clamping, and reperfusion injury. In this setting statins also have a protective effect, lowering all-cause mortality rate, atrial fibrillation, and stroke in the absence of any beneficial effect on postoperative infarction or renal failure.[107] The pleiotropic effect of statins could be the putative mechanism of this improvement of CMD.

CONCLUDING REMARKS

The mechanisms of myocardial ischemia are multiple and include disease of both the epicardial coronary arteries and the coronary microcirculation, and under certain circumstances these two vascular districts can be affected simultaneously. Microvascular dysfunction is caused by functional and/or structural abnormalities of intramural coronary arterioles, as well as by increased extravascular compression. Microvascular dysfunction often occurs in patients with normal coronary angiograms and can be detected only through the measurement of functional parameters that probe coronary physiology. These include the CFR and the IMR, which can be obtained using invasive or noninvasive techniques. Clinically, CMD has been classified into 4 types and may manifest itself as exercise-induced ischemia, ischemia at rest, or an acute coronary syndrome.

References

1. Camici PG, Crea F: Coronary microvascular dysfunction, *N Engl J Med* 356(8):830, 2007.
2. Pries AR, Badimon L, Bugiardini R, et al.: Coronary vascular regulation, remodelling, and collateralization: mechanisms and clinical implications on behalf of the Working Group on Coronary Pathophysiology and Microcirculation, *Eur Heart J* 36:3134–1346, 2015.
3. Deussen A, Ohanyan V, Jannasch A, et al.: Mechanisms of metabolic coronary flow regulation, *J Mol Cell Cardiol* 52(4):794, 2012.
4. Tomanek RJ: Structure–function of the coronary hierarchy, *Coronary Vasculature*, New York, 2013, Springer, pp 59.
5. Tune JD: Coronary circulation. In Granger ND, Granger J, editors: *Colloquium Series on Integrated Systems Physiology: From Molecule to Function*, San Rafael, CA, 2014, Morgan and Claypool, pp 1.
6. Crea F, Lanza GA, Camici PG: *Coronary Microvascular Dysfunction*, Milan, 2014, Springer Verlag Italia.
7. Westerhof N, Boer C, Lamberts RR, et al.: Cross-talk between cardiac muscle and coronary vasculature, *Physiol Rev* 86(4):1263, 2006.

8. Saitoh S, Zhang C, Tune JD, et al.: Hydrogen peroxide: a feed-forward dilator that couples myocardial metabolism to coronary blood flow, *Arterioscler Thromb Vasc Biol* 26(12):2614, 2006.
9. Liu Y, Bubolz AH, Mendoza S, et al.: H_2O_2 is the transferrable factor mediating flow-induced dilation in human coronary arterioles, *Circ Res* 108(5):566, 2011.
10. Beyer AM, Durand MJ, Hockenberry J, et al.: An acute rise in intraluminal pressure shifts the mediator of flow-mediated dilation from nitric oxide to hydrogen peroxide in human arterioles, *Am J Physiol Heart Circ Physiol* 307(11):H1587, 2014.
11. Beyer AM, Gutterman DD: Regulation of the human coronary microcirculation, *J Mol Cell Cardiol* 52(4):814, 2012.
12. Gutterman DD, Miura H, Liu Y: Redox modulation of vascular tone: focus of potassium channel mechanisms of dilation, *Arterioscler Thromb Vasc Biol* 25(4):671, 2005.
13. Sato A, Terata K, Miura H, et al.: Mechanism of vasodilation to adenosine in coronary arterioles from patients with heart disease, *Am J Physiol Heart Circ Physiol* 288(4):H1633, 2005.
14. Duncker DJ, Bache RJ: Regulation of coronary blood flow during exercise, *Physiol Rev* 88(3):1009, 2008.
15. Liu Y, Gutterman DD: Vascular control in humans: focus on the coronary microcirculation, *Basic Res Cardiol* 104(3):211, 2009.
16. Kuo L, Chilian WM, Davis MJ: Coronary arteriolar myogenic response is independent of endothelium, *Circ Res* 66(3):860, 1990.
17. Duncker DJ, Koller A, Merkus D, Canty Jr JM: Regulation of coronary blood flow in health and ischemic heart disease, *Prog Cardiovasc Dis* 57(5):409, 2015.
18. Davis MJ, Hill MA: Signaling mechanisms underlying the vascular myogenic response, *Physiol Rev* 79(2):387, 1999.
19. Davis MJ, Wu X, Nurkiewicz TR, et al.: Integrins and mechanotransduction of the vascular myogenic response, *Am J Physiol Heart Circ Physiol* 280(4):H1427, 2001.
20. Merkus D, Duncker DJ, Chilian WM: Metabolic regulation of coronary vascular tone: role of endothelin-1, *Am J Physiol Heart Circ Physiol* 283(5):H1915, 2002.
21. Zhang C, Knudson JD, Setty S, et al.: Coronary arteriolar vasoconstriction to angiotensin II is augmented in prediabetic metabolic syndrome via activation of AT1 receptors, *Am J Physiol Heart Circ Physiol* 288(5):H2154, 2005.
22. Berwick ZC, Dick GM, Tune JD: Heart of the matter: coronary dysfunction in metabolic syndrome, *J Mol Cell Cardiol* 52(4):848, 2012.
23. Downey JM: Extravascular coronary resistance. In Sperelakis N, editor: *Physiology and Pathophysiology of the Heart*, Boston, 1995, Kluwer, pp 1109.
24. Sun D, Huang A, Mital S, et al.: Norepinephrine elicits beta2-receptor-mediated dilation of isolated human coronary arterioles, *Circulation* 106(5):550, 2002.
25. Hein TW, Zhang C, Wang W, et al.: Heterogeneous beta2-adrenoceptor expression and dilation in coronary arterioles across the left ventricular wall, *Circulation* 110(17):2708, 2004.
26. Heusch G, Baumgart D, Camici P, et al.: Alpha-adrenergic coronary vasoconstriction and myocardial ischemia in humans, *Circulation* 101(6):689, 2000.
27. Feigl EO: The paradox of adrenergic coronary vasoconstriction, *Circulation* 76(4):737, 1987.
28. Heusch G: Reprint of: the paradox of alpha-adrenergic coronary vasoconstriction revisited, *J Mol Cell Cardiol* 52(4):832, 2012.
29. Broten TP, Miyashiro JK, Moncada S, et al.: Role of endothelium-derived relaxing factor in parasympathetic coronary vasodilation, *Am J Physiol Heart Circ Physiol* 262(5 Pt 2):H1579, 1992.
30. Camici PG, d'Amati G, Rimoldi O: Coronary microvascular dysfunction: mechanisms and functional assessment, *Nat Rev Cardiol* 12(1):48, 2015.
31. Gould KL, Johnson NP, Bateman TM, et al.: Anatomic versus physiologic assessment of coronary artery disease. Role of coronary flow reserve, fractional flow reserve, and positron emission tomography imaging in revascularization decision-making, *J Am Coll Cardiol* 62(18):1639, 2013.
32. Camici PG, Olivotto I, Rimoldi OE: The coronary circulation and blood flow in left ventricular hypertrophy, *J Mol Cell Cardiol* 52(4):857, 2012.
33. Olivotto I, Girolami F, Sciagra R, et al.: Microvascular function is selectively impaired in patients with hypertrophic cardiomyopathy and sarcomere myofilament gene mutations, *J Am Coll Cardiol* 58(8):839, 2011.
34. Maron MS, Olivotto I, Maron BJ, et al.: The case for myocardial ischemia in hypertrophic cardiomyopathy, *J Am Coll Cardiol* 54(9):866, 2009.
35. Crea F, Camici PG, Bairey Merz CN: Coronary microvascular dysfunction: an update, *Eur Heart J* 35(17):1101, 2014.
36. Pepine CJ, Anderson RD, Sharaf BL, et al.: Coronary microvascular reactivity to adenosine predicts adverse outcome in women evaluated for suspected ischemia results from the National Heart, Lung and Blood Institute WISE (Women's Ischemia Syndrome Evaluation) study, *J Am Coll Cardiol* 55(25):2825, 2010.
37. Spoladore R, Fisicaro A, Faccini A, et al.: Coronary microvascular dysfunction in primary cardiomyopathies, *Heart* 100(10):806, 2014.
38. Ong P, Athanasiadis A, Sechtem U: Patterns of coronary vasomotor responses to intracoronary acetylcholine provocation, *Heart* 99(17):1288, 2013.
39. Ong P, Athanasiadis A, Borgulya G, et al.: Clinical usefulness, angiographic characteristics, and safety evaluation of intracoronary acetylcholine provocation testing among 921 consecutive white patients with unobstructed coronary arteries, *Circulation* 129(17):1723, 2014.
40. Prior JO, Schindler TH, Facta AD, et al.: Determinants of myocardial blood flow response to cold pressor testing and pharmacologic vasodilation in healthy humans, *Eur J Nucl Med Mol Imaging* 34(1):20, 2007.
41. Levy AS, Chung JCS, Kroetsch JT, et al.: Nitric oxide and coronary vascular endothelium adaptations in hypertension, *Vasc Health Risk Manag* 5:1075, 2009.
42. Durand MJ, Gutterman DD: Diversity in mechanisms of endothelium-dependent vasodilation in health and disease, *Microcirculation* 20(3):239, 2013.
43. Bendall JK, Douglas G, McNeill E, et al.: Tetrahydrobiopterin in cardiovascular health and disease, *Antioxid Redox Signal* 20(18):3040, 2014.
44. Belin de Chantemele EJ, Stepp DW: Influence of obesity and metabolic dysfunction on the endothelial control in the coronary circulation, *J Mol Cell Cardiol* 52(4):840, 2012.
45. Thomas SR, Witting PK, Drummond GR: Redox control of endothelial function and dysfunction: molecular mechanisms and therapeutic opportunities, *Antioxid Redox Signal* 10(10):1713, 2008.
46. Evora PR, Evora PM, Celotto AC, et al.: Cardiovascular therapeutics targets on the NO-sGC-cGMP signaling pathway: a critical overview, *Curr Drug Targets* 13(9):1207, 2012.
47. Tsutsui M, Ohya Y, Sugahara K: Latest evidence in endothelium-derived hyperpolarizing factor research, *Circ J* 76(7):1599, 2012.
48. Eckly-Michel A, Martin V, Lugnier C: Involvement of cyclic nucleotide-dependent protein kinases in cyclic AMP-mediated vasorelaxation, *Br J Pharmacol* 122(1):158, 1997.
49. Lincoln TM, Cornwell TL: Intracellular cyclic GMP receptor proteins, *FASEB J* 7(2):328, 1993.
50. Carvajal JA, Germain AM, Huidobro-Toro JP, et al.: Molecular mechanism of cGMP-mediated smooth muscle relaxation, *J Cell Physiol* 184(3):409, 2000.
51. Jackson WF: Potassium channels in the peripheral microcirculation, *Microcirculation* 12(1):113, 2005.
52. Amberg GC, Bonev AD, Rossow CF, et al.: Modulation of the molecular composition of large conductance, Ca(2+) activated K(+) channels in vascular smooth muscle during hypertension, *J Clin Invest* 112(5):717, 2003.
53. Ohta H, Suzuki J, Akima T, et al.: Hemodynamic effect of endothelin antagonists in dogs with myocardial infarction, *J Cardiovasc Pharmacol* 31(Suppl 1):S255, 1998.
54. Johannsen UJ, Mark AL, Marcus ML: Responsiveness to cardiac sympathetic nerve stimulation during maximal coronary dilation produced by adenosine, *Circ Res* 50(4):510, 1982.
55. Gillespie MN, Booth DC, Friedman BJ, et al.: fMLP provokes coronary vasoconstriction and myocardial ischemia in rabbits, *Am J Physiol* 254(3 Pt 2):H481, 1988.
56. Clarke JG, Davies GJ, Kerwin R, et al.: Coronary artery infusion of neuropeptide Y in patients with angina pectoris, *Lancet* 1(8541):1057, 1987.
57. McFadden EP, Clarke JG, Davies GJ, et al.: Effect of intracoronary serotonin on coronary vessels in patients with stable angina and patients with variant angina, *N Engl J Med* 324(10):648, 1991.
58. Ito H: No-reflow phenomenon and prognosis in patients with acute myocardial infarction, *Nat Clin Pract Cardiovasc Med* 3(9):499, 2006.
59. Porto I, Belloni F, Niccoli G, et al.: Filter no-reflow during percutaneous coronary intervention of saphenous vein grafts: incidence, predictors and effect of the type of protection device, *EuroIntervent* 7(8):955, 2011.
60. Corbalan R, Larrain G, Nazzal C, et al.: Association of noninvasive markers of coronary artery reperfusion to assess microvascular obstruction in patients with acute myocardial infarction treated with primary angioplasty, *Am J Cardiol* 88(4):342, 2001.
61. Niccoli G, Burzotta F, Galiuto L, et al.: Myocardial no-reflow in humans, *J Am Coll Cardiol* 54(4):281, 2009.
62. Rajappan K, Rimoldi OE, Dutka DP, et al.: Mechanisms of coronary microcirculatory dysfunction in patients with aortic stenosis and angiographically normal coronary arteries, *Circulation* 105(4):470, 2002.
63. Paulus WJ, Tschöpe C: A novel paradigm for heart failure with preserved ejection fraction: comorbidities drive myocardial dysfunction and remodeling through coronary microvascular endothelial inflammation, *J Am Coll Cardiol* 62(4):263, 2013.
64. Garcia-Dorado D, Andres-Villarreal M, Ruiz-Meana M, et al.: Myocardial edema: a translational view, *J Mol Cell Cardiol* 52(5):931, 2012.
65. Jaffe R, Charron T, Puley G, et al.: Microvascular obstruction and the no-reflow phenomenon after percutaneous coronary intervention, *Circulation* 117(24):3152, 2008.
66. Bekkers SCAM, Yazdani SK, Virmani R, et al.: Microvascular obstruction: underlying pathophysiology and clinical diagnosis, *J Am Coll Cardiol* 55(16):1649, 2010.
67. Frangogiannis NG: The inflammatory response in myocardial injury, repair, and remodelling, *Nat Rev Cardiol* 11(5):255, 2014.
68. Hammer-Hansen S, Ugander M, Hsu L-Y, et al.: Distinction of salvaged and infarcted myocardium within the ischaemic area-at-risk with T2 mapping, *Eur Heart J Cardiovasc Imaging* 15(9):1048, 2014.
69. Morris PB, Ference BA, Jahangir E, et al.: Cardiovascular effects of exposure to cigarette smoke and electronic cigarettes: clinical perspectives from the Prevention of Cardiovascular Disease Section Leadership Council and Early Career Councils of the American College of Cardiology, *J Am Coll Cardiol* 66(12):1378, 2015.
70. Kaufmann PA, Gnecchi-Ruscone T, di Terlizzi M, et al.: Coronary heart disease in smokers: vitamin C restores coronary microcirculatory function, *Circulation* 102(11):1233, 2000.
71. Rooks C, Faber T, Votaw J, et al.: Effects of smoking on coronary microcirculatory function: a twin study, *Atherosclerosis* 215(2):500, 2011.
72. Varela-Carver A, Parker H, Kleinert C, et al.: Adverse effects of cigarette smoke and induction of oxidative stress in cardiomyocytes and vascular endothelium, *Curr Pharm Des* 16(23):2551, 2010.
73. Kaufmann PA, Gnecchi-Ruscone T, Schafers KP, et al.: Low density lipoprotein cholesterol and coronary microvascular dysfunction in hypercholesterolemia, *J Am Coll Cardiol* 36(1):103, 2000.
74. Naoumova RP, Kindler H, Leccisotti L, et al.: Pioglitazone improves myocardial blood flow and glucose utilization in nondiabetic patients with combined hyperlipidemia: a randomized, double-blind, placebo-controlled study, *J Am Coll Cardiol* 50(21):2051, 2007.
75. Brush Jr JE, Cannon III RO, Schenke WH, et al.: Angina due to coronary microvascular disease in hypertensive patients without left ventricular hypertrophy, *N Engl J Med* 319(20):1302, 1988.
76. Rimoldi O, Rosen SD, Camici PG: The blunting of coronary flow reserve in hypertension with left ventricular hypertrophy is transmural and correlates with systolic blood pressure, *J Hypertens* 32(12):2465, 2014.
77. Levy BI, Duriez M, Samuel JL: Coronary microvasculature alteration in hypertensive rats. Effect of treatment with a diuretic and an ACE inhibitor, *Am J Hypertens* 14(1):7, 2001.
78. Neglia D, Fommei E, Varela-Carver A, et al.: Perindopril and indapamide reverse coronary microvascular remodelling and improve flow in arterial hypertension, *J Hypertens* 29(2):364, 2011.
79. Di Carli MF, Charytan D, McMahon GT, et al.: Coronary circulatory function in patients with the metabolic syndrome, *J Nucl Med* 52(9):1369, 2011.
80. Schindler TH, Cardenas J, Prior JO, et al.: Relationship between increasing body weight, insulin resistance, inflammation, adipocytokine leptin, and coronary circulatory function, *J Am Coll Cardiol* 47(6):1188, 2006.
81. Murthy VL, Naya M, Foster CR, et al.: Association between coronary vascular dysfunction and cardiac mortality in patients with and without diabetes mellitus, *Circulation* 126(15):1858, 2012.
82. Lautamaki R, Airaksinen KE, Seppanen M, et al.: Insulin improves myocardial blood flow in patients with type 2 diabetes and coronary artery disease, *Diabetes* 55(2):511, 2006.
83. Schindler TH, Facta AD, Prior JO, et al.: Improvement in coronary vascular dysfunction produced with euglycaemic control in patients with type 2 diabetes, *Heart* 93(3):345, 2007.
84. Quinones MJ, Hernandez-Pampaloni M, Schelbert H, et al.: Coronary vasomotor abnormalities in insulin-resistant individuals, *Ann Intern Med* 140(9):700, 2004.
85. Lanza GA, Sestito A, Cammarota G, et al.: Assessment of systemic inflammation and infective pathogen burden in patients with cardiac syndrome X, *Am J Cardiol* 94(1):40, 2004.
86. Cosin-Sales J, Pizzi C, Brown S, et al.: C-reactive protein, clinical presentation, and ischemic activity in patients with chest pain and normal coronary angiograms, *J Am Coll Cardiol* 41(9):1468, 2003.
87. Recio-Mayoral A, Rimoldi OE, Camici PG, et al.: Inflammation and microvascular dysfunction in cardiac syndrome X patients without conventional risk factors for coronary artery disease, *JACC Cardiovasc Imaging* 6(6):660, 2013.
88. Pupita G, Maseri A, Kaski JC, et al.: Myocardial ischemia caused by distal coronary-artery constriction in stable angina pectoris, *N Engl J Med* 323(8):514, 1990.
89. Camici PG, Rimoldi OE: The clinical value of myocardial blood flow measurement, *J Nucl Med* 50(7):1076, 2009.
90. Sambuceti G, Marzilli M, Fedele S, et al.: Paradoxical increase in microvascular resistance during tachycardia downstream from a severe stenosis in patients with coronary artery disease: reversal by angioplasty, *Circulation* 103(19):2352, 2001.
91. Pursnani S, Korley F, Gopaul R, et al.: Percutaneous coronary intervention versus optimal medical therapy in stable coronary artery disease: a systematic review and meta-analysis of randomized clinical trials, *Circ Cardiovasc Interv* 5(4):476, 2012.
92. Boden WE, O'Rourke RA, Teo KK, et al.: Optimal medical therapy with or without PCI for stable coronary disease, *N Engl J Med* 356(15):1503, 2007.
93. Aarnoudse W, Van't Veer M, Pijls NH, et al.: Direct volumetric blood flow measurement in coronary arteries by thermodilution, *J Am Coll Cardiol* 50(24):2294, 2007.

94. Lee JM, Layland J, Jung JH, et al.: Integrated physiologic assessment of ischemic heart disease in real-world practice using index of microcirculatory resistance and fractional flow reserve: insights from the International Index of Microcirculatory Resistance Registry, *Circ Cardiovasc Intervent* 8(11), 2015. e002857.
95. Herzog BA, Husmann L, Valenta I, et al.: Long-term prognostic value of 13N-ammonia myocardial perfusion positron emission tomography added value of coronary flow reserve, *J Am Coll Cardiol* 54(2):150, 2009.
96. Ziadi MC, Dekemp RA, Williams KA, et al.: Impaired myocardial flow reserve on rubidium-82 positron emission tomography imaging predicts adverse outcomes in patients assessed for myocardial ischemia, *J Am Coll Cardiol* 58(7):740, 2011.
97. Murthy VL, Naya M, Foster CR, et al.: Improved cardiac risk assessment with noninvasive measures of coronary flow reserve, *Circulation* 124(20):2215, 2011.
98. Fukushima K, Javadi MS, Higuchi T, et al.: Prediction of short-term cardiovascular events using quantification of global myocardial flow reserve in patients referred for clinical 82Rb PET perfusion imaging, *J Nucl Med* 52(5):726, 2011.
99. Milo M, Nerla R, Tarzia P, et al.: Coronary microvascular dysfunction after elective percutaneous coronary intervention: correlation with exercise stress test results, *Int J Cardiol* 168(1):121, 2013.
100. van de Hoef TP, Bax M, Damman P, et al.: Impaired coronary autoregulation is associated with long-term fatal events in patients with stable coronary artery disease, *Circ Cardiovasc Intervent* 6(4):329, 2013.
101. van de Hoef TP, van Lavieren MA, Damman P, et al.: Physiological basis and long-term clinical outcome of discordance between fractional flow reserve and coronary flow velocity reserve in coronary stenoses of intermediate severity, *Circ Cardiovasc Intervent* 7(3):301, 2014.
102. Taqueti VR, Hachamovitch R, Murthy VL, et al.: Global coronary flow reserve is associated with adverse cardiovascular events independently of luminal angiographic severity and modifies the effect of early revascularization, *Circulation* 131(1):19, 2015.
103. Testa L, Van Gaal WJ, Biondi Zoccai GGL, et al.: Myocardial infarction after percutaneous coronary intervention: a meta-analysis of troponin elevation applying the new universal definition, *QJM* 102(6):369, 2009.
104. Mauri L, Cox D, Hermiller J, et al.: The PROXIMAL trial: proximal protection during saphenous vein graft intervention using the Proxis embolic protection system: a randomized, prospective, multicenter clinical trial, *J Am Coll Cardiol* 50(15):1442, 2007.
105. Merla R, Reddy NK, Wang FW, et al.: Meta-analysis of published reports on the effect of statin treatment before percutaneous coronary intervention on periprocedural myonecrosis, *Am J Cardiol* 100(5):770, 2007.
106. Croal BL, Hillis GS, Gibson PH, et al.: Relationship between postoperative cardiac troponin I levels and outcome of cardiac surgery, *Circulation* 114(14):1468, 2006.
107. Liakopoulos OJ, Choi YH, Haldenwang PL, et al.: Impact of preoperative statin therapy on adverse postoperative outcomes in patients undergoing cardiac surgery: a meta-analysis of over 30,000 patients, *Eur Heart J* 29(12):1548, 2008.

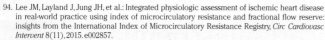

6 Precipitants of Myocardial Ischemia

Daniel Sedehi and Joaquin E. Cigarroa

INTRODUCTION

Myocardial ischemia occurs when the ability to supply oxygen and nutrients to the myocardium is exceeded by the myocardium's oxygen and nutrient requirements. The heart is primarily an aerobic organ and has a narrow threshold for a deficit in oxygen delivery. The myocardium, and consequently the coronary circulation, must be able to adapt quickly to meet the body's varying hemodynamic requirements. The development of acute ischemia sequentially adversely affects diastolic function, systolic function, and electrocardiographic changes and finally results in chest pain; a sequence referred to as *the ischemic cascade.*[1] In the presence of chronic ischemia, a patient may develop left ventricular (LV) systolic and diastolic dysfunction and elevation of LV diastolic pressure resulting in heart failure. A patient's clinical comorbidities, presenting clinical state, and hemodynamics determine the threshold for developing ischemia.

Myocardial Oxygen Demand

Myocardial oxygen demand is governed by three principal factors: heart rate, contractility, and wall tension. As the heart rate increases, the myocardial oxygen requirement increases, yet there is a concomitant decrease in diastolic filling period, which consequently decreases the available time for perfusion. As myocardial contractility increases, the requirement for oxygen and nutrients is also increased. Wall tension is the force generated by the myocardium at a given preload and afterload and may be calculated by the Laplace law (Fig. 6.1). Wall tension is affected by afterload, chamber size (i.e., radius), and wall thickness. Clinically, chamber dimensions are decreased by interventions that reduce LV preload whereas afterload is largely determined by systolic blood pressure. The impact of afterload (i.e., increased systolic blood pressure) on myocardial oxygen demand is greater than the impact of preload or heart rate. As afterload increases, the radius of the ventricle may increase and further elevate the pressure required by the ventricle to propel blood from the heart. As wall tension increases, myocardial oxygen demand increases.[2]

Assessment of these factors is essential in understanding an individual patient's potential for developing myocardial ischemia (Table 6.1). Moreover, each of these determinants of myocardial oxygen demand represents an important treatment target for reduction of ischemia (see Chapter 20).

Myocardial Oxygen Supply

Myocardial oxygen supply is determined by oxygen transport, oxygen delivery, and coronary arterial blood flow. Perturbations to any of these three components will decrease the ability to meet the metabolic requirements of the myocardium. Along with oxygen, the delivery of metabolic substrate to the myocardium is facilitated by normal coronary blood flow. In the normal resting state, the heart relies primarily on fatty acids, and to a lesser degree glucose, for facilitating aerobic metabolism. As supply diminishes and as demand increases—producing ischemia—the myocardium switches substrate utilization to lactate and glycogen.

Oxygen is transported in the blood bound to hemoglobin and dissociates from hemoglobin when delivered to tissues for oxidative metabolism. The transport of oxygen and the ability to deliver it to myocytes is impacted both by hemoglobin levels and factors that influence the oxygen dissociation curve (Fig. 6.2). The normal oxygen dissociation curve facilitates the binding of oxygen to hemoglobin in the lungs and the dissociation within the myocardial tissue where the carbon dioxide levels are higher and pH lower. Factors that shift the curve to the left decrease oxygen release in the tissues as the hemoglobin molecule has a higher affinity for oxygen; these include hypothermia, decrease in levels of 2,3-diphosphoglycerate, increase in pH (alkalosis), decrease in CO_2, and increases in carbon monoxide. In addition, acquired hemoglobinopathies such as methemoglobinemia shift the curve left with a net increase in the affinity for oxygen within the affected hemoglobin molecule.[3] Clinical states including hypothermia, acid/base disorders, anemia, hypoxemia, sepsis, and hemoglobinopathies can precipitate ischemia at lower thresholds, even in the absence of epicardial coronary artery disease (CAD). By decreasing delivery of oxygen to tissues, anemia results in reduced oxygen supply. At any level of hemoglobin, oxygen delivery is further influenced by factors that govern O_2 dissociation from hemoglobin as previously described (see Fig. 6.2).

Coronary blood flow regulation is essential for the heart to adapt its metabolic requirements and to receive adequate oxygen and nutrients. Coronary circulation is mediated by perfusion pressure (aortic diastolic to LV diastolic

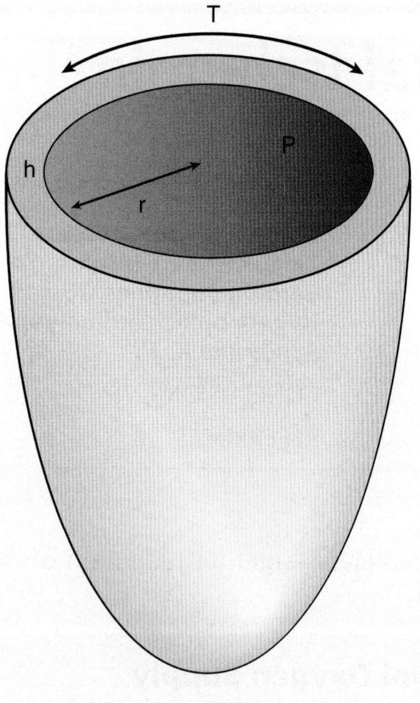

FIG. 6.1 Laplace law. Wall tension (*T*) increases directly with ventricular pressure (*P*) as well as with the radius of the ventricle (*r*). Conversely, the thickness of the wall is inversely related to wall tension. *(From Nadruz W. Myocardial remodeling in hypertension.* J Hum Hypertens. *2015;29(1):1–6.)*

TABLE 6.1 Myocardial O_2 Consumption Components

Total	
6–8 mL/min per 100 g	
Distribution	
Basal	20%
Electrical	1%
Volume work	15%
Pressure work	64%
Effects on MVO_2 of 50% Increase In	
Wall stress	25%
Contractility	45%
Pressure work	50%
Heart Rate	50%

Individual components are broken down into their relative contribution to myocardial oxygen consumption (MVO_2).
Adapted from Gould KL. Coronary Artery Stenosis. *New York: Elsevier; 1991.*

pressure), arterial tone (autoregulation), metabolic activity, sympathetic/parasympathetic activity, and the endothelium. The regulation of coronary blood flow occurs via neural pathways, metabolic mediators, myogenic control, and extravascular compressive forces (Table 6.2). Exogenous medications, including α- and β-adrenergic agonists/antagonists, adenosine, and dipyridamole, impact blood flow via coronary epicardial and resistance vessels.[4]

Coronary autoregulation maintains a relatively constant perfusion pressure over a broad range of aortic mean pressures (40 to 130 mm Hg).[5,6] The epicardial vessels do not contribute to resistance unless clinically significant stenoses are present. In the absence of coronary artery stenoses, the majority of resistance is provided by prearteriolar, arteriolar, and intramyocardial capillary vessels (Fig. 6.3). At rest, the capillaries are responsible for 25% of the microvascular resistance, which increases to 75% during periods of hyperemia.[7] In normal individuals, coronary flow can increase 3- to 5-fold under conditions of maximal hyperemia. This ability to augment coronary blood flow is termed *coronary flow reserve* (see Chapter 5). Abnormalities in coronary flow reserve occur in many pathologic states, including diabetes mellitus, hypertension, dyslipidemia, myocardial infarction, aortic stenosis, and idiopathic dilated cardiomyopathies.[8–11]

CLINICAL PREDISPOSITION

An individual's health and risk factors impact his/her ability to increase coronary blood flow to meet the substrate requirements of the myocardium. The coronary epicardial and resistance vessels must be able to dilate to augment coronary blood flow. Factors that inhibit the normal coronary flow reserve will increase the propensity for developing myocardial ischemia. The common underlying mechanisms include endothelial cell dysfunction and a decrease in myocardial capillary density. Common conditions that adversely impact endothelial cell function include increasing age, obesity, hypertension, dyslipidemia, diabetes mellitus, hyperhomocysteinemia, and in women a history of preeclampsia and/or a postmenopausal state.[12,13] In addition, risk factors including smoking, sedentary lifestyle, and poor nutrition also promote endothelial cell dysfunction.[12,14] These risk factors and clinical conditions decrease the production of vasodilators such as nitric oxide (NO) and prostacyclin while increasing the production of potent vasoconstrictors including endothelin-1. Over time, this produces a prothrombotic environment and stimulates the formation of atherosclerosis, which may precipitate ischemia. In the presence of endothelial dysfunction, stimuli that normally result in vasodilation may paradoxically cause coronary vasoconstriction and precipitate myocardial ischemia.

SPECIFIC ENVIRONMENTAL FACTORS

Hypoxemia

Individuals frequently develop hypoxemia secondary to medical conditions such as acute or chronic pulmonary diseases or exposure to high-altitude environments including airline travel and residing or visiting high-altitude locales. In addition to the direct effects of hypoxemia on oxygen delivery, individuals who are acutely hypoxemic develop tachycardia and an increase in rate pressure product. In the absence of epicardial CAD, the coronary physiology adapts to hypoxemia by epicardial coronary vasodilation and an increase in coronary flow reserve. In the presence of epicardial coronary disease, hypoxemia-induced epicardial coronary vasodilation may not occur; when studied in individuals with greater than 50% stenoses in at least one major epicardial vessel, vasoconstriction occurred, leading to a decrease in overall myocardial blood flow.[15,16] As a result, individuals with comorbidities such as hypertension may develop myocardial ischemia at a lower peak rate pressure product, which may limit their functional capacity. An understanding of the normal response to hypoxemia and the alterations that occur in patients with CAD is critical in directing patient management during critical illnesses to

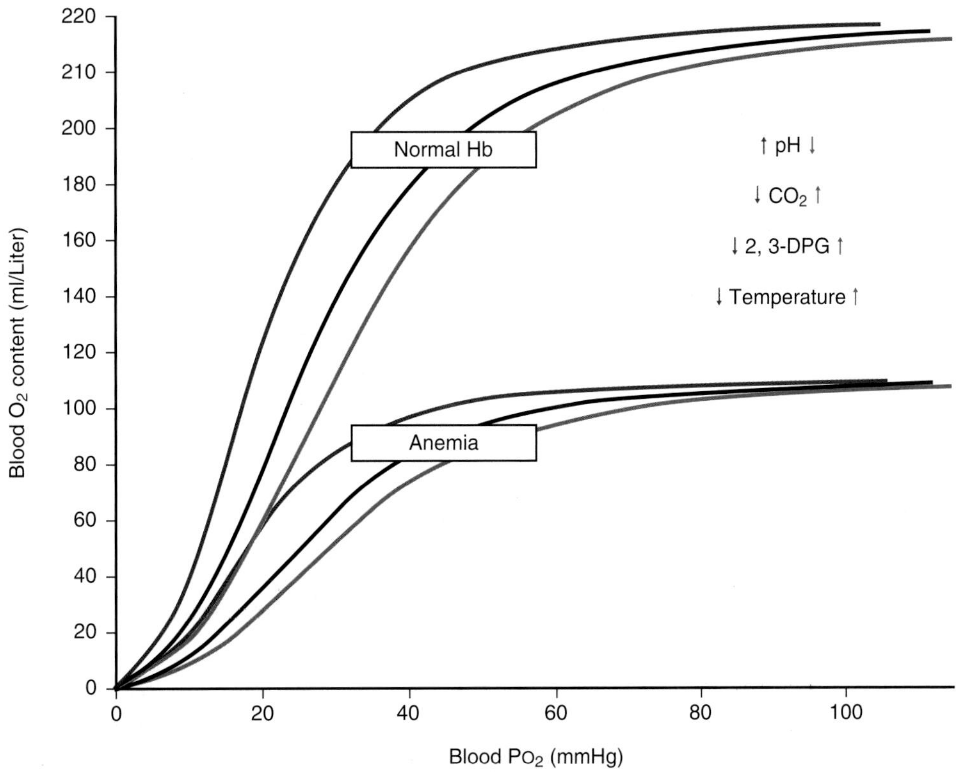

FIG. 6.2 Oxygen disassociation curve. Factors affecting the disassociation include pH, CO_2, 2,3-diphosphoglycerate (2,3-DPG), and temperature. Anemia decreases the overall oxygen-carrying capacity of blood. Po_2, partial pressure of oxygen. *(From Mairbaurl H. Red blood cells in sports: effects of exercise and training on oxygen supply by red blood cells.* Front Physiol. *2013;4:332.)*

TABLE 6.2 Net Effects of Myogenic Response, Metabolic Mediators, and Neurohormonal Input to Coronary Vascular Resistance, Both in Normal State and with Atherosclerosis

	NORMAL CORONARIES	ATHEROSCLEROSIS
Myogenic Response		
Pressure and flow-based dilation/constriction, resistance vessels	Dilation or constriction	Dilation or constriction
Metabolic Mediators		
Adenosine	Dilation of resistance vessels	Attenuated dilation
Sympathetic		
Norepinepherine		
α_1	Constriction	Constriction
β_2	Dilation	Attenuated dilation
Parasympathetic		
Acetylcholine	Dilation	Constriction of conduit vessels Attenuated dilation of resistance vessels

Adapted from Canty JM. Coronary blood flow and myocardial ischemia. In: Bonow RO et al. eds. Braunwald's Heart Disease. *Philadelphia: Elsevier; 2012.*

minimize the risk for myocardial ischemia. This should be assessed with an understanding of the impact the patient's overall clinical condition is having on the oxygen dissociation curve as this may also adversely impact the threshold for developing ischemia.

Hyperglycemia

The prevalence of diabetes mellitus is increasing and impacts a significant proportion of the general population. Individuals with metabolic syndrome or with diabetes mellitus have an increased incidence of myocardial ischemia and myocardial infarction. For patients hospitalized with acute illnesses, hyperglycemia in the absence of diabetes is often noted. The presence of hyperglycemia, independent of diabetes, is now known to adversely affect coronary physiology.[12,17] In a study of 104 patients without diabetes (fasting blood glucose of <126 mg/dL, hemoglobin A_{1c} <6.5%), cardiac catheterization and assessment of coronary blood flow, coronary artery diameter, and coronary vascular resistance were performed. Hyperglycemia did not impact endothelium-dependent epicardial vessel dilation but was associated with impaired endothelial function in resistance coronary vessels. In addition, hyperglycemia was associated with increased coronary vascular resistance.[18] These effects on coronary physiology may contribute to

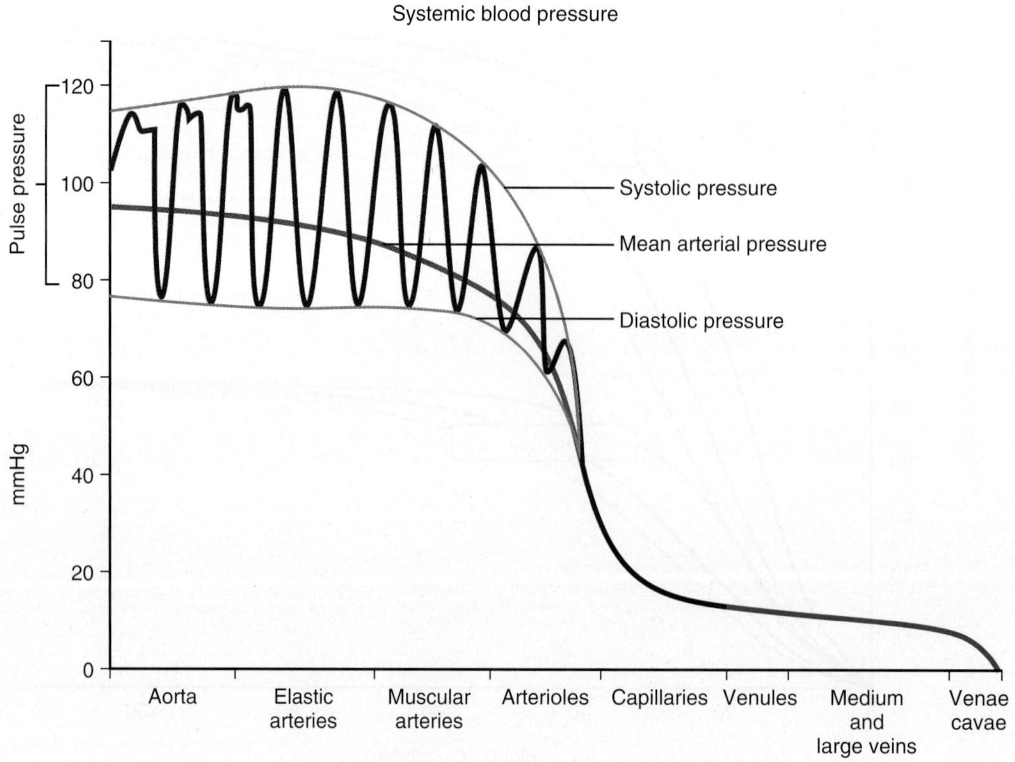

FIG. 6.3 Contributions to resistance within specific coronary vessels. Minimal resistance to flow exists within the epicardial vessels, whereas the majority of the resistance is seen in the arterioles and capillaries. *(From http://cnx.org/contents/A4QcTJ6a@3/Blood-Flow-Blood-Pressure-and-Resistance.)*

the increased risk for developing myocardial ischemia. Whether acute treatment of hyperglycemia decreases the risk of developing myocardial ischemia is unknown and requires further investigation. Diabetes, much like hypertension, plays a key role in the development of atherosclerosis, as well as myocardial ischemia. Diabetes mellitus leads to the development of oxygen free radicals, inflammation, and impaired vascular tone.[19–21] Hyperglycemia causes a downregulation of the endogenous nitric oxide synthase, inhibiting endogenous vasodilation via NO, as well as decreasing NO-related inhibition of platelet aggregation.[22,23] Insulin resistance leads to an increase in free fatty acids, thereby promoting free radical generation and inflammation. Diabetes also leads to an upregulation in endothelin-1 as well as angiotensin II, known vasoconstrictors and catalysts for atherogenesis.[24] Diabetes contributes to an alteration in collagen synthesis, leading to a weakened fibrous cap.[25] Along with its vascular effects, diabetes can elevate the prothrombotic nature of platelets, leading to further ischemic events.[19]

Hypercapnia

In the absence of respiratory disease, carbon dioxide, a product of aerobic cellular respiration, is maintained within a range of 35 to 45 mm Hg. Levels of carbon dioxide are known to impact the oxygen dissociation curve and coronary blood flow; the regional production of carbon dioxide is crucial to the metabolic control of myocardial blood flow.[26] Systemic hypercapnia is often accompanied by acidosis and changes in hemodynamic states. Together these often increase coronary blood flow, primarily via decreases in coronary vascular resistance.[27] Depending on the degree of sympathetic activation, the decrease in coronary vascular resistance may be blunted.[28] In addition, the ability of hemoglobin to bind oxygen and transport it to the tissue is impaired when systemic carbon dioxide is elevated and the patient has acidosis. Consequently, patients can develop ischemia at a lower peak rate pressure product or when the perfusion pressure is adversely impacted, especially in the presence of concomitant CAD.

Acidosis

The presence of acidosis shifts the oxygen dissociation curve to the right, which promotes the dissociation of oxygen from hemoglobin at the tissue level. In the presence of systemic acidosis, however, this decreases the oxygen-carrying capacity of hemoglobin and may contribute to a lower ischemic threshold. Furthermore, in vitro studies have shown that acidosis has a profound inhibitory effect on the production of cellular cyclic GMP synthesis, which is further impaired when coupled with the presence of hypoxemia.[29]

Hypothermia

Hypothermia is now commonly applied to out-of-hospital cardiac arrest patients who have been successfully resuscitated and who have impaired neurologic function. In canine models, both mild (32°C) and moderate (27°C) surface-induced hypothermia did not adversely impact coronary autoregulation.[30] Therapeutic hypothermia reduces heart rate, may decrease the magnitude of vasopressor requirements, and may minimally improve systolic function.[31] In contrast to the favorable hemodynamic effects, therapeutic hypothermia activates platelets and may be associated with an increase in the risk of stent thrombosis.[32] There is no evidence, however, that it changes the threshold for ischemia (see Fig. 6.2).

SPECIFIC CARDIOVASCULAR CONDITIONS

Hyperlipidemia

Elevated levels of low-density lipoprotein (LDL) confer an increased risk for atherosclerosis and myocardial ischemia, and treatment with lipid-modifying agents decreases this risk.[33–36] Mechanisms for the development of both ischemia and atherosclerosis are multiple, including inflammation-driven development of lipid-laden plaques, oxidation of LDL increasing inflammation, and decreased response to vasodilation through direct inhibition of endothelium-dependent vasodilation.[37–40] Improvements in levels and various treatments of hyperlipidemia have been shown to decrease recurrent ischemic events, furthering the understanding of the direct and indirect relationship between hyperlipidemia and myocardial ischemia.

Hypertension

Hypertension is an important contributor to myocardial ischemia[41–45] with effects on both myocardial oxygen demand and supply. Even without the longstanding adaptive mechanism of LV hypertrophy, hypertension itself leads to both endothelial dysfunction and a maladaptive response to appropriate endogenous nitrate-driven coronary vasodilation. Increased levels of angiotensin II directly affect atherosclerosis and endothelial dysfunction, through upregulation of proinflammatory cytokines such as interleukin-6, NF-κB, and reactive oxygen species.[46–48] Chronic hypertension disables normal endogenous mechanisms by which coronary arteries augment flow, mainly through endothelial NO and its effects on smooth muscles cells.[49–52] Management of hypertension, especially with inhibitors of the renin-angiotensin-aldos-terone system, has a significant impact in decreasing myocardial ischemia.

Hypotension

Systemic hypotension, with its many causes, leads to reduced tissue perfusion including that in the myocardium. A decrease in the coronary perfusion pressure occurs, which decreases myocardial oxygen delivery.[53–56] An increase in production of lactic acid further worsens delivery of oxygen to the myocardium.[57] This scenario is common in cardiogenic shock where worsening hypotension leads to an increase in systemic vasoconstriction, LV diastolic pressure, and worsening acidosis, which collectively decrease myocardial oxygen delivery. The presence of coexisting CAD will further impair myocardial tissue perfusion.[58]

Coronary Artery Disease

The development of CAD predisposes the patient to developing ischemia at lower peak rate pressure products, which may limit functional capacity. Daily experiences and activities including emotional stressors such as anger, tobacco use, and exercise can trigger ischemia.[59] Abnormalities in endothelial cell function may result in paradoxic vasoconstriction to stimuli including cold temperatures, exercise,

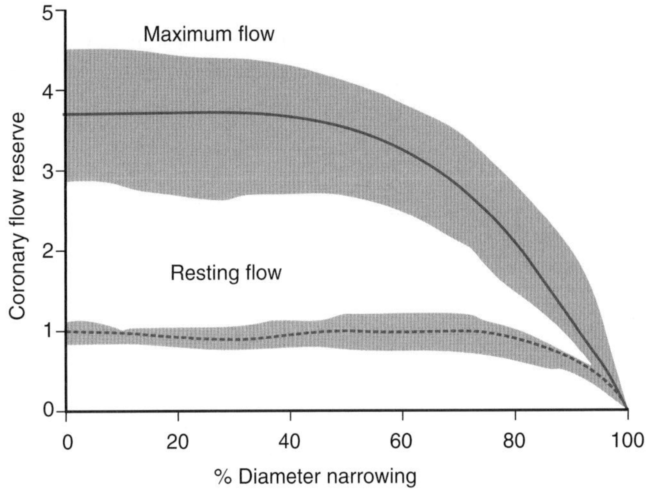

FIG. 6.4 Coronary flow reserve relative to percent of stenosis, shown in both resting and maximal flow states. At maximal flow, less narrowing is needed to produce a change in flow as compared with resting flow, which begins to decrease after 80% stenosis. *(Adapted from Gould KL, Lipscomb K, Hamilton GW. Physiologic basis for assessing critical coronary stenosis. Instantaneous flow response and regional distribution during coronary hyperemia as measures of coronary flow reserve.* Am J Cardiol. *1974;33:87–94.)*

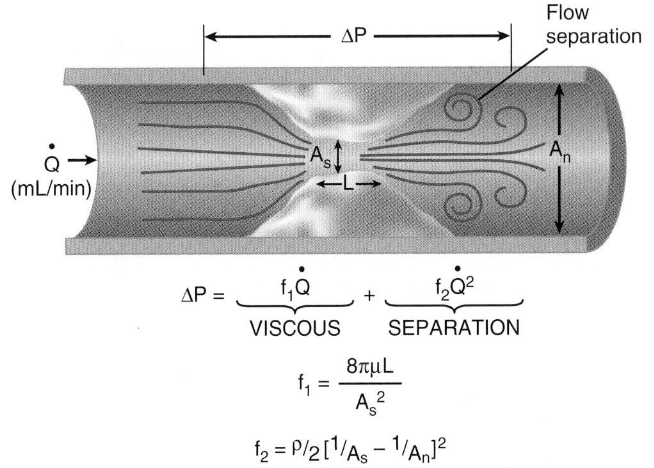

FIG. 6.5 The Bernoulli effect: fluid mechanics of a stenosis. The pressure drop across a stenosis can be predicted by the Bernoulli equation. It is inversely related to the minimum stenosis cross-sectional area and varies with the square of the flow rate as stenosis severity increases. *An,* Area of the normal segment; *As,* area of the stenosis; *f_1,* viscous coefficient; *f_2,* separation coefficient; *L,* stenosis length; *ΔP,* pressure drop; *Q̇* flow; *μ,* viscosity of blood; *ρ,* density of blood. *(From Canty JM, Duncker DJ. Coronary blood flow and myocardial ischemia. In: Mann DL et al. eds.* Braunwald's Heart Disease. *Philadelphia, Elsevier; 2015: Fig. 49.11.)*

hypoxemia, and emotional stressors, which can lead to angina. As coronary stenoses increase in severity, the coronary microcirculation dilates in an effort to maintain adequate blood flow (Fig. 6.4). The development of epicardial stenoses results in increased resistance to blood flow. The pressure gradient that develops across the lesion is described by the Bernoulli equation (Fig. 6.5). The pressure gradient is influenced by lesion length in a linear fashion but is exponentially increased by the reduction in cross-sectional area. Thus, small changes in cross-sectional area may have profound hemodynamic effects given that the pressure gradient is inversely proportional to the fourth power of the lumen reduction. Whereas resting blood flow is maintained at normal levels until epicardial coronary stenoses exceed approximately 85% of the normal vessel diameter, maximal

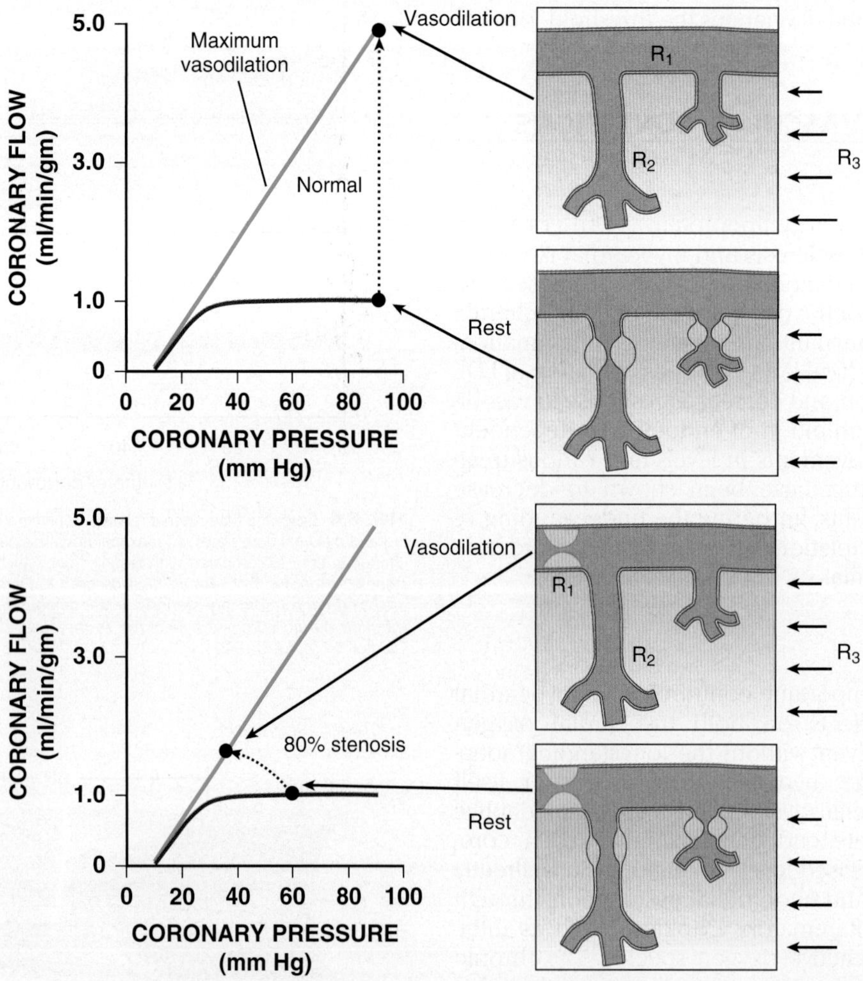

FIG. 6.6 Components of coronary vascular resistance. Without significant epicardial stenosis, the majority of the resistance is due to metabolic and autoregulatory mechanisms and extravascular compressive forces, which increase with flow from epicardium to endocardium. Significant epicardial stenoses contribute to resistance, and once above 80%, they play a majority role in the resistance within that coronary tree. *(From Canty JM. Coronary blood flow and myocardial ischemia. In: Bonow RO et al. eds.* Braunwald's Heart Disease. *Philadelphia: Elsevier; 2012:* Fig. *49.5.)*

hyperemic coronary blood flow is impaired once the epicardial stenoses exceed approximately 50% (Fig. 6.6).[60]

In the presence of CAD, many factors may impact the precipitation of myocardial ischemia including heart rate, blood pressure, myocardial wall tension, LV diastolic pressure, and clinical factors including hyperlipidemia, diabetes mellitus, and hypertension. Medical therapies directed toward decreasing heart rate and blood pressure and maintaining normal wall tension may favorably impact the patient, improving functional capacity by enhancing myocardial oxygen delivery while decreasing myocardial oxygen demand. In addition, medications that decrease epicardial vasoconstriction, including calcium-channel blockers and nitrates, are also beneficial by increasing coronary blood flow. Risk factor modifications, including treatment of hyperlipidemia, avoidance of smoking, mindfulness to decrease stress, and consistent cardioaerobic exercise, are also beneficial in preventing myocardial ischemia.

Valvular Heart Disease

Patients with aortic stenosis often complain of angina, even in the absence of CAD. These patients have multiple abnormalities including increased afterload secondary to the valvular lesion, LV hypertrophy, and abnormalities in coronary physiology. Factors impacting demand include heart rate, LV peak systolic pressure, inotropic state, and valve area. Factors impacting myocardial supply include diastolic filling time, wall thickness, and LV diastolic pressure. The first study to indicate a mechanism for the development of angina in this population was a study of coronary flow reserve.[61] Patients with aortic stenosis and LV hypertrophy without CAD underwent measurement of coronary flow reserve at the time of their operation and were compared with patients who did not have LV hypertrophy. In the aortic stenosis group with LV hypertrophy, the coronary flow reserve was reduced by greater than 50%. Subsequently, further insights into mechanisms of ischemia were identified by use of cardiac magnetic resonance and positron emission tomography to assess LV mass and myocardial blood flow at rest and during hyperemia.[62] Myocardial blood flow was reduced to a greater extent in the subendocardium than the subepicardium; the magnitude of reduction in blood flow was related to increasing severity of aortic stenosis. In addition, there was a strong correlation between diastolic filling time and coronary flow reserve. Thus, diastolic filling time and severity of aortic valve stenosis may be greater contributors to the threshold for ischemia than LV hypertrophy. Following aortic valve replacement, patients often have regression of LV hypertrophy, improvement in coronary flow reserve, and improvement in functional capacity with a reduction in angina.

Patients with aortic insufficiency may complain of angina and have demonstrable myocardial ischemia.[63] The etiology of coronary ischemia in the presence of severe aortic insufficiency has been attributed to a decrease in aortic diastolic pressure coupled with increase in LV end-diastolic pressure, which may decrease coronary blood flow. LV hypertrophy and LV dilation increase wall stress.[64,65] In a small study, myocardial ischemia was not found to correlate directly with hypertrophy or LV dilation, but was hypothesized to be more related to coronary flow dynamics in severe aortic regurgitation. Consideration for coronary steal with severe aortic insufficiency was postulated to be a significant contributing factor.[66] Any valvular lesion that impacts the ventricular geometry, preload, or afterload may decrease the threshold for developing myocardial ischemia.

Cardiomyopathies

Patients with idiopathic dilated cardiomyopathies are at increased risk for developing myocardial ischemia. Many factors impact this predisposition including the presence of comorbidities including hypertension, diabetes, and hyperlipidemia, as well as altered hemodynamics, including relative tachycardia and elevations in left atrial and LV pressures and secondary pulmonary hypertension. Changes in LV geometry including an increase in LV diastolic dimension adversely impact wall tension. Clinical studies have demonstrated that elevations in both left atrial and LV pressures predispose patients to develop ischemia. In addition to their effects on oxygen demand, elevations in left atrial and LV pressures adversely affect myocardial blood flow and coronary flow reserve, in part by reversing the endocardial/epicardial myocardial blood flow ratio.[67] In addition, when either LV diastolic or left atrial pressures are elevated, the coronary driving pressures shift from the difference between the aortic and right atrial pressure to the difference between the aortic and LV pressure. As the pressure in the left ventricle increases, the capillary resistance increases because the capillaries collapse secondary to the increase in pressure exerted by elevations in the LV diastolic pressure, and this results in a reduction in coronary blood flow.[68] In addition, patients with idiopathic dilated cardiomyopathies also have a reduction in capillary artery density and diameter that further impairs coronary flow reserve.[11] Given these abnormalities within the coronary circulation, efforts to optimize preload, reduce afterload, and lower heart rate are essential to reducing myocardial ischemia in these patients.

Hypertrophic Cardiomyopathy

Patients with hypertrophic cardiomyopathy and normal epicardial coronary arteries often complain of angina. Studies have demonstrated similarities to the mechanisms responsible for ischemia in patients with aortic stenosis. A unique difference in patients with hypertrophic cardiomyopathy is a decrease in capillary density relative to an increase in cardiac mass.[69] In these patients, a decrease in coronary flow reserve has been noted in several studies, particularly when studied during ventricular pacing.[70] During mild tachycardia with heart rates as high as 130 beats/min, the mild increase in LV end-diastolic pressure did not appear to dramatically alter coronary blood flow as evidenced by appropriately increased great cardiac vein flow. As pacing rates increased, the coronary blood flow decreased significantly, and the LV end-diastolic pressure increased significantly, leading to the hypothesis that the increased intracavitary pressure, coupled with decreased coronary flow reserve, precipitates myocardial ischemia.

Syndrome X

Some patients (predominantly premenopausal women) may complain of classic exertional angina and have evidence of myocardial ischemia by stress imaging studies, yet have angiographically normal arteries. Investigators have demonstrated abnormalities in endothelial cell function with the presence of paradoxic vasoconstriction and abnormal coronary blood flow reserve.[71] Impaired vasodilation occurs secondary to both endothelial-dependent and -independent factors.[72] Abnormalities in coronary blood flow reserve may be secondary to abnormalities in rheology and/or abnormalities in the coronary resistance vessels and capillaries. In a study of women with Syndrome X, resting coronary blood flow was increased and coronary autoregulation was abnormal. The abnormality in coronary autoregulation was demonstrated to be secondary to abnormalities in the coronary resistance vessels without differences in capillary density.[73] Treatments to increase the threshold for the development of angina and ischemia have focused on risk factor modification as well as medical therapies, including aminophylline, statins, β-blockers, angiotensin-converting enzyme inhibitors, and ranolazine.[74–78] (see Chapter 25).

CONCLUSIONS

Myocardial ischemia occurs when the myocardial demand for substrates exceeds that of supply. Although we often consider myocardial ischemia in the setting of critical CAD, it is clear that ischemia may occur with or without epicardial CAD. Understanding the emotional triggers, environmental and hemodynamic factors, and associated clinical conditions that may precipitate myocardial ischemia is critical for mitigating and/or treating patients with myocardial ischemia (Fig. 6.7). Among patients without severe stenoses that limit resting coronary blood flow, certain factors affecting coronary flow and perfusion pressure, including shear stress-induced plaque rupture and platelet aggregation, along with changes in oxygen-carrying capacity, can result in downstream ischemia. Increasing myocardial oxygen demand through an increase in heart rate, inotropy, and wall tension further potentiate this cascade, whether this be through the action of illicit substances, physiologic states, or severe infection and sepsis. Recognition and treatment of these factors are vital in decreasing downstream myocardial ischemia by rebalancing supply and demand.

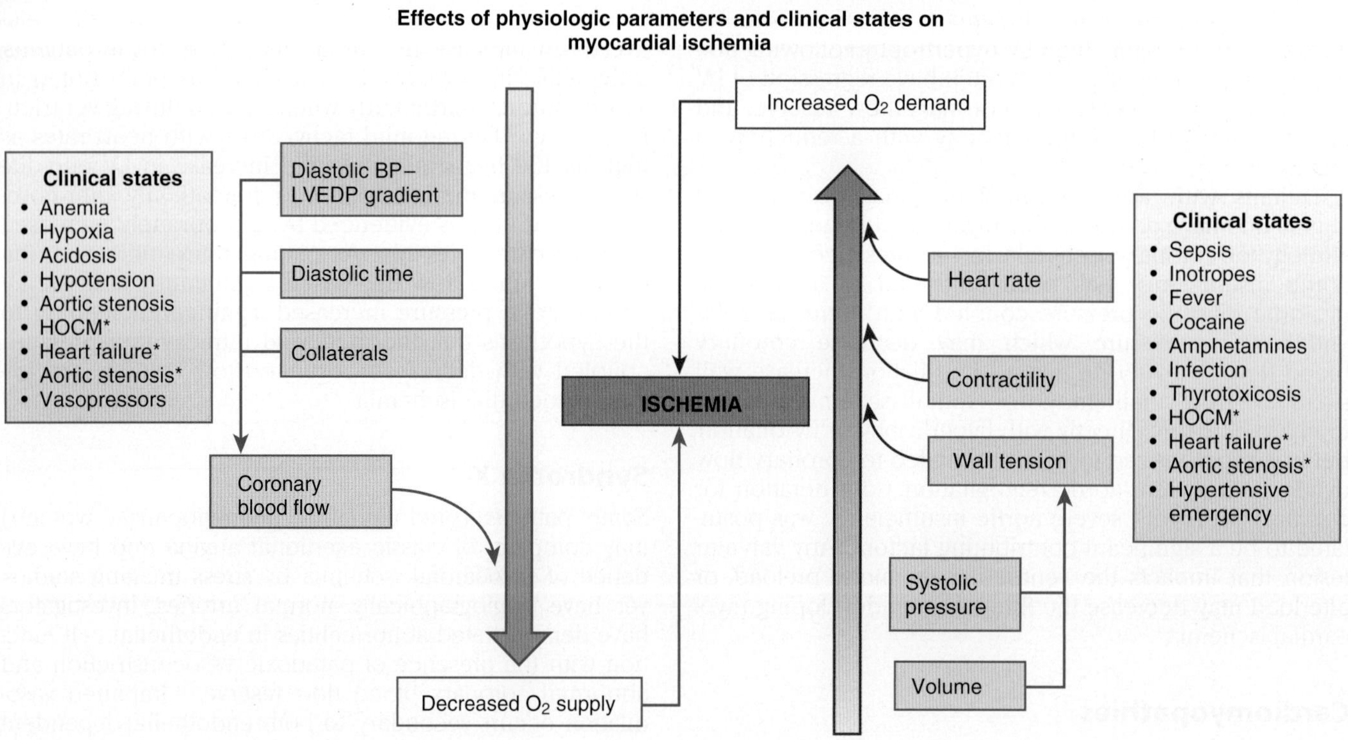

FIG. 6.7 Precipitants of myocardial ischemia. Hemodynamic consequences of clinical states and their effects on ischemia. * indicates that the condition affects both supply and demand. *BP*, Blood pressure; *HOCM*, hypertrophic obstructive cardiomyopathy; *LVEDP*, left ventricular end-diastolic pressure. *(Adapted from Morrow, Gersh, Braunwald. In: Zipes, Libby, Bonow, Braunwald, eds.* Chronic Coronary Artery Disease. Heart Disease. *7th ed. 2005.)*

References

1. Nesto RW, Kowalchuk GJ: The ischemic cascade: temporal sequence of hemodynamic, electrocardiographic and symptomatic expressions of ischemia, *Am J Cardiol* 59(7):23C–30C, 1987.
2. Sarnoff SJ, Braunwald E, Welch Jr GH, et al.: Hemodynamic determinants of oxygen consumption of the heart with special reference to the tension-time index, *Am J Physiol* 192(1):148–156, 1958.
3. Darling RCR: The effect of methemoglobin on the equilibrium between oxygen and hemoglobin, *Am J Physiol* 137:56–68, 1942.
4. Wilson RF, Wyche K, Christensen BV, et al.: Effects of adenosine on human coronary arterial circulation, *Circulation* 82(5):1595–1606, 1990.
5. Mosher P, Ross J Jr, McFate PA, et al.: Control of coronary blood flow by an autoregulatory mechanism, *Circ Res* 14:250–259, 1964.
6. Dole WP, Nuno DW: Myocardial oxygen tension determines the degree and pressure range of coronary autoregulation, *Circ Res* 59(2):202–215, 1986.
7. Jayaweera AR, Wei K, Coggins M, et al.: Role of capillaries in determining CBF reserve: new insights using myocardial contrast echocardiography, *Am J Physiol* 277(6 Pt 2):H2363–2372, 1999.
8. Borgquist R, Nilsson PM, Gudmundsson P, et al.: Coronary flow velocity reserve reduction is comparable in patients with erectile dysfunction and in patients with impaired fasting glucose or well-regulated diabetes mellitus, *Eur J Cardiovasc Prev Rehabil* 14(2):258–264, 2007.
9. Kamezaki F, Tasaki H, Yamashita K, et al.: Angiotensin receptor blocker improves coronary flow velocity reserve in hypertensive patients: comparison with calcium channel blocker, *Hypertens Res* 30(8):699–706, 2007.
10. Saraste A, Koskenvuo JW, Saraste M, et al.: Coronary artery flow velocity profile measured by transthoracic Doppler echocardiography predicts myocardial viability after acute myocardial infarction, *Heart* 93(4):456–457, 2007.
11. Tsagalou EP, Anastasiou-Nana M, Agapitos E, et al.: Depressed coronary flow reserve is associated with decreased myocardial capillary density in patients with heart failure due to idiopathic dilated cardiomyopathy, *J Am Coll Cardiol* 52(17):1391–1398, 2008.
12. Egashira K, Inou T, Hirooka Y, et al.: Effects of age on endothelium-dependent vasodilation of resistance coronary artery by acetylcholine in humans, *Circulation* 88(1):77–81, 1993.
13. Ciftci FC, Caliskan M, Ciftci O, et al.: Impaired coronary microvascular function and increased intima-media thickness in preeclampsia, *J Am Soc Hypertens* 8(11):820–826, 2014.
14. Al Suwaidi J, Higano ST, Holmes DR Jr, et al.: Obesity is independently associated with coronary endothelial dysfunction in patients with normal or mildly diseased coronary arteries, *J Am Coll Cardiol* 37(6):1523–1528, 2001.
15. Arbab-Zadeh A, Levine BD, Trost JC, et al.: The effect of acute hypoxemia on coronary arterial dimensions in patients with coronary artery disease, *Cardiology* 113(2):149–154, 2009.
16. Wyss CA, et al.: Influence of altitude exposure on coronary flow reserve, *Circulation* 108(10):1202–1207, 2003.
17. Fujimoto K, Hozumi T, Watanabe H, et al.: Acute hyperglycemia induced by oral glucose loading suppresses coronary microcirculation on transthoracic Doppler echocardiography in healthy young adults, *Echocardiography* 23(10):829–834, 2006.
18. Ichiki H, Hamasaki S, Nakasaki M, et al.: Relationship between hyperglycemia and coronary vascular resistance in non-diabetic patients, *Int J Cardiol* 141(1):44–48, 2010.
19. Beckman JA, Creager MA, Libby P: Diabetes and atherosclerosis: epidemiology, pathophysiology, and management, *JAMA* 287(19):2570–2581, 2002.
20. Williams SB, Cusco JA, Roddy MA, et al.: Impaired nitric oxide-mediated vasodilation in patients with non-insulin-dependent diabetes mellitus, *J Am Coll Cardiol* 27(3):567–574, 1996.
21. Johnstone MT, Creagor SJ, Scales KM, et al.: Impaired endothelium-dependent vasodilation in patients with insulin-dependent diabetes mellitus, *Circulation* 88(6):2510–2516, 1993.
22. Trovati M, Massucco P, Mattiello L, et al.: The insulin-induced increase of guanosine-3',5'-cyclic monophosphate in human platelets is mediated by nitric oxide, *Diabetes* 45(6):768–770, 1996.
23. Shige H, Ishikawa T, Suzukawa M, et al.: Endothelium-dependent flow-mediated vasodilation in the postprandial state in type 2 diabetes mellitus, *Am J Cardiol* 84(10):1272–1274, 1999. A9.
24. Christlieb AR, Janka HU, Kraus B, et al.: Vascular reactivity to angiotensin II and to norepinephrine in diabetic subjects, *Diabetes* 25(4):268–274, 1976.
25. Uemura S, Matsushita H, Li W, et al.: Diabetes mellitus enhances vascular matrix metalloproteinase activity: role of oxidative stress, *Circ Res* 88(12):1291–1298, 2001.
26. Crystal GJ: Carbon dioxide and the heart: physiology and clinical implications, *Anesth Analg* 121(3):610–623, 2015.
27. Case RB, Felix A, Wachter M, et al.: Relative effect of CO_2 on canine coronary vascular resistance, *Circ Res* 42(3):410–418, 1978.
28. Powers ER, Bannerman KS, Fitz-James I, et al.: Effect of elevations of coronary artery partial pressure of carbon dioxide (Pco_2) on coronary blood flow, *J Am Coll Cardiol* 8(5):1175–1181, 1986.
29. Agullo L, Garcia-Dorado D, Escalona N, et al.: Hypoxia and acidosis impair cGMP synthesis in microvascular coronary endothelial cells, *Am J Physiol Heart Circ Physiol* 283(3):H917–925, 2002.
30. London MJ, Sybert PE, Mangano DT, et al.: Surface-induced hypothermia: effects on coronary blood flow autoregulation and vascular reserve, *J Surg Res* 45(5):481–495, 1988.
31. Jacobshagen C, Pelster T, Pax A, et al.: Effects of mild hypothermia on hemodynamics in cardiac arrest survivors and isolated failing human myocardium, *Clin Res Cardiol* 99(5):267–276, 2010.
32. Straub A, Krajewski S, Hohmann JD, et al.: Evidence of platelet activation at medically used hypothermia and mechanistic data indicating ADP as a key mediator and therapeutic target, *Arterioscler Thromb Vasc Biol* 31(7):1607–1616, 2011.
33. Kannel WB, Castelli WP, Gordon T, et al.: Serum cholesterol, lipoproteins, and the risk of coronary heart disease. The Framingham study, *Ann Intern Med* 74(1):1–12, 1971.
34. Multiple Risk Factor Intervention Trial. Risk factor changes and mortality results. Multiple Risk Factor Intervention Trial Research Group, *JAMA* 248(12):1465–1477, 1982.
35. Cannon CP, Braunwald E, McCabe CH, et al.: Intensive versus moderate lipid lowering with statins after acute coronary syndromes, *N Engl J Med* 350(15):1495–1504, 2004.
36. Schwartz GG, Olsson AG, Ezekowitz MD, et al.: Effects of atorvastatin on early recurrent ischemic events in acute coronary syndromes: the MIRACL study: a randomized controlled trial, *JAMA* 285(13):1711–1718, 2001.
37. Steinbrecher UP, Parthasarathy S, Leake DS, et al.: Modification of low density lipoprotein by endothelial cells involves lipid peroxidation and degradation of low density lipoprotein phospholipids, *Proc Natl Acad Sci U S A* 81(12):3883–3887, 1984.
38. Steinberg D, Parthasarathy S, Carew TE, et al.: Beyond cholesterol. Modifications of low-density lipoprotein that increase its atherogenicity, *N Engl J Med* 320(14):915–924, 1989.
39. McNeill E, Channon KM, Greaves DR: Inflammatory cell recruitment in cardiovascular disease: murine models and potential clinical applications, *Clin Sci (Lond)* 118(11):641–655, 2010.
40. Ivan L, Antohe F: Hyperlipidemia induces endothelial-derived foam cells in culture, *J Recept Signal Transduct Res* 30(2):106–114, 2010.
41. Dunn FG, McLenachan J, Isles CG, et al.: Left ventricular hypertrophy and mortality in hypertension: an analysis of data from the Glasgow Blood Pressure Clinic, *J Hypertens* 8(8):775–782, 1990.
42. Dunn FG, Pringle SD: Left ventricular hypertrophy and myocardial ischemia in systemic hypertension, *Am J Cardiol* 60(17):19I–22I, 1987.
43. Murphy BP, Stanton T, Dunn FG: Hypertension and myocardial ischemia, *Med Clin North Am* 93(3):681–695, 2009.
44. Rakugi H, Yu H, Kamitani A, et al.: Links between hypertension and myocardial infarction, *Am Heart J* 132(1 Pt 2 Su):213–221, 1996.
45. Yamani MH, Massie BM: Hypertension, myocardial ischemia, and sudden death, *Curr Opin Cardiol* 9(5):542–550, 1994.
46. Kranzhofer R, Schmidt J, Pfeiffer CA, et al.: Angiotensin induces inflammatory activation of human vascular smooth muscle cells, *Arterioscler Thromb Vasc Biol* 19(7):1623–1629, 1999.
47. Kranzhofer R, Browatzki M, Schmidt J, et al.: Angiotensin II activates the proinflammatory transcription factor nuclear factor-kappaB in human monocytes, *Biochem Biophys Res Commun* 257(3):826–828, 1999.
48. Fukai T, Siegfried MR, Ushio-Fukai M, et al.: Modulation of extracellular superoxide dismutase expression by angiotensin II and hypertension, *Circ Res* 85(1):23–28, 1999.

49. Nitenberg A, Antony I, Aptecar E, et al.: Impairment of flow-dependent coronary dilation in hypertensive patients. Demonstration by cold pressor test induced flow velocity increase, *Am J Hypertens* 8(5 Pt 2):13S–18S, 1995.
50. Panza JA, Casino PR, Kilcoyne CM, et al.: Role of endothelium-derived nitric oxide in the abnormal endothelium-dependent vascular relaxation of patients with essential hypertension, *Circulation* 87(5):1468–1474, 1993.
51. Panza JA, Quyyumi AA, Brush JE Jr, et al.: Abnormal endothelium-dependent vascular relaxation in patients with essential hypertension, *N Engl J Med* 323(1):22–27, 1990.
52. Antony I, Lerebours G, Nitenberg A: Loss of flow-dependent coronary artery dilatation in patients with hypertension, *Circulation* 91(6):1624–1628, 1995.
53. Schmidt DH, Weiss MB, CAsarella WJ, et al.: Regional myocardial perfusion during atrial pacing in patients with coronary artery disease, *Circulation* 53(5):807–819, 1976.
54. Wilson JR, Martin JL, Untereker WJ, et al.: Sequential changes in regional coronary flow during pacing-induced angina pectoris: coronary flow limitation precedes angina, *Am Heart J* 107(2):269–277, 1984.
55. Hochman JS: Cardiogenic shock complicating acute myocardial infarction: expanding the paradigm, *Circulation* 107(24):2998–3002, 2003.
56. Menon V, Hochman JS: Management of cardiogenic shock complicating acute myocardial infarction, *Heart* 88(5):531–537, 2002.
57. Menon V, Slater JN, White HD, et al.: Acute myocardial infarction complicated by systemic hypoperfusion without hypotension: report of the SHOCK trial registry, *Am J Med* 108(5):374–380, 2000.
58. Hollenberg SM, Kavinsky CJ, Parrillo JE: Cardiogenic shock, *Ann Intern Med* 131(1):47–59, 1999.
59. Gabbay FH, Krantz DS, Kop WJ, et al.: Triggers of myocardial ischemia during daily life in patients with coronary artery disease: physical and mental activities, anger and smoking, *J Am Coll Cardiol* 27(3):585–592, 1996.
60. Gould KL, Lipscomb K, Hamilton GW: Physiologic basis for assessing critical coronary stenosis. Instantaneous flow response and regional distribution during coronary hyperemia as measures of coronary flow reserve, *Am J Cardiol* 33(1):87–94, 1974.
61. Marcus ML, Doty DB, Hiratzka LF, et al.: Decreased coronary reserve: a mechanism for angina pectoris in patients with aortic stenosis and normal coronary arteries, *N Engl J Med* 307(22):1362–1366, 1982.
62. Rajappan K, Rimoldi OE, Dutka DP, et al.: Mechanisms of coronary microcirculatory dysfunction in patients with aortic stenosis and angiographically normal coronary arteries, *Circulation* 105(4):470–476, 2002.
63. Segal J, Harvey WP, Hufnagel C: A clinical study of one hundred cases of severe aortic insufficiency, *Am J Med* 21(2):200–210, 1956.
64. Nitenberg A, Foult JM, Antony I, et al.: Coronary flow and resistance reserve in patients with chronic aortic regurgitation, angina pectoris and normal coronary arteries, *J Am Coll Cardiol* 11(3):478–486, 1988.
65. Kisanuki A, Matsushita R, Murayama T, et al.: Transesophageal Doppler echocardiographic assessment of systolic and diastolic coronary blood flow velocities at baseline and during adenosine triphosphate-induced coronary vasodilation in chronic aortic regurgitation, *Am Heart J* 133(1):71–77, 1997.
66. Aksoy S, Cam N, Guney MR, et al.: Myocardial ischemia in severe aortic regurgitation despite angiographically normal coronary arteries, *Tohoku J Exp Med* 226(1):69–73, 2012.
67. Domenech RJ: Regional diastolic coronary blood flow during diastolic ventricular hypertension, *Cardiovasc Res* 12(11):639–645, 1978.
68. Kaul S: Depressed myocardial blood flow reserve in nonischemic dilated cardiomyopathy: findings and explanations, *J Am Soc Echocardiogr* 26(3):288–289, 2013.
69. Pasternac A, Noble J, Streulens Y, et al.: Pathophysiology of chest pain in patients with cardiomyopathies and normal coronary arteries, *Circulation* 65(4):778–789, 1982.
70. Cannon III RO, Rosing DR, Maron BJ, et al.: Myocardial ischemia in patients with hypertrophic cardiomyopathy: contribution of inadequate vasodilator reserve and elevated left ventricular filling pressures, *Circulation* 71(2):234–243, 1985.
71. Egashira K, Inou T, Hirooka Y, et al.: Evidence of impaired endothelium-dependent coronary vasodilatation in patients with angina pectoris and normal coronary angiograms, *N Engl J Med* 328(23):1659–1664, 1993.
72. Bottcher M, Botker HE, Sonne H, et al.: Endothelium-dependent and -independent perfusion reserve and the effect of L-arginine on myocardial perfusion in patients with syndrome X, *Circulation* 99(14):1795–1801, 1999.
73. Rinkevich D, Belcik T, Gupta NC, et al.: Coronary autoregulation is abnormal in syndrome X: insights using myocardial contrast echocardiography, *J Am Soc Echocardiogr* 26(3):290–296, 2013.
74. Emdin M, Picano E, Lattanzi F, et al.: Improved exercise capacity with acute aminophylline administration in patients with syndrome X, *J Am Coll Cardiol* 14(6):1450–1453, 1989.
75. Fabian E, Varga A, Picano E, et al.: Effect of simvastatin on endothelial function in cardiac syndrome X patients, *Am J Cardiol* 94(5):652–655, 2004.
76. Lanza GA, Colonna G, Pasceri V, et al.: Atenolol versus amlodipine versus isosorbide-5-mononitrate on anginal symptoms in syndrome X, *Am J Cardiol* 84(7):854–856, 1999. A8.
77. Pauly DF, Johnson BD, Anderson RD, et al.: In women with symptoms of cardiac ischemia, nonobstructive coronary arteries, and microvascular dysfunction, angiotensin-converting enzyme inhibition is associated with improved microvascular function: a double-blind randomized study from the National Heart Lung and Blood Institute Women's Ischemia Syndrome Evaluation (WISE), *Am Heart J* 162(4):678–684, 2011.
78. Mehta PK, Goykhman P, Thomson LE, et al.: Ranolazine improves angina in women with evidence of myocardial ischemia but no obstructive coronary artery disease, *JACC Cardiovasc Imaging* 4(5):514–522, 2011.

SECTION III

CLINICAL EVALUATION

7 History and Physical Examination

Jonathan R. Enriquez and Shailja V. Parikh

INTRODUCTION

Despite continuing technological advances in cardiovascular medicine, the history and physical examination remain vital to establish an accurate diagnosis of chronic coronary artery disease (CAD). Whereas many patients may describe typical angina, providers cannot rely on these symptoms alone to diagnose ischemia because silent (asymptomatic) ischemia remains a common presentation, estimated to affect almost half of patients with CAD.[1] Conversely, some patients may endorse symptoms that closely mimic typical angina in the absence of significant CAD.[2] Thus appropriate integration of patient symptoms, demographics, clinical characteristics, and examination findings remains essential for the clinician to accurately determine the likelihood or classification of CAD and to assess comorbidities and sequelae.

Positive interactions during the interview and examination can also lay the foundation for establishing a healthy doctor-patient relationship, critical to allowing the patient to freely share his/her experiences, goals, and preferences with the provider. Formation of such trust may also increase the likelihood of adherence to the treatment plan.[3] This is of particular importance in the treatment of chronic coronary disease, which frequently relies on a multitude of medications and therapeutic lifestyle changes to improve symptoms and survival. Thus the following discussion of history-taking and physical examination may have important diagnostic and therapeutic implications for chronic CAD.

HISTORY

Typical Angina Pectoris

Typical anginal pain is characterized by its location, quality, duration, and exacerbating/alleviating factors. Angina can be retrosternal or diffuse in the chest, but it can also be felt in regions corresponding to the C7 through T4 dermatomes (eg, neck, jaw, and arms) because the sympathetic afferent nerves that signal myocardial ischemia also innervate these territories.[4] Typical angina may be pressure-like, squeezing, or heavy in quality. It is usually not sharp or stabbing, pleuritic, or positional.[5] Although the classic Levine sign (in which the patient places his/her fist over the chest to describe anginal pain) is often discussed, in a contemporary population this gesture had a low sensitivity (6%) for the detection of angina in patients admitted with chest discomfort.[6] Angina typically lasts for minutes rather than seconds in duration, and it may be exacerbated by physical exertion or mental/emotional stress and alleviated by rest and/or nitroglycerin.[7,8]

Atypical and Nonanginal Symptoms

Symptoms that do not fit the above classic features of typical angina are often referred to as atypical. Three categories of typical, atypical, and nonanginal symptoms are frequently used for clinical simplification (Table 7.1).[8] However, it is important to note that the presence of typical angina alone does not confirm the presence of CAD; conversely, atypical or nonanginal features alone do not exclude the possibility of CAD.[9] Nonetheless, some features may increase or

TABLE 7.1 Clinical Classification of Chest Pain

Typical Angina	**Retrosternal** chest discomfort Increased with **exertion or emotional** stress Relief with **rest or nitroglycerin**
Atypical Angina	Exhibits **2** of the above features
Noncardiac Chest Pain	Exhibits **0 or 1** of the above features

(Adapted from Fihn SD Gardin JM, Abrams J, et al. 2012 ACCF/AHA/ACP/AATS/PCNA/SCAI/STS Guideline for the diagnosis and management of patients with stable ischemic heart disease: a report of the American College of Cardiology Foundation/American Heart Association Task Force on Practice Guidelines, and the American College of Physicians, American Association for Thoracic Surgery, Preventive Cardiovascular Nurses Association, Society for Cardiovascular Angiography and Interventions, and Society of Thoracic Surgeons. J Am Coll Cardiol. *2012;60: e44–e164.)*

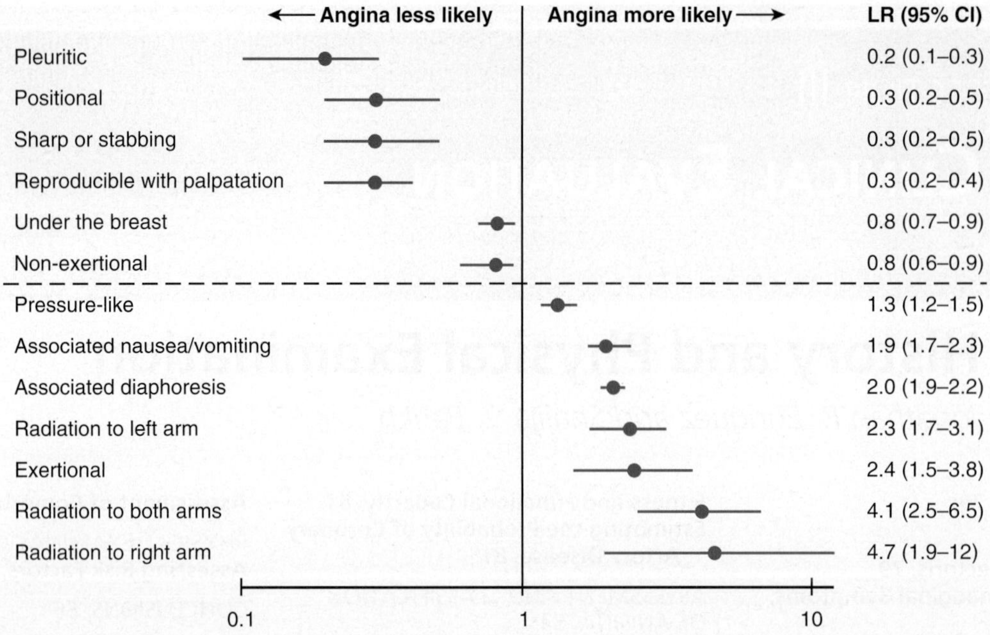

FIG. 7.1 Features of chest pain and likelihood of angina. Specific features of chest pain are listed to the *left* of the forest plot. Point estimates with 95% confidence intervals (CIs) depict likelihoods (LRs) of angina (logarithmic scale). Angina is indicated to be less likely to the left of unity and more likely to the right of unity. *(Data from Swap CJ, Nagurney JT. Value and limitations of chest pain history in the evaluation of patients with suspected acute coronary syndromes.* JAMA. *2005;294:2623–2629.)*

decrease the likelihood of chest pain being anginal in origin.[10,11] Symptoms and exam features with significant positive and negative likelihood ratios for angina are shown in Fig. 7.1.[12] Calculation of the posttest probability of CAD with likelihood ratios (LRs) is done as follows. First, estimate the pretest probability (P_{pre}) of CAD and convert the probability to odds (O_{pre}) with $O_{pre} = P_{pre}/(1 - P_{pre})$. Second, multiply that pretest odds (O_{pre}) of CAD by the LR to determine the posttest odds ($O_{post} = LR \times O_{pre}$). Finally, convert the posttest odds back to a probability, $P_{post} = O_{post}/(1 + O_{post})$.[13]

The LR with the lowest point estimate, making angina least likely, is pleuritic-type chest pain, followed by a positional component, pain being sharp/stabbing in quality, or reproducible with palpation. Angina is slightly less likely when pain is located under the breast or not associated with exertion. Although features such as association with exertion, radiation to the left arm, associated diaphoresis, nausea/vomiting, and pressure-like quality are classic/typical features of angina, these features did not lead to a large change in the probability of angina. Features with the highest LRs, which would theoretically most increase the probability of angina, were observed to be radiation to the right arm or both arms. Of note, the confidence intervals were wide for these latter two features, indicative of imprecision in the estimates of the LRs.

There are also other features of chest pain that have traditionally been accepted as useful in the differentiation of anginal versus nonanginal chest pain (eg, relief with nitroglycerin or gastrointestinal [GI] cocktails), but they may not have significant predictive value. In an analysis of 459 patients with chest pain at an urban teaching hospital, nitroglycerin relieved chest pain in 35% of patients who were found to have CAD as a cause of chest pain versus 41% of patients without CAD ($p > .20$). Similarly, relief of chest pain with a GI cocktail (often consisting of viscous lidocaine, an antacid, with/without other components) has also been documented to poorly differentiate symptoms of myocardial ischemia.[14,15] Some patients may not have chest pain during periods of ischemia, but instead only experience dyspnea or jaw, neck, or arm pain.[16] These symptoms without chest pain are often called *anginal equivalents*. Within each individual, specific anginal equivalents (ie, dyspnea, jaw pain, etc.) may characteristically recur with each subsequent episode of ischemia, and thus providers should inquire about similarities/differences to prior known anginal/ischemic episodes.

Gender Differences in Presentation

Historically, women have often been underrepresented in major clinical trials of CAD[17]; thus, characterization of CAD presentation in women has largely been derived from smaller analyses. However, compared with men, women have been reported to have higher prevalence of atypical chest pain features, including pain during rest, sleep, or mental stress, and associated neck/shoulder pain, nausea, fatigue, and dyspnea with ischemia.[17,18] The Women's Ischemic Syndrome Evaluation (WISE) study reported that as many as 65% of women with CAD may not exhibit "typical" anginal symptoms.[19] Some of these differences may be related to greater prevalence of coronary microvascular dysfunction, vasospasm, or heightened pain perception in women.[20,21] Further studies have suggested that gender differences in language or descriptors used may account for some of the reported differences in presentation, in that women may be more likely to describe their symptoms with other terms such as *discomfort*, *pressing*, *aching*, or *shortness of breath* when compared with men.[22,23]

Despite these reported gender differences, several studies have found that the presenting symptoms of CAD may be more similar than different between men and women.[23–25] In a meta-analysis of 74 studies involving more than 20,000 patients, women reported angina at a similar or slightly higher frequency than men did.[25] Even among many studies reporting gender differences in angina presentation, the most common descriptors used by both genders tended

TABLE 7.2 Probability of Coronary Artery Disease by Age, Gender, and Symptoms

AGE (YEARS)	NONANGINAL PAIN (%) Women	NONANGINAL PAIN (%) Men	ATYPICAL ANGINA (%) Women	ATYPICAL ANGINA (%) Men	TYPICAL ANGINA (%) Women	TYPICAL ANGINA (%) Men
30–39	5	18	10	29	28	59
40–49	8	25	14	38	37	69
50–59	12	34	20	49	47	77
60–69	17	44	28	59	58	84
70–79	24	54	37	69	68	89
>80	32	65	47	78	76	93

(Adapted from Genders TS, Steyerberg EW, Àlkadhi H, et al. A clinical prediction rule for the diagnosis of coronary artery disease: validation, updating, and extension. Eur Heart J. 2011;32(11):1316–1330.)

to be typical features such as "chest pain," "pressure," and "tightness."[22,23,26]

Fitness and Functional Capacity

Beyond inquiring about symptoms, assessing functional capacity during the history is important for assessing risk and prognosis. Multiple studies have confirmed a graded and inverse association between fitness level and mortality in patients with cardiovascular disease, independent of other risk factors. For example, in an analysis from the Duke database, patients who were able to exercise greater than 10 metabolic equivalents (METs) on a Bruce protocol without ischemia had 95% survival at 4 years; whereas those who could not achieve 4 METs had only 59% survival at 2 years.[27] In an analysis from the Veterans Affairs database, patients were divided into quintiles of exercise capacity. Patients in the lowest quintile of fitness (achieving <5 METs) had fourfold higher adjusted relative risk for mortality at 6 years compared with those in the highest quintile (>10.7 METs).[28] Furthermore, in an analysis of 9852 patients with known CAD from the Henry Ford Exercise Testing Project, each 1-MET increase in exercise capacity was associated with approximately 13% lower adjusted risk of mortality over the median follow-up of 11 years. Furthermore, patients with similar exercise capacity were found to have similar risk for mortality regardless of baseline revascularization status.[29]

Estimating the Probability of Coronary Artery Disease

Relying on the description of symptoms alone is insufficient to accurately diagnose CAD. Whereas a wide array of diagnostic testing modalities, including stress electrocardiography, echocardiography, myocardial perfusion imaging, magnetic resonance imaging, coronary computed tomography, and cardiac catheterization, are available, the indiscriminate application of these testing modalities can lead to potential misclassification of patients (as incorrectly having or not having CAD) due to imperfect test sensitivities/specificities. Moreover, mounting costs and risks for complications/adverse side effects of cardiac testing also remain important considerations. Therefore, prior to deciding on whether a diagnostic test should be used and/or selecting the most appropriate modality, providers must develop an estimate of the probability of CAD for each patient undergoing evaluation.

Categorizing symptoms into typical, atypical, and nonanginal pain can increase or decrease the likelihood of CAD; however, clinicians cannot accurately estimate the probability of CAD without first considering those symptoms in the context of the patient's age and gender. This concept was first illustrated by Diamond and Forrester in 1979[2] and was validated by similar findings from the Coronary Artery Surgery Study (CASS) trial.[30] The importance of age and gender in estimating the probability of CAD in a more contemporary multinational cohort is shown in Table 7.2. In patients presenting with typical anginal symptoms, the probability of significant CAD (>50% stenosis) can range from 28% to 93%, depending on age/gender. Likewise, the probability of CAD with nonanginal pain can range from 5% to 65%. Accordingly, many patients with nonanginal symptoms may still have higher probability for CAD than others with typical angina. For example, an 80-year-old man with *nonanginal* symptoms would have a 65% probability of CAD versus a 35-year-old woman with *typical angina* who would have a 28% probability of CAD (see Table 7.2).[31]

Incorporating comorbidities with age, gender, and symptoms can further improve determination of CAD probability. This was illustrated by investigators using the Duke Database of Cardiovascular Disease (Table 7.3).[8] For example, using Diamond–Forrester type classifications based on age/gender/symptoms alone, a 35-year-old man with typical angina would have a 59% probability of CAD; however, the likelihood of CAD would differ significantly between a healthy 35-year-old man with no cardiovascular risk factors and a 35-year-old man with diabetes, hyperlipidemia, and tobacco abuse. In the 35-year-old man with no risk factors, the probability of significant CAD (≥70% stenosis in a coronary artery) would be 30% versus 88% in the man with multiple risk factors. If patients had abnormal electrocardiograms at rest with significant ST- or T-wave changes or Q waves, probabilities of CAD would be higher.[32]

The Diamond-Forrester-type classifications and estimations from the Duke database can be of great utility in determining more precise probabilities of CAD; however, several limitations should be noted. These predictive models were developed from patients referred to university hospital settings; therefore, they may overestimate the probability of CAD for lower-risk primary care and/or community medical center populations. Additionally, these models may be less precise and overestimate probabilities of CAD in women when compared with the much lower prevalence of CAD observed in women in the WISE study.[33] Furthermore, these probabilities were derived from eras (the 1970s and 1980s) when risk factor burdens significantly differed from contemporary populations who have significantly less tobacco use, higher prevalence of obesity and diabetes, and higher prevalence of CAD in younger individuals.[31] Finally, these

TABLE 7.3 Probability of Coronary Artery Disease by Age, Gender, and Comorbidities

AGE (YEARS)	NONANGINAL PAIN (%) Women	NONANGINAL PAIN (%) Men	ATYPICAL ANGINA (%) Women	ATYPICAL ANGINA (%) Men	TYPICAL ANGINA (%) Women	TYPICAL ANGINA (%) Men
35	1–19	3–35	2–39	8–59	10–78	30–88
45	2–22	9–47	5–43	21–70	20–79	51–92
55	4–21	23–59	10–47	45–79	38–82	80–95
65	9–29	49–69	20–51	71–86	56–84	93–97

(Adapted from Fihn SD, Gardin JM, Abrams J, et al. 2012 ACCF/AHA/ACP/AATS/PCNA/SCAI/STS Guideline for the diagnosis and management of patients with stable ischemic heart disease: a report of the American College of Cardiology Foundation/American Heart Association Task Force on Practice Guidelines, and the American College of Physicians, American Association for Thoracic Surgery, Preventive Cardiovascular Nurses Association, Society for Cardiovascular Angiography and Interventions, and Society of Thoracic Surgeons. J Am Coll Cardiol. *2012;60:e44–e164.)*

reported probabilities tend to overestimate the prevalence of CAD across all age groups and genders when compared with studies that assess the prevalence of CAD by coronary computed tomographic angiography (CTA). This may be due to probability estimates traditionally being derived from patients undergoing clinically indicated evaluation with invasive cardiac catheterization (often after abnormal stress test results) who are more likely to have disease versus low- to intermediate-risk patients preferentially referred for noninvasive testing.[34]

ASSESSMENT AND CLASSIFICATION OF ANGINA

Assessment and classification of angina, including chronicity, severity, and burden of disease, are vital to determining the most appropriate treatment strategy. For example, one must ensure that an acute coronary syndrome is not present prior to instituting a treatment plan solely geared toward chronic stable CAD. Additionally, adequate assessment of the burden of symptoms and impairment in quality of life is necessary to tailor therapies to achieve adequate relief of symptoms.

Unstable angina is defined as angina that is new in onset, increasing in frequency, severity, or duration, or occurs at rest. A classification system of unstable angina was devised by Braunwald[35]; however, chronic stable angina is most often categorized by the Canadian Cardiovascular Society (CCS) classification system (Table 7.4), ranging from class 1 angina occurring only with strenuous, rapid, or prolonged exertion to class 4 angina with inability to do any activity without symptoms and/or angina at rest.[36]

As patients are often concerned with optimizing quality of life beyond longevity alone, further assessment of symptom-burden and health-related quality of life can be beneficial to understand the impact of CAD on patients' lives and to assess response to therapies.[37] Clinicians can use semiobjective quantitative measures such as how often the patient requires sublingual nitroglycerin and/or approximate walking distance achieved (eg, two blocks, 0.5 miles) before stopping due to angina. General health-related quality of life may be measured by survey instruments such as the Medical Outcomes Study 36-Item Short Form Health Survey (SF-36)[38]; whereas the Seattle Angina Questionnaire (SAQ)[39] is an example of a disease-specific quality of life instrument for CAD.

Historically, such surveys have been primarily used in research settings; however, with the advent of abbreviated survey versions[40] and a growing emphasis on patient-centered outcomes in clinical medicine,[41] there is potential for expanded use of such measures in clinical practice to supplement traditional history-taking for symptom assessment. The shortened version of the SAQ is a seven-question survey that can be completed at or prior to an office visit and may potentially improve efficiency of care. With the same questions asked the same way every time, the clinician may have more reproducible patient-centered data to aid clinical decision-making and potentially improve quality of care and health status.[40] Poorer health status in the SAQ domains of physical limitation, angina frequency, and quality of life is also associated with graded increases in risk for mortality and rehospitalization for acute coronary syndrome (Fig. 7.2).[42]

TABLE 7.4 Canadian Cardiovascular Society (CCS) Classifications of Angina

CCS CLASS	DESCRIPTION (SUMMARY)
I	Angina with strenuous, rapid, or prolonged exertion
II	Slight limitation of ordinary activity
III	Marked limitation of ordinary activity, such as walking 1 to 2 blocks or climbing 1 flight of stairs
IV	Angina at rest

(Adapted from Campeau L. Grading of angina pectoris [letter]. Circulation. *1976;54:522–523.*

Silent Ischemia and Infarction

A notable challenge in taking a history for chronic CAD is that significant CAD may be present without *any* associated symptoms or physical findings present. This phenomenon, described as silent myocardial ischemia or silent infarction, has been detected by various modalities including continuous ambulatory electrocardiographic monitoring, exercise tolerance testing, and stress imaging techniques (see Chapter 29, Screening for CAD in Asymptomatic Individuals). Silent ischemia has been described in asymptomatic individuals with and without known CAD.

Among asymptomatic individuals in the general population with no known CAD, the prevalence of silent ischemia has been estimated at 2% to 3%[43,44]; however, prevalence increases significantly with age and cardiovascular risk factors. In asymptomatic, apparently healthy individuals from the Baltimore Longitudinal Study of Aging, the prevalence of silent ischemia markedly increased with age, with evidence of silent ischemia present in less than 3% of those under 60 years of age but greater than 15% of those above 80 years of age.[45] In patients with diabetes, the risk of silent ischemia is particularly high. In a multicenter Italian study of 1899 asymptomatic diabetic patients less than or equal to 60 years of age, silent ischemia was present in at least 39%.[46] Silent ischemia/infarction can also occur in patients

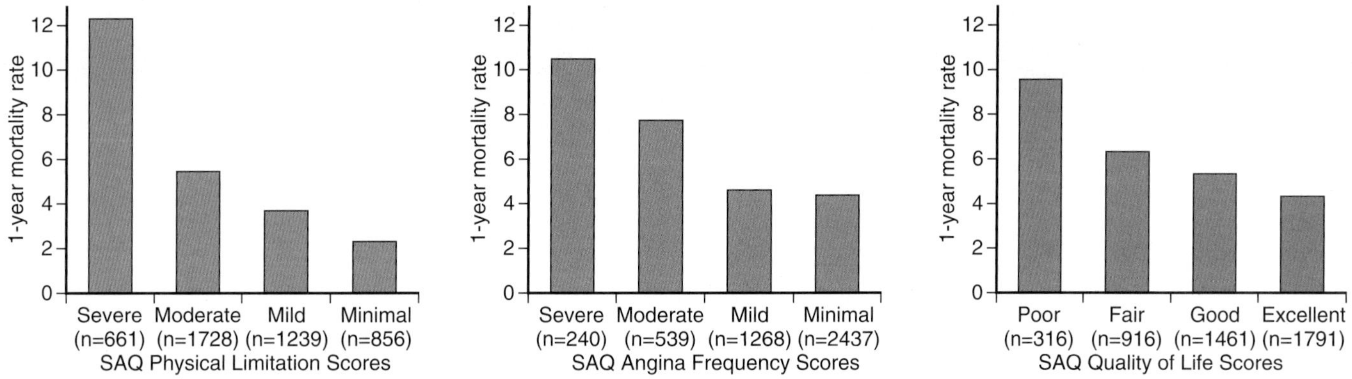

FIG. 7.2 One-year outcomes by Seattle Angina Questionnaire (SAQ) scores. Poorer health status in the domains of Physical Limitation, Angina Frequency, and Quality of Life is associated with graded increases in risk for 1-year mortality with coronary artery disease. *(Adapted from Spertus JA, Jones P, McDonell M, et al. Health status predicts long-term outcome in outpatients with coronary disease.* Circulation. *2002;106:43–49.)*

with a prior history of CAD and myocardial infarction. Approximately 30% to 43% of patients with prior myocardial infarction or angina have been reported to have silent ischemia.[1] Whereas it is estimated that almost half of patients with existing angina may have concomitant silent ischemia, with the application of adequate antiischemic therapies this may drop to approximately one-fourth to one-third of patients.[1]

Assessment of Comorbidities

Beyond assessing the patient's symptoms and functional capacity as previously described, it is also important to include in the history-taking an assessment of comorbidities and sequelae of chronic CAD to optimize secondary prevention therapy. The presence of traditional cardiovascular risk factors, such as history of hypertension, hyperlipidemia, diabetes mellitus, tobacco abuse, and dietary/exercise habits, should be inquired about and documented. Once these modifiable risk factors are identified, the clinician may then be able to address and potentially mitigate risk of future cardiovascular events. Global risk assessment for patients *without* known cardiovascular disease can be performed with the aid of various risk assessment tools, such as the 2013 American College of Cardiology/American Heart Association atherosclerotic cardiovascular disease (ASCVD) risk model, the Multi-Ethnic Study of Atherosclerosis (MESA) risk score, the Reynold risk score, or others.[47–49] For patients *with* chronic CAD or other atherosclerotic cardiovascular disease, global risk assessment models are not as well developed and the implications for clinical care are not as clear because these patients already have indications for secondary prevention medications (see Chapter 27 for discussion of global risk assessment in patients with Chronic CAD).

Potential sequelae of chronic CAD should be assessed during the history-taking. Symptoms such as dyspnea, orthopnea, paroxysmal nocturnal dyspnea, and edema may suggest congestive heart failure from left ventricular dysfunction. Palpitations or syncope may suggest atrial or ventricular arrhythmias. The prevalence of peripheral vascular disease in patients with CAD has been estimated to be two to three times higher versus those without CAD[50]; thus, inquiring about symptoms of claudication and cerebrovascular disease is important for comprehensive cardiovascular assessment.

PHYSICAL EXAMINATION

Whereas carotid, renal, or peripheral limb arterial stenoses can at times be detected on physical exam via ausculation and/or palpation, unfortunately, coronary stenoses cannot be detected in the same manner due to slower coronary artery filling predominantly occurring in diastole.[51] Thus, physical examination for chronic CAD is focused on asssessing risk factors and monitoring for sequelae of CAD. Notable risk factors, complications, and comorbidities of chronic coronary disease that should be assessed on physical examination are discussed hereafter (Table 7.5).

Assessing Risk Factors

Hypertension and Obesity

An accurate measurement of blood pressure requires that the patient rest for 5 minutes, and when the blood pressure is measured, s/he has both feet on the floor, legs uncrossed, back supported, and the arm maintained at the level of the heart.[52] Blood pressure should be measured in both arms. A disparity of 15 mm Hg or more is often due to subclavian artery stenosis and associated with increased risk for peripheral arterial disease, cerebrovascular disease, and cardiovascular death (hazard ratio 1.7, 95% confidence interval [CI], 1.1–2.5).[53] Body weight should be measured and weight indexed to height (kg/m^2) for calculation of the body mass index (BMI). Obesity is most often defined by a BMI greater than 30 kg/m^2; however, other metrics such as waist circumference and waist/hip ratio may also have clinical utility, as measures of central or visceral adiposity have been described to be predictors of cardiovascular risk beyond weight alone (see Chapter 19, Obesity and CAD). Although the relationship between obesity and CAD is nuanced, it is generally recommended to monitor and address obesity in the treatment of chronic CAD.[8]

Dyslipidemia

Several physical findings have been associated with dyslipidemia. Cutaneous xanthomas (and xanthelasma on the eyelids) are localized collections of lipid deposits within the skin, often associated with underlying lipid abnormalities (Figs. 7.3 and Fig. 7.4).[54,55] Correction of underlying dyslipidemia may at times result in improvement of xanthomas. Achilles tendon xanthomas have been reported to be a pathognomonic finding for familial hypercholesterolemia.

TABLE 7.5 Key Physical Examination Findings in Chronic Coronary Artery Disease

GOAL	CATEGORY	FINDINGS/COMMENTS
Assessing risk factors	Blood pressure	>15 mm Hg arm blood pressure disparity = increased risk for peripheral arterial disease (PAD) and cardiovascular death
	Weight	Body mass index >30 kg/m^2 = obesity
	Lipid abnormalities	Cutaneous xanthomas Xanthelasma on the eyelids Corneal arcus
	Diabetes mellitus	Acanthosis nigricans Skin tags
	Tobacco abuse and chronic obstructive pulmonary disease (COPD)	Odor of tobacco Staining of teeth, fingers, or nails Premature skin wrinkling Prolonged expiration, wheezing, distant breath sounds
	Miscellaneous	Ear lobe creases (Frank sign)
Assessing for complications	Congestive heart failure	Jugular venous distention, S_3, S_4, displaced point of maximal impulse, hepatomegaly, pulmonary/peripheral edema Ischemic mitral regurgitation Low-output cardiac failure
	Arrhythmias	Ectopy, atrial fibrillation
	PAD	Carotid bruits Peripheral pulses Peripheral skin discoloration or hair loss
Assessing for other causes of angina and dyspnea	Aortic stenosis	Late peaking systolic murmur Pulsus parvus et tardus
	Hypertrophic cardiomyopathy	Harsh crescendo-decrescendo systolic murmur dynamic with provocation
	Pulmonary hypertension	Loud P2, right S4, TR murmur, RV lift/heave

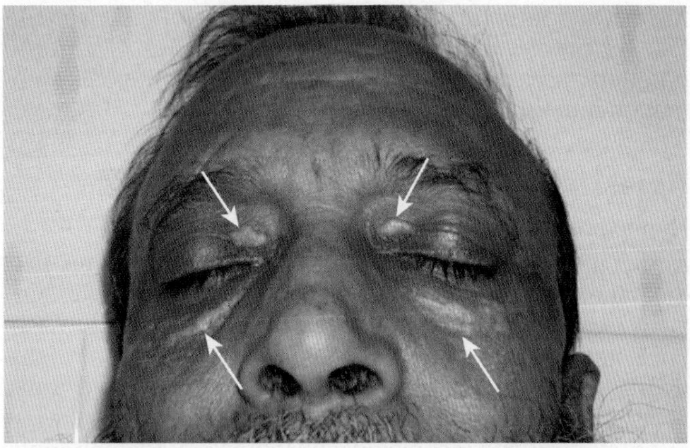

FIG. 7.3 Xanthelasma on bilateral upper and lower eyelids indicative of underlying lipid abnormalities. *(Reproduced from Dwivedi S, Jhamb R. Cutaneous markers of coronary artery disease.* World J Cardiol. *2010;2:262–269.)*

Moreover, the presence and degree of Achilles tendon xanthoma and width have been reported to correlate with risk of cardiovascular disease.[56,57]

Corneal arcus is a deposition of lipid-rich material in the peripheral cornea, which can be directly visualized without slit-lamp examination (Fig. 7.5). Corneal arcus may be indicative of dyslipidemia and has also been postulated to be a marker of atherosclerosis in some small studies; however, larger and more rigorous analyses, such as the Framingham Heart Study, which included more than 23,000 person-exams, found no significant increased risk for adverse cardiovascular events after adjustment for age and gender (hazard ratio, 1.17; 95% CI, 0.94–1.47, $p = .16$).[58,59]

Diabetes Mellitus and Insulin Resistance

Acanthosis nigricans is a darkening and thickening (pigmented hyperkeratosis) of the skin usually occurring on the neck and flexor surfaces (Fig. 7.6). It is most often associated with obesity and insulin resistance, although malignancy and other syndromes are also rare causes.[60] Weight loss may improve acanthosis in obese patients. Skin tags, also called *acrochordons*, are benign pedunculated growths commonly occurring on the neck, axillae, and groin, and are associated with diabetes and metabolic abnormalities. In a case-control comparison of individuals matched for age, gender, and BMI, the presence of three or more skin tags was associated with a threefold greater prevalence of diabetes mellitus (23.1% vs 8.5%, $p = .005$) compared with those without skin tags.[61] When compared with acanthosis nigricans, the presence of multiple skin tags (eight or more) may be more sensitive (although less specific) in identifying patients with insulin resistance and abnormal glucose metabolism.[62]

Tobacco Abuse and Chronic Obstructive Pulmonary Disease

As continued tobacco abuse increases risk for recurrent cardiovascular events and patients may at times attempt to conceal tobacco use,[63] detecting findings suggestive of tobacco use can identify an opportunity to reinforce the importance of cessation/abstaining to reduce risk. Nicotine staining on the teeth, fingers and/or nails, an odor of tobacco, or premature wrinkling of the skin may suggest current/former tobacco abuse. Furthermore, chronic obstructive pulmonary disease (COPD) has been reported to be a risk factor for cardiovascular mortality, independent of tobacco abuse.[64] Examination findings of prolonged expiration, wheezing, and distant breath sounds may suggest underlying COPD.[65]

Miscellaneous Physical Findings

It is worth mentioning that ear lobe creases (Fig. 7.7), also known as *Frank sign*,[66] have been reported in several studies to be a potential marker of increased risk for chronic CAD.[67] In a 2014 meta-analysis of 37 studies including over 31,000 patients, the authors concluded that the presence of ear lobe creases demonstrated a pooled sensitivity of 62% (95% CI, 56–67%), specificity 67% (95% CI, 61–73%), and

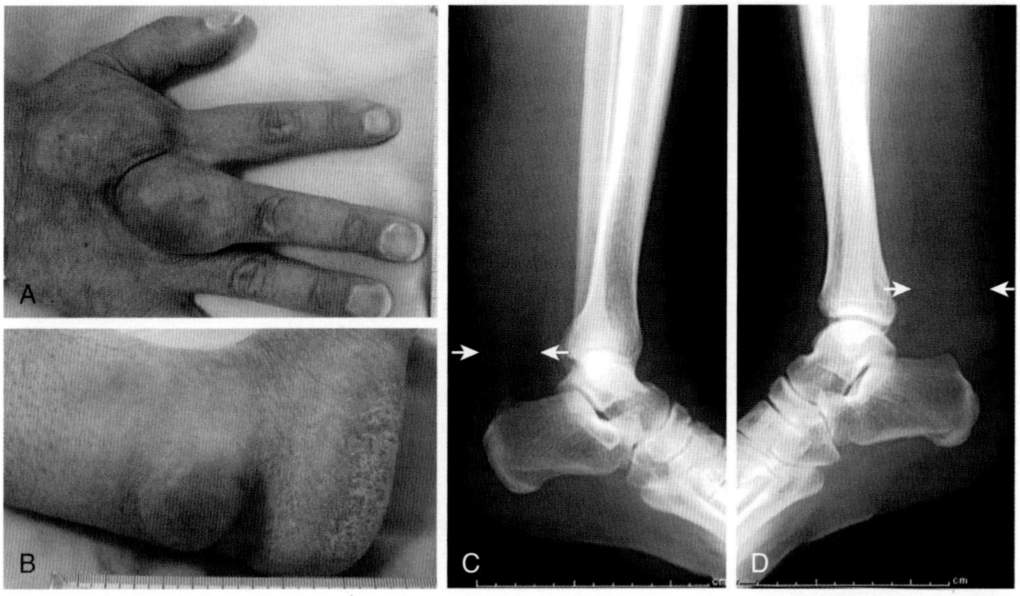

FIG. 7.4 Large tendon xanthomas on the hand **(A)** and Achilles tendon **(B)**, with radiographs (**C** and **D**) of the ankles showing severe Achilles tendon thickening in a patient with familial hyperlipidemia and severe coronary artery disease. *(Reproduced from Terasaki F, Morita H, Harada-Shiba M, et al. Familial hypercholesterolemia with multiple large tendinous xanthomas and advanced coronary artery atherosclerosis.* Intern Med. *2013;52(5):577–581.)*

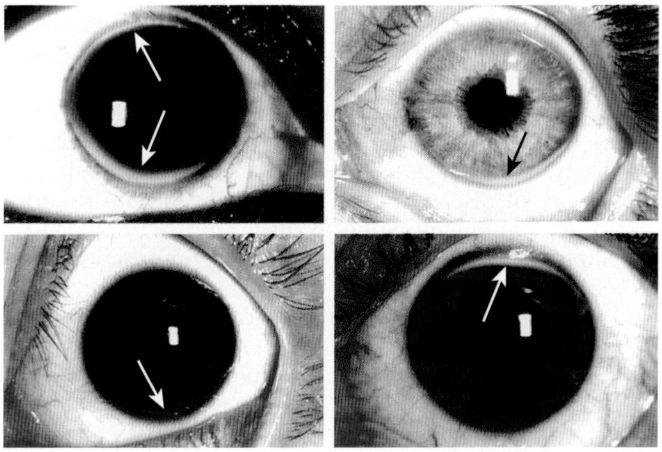

FIG. 7.5 Corneal arcus. Arcus deposits often begin at the 6 o'clock and 12 o'clock positions of the peripheral iris and progress circumferentially. *(Reproduced from Zech LA Jr, Hoeg JM. Correlating corneal arcus with atherosclerosis in familial hypercholesterolemia.* Lipids Health Dis. *2008;7:7.)*

odds ratio of 3.27 (95% CI, 2.47–4.32) for the presence of CAD.[68] The potential mediators of this association are not well understood. The prevalence of ear lobe creases and CAD both increase with age and diabetes; however, even after adjustment for demographics and traditional risk factors, ear lobe creases have been reported in some analyses to be independently associated with CAD.[66] Prior investigators have speculated that a mirrored atherosclerotic process may occur in both vascular beds. In the earlobes, it has been postulated that these vascular changes may lead to premature destruction of elastic fibers, which results in the formation of visible creases.[66]

Heart Failure

In an analysis of multicenter systolic heart failure trials between 1986 and 2005 including more than 25,000 patients, CAD was the cause of heart failure in 62% of patients.[69] CAD may also be a contributor in up to two-thirds of patients with diastolic heart failure[70]; thus examining for signs of heart failure is imperative in patients with CAD. Examination should include assessment for jugular venous distention, S_3 and S_4, displacement of the point of maximal impulse, hepatomegaly, and pulmonary/peripheral edema. Chronic CAD can also lead to heart failure by chronic ischemic

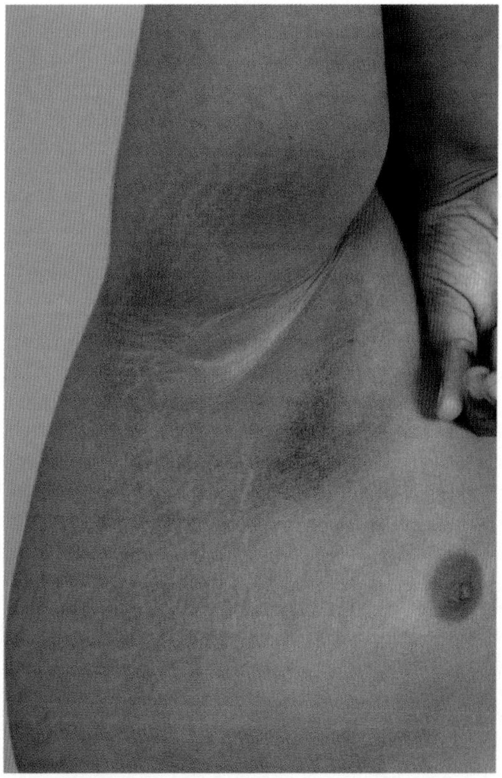

FIG. 7.6 Acanthosis nigricans in the axilla. Acanthosis is associated with insulin resistance and diabetes mellitus. *(From Couper J, Jones TW. Diabetes In: South M, ed: Practical Paediatrics, 7th ed. London: Elsevier Ltd. 2012;687–695.)*

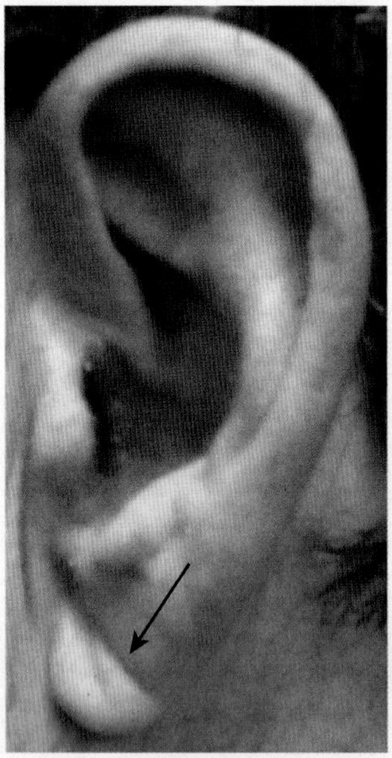

FIG. 7.7 Ear lobe crease, also called *Frank sign*, a potential marker of increased risk for coronary artery disease. *(Reproduced from Shmilovich H, Cheng VY, Rajani R, et al. Relation of diagonal ear lobe crease to the presence, extent, and severity of coronary artery disease determined by coronary computed tomography angiography.* Am J Cardiol. *2012;109:1283–1287.)*

mitral regurgitation, which is often appreciated as a holosystolic murmur radiating to the apex or axilla on auscultation. Regardless of the mechanism of heart failure in chronic CAD, the examiner should be vigilant for the development of advanced heart failure with low cardiac output and poor perfusion, manifested by hypotension, narrow pulse pressure, resting tachycardia, and cool extremities, which portends a grave prognosis if not urgently addressed.

Arrhythmias

A wide variety of atrial and ventricular arrhythmias, including premature ventricular contractions, atrial fibrillation, ventricular tachycardia/fibrillation, varying degrees of heart block, and others, may be seen in chronic ischemic heart disease. Examination findings of irregularities in the rhythm or severe bradycardia or tachycardia should prompt further evaluation, usually with a 12-lead electrocardiogram as the subsequent step.

Cardiac Auscultation and Palpation

Because aortic stenosis, hypertrophic cardiomyopathy, and pulmonary hypertension may all present with angina and dyspnea as the initial symptoms, it is also important to auscultate and palpate for evidence of these conditions. Severe aortic valve stenosis classically demonstrates a mid- to late-peaking systolic murmur radiating to the carotids with pulsus parvus et tardus and a soft A2. Hypertrophic cardiomyopathy may exhibit a harsh crescendo-decrescendo systolic murmur that increases with Valsalva or rising to standing and diminishes with squatting due to dynamic left ventricular outflow tract obstruction. A second murmur of mitral regurgitation from systolic anterior motion of the mitral valve may also be appreciated. Patients with pulmonary arterial hypertension may have a loud P2, a right-sided S_4, a murmur of tricuspid regurgitation, or a right ventricular lift/heave on palpation of the chest.[71]

Peripheral Arterial Disease

Coronary and peripheral arterial disease frequently coexist with approximately 15% to 40% of patients having concomitant diseases.[72] Thus, it remains important to examine for evidence of noncoronary atherosclerosis in patients with chronic CAD. Carotid arteries should be auscultated to assess for bruits, which are associated with increased risk for atherosclerotic cardiovascular events, although not necessarily specific for a focal stenosis in the auscultated territory.[73] Abdominal palpation alone should not be relied on to diagnose or exclude the presence of aortic aneurysm because sensitivity/specificity are inadequate.[74] The peripheral pulses (eg, radial, femoral, dorsalis pedis, posterior tibialis) should be palpated. Diminished pulses, as well as skin discoloration, hair loss, or mottled appearance of the skin, may signify peripheral arterial disease.

CONCLUSIONS

During the history and physical examination, the provider has a daunting task of collecting and sorting through a potential plethora of subjective information and physical findings to form an accurate assessment of the presence, severity, comorbidities, and complications of CAD, while simultaneously working to build the patient-provider relationship. Each encounter presents unique challenges and opportunities from both the physician and patient perspectives, with increasing constraints from time and technology in many contemporary healthcare settings. Using established prediction tools that integrate demographics and symptoms, with or without risk factors, along with provider knowledge of the predictive value of various symptoms, will likely allow for greater accuracy in the estimation of probability of disease, rather than relying on the description of typical angina alone to diagnose CAD. Assessment of symptom-burden, functional capacity, comorbidities, and monitoring for complications during the history and physical exam are prerequisite elements for the development of a comprehensive treatment plan to optimize quality of life and outcomes in patients with chronic CAD.

References

1. Cohn PF, Fox KM, Daly C: Silent myocardial ischemia, *Circulation* 108:1263–1277, 2003.
2. Diamond GA, Forrester JS: Analysis of probability as an aid in the clinical diagnosis of coronary-artery disease, *N Engl J Med* 300:1350–1358, 1979.
3. Kerse N, Buetow S, Mainous III AG, et al.: Physician-patient relationship and medication compliance: a primary care investigation, *Ann Fam Med* 2:455–461, 2004.
4. Crea F, Gaspardone A, Kaski JC, et al.: Relation between stimulation site of cardiac afferent nerves by adenosine and distribution of cardiac pain: results of a study in patients with stable angina, *J Am Coll Cardiol* 20:1498–1502, 1992.
5. Lee TH, Cook EF, Weisberg M, et al.: Acute chest pain in the emergency room. Identification and examination of low-risk patients, *Arch Intern Med* 145:65–69, 1985.
6. Marcus GM, Cohen J, Varosy PD, et al.: The utility of gestures in patients with chest discomfort, *Am J Med* 120:83–89, 2007.
7. Deanfield JE, Shea M, Kensett M, et al.: Silent myocardial ischaemia due to mental stress, *Lancet* 2:1001–1005, 1984.
8. Fihn SD, Gardin JM, Abrams J, et al.: 2012 ACCF/AHA/ACP/AATS/PCNA/SCAI/STS Guideline for the diagnosis and management of patients with stable ischemic heart disease: a report of the American College of Cardiology Foundation/American Heart Association Task Force on Practice Guidelines, and the American College of Physicians, American Association for Thoracic Surgery, Preventive Cardiovascular Nurses Association, Society for Cardiovascular Angiography and Interventions, and Society of Thoracic Surgeons, *J Am Coll Cardiol* 60:e44–e164, 2012.
9. Canto JG, Fincher C, Kiefe CI, et al.: Atypical presentations among Medicare beneficiaries with unstable angina pectoris, *Am J Cardiol* 90:248–253, 2002.
10. Amsterdam EA, Wenger NK, Brindis RG, et al.: 2014 AHA/ACC Guideline for the Management of Patients with Non-ST-Elevation Acute Coronary Syndromes: a report of the American College of Cardiology/American Heart Association Task Force on Practice Guidelines, *J Am Coll Cardiol* 64:e139–228, 2014.
11. Henrikson CA, Howell EE, Bush DE, et al.: Chest pain relief by nitroglycerin does not predict active coronary artery disease, *Ann Intern Med* 139:979–986, 2003.
12. Swap CJ, Nagurney JT: Value and limitations of chest pain history in the evaluation of patients with suspected acute coronary syndromes, *JAMA* 294:2623–2629, 2005.
13. McGee S: Simplifying likelihood ratios, *J Gen Intern Med* 17:646–649, 2002.
14. Servi RJ, Skiendzielewski JJ: Relief of myocardial ischemia pain with a gastrointestinal cocktail, *Am J Emerg Med* 3:208–209, 1985.

15. Wrenn K, Slovis CM, Gongaware J: Using the "GI cocktail": a descriptive study, *Ann Emerg Med* 26:687–690, 1995.
16. Arnold JR: Blockpnea and silent myocardial ischemia, *Am J Cardiol* 90:346, 2002.
17. Douglas PS, Ginsburg GS: The evaluation of chest pain in women, *N Engl J Med* 334:1311–1315, 1996.
18. Tamura A, Naono S, Torigoe K, et al.: Gender differences in symptoms during 60-second balloon occlusion of the coronary artery, *Am J Cardiol* 111:1751–1754, 2013.
19. Pepine CJ, Balaban RS, Bonow RO, et al.: Women's Ischemic Syndrome Evaluation: current status and future research directions: report of the National Heart, Lung and Blood Institute workshop: October 2–4, 2002: Section 1: diagnosis of stable ischemia and ischemic heart disease, *Circulation* 109:e44–e46, 2004.
20. Cannon III RO, Camici PG, Epstein SE: Pathophysiological dilemma of syndrome X, *Circulation* 85:883–892, 1992.
21. Kaski JC, Rosano GM, Collins P, et al.: Cardiac syndrome X: clinical characteristics and left ventricular function. Long-term follow-up study, *J Am Coll Cardiol* 25:807–814, 1995.
22. Philpott S, Boynton PM, Feder G, et al.: Gender differences in descriptions of angina symptoms and health problems immediately prior to angiography: the ACRE study. Appropriateness of Coronary Revascularisation study, *Soc Sci Med* 52:1565–1575, 2001.
23. Kreatsoulas C, Shannon HS, Giacomini M, et al.: Reconstructing angina: cardiac symptoms are the same in women and men, *JAMA Intern Med* 173:829–831, 2013.
24. Canto JG, Goldberg RJ, Hand MM, et al.: Symptom presentation of women with acute coronary syndromes: myth vs reality, *Arch Intern Med* 167:2405–2413, 2007.
25. Hemingway H, Langenberg C, Damant J, et al.: Prevalence of angina in women versus men: a systematic review and meta-analysis of international variations across 31 countries, *Circulation* 117:1526–1536, 2008.
26. Kimble LP, McGuire DB, Dunbar SB, et al.: Gender differences in pain characteristics of chronic stable angina and perceived physical limitation in patients with coronary artery disease, *Pain* 101:45–53, 2003.
27. McNeer JF, Margolis JR, Lee KL, et al.: The role of the exercise test in the evaluation of patients for ischemic heart disease, *Circulation* 57:64–70, 1978.
28. Myers J, Prakash M, Froelicher V, et al.: Exercise capacity and mortality among men referred for exercise testing, *N Engl J Med* 346:793–801, 2002.
29. Hung RK, Al-Mallah MH, McEvoy JW, et al.: Prognostic value of exercise capacity in patients with coronary artery disease: the FIT (Henry Ford ExercIse Testing) project, *Mayo Clin Proc* 89: 1644–1654, 2014.
30. Chaitman BR, Bourassa MG, Davis K, et al.: Angiographic prevalence of high-risk coronary artery disease in patient subsets (CASS), *Circulation* 64:360–367, 1981.
31. Genders TS, Steyerberg EW, Alkadhi H, et al.: A clinical prediction rule for the diagnosis of coronary artery disease: validation, updating, and extension, *Eur Heart J* 32:1316–1330, 2011.
32. Pryor DB, Harrell Jr FE, Lee KL, et al.: Estimating the likelihood of significant coronary artery disease, *Am J Med* 75:771–780, 1983.
33. Shaw LJ, Bairey Merz CN, Pepine CJ, et al.: Insights from the NHLBI-Sponsored Women's Ischemia Syndrome Evaluation (WISE) Study: Part I: gender differences in traditional and novel risk factors, symptom evaluation, and gender-optimized diagnostic strategies, *J Am Coll Cardiol* 47: S4–S20, 2006.
34. Cheng VY, Berman DS, Rozanski A, et al.: Performance of the traditional age, sex, and angina typicality-based approach for estimating pretest probability of angiographically significant coronary artery disease in patients undergoing coronary computed tomographic angiography: results from the multinational coronary CT angiography evaluation for clinical outcomes: an international multicenter registry (CONFIRM), *Circulation* 124:2423–2432, 2011. 1–8.
35. Braunwald E: Unstable angina. A classification, *Circulation* 80:410–414, 1989.
36. Campeau L: Grading of angina pectoris [letter], *Circulation* 54:522–523, 1976.
37. Thompson DR, Yu CM: Quality of life in patients with coronary heart disease—I: assessment tools, *Health Qual Life Outcomes* 1:42, 2003.
38. Ware Jr JE, Sherbourne CD: The MOS 36-item short-form health survey (SF-36). I. Conceptual framework and item selection, *Medical Care* 30:473–483, 1992.
39. Spertus JA, Winder JA, Dewhurst TA, et al.: Development and evaluation of the Seattle Angina Questionnaire: a new functional status measure for coronary artery disease, *J Am Coll Cardiol* 25:333–341, 1995.
40. Chan PS, Jones PG, Arnold SA, et al.: Development and validation of a short version of the Seattle Angina Questionnaire, *Circ Cardiovasc Qual Outcomes* 7:640–647, 2014.
41. Barry MJ, Edgman-Levitan S: Shared decision making—pinnacle of patient-centered care, *N Engl J Med* 366:780–781, 2012.
42. Spertus JA, Jones P, McDonell M, et al.: Health status predicts long-term outcome in outpatients with coronary disease, *Circulation* 106:43–49, 2002.
43. Froelicher VF, Thompson AJ, Longo Jr MR, et al.: Value of exercise testing for screening asymptomatic men for latent coronary artery disease, *Prog Cardiovasc Dis* 18:265–276, 1976.
44. Thaulow E, Erikssen J, Sandvik L, et al.: Initial clinical presentation of cardiac disease in asymptomatic men with silent myocardial ischemia and angiographically documented coronary artery disease (the Oslo Ischemia Study), *Am J Cardiol* 72:629–633, 1993.
45. Fleg JL, Gerstenblith G, Zonderman AB, et al.: Prevalence and prognostic significance of exercise-induced silent myocardial ischemia detected by thallium scintigraphy and electrocardiography in asymptomatic volunteers, *Circulation* 81:428–436, 1990.
46. Scognamiglio R, Negut C, Ramondo A, et al.: Detection of coronary artery disease in asymptomatic patients with type 2 diabetes mellitus, *J Am Coll Cardiol* 47:65–71, 2006.
47. Goff Jr DC, Lloyd-Jones DM, Bennett G, et al.: 2013 ACC/AHA guideline on the assessment of cardiovascular risk: a report of the American College of Cardiology/American Heart Association Task Force on Practice Guidelines, *Circulation* 129:S49–S73, 2014.
48. McClelland RL, Jorgensen NW, Budoff M, et al.: 10-year coronary heart disease risk prediction using coronary artery calcium and traditional risk factors: derivation in the MESA (Multi-Ethnic Study of Atherosclerosis) with validation in the HNR (Heinz Nixdorf Recall) Study and the DHS (Dallas Heart Study), *J Am Coll Cardiol* 66:1643–1653, 2015.
49. Ridker PM, Buring JE, Rifai N, et al.: Development and validation of improved algorithms for the assessment of global cardiovascular risk in women: the Reynolds Risk Score, *JAMA* 297:611–619, 2007.
50. Criqui MH, Denenberg JO, Langer RD, et al.: The epidemiology of peripheral arterial disease: importance of identifying the population at risk, *Vasc Med* 2:221–226, 1997.
51. Bache RJ, Cobb FR: Effect of maximal coronary vasodilation on transmural myocardial perfusion during tachycardia in the awake dog, *Circ Res* 41:648–653, 1977.
52. Pickering TG, Hall JE, Appel LJ, et al.: Recommendations for blood pressure measurement in humans and experimental animals: part 1: blood pressure measurement in humans: a statement for professionals from the Subcommittee of Professional and Public Education of the American Heart Association Council on High Blood Pressure Research, *Circulation* 111:697–716, 2005.
53. Clark CE, Taylor RS, Shore AC, et al.: Association of a difference in systolic blood pressure between arms with vascular disease and mortality: a systematic review and meta-analysis, *Lancet* 379:905–914, 2012.
54. Cruz Jr PD, East C, Bergstresser PR: Dermal, subcutaneous, and tendon xanthomas: diagnostic markers for specific lipoprotein disorders, *J Am Acad Dermatol* 19:95–111, 1988.
55. Dwivedi S, Jhamb R: Cutaneous markers of coronary artery disease, *World J Cardiol* 2:262–269, 2010.
56. Zech Jr LA, Hoeg JM: Correlating corneal arcus with atherosclerosis in familial hypercholesterolemia, *Lipids Health Dis* 7:7, 2008.
57. Oosterveer DM, Versmissen J, Yazdanpanah M, et al.: Differences in characteristics and risk of cardiovascular disease in familial hypercholesterolemia patients with and without tendon xanthomas: a systematic review and meta-analysis, *Atherosclerosis* 207:311–317, 2009.
58. Fernandez A, Sorokin A, Thompson PD: Corneal arcus as coronary artery disease risk factor, *Atherosclerosis* 193:235–240, 2007.
59. Fernandez AB, Keyes MJ, Pencina M, et al.: Relation of corneal arcus to cardiovascular disease (from the Framingham Heart Study data set), *Am J Cardiol* 103:64–66, 2009.
60. Schilling WH, Crook MA: Cutaneous stigmata associated with insulin resistance and increased cardiovascular risk, *Int J Dermatol* 53:1062–1069, 2014.
61. Rasi A, Soltani-Arabshahi R, Shahbazi N: Skin tag as a cutaneous marker for impaired carbohydrate metabolism: a case-control study, *Int J Dermatol* 46:1155–1159, 2007.
62. Sudy E, Urbina F, Maliqueo M, et al.: Screening of glucose/insulin metabolic alterations in men with multiple skin tags on the neck, *J Dtsch Dermatol Ges* 6:852–855, 2008.
63. Stuber J, Galea S: Who conceals their smoking status from their health care provider? *Nicotine Tob Res* 11:303–307, 2009.
64. Sin DD, Wu L, Man SF: The relationship between reduced lung function and cardiovascular mortality: a population-based study and a systematic review of the literature, *Chest* 127: 1952–1959, 2005.
65. Broekhuizen BD, Sachs AP, Oostvogels R, et al.: The diagnostic value of history and physical examination for COPD in suspected or known cases: a systematic review, *Fam Pract* 26: 260–268, 2009.
66. Shmilovich H, Cheng VY, Rajani R, et al.: Relation of diagonal ear lobe crease to the presence, extent, and severity of coronary artery disease determined by coronary computed tomography angiography, *Am J Cardiol* 109:1283–1287, 2012.
67. Griffing G: Images in clinical medicine. Frank's sign, *N Engl J Med* 370:e15, 2014.
68. Lucenteforte E, Romoli M, Zagli G, et al.: Ear lobe crease as a marker of coronary artery disease: a meta-analysis, *Intl J Cardiol* 175:171–175, 2014.
69. Gheorghiade M, Sopko G, De Luca L, et al.: Navigating the crossroads of coronary artery disease and heart failure, *Circulation* 114:1202–1213, 2006.
70. Vasan RS, Benjamin EJ, Levy D: Prevalence, clinical features and prognosis of diastolic heart failure: an epidemiologic perspective, *J Am Coll Cardiol* 26:1565–1574, 1995.
71. Colman R, Whittingham H, Tomlinson G, et al.: Utility of the physical examination in detecting pulmonary hypertension. A mixed methods study, *PloS One* 9, 2014: e108499.
72. Dieter RS, Tomasson J, Gudjonsson T, et al.: Lower extremity peripheral arterial disease in hospitalized patients with coronary artery disease, *Vasc Med* 8:233–236, 2003.
73. Wolf PA, Kannel WB, Sorlie P, et al.: Asymptomatic carotid bruit and risk of stroke. The Framingham study, *JAMA* 245:1442–1445, 1981.
74. Lederle FA, Simel DL: The rational clinical examination. Does this patient have abdominal aortic aneurysm? *JAMA* 281:77–82, 1999.

8 Lipid Measurements

Anand Rohatgi

INTRODUCTION

Atheromatous plaque in arterial wall is the pathologic substrate for myocardial infarction and ischemic stroke and is intimately related to the deposition of oxidized lipids from the circulation into the subintimal space, initiating a vicious cycle of local inflammation, macrophage foam cell formation, and smooth muscle recruitment. The measurement of circulating lipids has led to significant improvements not only in understanding the pathophysiology of atherosclerotic cardiovascular disease (ASCVD) but also in improving risk prediction and management of ASCVD.

TRADITIONAL LIPOPROTEIN MEASUREMENTS

The three major classes of lipoproteins are low-density lipoprotein (LDL), very low-density lipoprotein (VLDL), and high-density lipoprotein (HDL).[1] Apolipoprotein B (apoB) is the main protein constituent of atherogenic lipoproteins, including LDL, VLDL, intermediate-density lipoprotein (IDL), lipoprotein(a), and chylomicrons, and it serves as the primary ligand for the LDL receptor and scavenger receptors in arterial macrophages and other tissues types. LDL cholesterol (LDL-C) is the most abundant apoB-containing lipid, accounting for 60% to 70% of the total serum cholesterol. VLDL consists of triglycerides and most of the remaining atherogenic apoB-containing cholesterol. IDL is similar to LDL and also contains apoB and triglycerides. Chylomicrons are very large particles that carry dietary cholesterol and triglycerides from the intestine to the liver. In contrast, HDL cholesterol (HDL-C) contains apolipoprotein A-I (apoA-I), which is considered atheroprotective, and makes up approximately 20% to 30% of the total serum cholesterol pool. Total cholesterol, HDL-C, and triglycerides are directly measured enzymatically, and LDL-C is typically calculated using the Friedewald formula (Fig. 8.1).[2] The overall burden of atherogenic lipoproteins can be assessed as non-HDL-C, calculated by simply subtracting HDL-C from total cholesterol (see Fig. 8.1).[3]

Total and Low-Density Lipoprotein Cholesterol

Genetic and intervention studies in humans reveal an overwhelming consistency in the relationship between LDL-C (or total cholesterol) levels and both incident ASCVD in those free of ASCVD and recurrent events in those with established ischemic heart disease (Fig. 8.2).[4,5] Studies have revealed an absence of atheromatous plaques and clinically evident coronary disease in populations where LDL-C is maintained under 100 mg/dL (2.6 mmol/L) (or total cholesterol < 150 mg/dL [3.9 mmol/L]).[6] LDL-C levels above 190 mg/dL (4.9 mmol/L) suggest a genetic disorder such as familial hypercholesterolemia and increased short-term ASCVD risk.[7] Total cholesterol is directly measured and was the primary lipid studied in the original cholesterol investigations. Current American and European ASCVD risk algorithms use total cholesterol as the measure of atherogenic lipoprotein.[3,7] Total and LDL-C levels can be lowered by a variety of interventions, including reduced dietary intake of trans and saturated fats, increased dietary intake of soluble fiber, and pharmacotherapies such as statins, bile acid sequestrants, nicotinic acid, cholesterol absorption inhibitors, and proprotein convertase subtilisin kexin type 9 (PCSK9) inhibitors (Table 8.1).[8]

High-Density Lipoprotein Cholesterol

HDL-C is the other major lipid used in validated risk scoring algorithms. Observational studies show consistent relationships between low HDL-C (< 40 mg/dL) (1 mmol/L) and increased ASCVD risk (Fig. 8.3).[9] HDL-C levels have a significant inherited component and are typically higher in women and in those of African descent. Low HDL-C levels are associated with smoking, insulin resistance, hypertriglyceridemia, and physical inactivity. Low HDL-C is one of the five components of the metabolic syndrome and is often part of a lipid triad that includes high triglycerides and small dense LDL particles.[10] HDL-C levels below 40 mg/dL (1 mmol/L) in men and below 50 mg/dL (1.3 mmol/L) in women are considered major ASCVD risk markers; however there is insufficient evidence to support raising HDL-C as a treatment target.[3,7] Lifestyle interventions that are associated with increases in HDL-C include smoking cessation, weight loss, reduced carbohydrate consumption, increased physical activity, and moderate alcohol consumption.[8] Nicotinic acid is the most potent clinically available pharmacotherapy that raises HDL-C levels, with differential and weaker effects seen after administration of fibrates and statins (see Table 8.1).[19] However, as noted

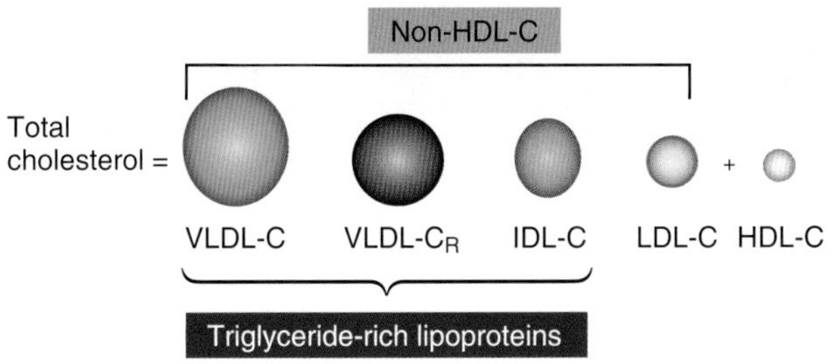

LDL-C = Total cholesterol – HDL-C – Triglyceride/5 (Friedewald)

Non-HDL-C = Total cholesterol – HDL-C

FIG. 8.1 Calculation of low-density lipoprotein cholesterol (LDL-C), and non-high-density lipoprotein cholesterol (HDL-C). In the Friedewald formula for calculating LDL-C, triglycerides are divided by 5 if using mg/dL and by 2.22 if using mmol/L. *(Data from Friedewald WT, Levy RI, Fredrickson DS. Estimation of the concentration of low-density lipoprotein cholesterol in plasma, without use of the preparative ultracentrifuge.* Clin Chem. *1972;18(6):499–502 and Grundy SM, Cleeman JI, Merz CN, et al. Implications of recent clinical trials for the National Cholesterol Education Program Adult Treatment Panel III guidelines.* Circulation. *2004;110:227–239.)*

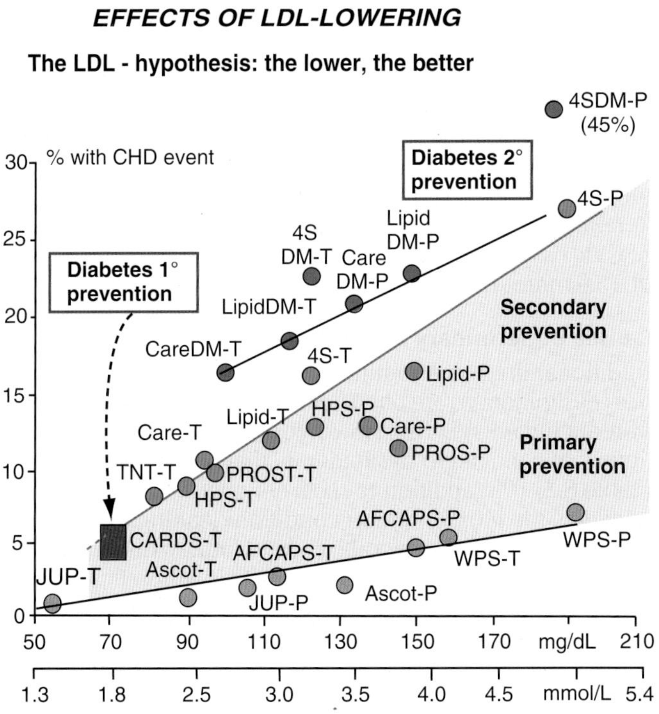

FIG. 8.2 The log-linear relationship of low-density lipoprotein cholesterol (LDL-C) and coronary heart disease from statin trials. *CPPT,* Coronary Primary Prevention Trial; *FHS,* Framingham Health Study; *LRCP,* Lipid Research Clinics Prevalence Mortality Follow-Up Study; *MRFIT,* Multiple Risk Factor Intervention Trial. *CHD,* Coronary heart disease. *(Figure Opie LH, 2012; modified from Fisher M. Diabetes and atherogenesis.* Heart. *2004;90:336–340 by addition of new trials. As modified in Opie LH, Gersh BJ.* Drugs for the Heart. *8th ed. Philadelphia: Elsevier; 2013:411.)*

above, raising HDL-C has not been proven to be a valid therapeutic approach to improve ASCVD outcomes.[33–34]

Triglycerides

Triglycerides are fatty acids that contain most of the fat stored by the body and are derived from dietary sources and metabolism of fat depots. A fasting triglyceride level above 150 mg/dL (1.7 mmol/L) is considered dyslipidemia and is a component of the metabolic syndrome. Hypertriglyceridemia is defined as a fasting level above 200 mg/dL (2.3 mmol/L) and is associated with increased ASCVD risk.[11] Increasing triglyceride levels reflect enrichment of circulating levels of triglyceride-rich lipoproteins; of which VLDL is the most common, followed by IDL and chylomicrons.[11]

The relationship between hypertriglyceridemia and ASCVD risk has been controversial. Adjustment for HDL-C and non-HDL-C levels partially attenuates the association between triglyceride levels and incident events in some but not all studies.[11] In contrast, Mendelian randomization studies suggest that triglyceride-rich lipoproteins or their remnants are causally related to increased risk of ischemic heart disease.[12–15] Elevated triglyceride levels are associated with an atherogenic dyslipidemia comprised of cholesterol enrichment of triglyceride-rich lipoproteins, increased small dense LDL particles, and low HDL-C, which may also contribute to the increased risk seen with hypertriglyceridemia, especially among those with metabolic syndrome or diabetes.[16] Lastly, the increased ASCVD risk seen with elevated triglycerides seems to be disproportionately higher in women than in men.[16,17]

Triglyceride levels can rise significantly following a fatty meal; therefore it is usually recommended to measure fasting triglyceride levels; however nonfasting triglyceride levels above 200 mg/dL (2.3 mmol/L) are also associated with increased risk and may be a better predictor than fasting levels (Fig. 8.4).[18] In fact, several of the Mendelian randomization studies mentioned above assessed nonfasting triglyceride levels and demonstrated causality with incident ischemic heart disease. Elevations in nonfasting triglycerides reflect increased exposure to atherogenic triglyceride-rich lipoproteins in the circulation.

Hypertriglyceridemia, like low HDL-C, is also seen with hyperglycemia and increased insulin resistance, obesity, alcohol intake, physical inactivity, and carbohydrate intake. When triglyceride levels are above 400 mg/dL (4.5 mmol/L), the levels of triglyceride-rich lipoproteins such as VLDL and IDL are elevated and the calculated LDL-C is not valid. Therefore, non-HDL-C should be calculated (see the section on non-HDL-C) when triglycerides are above 200 to 400 mg/dL (2.3 to 4.5 mmol/L).[3,19]

Fibrates, high-dose nicotinic acid, and high-dose omega-3 fatty acids are the most potent triglyceride-lowering agents (see Table 8.1).[19] Most other lipid-lowering drug classes modestly lower triglyceride levels, with the exception of bile acid sequestrants, which can raise levels. The evidence to support targeting triglyceride levels to reduce ASCVD risk is inconsistent.[16] In two randomized controlled trials, adding fenofibrate to statin therapy did not improve outcomes compared with statin alone in the overall trial populations,[19a,19b] but did show a benefit in the subgroups defined by high triglyceride and low HDL-C at baseline.[19c] Monotherapy with gemfibrozil in high-risk patients improved outcomes,[19d] but a meta-analysis of all fibrate trials revealed no improvement in cardiovascular mortality and a nonsignificant trend toward increased noncardiovascular deaths.[20] The evidence for nicotinic acid is remarkably similar to that of fibrates: older studies without statin background therapy suggested benefit but more contemporary trials with background statin therapy have been negative.[16] Similar to the fibrate trials, subgroups defined by high triglyceride and low HDL-C seemed to benefit from high-dose nicotinic acid.[16] Omega-3 fatty acids have been studied using various formulations and various doses of the active ingredients.[16] A randomized controlled trial in Japanese patients showed improvement in a composite ASCVD endpoint in those allocated to pure ethyl ester in addition to

TABLE 8.1 Interventions Affecting Lipid Levels

LIPID-MODIFYING THERAPIES	LDL-C	NON-HDL-C	HDL-C	TRIGLYCERIDES	LP(a)
Statins	↓ 18–55%	↓ 15–51%	↑ 5–15%	↓ 7–30%	↔
Bile-acid sequestrants	↓ 15–30%	↓ 4–16%	↑ 3–5%	↑ 0–10%	
Cholesterol absorption inhibitors	↓ 13–20%	↓ 14–19%	↑ 3–5%	↓ 5–11%	
PCSK9 inhibitors	↓ 61–62%	↓ 52%	↑ 5–7%	↓ 12–17%	↓ 25%
ApoB antisense	↓ 25–37%		↑ 2–15%	↓ 9–26%	↓ 21–33%
MTP inhibitor	↓ 44–50%	↓ 44–50%	↓ 12–↑1%	↓ 29–45%	↓ 15–19%
Nicotinic acid	↓ 5–25%	↓ 8–23%	↑ 15–35%	↓ 20–50%	↓ 20–40%
Fibric acids	↓ 5–↑20%	↓ 5–19%	↑ 10–20%	↓ 20–50%	
Long-chain omega-3 fatty acids	↓6–↑25%	↓5–14%	↓ 5–↑7%	↓ 19–44%	

HDL-C, high-density lipoprotein cholesterol; *LDL-C*, low-density lipoprotein cholesterol; *Lp*, lipoprotein; *MTP*, microsomal triglyceride transfer protein; *PCSK9*, proprotein convertase subtilisin kexin type 9.
Adapted from Jacobson TA, Ito MK, Maki KC, et al. National Lipid Association recommendations for patient-centered management of dyslipidemia: part 1 — executive summary. J Clin Lipidol. *2014;8(5):473–488.*

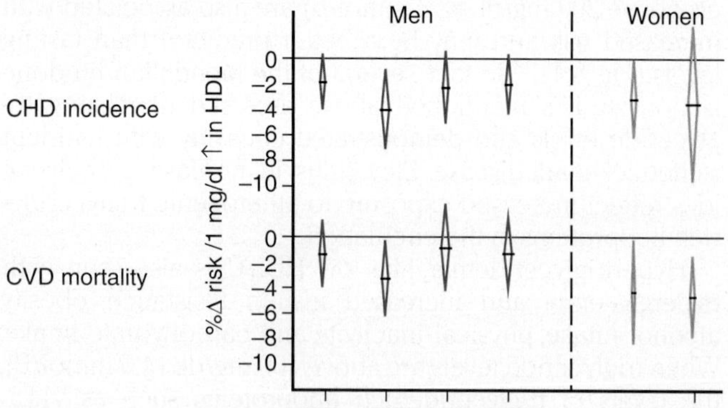

FIG. 8.3 High-density lipoprotein (HDL) cholesterol and coronary heart disease (CHD) risk. Results from four American cohorts. *CPPT*, Coronary Primary Prevention Trial; *CVD*, cardiovascular disease; *FHS*, Framingham Health Study; *LRCF*, Lipid Research Clinics Prevalence Mortality Follow-Up Study; *MRFIT*, Multiple Risk Factor Intervention Trial. *(Adapted from Gordon DJ, Probstfield JL, Garrison RJ, et al. High-density lipoprotein cholesterol and cardiovascular disease. Four prospective American studies.* Circulation. *1989;79:8–15.)*

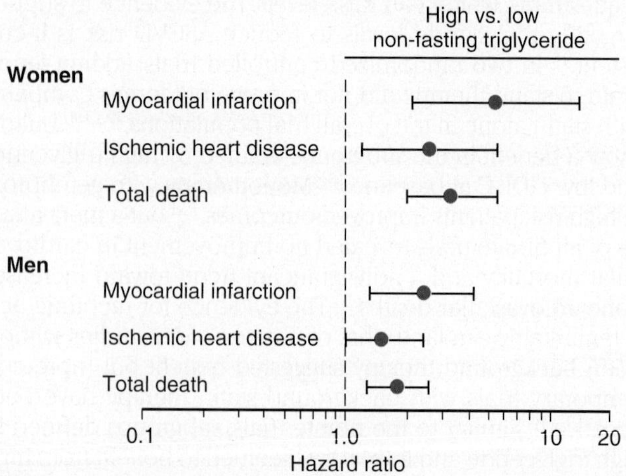

FIG. 8.4 Nonfasting triglyceride levels and incident cardiovascular events. Hazard ratios and 95% confidence intervals displayed for nonfasting triglyceride levels > 442 mg/dL (5 mmol/L) versus < 88.5 mg/dL (1 mmol/L). *(Data from Nordestgaard BG, Benn M, Schnohr P, et al. Nonfasting triglycerides and risk of myocardial infarction, ischemic heart disease, and death in men and women.* JAMA. *2007;298(3):299–308.)*

background statin therapy, with a magnified effect in those with high triglyceride and low HDL-C.[16] However, a subsequent meta-analysis of omega-3 fatty acids failed to show a consistent improvement in any cardiovascular endpoint.[21] Ongoing randomized trials of high-dose omega-3 fatty acids among those with elevated triglycerides and ASCVD risk will provide more direct guidance on the role of omega-3 therapies in reducing triglycerides to reduce ASCVD risk. Regardless of ASCVD risk, triglyceride levels should be kept below 500 mg/dL (5.6 mmol/L) to avoid the risk of pancreatitis.[11]

Causes of Secondary Dyslipidemia

Traditional lipids are routinely measured and abnormal values (dyslipidemia) are often acted upon directly with the goal of reducing ASCVD risk. However, there are common conditions that can lead to dyslipidemia that should be evaluated (Table 8.2).[19] In addition to diets enriched in trans and saturated fats, the most common conditions leading to increased LDL-C levels include hypothyroidism, kidney disease, menopause, and medications including thiazide diuretics, fibrates, and glucocorticoids. With respect to triglycerides, in addition to diets with high glycemic loads, other common conditions leading to elevated levels include excess alcohol intake, diabetes, nephrotic syndrome, β-blockers, hormone replacement therapy, atypical antipsychotic drugs, and other conditions that also raise LDL-C levels (see Table 8.2). Addressing these causes first can often lead to improvements or resolution of the dyslipidemias without lipid-modifying therapies.

Non-High-Density Lipoprotein Cholesterol

Non-HDL-C is calculated easily by subtracting HDL-C from total cholesterol and represents the cholesterol in all apoB-containing atherogenic lipoproteins, including LDL, VLDL, and IDL (see Fig. 8.1).[3,19] Typically, thresholds for defining treatment and goals for non-HDL-C are 30 mg/dL (0.77 mmol/L) higher than those for LDL-C; therefore ideal non-HDL-C levels are below 130 mg/dL (3.3 mmol/L) for primary prevention. Non-HDL-C predicts ASCVD risk similarly or better than LDL-C (Fig. 8.5).[22] In contrast to calculated LDL-C, non-HDL-C is not sensitive to elevated triglycerides and can be measured in the nonfasting state; therefore it is a better measure of atherogenic lipids in those with elevated triglyceride levels

TABLE 8.2 Causes of Secondary Dyslipidemia

	ELEVATED LDL-C	ELEVATED TRIGLYCERIDES	LOW HDL-C
Diseases			
Hypothyroidism	+	+	+
Chronic kidney disease	+	+	+
Nephrotic syndrome	+	+	+
Autoimmune disorders	+	+	+
Menopause	+	+	+
Polycystic ovary syndrome	+	+	
Pregnancy	+	+	
HIV infection	+	+	+
Obstructive liver disease	+		
Diabetes		+	+
Metabolic syndrome		+	+
Excessive alcohol intake		+	
Drugs			
Thiazide diuretics	+	+	
Glucocorticoids	+	+	
Anabolic steroids	+		+
Fibric acids	+		
Omega-3 fatty acids containing docosahexanoic acid	+		
Thiazolidinediones	+	+ (rosiglitazone only)	
Immunosuppressive drugs	+	+	
Oral estrogens		+	
Tamoxifen		+	
Raloxifene		+	
Retinoids		+	
β-blockers		+	+
Atypical antipsychotics		+	
Protease inhibitors		+	
Bile acid sequestrants		+	
Cyclophosphamide		+	

HDL-C, high-density lipoprotein cholesterol; *HIV,* human immunodeficiency virus; *LDL-C,* low-density lipoprotein cholesterol.
Adapted from Jacobson TA, Ito MK, Maki KC, et al. National Lipid Association recommendations for patient-centered management of dyslipidemia: part 1 — executive summary. J Clin Lipidol. *2014;8(5):473–488.*

(~ above 200 mg/dL; 2.3 mmol/L). Elevations in non-HDL-C reflect increasing levels of atherogenic remnant lipoproteins and often occur with worsening hyperglycemia and insulin resistance, obesity, physical inactivity, and increased carbohydrate and alcohol intake. Lastly, non-HDL-C is significantly associated with ASCVD risk among those on statins as well as among those at high risk[22]; therefore non-HDL-C is an easy measure of residual risk that can be lowered by intensifying lifestyle change and/or lipid-lowering therapy.

MEASUREMENT OF ADVANCED LIPOPROTEINS

Apolipoprotein B and Apolipoprotein A-I

ApoB and apoA-I levels are most commonly measured by the vertical auto profile (VAP) or by nuclear magnetic resonance (NMR) spectroscopy, but they can also be measured with immunoassay. There is significant variability among the tests; apolipoprotein levels are highest using immunoassays and lowest using VAP.[23] ApoB is carried by all atherogenic lipoproteins in a 1:1 fashion such that every LDL, VLDL, and IDL particle contains one apoB lipoprotein.[19] Thus it is the most direct measure of atherogenic lipoproteins but is not part of routine laboratory assessment. Like non-HDL-C, apoB levels are not affected by the nonfasting state or by hypertriglyceridemia. Maintaining levels below 80 to 90 mg/dL is recommended for patients with ASCVD who are taking lipid-lowering therapy.[3,19] ApoB levels consistently outperform LDL-C in risk prediction, whereas direct comparisons with non-HDL-C are mixed.[1] Among patients on lipid-lowering therapies, the relationship between atherogenic cholesterol and apoB changes, such that there are larger decreases in cholesterol than apoB. However, given that assays measuring apoB have not been standardized, and non-HDL-C performs as well or almost as well as apoB and is not associated with additional cost, it remains unclear what role apoB measurement should play in ASCVD risk prediction or management. In summary, given that LDL-C and non-HDL-C are part of routine laboratory assessments and inexpensive to measure, the added value of apoB measurements is probably too small to merit the cost.

ApoA-I is the main protein carried by HDL particles and is considered to have antiatherogenic properties by participating in the removal of cholesterol from the arterial wall and transport to the liver for excretion into the bile and out of the body. Unlike apoB, apoA-I does not have a 1:1 ratio with HDL particles and is therefore not an exact reflection of all circulating HDL particles.[24] Many studies have supported an independent inverse association between apoA-I levels and incident ASCVD events; however individual-level meta-analyses revealed a failure of apoA-I to improve risk prediction performance when accounting for traditional lipids.[25] Similarly, the ratio apoB/apoA-I is also associated with cardiovascular disease (CVD) but does not consistently perform better than traditional lipids and non-HDL-C in terms of improving discrimination and reclassification.[26] Given the variability across measurement techniques, limited availability, and minimal to no improvements in risk prediction beyond non-HDL-C or other combinations of traditional lipids, the value of measuring the apolipoproteins for risk prediction remains unclear.

Lipoprotein(a)

Lipoprotein(a) [Lp(a)] is a complex LDL-like lipoprotein particle containing one apoB surrounding a core of cholesteryl ester, triglyceride, and phospholipid. It differs from LDL in that the apoB protein is covalently linked to a highly glycosylated protein called apolipoprotein(a) that resembles plasminogen.[27] Lp(a) consists of many isoforms of varying sizes of apo(a) that are determined by the number of Kringle repeats in the apo(a) domain. Circulating levels of Lp(a) are heavily influenced by genetically determined numbers of

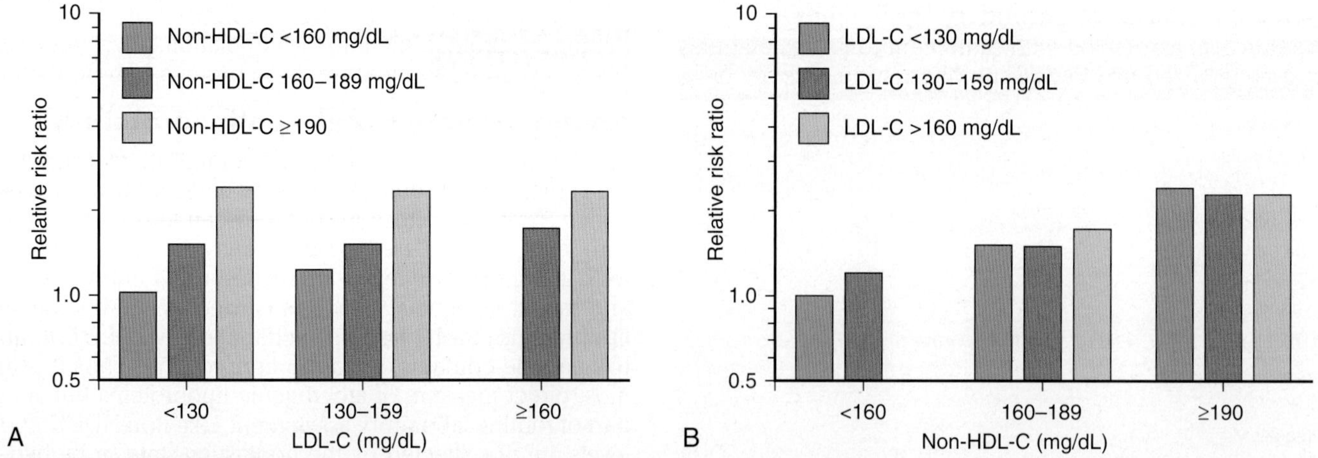

FIG. 8.5 Non-high-density lipoprotein cholesterol (HDL-C), low-density lipoprotein cholesterol (LDL-C), and cardiovascular events from the Framingham cohort and Framingham offspring studies. Cardiovascular events defined as incident fatal and nonfatal myocardial infarction, acute coronary syndrome, and sudden cardiovascular death (*N* = 990/5794). **(A)** The relative risk ratio of increasing categories of non-HDL-C within groups of LDL-C. **(B)** The same data, but the relative risk ratio of increasing categories of LDL-C is displayed within groups of non-HDL-C. For both **A** and **B**, the reference group is LDL-C < 130 mg/dL (3.4 mmol/L) and non-HDL-C < 160 mg/dL (4.1 mmol/L). *(Adapted from Liu J, Sempos CT, Donahue RP, et al. Non-high-density lipoprotein and very-low-density lipoprotein cholesterol and their risk predictive values in coronary heart disease.* Am J Cardiol. *2006;98(10):1363–1368 [Fig. 1, Table 4].)*

Kringle repeats and consequent apo(a) size, with smaller size correlating with higher Lp(a) levels.[27] Environment and lifestyle have little effect on circulating levels.[28] Measurement of Lp(a) levels in humans has been complicated by the inability of earlier methods to account for isoform size and a lack of standardization of reference calibrators.[27] In 2016, the World Health Organization Committee of Biological Standards accepted a reference standard for use in assay calibrators in nmol/L, which circumvents the problems associated with size variability of apo(a).[27] In addition, use of a specific assay with a 5-calibrator system has been certified for lack of significant bias based on apo(a) isoform size.

Most studies have revealed direct relationships between increasing Lp(a) levels and CV risk, specifically myocardial infarction and stroke.[29] Furthermore, Mendelian randomization studies support Lp(a) as a causal risk factor for clinical atherosclerotic events. In one study, genetically elevated Lp(a) levels were associated with a hazard ratio of 1.22 [95% confidence interval (CI) 1.09–1.37] per doubling of Lp(a) level.[30] Another study identified two genetic variants that strongly correlated with increased Lp(a) levels and were associated with a combined odds ratio of 2.57 (95% CI 1.80–3.67) for coronary disease, findings that were replicated in other cohorts.[31] These studies support the notion that elevated Lp(a) likely represents an inherited risk for ASCVD and may be useful to measure in those without traditional ASCVD risk factors but a family history of premature ASCVD, to help further stratify risk. Lp(a) measurement may also help clarify etiology in those developing ASCVD without significant risk factors or recurrent ASCVD despite statin treatment. However, several but not all studies have observed that the increased risk associated with elevated Lp(a) is diminished among those on statin treatment with significant LDL-C lowering,[27] limiting clinical usefulness of the test among those already on lipid-lowering treatment.

The threshold of increased risk seen in many studies correlates with approximately the 75th percentile from Caucasian population-based cohorts, or approximately 30 mg/dL (75 nmol/L) (Fig. 8.6).[30] Interestingly, Lp(a) levels vary significantly by ethnicity, with individuals of African descent having the highest values and South Asians having values between Africans and Caucasians.[28] Most studies correlating Lp(a) with CV risk have been performed in Caucasians; therefore, it remains unknown what the appropriate threshold level for increased risk will be in non-Caucasian populations. It is important to note that Lp(a) levels should be measured with isoform-insensitive assays and that validated reference standards do not exist currently.[27]

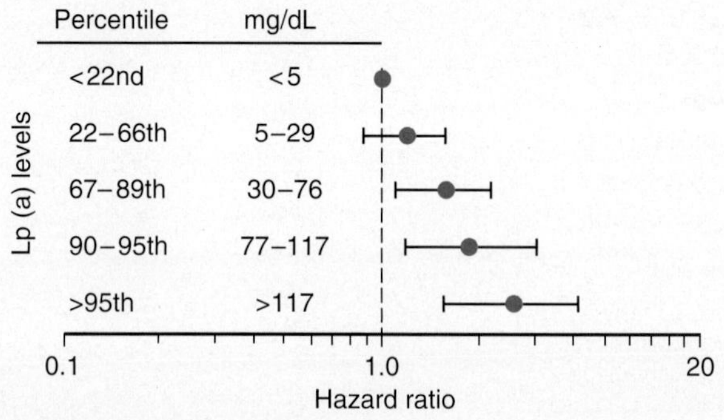

FIG. 8.6 Lipoprotein (Lp)(a) levels and risk of myocardial infarction in the Copenhagen City Heart Study. Multivariable-adjusted hazard ratios and 95% confidence intervals are displayed for increasing levels of Lp(a) and incident myocardial infarction (*N* = 7524), with < 22nd% as the referent group. *(Data from Kamstrup PR, Tybjaerg-Hansen A, Steffensen R, et al. Genetically elevated lipoprotein(a) and increased risk of myocardial infarction.* JAMA. *2009;301(22):2331–2339.)*

The strategy to lower Lp(a) levels to reduce ASCVD risk has been bolstered by genetic studies establishing Lp(a) as a causal risk factor for ASCVD. Nicotinic acid is the most potent Lp(a)-lowering drug that is clinically available, reducing Lp(a) levels by 20% to 40% (see Table 8.1).[32] However, in a large randomized controlled trial of extended-release high-dose nicotinic acid, there was no benefit of adding it to statin therapy, despite a 21% reduction in Lp(a) and other favorable lipid changes.[33] A second large randomized trial of extended-release high-dose nicotinic acid in addition to statin therapy also did not improve ASCVD outcomes,[34] limiting enthusiasm for the use of nicotinic acid as a clinically useful Lp(a)-lowering agent. Statins significantly lower LDL-C and apoB levels but, intriguingly, have no consistent effect on Lp(a) levels.[32] ApoB antisense oligonucleotides and microsomal triglyceride transfer protein inhibitors are clinically available for treatment in patients with homozygous familial hypercholesterolemia and are associated with 17% to 26%

reductions in Lp(a) levels (see Table 8.1).[32] Unfortunately, they are also associated with significant toxicities that may limit generalized use. PCSK9 inhibitors have recently been approved for clinical use and are associated with approximately a 25% reduction in Lp(a) levels.[32] Ongoing outcome trials will determine if reductions in Lp(a) by PCSK9 inhibition is associated with CV benefit.

Lipoprotein Particle Size and Concentration

Each of the lipoprotein classes (LDL, VLDL, IDL, HDL) is comprised of subclasses of varying sizes. In addition to measuring the total cholesterol content of these particles, advanced techniques can also measure the size and total concentration of each lipoprotein class. The most common methods include density gradient rapid ultracentrifugation, NMR spectroscopy, gel electrophoresis, and ion mobility. However, agreement across methods varies, making direct comparisons challenging.[35–37]

LDL and HDL size-based subclasses have yielded inconsistent relationships with CVD, in part due to varying adjustments for cardiometabolic status.[38] Small LDL particles are the most atherogenic, and many but not all studies have shown associations with increased ASCVD risk. However, incorporation of total LDL particle number attenuates this association in some studies, and it remains unclear whether measurement of small LDL improves risk prediction beyond traditional lipid measurements, including non-HDL-C. Similarly, although increased total LDL particle number has been associated with increased ASCVD risk in many studies, the risk prediction afforded by LDL particle number has not been superior to non-HDL-C or apoB.[39] In a large population-based cohort (MESA), when LDL particle number was discordant and higher than LDL-C, only LDL particle number predicted ASCVD risk,[40] suggesting that increased numbers of atherogenic particles, independent of cholesterol load, confer increased risk. However, in this analysis, there was no direct comparison with non-HDL-C or apoB, which also reflect increased levels of atherogenic particles. With regard to HDL particle subclasses, large HDL particles reflect mature HDL capable of transporting circulating cholesterol back to the liver and have been associated with lower risk in several studies. However, large HDL particles are highly correlated with HDL-C levels, and associations with ASCVD are attenuated when accounting for adiposity and insulin resistance.[41–43] In addition, extremely elevated HDL-C and HDL size have been paradoxically directly associated with increased CV events, suggesting dysfunctional HDL particles at the upper extremes of HDL-C concentration and size.[41–43] In contrast, higher total HDL particle number is more consistently correlated with reduced ASCVD risk, even with adjustment for HDL-C and at the extremes, and abolishes the association between HDL-C and CV events.[41–44] However, it remains unclear at this stage whether measurement of lipoprotein particle composition adds to ASCVD risk assessment beyond traditional lipids and risk factors.

NOVEL LIPID TESTS

Measurement of circulating cholesterol content, particle concentration, and particle composition of LDL and HDL do not directly interrogate the most proximate lipid processes related to arterial atherosclerosis: influx of cholesterol derived from oxidized apoB-containing lipoproteins from the circulation, and efflux of cholesterol to apoA-I-containing lipoproteins out into the circulation. Novel tests have been developed to measure these processes more directly, and ongoing studies are testing the clinical relevance of these assays for risk prediction and as targets of therapy.

Oxidized Low-Density Lipoprotein

Although increased circulating LDL leads to increased uptake in the arterial wall, it is the oxidized forms of LDL (ox-LDL) that induce cholesterol accumulation into monocytes/macrophages and subsequent atheroma formation.[45] Ox-LDL directly promotes atherosclerosis by driving foam cell formation, endothelial dysfunction, smooth muscle cell migration and proliferation, and platelet activation.[46]

Small but significant amounts of ox-LDL are measureable in the blood. Three different enzyme-linked immunosorbent assays using various murine monoclonal antibodies have been tested in human research studies but none is commercially available for clinical use.[47] These three antibody assays detect different epitopes on ox-LDL and results cannot be easily compared. At least one of these assays detects oxidized phospholipid on apoB particles and strongly correlates with circulating Lp(a) levels (r = 0.8 to 0.9), limiting the ability to determine associations with ASCVD specific to ox-LDL. Ox-LDL levels are higher in those with existing coronary and peripheral arterial disease and rise acutely after myocardial and cerebral infarctions, as well as after coronary revascularization.[47] However, ox-LDL levels have not been consistently shown to correlate with burden of atherosclerosis or improve risk prediction of incident events.[47] It remains to be seen whether development of more standardized assays for ox-LDL measurement may lead to a clinically useful ox-LDL test.

Cholesterol Efflux

Most lipid testing has focused on the influx of atherogenic circulating lipids into arterial walls and progression of atherosclerotic plaques. HDL promotes efflux of cholesterol out of the arterial wall into the circulation, and its circulating cholesterol content (HDL-C) has been assumed to reflect this antiatherosclerotic process.[48] Low levels of HDL-C have been associated with incident ASCVD in multiple studies;[9] however low HDL-C is part of the metabolic syndrome profile and reflects increased insulin resistance. Accounting for insulin resistance through measures of adiposity, hypertriglyceridemia, and hyperglycemia abolish or significantly weaken the CV risk associated with low HDL-C.[49] In addition, several randomized controlled trials of therapies raising HDL-C have failed to improve outcomes, further highlighting the limitations of using HDL-C as a sole therapeutic target.[49]

In an effort to more directly measure HDL function, assays measuring cholesterol efflux have been developed and tested in humans.[50] The concept involves quantifying the amount of labeled cholesterol that effluxes out of standardized macrophages into apoB-depleted serum or plasma containing mostly apoA-I lipoproteins (the main protein associated with HDL) (Fig. 8.7).[48] In a large study, efflux was inversely associated with prevalent coronary disease at the time of coronary angiography.[51] Subsequently, several large cohorts have revealed consistent associations between low baseline efflux and increased risk of both incident and recurrent ASCVD (Fig. 8.8).[44,52,53] These associations are independent of HDL-C and HDL particle concentrations, as

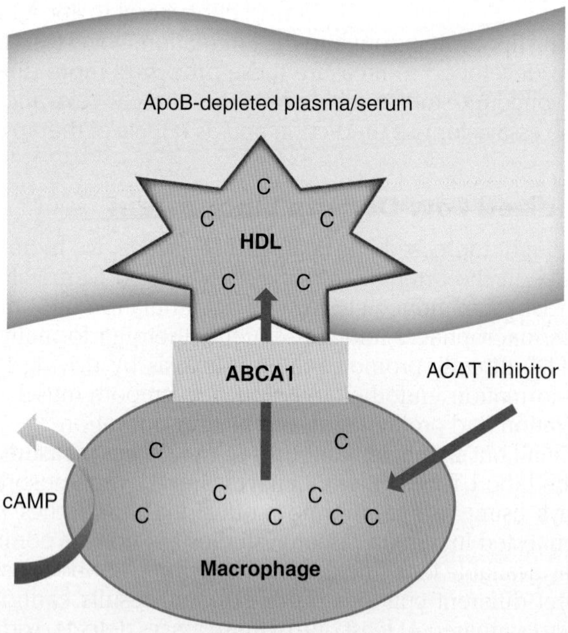

FIG. 8.7 Macrophage-specific cholesterol efflux. Macrophages are labeled with cholesterol and incubated with apolipoprotein B-depleted plasma or serum. The amount of labeled cholesterol *(C)* that moves from the cells to the acceptor as a fraction of the total labeled cholesterol in the cells is quantified as cholesterol efflux.

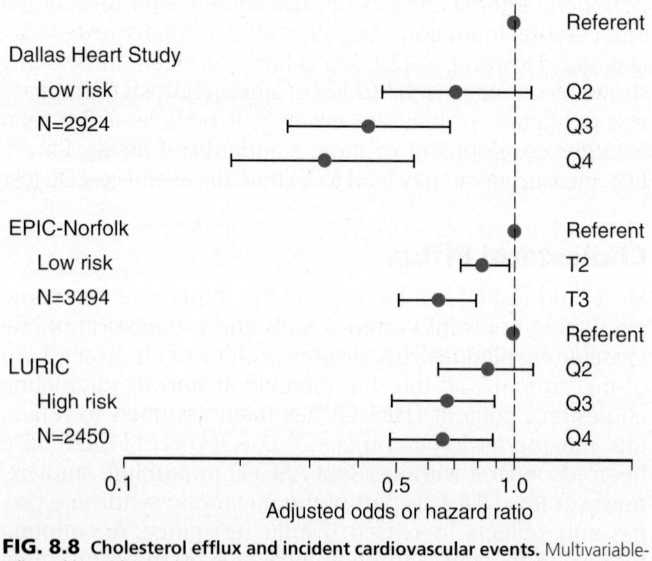

FIG. 8.8 Cholesterol efflux and incident cardiovascular events. Multivariable-adjusted hazards or odds ratios with 95% confidence intervals displayed for increasing levels of cholesterol efflux with the lowest group as the referent. *EPIC*, European Prospective Investigation of Cancer; *LURIC*, Ludwigshafen Risk and Cardiovascular Health study; *Q*, quartile; *T*, tertile.[44,52,53]

well as measures of insulin resistance and inflammation. In these studies, the association between HDL-C and CV events was attenuated when accounting for efflux. These assays remain in development as they are cell-based and have not been standardized with reference ranges. However, a recent report on the additive risk prediction utility of cholesterol efflux beyond other emerging risk factors such as coronary calcium, family history, and C-reactive protein suggests that perhaps this HDL function marker may be clinically useful.[54]

LIPID TARGETS ON TREATMENT

Statins significantly lower ASCVD risk in both primary and secondary prevention populations and are the first choice in terms of lipid-modifying therapy for risk reduction.[3,7] The main targets of statins have been LDL-C and non-HDL-C as they best reflect reductions in risk in randomized controlled trials of statins.[55] Some guidelines suggest that an optional goal is to target apoB when LDL-C and non-HDL-C goals have been met, particularly in those with diabetes or elevated triglyceride levels.[1,3,19,56] Direct comparisons of LDL-C and non-HDL-C as treatment targets in an individual-level meta-analysis pooling eight primary and secondary prevention statin trials reveal incremental risk reduction when directly targeting non-HDL-C to < 130 mg/dL (3.3 mmol/L) versus targeting LDL-C to < 100 mg/dL (2.6 mmol/L).[57] Compared with those achieving both LDL-C and non-HDL-C targets, those who did not achieve the non-HDL-C target of < 130 mg/dL (3.3 mmol/L) had 20% to 30% increased risk regardless of achieved LDL-C. In this meta-analysis, statin-induced change in non-HDL-C explained 64% of the treatment benefit, compared with 54% explained by change in apoB and only 50% explained by change in LDL-C. These observations of clear superiority of non-HDL-C over LDL-C, along with the ease and no added cost of calculating non-HDL-C versus measuring apoB, clearly make non-HDL-C a primary lipid target for statin therapy.

Other traditional and advanced lipoprotein measures have not been proven to be better than non-HDL-C as treatment targets to reduce ASCVD. Elevated triglycerides and low HDL-C are components of the metabolic syndrome and reflect increased atherosclerotic and cardiometabolic risk.[10] However, pharmacotherapies targeting these lipoproteins, when given in combination with statin therapy, have not consistently been shown to reduce ASCVD despite significant reductions in triglycerides[58] or increases in HDL-C.[59] High triglycerides and low HDL-C translate into increased triglyceride-rich lipoproteins; therefore non-HDL-C can be used to track efficacy of lifestyle measures to improve this profile. Similarly, because abnormal levels of most advanced lipoprotein tests usually reflect increased insulin resistance, non-HDL-C is an adequate surrogate without added expense to follow lifestyle measures to improve the insulin-resistant state. Lastly, there is insufficient current evidence to support lowering Lp(a) as a treatment target.[32] In the Atherothrombosis Intervention in. Metabolic Syndrome with Low HDL/High Triglycerides and Impact on Global Health Outcomes (AIM-HIGH) trial, reduction of Lp(a) levels with extended-release niacin was not associated with improved outcomes.[60] In summary, most lipid measures, whether traditional or advanced, may provide improved baseline risk estimation but none is considered to be better than non-HDL-C as a treatment target for statins or any other lipid-modifying therapy to reduce ASCVD risk.

Treatment Targets Versus Fixed-Dose Statins

The 2013 American College of Cardiology/American Heart Association (ACC/AHA) Cholesterol Guidelines recommend fixed-dose high- or medium-potency statins for high- or intermediate-risk individuals, respectively, and suggest abandoning lipid treatment targets.[7] Prior Adult Treatment Panel lipid guidelines[6] and other current guidelines continue to emphasize lipid treatment goals, with statins as first-line therapies.[3,19,56] The divergence of the ACC/AHA guidelines is in part related to an ongoing debate on whether evidence from randomized controlled trials or observations from epidemiologic studies should dictate management strategies. The vast majority of randomized controlled trials

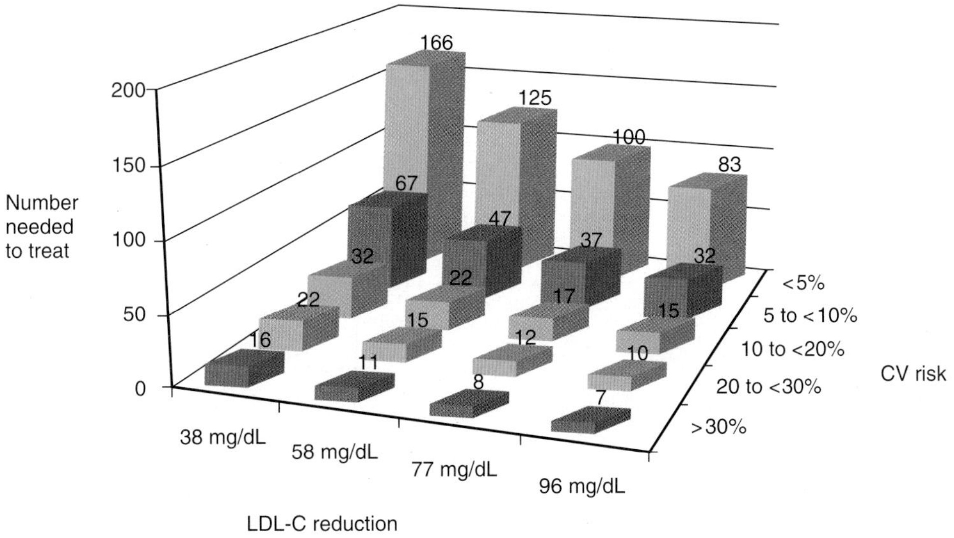

FIG. 8.9 Number needed to treat with statins by low-density lipoprotein cholesterol (LDL-C) reduction and cardiovascular risk. *(Data extrapolated from Cholesterol Treatment Trialists' Collaboration meta-analysis.* Lancet. *2012;380(9841):581–590.)*

have tested fixed-dose statins and have shown reductions in ASCVD events compared with placebo or high- versus medium-potency statins.[4] Treatment to a target LDL-C or non-HDL-C as a strategy has not been tested for hard outcomes in a large trial. This forms the basis of the 2013 ACC/AHA recommendations, which emphasized the randomized controlled trial evidence, in part to highlight the benefit of initiating and maintaining high-potency statins in high-risk individuals, regardless of baseline or on-treatment LDL-C levels. At the time of the 2013 ACC/AHA guidelines, no nonstatin therapy had been shown to reduce hard ASCVD risk in addition to statins, further strengthening the position to use only fixed-dose statins.

However, randomized trials of statins and genetic epidemiology studies reveal a consistent log-linear relationship between baseline and on-treatment LDL-C levels and ASCVD risk with no apparent floor.[5,61] Whereas there has been little debate whether the high-risk person who achieves a 50% reduction in LDL-C to 60 mg/dL (1.6 mmol/L) on high-potency statin has achieved effective risk reduction, there continues to be debate about whether a person with lower starting LDL-C levels closer to recommended goals of 70 to 100 mg/dL (1.8 to 2.6 mmol/L) will also benefit from high- versus medium-potency statin. Meta-analyses of all the randomized trials suggest that statins at fixed doses as assigned in the trials result in consistent risk reductions across the spectrum of baseline LDL-C levels, even as low as 50 mg/dL (1.3 mmol/L).[61] Less commonly in the current era, some individuals have baseline LDL-C levels above 160 mg/dL (4.1 mmol/L) and treatment with high-potency statin may get their LDL-C to 80 to 90 mg/dL (2.0 to 2.3 mmol/L), and the question then becomes whether there would be incremental benefit in further LDL-C lowering.

An essential concept surrounding these debates is the number needed to treat (NNT) to prevent one event. In contrast to relative risk reduction, which is remarkably consistent for statins across the spectrum of baseline risk and lipid levels,[4] the NNT is based on the absolute risk reduction, which varies by baseline risk and the magnitude of lipid-lowering achieved. As an example, extrapolating published data from the meta-analysis by the Cholesterol Treatment Trialists' (CTT) Collaboration,[61] the NNT is markedly higher in those at lower versus higher risk (< 10% vs > 10%) (Fig. 8.9). Furthermore, in the low-risk group, the high NNT is significantly lowered (improved) with larger reductions in LDL-C. A separate published analysis of the same data suggests a similar pattern: the NNT is highest in those at low risk and low baseline LDL-C/non-HDL-C levels.[62] In this analysis, fixed-dose statin (vs treatment target) resulted in a more favorable NNT in those with LDL-C levels below ~100 mg/dL (2.6 mmol/L). In contrast, an LDL target < 70 mg/dL (< 1.8 mmol/L) (vs fixed-dose statin) resulted in a lower NNT in those with LDL-C levels > 160 mg/dL (4.1 mmol/L) (Fig. 8.10).

Several other points regarding lipid testing among patients already receiving lipid modifying therapy merit comment. The 2015 Improved Reduction of Outcomes: Vytorin Efficacy International Trial (IMPROVE-IT) study was the first randomized controlled clinical trial to show that a nonstatin drug, ezetimibe, in addition to statin, reduced the risk of prespecified major ASCVD events when compared with statin therapy alone.[63] In this high-risk cohort of patients with acute coronary syndrome, the achieved LDL-C was 54 mg/dL (1.4 mmol/L) in the simvastatin+ezetimibe group versus 70 mg/dL (1.8 mmol/L) in the simvastatin monotherapy group, resulting in a 2% absolute reduction in the primary combined endpoint (32.7% vs 34.7%, $p = 0.016$). There was also a 2% absolute reduction in the hard endpoints of nonfatal and fatal myocardial infarction (MI) or stroke (20.4% vs 22.2%, hazard ratio 0.90, 95%CI 0.84–0.96, $p = 0.003$). The reduction in events with ezetimibe+statin correlated with a further 24% LDL-C lowering. Moreover, the findings are consistent with the log-linear relationship between LDL-C and ASCVD from previous statin trials and raise the possibility that achieved LDL-C may still be useful as therapeutic target.

PCSK9-inhibitors also significantly lower LDL-C in addition to statin therapy (see Table 8.1).[64,65] If this novel class of lipid drugs is confirmed to reduce CV events, as preliminary data suggest,[64,65] the case for targeting the lowest possible LDL-C/non-HDL-C will become stronger. Lastly, lipid testing on therapy may reveal continued or new elevations of non-HDL-C, indicating lack of adherence to drug therapy and lifestyle recommendations and/or the development of new disorders such as diabetes, hypothyroidism, or nephrotic syndrome.

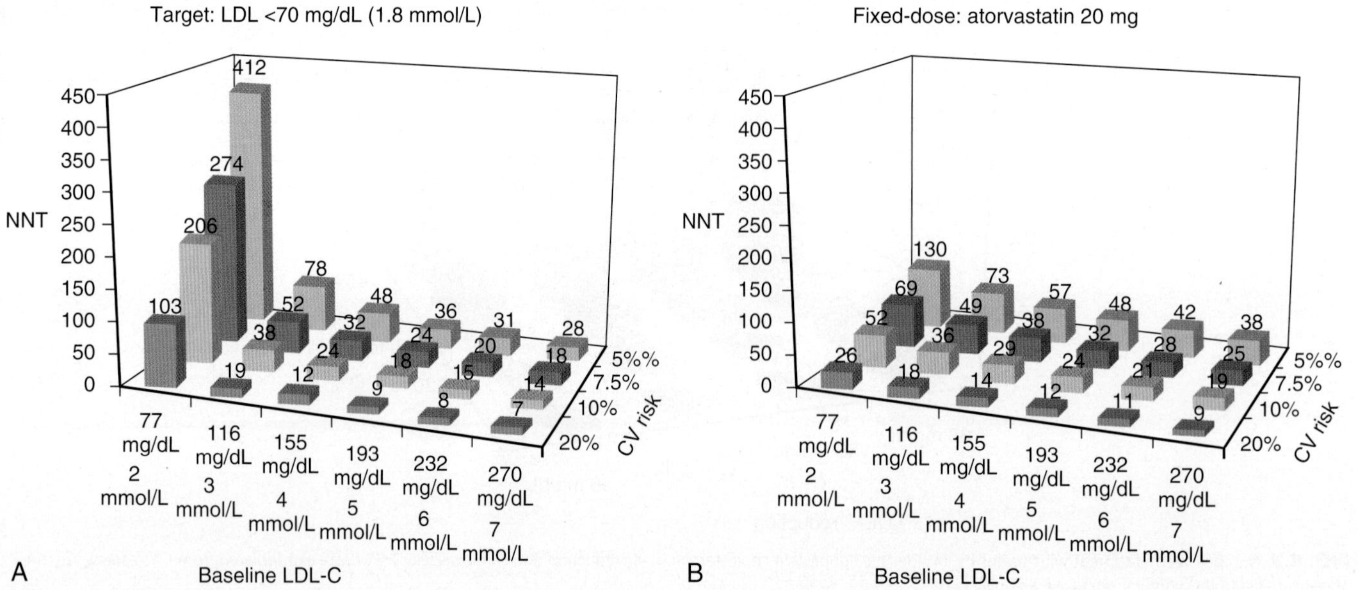

FIG. 8.10 Number needed to treat (NNT) with statins by baseline low-density lipoprotein-cholesterol (LDL-C) and cardiovascular risk. **(A)** NNT based on target LDL < 70 mg/dL (1.8 mmol/L). **(B)** NNT based on fixed-dose atorvastatin, 20 mg. *(Data extrapolated from Tables 1 and 4 in Soran H, Schofield JD, Durrington PN. Cholesterol, not just cardiovascular risk, is important in deciding who should receive statin treatment.* Eur Heart J. *2015;36(43):2975–2983.)*

SUMMARY AND GUIDELINE RECOMMENDATIONS

The concept that abnormal lipids contribute significantly to ASCVD risk has been firmly in place since as early as the 1950s. Total cholesterol and low HDL-C are the standard lipids used in risk prediction algorithms to determine need for statins and other risk-reducing measures. Lipid targets have focused on specific LDL-C and non-HDL-C thresholds, but the NNT to prevent one event varies on baseline risk, starting lipid levels, and degree of lipid-lowering. With respect to lipid targets, non-HDL-C is superior to LDL-C in predicting residual risk and does not require fasting status. Many advanced lipoprotein measures incrementally improve risk prediction but typically reflect insulin-resistant states, are not current targets of therapy, and do not perform sufficiently better than non-HDL-C across broad populations. Randomized controlled trials of statins strongly suggest that high-risk individuals benefit from high-potency statins, regardless of baseline or on-treatment LDL-C/non-HDL-C levels. The results of the IMPROVE-IT trial[63] and preliminary results from trials of several PCSK9-inhibitors[64-65] suggest a role of additional LDL-C/non-HDL-C lowering in addition to statin therapy.

References

1. Expert Dyslipidemia Panel of the International Atherosclerosis Society Panel Members: An International Atherosclerosis Society Position Paper: global recommendations for the management of dyslipidemia-full report, *J Clin Lipidol* 8(1):29–60, 2014.
2. Friedewald WT, Levy RI, Fredrickson DS: Estimation of the concentration of low-density lipoprotein cholesterol in plasma, without use of the preparative ultracentrifuge, *Clin Chem* 18(6):499–502, 1972.
3. Perk J, De Backer G, Gohlke H, et al.: European Guidelines on cardiovascular disease prevention in clinical practice (version 2012). The Fifth Joint Task Force of the European Society of Cardiology and Other Societies on Cardiovascular Disease Prevention in Clinical Practice (constituted by representatives of nine societies and by invited experts), *Eur Heart J* 33(13):1635–1701, 2012.
4. Cholesterol Treatment Trialists C, Baigent C, Blackwell L, et al.: Efficacy and safety of more intensive lowering of LDL cholesterol: a meta-analysis of data from 170,000 participants in 26 randomised trials, *Lancet* 376(9753):1670–1681, 2010.
5. Ference BA, Majeed F, Penumetcha R, et al.: Effect of naturally random allocation to lower low-density lipoprotein cholesterol on the risk of coronary heart disease mediated by polymorphisms in NPC1L1, HMGCR, or both. A 2 × 2 factorial Mendelian randomization study, *J Am Coll Cardiol* 65(15):1552–1561, 2015.
6. National Cholesterol Education Program (NCEP) Expert Panel on Detection, Evaluation, and Treatment of High Blood Cholesterol in Adults. Third Report of the National Cholesterol Education Program (NCEP) Expert Panel on Detection, Evaluation, and Treatment of High Blood Cholesterol in Adults (Adult Treatment Panel III) final report, *Circulation* 106(25):3143–3421, 2002.
7. Stone NJ, Robinson JG, Lichtenstein AH, et al.: 2013 ACC/AHA guideline on the treatment of blood cholesterol to reduce atherosclerotic cardiovascular risk in adults: a report of the American College of Cardiology/American Heart Association Task Force on Practice Guidelines, *Circulation* 129(25 Suppl 2):S1–S45, 2014.
8. European Association for Cardiovascular Prevention & Rehabilitation, Reiner Z, Catapano AL, et al.: ESC/EAS Guidelines for the management of dyslipidaemias: the Task Force for the management of dyslipidaemias of the European Society of Cardiology (ESC) and the European Atherosclerosis Society (EAS), *Eur Heart J* 32(14):1769–1818, 2011.
9. Gordon DJ, Probstfield JL, Garrison RJ, et al.: High-density lipoprotein cholesterol and cardiovascular disease. Four prospective American studies, *Circulation* 79(1):8–15, 1989.
10. Grundy SM, Cleeman JI, Daniels SR, et al.: Diagnosis and management of the metabolic syndrome: an American Heart Association/National Heart, Lung, and Blood Institute Scientific Statement, *Circulation* 112(17):2735–2752, 2005.
11. Hegele RA, Ginsberg HN, Chapman MJ, et al.: The polygenic nature of hypertriglyceridaemia: implications for definition, diagnosis, and management, *Lancet Diabetes Endocrinol* 2(8):655–666, 2014.
12. Varbo A, Benn M, Tybjaerg-Hansen A, et al.: Remnant cholesterol as a causal risk factor for ischemic heart disease, *J Am Coll Cardiol* 61(4):427–436, 2013.
13. Jorgensen AB, Frikke-Schmidt R, West AS, et al.: Genetically elevated non-fasting triglycerides and calculated remnant cholesterol as causal risk factors for myocardial infarction, *Eur Heart J* 34(24):1826–1833, 2013.
14. Do R, Willer CJ, Schmidt EM, et al.: Common variants associated with plasma triglycerides and risk for coronary artery disease, *Nat Genet* 45(11):1345–1352, 2013.
15. Jorgensen AB, Frikke-Schmidt R, Nordestgaard BG, et al.: Loss-of-function mutations in APOC3 and risk of ischemic vascular disease, *N Engl J Med* 371(1):32–41, 2014.
16. Brinton EA: Management of hypertriglyceridemia for prevention of atherosclerotic cardiovascular disease, *Endocrinol Metab Clin North Am* 45(1):185–204, 2016.
17. Liu J, Zeng FF, Liu ZM, et al.: Effects of blood triglycerides on cardiovascular and all-cause mortality: a systematic review and meta-analysis of 61 prospective studies, *Lipids Health Dis* 12:159, 2013.
18. Nordestgaard BG, Benn M, Schnohr P, et al.: Nonfasting triglycerides and risk of myocardial infarction, ischemic heart disease, and death in men and women, *JAMA* 298(3):299–308, 2007.
19. Jacobson TA, Ito MK, Maki KC, et al.: National Lipid Association recommendations for patient-centered management of dyslipidemia: part 1 — executive summary, *J Clin Lipidol* 8(5):473–488, 2014.
19a. Keech A, Simes RJ, Barter P, et al.: Effects of long-term fenofibrate therapy on cardiovascular events in 9795 people with type 2 diabetes mellitus (the FIELD study): randomised controlled trial, *Lancet* 366:1849–1861, 2005.
19b. ACCORD study group, et al.: Effects of combination lipid therapy in type 2 diabetes mellitus, *N Engl J Med* 362:1563–1574, 2010.
19c. Scott R, O'Brien R, Fulcher G, et al.: Effects of fenofibrate treatment on cardiovascular disease risk in 9,795 individuals with type 2 diabetes and various components of the metabolic syndrome: the Fenofibrate Intervention and Event Lowering in Diabetes (FIELD) study, *Diabetes Care* 32:493–498, 2009.
19d. Rubins HB, Robins SJ, Collins, et al.: Diabetes, plasma insulin, and cardiovascular disease: subgroup analysis from the Department of Veterans Affairs high-density lipoprotein intervention trial (VA-HIT), *Arch Intern Med* 162:2597–2604, 2002.
20. Jun M, Foote C, Lv J, et al.: Effects of fibrates on cardiovascular outcomes: a systematic review and meta-analysis, *Lancet* 375(9729):1875–1884, 2010.
21. Rizos EC, Ntzani EE, Bika E, et al.: Association between omega-3 fatty acid supplementation and risk of major cardiovascular disease events: a systematic review and meta-analysis, *JAMA* 308(10):1024–1033, 2012.
22. Robinson JG, Wang S, Smith BJ, et al.: Meta-analysis of the relationship between non-high-density lipoprotein cholesterol reduction and coronary heart disease risk, *J Am Coll Cardiol* 53(4):316–322, 2009.
23. Grundy SM, Vega GL, Tomassini JE, et al.: Comparisons of apolipoprotein B levels estimated by immunoassay, nuclear magnetic resonance, vertical auto profile, and non-high-density lipoprotein cholesterol in subjects with hypertriglyceridemia (SAFARI Trial), *Am J Cardiol* 108(1):40–46, 2011.
24. Silva RA, Huang R, Morris J, et al.: Structure of apolipoprotein A-I in spherical high density lipoproteins of different sizes, *Proc Natl Acad Sci U S A* 105(34):12176–12181, 2008.
25. Emerging Risk Factors Collaboration, Di Angelantonio E, Gao P, et al.: Lipid-related markers and cardiovascular disease prediction, *JAMA* 307(23):2499–2506, 2012.

26. Emerging Risk Factors Collaboration, Di Angelantonio E, Sarwar N, et al.: Major lipids, apolipoproteins, and risk of vascular disease, *JAMA* 302(18):1993–2000, 2009.
27. Marcovina SM, Albers JJ: Lipoprotein (a) measurements for clinical application, *J Lipid Res* 57(4):526–537, 2016.
28. Enkhmaa B, Anuurad E, Berglund L: Lipoprotein(a): impact by ethnicity, environmental and medical conditions, *J Lipid Res*, 2015. Dec 4. pii: jlr.R051904.
29. Nordestgaard BG, Chapman MJ, Ray K, et al.: Lipoprotein(a) as a cardiovascular risk factor: current status, *Eur Heart J* 31(23):2844–2853, 2010.
30. Kamstrup PR, Tybjaerg-Hansen A, Steffensen R, et al.: Genetically elevated lipoprotein(a) and increased risk of myocardial infarction, *JAMA* 301(22):2331–2339, 2009.
31. Clarke R, Peden JF, Hopewell JC, et al.: Genetic variants associated with Lp(a) lipoprotein level and coronary disease, *N Engl J Med* 361(26):2518–2528, 2009.
32. van Capelleveen JC, van der Valk FM, Stroes ES: Current therapies for lowering lipoprotein(a), *J Lipid Res*, 2015. Dec 4. pii: jlr.R053066.
33. Boden WE, Probstfield JL, Anderson T, et al.: Niacin in patients with low HDL cholesterol levels receiving intensive statin therapy, *N Engl J Med* 365(24):2255–2267, 2011.
34. Group HTC, Landray MJ, Haynes R, et al.: Effects of extended-release niacin with laropiprant in high-risk patients, *N Engl J Med* 371(3):203–212, 2014.
35. Chung M, Lichtenstein AH, Ip S, et al.: Comparability of methods for LDL subfraction determination: a systematic review, *Atherosclerosis* 205(2):342–348, 2009.
36. Williams PT, Zhao XQ, Marcovina SM, et al.: Comparison of four methods of analysis of lipoprotein particle subfractions for their association with angiographic progression of coronary artery disease, *Atherosclerosis* 233(2):713–720, 2014.
37. Sninsky JJ, Rowland CM, Baca AM, et al.: Classification of LDL phenotypes by 4 methods of determining lipoprotein particle size, *J Investig Med* 61(6):942–949, 2013.
38. Krauss RM: Lipoprotein subfractions and cardiovascular disease risk, *Curr Opin Lipidol* 21(4):305–311, 2010.
39. Greenland P, Alpert JS, Beller GA, et al.: 2010 ACCF/AHA guideline for assessment of cardiovascular risk in asymptomatic adults: a report of the American College of Cardiology Foundation/American Heart Association Task Force on Practice Guidelines, *J Am Coll Cardiol* 56(25): e50–e103, 2010.
40. Otvos JD, Mora S, Shalaurova I, et al.: Clinical implications of discordance between low-density lipoprotein cholesterol and particle number, *J Clin Lipidol* 5(2):105–113, 2011.
41. Parish S, Offer A, Clarke R, et al.: Lipids and lipoproteins and risk of different vascular events in the MRC/BHF Heart Protection Study, *Circulation* 125(20):2469–2478, 2012.
42. Mackey RH, Greenland P, Goff Jr DC, et al.: High-density lipoprotein cholesterol and particle concentrations, carotid atherosclerosis, and coronary events: MESA (Multi-Ethnic Study of Atherosclerosis), *J Am Coll Cardiol* 60(6):508–516, 2012.
43. van der Steeg WA, Holme I, Boekholdt SM, et al.: High-density lipoprotein cholesterol, high-density lipoprotein particle size, and apolipoprotein A-I: significance for cardiovascular risk: The IDEAL and EPIC-Norfolk Studies, *J Am Coll Cardiol* 51(6):634–642, 2008.
44. Rohatgi A, Khera A, Berry JD, et al.: HDL cholesterol efflux capacity and incident cardiovascular events, *N Engl J Med* 371(25):2383–2393, 2014.
45. Yoshida H, Kisugi R: Mechanisms of LDL oxidation, *Clin Chim Acta* 411(23–24):1875–1882, 2010.
46. Pirillo A, Norata GD, Catapano AL: LOX-1, OxLDL, and atherosclerosis, *Mediators Inflamm* 2013:152786, 2013.
47. Trpkovic A, Resanovic I, Stanimirovic J, et al.: Oxidized low-density lipoprotein as a biomarker of cardiovascular diseases, *Crit Rev Clin Lab Sci* 52(2):70–85, 2015.
48. Rader DJ, Alexander ET, Weibel GL, et al.: The role of reverse cholesterol transport in animals and humans and relationship to atherosclerosis, *J Lipid Res* 50(Suppl):S189–S194, 2009.
49. Rader DJ, Hovingh GK: HDL and cardiovascular disease, *Lancet* 384(9943):618–625, 2014.
50. Rohatgi A: High-density lipoprotein function measurement in human studies: focus on cholesterol efflux capacity, *Prog Cardiovasc Dis* 58(1):32–40, 2015.
51. Khera AV, Cuchel M, de la Llera-Moya M, et al.: Cholesterol efflux capacity, high-density lipoprotein function, and atherosclerosis, *N Engl J Med* 364(2):127–135, 2011.
52. Ritsch A, Scharnagl H, Marz W: HDL cholesterol efflux capacity and cardiovascular events, *N Engl J Med* 372(19):1870–1871, 2015.
53. Saleheen D, Scott R, Javad S, et al.: Association of HDL cholesterol efflux capacity with incident coronary heart disease events: a prospective case-control study, *Lancet Diabetes Endocrinol* 3(7):507–513, 2015.
54. Mody P, Joshi PH, Khera A, et al.: Cholesterol efflux capacity and cardiovascular risk prediction beyond coronary calcium, family history and C-reactive protein, *J Am Coll Cardiol* 67(21):2480–2487, 2016.
55. Briel M, Ferreira-Gonzalez I, You JJ, et al.: Association between change in high density lipoprotein cholesterol and cardiovascular disease morbidity and mortality: Systematic review and meta-regression analysis, *BMJ* 338:b92, 2009.
56. Anderson TJ, Gregoire J, Hegele RA, et al.: 2012 update of the Canadian Cardiovascular Society guidelines for the diagnosis and treatment of dyslipidemia for the prevention of cardiovascular disease in the adult, *Can J Cardiol* 29(2):151–167, 2013.
57. Boekholdt SM, Arsenault BJ, Mora S, et al.: Association of LDL cholesterol, non-HDL cholesterol, and apolipoprotein B levels with risk of cardiovascular events among patients treated with statins: a meta-analysis, *JAMA* 307(12):1302–1309, 2012.
58. Ginsberg HN, Elam MB, Lovato LC, et al.: Effects of combination lipid therapy in type 2 diabetes mellitus, *N Engl J Med* 362(17):1563–1574, 2010.
59. Mani P, Rohatgi A: Niacin therapy, HDL cholesterol, and cardiovascular disease: is the HDL hypothesis defunct? *Curr Atheroscler Rep* 17(8):521, 2015.
60. Albers JJ, Slee A, O'Brien KD, et al.: Relationship of apolipoproteins A-1 and B, and lipoprotein(a) to cardiovascular outcomes: the AIM-HIGH trial (Atherothrombosis Intervention in Metabolic Syndrome with Low HDL/High Triglyceride and Impact on Global Health Outcomes), *J Am Coll Cardiol* 62(17):157–159, 2013.
61. Cholesterol Treatment Trialists (CTT) Collaborators, Mihaylova B, Emberson J, et al.: The effects of lowering LDL cholesterol with statin therapy in people at low risk of vascular disease: meta-analysis of individual data from 27 randomised trials, *Lancet* 380(9841):581–590, 2012.
62. Soran H, Schofield JD, Durrington PN: Cholesterol, not just cardiovascular risk, is important in deciding who should receive statin treatment, *Eur Heart J* 36(43):2975–2983, 2015.
63. Cannon CP, Blazing MA, Giugliano RP, et al.: Ezetimibe added to statin therapy after acute coronary syndromes, *N Engl J Med* 372(25):2387–2397, 2015.
64. Sabatine MS, Giugliano RP, Wiviott SD, et al.: Efficacy and safety of evolocumab in reducing lipids and cardiovascular events, *N Engl J Med* 372(16):1500–1509, 2015.
65. Robinson JG, Farnier M, Krempf M, et al.: Efficacy and safety of alirocumab in reducing lipids and cardiovascular events, *N Engl J Med* 372(16):1489–1499, 2015.

9 Standard and Novel Biomarkers

Stefan Blankenberg and Tanja Zeller

INTRODUCTION

Several diagnostic tools exist to clinically assess the prevalence and severity of coronary heart disease and to enhance the ability to identify the "vulnerable" patient at risk of developing cardiovascular events. In addition, the assessment of biomarkers is one option to improve the diagnosis of disease, to better identify high-risk individuals, to improve prognostication, and to optimize the selection of and response to chronic artery disease treatment. The major strength of biomarker assessment in chronic coronary artery disease (CAD) constitutes the improved prognostication and monitoring of disease.

The term biomarker (i.e., biologic marker) was introduced approximately 30 years ago indicating a measurable and quantifiable biological parameter (e.g. specific enzyme concentration, specific hormone concentration, specific gene phenotype distribution in a population, presence of biological substances) which serve as indices for health- and physiology-related assessments, such as disease risk, psychiatric disorders, environmental exposure and its effects, disease diagnosis, metabolic processes, substance abuse, pregnancy, cell line development, epidemiologic studies, etc.[1]

This term was further developed and the definition standardized as

> *"a characteristic that is objectively measured and evaluated as an indicator of normal biological processes, pathogenic processes, or pharmacologic responses to a therapeutic intervention."*[2]

A biomarker can be determined as a biosample (blood-, urinary-, or tissue-borne); it may be a recording like blood pressure, electrocardiogram (ECG), stress test, or Holter; or it can constitute an imaging test (echocardiogram, magnetic resonance imaging [MRI], or computed tomography [CT] scan). This chapter focuses on the impact of blood-borne biomarkers in chronic CAD.

There are several main practical considerations for the use of blood-borne biomarkers in stable CAD (Box 9.1). First, biomarkers might help to identify the prevalence of a disease in addition to clinical assessment, ECG, stress test, and imaging tests such as echocardiography or CT scan. However, the diagnostic accuracy of blood-borne biomarkers in identifying or validating chronic CAD is rather weak. Second, biomarkers may help to improve prognostication in diseased individuals as some biomarkers are strongly related to future cardiovascular events. Third, biomarkers may support treatment selection in CAD patients. Fourth, biomarkers might serve as indicators for disease progression and, finally, biomarkers might be used to monitor treatment success, although the use of biomarkers for the monitoring of disease progression and treatment success has not been successfully proven so far.

The advent of new molecular technologies such as gene sequencing or reliable determination of noncoding RNAs allows the identification of novel biomarkers related to a disease. These novel biomarkers, which have not entered the clinical routine so far, might have the potential for more accurate disease-related application.

The overall expectation of a biomarker for chronic cardiovascular disease (CVD) is to enhance the ability of the clinician to optimally manage the patient (Fig. 9.1). For instance, in a person with chronic or atypical chest pain, a biomarker may be expected to facilitate the identification of patients with chest pain of ischemic etiology leading to the clinical

BOX 9.1 Biomarker Criteria: What Makes a Biomarker Useful?

1. Provides additional information to already established clinical parameters
2. Objectively measurable and quantifiable biologic parameter
3. Measurable in an accurate and standardized way with low intra-individual variability
4. Indicator of health and physiology-related assessments
5. Tested in prospective studies to validate its prognostic and diagnostic efficacy
6. Able to
   - identify individuals at high risk
   - identify disease prevalence in addition to clinical assessment
   - improve prognostication in healthy and diseased individuals
   - provide information that could lead to a change in therapeutic strategies and support treatment selection
   - monitor treatment success
   - assist the clinician for optimal patient management
   - assess response to therapy
7. Easily accessible, measurable, cost-effective

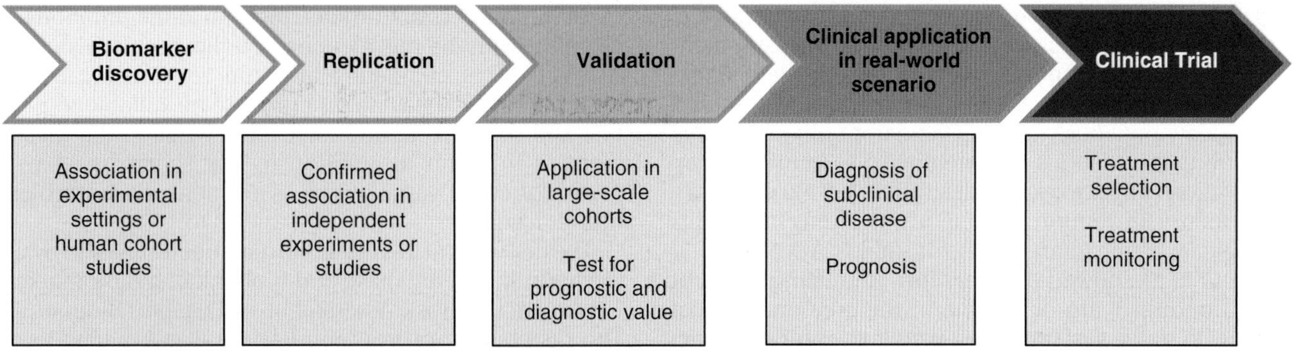

FIG. 9.1 Workflow and qualification of establishing a biomarker for chronic coronary artery disease.

symptom of angina. In a patient with CAD, a biomarker may assess the likelihood of a future event and response to therapy.

The clinical value of a biomarker is related to its accuracy, its standardized determination including reproducibility, its accessibility, and direct interpretation of the biomarker results for clinicians. The interpretation should include consistent prediction in multiple studies and the capacity to improve patient management. Changes in biomarker levels should lead to clinically relevant consequences (see Fig. 9.1).

To date, cardiovascular risk assessment has been predominantly based on classic risk factors. However, particularly in diseased individuals, the classic risk factors do not fully explain the risk of repeated events. Most of these factors are modifiable, and intervention is likely to reduce the risk of CVD. To improve risk estimation beyond what is possible with classic risk factors, many biomarkers have now been related to cardiovascular risk in secondary prevention. It seems that biomarkers of inflammation like C-reactive protein (CRP), biomarkers of hemodynamics like B-type natriuretic peptide (BNP) and the N-terminal fragment of its prohormone, NT-proBNP, and—most recently—markers reflecting cardiac micronecrosis such as cardiac troponins measured with high-sensitivity assays have most consistently improved risk estimates and led to interventions.

Various biomarkers have been postulated to improve risk prediction and patient care in stable CAD patients. Only a few biomarkers have undergone rigorous evaluation regarding whether or not they add prognostic information beyond that which is already obtained by simpler clinical methods and classic risk factors (see Fig. 9.1). These extensively studied biomarkers are cardiac troponin I or T, CRP, and BNP. In addition, multiple studies have tested their interaction with different therapeutic strategies.

In general, biomarkers that are currently discussed to support management in chronic CAD reflect different pathophysiologic processes such as cardiac micronecrosis and hemodynamics, as well as more general processes such as inflammation, vascular function, renal function, and lipid disorders.

This chapter provides an overview about established and novel biomarkers in chronic CAD and describes the molecular basis of biomarker discovery and selection and the practical considerations that are a prerequisite to their clinical use.

BIOMARKERS OF MYOCARDIAL INJURY

Cardiac Troponin

Myocardial injury occurs when there is a disruption of normal cardiac myocyte membrane integrity. This results in the release of intracellular components into the extracellular space, including detectable levels of a variety of biologically active cytosolic and structural proteins, such as cardiac troponins. Myocardial injury has traditionally been considered to be an irreversible process (cell death), occurring mainly during an acute pathologic cardiac condition like an acute coronary ischemic event or acute myocarditis.[3] The advent of more sensitive methods allows troponin determination in apparently stable cardiac healthy conditions.

Cardiac troponins I and T are regulatory proteins that control the calcium-mediated interaction of actin and myosin during contraction. These proteins are products of specific genes and therefore have the potential to be unique for the heart. Studies performed with cardiac troponin I have failed to locate any troponin I outside of the heart at any stage of neonatal development. In contrast, cardiac troponin T is expressed to a minor extent in skeletal muscle.[4] Data indicate that there are at least some patients with skeletal muscle disease who have detectable levels of cardiac troponins. This implies that skeletal muscle injury can, in some patients, be the source for elevations of troponin detected in the blood,[5] even in a healthy state.

Assays to Measure Cardiac Troponins

Cardiac troponins I and T are specific markers for myocardial injury. However, there are variations in the sensitivity and specificity of various immunoassays. This is related to a lack of standardization, the presence of modified cardiac troponin I and troponin T in "serum" or "plasma", and variations in antibody cross-reactivities to the various detectable forms of troponin I that result from their degradation. Because each assay relies on specific conditions, one cannot extrapolate a value from one assay to another. Older assays are less sensitive than newer assays. The former are referred to as *conventional* or *sensitive* assays and the latter are referred to as *high-sensitivity*[6] assays.[7,8] One criterion for calling an assay high sensitivity is the proportion of apparently healthy individuals in whom the assay is capable of detecting troponin.[9] All individuals have small amounts of measurable troponin levels in their blood.[10] Most conventional or sensitive assays detect troponin levels only in very few normal individuals, whereas some high-sensitivity assays detect troponin in nearly 100% of normal individuals.[7,8,11–14] Both the analytical performance of the assay and instrumentation and differences in the reference populations likely contribute to reported variability between assays (as reviewed by Jaffe[3]).

The highly sensitive assays have tremendous potential for clinical practice. Compared with sensitive troponin assays, high-sensitivity troponin assays enhance the accuracy and speed of the diagnosis, improve outcome, and are cost-effective.[15] High-sensitivity assays that allow the measurement of very low cardiac troponin levels in patients with stable heart disease are now available for clinical and research use. These low, previously undetectable troponin levels have shown strong associations with incidents, i.e., future myocardial infarction (MI), stroke, and death, in a variety of primary and secondary prevention populations, including in patients with stable ischemic heart disease or stable CAD.[16–18]

Omland et al. showed that very low circulating levels of cardiac troponin T are detectable in the great majority of patients with stable CAD and preserved left ventricular function. Multiple conventional risk factors were associated with higher troponin T levels in this population, and very low circulating levels of troponin T had a graded relationship with the incidence of cardiovascular death and heart failure (HF). Moreover, the authors presented insights into the levels well below the limit of detection of previous assays and below the 99th percentile in apparently healthy blood donors. Even in this range, troponin levels were strongly associated with the incidence of cardiovascular death and HF; however, the levels were not independently associated with the incidence of MI.[18]

When applying a high-sensitivity troponin I test in the same study population, Omland et al. demonstrated that small elevations were associated with the incidence of cardiovascular death or HF in patients with stable CAD and provide additional prognostic information to conventional risk markers and prognostic cardiovascular biomarkers, including troponin T. Interestingly, the correlation between troponin I and troponin T levels was of only moderate strength, suggesting that mechanisms of release and/or degradation may potentially differ between the troponins in the chronic setting. Furthermore, troponin I, but not troponin T, was significantly and independently associated with both prior acute MI (AMI) and the incidence of subsequent AMI. Chronic, low-grade elevation of troponin I and troponin T in patients with stable CAD may potentially reflect different pathophysiologic determinants and suggest different therapeutic responses.[17]

Everett et al. showed in their study involving patients with both type 2 diabetes and stable ischemic heart disease that baseline cardiac troponin T levels above the upper limit of normal were associated with approximately a doubling of the risks of MI, stroke, HF, death from cardiovascular causes, and death from any cause. Nearly 40% of the patients had high-sensitivity cardiac troponin T levels at baseline that were above the upper reference limit used to define myocardial injury. The incidence of the primary composite endpoint of death from cardiovascular causes, MI, or stroke at 5 years in this group was 27%, which was double the rate in the group with normal baseline troponin T levels. Similar results were seen with respect to other important outcomes, such as the secondary composite outcome of death from any cause, MI, stroke, or HF. The relationship between troponin T levels and the subsequent risk of MI, stroke, HF, death from cardiovascular causes, and death from any cause suggests that high-sensitivity cardiac troponin T level is a powerful prognostic marker in patients who have both type 2 diabetes and stable ischemic heart disease.[16]

The newly established technologies allow precise measurement of low circulating troponin levels even in the general population.[10] This biomarker is of particular importance, as it is cardiac specific and directly reflects pathologic cardiac conditions. Cardiac troponin concentrations also correlate with the prevalence of cardiovascular risk factors. Assessment of circulating troponin levels using a robust, highly sensitive assay might therefore be suitable to predict first and subsequent adverse events. Whether the measurement of troponin in addition to risk scoring systems[19] is useful for cardiovascular risk assessment will be subject to further research.

The first steps in this direction have been analysed by using the harmonized database and biobank of the Biomarker for Cardiovascular Risk Assessment in Europe (BiomarCaRE). The distribution of troponin I levels was evaluated on an individual level, assayed using a highly sensitive method in population cohorts across Europe. The association with cardiovascular mortality, first nonfatal and fatal cardiovascular events, and overall mortality has been characterized, and the predictive value beyond the variables used in the European Society of Cardiology Systematic COronary Risk Evaluation (ESC SCORE) has been determined. The application of high-sensitivity cardiac troponin I has the potential to improve risk prediction of cardiac death in the general population. A potentially clinically relevant cut-off value was applied. The results of the BiomarCaRE study indicate conditions in which the determination of troponin I concentrations provides additional prognostic information to established risk models. Troponin I determination might support the selection of those individuals who would benefit most from preventive strategies.[19] However, the direct interaction between troponin elevation and preventive treatment strategies in particular in diseased individuals still has to be proven.

BIOMARKERS OF VASCULAR FUNCTION AND NEUROHUMORAL ACTIVITY

B-Type Natriuretic Peptide

BNP is a natriuretic peptide hormone with vasoactive functions and is involved in volume homeostasis and cardiovascular remodeling.[20] Both BNP and NT-proBNP are robust markers of neurohormonal activation. BNP is produced from larger precursor molecules, prepro-BNP(1-134) and pro-BNP(1-108), pro-BNP is then cleaved into the active moiety BNP(1-32) and an inactive part, NT-proBNP(1-76).[21] Although this simple model of the cleavage pattern is widely described, the cleavage mechanisms seem to be more complex and dependent on different factors. A number of reports have demonstrated high-molecular-weight material, apparently unprocessed proBNP forms, circulating in healthy as well as in diseased individuals, even in almost equal amounts as processed BNP.[22] proBNP is a glycoprotein including several glycosylation sites within the protein. The glycosylation status seems to be crucial for further proBNP processing, in particular at the glycosylation sites near the region of cleavage. Molecular studies have shown an O-glycosylation-dependent inhibition of proBNP processing, which could be one possible explanation for the presence of higher levels of unprocessed proBNP in biologic samples.[23] In addition, NT-proBNP in human blood is also glycosylated, which can negatively influence the recognition of NT-proBNP by antibodies targeting the central part of the molecule[23] and thus might not be easily accessible by standard assays. These data are of clinical interest, as they indicate the existence of different high-molecular-weight and low-molecular-weight forms of BNP in biologic material.

Consequently, assays to detect BNP/NT-proBNP need to be able to clearly distinguish between these various circulating forms of BNP.

Several other mechanisms also contribute to an increase in BNP levels such as cardiac hypertrophy, or increased muscle mass in left ventricular hypertrophy. By binding to its receptor (natriuretic peptide A receptor), BNP mediates natriuresis, vasodilatation, and renin inhibition, as well as anti-ischemic effects.[21] Clearance of BNP is mediated mainly via the natriuretic peptide C (clearance) receptor and the widely distributed enzyme neprilysin. Although functionally inactive, NT-proBNP has a longer half-life compared to BNP (1–2 h vs. 20 min), resulting in higher circulating levels. The longer in vivo half-life and enhanced in vitro stability are clear advantages, particularly in settings such as general practice where samples are shipped to hospital laboratories for analysis.

The main source of circulating BNP is the ventricular myocardium where it is produced in response to dilatation and pressure overload, and released into the circulation.[24] This reflection of myocardial stretch makes BNP an excellent marker for diagnosis[25,26] and an important surrogate for severity of HF.[26] As markers for myocardial stretch, and the fact that therapy of HF modulates levels of BNP and NT-proBNP, these biomarkers are recommended for the assessment of diagnosis, prognosis, and treatment success in HF by all major cardiovascular societies.[26]

A large body of data provide evidence that BNP production is stimulated by hypoxia and ischemia itself, processes which may result in myocyte stress under ischemic conditions despite constancy in measurable hemodynamic parameters.[27]

For patients with HF with reduced ejection fraction (HFrEF), impressive data have been generated for BNP in the prediction of outcome. In particular, patients with persistently high BNP levels are at high risk for adverse outcomes. In chronic HF, higher levels of BNP are associated with increased cardiovascular and all-cause mortality, independent of age, New York Heart Association class, previous MI, and left ventricular ejection fraction (LVEF).[28] BNP is also associated with re-admission for HF and outcomes after presentation to the emergency department for HF, a setting in which traditional risk factors do not have any prognostic value.[28] In HF with preserved ejection fraction (HFpEF), BNP has also been shown to be an important prognostic marker in patients for predicting mortality.[21]

In addition to its use for HF diagnosis and prognosis, NT-proBNP has also been recognized as a marker of long-term mortality in patients with stable coronary disease. Kragelund et al.[29] showed, in over 1000 coronary heart disease (CHD) patients, including a high proportion of patients with suspected HF, that NT-proBNP levels were significantly higher in patients who died from any cause after a median follow-up of 9 years. Patients with high NT-pro-BNP levels were older, had a lower LVEF and a lower creatinine clearance rate, and were more likely to have a history of MI, clinically significant CAD, and diabetes.[29] In another large study whose aim was to examine the predictive value of BNP in CAD for long-term cardiovascular outcome, Schnabel et al.[27] prospectively analyzed BNP levels in patients with stable angina. BNP levels were significantly increased in patients with future cardiovascular events. Patients with high levels of BNP had an elevated risk for cardiovascular events, even after adjustment for potential confounders such as age, gender, body mass index (BMI), CRP, and HDL-C (Fig. 9.2).[27] These data provide clear and independent evidence that BNP is a strong prognostic marker that provides additional information above and beyond that provided by classic risk factors.

In the studies of Kargelund and Schnabel,[29,30] a high proportion of clinically suspected HF patients—and thus high-risk stable CAD patients—were present. Thus, the association between BNP and mortality might be explained mainly by the ability of BNP to predict HF. To further examine whether BNP can act as a prognostic indicator in patients with low-risk stable CAD and to investigate whether BNP levels might also relate to

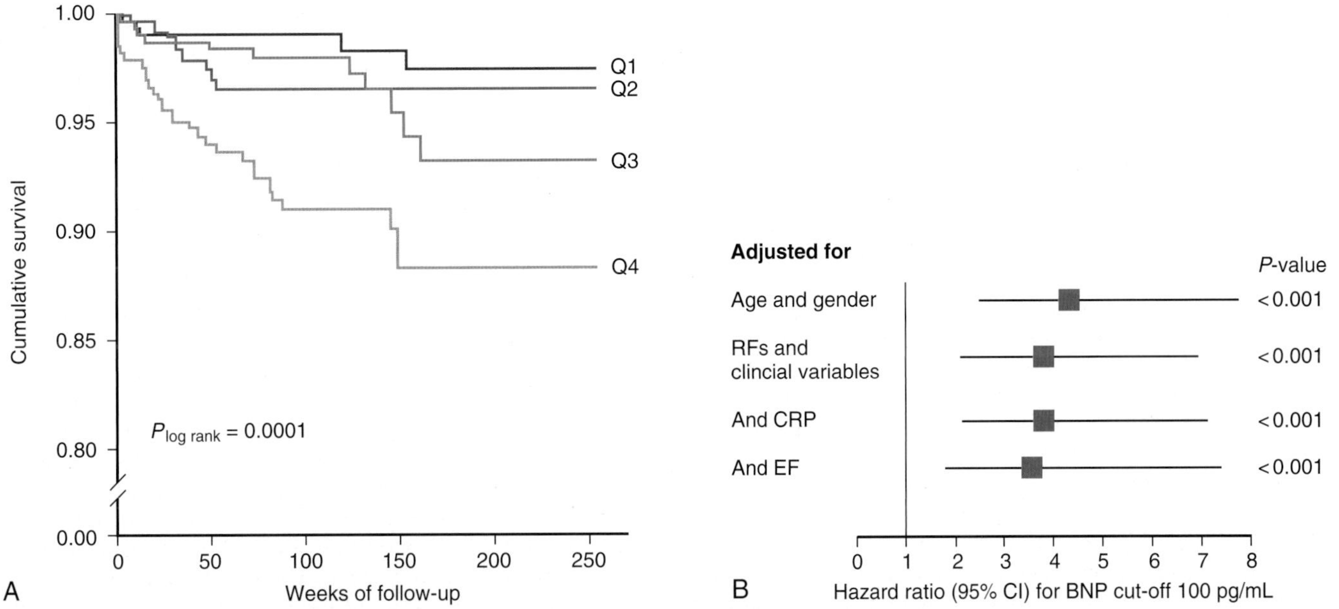

FIG. 9.2 Evidence for the predictive value of B-type natriuretic peptide in coronary artery disease for long-term cardiovascular outcome. Patients with high levels of BNP showed an elevated risk for cardiovascular events (A), even after adjustment for potential classical confounders (B). *BNP*, B-type natriuretic peptide; *CI*, confidence interval; *CRP*, C-reactive protein; *EF*, ejection fraction; *RF*, reduction factor. *(From Schnabel R, Lubos E, Rupprecht HJ, et al. B-type natriuretic peptide and the risk of cardiovascular events and death in patients with stable angina: results from the AtheroGene study.* J Am Coll Cardiol. *2006;47:552–558.)*

incidence of coronary ischemic events, plasma BNP and NT-proBNP levels were measured in a subcohort of the Prevention of Events with Angiotensin-Converting Enzyme Inhibition (PEACE) trial, including patients with stable CAD and preserved systolic function.[31] Both BNP and NT-proBNP showed predictive value for incidence of cardiovascular death, congestive HF, and stroke, but not for MI. After adjustment for classic risk factors, both peptides were still predictive for HF but only NT-proBNP remained predictive for cardiovascular death and stroke. Importantly, even after adjustment for the incidence of HF, NT-proBNP remained a significant predictor of cardiovascular mortality.[31] Accordingly, both BNP peptides added strong prognostic information to classic risk factors in both high- and low-risk patients with stable CAD.

Although persuasive evidence exists that NT-proBNP and BNP strongly predict outcome in individuals with chronic CAD, the determination of these natriuretic markers is currently not established in the clinical routine of stable ischemic heart disease assessment. This is explained by the lack of treatment consequences in individuals with chronic CAD who have elevated NT-proBNP or BNP levels. Nevertheless, elevated natriuretic peptide levels in these patients should prompt detailed diagnostic efforts to exclude the presence of HF.

Atrial Natriuretic Peptide

Similar to BNP, atrial or A-type natriuretic peptide (ANP) is a hormone that is released from myocardial cells in response to volume expansion and increased wall stress.[32] ANP circulates primarily as a 28–amino acid polypeptide predominately synthesized and secreted by atrial cardiomyocytes in healthy individuals. In HF, ANP is also produced by ventricular cardiomyocytes. ANP is derived from a precursor molecule of 126 amino acids, called proANP, and is cleaved into a 98–amino acid N-terminal fragment (NT-proANP) and the active ANP. NT-proANP has a much longer half-life than active ANP and has therefore been proposed as a more reliable analyte for measurement than ANP.[33] Further fragmentation of proANP results in a mid-regional ANP molecule (MR-proANP), which is even more stable than the N- or C-terminal part of the precursor.[34]

Just like the related B-type natriuretic peptides, an increase in ANP and its cleavage associates with HF. The Leicester Acute Myocardial Infarction Peptide (LAMP) study demonstrated that MR-proANP is a powerful predictor of death in post-MI patients.[35] This was especially evident in patients with an elevated NT-proBNP, indicating that the combination of both A- and B-type natriuretic peptides gives added prognostic information above existing clinical characteristics.[35] The Gruppo Italiano per lo Studio della Sopravvivenza nell'Infarto Miocardico Heart Failure (GISSI-HF) trial provided evidence that measurement of MR-proANP provided prognostic information independently of NT-proBNP.[36] Natriuretic peptides and other vasoactive peptides were measured in 1237 patients with chronic stable HF at randomization and at 3 months. The addition of MR-proANP improved classification for mortality when added to models based on clinical risk factors alone (net reclassification improvement [NRI] = 0.12) or together with NT-proBNP (NRI = 0.06). Increases in MR-proANP levels were associated with mortality (hazard ratio 1.38, 95% confidence interval [CI] 0.99–1.93 and hazard ratio 1.58, 95% CI 1.13–2.21, in the middle and highest versus the lowest tertiles, respectively).[36,37]

Although data on the value of ANP and its amino- and mid-terminal fragments in chronic coronary disease are available, more data are needed to define the clinical utility of MR-proANP measurements in patients with stable angina pectoris and chronic CAD.

Adrenomedullin

Adrenomedullin (ADM) is a peptide that was originally isolated from human pheochromocytoma cells; it has an amino acid sequence that is similar to human calcitonin gene-related peptide, a potent vasodilator.[32] In addition to the strong vasodilatory effects on the vasculature, ADM enhances myocardial contractility via a cyclic adenosine monophosphate-independent mechanism (reviewed by Colucci[38]). Although not cardiac-specific, ADM exerts various effects on the cardiovascular system, i.e., induction of hypotension and bronchodilatation or enhancement of renal perfusion.

ADM is derived from a 185–amino acid precursor peptide (preproADM), which is processed into another biologically active peptide termed *proadrenomedullin N-terminal 20 peptide* (PAMP). This peptide fragment has a suggested hypotensive effect and two peptides flanking ADM: one mid-regional part of proADM (proADM 45–92) and the COOH terminus of the molecule (proADM 153–185).[39]

Earlier studies investigating the active form of ADM showed that ADM plasma levels are elevated in patients with chronic HF and increase with disease severity.[41] Because active ADM immediately binds to receptors in the vicinity of its production and has a short half-life (22 min), reliable measurement of active ADM in the circulation is difficult. Therefore, novel immunoassays measuring the stable mid-regional part of proADM (MR-proADM) have been developed[39] and are currently used to assess MR-proADM levels.

In hypertensive African Americans, MR-proADM is correlated with pulse pressure, left ventricular (LV) mass, and albuminuria (reviewed by Neumann et al.[40]). In patients with HF, ADM was an independent predictor of mortality and added further prognostic value to established biomarkers, e.g., NT-proBNP.[40] In the Biomarkers in Acute Heart Failure (BACH) trial, which investigated the prognostic value of MR-proADM in patients with acute HF, the peptide predicted survival over a period of 90 days superior to BNP and NT-proBNP.[41] Using cut-off values, the accuracy to predict 90-day survival was 73% for MR-proADM, 62% for BNP, and 64% for NT-proBNP (difference $p < 0.001$). Even in the adjusted multivariable Cox regression, MR-proADM carried independent prognostic value.

The prognostic impact of MR-proADM on future fatal and nonfatal cardiovascular events in patients with symptomatic CAD was assessed in the AtheroGene study.[42] Individuals presenting with stable angina pectoris had comparable MR-proADM levels to levels in those with acute coronary events. Individuals who suffered a subsequent cardiovascular event had elevated MR-proADM levels at baseline in both groups. Baseline MR-proADM levels were independently associated with future cardiovascular events, and MR-proADM added information beyond that obtained from classic risk models. The additional use of MR-proADM for risk stratification in patients with known stable coronary heart disease was also shown in the Long-Term Intervention with Pravastatin in Ischemic Disease (LIPID) study.[43] Here, baseline levels of MR-proADM predicted major CHD events (nonfatal MI or CHD death and all-cause mortality) after 1 year. An increase in MR-proADM levels after 1 year was associated with an increased risk of subsequent CHD events, nonfatal MI, HF, and all-cause mortality. Adjustment for baseline BNP levels did not change the significance of these associations.

Concerning its prognostic value in post-MI patients, MR-proADM was also a powerful predictor of adverse outcome and was correlated with future cardiovascular events in patients with symptomatic CAD and acute chest pain. In the LAMP Study, MR-proADM was increased in post-MI patients[35] who suffered death or HF, and MR-proADM levels were significant independent predictors of death and HF in these patients. MR-proADM levels provided even stronger risk stratification in those patients who had NT-proBNP levels above the median, indicating that MR-proADM represents a powerful and clinically useful marker for prognosis of death and HF after AMI, comparable to or in combination with NT-proBNP.

Growth Differentiation Factor-15

Growth differentiation factor-15 (GDF-15), also known as *serum macrophage inhibitory cytocine-1* (MIC-1), is a member of the transforming growth factor (TGF-ß) cytokine superfamily, which has been discussed in the last decade as a novel emerging biomarker for CVD and other diseases such as cancer.[44] Under physiologic conditions, GDF-15 is solely expressed in the placenta, but its expression pattern is increased under various pathophysiologic conditions.[45] GDF-15 has been shown to be associated with oxidative stress, inflammation, and stress induced by biomechanical stretching of the heart.[46] In an experimental mouse model, Kempf et al. showed endogenous GDF-15 to be significantly involved in cardiac protection in ischemia or reperfusion injury.[46] However, the pathophysiologic role of GDF-15 in different pathologic disease states and its regulatory mechanism are still controversial.[45]

In diseased patients suffering from HF, GDF-15 measurement improved the prediction of mortality and an adverse outcome.[47] Interestingly, GDF-15 levels seem to better correlate with diastolic dysfunction than NT-proBNP levels and thus add incremental information to NT-proBNP in a population at risk.[47] Brown et al. described increased plasma levels of GDF-15 as a predictor for cardiovascular events in patients in a case-control study in healthy women.[48] Interestingly, GDF-15 was also reported to be a prognostic marker in non-ST-segment elevation MI (NSTEMI) or ST-segment elevation MI (STEMI).[49] GDF-15 has also been evaluated as a prognostic tool in stable CAD. In the AtheroGene study, GDF-15 was associated with coronary heart disease mortality, but not MI, after adjustment for confounders.[49] In the Heart and Soul study, GDF-15 was independently associated with increased risk of cardiovascular events.[50] GDF-15 levels have also been implicated as a marker for patients at risk of death and HF rehospitalization in both HFrEF and HFpEF.[51] To date, this marker constitutes a powerful risk predictor in various clinical conditions, but without direct clinical applicability. Whether the determination of GDF-15 in chronic CAD might help to improve treatment strategies has not yet been tested.

BIOMARKERS OF RENAL FUNCTION

It has been well proven that impairment of renal function is strongly associated with CAD and cardiovascular mortality.[6,52] Beyond shared risk factors, decreased renal function affects the cardiovascular system through numerous mechanisms, e.g., increased aldosterone activity,[53] enhanced proinflammation,[54] and platelet activation.[55] These mechanisms lead to an acceleration of the development and progression of CAD, resulting in a poor prognosis of patients with decreased renal function. In addition to manifest chronic kidney disease,[56] slight impairment of renal function is also associated with increased coronary risk.[57,58] Therefore, biomarkers for the identification and exact quantification of different stages of renal dysfunction are essential for risk stratification, prevention, and therapies of CAD.

Estimated Glomerular Filtration Rate

The estimated glomerular filtration rate (eGFR) is the most relevant parameter for assessment of renal function in clinical practice. Different equations for the estimation of GFR have been developed during the past decades. Today, the eGFR equation of the Chronic Kidney Disease Epidemiology Collaboration (CKD-EPI)[56] is the best validated equation in terms of accuracy and risk prediction, especially in individuals with normal or only mildly reduced GFR.[56] Thus, the CKD-EPI equation is currently replacing other eGFR equations such as the Cockcroft-Gault equation or the Modification of Diet in Renal Disease (MDRD) equation. Despite several limitations, serum creatinine remains the most commonly used renal marker for estimation of GFR.

Numerous large studies have shown a substantial increase of cardiovascular risk in relation to eGFR decline toward 60 mL/min per 1.73 m^2 or below.[6] Individuals with an eGFR less than 60 mL/min per 1.73 m^2 are defined as high cardiovascular risk. Although those individuals are exposed to more adverse effects by the use of cardiovascular drugs or iodinated contrast agents compared to individuals with a preserved renal function, the benefit of an intensive treatment of CVD outweighs this substantially in patients with decreased renal function.[59,60] Therefore, a baseline and annual measurement of creatinine and assessment of renal function with eGFR is recommended for all patients with known or suspected CAD.[61]

Cystatin C

As serum creatinine measurements have limitations due to variations in creatinine production, secretion, and extrarenal excretion influenced by age, gender, muscle metabolism, and renal reserve, potentially more robust renal markers have been evaluated. Of these, cystatin C is the best validated and most widespread renal marker beside serum creatinine. Cystatin C is produced by all nucleated cells at a relatively constant rate, is filtered at the glomerulus, and is not reabsorbed in the tubules. Due to fewer variations influenced by age, gender, muscle mass, diet, or other factors, impaired cystatin C concentration better detects particularly mild decreases of renal function.[62] In a large cohort of patients with CAD and normal or only mildly reduced renal function, cystatin C was a potent predictor of cardiovascular mortality beyond classic risk factors.[63]

In terms of GFR prediction, the use of cystatin C for estimation of eGFR with cystatin C–based eGFR equations has similar accuracy compared to the use of creatinine-based eGFR equations.[62] The combined CKD-EPI eGFR equation using both serum creatinine and cystatin C has been shown to be more exact for estimation of GFR than eGFR equations based on either of these markers alone.[56] In terms of cardiovascular risk prediction, eGFR calculated with the cystatin C–based or combined CKD-EPI equation was shown to be more strongly associated with the cardiovascular prognosis than eGFR calculated with serum creatinine–based equations both in a cohort of HF patients and in a cohort of patients with CAD.[64,65]

Measurement of cystatin C in addition to serum creatinine and assessment of eGFR with the combined CKD-EPI equation can be helpful as a confirmatory test in patients with a creatinine-based GFR estimation of 45 to 75 mL/min per 1.73 m^2 to identify, or exclude more accurately, the cardiovascular high-risk setting of reduced renal function with a GFR less than 60 mL/min per 1.73 m^2, which requires the most intensive treatment of cardiovascular risk factors.

LIPID BIOMARKERS

More than a century ago the German chemist Adolf Windaus described a far higher amount of cholesterol in atherogenic plaques of human aortas compared to healthy aortas. Since then, numerous studies have demonstrated a key role of atherogenic cholesterol-containing lipoprotein particles, particularly low-density lipoprotein cholesterol (LDL-C), for the development of CAD.[66]

Although there is a large diversity of measurable lipoproteins and various lipoprotein ratios have been evaluated, the strong evidence of lipid-lowering therapy established through many randomized controlled trials is almost entirely based on total cholesterol and LDL-C. (See Chapter 8 for more on lipid biomarkers.)

Recommendations for Lipid Profile Measurement

A lipid profile including total cholesterol (TC), high-density lipoprotein cholesterol (HDL-C), LDL-C, and triglycerides (TGs) should be assessed in all patients with suspected or known stable CAD. In those patients with established diagnosis of CAD the lipid profile should be reassessed in an intervallic manner in order to control the efficacy of lipid-lowering therapy and to evaluate dose adjustments in the case of LDL-C goal-directed therapy. Without clear evidence for the duration of intervals of reassessment, annual measurements of the lipid profile are recommended.[61]

Whereas measurement of lipids at a fasting status was common for decades, the 2016 joint consensus statement from the European Atherosclerosis Society and European Federation of Clinical Chemistry and Laboratory Medicine recommended the routine use of nonfasting lipid profiles to improve patient compliance and simplify the processes of lipid testing.[67] This recommendation is based on well-proven data indicating that the changes of lipid parameters 1 to 6 hours after a common meal are not clinically relevant. A fasting measurement of the lipid profile is only recommended in the case of very high nonfasting TG levels (> 440 mg/dL according to ESC recommendations, > 500 mg/dL according to American Heart Association [AHA]/American College of Cardiology [ACC] recommendations).

Low-Density Lipoprotein Cholesterol

Epidemiologic, genetic, mechanistic, and intervention studies have proven the causal role of LDL-C in the genesis of CAD. In patients with CAD, an LDL-C reduction with statins of 1 mmol/L (38.7 mg/dL) results in a 20% to 25% relative risk reduction of major vascular events irrespective of baseline LDL-C.[68] Furthermore, several studies have shown a lower progression and even regression of CAD with significant percent diameter stenosis decrease and minimum lumen diameter increase under intensive LDL-C reduction by high-dose statin therapy.[69]

Neither treatment to a specific LDL-C target nor comparison of different LDL-C treatment targets has been investigated by randomized controlled trials. The vast majority of randomized controlled trials proving a risk reduction in patients with CAD used a fixed-dose statin therapy. Based on this evidence the latest ACC/AHA guidelines do not recommend any specific LDL-C targets or titrating lipid-lowering therapy to LDL-C goals, but do recommend high-intensity statin therapy in all patients with known CAD regardless of specific LDL-C targets. In contrast, the ESC guidelines recommend statin therapy for all patients with CAD with a treatment target of LDL-C less than 1.8 mmol/L (< 70 mg/dL) or at least 50% reduction from baseline LDL-C if the target level cannot be achieved. Despite different recommendations regarding the strategies of lipid-lowering therapy for patients with known CAD, both the ESC guidelines and ACC/AHA guidelines recommend at least annual measurements of LDL-C to evaluate the adherence and response to lipid-lowering therapy.[61,70] LDL-C can be determined using the Friedewald formula, if TGs are less than 400 mg/dL, or measured directly irrespective of TG levels.

High-Density Lipoprotein Cholesterol

An inverse correlation of HDL-C levels and the risk of CAD has been found by numerous epidemiologic studies. Several protective mechanisms of HDL-C have been described.[71] Despite the strong correlation of HDL-C levels and CAD, no causation between HDL-C and the genesis of CAD or atherosclerosis has been established. Of particular importance, Mendelian randomization studies have not shown an association between genetic mechanisms that raise HDL-C levels and the risk of CVD.[72] Furthermore, clinical trials investigating HDL-C-raising therapies such as niacin or cholesteryl ester transfer protein inhibitors have failed to improve cardiovascular outcomes.[73,74] In the setting of secondary prevention, both the AHA/ACC and ESC guidelines do not specify HDL-C levels as treatment targets for patients with CAD. In the setting of primary prevention or suspected CAD, measurement of HDL-C is recommended for risk estimation and can be used for decision-making in individuals with a cardiovascular risk at the threshold for intensive risk factor modification, where these individuals qualify for more intensive advice in the case of low HDL-C levels.[75] Low HDL-C levels are defined as less than 1.0 mmol/L (< 40 mg/dL) in men and less than 1.2 mmol/L (< 45 mg/dL) in women.

Markers of functional properties of HDL as cholesterol efflux capacity and not solely HDL-C levels are promising and might be established as relevant biomarkers and treatment targets.[76]

Triglycerides

Elevated levels of TGs are associated with CVD with an increased risk for fasting levels of greater than 1.7 mmol/L

(> 150 mg/dL). Compared to hypercholesterolemia as a cardiovascular risk factor, the association of TGs and CVD is far weaker. However, evidence suggesting a causal role of TGs in the genesis of coronary heart disease was recently presented.[77,78] Because clinical trials with triglyceride-reducing therapies such as fibrates, nicotinic acid, and fish oil have failed to show a cardiovascular risk reduction, guidelines do not specify treatment targets for patients with CAD.[61] Irrespective of the presence of CVD the ACC/AHA guidelines recommend an evaluation for secondary causes of hyperlipidemia in the case of very high TG levels (≥ 500 mg/dL [≥ 5.7 mmol/L]), e.g., high alcohol intake, nephrotic syndrome, hypothyroidism, or poorly controlled diabetes.[70]

Lipoprotein(a)

Beyond the role of a cardiovascular risk factor, genetic studies indicate a causal role of lipoprotein(a) (Lp[a]) for CVD, particularly CAD.[79,80] Plasma levels of Lp(a) are genetically determined, remain relatively constant throughout life without significant response to lifestyle changes, and vary strongly between ethnicities, with the lowest levels in Caucasians and highest levels in African Americans.[81] A strong inverse correlation between the size of the apo(a) isoforms and Lp(a) levels has been shown.[82] Therefore, assays for Lp(a) measurements are recommended to be isoform insensitive.[81] Several substances, such as some fibrates or niacin, have been shown to moderately reduce Lp(a) levels by a maximum of 30% to 35%. However, no clinical trials have shown cardiovascular risk reduction for selective Lp(a) reduction. Instead of broad screening for elevated Lp(a) levels in the general population, Lp(a) should be measured once only in selected individuals. For patients with CAD, measurement of Lp(a) is recommended in those with a premature CAD, in those with a family history of premature CVD and/or elevated Lp(a), and in those with recurrent vascular events despite intensive statin treatment.[81] Reassessment of Lp(a) levels is only necessary in patients who receive Lp(a)-reducing treatment such as niacin or lipid apheresis.

INFLAMMATORY BIOMARKERS

High-Sensitivity C-Reactive Protein

CRP is a sensitive marker of inflammation and tissue damage. Phylogenetically conserved, CRP plays a role in the response to inflammation. Produced in the liver, levels of CRP rapidly rise nonspecifically during acute phase reactions, such as infections. CRP directly binds highly atherogenic oxidized LDL-C and is present within lipid-laden plaques,[83] thereby triggering the immune response.

CRP has received widespread interest in CVD, although controversy remains regarding its clinical value as a potential proinflammatory mediator. Data from several epidemiologic studies indicate a significant association between elevated serum or plasma levels of CRP and the prevalence of underlying atherosclerosis, the risk of recurrent cardiovascular events among patients with established disease, and the incidence of first cardiovascular events among individuals at risk for atherosclerosis.[84,85]

In addition, a number of drugs used in the treatment of CVD, such as statins, reduce serum CRP levels. The potential interaction of CRP levels with statin therapy has been retrospectively and prospectively tested in various clinical trials. The Pravastatin or Atorvastatin Evaluation and Infection Therapy–Thrombolysis in Myocardial Infarction 22 (PROVE-IT–TIMI 22) and Reversal of Atherosclerosis with Aggressive Lipid Lowering (REVERSAL) trials showed that intensive statin therapy achieved a greater reduction in high-sensitivity C-reactive protein (hs-CRP) levels and, together with LDL-C, were associated with a greater reduction in the number of clinical events and progression of atherosclerotic plaque burden. Statins reduced hs-CRP and LDL-C levels by 38% and 35%, respectively.[83] Confirmation of these data could be shown in the Aggrastat to Zocor (A to Z) trial, in which on-treatment hs-CRP levels were independently associated with long-term survival.[83] The Justification for the Use of Statins in Primary Prevention: An Intervention Trial Evaluating Rosuvastatin (JUPITER) study prospectively tested the impact of rosuvastatin therapy in cardiovascular risk individuals with LDL levels below 130 mg/dL and CRP above 2 mg/L. In this trial of apparently healthy individuals without hyperlipidemia but with elevated hs-CRP levels, rosuvastatin significantly reduced the incidence of major cardiovascular events.[86] These data provide the possibility that reduced inflammation contributes to the beneficial effects of these medications.

The question of whether CRP is causally linked with CAD (and thus lowering CRP should also reduce CAD risk), or just a marker of underlying atherosclerosis, has been investigated in Mendelian randomization studies. These approaches allow the drawing of conclusions about the causality underlying the relationship between biomarker and diseases. Mendelian randomization studies investigate the impact of genetic variations, which influence circulating biomarker levels like CRP concentration, on future cardiovascular events. Several such Mendelian randomization studies investigating CRP and cardiovascular events have convincingly excluded a causal role of CRP for CAD.[87,88] In contrast, Mendelian randomization studies targeting the LDL hypothesis have proven the causal role of LDL-C for incident cardiovascular events. Despite the consistent epidemiologic evidence, there is, at present, no established role for routine measurement of hs-CRP in patients with CVD.[89]

Various studies described the association between CRP and outcome in patients with stable angina and chronic CAD. Hs-CRP levels were, among other inflammatory markers, significantly higher in those patients who died of cardiac events during follow-up and were predictive of death.[90,91] This association was not observed in statin-treated individuals. However, in patients without statin medication, cardiac mortality was low when the patients had low hs-CRP levels but was high in individuals with elevated hs-CRP levels. These patients had a 2.3-fold risk increase for fatal coronary events, independent of LDL-C levels.[90] In the PEACE trial, the ability of hs-CRP to predict outcomes in patients with stable CAD and a preserved ejection fraction was further tested. In over 3700 patients, hs-CRP levels were measured and patients were followed up over a median of 4.8 years for cardiovascular death, MI, or stroke.[92] Higher hs-CRP levels were associated with a significantly increased risk of cardiovascular death, MI, and stroke, even at average levels > 1 mg/L. Elevated hs-CRP levels were also found to be an independent predictor for incident HF and diabetes. Thus, in patients with stable CAD, hs-CRP levels were a strong predictor of cardiovascular death, MI, stroke, new HF, and new diabetes, independent of baseline characteristics and treatments.[92]

Despite being associated with incident cardiovascular events in patients with chronic CAD, the strength of the CRP association is not comparable to that of cardiac specific biomarkers such as troponin or NT-proBNP. For example, in the Heart Outcomes Prevention Evaluation (HOPE) Study, which evaluated several biomarkers in a setting of high-risk individuals, data showed that classic risk factor models do not gain accuracy by including inflammatory markers for the prediction of future cardiovascular events. The value for risk prediction attributable to CRP was modest, whereas plasma NT-proBNP levels strongly predicted future fatal and nonfatal cardiac events and, significantly, added information above classic risk factors.[93] Furthermore, no interaction between CRP levels and ramipril therapy was observed.

At this stage, the clinical use of CRP determination in patients with established chronic CAD is not fully proven and has not been included in guideline recommendations.

Interleukin-6

Whereas the association between inflammation and the development of atherosclerotic disease is well known, proving causation for any particular biomarker of inflammation has been difficult. Interleukin (IL)-6 signals a downstream proinflammatory response by activating membrane-bound IL-6 receptors on the cell surface. IL-6 receptors appear to play a direct causal role in the development of CHD and have been discussed as a target for therapeutic interventions to prevent CHD. Two large meta-analyses have confirmed the crucial role of IL-6 in the generation of inflammation and the associated risk of CHD.[94,95] These studies demonstrated an association between IL-6 levels and CHD in a dose-dependent manner. Taken together, these results provide evidence supporting a causal role of IL-6 in the development of CHD and suggest it as a target for therapeutic interventions to prevent CHD.[96]

Multiple Marker Strategies

The simultaneous measurement and analysis of several biomarkers might add more clinically useful information, as a broader picture of the different pathophysiologic aspects could be reflected upon and thus would be more informative. Several studies have evaluated the performance of these multimarker strategies in individuals with chronic CAD.

The incremental value of simultaneously measured markers reflecting acute-phase reaction, proinflammatory pathways, endothelial cell activation, and vascular function, compared to classic risk factors, was assessed in the secondary prevention setting of the HOPE Study. Among others, hs-CPR, IL-6, and NT-proBNP were analyzed with regard to the endpoints of MI, stroke, and cardiovascular death.[93] Inflammatory markers such as CRP and IL-6 added only limited additional prognostic information above classic risk factors (although individually significantly related to cardiovascular risk), whereas the inclusion of NT-proBNP improved the prediction of future cardiac events, resulting in significant incremental prognostic information.[93]

Another multimarker approach for risk prediction in CAD selected more novel biomarkers reflecting inflammation (CRP, GDF-15), lipid metabolism (apolipoproteins), renal function (cystatin C and creatinine), and cardiovascular function and remodeling (including natriuretic peptides and MR-proADM), representing multiple pathways of CAD.[30] This comparative analysis revealed Nt-proBNP, MR-proADM, cystatin C, and MR-proANP as the most informative biomarkers offering incremental predictive ability over classic risk factors. The combination of these biomarkers was most strongly related to outcome, and added incremental risk information to classic risk factor models. However, the combination did not enhance risk stratification or reclassification compared to the strongest single biomarkers, NT-proBNP and GDF-15.[30] Supporting these data, a multimarker approach in the PEACE trial including stable CAD patients at low risk assessed the markers MR-proANP and MR-proADM, as well as endothelin and copeptin. After adjustment for clinical cardiovascular risk predictors and LVEF, elevated levels of MR-proANP, MR-proADM, and CT-proET-1 were independently associated with the risk of cardiovascular death or HF. These three biomarkers also significantly improved metrics of discrimination when added to a clinical model.[97]

In the LIPID study the predictive power of biomarkers reflecting hemodynamics, micronecrosis, inflammation, coagulation, lipids, neurohumoral activity, and renal function was examined beyond classic risk factor models.[98] Furthermore, the investigators addressed whether changes in concentrations of these biomarkers over 12 months affected the risk of subsequent CHD events. All baseline biomarkers measured—except lipoprotein-associated phospholipase A2 (Lp-PLA2) activity and Lp(a)—were associated with outcome. The strongest prediction was observed for BNP and sensitive troponin I baseline concentrations. The prediction strength of these biomarkers was also strong compared with classic risk factors and other clinical features. Of all variables assessed, only a history of MI was a stronger predictor than troponin I or BNP. The other biomarkers—cystatin C, MR-proADM, D-dimer, and CRP—had significant but lesser prognostic value. The major finding was that changes in levels of troponin I and BNP in addition to their baseline levels predicted higher or lower CHD risk. These associations were observed irrespective of whether patients were randomized to pravastatin or placebo. Thus, both of these markers can be considered to reflect aggregate therapeutic and environmental effects. Despite evidence that some biomarkers can add information concerning prediction of the risk of CVD and associated events, apart from their diagnostic value in acute MI (troponin) and HF (particularly BNP) the direct clinical benefit of their assessment in usual clinical practice has not been well defined.

In summary, the data of most multiple marker studies suggest that combining biomarkers reflecting different cardiovascular processes in a panel can be helpful for improved risk prediction in chronic CAD and repeated biomarker measures such as troponin or BNP, and their level changes might directly translate into risk prediction.

NOVEL, OMICS-BASED BIOMARKERS

To improve risk estimation above and beyond established risk scores and to advance therapy decision-making and guidance, novel[94] biomarkers are of considerable interest. The implementation of these new biomarkers into clinical practice is under development, with intensive research efforts ongoing, and represents an important area in biomedical research.

High-throughput technologies that allow the measurement of large panels of markers on a genome-wide scale—often

TABLE 9.1 Omics Approaches for the Discovery of Novel Biomarkers

OMICS APPROACH	APPLICATION
Genomics	Assessment of genomic variations across the genome Measured by microarrays and sequencing Association of genomic variants and disease traits Mainly SNPs
Transcriptomics	Assessment of all RNA transcripts Measured by microarrays and sequencing Association of transcripts and disease traits Mainly mRNA and noncoding RNAs
Metabolomics	Assessment of all low-molecular-mass metabolites Measured mainly by mass spectrometry and NMR Targeted and nontargeted approaches Association of metabolites and disease traits
Proteomics	Assessment of all proteins and peptides Measured mainly by mass spectrometry Association of peptides and disease traits
Lipidomics	Assessment of the complete collection of lipids Measured mainly by mass spectrometry and NMR Association of lipids and disease traits

mRNA, Messenger RNA; *NMR*; nuclear magnetic resonance technology; *SNPs*, single nucleotide polymorphisms.

referred to as *omics approaches*—are making it possible to discover novel biomarker profiles.[99] Improvements in these technologies have allowed researchers to interrogate genes (genomics), gene transcripts (transcriptomics), proteins (proteomics), metabolites (metabolomics), and lipids (lipidomics) for biomarker discovery (Table 9.1). Advantages of the omics technologies over traditional approaches include their broad applicability not only to circulating proteins but also to other molecules such as RNA and metabolites, as well as their ability to analyze very large numbers of molecules simultaneously.[100] Thereby, the identification of novel biomarkers can shed light onto molecular and pathophysiologic mechanisms and pathways and can identify biomarkers causally involved in chronic CVDs. In the following section we will provide an overview of emerging and potential omics-based biomarkers.

Genomic Biomarkers

Genomic (see Chapter 3) variations, mainly the so-called single nucleotide polymorphisms (SNPs), are dominant markers of the genetic variability in humans, and a multitude of genome-wide association studies (GWAS) have explored the influence of these genomic variations on CVDs. A GWAS is a gene-mapping study that assesses evidence of association between genomic variants and disease status or clinical phenotypes across the genome. By design, GWAS provide an unbiased survey of the effects of genomic variants. The performance of GWAS became feasible by the advent of high-throughput genotyping microarray platforms that allow millions of genotypes to be assessed in a single experiment and, more currently, by sequencing approaches including exome and whole genome sequencing covering the entire genome. However, the power of detection depends directly on the sample size of the study population, the minor allele frequency of the SNP, the strength of linkage disequilibrium between SNPs, and the effect sizes of the alleles.[101] As larger sample sizes increase the power, emphasis has increased on meta-analyses of GWAS results of many individual studies.[101] These meta-analyses mainly include the Coronary ARtery DIsease Genome wide Replication and Meta-analysis (CARDIoGRAM), the Coronary Artery Disease (C4D) consortia, and the joint CARDIoGRAMplusC4D consortium and have tagged over 56 SNPs so far as associated with CVD with high statistical significance.[102] The pathophysiologic pathways covered by the identified regions include, among others, inflammation, lipid metabolism, vascular remodeling, and nitric oxide (NO)/cyclic guanosine monophosphate (cGMP) signaling.[102]

The most prominent genomic region with the highest population-attributable risk identified so far is located on chromosome 9p21.3. It is particularly striking that this genomic region contains no annotated genes, and SNPs that tag this region are not associated with any established risk factor for CAD.[101] However, this locus encodes different transcripts of the long noncoding RNA ANRIL that function in vascular disease.[103] The top associated SNPs are found adjacent to the last exon of ANRIL, and mechanistic studies have shown that the 9p21 risk allele disrupts an inhibitory STAT1 binding site, leading to upregulation of ANRIL expression.[104] These data suggest that genetic variants, by an influence on gene expression, might function as genetic biomarkers. Another prominent marker that resulted from genomics analyses on cholesterol levels is the proprotein convertase subtilisin/kexin type 9 (PCSK9). PCSK9 functions in LDL-C metabolism leading to the degradation of LDL-C receptors. Gain-of-function and loss-of-function mutations in the PCSK9 gene lead to strong alterations in LDL-C levels and thereby a change in risk for CVD.[102] Therefore, PCSK9 inhibitors are promising subjects of current therapeutic concepts.

The enormous progress made in the field of genomic cardiovascular research leads inevitably to the question of whether genomic variants have the power to serve as genetic markers and substantially improve the predication of clinically important cardiovascular outcomes and therapy discrimination.[101] As most of the single genetic variants typically explain only a modest fraction of the variance, an aggregated multilocus genetic risk score might improve risk prediction.[105] Basically, the generation of a genetic risk score involves summarizing information across multiple SNPs, e.g., by summing the number of risk-conferring alleles (0, 1, or 2) across all loci.[105]

Efforts on genetic risk scores have evaluated the ability of validated lipid-modulating SNPs, SNPs associated to type 2 diabetes, hypertension, coronary heart disease, and CVD.[101,105] Studies assessing genetic risk scores for the prediction of incident CVD used CAD-associated SNPs and identified a 24-SNP, as well as a 46-SNP risk score.[106,107] In both studies the genetic risk score showed an association with incident CAD. However, although the risk score models significantly improved risk reclassification beyond traditional risk factors, discrimination was not improved. Similarly, the evaluation of genetic risk scores in secondary prevention indicated that genetic risk scores are not successful in predicting new cardiovascular events in individuals with previous CAD.[108]

Evidently, genomics have yielded several key insights into putative causes and mechanisms of CVD. However, currently, no genetic marker or genetic risk score is ready for widespread use as a risk marker in stable CAD.

Transcriptomic Biomarkers

Technical advances in the field of transcriptomics—the simultaneous study of RNA transcripts and their expression patterns at a genome-wide level—harbor the potential to gain a better understanding of complex biologic systems as well as the potential for identification and development of novel biomarkers. Transcriptomic approaches include microarray-based methods, where tens of thousands of transcripts are simultaneously analyzed by chemically labeling RNA molecules and subsequent hybridization to probes on the microarray. With the novel RNA sequencing technologies, a population of RNA is converted to a cDNA library, which is subsequently sequenced in a high-throughput base-by-base manner to obtain short sequences, providing a much better and deeper coverage for detection of low abundance transcripts.

In the cardiovascular biomarker field, recent advances have identified several transcriptomics-based biomarkers that have the potential for translation as clinically useful biomarkers in chronic CAD.

Growth Differentiation Factor-15

A biomarker initially identified by transcriptomics analyses is GDF-15, a distant member of the TGF-β cytokine superfamily. GDF-15 is a stress-responsive cytokine expressed in the cardiovascular system. Microarray analyses showed that the GDF-15 gene was highly upregulated in NO-treated cardiomyocytes, under oxidative stress, in pressure overloaded left ventricles of mice with aortic stenosis, and in a mouse model of dilated cardiomyopathy.[109] Its value as a circulating biomarker for chronic CAD has been outlined previously.

Soluble ST2

Another example of a transcriptomics-based biomarker is soluble source of tumorigenicity 2 (sST2). Weinberg et al.[109] identified the *ST2* gene (also called *receptor of IL-33*) as upregulated in cardiac myocytes subjected to mechanical stress by microarray analysis. Soluble ST2 is a secreted receptor belonging to the IL-1 receptor family that regulates inflammation and immunity[110] and is involved in cardiac stress response and remodeling.[111] Soluble ST2 in complex with IL-33 has been implicated in the pathogenesis of CAD, mainly HF. Increased sST2 levels and thus impaired IL-33/ST2L signaling lead to cardiac hypertrophy, fibrosis, worsening left ventricular function, and arterial hypertension[112,113] and were also shown to be related to increased events of HF.[114] In the Framingham Heart Study, measurements of soluble ST2 showed clear gender differences, an increase with age, and increased levels in association with diabetes and hypertension,[112] and sST2 added prognostic value to standard risk factors with regard to cardiovascular events and HF and was related to an adverse outcome in patients diagnosed with chronic HF.[110,114] In combination with additional biomarkers (MR-proADM, high-sensitivity Troponin T [hsTnT], combined free light chains [cFLC], and hs-CRP), sST2 provided an even more incremental prognostic value in a dichotomized analysis in patients with HF. Thus, sST2 in combination with additional markers has potential as a clinically valuable marker.[111]

GDF-15 and ST2 are clear examples of how an initial transcriptomics analysis identified a target as a cardiac biomarker that is on its way to validation and clinical application.

Expression Signatures

Grouping several messenger RNAs (mRNAs) into a combined set can reflect a broader picture of the pathophysiologic mechanisms and pathways, and thus assist in the understanding of disease pathobiology, and might be useful for prioritizing novel therapeutic targets for treating the disease. Consequently, the combination of different mRNAs with a gene expression signature might prove to be a powerful biomarker for CAD. To date, a number of studies have been published examining whole blood gene expression profiling to identify individuals at risk of CAD.

Aiming to investigate the extent to which gene expression patterns in peripheral blood can mirror the severity of CAD, Sinnaeve et al.[115] identified and subsequently tested a signature of 160 genes in angiographically documented CAD. Molecular pathways covered by these 160 genes included angiogenesis, the inflammatory response, apoptosis, cell adhesion, cell growth, cell cycle arrest, cell-cell communication, lipid homeostasis, and the immune response. Similarly, a total of 35 genes showed differential expression in whole blood of CHD individuals with alterations in pathways of hematopoiesis, ubiquitination, apoptosis, and innate immune response pathways.[116]

In the Personalized Risk Evaluation and Diagnosis in the Coronary Tree (PREDICT) study, a whole blood 23-gene expression score was developed and validated for the assessment of obstructive CAD in nondiabetic patients.[117] This score was further evaluated in the multicenter Cardiovascular OutcoMes for People Using Anticoagulation StrategieS (COMPASS) study with regard to the diagnostic accuracy in symptomatic patients referred for myocardial perfusion.[118] This gene expression score was a significant predictor of CAD and resulted, at a predefined threshold, in a high sensitivity and high negative predictive value, making this score extremely promising and one of the best examples of the value of transcriptomics-based biomarkers in the cardiovascular field today.

However, when comparing the genes identified in these different studies, it becomes obvious that there is little overlap and that the effect sizes of the genes were small. A number of reasons might explain these discrepancies. First, multiplex tests are often complex, containing multiple sample processing steps, operators, machines, and types of reagents, which can affect assay variability. Secondly, the lack of concordance in the clinical phenotype or differences in disease definition can be a major contributor to different study results; for instance, the use of different or no control groups can result in decreased power to detect true findings. Furthermore, the large variety of available gene expression technologies can lead to different results across studies. Therefore—as for any biomarker discovery approach—harmonized definitions in phenotypes and disease entities, the use of standardized control groups, and technical, as well as clinical, validation in different technological settings and in independent cohorts are prerequisites for the clinical implementation of transcriptomics biomarkers.

Noncoding RNA

RNA has long been considered as the messenger molecule between genes and proteins, where RNA is transcribed from DNA to mRNA and subsequently translated into a protein.[105] In recent years, however, noncoding RNA (ncRNA) species (besides transfer and ribosomal RNA) have been characterized, including microRNAs (miRNAs),[119] long noncoding RNAs (lncRNAs),[104] and most currently circular RNAs (circRNAs).[120] ncRNAs can be small molecules between 20 and 23 nt in length (miRNAs), molecules longer than 200 nt (lncRNAs), or can form covalently closed, circular RNA molecules (circRNAs).[120] ncRNAs have in common that they are nonprotein coding transcripts with regulatory functions within important cellular and developmental processes and disease pathologies. ncRNAs fulfill several criteria to be considered as potential biomarkers: (1) some are quantitatively altered in CVD, (2) they show organ- and cell-specific expression patterns and thus can act as indicators of pathogenic processes,[121] (3) they are easily accessible, and (4) they withstand conditions such as longtime storage, multiple freeze/thaw cycles, and different pH values, and show a high degree of stability in body fluids.[122] The release of ncRNAs into extracellular compartments, in particular into the bloodstream, represents the possibility of noninvasively detecting and using them as disease biomarkers. In the CVD setting, numerous studies have explored ncRNAs as circulating biomarkers, putting them on the verge of implementation in clinical disease evaluation.[123]

microRNAs

miRNAs are the best investigated ncRNAs so far. Since their discovery in 1993,[124] approximately 1800 miRNAs have been annotated (see http://www.mirbase.org/). miRNAs are produced by all cell types and interact mainly with the 3′ untranslated region of protein-coding genes, thereby inhibiting the translational process.

The potential of circulating miRNAs as cardiovascular biomarkers has been widely studied. For example, in patients with stable CAD, reduced levels of miR-126 and members of miR-17-92a have been detected. In patients with CHD, lower levels of miR-145-5p cluster were found.[100] In another study, assessing the value for discrimination of unstable angina pectoris and stable CAD, higher levels of miRNA-21, miRNA-133a/b, and miRNA-199a, and lower levels of miRNA-145 and miRNA-155, were suggested.[125] As only small cohort sizes have been investigated, validation in larger cohorts is necessary. However, in agreement with this study, lower levels of miRNA-145 and miRNA-155 showed an inverse correlation with CAD severity scores (Gensini and Synergy between percutaneous coronary intervention with Taxus and cardiac surgery [SYNTAX]).[125]

In a large study investigating the value of miRNAs for stratification of subsequent coronary events among patients with CAD, eight miRNAs, previously shown to facilitate diagnosis of acute coronary syndrome, were investigated.[126] The analyses indicated that, in particular, miR-132 and miR-140-3p, as well as miR-201, precisely predicted cardiovascular death.

Similarly, in HF patients the potential of miRNAs as circulating biomarkers has been assessed. For example, a screening of circulating miRNAs in patients with HF identified 186 circulating miRNAs.[123] Of these, miR-423-5p, miR-320a, miR-22, and miR-92b were upregulated in HF patients compared with healthy controls. A subsequently successfully developed score consisting of these miRNAs was able to discriminate HF patients from healthy controls. A significant association between this miRNA score and several established HF parameters such as NT-proBNP, wide QRS complex, and LV dilatation was found.[123] These miRNAs had also been identified in additional studies on HF,[127–129] indicating a specific role in the underlying molecular pathways of HF. Similar to the research on single miRNAs, several studies assessed the potential of miRNA signatures as biomarkers for CAD, mainly including miR-126, miR-223, and miR-197.[130,131]

The results presented here emphasize the great potential of miRNAs as emerging CAD biomarkers. However, there is still a need for more, larger epidemiologic and clinical studies evaluating and validating these miRNA results.

lncRNAs

lncRNAs are transcribed from either intergenic regions, from introns of protein-coding sequences, or from an antisense strand of genes.[104] In contrast to miRNA sequences, the primary sequence of lncRNAs is only poorly conserved. The number of lncRNAs within cells is believed to be approximately 9000.[132] However, the number of lncRNAs that have been studied in CAD is still very limited. In total, eight different transcripts have been assessed as potential biomarkers, with promising results.[125,133] A 2015 transcriptomics analysis of HF patients showed the potential of lncRNAs as biomarkers in CAD.[133] Higher levels of LIPCAR (long intergenic noncoding RNA predicting cardiac remodeling) were associated with a higher risk of cardiovascular mortality in HF patients in addition to traditional risk factors. Other lncRNAs, including aHIF, ANRIL, KCNQ1OT1, MIAT, and MALAT1, have also been reported as potential biomarkers in HF. Of particular interest is the lcRNA ANRIL. ANRIL is encoded on chromosome 9p21, the genomic region, which had been identified as the most significant susceptibility locus of CAD by GWAS (see the section on Genomics Biomarkers). The 9p21 region is a region with no protein-coding genes annotated, and for a long time the effector within this region was unknown. Identification of ANRIL provided possible functional links to the 9p21 region. Genetic variants (SNPs) identified by GWAS disrupt the binding site for the transcriptional factor STAT1 in the ANRIL gene, leading to an upregulation of ANRIL.[104] Further studies focusing on the mechanistic role of ANRIL, showed an involvement in cell viability, proliferation, adhesion, and apoptosis.[104]

In 2015, lncRNA CoroMarker[134] and LncPPARδδ[135] were identified as predictive biomarkers for CAD. Despite this progress, the cellular origin of circulating lncRNAs is often unclear[136] and little knowledge on the causal involvement in the underlying disease is currently available.

Circular RNAs

Even though the existence of circRNAs has been known for some time, this class of ncRNAs has only recently gained interest as potential biomarkers.[120] Due to their circular state, these RNA molecules are highly stable and show an evolutionary conservation. circRNAs can be reproducibly detected at high levels in peripheral blood and other body fluids. A 2016 study revealed over 9000 candidate circRNAs detected in heart tissue.[137] However, their regulation in CAD still remains mainly unexplored and upcoming studies will have to further explore the potential of circRNAs as clinically relevant biomarkers.

As already reported for the assessment of mRNA/gene expression biomarkers, research on ncRNAs also needs to deal with a range of current challenges due to preanalytical and analytical factors influencing data quality.

Similar to any other biomarkers the use of standardized control groups, independent large-scale technical groups, and clinical validation groups is necessary. In addition, other factors have been shown to influence ncRNA levels. In particular, antiplatelet medication, heparin, and statin treatment might influence circulating miRNA levels and release kinetics.[125] A major limitation in ncRNA biomarker research is the current lack of standardization of sample isolation,[138] processing, and detection techniques,[139] as well as endogenous and exogenous controls for data normalization. As alterations and material-dependent stabilities of ncRNA levels in different materials such as plasma, serum, urine, and cells have been found[140] the choice of material also needs to be carefully considered.

Metabolomic Biomarkers

Metabolomics is based on profiling all low-molecular-mass metabolites present in biologic samples. Most metabolites are lipids (such as phospholipids, glycerophospholipids, sphingolipids), acylcarnitines, amino acids, biogenic amines, hormones, bile acids, or fatty acids. Compared with other omics technologies, there are fewer metabolites (3×10^3) than there are genes (2×10^4), transcripts ($> 10^6$), proteins ($> 10^6$), and posttranslational modified proteins ($> 10^7$).[141] Current metabolomics approaches can assess several hundreds of molecules, depending on the platform, but no single technology can measure the complete metabolome. For detection of novel metabolites or differences among samples, nontargeted approaches are used that are performed by nuclear magnetic resonance or mass spectrometry, whereas targeted approaches use prespecified panels of metabolites (e.g., the metabolon panel, or the Biocrates metabolite kit). The assessment of a particular isolated metabolite will not be fully informative and makes a correct interpretation difficult. However, metabolite profiles (such as a group of metabolites) may greatly improve the interpretation of an altered metabolomics pathway, in particular when combined with other omics results.[142]

With respect to CAD, metabolomics approaches have led to the identification of metabolites in several pathways with potential as novel clinical biomarkers.[143,144] Metabolites derived from dietary choline and L-carnitine have been described as playing a role in aortic lesion formation in mice and risk of CAD in humans.[145] Evaluating the discriminative capabilities of metabolites for CAD, Shah et al.,[146] using principle component analyses, identified branched-chain amino acid metabolites and urea cycle metabolites in association with CAD. Of particular interest is a 2016 study that integrated targeted metabolomics with an unbiased genetic screen and identified loci on chromosomes 2q34 and 5q14.1 as being associated with plasma levels of metabolites related to betaine metabolism, as well as a decreased risk of CAD.[145] These data suggest that glycine metabolism and the urea cycle are potential metabolic pathways involved in CAD.

Although in its infancy with regard to biomarkers for CAD, metabolomics approaches have a great potential in identifying and clinically utilizing metabolites in the near future.

Others: Proteomic and Lipidomic Biomarkers

There are several other areas of omics studies for which there is growing interest in the field of CAD biomarkers. One area is proteomics, the analysis of the protein repertoire of a given cell type mainly based on mass spectrometry technologies. Proteomics uniquely offers insights into diseases because proteins and their bioenzymatical functions largely determine the phenotypic diversity. It has been estimated that more than 300,000 human polypeptide species are represented in the human plasma proteome. Of particular interest in proteomics biomarker research are posttranslational modifications, that is, alterations in proteins (such as phosphorylation, acetylation, or ubiquitinylation) introduced covalently and/or enzymatically during or after the translation, which regulate activity, stability, and folding of proteins.

Compared to other omics approaches described previously, only a small amount of proteomics studies targeting CAD have been performed to date. For example, in urinary samples, over 100 peptides were discovered in HF individuals with reduced ejection fraction. The combination of all markers accurately discriminated between HF patients and controls, indicating that the urinary proteome might help to improve the diagnosis and prognosis of HF.[147] In addition, some posttranslational modifications, such as glycosylation, have already been evaluated as potential biomarkers in CAD.[100]

Lipidomics, the assessment of the complete collection of lipids, can also be determined by mass spectrometry or nuclear magnetic resonance technologies and is another emerging omics field. Plasma lipids are solubilized and dispersed through their association with specific groups of proteins, e.g., with albumin or plasma lipoproteins.[148] The structural diversity of lipids is mirrored by the enormous variation in their physiologic function.[148] As lipids such as HDL-C, LDL-C, and Lp(a) are important molecules involved in the physiology of CAD, the examination of all forms of lipids and lipid metabolism is of utmost interest in CAD biomarker research.

In a large study of CAD subjects with long term follow-up, distinct ceramide species (a family of waxy lipid molecules) were significantly associated with fatal outcome,[148] providing evidence that ceramides may be useful biomarkers independently of traditional risk factors. Interestingly, this study also investigated the effect of lipid-lowering therapy on lipid levels. Simvastatin lowered plasma ceramides broadly by approximately 25%, but no changes in ceramides were observed in the ezetimibe group. PCSK9 deficiency was significantly associated with lowered LDL-C (-13%) accompanied by a significant 20% reduction in CAD outcome risk-related ceramides.[149]

An overview of all biomarkers related to chronic CAD is provided in Fig. 9.3.

CONCLUSIONS

In recent years, biomarker research has improved risk stratification in CAD patients. Although the use of established markers such as NT-proBNP and cardiac troponins is recommended in the guidelines for diagnosis of HF and acute coronary syndrome, the biomarker determination in stable angina and chronic CAD patients is—apart from the determination of lipid profiles—not recommended in clinical routine.

Several emerging biomarkers have been identified, including gene expression signatures and noncoding RNAs, and a few are on their way to being translated into clinical utility. However, several aspects deserve more detailed care, ranging from appropriate study design and material to analytical methods, standardizations, and, most importantly, validation in independent and large-scale studies.

To reach clinical application of a biomarker, the central questions about the clinical potential need to be evaluated as outlined by Morrow and de Lemos:[150]

(1) Can the clinician measure the biomarker?
(2) Does the biomarker add new information?
(3) Does the biomarker help the clinician to manage patients?

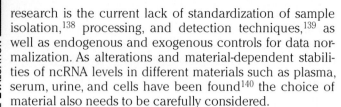

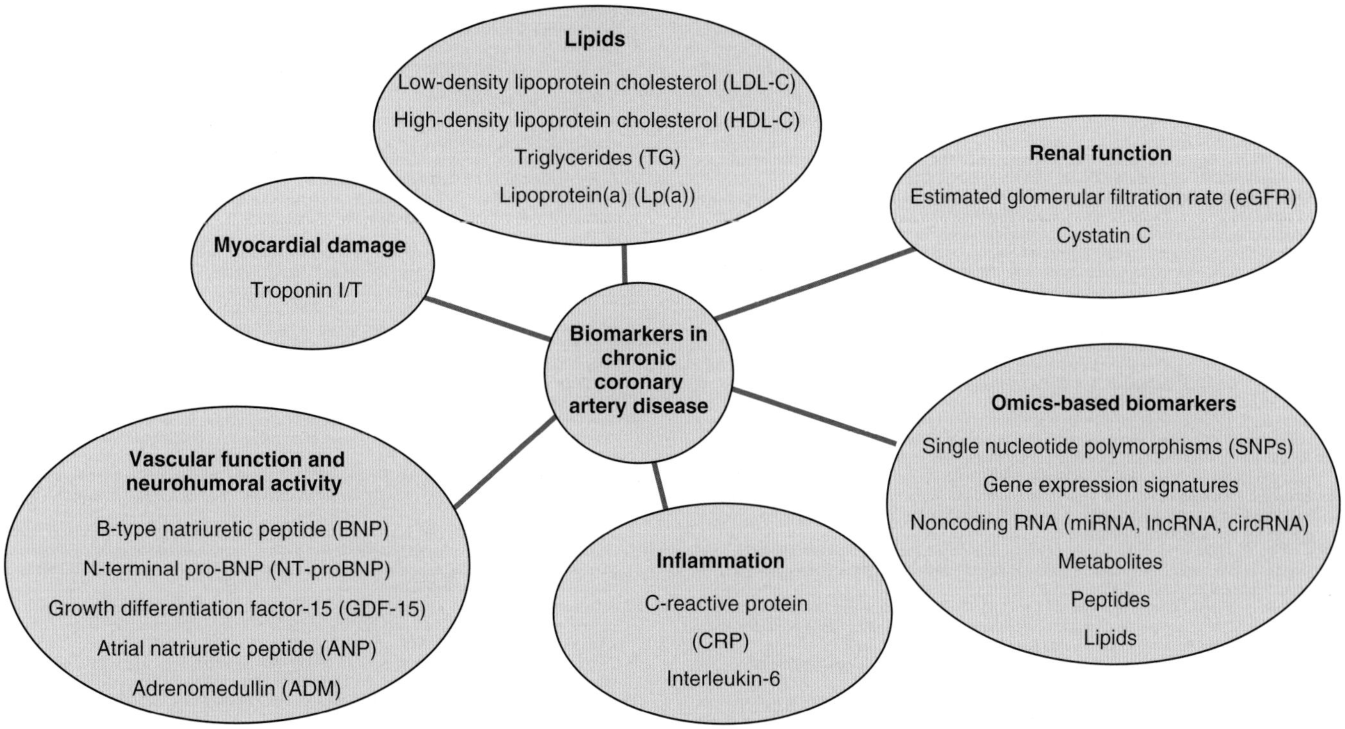

FIG. 9.3 Established and novel biomarkers in chronic coronary artery disease. *circRNA*, Circular RNA; *lncRNA*, long noncoding RNA; *miRNA*, microRNA.

References

1. Medicine USNLo: Medical Subject Headings. https://www.nlm.nih.gov/mesh/.
2. Biomarkers Definitions Working Group: Biomarkers and surrogate endpoints: preferred definitions and conceptual framework, *Clin Pharmacol Ther* 69:89, 2001.
3. Jaffe AS: Troponins as biomarkers of cardiac injury. http://www.uptodate.com/contents/troponins-as-biomarkers-of-cardiac-injury?source=preview&search=Troponin&anchor=H36#H1.
4. Gravning J, Smedsrud MK, Omland T, et al.: Sensitive troponin assays and N-terminal pro-B-type natriuretic peptide in acute coronary syndrome: prediction of significant coronary lesions and long-term prognosis, *Am Heart J* 165:716, 2013.
5. Jaffe AS, Vasile VC, Milone M, et al.: Diseased skeletal muscle: a noncardiac source of increased circulating concentrations of cardiac troponin T, *J Am Coll Cardiol* 58:1819, 2011.
6. Go AS, Chertow GM, Fan D, et al.: Chronic kidney disease and the risks of death, cardiovascular events, and hospitalization, *N Engl J Med* 351:1296, 2004.
7. Kavsak PA, MacRae AR, Yerna MJ, Jaffe AS: Analytic and clinical utility of a next-generation, highly sensitive cardiac troponin I assay for early detection of myocardial injury, *Clin Chem* 55:573, 2009.
8. Giannitsis E, Kurz K, Hallermayer K, et al.: Analytical validation of a high-sensitivity cardiac troponin T assay, *Clin Chem* 56:254, 2010.
9. Apple FS: A new season for cardiac troponin assays: it's time to keep a scorecard, *Clin Chem* 55:1303, 2009.
10. Apple FS, Ler R, Murakami MM: Determination of 19 cardiac troponin I and T assay 99th percentile values from a common presumably healthy population, *Clin Chem* 58:1574, 2012.
11. Wilson SR, Sabatine MS, Braunwald E, et al.: Detection of myocardial injury in patients with unstable angina using a novel nanoparticle cardiac troponin I assay: observations from the PROTECT-TIMI 30 Trial, *Am Heart J* 158:386, 2009.
12. Venge P, Johnston N, Lindahl B, James S: Normal plasma levels of cardiac troponin I measured by the high-sensitivity cardiac troponin I access prototype assay and the impact on the diagnosis of myocardial ischemia, *J Am Coll Cardiol* 54:1165, 2009.
13. Januzzi Jr JL, Bamberg F, Lee H, et al.: High-sensitivity troponin T concentrations in acute chest pain patients evaluated with cardiac computed tomography, *Circulation* 121:1227, 2010.
14. Diamond GA, Kaul S: How would the Reverend Bayes interpret high-sensitivity troponin? *Circulation* 121:1172, 2010.
15. Neumann JT, Sorensen NA, Schwemer T, et al.: Diagnosis of myocardial infarction using a high-sensitivity troponin I 1-hour algorithm, *JAMA Cardiol* 1:397, 2016.
16. Everett BM, Brooks MM, Vlachos HE, et al.: Troponin and cardiac events in stable ischemic heart disease and diabetes, *N Engl J Med* 373:610, 2015.
17. Omland T, Pfeffer MA, Solomon SD, et al.: Prognostic value of cardiac troponin I measured with a highly sensitive assay in patients with stable coronary artery disease, *J Am Coll Cardiol* 61:1240, 2013.
18. Omland T, de Lemos JA, Sabatine MS, et al.: A sensitive cardiac troponin T assay in stable coronary artery disease, *N Engl J Med* 361:2538, 2009.
19. Blankenberg S, Salomaa V, Makarova N, et al.: Troponin I and cardiovascular risk prediction in the general population: the BiomarCaRE consortium, *Eur Heart J* 37:2428, 2016.
20. Wang TJ, Larson MG, Levy D, et al.: Plasma natriuretic peptide levels and the risk of cardiovascular events and death, *N Engl J Med* 350:655, 2004.
21. Mahadavan G, Nguyen TH, Horowitz JD: Brain natriuretic peptide: a biomarker for all cardiac disease? *Curr Opin Cardiol* 29:160, 2014.
22. Seferian KR, Tamm NN, Semenov AG, et al.: The brain natriuretic peptide (BNP) precursor is the major immunoreactive form of BNP in patients with heart failure, *Clin Chem* 53:866, 2007.
23. Semenov AG, Postnikov AB, Tamm NN, et al.: Processing of pro-brain natriuretic peptide is suppressed by O-glycosylation in the region close to the cleavage site, *Clin Chem* 55:489, 2009.
24. Halim SA, Newby LK, Ohman EM: Biomarkers in cardiovascular clinical trials: past, present, future, *Clin Chem* 58:45, 2012.
25. Maisel AS, Krishnaswamy P, Nowak RM, et al.: Rapid measurement of B-type natriuretic peptide in the emergency diagnosis of heart failure, *N Engl J Med* 347:161, 2002.
26. Ponikowski P, Voors AA, Anker SD, et al.: 2016 ESC guidelines for the diagnosis and treatment of acute and chronic heart failure: the Task Force for the diagnosis and treatment of acute and chronic heart failure of the European Society of Cardiology (ESC). Developed with the special contribution of the Heart Failure Association (HFA) of the ESC, *Eur J Heart Fail* 18:891, 2016.
27. Schnabel R, Lubos E, Rupprecht HJ, et al.: B-type natriuretic peptide and the risk of cardiovascular events and death in patients with stable angina: results from the AtheroGene study, *J Am Coll Cardiol* 47:552, 2006.
28. de Lemos JA, McGuire DK, Drazner MH: B-type natriuretic peptide in cardiovascular disease, *Lancet* 362:316, 2003.
29. Kragelund C, Gronning B, Kober L, et al.: N-terminal pro-B-type natriuretic peptide and long-term mortality in stable coronary heart disease, *N Engl J Med* 352:666, 2005.
30. Schnabel RB, Schulz A, Messow CM, et al.: Multiple marker approach to risk stratification in patients with stable coronary artery disease, *Eur Heart J* 31:3024, 2010.
31. Omland T, Sabatine MS, Jablonski KA, et al.: Prognostic value of B-type natriuretic peptides in patients with stable coronary artery disease: the PEACE Trial, *J Am Coll Cardiol* 50:205, 2007.
32. van Kimmenade RR, Januzzi Jr JL: Emerging biomarkers in heart failure, *Clin Chem* 58:127, 2012.
33. Morgenthaler NG, Struck J, Thomas B, Bergmann A: Immunoluminometric assay for the midregion of pro-atrial natriuretic peptide in human plasma, *Clin Chem* 50:234, 2004.
34. Katan M, Fluri F, Schuetz P, et al.: Midregional pro-atrial natriuretic peptide and outcome in patients with acute ischemic stroke, *J Am Coll Cardiol* 56:1045, 2010.
35. Khan SQ, Dhillon O, Kelly D, et al.: Plasma N-terminal B-type natriuretic peptide as an indicator of long-term survival after acute myocardial infarction: comparison with plasma midregional pro-atrial natriuretic peptide: the LAMP (Leicester Acute Myocardial Infarction Peptide) study, *J Am Coll Cardiol* 51:1857, 2008.
36. Masson S, Latini R, Carbonieri E, et al.: The predictive value of stable precursor fragments of vasoactive peptides in patients with chronic heart failure: data from the GISSI-heart failure (GISSI-HF) trial, *Eur J Heart Fail* 12:338, 2010.
37. Colucci WS, Chen HH: Natriuretic peptide measurement in heart failure. http://www.uptodate.com/contents/natriuretic-peptide-measurement-in-heart-failure?source=machineLearning&search=BNP&selectedTitle=1%7E150&sectionRank=1&anchor=H4#H4.
38. Colucci WS: Nitric oxide, other hormones, cytokines, and chemokines in heart failure. http://www.uptodate.com/contents/nitric-oxide-other-hormones-cytokines-and-chemokines-in-heart-failure?source=machineLearning&search=adrenomedullin&selectedTitle=1%7E10&sectionRank=1&anchor=H14#H14.
39. Neumann JT, Tzikas S, Funke-Kaiser A, et al.: Association of MR-proadrenomedullin with cardiovascular risk factors and subclinical cardiovascular disease, *Atherosclerosis* 228:451, 2013.
40. Morgenthaler NG, Struck J, Alonso C, Bergmann A: Measurement of midregional proadrenomedullin in plasma with an immunoluminometric assay, *Clin Chem* 51:1823, 2005.
41. Maisel A, Mueller C, Nowak R, et al.: Mid-region pro-hormone markers for diagnosis and prognosis in acute dyspnea: results from the BACH (Biomarkers in Acute Heart Failure) trial, *J Am Coll Cardiol* 55:2062, 2010.
42. Wild PS, Schnabel RB, Lubos E, et al.: Midregional proadrenomedullin for prediction of cardiovascular events in coronary artery disease: results from the AtheroGene study, *Clin Chem* 58:226, 2012.
43. Funke-Kaiser A, Mann K, Colquhoun D, et al.: Midregional proadrenomedullin and its change predicts recurrent major coronary events and heart failure in stable coronary heart disease patients: the LIPID study, *Int J Cardiol* 172:411, 2014.
44. Klok FA, Surie S, Kempf T, et al.: A simple non-invasive diagnostic algorithm for ruling out chronic thromboembolic pulmonary hypertension in patients after acute pulmonary embolism, *Thromb Res* 128:21, 2011.
45. Corre J, Hebraud B, Bourin P: Concise review: growth differentiation factor 15 in pathology: a clinical role? *Stem Cells Transl Med* 2:946, 2013.
46. Kempf T, Eden M, Strelau J, et al.: The transforming growth factor-beta superfamily member growth-differentiation factor-15 protects the heart from ischemia/reperfusion injury, *Circ Res* 98:351, 2006.
47. Baessler A, Strack C, Rousseva E, et al.: Growth-differentiation factor-15 improves reclassification for the diagnosis of heart failure with normal ejection fraction in morbid obesity, *Eur J Heart Fail* 14:1240, 2012.

48. Brown DA, Breit SN, Buring J, et al.: Concentration in plasma of macrophage inhibitory cytokine-1 and risk of cardiovascular events in women: a nested case-control study, *Lancet* 359:2159, 2002.
49. Kempf T, Sinning JM, Quint A, et al.: Growth-differentiation factor-15 for risk stratification in patients with stable and unstable coronary heart disease: results from the AtheroGene study, *Circ Cardiovasc Genet* 2:286, 2009.
50. Schopfer DW, Ku IA, Regan M, Whooley MA: Growth differentiation factor 15 and cardiovascular events in patients with stable ischemic heart disease (The Heart and Soul Study), *Am Heart J* 167:186–192, 2014.e1.
51. Chan MM, Santhanakrishnan R, Chong JP, et al.: Growth differentiation factor 15 in heart failure with preserved vs. reduced ejection fraction, *Eur J Heart Fail* 18:81, 2016.
52. Chronic Kidney Disease Prognosis Consortium, Matsushita K, van der Velde M, et al.: Association of estimated glomerular filtration rate and albuminuria with all-cause and cardiovascular mortality in general population cohorts: a collaborative meta-analysis, *Lancet* 375:2073, 2010.
53. Mule G, Nardi E, Guarino L, et al.: Plasma aldosterone and its relationship with left ventricular mass in hypertensive patients with early-stage chronic kidney disease, *Hypertens Res* 38:276, 2015.
54. Barnes PJ, Karin M: Nuclear factor-kappaB: a pivotal transcription factor in chronic inflammatory diseases, *N Engl J Med* 336:1066, 1997.
55. Gremmel T, Muller M, Steiner S, et al.: Chronic kidney disease is associated with increased platelet activation and poor response to antiplatelet therapy, *Nephrol Dial Transplant* 28:2116, 2013.
56. Inker LA, Schmid CH, Tighiouart H, et al.: Estimating glomerular filtration rate from serum creatinine and cystatin C, *N Engl J Med* 367:20, 2012.
57. Manjunath G, Tighiouart H, Ibrahim H, et al.: Level of kidney function as a risk factor for atherosclerotic cardiovascular outcomes in the community, *J Am Coll Cardiol* 41:47, 2003.
58. Reis SE, Olson MB, Fried L, et al.: Mild renal insufficiency is associated with angiographic coronary artery disease in women, *Circulation* 105:2826, 2002.
59. Shepherd J, Kastelein JJ, Bittner V, et al.: Intensive lipid lowering with atorvastatin in patients with coronary heart disease and chronic kidney disease: the TNT (Treating to New Targets) study, *J Am Coll Cardiol* 51:1448, 2008.
60. James S, Budaj A, Aylward P, et al.: Ticagrelor versus clopidogrel in acute coronary syndromes in relation to renal function: results from the Platelet Inhibition and Patient Outcomes (PLATO) trial, *Circulation* 122:1056, 2010.
61. Task Force M, Montalescot G, Sechtem U, et al.: 2013 ESC guidelines on the management of stable coronary artery disease: the Task Force on the management of stable coronary artery disease of the European Society of Cardiology, *Eur Heart J* 34:2949, 2013.
62. Shlipak MG, Mattes MD, Peralta CA: Update on cystatin C: incorporation into clinical practice, *Am J Kidney Dis* 62:595, 2013.
63. Keller T, Messow CM, Lubos E, et al.: Cystatin C and cardiovascular mortality in patients with coronary artery disease and normal or mildly reduced kidney function: results from the AtheroGene study, *Eur Heart J* 30:314, 2009.
64. Manzano-Fernandez S, Flores-Blanco PJ, Perez-Calvo JI, et al.: Comparison of risk prediction with the CKD-EPI and MDRD equations in acute decompensated heart failure, *J Card Fail* 19:583, 2013.
65. Waldeyer C, Karakas M, Scheurle C, et al.: The predictive value of different equations for estimation of glomerular filtration rate in patients with coronary artery disease—results from the AtheroGene study, *Int J Cardiol* 221:908, 2016.
66. Goldstein JL, Brown MS: A century of cholesterol and coronaries: from plaques to genes to statins, *Cell* 161:161, 2015.
67. Nordestgaard BG, Langsted A, Mora S, et al.: Fasting is not routinely required for determination of a lipid profile: clinical and laboratory implications including flagging at desirable concentration cut-points—a joint consensus statement from the European Atherosclerosis Society and European Federation of Clinical Chemistry and Laboratory Medicine, *Eur Heart J* 37:1944, 2016.
68. Baigent C, Keech A, Kearney PM, et al.: Efficacy and safety of cholesterol-lowering treatment: prospective meta-analysis of data from 90,056 participants in 14 randomised trials of statins, *Lancet* 366:1267, 2005.
69. Ballantyne CM, Raichlen JS, Nicholls SJ, et al.: Effect of rosuvastatin therapy on coronary artery stenoses assessed by quantitative coronary angiography: a study to evaluate the effect of rosuvastatin on intravascular ultrasound-derived coronary atheroma burden, *Circulation* 117:2458, 2008.
70. Stone NJ, Robinson JG, Lichtenstein AH, et al.: 2013 ACC/AHA guideline on the treatment of blood cholesterol to reduce atherosclerotic cardiovascular risk in adults: a report of the American College of Cardiology/American Heart Association Task Force on Practice Guidelines, *Circulation* 129: S1, 2014.
71. Natarajan P, Ray KK, Cannon CP: High-density lipoprotein and coronary heart disease: current and future therapies, *J Am Coll Cardiol* 55:1283, 2010.
72. Voight BF, Peloso GM, Orho-Melander M, et al.: Plasma HDL cholesterol and risk of myocardial infarction: a Mendelian randomisation study, *Lancet* 380:572, 2012.
73. AIM-HIGH Investigators, Boden WE, Probstfield JL, et al.: Niacin in patients with low HDL cholesterol levels receiving intensive statin therapy, *N Engl J Med* 365:2255, 2011.
74. Schwartz GG, Olsson AG, Abt M, et al.: Effects of dalcetrapib in patients with a recent acute coronary syndrome, *N Engl J Med* 367:2089, 2012.
75. Authors/Task Force Members, Piepoli MF, Hoes AW, et al.: 2016 European guidelines on cardiovascular disease prevention in clinical practice: the Sixth Joint Task Force of the European Society of Cardiology and Other Societies on Cardiovascular Disease Prevention in Clinical Practice (constituted by representatives of 10 societies and by invited experts): developed with the special contribution of the European Association for Cardiovascular Prevention & Rehabilitation (EACPR), *Eur J Prev Cardiol* 23, 2016. NP1.
76. Rosenson RS: The high-density lipoprotein puzzle: why classic epidemiology, genetic epidemiology, and clinical trials conflict? *Arterioscler Thromb Vasc Biol* 36:777, 2016.
77. Myocardial Infarction Genetics, CARDIoGRAM Exome Consortia Investigators, Stitziel NO, et al.: Coding variation in ANGPTL4, LPL, and SVEP1 and the risk of coronary disease, *N Engl J Med* 374:1134, 2016.
78. Holmes MV, Asselbergs FW, Palmer TM, et al.: Mendelian randomization of blood lipids for coronary heart disease, *Eur Heart J* 36:539, 2015.
79. Kamstrup PR, Tybjaerg-Hansen A, Steffensen R, Nordestgaard BG: Genetically elevated lipoprotein(a) and increased risk of myocardial infarction, *JAMA* 301:2331, 2009.
80. Clarke R, Peden JF, Hopewell JC, et al.: Genetic variants associated with Lp(a) lipoprotein level and coronary disease, *N Engl J Med* 361:2518, 2009.
81. Nordestgaard BG, Chapman MJ, Ray K, et al.: Lipoprotein(a) as a cardiovascular risk factor: current status, *Eur Heart J* 31:2844, 2010.
82. Kraft HG, Lingenhel A, Kochl S, et al.: Apolipoprotein(a) kringle IV repeat number predicts risk for coronary heart disease, *Arterioscler Thromb Vasc Biol* 16:713, 1996.
83. Yousuf O, Mohanty BD, Martin SS, et al.: High-sensitivity C-reactive protein and cardiovascular disease: a resolute belief or an elusive link? *J Am Coll Cardiol* 62:397, 2013.
84. Pearson TA, Mensah GA, Alexander RW, et al.: Markers of inflammation and cardiovascular disease: application to clinical and public health practice: a statement for healthcare professionals from the Centers for Disease Control and Prevention and the American Heart Association, *Circulation* 107:499, 2003.
85. Zacho J, Tybjaerg-Hansen A, Jensen JS, et al.: Genetically elevated C-reactive protein and ischemic vascular disease, *N Engl J Med* 359:1897, 2008.
86. Ridker PM, Danielson E, Fonseca FA, et al.: Rosuvastatin to prevent vascular events in men and women with elevated C-reactive protein, *N Engl J Med* 359:2195, 2008.
87. Elliott P, Chambers JC, Zhang W, et al.: Genetic loci associated with C-reactive protein levels and risk of coronary heart disease, *JAMA* 302:37, 2009.
88. Jansen H, Samani NJ, Schunkert H: Mendelian randomization studies in coronary artery disease, *Eur Heart J* 35:1917, 2014.
89. Morrow DA: C-reactive protein in cardiovascular disease. http://www.uptodate.com/contents/c-reactive-protein-in-cardiovascular-disease?source=machineLearning&search=C-reactive+protein&selectedTitle=2%7E150&sectionRank=1&anchor=H5#H5.
90. Bickel C, Rupprecht HJ, Blankenberg S, et al.: Relation of markers of inflammation (C-reactive protein, fibrinogen, von Willebrand factor, and leukocyte count) and statin therapy to long-term mortality in patients with angiographically proven coronary artery disease, *Am J Cardiol* 89:901, 2002.
91. Koenig W: High-sensitivity C-reactive protein and atherosclerotic disease: from improved risk prediction to risk-guided therapy, *Int J Cardiol* 168:5126, 2013.
92. Sabatine MS, Morrow DA, Jablonski KA, et al.: Prognostic significance of the Centers for Disease Control/American Heart Association high-sensitivity C-reactive protein cut points for cardiovascular and other outcomes in patients with stable coronary artery disease, *Circulation* 115:1528, 2007.
93. Blankenberg S, McQueen MJ, Smieja M, et al.: Comparative impact of multiple biomarkers and N-terminal pro-brain natriuretic peptide in the context of conventional risk factors for the prediction of recurrent cardiovascular events in the Heart Outcomes Prevention Evaluation (HOPE) Study, *Circulation* 114:201, 2006.
94. IL6R Genetics Consortium Emerging Risk Factors Collaboration, Sarwar N, Butterworth AS, et al.: Interleukin-6 receptor pathways in coronary heart disease: a collaborative meta-analysis of 82 studies, *Lancet* 379:1205, 2012.
95. Interleukin-6 Receptor Mendelian Randomisation Analysis Consortium: The interleukin-6 receptor as a target for prevention of coronary heart disease: a Mendelian randomisation analysis, *Lancet* 379:1214, 2012.
96. Wilson PW: Overview of the risk equivalents and established risk factors for cardiovascular disease. http://www.uptodate.com/contents/overview-of-the-risk-equivalents-and-established-risk-factors-for-cardiovascular-disease?source=machineLearning&search=il-6&selectedTitle=2%7E150&sectionRank=1&anchor=H835935#H835935.
97. Sabatine MS, Morrow DA, de Lemos JA, et al.: Evaluation of multiple biomarkers of cardiovascular stress for risk prediction and guiding medical therapy in patients with stable coronary disease, *Circulation* 125:233, 2012.
98. Tonkin AM, Blankenberg S, Kirby A, et al.: Biomarkers in stable coronary heart disease, their modulation and cardiovascular risk: the LIPID biomarker study, *Int J Cardiol* 201:499, 2015.
99. Valdes AM, Glass D, Spector TD: Omics technologies and the study of human ageing, *Nat Rev Genet* 14:601, 2013.
100. Hoefer IE, Steffens S, Ala-Korpela M, et al.: Novel methodologies for biomarker discovery in atherosclerosis, *Eur Heart J* 36:2635, 2015.
101. Zeller T, Blankenberg S, Diemert P: Genomewide association studies in cardiovascular disease—an update 2011, *Clin Chem* 58:92, 2012.
102. Kessler T, Vilne B, Schunkert H: The impact of genome-wide association studies on the pathophysiology and therapy of cardiovascular disease, *EMBO Mol Med* 8:688, 2016.
103. Chen HH, Almontashiri NA, Antoine D, Stewart AF: Functional genomics of the 9p21.3 locus for atherosclerosis: clarity or confusion? *Curr Cardiol Rep* 16:502, 2014.
104. Boon RA, Jae N, Holdt L, Dimmeler S: Long noncoding RNAs: from clinical genetics to therapeutic targets? *J Am Coll Cardiol* 67:1214, 2016.
105. Smith JA, Ware EB, Middha P, et al.: Current applications of genetic risk scores to cardiovascular outcomes and subclinical phenotypes, *Curr Epidemiol Rep* 2:180, 2015.
106. Tikkanen E, Havulinna AS, Palotie A, et al.: Genetic risk prediction and a 2-stage risk screening strategy for coronary heart disease, *Arterioscler Thromb Vasc Biol* 33:2261, 2013.
107. Ganna A, Magnusson PK, Pedersen NL, et al.: Multilocus genetic risk scores for coronary heart disease prediction, *Arterioscler Thromb Vasc Biol* 33:2267, 2013.
108. Weijmans M, de Bakker PI, van der Graaf Y, et al.: Incremental value of a genetic risk score for the prediction of new vascular events in patients with clinically manifest vascular disease, *Atherosclerosis* 239:451, 2015.
109. Siemelink MA, Zeller T: Biomarkers of coronary artery disease: the promise of the transcriptome, *Curr Cardiol Rep* 16:513, 2014.
110. Sinning C, Zengin E, Zeller T, et al.: Candidate biomarkers in heart failure with reduced and preserved ejection fraction, *Biomarkers* 20:258, 2015.
111. Jackson CE, Haig C, Welsh P, et al.: The incremental prognostic and clinical value of multiple novel biomarkers in heart failure, *Eur J Heart Fail*, 2016. http://dx.doi.org/10.1002/ejhf.543.
112. Coglianese EE, Larson MG, Vasan RS, et al.: Distribution and clinical correlates of the interleukin receptor family member soluble ST2 in the Framingham Heart Study, *Clin Chem* 58:1673, 2012.
113. Ho JE, Larson MG, Ghorbani A, et al.: Soluble ST2 predicts elevated SBP in the community, *J Hypertens* 31:1431, 2013.
114. Wang TJ, Wollert KC, Larson MG, et al.: Prognostic utility of novel biomarkers of cardiovascular stress: the Framingham Heart Study, *Circulation* 126:1596, 2012.
115. Sinnaeve PR, Donahue MP, Grass P, et al.: Gene expression patterns in peripheral blood correlate with the extent of coronary artery disease, *PloS One* 4:e7037, 2009.
116. Joehanes R, Ying S, Huan T, et al.: Gene expression signatures of coronary heart disease, *Arterioscler Thromb Vasc Biol* 33:1418, 2013.
117. Elashoff MR, Wingrove JA, Beineke P, et al.: Development of a blood-based gene expression algorithm for assessment of obstructive coronary artery disease in non-diabetic patients, *BMC Med Genomics* 4:26, 2011.
118. Thomas GS, Voros S, McPherson JA, et al.: A blood-based gene expression test for obstructive coronary artery disease tested in symptomatic nondiabetic patients referred for myocardial perfusion imaging the COMPASS study, *Circ Cardiovasc Genet* 6:154, 2013.
119. Kaudewitz D, Zampetaki A, Mayr M: MicroRNA biomarkers for coronary artery disease? *Curr Atheroscler Rep* 17:70, 2015.
120. Memczak S, Papavasileiou P, Peters O, Rajewsky N: Identification and characterization of circular RNAs as a new class of putative biomarkers in human blood, *PloS One* 10:e0141214, 2015.
121. van Rooij E: The art of microRNA research, *Circ Res* 108:219, 2011.
122. Mitchell PS, Parkin RK, Kroh EM, et al.: Circulating microRNAs as stable blood-based markers for cancer detection, *Proc Natl Acad Sci U S A* 105:10513, 2008.
123. Schulte C, Zeller T: MicroRNA-based diagnostics and therapy in cardiovascular disease—summing up the facts, *Cardiovasc Diagn Ther* 5:17, 2015.
124. Lee RC, Feinbaum RL, Ambros V: The C. elegans heterochronic gene lin-4 encodes small RNAs with antisense complementarity to lin-14, *Cell* 75:843, 1993.
125. Busch A, Eken SM, Maegdefessel L: Prospective and therapeutic screening value of non-coding RNA as biomarkers in cardiovascular disease, *Ann Transl Med* 4:236, 2016.
126. Karakas M, Schulte C, Appelbaum S, et al.: Circulating microRNAs strongly predict cardiovascular death in patients with coronary artery disease—results from the large AtheroGene study, *Eur Heart J*, 2016. http://dx.doi.org/10.1093/eurheartj/ehw250.
127. Ellis KL, Cameron VA, Troughton RW, et al.: Circulating microRNAs as candidate markers to distinguish heart failure in breathless patients, *Eur J Heart Fail* 15:1138, 2013.
128. Luo P, He T, Jiang R, Li G: MicroRNA-423-5p targets O-GlcNAc transferase to induce apoptosis in cardiomyocytes, *Mol Med Rep* 12:1163, 2015.

129. Luo P, Zhang W: MicroRNA4235p mediates H_2O_2-induced apoptosis in cardiomyocytes through OGlcNAc transferase, *Mol Med Rep* 14:857, 2016.
130. Zampetaki A, Willeit P, Tilling L, et al.: Prospective study on circulating microRNAs and risk of myocardial infarction, *J Am Coll Cardiol* 60:290, 2012.
131. Schulte C, Molz S, Appelbaum S, et al.: miRNA-197 and miRNA-223 predict cardiovascular death in a cohort of patients with symptomatic coronary artery disease, *PloS One* 10:e0145930, 2015.
132. Pennisi E: Genomics. ENCODE project writes eulogy for junk DNA, *Science* 337:1159, 2012.
133. Archer K, Broskova Z, Bayoumi AS, et al.: Long non-coding RNAs as master regulators in cardiovascular diseases, *Int J Mol Sci* 16:23651, 2015.
134. Yang Y, Cai Y, Wu G, et al.: Plasma long non-coding RNA, CoroMarker, a novel biomarker for diagnosis of coronary artery disease, *Clin Sci (Lond)* 129:675, 2015.
135. Cai Y, Yang Y, Chen X, et al.: Circulating "LncPPARdelta" from monocytes as a novel biomarker for coronary artery diseases, *Medicine* 95:e2360, 2016.
136. Skroblin P, Mayr M: "Going long": long non-coding RNAs as biomarkers, *Circ Res* 115:607, 2014.
137. Werfel S, Nothjunge S, Schwarzmayr T, et al.: Characterization of circular RNAs in human, mouse and rat hearts, *J Mol Cell Cardiol* 98:103, 2016.
138. Hantzsch M, Tolios A, Beutner F, et al.: Comparison of whole blood RNA preservation tubes and novel generation RNA extraction kits for analysis of mRNA and MiRNA profiles, *PloS One* 9:e113298, 2014.
139. Schwarzenbach H, da Silva AM, Calin G, Pantel K: Data normalization strategies for microRNA quantification, *Clin Chem* 61:1333, 2015.
140. Chen X, Ba Y, Ma L, et al.: Characterization of microRNAs in serum: a novel class of biomarkers for diagnosis of cancer and other diseases, *Cell Res* 18:997, 2008.
141. Atzler D, Schwedhelm E, Zeller T: Integrated genomics and metabolomics in nephrology, *Nephrol Dial Transplant* 29:1467, 2014.
142. Marcinkiewicz-Siemion M, Ciborowski M, Kretowski A, et al.: Metabolomics—A wide-open door to personalized treatment in chronic heart failure? *Int J Cardiol* 219:156, 2016.
143. Roberts LD, Gerszten RE: Toward new biomarkers of cardiometabolic diseases, *Cell Metab* 18:43, 2013.
144. Wang Z, Klipfell E, Bennett BJ, et al.: Gut flora metabolism of phosphatidylcholine promotes cardiovascular disease, *Nature* 472:57, 2011.
145. Hartiala JA, Tang WH, Wang Z, et al.: Genome-wide association study and targeted metabolomics identifies sex-specific association of CPS1 with coronary artery disease, *Nat Commun* 7:10558, 2016.
146. Shah SH, Bain JR, Muehlbauer MJ, et al.: Association of a peripheral blood metabolic profile with coronary artery disease and risk of subsequent cardiovascular events, *Circ Cardiovasc Genet* 3:207, 2010.
147. Rossing K, Bosselmann HS, Gustafsson F, et al.: Urinary proteomics pilot study for biomarker discovery and diagnosis in heart failure with reduced ejection fraction, *PloS One* 11:e0157167, 2016.
148. Quehenberger O, Dennis EA: The human plasma lipidome, *N Engl J Med* 365:1812, 2011.
149. Tarasov K, Ekroos K, Suoniemi M, et al.: Molecular lipids identify cardiovascular risk and are efficiently lowered by simvastatin and PCSK9 deficiency, *J Clin Endocrinol Metab* 99:E45, 2014.
150. Morrow DA, de Lemos JA: Benchmarks for the assessment of novel cardiovascular biomarkers, *Circulation* 115:949, 2007.

10 ECG and Standard Exercise Stress Testing

George Rodgers and Kristopher Heinzman

INTRODUCTION

The 12-lead electrocardiogram (ECG) has remained the standard initial evaluation tool in patients with suspected or known ischemic and electrophysiologic cardiac conditions for more than half a century. With the first description of the string galvanometer by Einthoven in the early part of the 20th century, the electrical activity of the human heart could be directly represented in an interpretable format.[1] Advances in ECG technology and clinical interpretation have allowed this simple test to remain an important tool in the evaluation of patients with acute ischemia, arrhythmias, genetic abnormalities, and chronic coronary artery disease (CAD).

Advances in technology have also brought multiple new tools for evaluating cardiac structure and function such as echocardiography and magnetic resonance imaging. However, the ECG remains the most widely used procedure for evaluating cardiac status, and competent ECG interpretation allows for a cost-effective method to avoid overtesting and to facilitate the early recognition of potentially dangerous conditions.

INDICATIONS FOR ELECTROCARDIOGRAPHIC TESTING

The American College of Cardiology/American Heart Association (ACC/AHA) guidelines for electrocardiography outline the appropriate use of the ECG in patients with known coronary disease[2] (Table 10.1). Class I indications are given to patients undergoing initial evaluation, those prescribed ongoing pharmacologic therapy known to produce ECG changes, and those with new signs or symptoms (Box 10.1). Coronary disease is a chronic condition, and patients are known to have clinical progression in the absence of symptoms or exacerbations. The guidelines suggest that periodic ECG evaluation of patients with chronic cardiac conditions is warranted. In the absence of symptoms, this interval should be no more frequent than every 4 months and likely no longer than yearly.[2] The most appropriate interval varies by individual patient depending on age, severity of disease, and known natural progression.[2] ECG evaluation is appropriate in all patients with known coronary disease undergoing preoperative evaluation.[3]

Intraventricular Conduction Delays

Intraventricular conduction delays (IVCDs) and bundle branch blocks (BBBs) can be seen in patients without known cardiovascular disease (CVD) (isolated BBB) and in those with nonischemic or ischemic cardiomyopathies.[4,5] Criteria for defining these conduction disturbances have been well established.[6] Some patients with BBB will have rate-related or intermittent episodes of BBB, which may progress to permanent BBB over time.

In multiple studies, the presence of a right BBB (RBBB) has not been associated with an increased risk of overall mortality, cardiovascular mortality, or CVD.[7,8] However, multiple population-based longitudinal studies have shown that the presence of a left BBB (LBBB) is associated with CVD including future high-grade atrioventricular block and increased cardiovascular mortality.[5,8] More recently, these findings have been extended to patients with incomplete LBBB and nonspecific IVCD.

Despite these clinical findings, the presence of an RBBB and not an LBBB has been recently found to be associated with large anteroseptal scarring in patients with cardiomyopathy of both ischemic and nonischemic etiology.[9] This is consistent with necropsy studies evaluating the blood supply of the conduction system.[10] Whereas the right bundle is supplied solely by septal perforators originating from the left anterior descending artery, the left bundle has dual blood supply in 90% of cases with the septal perforators feeding the anterior fascicle of the left bundle and the right coronary artery feeding the posterior fascicle via the posterior descending artery[10] (Fig. 10.1). The anterior and posterior fascicles of the left bundle each have a dual blood supply in up to 50% of cases. For this reason, despite the common misconception, new complete LBBB is rarely seen as a complication of acute anterior infarction and, when seen, is usually indicative of massive infarction.[11]

TABLE 10.1 American College of Cardiology/American Heart Association Guidelines for Electrocardiograms (ECGs) in Patients with Known Cardiovascular Disease or Dysfunction

INDICATION	CLASS I (INDICATED)	CLASS II (EQUIVOCAL)	CLASS III (NOT INDICATED)
Baseline or initial evaluation	All patients	None	None
Response to therapy	Patients in whom prescribed therapy is known to produce changes on the ECG that correlate with therapeutic responses or disease progression. Patients in whom prescribed therapy may produce adverse effects that may be predicted from or detected by changes on the ECG.	None	Patients receiving pharmacologic or nonpharmacologic therapy not known to produce changes on the ECG or to affect conditions that may be associated with such changes.
Follow-up evaluation	Patients with a change in symptoms, signs, or laboratory findings related to cardiovascular status. Patients with an implanted pacemaker or antitachycardia device. Patients with new signs or symptoms related to cardiovascular function. Patients with cardiovascular disease, even in the absence of new symptoms or signs, after an interval of time appropriate for the condition or disease.	None	Adult patients whose cardiovascular condition is usually benign and unlikely to progress (e.g., patients with asymptomatic mild mitral valve prolapse, mild hypertension, or premature contractions in absence of organic heart disease). Adult patients with chronic stable heart disease seen at frequent intervals (e.g., 4 months).
Before surgery	All patients with known cardiovascular disease or dysfunction, except as noted under class II.	Patients with hemodynamically insignificant congenital or acquired heart disease, mild systemic hypertension, or infrequent premature complexes in absence of organic heart disease.	None

BOX 10.1 Indications for Electrocardiographic Testing

Specific Conditions
- Chamber enlargement or hypertrophy
- Resolution or alteration of Arrhythmia or conduction disturbances
- Electrolyte abnormalities
- Pericarditis
- Endocarditis
- Myocarditis
- Transplant rejection
- Infiltrative cardiomyopathy

New Symptoms
- Syncope or near-syncope
- Change in anginal pattern
- Chest pain
- New or worsened dyspnea
- Extreme fatigue or weakness
- Palpitations

Physical Exam Findings
- Signs of congestive heart failure
- New organic murmur or friction rub
- Accelerating or poorly controlled systemic hypertension
- Findings suggestive of pulmonary hypertension
- Recent stroke
- Inappropriate heart rate
- Unexplained fever in known valvular disease

Cardiac Medications

Amiodarone Dronedarone Digoxin	ECG at baseline and every 6 months thereafter
Flecainide Propafenone Sotalol	ECG at baseline, 2–3 weeks postinitiation, and every 6 months thereafter
Dofetilide	ECG every 3 months after inpatient initiation

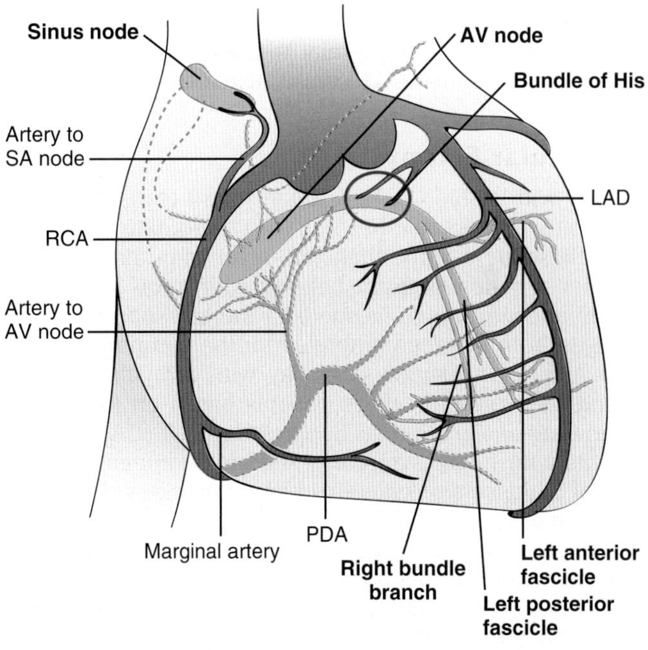

FIG. 10.1 Schematic diagram of the blood supply to the cardiac conduction system. The first septal perforators can be seen supplying the distal portion of the atrioventricular (AV) node and then the right bundle branch. In this depiction, both the anterior and posterior fascicles of the left bundle have a dual blood supply from the left anterior descending (LAD) and posterior descending artery (PDA) systems. *RCA*, Right coronary artery; *SA*, sinoatrial. *(Redrawn from Levine HJ.* Clinical Cardiovascular Physiology. *New York: Grune and Stratton; 1976.)*

One of the most significant effects of IVCD in patients with coronary disease is the challenge that it presents with interpretation of acute ischemic changes and stress ECG changes. Stress ECG alone has a very poor diagnostic accuracy in the presence of LBBB.[12] However, important prognostic information can still be gathered from exercise performance when combined with an imaging modality to evaluate for ischemia such as two-dimensional echocardiography or myocardial perfusion imaging.[12,13] In one large single-institution experience, among patients with a positive exercise stress echocardiogram, those with underlying LBBB had a significantly higher future mortality rate than those with an RBBB or no conduction abnormality (4.5% per year vs 2.5% per year and 1.9% per year, respectively). Additionally, those patients with a normal stress echocardiogram showed a similar mortality with and without LBBB.[14]

Whereas the presence of LBBB with known coronary disease clearly is associated with an increase in the risk of cardiovascular events, the presence of LBBB does not increase the probability of coronary disease itself. In a study of patients without known coronary disease referred for coronary computed tomography angiography (CCTA), 106 patients with presumed new LBBB were compared with 303 matched controls and found to have no significant difference in the presence of obstructive coronary disease.[15] This study also found comparable image quality in LBBB patients and non-LBBB controls, suggesting that CCTA is a reasonable diagnostic test in patients with LBBB.

The clinical scenario most often seen in chronic coronary patients is a new-onset BBB in the absence of symptoms. There are no consensus guidelines for how these patients should be evaluated. The evidence would suggest that the most likely etiology is a chronic degenerative/fibrotic process affecting the conduction system rather than new ischemia. However, it may be reasonable to consider noninvasive evaluation of cardiac function and in selected patients, screening for ischemia. Additionally, increasing the frequency of routine ECG testing is also reasonable.

Ventricular Ectopy

Patients with stable CAD are often found to have premature ventricular ectopic beats (PVCs) on routine ECG. Most times these are asymptomatic; however some patients will experience palpitations. In patients with a low burden of ectopy and no symptoms, medical therapy should not be changed from that recommended for the coronary disease itself. Attempts to suppress ectopy with arrhythmic drugs should be avoided in these patients based on the results of the Cardiac Arrhythmias Suppression Trial (CAST).[16] For patients with minor symptoms, starting or increasing dosages of β-blockers or calcium-channel blockers should be considered.

Patients with high burdens of ventricular ectopy may have decreased systolic function.[17,18] An exact burden cutoff has not been elucidated to date; however studies have shown that a range of PVC burden from 13% to 24% of total beats is independently associated with development of cardiomyopathy.[19,20] In addition, successful elimination of the ectopy through ablation can result in significant improvement and even normalization of systolic function.[19,20] The link between a high burden of ectopy and cardiomyopathy has been extended to patients with chronic coronary disease. In a small single-center study of patients with CAD and high ectopy burden, PVC ablation decreased PVC burden from 22% to 2.6%. The mean left ventricular ejection fraction (LVEF) improved in these patients from 38% to 51%, significantly better than in a control population without ablation that showed no change in systolic function.[21] This more aggressive strategy may eliminate the need for implantable cardioverter-defibrillators (ICDs) in some patients. In

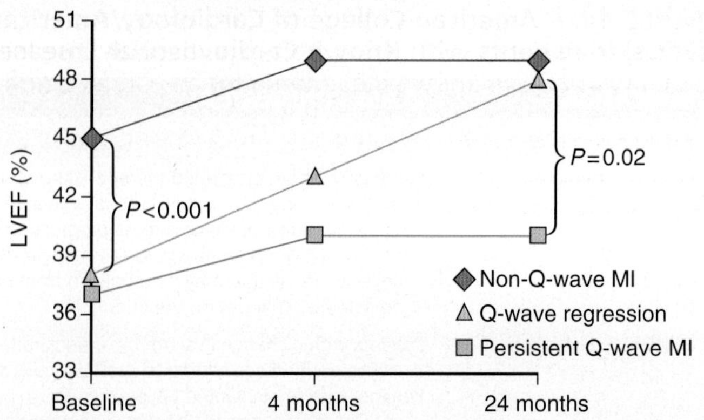

FIG. 10.2 Patients with Q-wave regression displayed significantly larger left ventricular ejection fraction (LVEF) improvement at 24 months compared with both persistent Q waves found on electrocardiogram and with non-Q-wave myocardial infarction patients. *(Adapted from Delewi R, Ijff G, van de Hoef TP, et al. Pathological Q waves in myocardial infarction in patients treated by primary PCI.* JACC Cardiovasc Imaging. *2013;6(3):324–331.)*

a study of 66 patients (including 11 with known coronary disease) undergoing PVC suppression with ablation who met current guidelines for ICD implantation before therapy, 64% no longer had an indication based on improvement in LVEF (including 10 of the 11 patients with prior myocardial infarction).[22]

Whereas most patients with PVCs should still be managed based on symptoms only, further attention should be paid to the patient with very frequent ventricular ectopy. Evidence shows these patients are at higher risk of developing cardiomyopathy and that elimination of the ectopy can reverse left ventricular dysfunction, even among those with an ischemic etiology. As there are no specific guidelines addressing management of PVCs in patients with CAD, we recommend ambulatory Holter monitoring and assessment of LV function in patients with a high burden of ectopy by history or ECG.

Persistent and New Q Waves

As mentioned previously, ECGs should be obtained at baseline and at regular intervals in patients with chronic CAD. CAD patients will often have evidence of prior infarction or conduction system disease at baseline. These baseline ECGs are important to use as a comparison when patients present with new symptoms.

Pathologic Q waves are considered the classic ECG sign of necrotic myocardium and are seen in the late progression of myocardial infarction (MI).[23] In the modern era of reperfusion therapy however, many patients who are found to have Q waves on presenting ECGs can have partial or complete resolution over time.[24,25] Compared with patients with persistent Q waves, those with eventual Q wave regression have significantly improved LVEF[26] (Fig. 10.2).

When routine ECGs are performed in patients with coronary disease, occasionally one will find evidence of new MI in patients who have had no apparent symptoms. This evaluation and management of apparent "silent" MI is not directly addressed in current practice guidelines. Clearly a careful history should be obtained, focusing on symptoms that may have been atypical for the patient and symptoms that may point to crescendo angina or congestive heart failure. In our opinion, in the absence of symptoms the finding of new Q waves on routine ECG does not require an evaluation for ischemia, but should trigger consideration for reassessment of LV function. This is particularly true for patients who have not yet met criteria for an ICD as a new infarction may now place them at increased risk of sudden death. If new LV dysfunction is seen, it is reasonable to consider an assessment for ischemic and viable myocardium even in the absence of symptoms, as revascularization may improve LV function.

Many other ECG abnormalities may be seen, from nonspecific ST changes to LV hypertrophy, which have been associated with increased risk of coronary events in the non-CVD and hypertensive populations. The potential effect on long-term prognosis in patients already diagnosed with coronary disease is not well understood. However, given that each of these findings alone changes classic risk models only modestly, it is unlikely that these findings in patients with known coronary disease on optimal medical therapy significantly modifies their future risk of coronary events. It is again our opinion that these findings should trigger a reevaluation of potential symptoms and possibly a reassessment of LV function.

EXERCISE TREADMILL TESTING

Historical Perspective

In 1941 Masters and Jaffe reported the combination of Masters' two-step stress test with the ECG to obtain objective evidence of angina pectoris.[27] Because many patients could not perform the Masters two-step stress test, Bruce and colleagues devised a more accessible version of the stress test using the motorized treadmill with inclination in 1956.[28] His eponymous protocol has been included in over 15,000 scholarly articles and remains the most common and most studied protocol today.

More definitive diagnostic procedures and treatment were developed soon afterward. Coronary angiography was introduced in 1958 and coronary artery bypass (CABG) surgery in 1967. Since the early days of stress testing, other modalities of imaging have accompanied stress ECG, especially myocardial perfusion imaging and echocardiography. The combination of imaging with the stress ECG has improved the sensitivity and specificity of the test[29] (see Chapters 11, 12, and 15). Categorically, these are functional or physiologic tests that depend on their ability to produce objective evidence of myocardial ischemia.

The objectives of stress ECG need to be evaluated in the context of a cost-sensitive environment. The first consideration is the diagnostic value of determining obstructive CAD, more precisely the confirmation that a patient's symptoms of chest discomfort are due to angina pectoris. The second is risk stratification and the prognostic value of stress ECG. The stress ECG may appropriately identify patients at high risk for MI and other major adverse cardiac events. Thus the clinician may better determine which patient might derive incremental benefit from revascularization. Finally, one may use stress ECG to objectively determine the efficacy of a treatment regimen whether it is revascularization or medical therapy.

This section will describe the role of stress ECG in CAD; it will also review the physiology of exercise and the pathophysiology of myocardial ischemia and describe the performance of the test and the interpretation of its outcomes.

The Physiology of Exercise

Exercise, and for that matter any activity that requires the contractions of muscles, requires energy. This energy is predominantly derived from oxidative metabolism to generate adenosine triphosphate. Fundamentally, the process requires efficient delivery of oxygen to the tissues. At any moment, the total body uptake of oxygen is defined as VO_2. The Fick equation describes the relationship between cardiac output (CO) and the extraction of oxygen at the tissue level (arteriovenous oxygen difference). $VO_2 = CO \times a\text{–}vO_2$ difference.[30]

The VO_2, or total body oxygen requirement at rest, is described as 1 MET (metabolic equivalent). This is estimated at 3.5 mL O_2/kg body wt. per min. Thus any physiologic activity or exercise can be described as a multiple of this basal metabolic unit. Whereas 1 MET corresponds to complete rest, 5 METs of energy is the equivalent of walking one block or climbing one flight of stairs.

During exercise, VO_2 increases. In other words, the person who is exercising requires more oxygen to supply energy for exercising muscles. In order to accomplish this, CO (the product of heart rate [HR] × stroke volume) may increases fourfold to sixfold, HR may increase twofold to threefold, and stroke volume may increase by 50%. At approximately 40% of maximum VO_2 the increase in stroke volume plateaus due to a progressive decrease in diastolic filling time.[31] By definition, VO_2 max is the maximum achievable VO_2 and is related to age, sex, physical fitness, and cardiac status. O_2 extraction in the periphery may increase as much as threefold during exercise, and the maximum O_2 extraction is estimated at 15–17 mL O_2/100 mL blood as the physiologic limit. VO_2 peak describes the symptom-limited maximum of a given patient undergoing exercise while testing and is commonly expressed as the patient's maximum exercise capacity or aerobic limit.

Aerobic exercise (high-repetition/low-resistance exercise) involves vigorous muscle activity (multiple cycles of muscular contraction and relaxation). Oxidative metabolites are generated in these large working muscles. The metabolites cause dilation of local arterioles, which increases the blood flow to the exercising muscles up to fourfold. Massive dilation of these vessels decreases vascular resistance, which contributes to the increase in stroke volume. With upright exercise such as jogging or fast walking, large muscle groups lead to an increase in sympathetic tone and a relative decrease in vagal tone. This increase in sympathetic tone increases HR and myocardial contractility. This also causes a shunting of blood from the renal, splanchnic, and cutaneous vascular beds supplying large muscles. This circulatory shunting increases the venous return and further contributes to an increase in CO through the Starling mechanism. During exercise, systolic pressure increases gradually, driven by an increase in CO, and diastolic pressure remains constant or decreases slightly.[30]

Dynamic arm exercise results in a similar hemodynamic response but HR and systolic blood pressure tend to be higher. During exercise, the myocardium experiences a marked increase in oxygen demand. This demand is driven by HR, blood pressure, LV contractility, wall thickness, and cavity size. The rate–pressure product (maximum HR × maximal systolic blood pressure achieved during exercise) is an excellent index of the O_2 demand (see Chapter 6). Myocardial ischemia develops when the demand for oxygen is not met. The main goal of stress testing is to elicit myocardial ischemia under a controlled condition.[30]

BOX 10.2 Indications for Stress Electrocardiogram (ECG)

1. Diagnosis of coronary artery disease in patients with an intermediate pretest probability of ischemic heart disease who have an interpretable ECG and at least moderate physical functioning capability
2. Risk assessment in patients with stable ischemic heart disease who are able to exercise to an adequate workload and have an interpretable ECG
3. Patients with known stable ischemic heart disease who have new or worsening symptoms not consistent with unstable angina and have at least moderate physical functioning capability and interpretable ECG
4. Determination of the efficacy of a treatment regimen in patients with known stable ischemic heart disease who are able to exercise to an adequate workload and have an interpretable ECG

Adapted from Fihn, SD, Gardin, JM, Abrams J, et al. 2012 ACCF/AHA/ACP/AATS/PCNA/SCAI/STS Guideline for the diagnosis and management of patients with stable ischemic heart disease: a report of the American College of Cardiology Foundation/American Heart Association Task Force on Practice Guidelines, and the American College of Physicians, American Association for Thoracic Surgery, Preventive Cardiovascular Nurses Association, Society for Cardiovascular Angiography and Interventions, and Society of Thoracic Surgeons. *Circulation.* 2012;60:126;e44–164 and Greenland P, Alpert JS, Beller GA, et al. 2010 ACCF/AHA guideline for assessment of cardiovascular risk in asymptomatic adults: a report of the American College of Cardiology Foundation/American Heart Association Task Force on Practice Guidelines. *Circulation.* 2010;112,e584–636.

TECHNICAL ASPECTS OF STRESS TESTING

Subject Preparation

Perhaps the most important aspect of stress testing is patient selection. As discussed in more detail in the next section, stress testing performs optimally as a diagnostic test when patients with intermediate likelihood of disease are selected (Box 10.2). Furthermore, the patient must be physically capable of performing treadmill exercise and the ECG must be interpretable for ischemic changes.

The most common forms of stress testing are the graded motorized treadmill and the cycle ergometer (stationary bicycle). The cycle ergometer is more commonly used outside the United States; it has the advantage of less expense and requires less laboratory space. Furthermore the cycle ergometer allows for easier access to the patient's arms and torso for measuring blood pressures and recording the ECG during exercise. However, subjects inexperienced in cycling tend to fatigue before they reach their true VO_2 max due to leg fatigue. Inexperienced subjects achieve 10% to 20% lower VO_2 max on the cycle ergometer than on treadmill exercise.[32] Dynamic arm exercise is another variety of aerobic stress available for patients who cannot perform adequate leg exercise; however, this modality is rarely used in clinical practice (Box 10.3). The graded treadmill is the most common modality used in the United States. There are a variety of protocols available, but the Bruce protocol (Table 10.2) is by far the most common and best studied protocol in practice today.

Most people can perform the Bruce protocol stress test. Some individuals have never exercised on a treadmill. A brief demonstration of the treadmill exercise is highly recommended before allowing a patient to initiate the test.[33,34]

Patient Selection

The subject must be physically able to exercise (Box 10.4). The patient should first be interviewed and examined to

BOX 10.3 Exercise Modalities and Protocols

1. Bruce protocol: standard graded motorized treadmill stress testing
2. Modified Bruce protocol: standard graded motorized treadmill stress testing to accommodate patients with limited physical functional capacity
3. Cycle ergometer: utilizes bicycle type exercise
4. Arm cycle ergometry: utilizes upper extremity exercise
5. Cardiopulmonary exercise testing: combines stationary cycle or motorized treadmill exercise with direct determination of oxygen uptake (VO_2)

TABLE 10.2 Bruce Protocol

STAGE	TIME (MIN)	SPEED (MPH)	GRADE (%)	METS
Rest	0:00	0.0	0	1.0
1	3:00	1.7	10	4.6
2	3:00	2.5	12	7.0
3	3:00	3.4	14	10.1
4	3:00	4.2	16	12.9

The modified Bruce protocol uses initial low-level 3-min stages at a speed of 1.7 MPH and grade 0% and 5%, respectively, and then continues to the full Bruce protocol.

From American College of Sports Medicine Guidelines for Exercise Testing and Prescription. *9th ed. Philadelphia: Lippincott, Williams and Wilkins; 2013.*

BOX 10.4 The Patient Assessment for Exercise

History

1. Medical diagnoses and past medical history: a variety of diagnoses should be reviewed, including cardiovascular disease (known existing coronary artery disease [CAD], previous myocardial infarction, or coronary revascularization); arrhythmias, syncope or presyncope; pulmonary disease, including asthma, emphysema, bronchitis, or recent pulmonary embolism; cerebral vascular disease, including stroke; peripheral artery disease; current pregnancy; musculoskeletal, neuromuscular, and joint disease
2. Symptoms: angina; chest, jaw, or arm discomfort; shortness of breath; palpitations, especially if associated with physical activity, eating a large meal, emotional upset, or exposure to cold
3. Risk factors for atherosclerotic disease: hypertension, diabetes, obesity, dyslipidemia, smoking; if the patient is without known CAD, determine the pretest probability of CAD (see Chapter 7)
4. Recent illness, hospitalization, or surgical procedure
5. Medication dose and schedule (particularly β-blockers)
6. Ability to perform physical activity

Physical Examination

1. Pulse rate and regularity
2. Resting blood pressure while sitting and standing
3. Auscultation of lungs, with specific attention to uniformity of breath sounds in all areas, particularly in patients with shortness of breath or history of heart failure or pulmonary disease
4. Auscultation of the heart, with particular attention in patients with heart failure or valvular disease
5. Examination related to orthopedic, neurologic, or other medical conditions that might limit exercise

Adapted from Balady GJ, Morise AP. Exercise testing. In: *Braunwald's Heart Disease.* Mann DL, Zipes DP, Libby P, et al, eds. 10th ed. 2015, Philadelphia, Elsevier: 157.

BOX 10.5 Contraindications to Exercise Testing

Absolute Contraindications
- Acute myocardial infarction (within 2 days)
- High-risk unstable angina
- Uncontrolled cardiac arrhythmia with hemodynamic compromise
- Symptomatic severe aortic stenosis
- Decompensated heart failure
- Acute pulmonary embolism or pulmonary infarction
- Acute myocarditis or pericarditis
- Physical disability precluding safe and adequate testing

Relative Contraindications
- Known left main coronary artery stenosis
- Moderate aortic stenosis with uncertain relationship to symptoms
- Atrial tachyarrhythmias with uncontrolled ventricular rates
- Acquired complete heart block
- Hypertrophic cardiomyopathy with a severe resting gradient
- Mental impairment with limited ability to cooperate

From Fletcher GF, Ades PA, Kligfield P, et al. Exercise standards for testing and training: a scientific statement from the American Heart Association. *Circulation.* 2013;128:873–934.

ensure that he or she does not have an important contraindication to exercise (Box 10.5).

During the interview the clinician should inquire about the patient's symptoms of chest pain, in particular its characteristics.[35] A risk calculator (see Chapter 7) may be used[36–38] to assist the clinician in making a more objective assessment of the patient's pretest probability. The clinician should further ask the patient about prior heart conditions or procedures—especially CAD, heart failure, history of pacemaker or ICD implantation, prior percutaneous coronary intervention (PCI) or CABG, and serious valve conditions (in particular aortic stenosis). On a brief physical exam the clinician should evaluate the patient for evidence of important contraindications such as decompensated heart failure or aortic stenosis.

LV hypertrophy with strain pattern may distort ST-segments and present difficulty in distinguishing ischemic ST depression during ECG stress testing. Certain distinguishing characteristics of LV hypertrophy with strain (e.g., the association with increased R-wave voltage and asymmetry of inverted T waves) may help,[39] but in general significant LV hypertrophy with strain decreases the diagnostic accuracy of stress ECG.[40] Although LV hypertrophy with strain is not a contraindication for stress ECG, the clinician may decide to combine stress with an imaging modality as an alternative to stress ECG if the ST strain pattern is deemed sufficiently pronounced[41] (See Chapters 11, 12, and 15).

Certain medications may affect the stress ECG. In particular digoxin is known to cause ST depression on the resting ECG and may lead to false-positive test results. β-Blockers may significantly reduce the HR response to exercise and result in an inadequate and nondiagnostic study. The decision on how to manage the patient who is currently on β-blockers depends entirely on the objectives of the stress test. If the objective is to diagnose obstructive CAD, the clinician should advise the patient not to take the β-blockers before the test so that the patient has the opportunity to achieve an adequate HR response. However, if the patient is known to have obstructive CAD and the objective of the stress test is to assess risk or to determine the efficacy of the patient's medical regimen that includes a β-blocker, the patient should be instructed to take all medications before the stress test as prescribed. In this scenario one can objectively determine the patient's ischemic threshold.[30]

TABLE 10.3 Borg Scale of Perceived Exertion

PERCEPTION OF EXERTION	BORG SCALE	EXAMPLES
None	6	Reading a book
Very, very light	7–8	Tying shoes
Very light	9–10	Folding clothes
Fairly light	11–12	Easy walking
Somewhat hard	13–14	Brisk walking
Hard	15–16	Bicycling, swimming
Very hard	17–18	Highest level sustainable
Very, very hard	19–20	Highest level unsustainable, finishing kick in a race

BOX 10.6 Patient Monitoring During Exercise Testing

During the Exercise
- Twelve-lead electrocardiogram (ECG) during the last minute of each stage or at least every 3 min
- Blood pressure during the last minute at each stage or at least every 3 min
- Symptom rating scales as appropriate for the test indication in laboratory protocol

During the Recovery Period
- Monitoring for a minimum of 6 min after exercise in a sitting or supine position or until near-baseline heart rate, blood pressure, ECG, and symptoms are measured or reached. An active cool down may be included in the recovery period, particularly following high levels of exercise, to minimize the postexercise hypotensive effects of venous pooling in the lower extremities.
- Twelve-lead ECG every minute
- Heart rate and blood pressure immediately after exercise and then every 1 or 2 min thereafter until near-baseline measures are reached
- Symptomatic ratings every minute as long as symptoms persist after exercise. Patient should be observed until all symptoms have resolved/returned to baseline levels.

Adapted from Balady GJ, Morise AP. Exercise testing. In: *Braunwald's Heart Disease.* Mann DL, Zipes DP, Libby P, et al, eds. 10th ed. 2015, Philadelphia, Elsevier: 157.

Monitoring During Exercise

ECG leads are placed in a 12-lead "torso" configuration on the individual and secured to accommodate the exercising patient. Care should be taken to ensure proper skin preparation as the ECG leads are applied. A resting ECG should be performed while the patient is standing. A blood pressure cuff is placed on one arm so that blood pressure can be monitored at rest as well as at the end of each 3-min stage of exercise. Finally, the patient's symptoms are monitored. Some clinicians use the Borg Scale of Exercise (Table 10.3) to quantify the subjective experience of exertion.[30] Patients are asked to report whether they feel a pressure-like substernal chest discomfort during exercise, to grade its severity, and to determine whether it is limiting the ability to proceed or not (Box 10.6).

Termination of the Test

The goals of stress testing are twofold: the patient exercises to his/her maximum capacity (exhaustion) and exceeds 85% of the maximum age-predicted maximum HR (MAPHR) and/or the patient objectively demonstrates myocardial ischemia with characteristic ST depression.

The MAPHR is traditionally calculated as 220 minus the patient's age in years (MAPHR = 220 – age).

The maximum achievable workload (determined by the duration of exercise on the test) represents the patient's exercise capacity, which is an important prognostic factor. Whereas cardiopulmonary testing employs ventilator gas exchange analysis to determine actual VO_2,[42] most stress labs estimate the METs performed from time on the treadmill. The patient's work performance can be evaluated against an expected result based on age.

$$\text{Men: predicted METs} = 18 - 0.15 \times \text{age (years)}$$

$$\text{Women: predicted METs} = 14.7 - 0.13 \times \text{age (years)}$$

The O_2 demand is estimated by the double product of the maximum HR achieved × the maximum systolic pressure achieved.

Technically, a *maximal stress study* is one in which the patient achieves his/her predicted maximal HR [MAPHR = 220 – age (years)]. However, a *diagnostically adequate* test is one in which the patient achieves or exceeds 85% MAPHR with exercise. This is one of the primary goals of the test. Thus a *submaximal study* is one in which the patient is unable to achieve this goal. Patients who perform a submaximal stress test should typically achieve a double product (maximum HR × maximum systolic pressure) greater than 20,000. A *diagnostic test* however may result before the patient achieves his/her MAPHR, if he/she reports limiting angina and ischemic ECG changes. An *inadequate study* is one in which the patient fails to achieve 85% of his/her predicted maximum HR and fails to demonstrate ischemic ECG changes. If the patient performs a stress ECG test in which 85% MAPHR is not achieved and exhibits no ischemic ECG changes, the test is considered *nondiagnostic*. Patients who cannot achieve greater than 80% of their MAPHR (and who are not taking β-blockers or other negative chronotropic medications) may have chronotropic insufficiency.[30] In general, the stress test should continue until the patient is exhausted (Borg scale ≥17). This represents the patient's maximum exercise capacity as measured in minutes on the Bruce protocol, and this time is an important component of the Duke treadmill score (see hereafter).

Patient safety is of utmost importance and the test may need to be terminated prematurely (Box 10.7). The supervising professional should maintain close observation of the patient as he/she exercises and should be prepared to stop the treadmill the moment that the patient appears unstable so that the patient does not sustain injury. Furthermore, a stress ECG test should be terminated if the patient exhibits 2 mm horizontal ST depression in one or more leads and/or a drop of 10 mm Hg in systolic pressure after an initial rise whether or not the patient reports symptoms.[43]

BOX 10.7 Indications for Terminating an Exercise Test

Absolute Indications

- ST-elevation (> 1.0 mm) in leads without Q waves (other than aVR, aVL, or V1)
- Drop in systolic blood pressure of > 10 mm Hg, despite an increase in workload, when accompanied by any other evidence of ischemia
- Moderate to severe angina
- Central nervous system symptoms (e.g. ataxia, dizziness, or near-syncope)
- Signs of poor perfusion (cyanosis or pallor)
- Sustained ventricular tachycardia or other arrhythmia that interferes with normal maintenance of cardiac output during exercise
- Technical difficulties monitoring the electrocardiogram
- Patient's request to stop

Relative Indications

- Marked ST displacement (> 2 mm horizontal or downsloping) in a patient with suspected ischemia
- Drop in systolic blood pressure > 10 mm Hg (persistently below baseline), despite an increase in workload, in the absence of other evidence of ischemia
- Increasing chest pain
- Fatigue, shortness of breath, wheezing, leg cramps, or claudication
- Arrhythmias other than sustained ventricular tachycardia, including multifocal ectopy, ventricular triplets, supraventricular tachycardia, atrioventricular heart block, or bradycardia arrhythmias
- Exaggerated hypertensive response (systolic blood pressure > 250 mm Hg and/or diastolic blood pressure > 115 mm Hg)
- Development of a bundle branch block that cannot be distinguished from ventricular tachycardia

From Fletcher GF, Ades PA, Kligfield P, et al. Exercise standards for testing and training: a scientific statement from the American Heart Association. *Circulation*. 2013;128:873–934.

Supervision of the Test

The ACC/AHA Clinical Statement on Stress Testing addresses competency in stress testing and specifically the qualifications and competency for those who would supervise the stress test.[44] The authors describe three categories of supervision: personal supervision, in which the supervising professional is at the patient's side; direct supervision, in which the supervising professional is within immediate access and available if a problem arises but not necessarily physically in the stress lab; and general supervision, in which the supervising professional has a more general role of oversight and is not immediately available. The authors are of the opinion that exercise physiologists, stress techs, RNs, PAs, and NPs, with appropriate training, can competently personally supervise the test, while the cardiologist or other physician remains immediately available in case of an emergency (direct supervision).[44] For patients screened and found to be appropriate (with no contraindications) for the test, the risk of sudden cardiac arrest during stress testing is extremely low (1 in 10,000).[45] In fact, the most common cause of liability or lawsuits generated as a result of a mishap during stress testing involves mechanical falls in which the patient is physically injured. Thus great care should be taken to make sure that the patient is safe and understands procedures for emergency stopping and that safety handrails are available during the exercise to mitigate these issues.[46]

STRESS TESTING IN PATIENTS WITH CORONARY ARTERY DISEASE

The stress ECG is a very useful diagnostic tool in CAD. In the appropriate context, it can provide valuable diagnostic

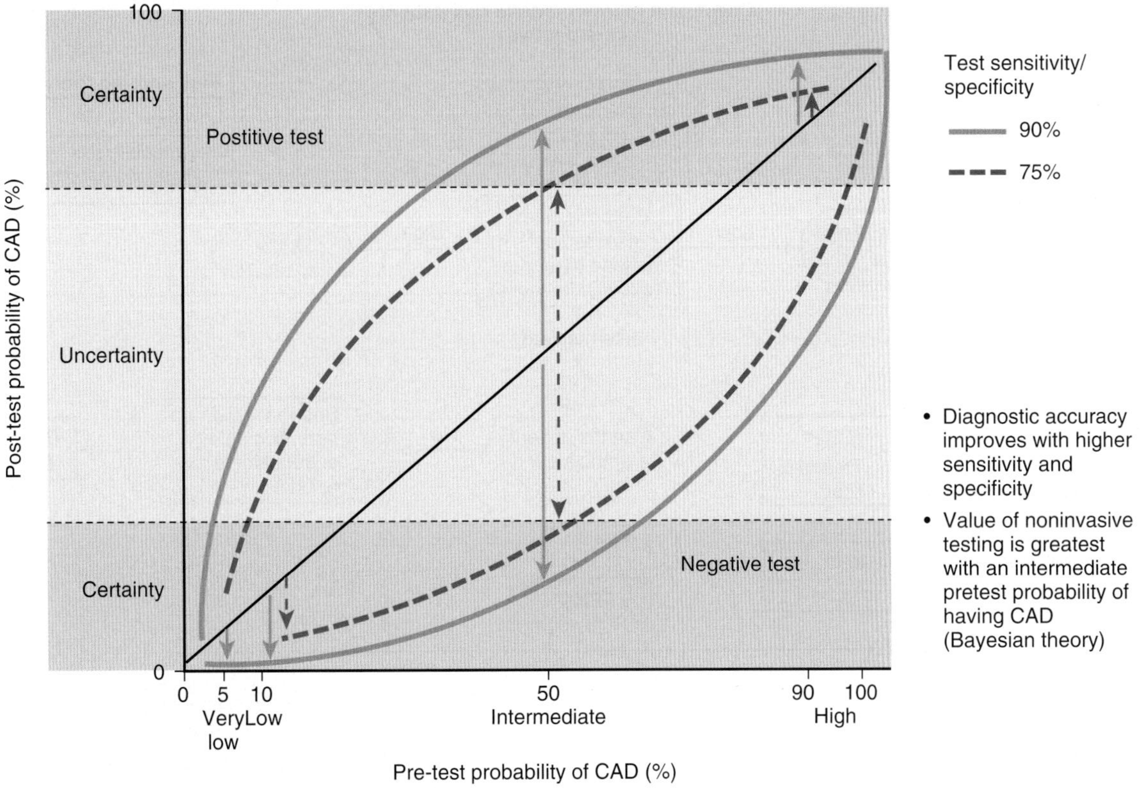

FIG. 10.3 The relation between pretest and posttest probability. Diagnostic accuracy improves with a test with a higher sensitivity and specificity. Bayesian theory has shown that the value of noninvasive testing is greatest in patients with an intermediate pretest probability of having coronary artery disease. *(From Weustink AC, de Feyter PJ. The role of multi-slice computed tomography in stable angina management: a current perspective.* Neth Heart J. *2011;19(7–8):336–343.)*

and prognostic information regarding CAD. As with any test, it has its limitations. It also has distinct advantages in that it provides a wealth of physiologic information in a standardized and controlled environment. Furthermore, it is relatively inexpensive and most patients can perform graded treadmill exercise.[47–49]

Fundamentally, the stress ECG attempts to induce myocardial ischemia in a safe and standardized fashion. It captures multiple important physiologic and ECG parameters in the process. Components of the Duke treadmill score, for example, exercise capacity (duration on the treadmill), reproduction of symptoms, and detection of ischemic ECG changes, are recorded.[50]

The clinician must be clear on the objectives of the test. Stress ECG can potentially detect only obstructive coronary atherosclerotic lesions that are flow limiting (i.e., ≧75% diameter stenosis) or severe microvascular abnormalities associated with exercise-induced ischemia. The more severely narrowed a coronary artery is and the more myocardium at risk (based on proximal location and number of severe lesions involved), the more likely the stress ECG is to register a positive result. Several important studies have compared stress ECG outcomes to the gold standard of coronary angiography. These studies are subject to selection bias, because clinicians regarded the patients in these studies as having a higher pretest probability sufficient to warrant a cardiac catheterization. The sensitivity of the stress ECG (the percentage of patients with actual obstructive CAD who have a positive stress test) is ~70%. The specificity of the stress ECG (the percentage of patients without obstructive CAD who have a negative test) is 75% to 80%.[51] Clearly the test performs better with optimal patient selection. According to the Bayes theorem, the pretest probability significantly affects the posterior probability or outcome of the test.[52] If many low-risk patients (low pretest probability) undergo stress ECG, an excessive number of false-positive results are likely, whereas if patients with a very high pretest probability are tested, the false-negative result may be high[53] (Fig. 10.3). Accordingly, stress ECG is most likely to provide clinically useful diagnostic information in those patients at intermediate pretest probability of disease.

Often the objective of the stress ECG is to determine whether the patient's symptoms of chest discomfort are due to obstructive CAD. The presumed implication is that if the patient who has these symptoms is found to have one or more flow-limiting coronary lesions, he or she could potentially benefit from revascularization with either PCI or CABG.

Several probabilistic tools/calculators have sought to aid the clinician in assessing a patient's pretest probability of obstructive CAD (see Chapter 7). They incorporate the important characteristics of angina[35] as well as age, gender, and other risk factors. One well known algorithm is the Duke chest pain score. This calculator tool derived its fundamental information from the results of a retrospective study and was then applied prospectively to test its validity. This calculator generates a probability score that evaluates the likelihood an individual patient's symptoms correlate with significant obstructive CAD. Thus using the Duke chest pain calculator one could determine that a particular patient has a very low probability (low pretest probability) and probably should not undergo a stress ECG in his or her initial diagnostic evaluation. On the other hand, if a patient is found to have a very high probability of having significant obstructive CAD (e.g., a Duke chest pain score >85%), the stress ECG is not likely to provide any further incremental value for that patient and he or she should more likely go directly to catheterization.

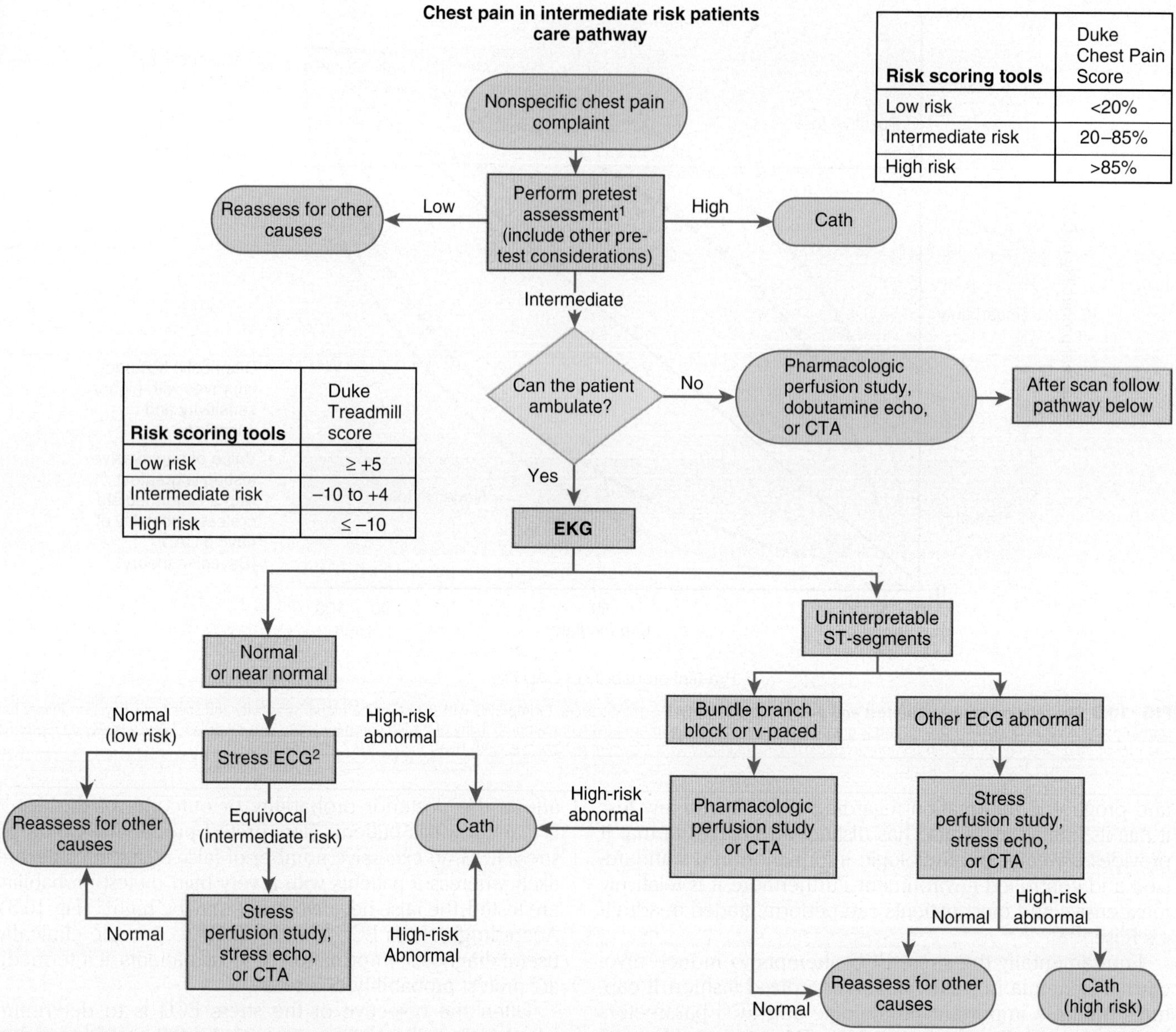

FIG. 10.4 Algorithm for stress electrocardiogram (ECG) for chest pain evaluation. The clinician first determines the patient's pretest probability based on the patient's traditional risk factors and characteristics of chest pain. The Duke chest pain score may be used for this purpose. Patients with low pretest probability would not likely benefit from further ischemic evaluation and should be assessed for other etiologies of chest pain. Patients with very high pretest probability for angina due to obstructive coronary artery disease are ordinarily best served with coronary angiography. Those with intermediate pretest probability are best served by noninvasive evaluation for inducible myocardial ischemia. If the patient can exercise and has an interpretable resting ECG, he or she should undergo stress ECG. Those who do not meet these criteria may undergo pharmacologic stress testing with cardiac imaging. The results of the stress ECG may be evaluated with the Duke treadmill score. Patients with a low risk (≥ 5) likely do not have obstructive CAD and have a very favorable prognosis for absence of cardiac events. Those with high-risk Duke treadmill score (≤ 10) most likely have significant obstructive CAD and should undergo coronary angiography. Those with an intermediate Duke treadmill score (4 to −10) should undergo stress testing with cardiac imaging.

As mentioned previously, the patients best served by stress ECG are those who have an intermediate likelihood of having obstructive CAD (pretest probability between 20% and 85%)[37,38] (Fig. 10.4).

ST Depression

Positive ischemic changes are defined as at least 1 mm (or 0.1mV) horizontal or downsloping ST depression in three consecutive beats in one or more ECG leads. The PQ line is used as the isoelectric line and the ST depression is measured at 60 ms (to 80 ms) beyond the J point. ST-segment depression greater than 2 mm is a criterion for termination of the test. Upsloping ST depression is not considered a positive (ischemic) response.[30] Pathophysiologically, ST depression represents subendocardial ischemia (Fig. 10.5).

Unlike ST elevation in the case of ST-segment elevation MI (STEMI), the particular leads exhibiting ischemic ST depression are a poor predictor of the anatomic region of ischemia. The lateral leads (I, aVL, and V6) are the most likely leads to exhibit ischemic changes; however, one may subsequently find that the significant lesions may be found in the left anterior descending (LAD) artery (anterior distribution) or the right coronary artery (inferior distribution).

ST Elevation

ST elevation during stress ECG is an abnormal and fairly unusual response. Most commonly it is seen in the presence of pathologic Q waves, where it may suggest an LV aneurysm or periinfarction ischemia. In this case a stress test with nuclear perfusion imaging may help further

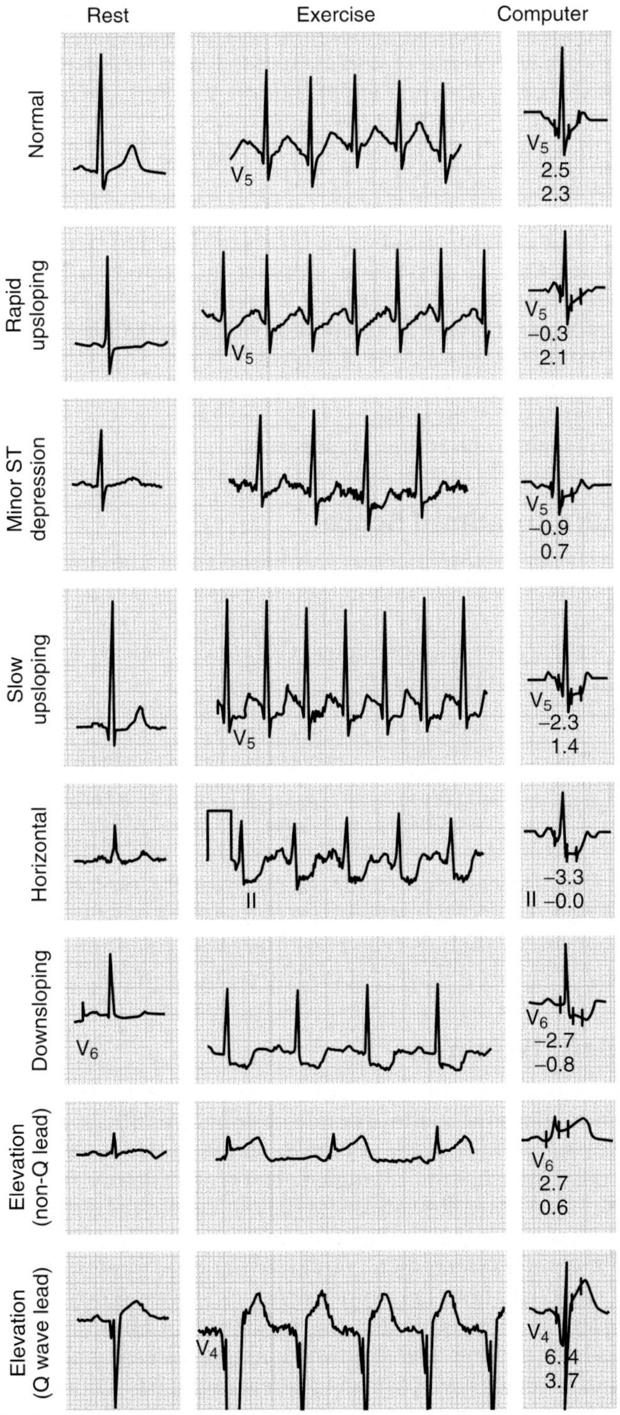

FIG. 10.5 Eight typical exercise electrocardiographic patterns at rest and at peak exertion during stress testing. The computer-process incrementally average beat corresponds with raw data taken at the same time point during exercise and is illustrated in the **last column.** The patterns represent worsening electrocardiographic responses during exercise. In the column of computer-average beats, ST80 displacement **(top number)** indicates the magnitude of the ST-segment displacement 80 ms after the J point relative to the PQ junction or E point. ST-segment slope measurement **(bottom number)** indicates the ST-segment slope and at a fixed time point after the J point to the ST80 measurement. At least three non-computer-processed average complexes with a stable baseline should meet the criteria for abnormality before the exercise electrocardiographic result can be considered abnormal. Normal and rapidly upsloping ST-segment responses typically occur with exercise. J point depression with rapidly upsloping ST-segments is a common response in an older, apparently healthy person. Minor ST-segment depression can occasionally occur at submaximal workload in patients with coronary artery disease (CAD); in this figure, the ST-segment is depressed 0.09 mV (0.9 mm) 80 ms after the J point. A slow upsloping ST-segment pattern may suggest an ischemic response in patients with known CAD or in those with a high pretest clinical risk for CAD. Criteria for slow upsloping ST-segment depression include J point and ST80 depression of ≥ 0.15 mV and an ST-segment slope greater than 1.0 mV/s. This pattern may also proceed to horizontal or downsloping ST-segment depression that will occur during recovery. Classic criteria for myocardial ischemia include horizontal ST-segment depression observed when both the J point and ST80 depression are > 0.1 mV and the ST-segment slope is within the range of 1.0 mV/s. Downsloping ST-segment depression occurs when the J point and ST80 depression are 0.1 mV and the ST-segment slope is −1.0 mV/s. ST-segment elevation in the non-Q-wave infarct lead occurs when the J point and ST60 are > 1.0 mV and it represents a severe ischemic response. ST-segment elevation in infarct territory (Q-wave lead) indicates a severe wall motion abnormality and, in most cases, is not considered an ischemic response. *(From Chaitman BR. Exercise electrocardiographic stress testing. In: Beller GA, ed.* Chronic Ischemic Heart Disease. *In: Braunwald E, series ed.* Atlas of Heart Diseases. *Vol 5. Philadelphia: Current Medicine; 1995:2.1–2.30.)*

evaluate this finding. In the absence of pathologic Q waves, ST elevation suggests transmural ischemia and is more likely associated with significant proximal CAD (e.g., proximal LAD) or coronary spasm. In particular, there is growing evidence that ST elevation in lead aVR of ≥ 1 mm (0.1 mV) is a potential indicator of significant left main or proximal LAD disease.[54–56]

Bundle Branch Block

LBBB on the resting ECG is a contraindication to ECG stress testing because ischemic ST changes cannot be interpreted.

In 0.5% of stress testing cases a BBB develops during exercise. If LBBB develops with a HR greater than 125 beats/min the finding is of no consequence regarding CAD. However, if LBBB appears during exercise before HR of 125 beats/min, it has prognostic significance for future major adverse cardiac events (MACEs). Exercise-induced RBBB is not associated with increased risk of MACE. Ischemic changes in leads II, III, aVF and I, aVL, and V6 may be interpreted in the setting of RBBB, but ECG leads V1 to V4 cannot be interpreted.[57,58]

T-Wave Changes

In general T-wave changes (including inversion or pseudonormalization) have no diagnostic relevance. However more refined analytical technics using signal averaging may reveal increased risk for ventricular arrhythmias.

Arrhythmias

Isolated PVCs are observed in approximately 20% of stress tests and have no diagnostic importance. However, frequent PVCs and nonsustained VT, although rarely seen (2–3% of cases), may have prognostic importance. PVCs with an RBBB morphology in particular suggest an increased risk for MACE.

Exercise-induced supraventricular arrhythmias, for example, supraventricular tachycardia or atrial fibrillation, are not predictive of ischemia. These findings may however predict the appearance of supraventricular tachycardia or atrial fibrillation at a later date.[59,60]

PROGNOSIS

The stress ECG is also a strong prognostic tool. The more flow-limiting lesions that a patient has and the more proximal the disease, the more myocardium is at risk and the more likely the stress ECG is to be positive. Furthermore, as more myocardium is at risk due to widespread and severe coronary disease, the more physiologic parameters are adversely affected in this functional test.

Exercise Capacity

Exercise capacity has been found to be a strong predictor of future MACEs. Bourque et al.[61] found that the ability of a patient to achieve greater than 10 METs of exercise had a strong negative predictive value for MACE and the absence of significant (> 10%) LV ischemia.[61–63] In contrast, patients with severe disease are limited in their capacity to exercise. This is observed in several ways. First, the duration of the test is limited. It is often limited because of anginal symptoms but also because of the patient's diminished capacity to perform work. In some patients this diminished capacity to perform work is due to an inability (in the absence of β-blockers) to appropriately increase their HR during exercise. This finding, termed *chronotropic insufficiency*, is a strong predictor of adverse cardiac events.[64–67]

Alternatively some patients may have diminished capacity to perform exercise due to widespread ischemia that decreases LV stroke volume and therefore decreases CO and thus the ability to perform cardiac work. In the extreme, widespread myocardial ischemia may be reflected in a drop in systolic blood pressure (defined as a drop of 10 mm Hg in systolic blood pressure from the resting systolic blood pressure). Indeed, exercise-induced hypotension is associated with a poor prognosis and a higher likelihood that the patient may have left main disease or severe three-vessel CAD. Regardless of the underlying physiologic mechanism, patients who are unable to exercise to the goal of 85% of predicted maximum HR are considered at higher risk for cardiac events.[47–49]

Heart Rate Response

Early HR acceleration suggests deconditioning. However atrial fibrillation may confuse this issue. Furthermore, early HR acceleration may indicate anemia or significant LV systolic dysfunction.[68] During recovery, vagal tone increases and sympathetic tone decreases. This leads to a gradual decrease in HR in healthy individuals. An abnormal recovery (slower than usual to return to baseline resting HR) would suggest poor conditioning.[69]

An abnormal response would be:

< 12 beats/min after 1 min of recovery while standing
< 18 beats/min after 1 min of recovery while sitting
< 42 beats/min after 2 min of recovery while sitting.

Blood Pressure Response

The systolic blood pressure normally increases at least to greater than 140 mm Hg with maximal exercise. The double product (maximal HR × maximal SBP) normally exceeds 20,000. A systolic blood pressure that does not exceed 140 mm Hg and a double product that does not exceed 10,000 suggest a poor prognosis.

A drop in systolic blood pressure greater than 10 mm Hg after an initial rise indicates a very poor prognosis. One must however be aware of a pseudodrop in systolic blood pressure in the case of an anxious patient whose systolic blood pressure was excessively elevated at rest but "settled down" once the test began.[43,70] An excessive increase in systolic blood pressure above 220 mm Hg suggests hypertension that has previously gone undiagnosed.

ECG Changes

The time during the exercise phase at which significant ST depression appears is very important and may be referred to as *the ischemic threshold*. Duration of exercise relates to performance of work and therefore O_2 demand. Ischemia that appears with a low workload (within 6 min) corresponds to a poor prognosis and high likelihood of significant left main, proximal LAD, and/or three-vessel disease.

Important factors that relate ST depression to the probability of significant disease are:

1. A shorter time to induce significant ST depression
2. The duration of ischemic changes (the number of minutes that ST depression persists in recovery). Typically, ST depression lasts at least 2 min before the ST depression normalizes. ST depression lasting longer than 5 min would suggest a poor prognosis.
3. Number of leads exhibiting ST depression
4. Depth of ST depression
5. Elevation rather than depression

Duke Treadmill Score

The Duke treadmill score combines and balances several important testing parameters. It provides a quantifiable means to determine the likelihood that a positive result reflects significant obstructive CAD and serves as an important prognostic indicator.[50]

The Duke treadmill score = Duration of exercise in minutes (on Bruce protocol) − {5 × (ST depression)} − {4 × (angina variable)}

ST depression: Measured in mm

Angina variable: 0 = No Angina; 1 = Mild Angina; 2 = Limiting Angina

Exercise capacity (time on the exercise protocol) and the degree of ST depression are perhaps the most important prognostic variables (Fig. 10.6). The Duke treadmill score is prognostically relevant for both men and women.[71]

Silent Ischemia

Often patients will meet ECG criteria for ischemia during treadmill testing in the absence of symptoms. This is referred to as *silent myocardial ischemia,* which is also a term used to describe ischemic changes seen on ambulatory ECG (not discussed here). Review of the data related to the prognostic significance of this finding is mixed as it spans eras of significant changes in medical and interventional therapy.[72]

Early data from the Coronary Artery Surgery Study (CASS) registry in 1988 evaluated the incidence of MI and sudden death in patients with known coronary disease and symptomatic versus asymptomatic exercise-induced ischemia.[73] In the study, 424 patients with asymptomatic ST changes during exercise testing were compared with 456 patients with ST changes and angina. At 7-year follow-up there were similar rates of both MI (20% vs 18%) and sudden cardiac death (9% vs 7%). There was no significant difference between the two groups and both groups had significantly higher adverse event rates than matched controls over the same period. This suggests that patients with evidence of ischemia but without symptoms were at the same risk as those who experienced angina (Fig. 10.7).

A more recent study from 2003 evaluated 356 patients after coronary intervention with exercise myocardial perfusion scans:[74] 23% of patients tested showed evidence of target vessel ischemia and 62% of these patients had no symptoms. Over 4 years of follow-up, the finding of silent ischemia predicted higher rates of cardiac death, MI, or revascularization than no ischemia but a better outcome than symptomatic ischemia.

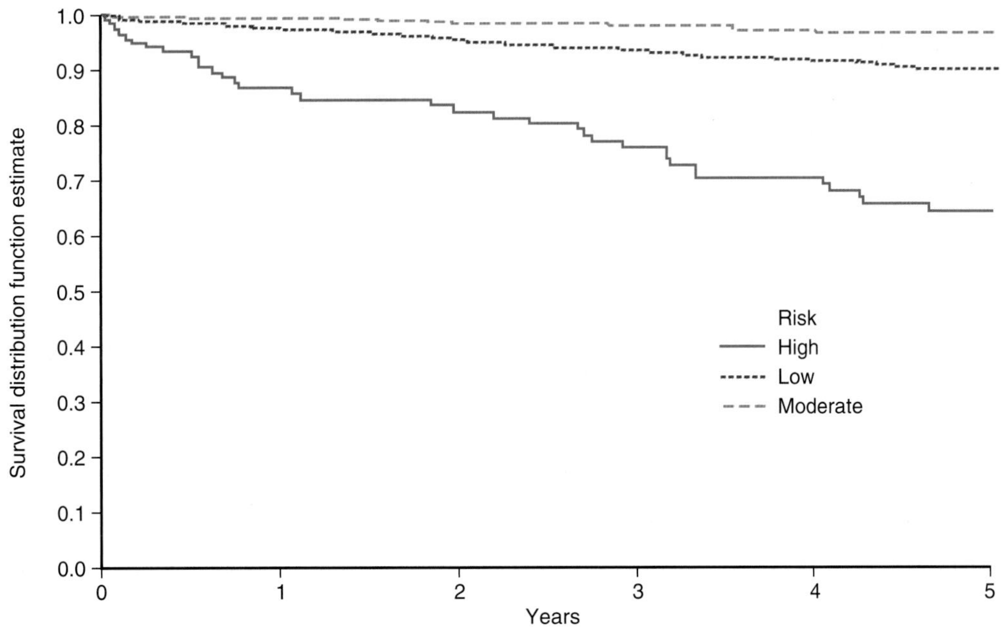

FIG. 10.6 The prognostic value of the Duke treadmill score (DTS) is illustrated in these Kaplan-Meier survival curves of patients with low- (DTS ≥ +5), intermediate- (DTS ≤ +4 to −10), and high-risk (< −10) for cardiovascular events. *(From Shaw LJ, Peterson ED, Shaw LK, et al. Use of a prognostic treadmill score in identifying CAD subgroups.* Circulation. *1998;98:1622–1630.)*

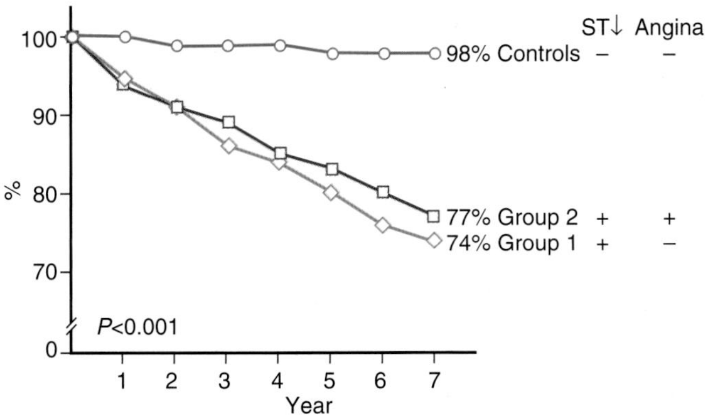

FIG. 10.7 Cumulative 7-year probability of remaining free of myocardial infarction and sudden death among patients with ischemic changes on stress testing with or without symptoms. *(Adapted from Weiner DA, Ryan TJ, McCabe CH, et al. Risk of developing an acute myocardial infarction or sudden coronary death in patients with exercise-induced silent myocardial ischemia. A report from the Coronary Artery Surgery Study (CASS) registry.* Am J Cardiol. *1988;62:1155–1158.)*

With evidence showing that silent ischemia predicts poor outcomes, it is not surprising that studies have evaluated the effect of revascularization targeting silent ischemia on these outcomes. The Asymptomatic Cardiac Ischemia Pilot (ACIP) study tested percutaneous transluminal coronary angioplasty (PTCA) and CABG versus medical therapy in patients with silent ischemia seen on ambulatory ECG and an abnormal exercise tolerance test.[75] All patients were without symptoms at the time of ischemic changes and one-third had no angina symptoms whatsoever. Patients randomized to revascularization had a significant improvement in silent ischemia elimination (55% vs 40%) and lower rates of a composite including death, MI, revascularization, and unstable angina than those randomized to medical therapy.

More recently in 2012, a post hoc analysis of the Clinical Outcomes Utilizing Revascularization and Aggressive Drug Evaluation (COURAGE) trial evaluated potential differences in the patients with known CAD treated with either optimal medical therapy (OMT) or PCI.[76] Of the 2280 patients in the trial, 283 (12%) had no history of anginal symptoms. Compared to patients with symptoms, those with silent myocardial ischemia had fewer revascularizations regardless of treatment assignment (27% vs 16%) and fewer hospitalizations for acute coronary syndrome (12% vs 7%). Among patients with silent ischemia, no significant difference was seen in the outcomes of death, MI, or hospitalization for acute coronary syndrome between those assigned to OMT or PCI.

Taking a different approach, in 2004 the Aggressive Diagnosis of Restenosis (ADORE) trial enrolled 342 patients after PCI to test a strategy of routine stress testing regardless of symptoms versus a selective approach in which testing was performed only when clinically indicated.[77] Measured outcomes, which included exercise capacity, functional status, and quality of life scores, showed no difference at 9 months between the two groups.

Results of ADORE and of OMT versus PCI trials in the era of modern medical therapy support the AHA/ACC guidelines recommendations against routine stress testing in asymptomatic patients after revascularization in the abscess of clear indications. Stress tests are occasionally performed for indications other than angina such as preoperative evaluation. When silent ischemia is found on these studies the decision on how to proceed is more difficult. It is necessary to consider the characteristics of the patient and the reason the test was ordered before making a decision on how to proceed. Based on recent data, continuing OMT alone may represent the most appropriate strategy for the majority of patients with silent ischemia.

THERAPEUTIC EFFICACY

Another strategy for the use of stress ECG in patients with known obstructive CAD is to objectively determine the efficacy of medical therapy. By utilizing the objective measures of a stress ECG, the ischemic threshold can be compared before and after therapy and thus a quantifiable measure of treatment efficacy can be obtained. In addition, the

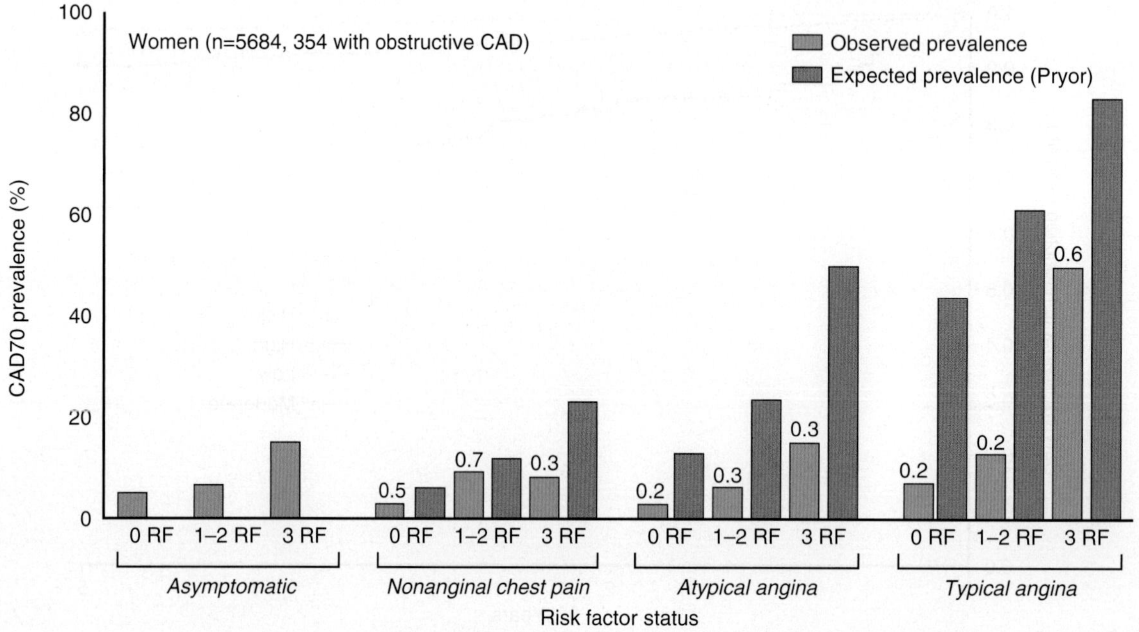

FIG. 10.8 Pretest probability in women. These results are based on a registry of over 14,000 patients. Observed prevalence and expected prevalence of angiographically confirmed greater than or equal to 70% stenotic coronary artery disease (CAD 70) in the study's women. Expected prevalence was calculated using the algorithm described by Pryor et al., which incorporates sex, age, angina typicality, history of prior myocardial infarction, presence of Q waves on resting electrocardiogram (ECG), and presence of three risk factors (RFs): diabetes, dyslipidemia, and active smoking. Study patients were assumed to have no Q waves on resting ECG. Within each system category, patients were subgrouped by number of RFs. In all groups, expected prevalence was higher than observed prevalence. The differences were particularly dramatic in patients with atypical angina or typical angina and less than three RFs, for whom observed-to-expected ratios were less than 0.4. *(From Cheng VY, Berman DS, Rozanski A, et al. Performance of the traditional age, sex, and angina typicality-based approach for estimating pretest probability of Angiographically significant coronary artery disease in patients undergoing coronary computed tomography angiography: results from the multinational Coronary CT Angiography Evaluation for Clinical Outcomes: An International Multicenter Registry (CONFIRM). Circulation. 2011;124:2423–2432, 1–8.)*

threshold of symptoms, ischemic ST-segment changes, and duration on the treadmill may be helpful parameters to establish a new ischemic threshold in patients on medical therapy and to provide recommendations on the intensity of exercise (i.e., exercise prescription).

Women

The subjects in most studies evaluating the sensitivity and specificity of the stress ECG have been predominantly male. A meta-analysis of these studies revealed a sensitivity of 68% and a specificity of 77%. In contrast studies in women suggested a substantially lower sensitivity of 31% with a specificity of 71%.[71] There is a relatively low prevalence of disease especially in premenopausal women. Cheng et al.[78] (Fig. 10.8) used CCTA to evaluate CAD prevalence among women and found that age, angina characteristics, and three or more traditional Framingham risk factors allowed for stratification into low-, intermediate-, and high-risk cohorts. Subsequent studies of women with intermediate risk of CAD revealed a sensitivity of 61% and a specificity of 70% of stress ECG.[71]

Importantly, it has been observed that ST depression on stress ECG is not as reliable a diagnostic variable for women compared with men.[71] This is particularly true when a woman has ST depression on her baseline ECG.

Exercise capacity is a very important predictor of obstructive CAD and adverse cardiac events in women.[79] The Duke treadmill score provides similar prediction of events in women compared with men.[80] Because the stress ECG has a strong negative predictive value for women who can exercise and who have a normal resting ECG, ACC/AHA guidelines recommend stress ECG as the first functional test to consider in women with intermediate risk.[30]

PREOPERATIVE EVALUATION FOR NONCARDIAC SURGERY

Asymptomatic patients with known CAD who are active (able to perform at least 4 METs, e.g., light housework) are generally felt to be reasonable candidates for surgery.[81] However, in patients who have a previously undiagnosed chest pain syndrome, a stress ECG may be helpful. One may use the stress ECG to objectively determine the ischemic threshold in symptomatic patients with known CAD. One might use more caution or consider intensifying medical therapy before surgery if the patient develops myocardial ischemia at a relatively low workload. Finally, one might consider preoperative evaluation with stress ECG in patients who have no symptoms but are generally very sedentary (< 4 METs). However, these patients may not be capable of performing an adequate stress test and a pharmacologic stress test may be a better option.

CONCLUSIONS

The 12-lead ECG remains an essential tool for evaluation of patients with suspected acute and chronic CAD and the various arrhythmias that accompany CAD. Even in an era of advanced imaging technology, the stress ECG retains its position as the most cost-effective means to evaluate most patients with known and intermediate probability for CAD. Thus these relatively simple and inexpensive tests are likely to remain in the clinician's diagnostic armamentarium for years to come.

References

1. Einthoven W: Un nouveau galvanometre, *Arch Neerl Sci Exactes Nat* 625–630, 1901.
2. Schlant RC, Adolph RJ, DiMarco JP, et al.: Guidelines for electrocardiography. A report of the American College of Cardiology/American Heart Association Task Force on Assessment of Diagnostic and Therapeutic Cardiovascular Procedures (Committee on Electrocardiography), *J Am Coll Cardiol* 19:473–481, 1992.
3. Fleisher LA, Beckman JA, Brown KA, et al.: ACC/AHA 2007 guidelines on perioperative cardiovascular evaluation and care for noncardiac surgery: a report of the American College of Cardiology/American Heart Association Task Force on Practice Guidelines (Writing Committee to Revise the 2002 Guidelines on Perioperative Cardiovascular Evaluation for Noncardiac Surgery): developed in collaboration with the American Society of Echocardiography, American Society of Nuclear Cardiology, Heart Rhythm Society, Society of Cardiovascular Anesthesiologists, Society for Cardiovascular Angiography and Interventions, Society for Vascular Medicine and Biology, and Society for Vascular Surgery, *Circulation* 116:e418–e499, 2007.
4. Freedman RA, Alderman EL, Sheffield LT, et al.: Bundle branch block in patients with chronic coronary artery disease: angiographic correlates and prognostic significance, *J Am Coll Cardiol* 10:73–80, 1987.
5. Schneider JF, Thomas Jr HE, Kreger BE, et al.: Newly acquired left bundle-branch block: the Framingham study, *Ann Intern Med* 90:303–310, 1979.
6. Surawicz B, Childers R, Deal BJ, et al.: AHA/ACCF/HRS recommendations for the standardization and interpretation of the electrocardiogram: part III: intraventricular conduction disturbances: a scientific statement from the American Heart Association Electrocardiography and Arrhythmias Committee, Council on Clinical Cardiology; the American College of Cardiology Foundation; and the Heart Rhythm Society. Endorsed by the International Society for Computerized Electrocardiology, *J Am Coll Cardiol* 53:976–981, 2009.
7. Rotman M, Triebwasser JH: A clinical and follow-up study of right and left bundle branch block, *Circulation* 51:477–484, 1975.
8. Fahy GJ, Pinski SL, Miller DP, et al.: Natural history of isolated bundle branch block, *Am J Cardiol* 77:1185–1190, 1996.
9. Strauss DG, Loring Z, Selvester RH, et al.: Right, but not left, bundle branch block is associated with large anteroseptal scar, *J Am Coll Cardiol* 62:959–967, 2013.
10. Frink RJ, James TN: Normal blood supply to the human His bundle and proximal bundle branches, *Circulation* 47:8–18, 1973.
11. Brilakis ES, Wright RS, Kopecky SL, et al.: Bundle branch block as a predictor of long-term survival after acute myocardial infarction, *Am J Cardiol* 88:205–209, 2001.
12. Biagini E, Shaw LJ, Poldermans D, et al.: Accuracy of non-invasive techniques for diagnosis of coronary artery disease and prediction of cardiac events in patients with left bundle branch block: a meta-analysis, *Eur J Nucl Med Mol Imaging* 33:1442–1451, 2006.
13. Rowe DW, Oquendo I, Depuey EG, et al.: The noninvasive diagnosis of coronary artery disease in patients with left bundle-branch block, *Tex Heart Inst J* 9:397–406, 1982.
14. Supariwala AA, Po JR, Mohareb S, et al.: Prevalence and long-term prognosis of patients with complete bundle branch block (right or left bundle branch) with normal left ventricular ejection fraction referred for stress echocardiography, *Echocardiography* 32:483–489, 2015.
15. Clerc OF, Possner M, Maire R, et al.: Association of left bundle branch block with obstructive coronary artery disease on coronary CT angiography: a case-control study, *Eur Heart J Cardiovasc Imaging* 17(7):765–771, 2016.
16. Pratt CM, Moye LA: The cardiac arrhythmia suppression trial. Casting suppression in a different light, *Circulation* 91:245–247, 1995.
17. Takemoto M, Yoshimura H, Ohba Y, et al.: Radiofrequency catheter ablation of premature ventricular complexes from right ventricular outflow tract improves left ventricular dilation and clinical status in patients without structural heart disease, *J Am Coll Cardiol* 45:1259–1265, 2005.
18. Sekiguchi Y, Aonuma K, Yamauchi Y, et al.: Chronic hemodynamic effects after radiofrequency catheter ablation of frequent monomorphic ventricular premature beats, *J Cardiovasc Electrophysiol* 16:1057–1063, 2005.
19. Baman TS, Lange DC, Ilg KJ, et al.: Relationship between burden of premature ventricular complexes and left ventricular function, *Heart Rhythm* 7:865–869, 2010.
20. Penela D, Van Huls Van Taxis C, Aguinaga L, et al.: Neurohormonal, structural, and functional recovery pattern after premature ventricular complex ablation is independent of structural heart disease status in patients with depressed left ventricular ejection fraction: a prospective multicenter study, *J Am Coll Cardiol* 62:1195–1202, 2013.
21. Sarrazin JF, Labounty T, Kuhne M, et al.: Impact of radiofrequency ablation of frequent post-infarction premature ventricular complexes on left ventricular ejection fraction, *Heart Rhythm* 6:1543–1549, 2009.
22. Penela D, Acosta J, Aguinaga L, et al.: Ablation of frequent PVC in patients meeting criteria for primary prevention ICD implant: safety of withholding the implant, *Heart Rhythm* 12:2434–2442, 2015.
23. Raunio H, Rissanen V, Romppanen T, et al.: Changes in the QRS complex and ST segment in transmural and subendocardial myocardial infarctions. A clinicopathologic study, *Am Heart J* 98:176–184, 1979.
24. Clemmensen P, Grande P, Saunamaki K, et al.: Evolution of electrocardiographic and echocardiographic abnormalities during the 4 years following first acute myocardial infarction, *Eur Heart J* 16:1063–1069, 1995.
25. Albert DE, Califf RM, LeCocq DA, et al.: Comparative rates of resolution of QRS changes after operative and nonoperative acute myocardial infarcts, *Am J Cardiol* 51:378–381, 1983.
26. Delewi R, Ijff G, van de Hoef TP, et al.: Pathological Q waves in myocardial infarction in patients treated by primary PCI, *JACC Cardiovasc Imaging* 6:324–331, 2013.
27. Master AM, Jaffe H: The electrocardiographic changes after exercise in patients with angina pectoris, *J Mt Sinai Hosp*7, 1941.
28. Bruce RA: Evaluation of functional capacity and exercise tolerance of cardiac patients, *Mod Concepts Cardiovasc Dis* 25:321–326, 1956.
29. Senior R, Monaghan M, Becher H, et al.: Stress echocardiography for the diagnosis and risk stratification of patients with suspected or known coronary artery disease: a critical appraisal. Supported by the British Society of Echocardiography, *Heart* 91:427–436, 2005.
30. Fletcher GF, Ades PA, Kligfield P, et al.: Exercise standards for testing and training: a scientific statement from the American Heart Association, *Circulation* 128:873–934, 2013.
31. Vella CA, Robergs RA: A review of the stroke volume response to upright exercise in healthy subjects, *Br J Sports Med* 39:190–195, 2005.
32. Myers J, Buchanan N, Walsh D, et al.: Comparison of the ramp versus standard exercise protocols, *J Am Coll Cardiol* 17:1334–1342, 1991.
33. *American College of Sports Medicine Guidelines for Exercise Testing and Prescription*, Wolters Kluwer Health/Lippincott Williams & Wilkins, Philadelphia, 2013.
34. Myers J, Arena R, Franklin B, et al.: Recommendations for clinical exercise laboratories: a scientific statement from the American Heart Association, *Circulation* 119:3144–3161, 2009.
35. Diamond GA, Forrester JS: Analysis of probability as an aid in the clinical diagnosis of coronary-artery disease, *N Engl J Med* 300:1350–1358, 1979.
36. Chaitman BR, Bourassa MG, Davis K, et al.: Angiographic prevalence of high-risk coronary artery disease in patient subsets (CASS), *Circulation* 64:360–367, 1981.
37. Pryor DB, Harrell Jr FE, Lee KL, et al.: Estimating the likelihood of significant coronary artery disease, *Am J Med* 75:771–780, 1983.
38. Pryor DB, Shaw L, McCants CB, et al.: Value of the history and physical in identifying patients at increased risk for coronary artery disease, *Ann Intern Med* 118:81–90, 1993.
39. Vankatesan S: *Braunwald's Heart Disease*, ed 3, 1992, p 125.
40. Ellestad MH, Savitz S, Bergdall D, et al.: The false positive stress test. Multivariate analysis of 215 subjects with hemodynamic, angiographic and clinical data, *Am J Cardiol* 40:681–685, 1977.
41. Marwick TH, Torelli J, Harjai K, et al.: Influence of left ventricular hypertrophy on detection of coronary artery disease using exercise echocardiography, *J Am Coll Cardiol* 26:1180–1186, 1995.
42. Balady GJ, Arena R, Sietsema K, et al.: Clinician's guide to cardiopulmonary exercise testing in adults: a scientific statement from the American Heart Association, *Circulation* 122:191–225, 2010.
43. Le VV, Mitiku T, Sungar G, et al.: The blood pressure response to dynamic exercise testing: a systematic review, *Prog Cardiovasc Dis* 51:135–160, 2008.
44. Rodgers GP, Ayanian JZ, Balady G, et al.: American College of Cardiology/American Heart Association Clinical Competence Statement on Stress Testing. A Report of the American College of Cardiology/American Heart Association/American College of Physicians–American Society of Internal Medicine Task Force on Clinical Competence, *Circulation* 102:1726–1738, 2000.
45. Skalski J, Allison TG, Miller TD: The safety of cardiopulmonary exercise testing in a population with high-risk cardiovascular diseases, *Circulation* 126:2465–2472, 2012.
46. Magulamurti S. Personal communication with the author re: exercise testing in coronary disease.
47. Peterson PN, Magid DJ, Ross C, et al.: Association of exercise capacity on treadmill with future cardiac events in patients referred for exercise testing, *Arch Intern Med* 168:174–179, 2008.
48. Keteyian SJ, Brawner CA, Savage PD, et al.: Peak aerobic capacity predicts prognosis in patients with coronary heart disease, *Am Heart J* 156:292–300, 2008.
49. Kim ES, Ishwaran H, Blackstone E, et al.: External prognostic validations and comparisons of age- and gender-adjusted exercise capacity predictions, *J Am Coll Cardiol* 50:1867–1875, 2007.
50. Shaw LJ, Peterson ED, Shaw LK, et al.: Use of a prognostic treadmill score in identifying diagnostic coronary disease subgroups, *Circulation* 98:1622–1630, 1998.
51. Gibbons RJ, Balady GJ, Bricker JT, et al.: ACC/AHA 2002 guideline update for exercise testing: summary article: a report of the American College of Cardiology/American Heart Association Task Force on Practice Guidelines (Committee to Update the 1997 Exercise Testing Guidelines), *Circulation* 106:1883–1892, 2002.
52. Rifkin RD, Hood Jr WB: Bayesian analysis of electrocardiographic exercise stress testing, *N Engl J Med* 297:681–686, 1977.
53. Weustink AC, de Feyter PJ: The role of multi-slice computed tomography in stable angina management: a current perspective, *Neth Heart J* 19:336–343, 2011.
54. Vorobiof G, Ellestad MH: Lead aVR: dead or simply forgotten? *JACC Cardiovasc Imaging* 4:187–190, 2011.
55. Polizos G, Ellestad MH: Significance of lead strength during exercise testing, *Ann Noninvasive Electrocardiol* 12:59–63, 2007.
56. Ellestad MH: Unconventional electrocardiographic signs of ischemia during exercise testing, *Am J Cardiol* 102:949–953, 2008.
57. Stein R, Nguyen P, Abella J, et al.: Prevalence and prognostic significance of exercise-induced right bundle branch block, *Am J Cardiol* 105:677–680, 2010.
58. Stein R, Ho M, Oliveira CM, et al.: Exercise-induced left bundle branch block: prevalence and prognosis, *Arq Bras Cardiol* 97:26–32, 2011.
59. Morise AP: Exercise testing in nonatherosclerotic heart disease: hypertrophic cardiomyopathy, valvular heart disease, and arrhythmias, *Circulation* 123:216–225, 2011.
60. Eckart RE, Field ME, Hruczkowski TW, et al.: Association of electrocardiographic morphology of exercise-induced ventricular arrhythmia with mortality, *Ann Intern Med* 149:451–460, 2008. W82.
61. Bourque JM, Holland BH, Watson DD, et al.: Achieving an exercise workload of > or = 10 metabolic equivalents predicts a very low risk of inducible ischemia: does myocardial perfusion imaging have a role? *J Am Coll Cardiol* 54:538–545, 2009.
62. Bourque JM, Charlton GT, Holland BH, et al.: Prognosis in patients achieving >/=10 METs on exercise stress testing: was SPECT imaging useful? *J Nucl Cardiol* 18:230–237, 2011.
63. Bourque JM, Beller GA: Value of exercise ECG for risk stratification in suspected or known CAD in the era of advanced imaging technologies, *JACC Cardiovasc Imaging* 8:1309–1321, 2015.
64. Brubaker PH, Kitzman DW: Chronotropic incompetence: causes, consequences, and management, *Circulation* 123:1010–1020, 2011.
65. Dobre D, Zannad F, Keteyian SJ, et al.: Association between resting heart rate, chronotropic index, and long-term outcomes in patients with heart failure receiving beta-blocker therapy: data from the HF-ACTION trial, *Eur Heart J* 34:2271–2280, 2013.
66. Maddox TM, Ross C, Ho PM, et al.: The prognostic importance of abnormal heart rate recovery and chronotropic response among exercise treadmill test patients, *Am Heart J* 156:736–744, 2008.
67. Khan MN, Pothier CE, Lauer MS: Chronotropic incompetence as a predictor of death among patients with normal electrograms taking beta blockers (metoprolol or atenolol), *Am J Cardiol* 96:1328–1333, 2005.
68. Chaitman BR: Should early acceleration of heart rate during exercise be used to risk stratify patients with suspected or established coronary artery disease? *Circulation* 115:430–431, 2007.
69. Johnson NP, Goldberger JJ: Prognostic value of late heart rate recovery after treadmill exercise, *Am J Cardiol* 110:45–49, 2012.
70. Weiss SA, Blumenthal RS, Sharrett AR, et al.: Exercise blood pressure and future cardiovascular death in asymptomatic individuals, *Circulation* 121:2109–2116, 2010.
71. Kohli P, Gulati M: Exercise stress testing in women: going back to the basics, *Circulation* 122:2570–2580, 2010.
72. Conti CR, Bavry AA, Petersen JW: Silent ischemia: clinical relevance, *J Am Coll Cardiol* 59:435–441, 2012.
73. Weiner DA, Ryan TJ, McCabe CH, et al.: Risk of developing an acute myocardial infarction or sudden coronary death in patients with exercise-induced silent myocardial ischemia. A report from the Coronary Artery Surgery Study (CASS) registry, *Am J Cardiol* 62:1155–1158, 1988.
74. Zellweger MJ, Weinbacher M, Zutter AW, et al.: Long-term outcome of patients with silent versus symptomatic ischemia six months after percutaneous coronary intervention and stenting, *J Am Coll Cardiol* 42:33–40, 2003.
75. Bourassa MG, Pepine CJ, Forman SA, et al.: Asymptomatic Cardiac Ischemia Pilot (ACIP) study: effects of coronary angioplasty and coronary artery bypass graft surgery on recurrent angina and ischemia. The ACIP investigators, *J Am Coll Cardiol* 26:606–614, 1995.
76. Gosselin G, Teo KK, Tanguay JF, et al.: Effectiveness of percutaneous coronary intervention in patients with silent myocardial ischemia (post hoc analysis of the COURAGE trial), *Am J Cardiol* 109:954–959, 2012.
77. Eisenberg MJ, Blankenship JC, Huynh T, et al.: Evaluation of routine functional testing after percutaneous coronary intervention, *Am J Cardiol* 93:744–747, 2004.
78. Cheng VY, Berman DS, Rozanski A, et al.: Performance of the traditional age, sex, and angina typicality-based approach for estimating pretest probability of angiographically significant coronary artery disease in patients undergoing coronary computed tomographic angiography: results from the multinational Coronary CT Angiography Evaluation for Clinical Outcomes: An International Multicenter Registry (CONFIRM), *Circulation* 124:2423–2432, 2011. 1–8.
79. Robert AR, Melin JA, Detry JM: Logistic discriminant analysis improves diagnostic accuracy of exercise testing for coronary artery disease in women, *Circulation* 83:1202–1209, 1991.
80. Alexander KP, Shaw LJ, Shaw LK, et al.: Value of exercise treadmill testing in women, *J Am Coll Cardiol* 32:1657–1664, 1998.
81. American College of Cardiology Foundation/American Heart Association Task Force on Practice Guidelines, American Society of Echocardiography, American Society of Nuclear Cardiology, et al.: 2009 ACCF/AHA focused update on perioperative beta blockade incorporated into the ACC/AHA 2007 guidelines on perioperative cardiovascular evaluation and care for noncardiac surgery, *J Am Coll Cardiol* 54:e13–e118, 2009.

11 Echocardiography

Rajdeep S. Khattar and Roxy Senior

INTRODUCTION

Over many decades, echocardiography has evolved considerably to provide a comprehensive assessment of cardiac structure and function in a truly bedside manner.[1] Echocardiography is a readily available technique that is portable, inexpensive, and free from radiation. Echocardiographic imaging modalities now include M-mode, two-dimensional, flow Doppler, color flow mapping, tissue Doppler, contrast, three-dimensional, and speckle-tracking strain imaging. Echocardiography may also be applied in conjunction with exercise or pharmacologic stress in the diagnostic evaluation of coronary artery disease (CAD) and for certain noncoronary conditions. In addition, echocardiography may be performed via the transesophageal route, not only for diagnostic purposes, but increasingly for imaging guidance during cardiac structural interventions under general anaesthesia. Consequently, the indications for echocardiography are wide ranging, leading to the publication of numerous international guidelines for standardization of methodologies and appropriate use of the technique in various cardiac conditions.[2–5]

In this chapter, the clinical application of echocardiography will be divided into three broad categories as follows: (1) detection of CAD, (2) assessment of left ventricular (LV) dysfunction, and (3) delineation of structural complications.

DETECTION OF CORONARY ARTERY DISEASE

Pathophysiology of Myocardial Ischemia

The pathophysiologic changes that occur as a consequence of interruption in coronary blood flow are described by the ischemic cascade as shown in Fig. 11.1. Resting blood flow may be preserved until a coronary artery stenosis approaches 90% diameter narrowing. At lesser degrees of stenosis, although resting flow is normal, coronary flow reserve (CFR) may be reduced such that when there is an increase in oxygen demand with exercise, there is an inability to increase blood flow adequately to meet the metabolic requirements, leading to a supply-demand mismatch and subsequent myocardial ischemia. The inadequate increase in blood flow in the stenosed coronary artery bed leads to a sequential reduction in myocardial perfusion, diastolic dysfunction, reduced myocardial systolic strain, visible regional wall motion abnormality (WMA), electrocardiogram (ECG) changes, and finally symptoms. These changes are reversible with cessation of exercise. In addition to coronary artery stenosis severity, blood flow to the myocardium may be affected by location of the stenosis, lesion length, number of lesions, and comorbidities such as hypertension and diabetes affecting intrinsic CFR.

Regional Wall Motion Changes in Myocardial Ischemia and Infarction

The echocardiographic hallmark of underlying CAD is the presence of resting or stress-induced regional WMA. Normal LV wall motion consists of endocardial thickening that occurs in a relatively synchronous manner in all myocardial walls leading to a decrease in cavity size. These changes are greater in magnitude at the base of the LV and less so moving toward the apex. Normal myocardial contraction depends predominantly on endocardial rather than epicardial contraction because the velocity and magnitude of contraction are greater in the subendocardial rather than subepicardial layers. Consequently, impaired function of the subendocardial muscle fibers has a disproportionate impact on overall wall thickening and LV systolic function. It has been shown that ischemia or infarction of the inner 20% of the myocardial wall leads to an absence of visible contraction in that region. This means that even nontransmural ischemia or infarction results in malfunction of the entire wall that is indistinguishable from that seen with transmural involvement.

If a prolonged period of ischemia has occurred due to transient occlusion with minimal infarction and restoration of blood flow, recovery of function within the affected myocardial segment may be delayed due to myocardial stunning. Repetitive episodes of demand ischemia may also lead to myocardial stunning. Echocardiographically, myocardial stunning manifests as a persistent regional WMA soon after restoration of blood flow, followed by recovery of contraction within a few days up to a few weeks later.

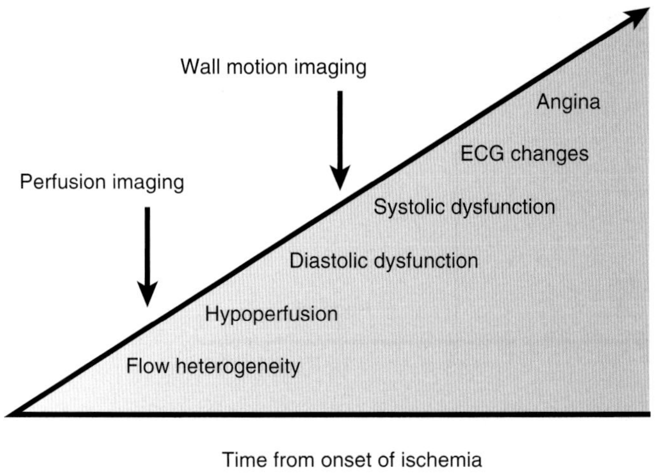

FIG. 11.1 **Pathophysiology of myocardial ischemia—the ischemic cascade.** *ECG*, Electrocardiogram.

If complete coronary artery occlusion occurs and flow is not restored, myocardial infarction (MI) and necrosis may ensue leading to persistent regional WMA and LV dysfunction. The extent of myocardial damage depends on the duration of complete coronary artery occlusion. If flow can be restored within 60 minutes, myocardial loss may be minimized. If flow can be restored within 4 hours there may be varying degrees of nontransmural or partial thickness infarction involving the subendocardial layers. A complete absence of blood flow for 4 to 6 hours tends to result in irreversible, transmural myocardial damage. The location of the regional WMA is a good indicator of the coronary artery territory involved in the infarction. However, the size of the WMA on echocardiography may overestimate infarct size both in terms of thickness of infarction due to tethering of the adjacent noninfarcted walls.

In some patients with LV dysfunction due to CAD, there may be areas of chronically dysfunctional myocardium that result from a state of chronic low blood flow, enough to sustain viability to the affected myocardium, but causing repetitive ischemia and stunning. These areas of so-called hibernating myocardium have the ability to regain contractile function following revascularization and are therefore important to identify.

Resting Echocardiography

A resting echocardiogram may be helpful in the diagnosis of CAD if performed during symptoms. If a WMA is identified during chest pain and then resolves with relief of symptoms, this is very good evidence that the chest pain is due to myocardial ischemia. Equally, even in the absence of symptoms, the detection of a regional area of akinesia at rest is suggestive of silent CAD and previous MI, particularly if associated with increased echogenicity and thinning of the myocardium (Video 11.1). In the absence of symptoms, a normal resting echocardiogram adds little in establishing whether the patient has underlying CAD. Importantly, however, there are a number of other cardiac causes of chest pain, such as severe aortic stenosis, hypertrophic cardiomyopathy, mitral valve prolapse, and right ventricular pathology which may be excluded by echocardiography. Transthoracic echocardiography may also be useful in the evaluation of chest pain in the acute setting for differentiating MI, aortic dissection, pulmonary embolism, or acute pericarditis and pericardial effusion.

Stress Echocardiography

In view of the limited diagnostic accuracy of exercise electrocardiography, cardiac imaging-based investigations are gradually superseding its use in clinical practice.[6–9] Moreover, approximately 20% to 30% of patients are unable to exercise adequately because of comorbidities such as osteoarthritis, chronic pulmonary disease, and peripheral vascular disease.

The technique of stress echocardiography became clinically applicable in the 1980s when two-dimensional echocardiography was used in conjunction with physiologic exercise or pharmacologic stress agents to provoke ischemia. Since then, with continued technological advances in image quality, particularly the introduction of intravenous ultrasound contrast agents, stress echocardiography has evolved into a safe, accurate, and well-established technique for the diagnostic and prognostic evaluation of suspected cardiac chest pain.[10–13]

Exercise Echocardiography

Physiologic exercise is the preferred method of stress testing for ambulant patients, and this can be achieved either by treadmill exercise or bicycle ergometry. For treadmill exercise, the Bruce protocol is most commonly used and the exercise time or workload achieved per se provides useful clinical and prognostic information.[14] Imaging under these circumstances is performed at rest and immediately after exercise, allowing a time interval of approximately 60 to 90 seconds in which to acquire the poststress images. Upright or semisupine bicycle ergometry offers the advantage of imaging at any time during exercise, rather than immediately postexercise as with treadmill exercise. However, the test may be limited by suboptimal patient position for image acquisition or leg fatigue preventing the attainment of target heart rate and potential cardiac symptoms. Treadmill exercise tends to evoke a higher workload and peak heart rate than does bicycle ergometry and therefore may be preferable for ischemia testing. However, bicycle exercise may be more suitable if additional Doppler-derived information is required, for example, on valve function, filling pressures, or pulmonary artery (PA) pressure.

Pharmacologic Stress Echocardiography

A pharmacologic approach to stress testing, using inotropic or vasodilator stress agents in conjunction with echocardiography, is a suitable alternative for those unable to exercise and provides similar diagnostic accuracy to exercise echocardiography. Pharmacologic stress testing avoids the challenges of image acquisition posed by exercise such as hyperventilation and excessive chest wall movement. Moreover, the stress images can be obtained at a constant and controlled heart rate at peak stress without undue time pressure.

1. Dobutamine Stress Echocardiography

Dobutamine, a synthetic catecholamine, is the most widely used stressor agent and acts by stimulating α-1, β-1, and β-2 adrenoceptors. This leads to an increase in heart rate, blood pressure (BP), and inotropic activity, thereby increasing myocardial oxygen demand. The protocol for dobutamine stress echocardiography uses a weight-adjusted, graded intravenous dobutamine infusion[15,16] (Fig. 11.2). Echocardiographic images are acquired at rest, mid-dose, peak dose, and recovery; heart rate, BP, and cardiac rhythm are monitored

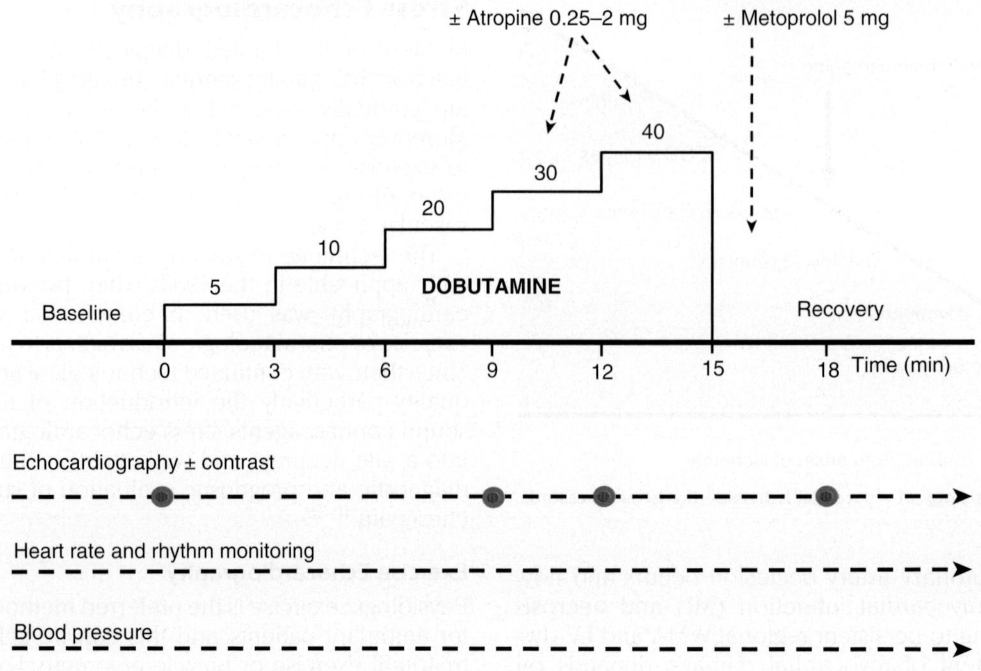

FIG. 11.2 Protocol for dobutamine stress echocardiography. If resting wall motion is normal, dobutamine is started at a dose of 10 μg/kg per min, but if there is a regional wall motion abnormality, assessment of myocardial viability may be indicated starting at a dose of 5 μg/kg per min. Red dots represent the time points for image acquisition.

throughout the study. The increase in systolic BP is less with dobutamine compared to exercise. Endpoints of the test include achievement of 85% of age-predicted target heart rate; development of cardiac symptoms or ischemia, arrhythmias, hypotension, or severe hypertension; and intolerable side effects to dobutamine. If target heart rate has not been achieved at maximal dobutamine stress, intravenous atropine may be given in divided doses to a maximum dose of 2 mg. On rare occasions, short-acting intravenous β-blockade may be needed to reverse the effects of dobutamine.

Achievement of target heart rate is an important goal of ischemia testing with dobutamine, and therefore any rate-limiting medications should be withheld for at least 48 hours to avoid a nondiagnostic test. Among those with reportedly normal dobutamine stress echocardiograms, a suboptimal heart rate response is associated with a higher cardiac event rate.

The use of dobutamine is associated with side effects such as headache, tremor, palpitations, nausea, urinary urgency, and anxiety, but with prior counselling and reassurance these are adequately well tolerated and do not usually lead to premature termination of the test. A minority of patients develop a reflex vagal response to dobutamine leading to hypotension and a fall in heart rate. Every test carries a definite, albeit minor, risk and exercise is generally safer than pharmacologic stress. For dobutamine stress echocardiography, ventricular arrhythmias, prolonged ischemia, and MI have a reported incidence of approximately 1 in 1000 with an incidence of death of 1 in 5000.[17] In experienced hands, dobutamine stress echocardiography can be safely performed in patients with LV dysfunction, aortic and cerebral aneurysms, and implantable cardioverter defibrillators.

2. Vasodilator Stress Echocardiography

Vasodilator stress echocardiography is typically performed with either dipyridamole or adenosine.[10,12,18] Dipyridamole stimulates A_{2A} adenosinergic receptors present on the endothelial and smooth muscle cells of coronary arterioles. This leads to an increase in endogenous adenosine levels by the inhibition of cellular uptake of adenosine and the prevention of its breakdown by adenosine deaminase. Adenosine is a coronary arteriolar vasodilator that causes hyperemia in myocardial segments with normal vasodilatory reserve, ie, without significant epicardial stenoses or impairment in microvascular function. In contrast, segments with impaired vasodilatory reserve may become ischemic after administration of adenosine, due to a coronary steal phenomenon, where blood flow is preferentially directed to segments with normal epicardial and microvascular resistance (e-Figs. 11.1 and 11.2).

The dipyridamole protocol consists of an intravenous infusion of 0.84 mg/kg over 10 min, in two separate doses. A dose of 0.56 mg/kg is given over 4 min, followed by echocardiographic imaging, and if no sign of ischemia, an additional 0.28 mg/kg is given over 2 min. If no endpoint is reached, atropine is added. The same overall dose of 0.84 mg/kg can also be given over 6 min. All caffeine-containing foods should be avoided for 12 hours before testing, and all theophylline-containing drugs should be discontinued for at least 24 hours. The peak vasodilatory effect of dipyridamole is obtained 4 to 8 minutes after the end of the infusion, and the half-life is approximately 6 hours. The dipyridamole dose usually employed for stress echocardiography (0.84 mg/kg) causes a 3- to 4-fold increase in coronary blood flow in normals over resting values. Vasodilator stress usually produces a mild decrease in BP and a mild increase in heart rate. Therefore, atropine is frequently required to achieve target heart rate and thereby increase myocardial oxygen demand. Aminophylline should be available for immediate use in case an adverse dipyridamole-related event occurs and be routinely infused at the end of the test.

Adenosine can be used in a similar manner and is typically infused at a maximum dose of 140 μg/kg per min over 6 min. Imaging is performed prior to and after starting the adenosine infusion, and, compared with dipyridamole, adenosine has the advantage of a shorter half-life.

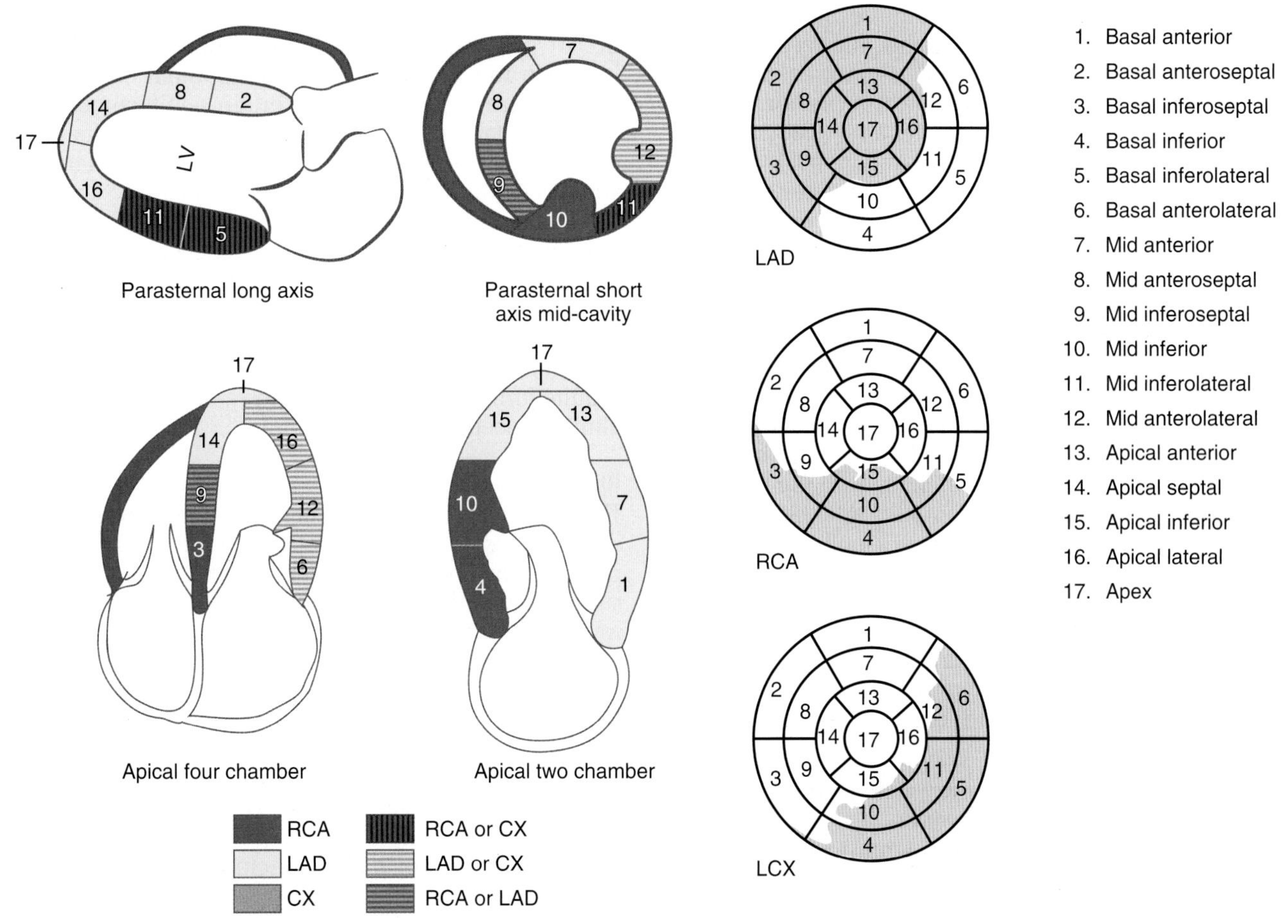

FIG. 11.3 Echocardiographic images, bullseye plot, and coronary artery distribution using the 17-segment left ventricular model for assessment of regional wall motion. *LAD*, Left anterior descending artery; *LCX*, left circumflex artery; *LV*, left ventricle; *RCA*, right coronary artery.

Combined with wall motion assessment, dedicated imaging of the left anterior descending (LAD) coronary artery during vasodilator stress may be performed to provide an assessment of CFR (e-Fig. 11.3). The ratio of hyperemic peak to basal peak diastolic coronary flow Doppler velocities represents CFR, and this parameter has been shown to provide additive prognostic value over and above wall motion assessment.[19,20] However, the technique is not widely used because of protocol complexity and challenging imaging of the LAD.

Minor, but limiting, side effects preclude the achievement of maximal pharmacologic stress in less than 5% of patients given dipyridamole. Approximately two-thirds of patients studied with the high-dose dipyridamole protocol experience minor side effects such as flushing and headache that usually resolve following administration of aminophylline at the end of testing. On rare occasions, dipyridamole-induced ischemia requires the administration of nitrates. Major life-threatening complications, including MI, complete heart block, asystole, ventricular tachycardia, or pulmonary edema, occur in approximately 1 in 1000 cases. Adenosine has a similar side-effect profile to dipyridamole, but may be safer because of the shorter duration of action. Both agents are contraindicated in patients with significant conduction disease and reactive airways obstruction. Under these circumstances, dobutamine may be the pharmacologic stressor agent of choice. Conversely, vasodilator stress may be a safer option in those with a predisposition to atrial or ventricular tachyarrhythmias. In general, the choice of pharmacologic stressor agent is governed by operator preference and familiarity.

3. Pacing-Induced Stress Echocardiography

In those with a permanent pacemaker, it may not be possible to provoke an adequate heart rate response with exercise or dobutamine-atropine stress. Stress testing can be performed by programming the pacing rate to increase every 2 to 3 minutes until target heart rate is achieved. This technique can be used in conjunction with dobutamine to further increase inotropic activity and myocardial oxygen consumption. Transesophageal atrial pacing stress echocardiography is an alternative method to exercise or pharmacologic stress testing, but has not gained popularity.

Analysis of Regional Wall Motion

Most commonly, analysis of regional wall motion is qualitative, based on visual assessment of myocardial thickening rather than motion, which may be influenced by pushing and pulling forces. Normal wall motion consists mainly of endocardial thickening representing a 35% to 40% increase in wall thickness from diastole with varying reductions in endocardial thickening seen in ischemia. The analysis is aided by dividing the LV into myocardial segments. For the purposes of wall motion analysis, a 16-segment model was previously used, but a 17-segment model is now recommended in which the additional segment represents the true apex.[21] This allows comparison with myocardial perfusion studies using nuclear imaging and cardiac magnetic resonance (CMR) imaging, which have traditionally included a true apical segment. (Fig. 11.3). A visual assessment of each individual segment is made in multiple views, ascribing a wall motion score such that normokinesis = 1, hypokinesis = 2, akinesis = 3, and dyskinesis = 4. The total score of the segments can then be divided by the number of segments analyzed to derive a wall motion score index. A completely normal LV at rest has a score index of 1.0. In the context of previous MI, the wall motion score index at rest provides a very good approximation of the location and size of MI and global LV systolic function. With normal resting wall motion and stress-induced reversible ischemia, the wall motion score index during stress represents the location, extent, and severity of ischemia. This approach helps to identify the coronary artery territory responsible for the regional WMA. Involvement of the anterior septum and anterior wall signifies disease in the LAD artery and its branches (Video 11.2), whereas abnormalities of the inferior wall tend to indicate right CAD in the majority of cases (Video 11.3). There can be substantial overlap in blood supply to the inferolateral wall by the right coronary and left circumflex arteries, and similarly with the anterolateral walls by the LAD and left circumflex arteries. Dilatation of the LV cavity with stress often indicates multivessel disease (Video 11.4). The ischemic threshold may also be assessed by determining the heart rate at which regional WMAs were detected, and this has been shown to correlate with the number of stenosed coronary arteries.

The use of ultrasound contrast agents has helped to improve image quality and observer variability (see following discussion). Most studies are unequivocally negative or positive, but there are sometimes borderline cases in which the image quality is suboptimal or wall motion changes are subtle and of uncertain significance. The most important factor in minimizing variability and maintaining diagnostic accuracy is appropriate and rigorous training in stress echocardiography.

Quantitative methods have been sought to make the findings more tangible and improve reporting by less experienced physicians. Automated endocardial border detection using integrated back scatter, tissue Doppler assessment of myocardial displacement, velocity, strain and strain rate, and real-time three-dimensional imaging have been studied but require further simplification and validation in order to gain clinical acceptance.

BOX 11.1 Indications for Stress Echocardiography for the Assessment of Coronary Artery Disease

Universal Indications

- Intermediate pretest probability of CAD
- Abnormal resting ECG (ST/T wave changes, LBBB)
- Inconclusive exercise ECG because of equivocal ST changes
- Suspicion of a false-positive exercise ECG
- Functional assessment of an equivocal coronary artery stenosis
- Evaluation of cardiac etiology of exertional dyspnea
- Risk stratification in known CAD
- Preoperative risk assessment for noncardiac surgery

Pharmacologic Stress Indications

- Inability to exercise
- Submaximal exercise ECG
- Assessment of myocardial viability—dobutamine

CAD, Coronary artery disease; *ECG*, electrocardiogram; *LBBB*, left bundle branch block.

Indications

The indications for stress echocardiography are summarized in Box 11.1. Appropriateness criteria for stress echocardiography have also been established.[11] Dobutamine stress echocardiography is indicated for the assessment of myocardial viability in those with resting akinetic regions, as discussed later.

Safety and Feasibility

Advances in imaging technology, in particular the introduction of harmonic imaging and use of ultrasound contrast agents, have significantly improved endocardial definition (Fig. 11.4). Accordingly, stress echocardiography is now feasible in over 95% of patients including those with morbid obesity.[22]

Diagnostic Accuracy

A large evidence base shows that all forms of exercise and pharmacologic stress echocardiography are more accurate than the treadmill exercise ECG, with sensitivities, specificities, and overall diagnostic accuracies approximating to 80% to 90%.[10] The normalcy rate of stress echocardiography is approximately 90% to 95%.[1]

False-negative studies may be due to suboptimal stress, use of β-blockers, single-vessel disease, and hyperdynamic states. False-positive studies can be due to reduced CFR and ischemia in the absence of epicardial CAD. This may include patients with significant LV hypertrophy, diabetes mellitus, myocarditis, cardiomyopathies, and syndrome X. Exercise may result in worsening regional and global

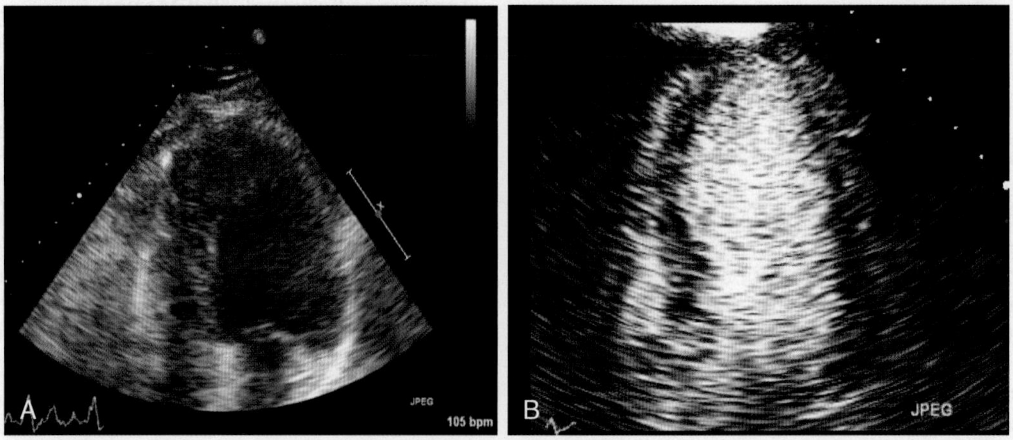

FIG. 11.4 Contrast echocardiography for left ventricular opacification. **(A)** Apical four-chamber view showing poor endocardial definition of the left ventricular myocardium with harmonic imaging. **(B)** The same apical four-chamber view with contrast-enhanced imaging clearly showing the endocardium, allowing a proper assessment of regional wall motion and ejection fraction.

systolic function in myopathic ventricles in the absence of ischemia (Video 11.5). Abnormal septal motion due to left bundle branch block (LBBB), ventricular pacing, or following cardiac surgery may also confound the interpretation of regional wall changes with stress. In addition, septal dyssynchrony may lead to worsening septal perfusion and wall thickening at higher heart rates in the absence of coronary artery obstruction.

Prognostic Value

Stress echocardiography provides independent prognostic information over and above clinical risk factors and stress test parameters for the prediction of all-cause mortality, cardiac death, and composite endpoints[23] (e-Fig. 11.4). A normal stress echocardiogram yields an annual event rate of less than 1%,[24] similar to that of an age- and sex-matched normal population. Under these circumstances, further diagnostic evaluation is rarely needed and, in particular, coronary angiography can be avoided. A positive stress echocardiogram carries a risk of nonfatal MI and all-cause death over subsequent years of over 10%, and certain stress echo parameters help to further stratify risk. These include the location, extent, and severity of stress-induced WMA, low ischemic threshold, LV hypertrophy, resting ejection fraction (EF), and peak wall motion score index. False-positive stress echocardiograms have also been associated with a higher risk of events, indicating the limitations of coronary angiography as a gold standard.[25]

Cost-Effectiveness Versus Exercise Electrocardiography

Compared to exercise electrocardiography, stress echocardiography identifies more patients as low risk and fewer as intermediate and high risk. Although initial procedural costs are greater, stress echocardiography leads to a lower cost of additional downstream procedures when compared with exercise electrocardiography, with lower rates of coronary angiography and revascularization. Consequently, exercise echocardiography has been shown to be a cost-effective alternative to exercise electrocardiography.[26,27] Similar results have been shown in patients presenting with troponin-negative chest pain (e-Fig. 11.5).[28]

Comparison with Alternative Imaging Techniques

Perfusion scintigraphy is a long-established technique for ischemia testing and is the main diagnostic alternative to stress echocardiography. The overall diagnostic accuracies of the two techniques and prognostic value are similar; there is a nonsignificant trend toward higher sensitivity with perfusion scintigraphy, but higher specificity with stress echocardiography.[12] The two techniques have broadly similar clinical applications and the choice of test depends mainly on availability and expertise. Although stress echocardiography is operator dependent and more subjective, it has the benefits of lower cost, widely available equipment, truly bedside nature, and no exposure to radiation. In contrast with radionuclide imaging, echocardiographic images can be obtained anywhere along the continuum from rest to peak physiologic stress. Moreover, stress echocardiography has the major advantage of excluding other causes of cardiac symptoms such as valvular disease, cardiomyopathies, pericardial disease, and congenital heart defects. CMR imaging allows the assessment of myocardial perfusion or wall motion with good accuracy. The advantages of the technique are related to high image quality and the absence of ionizing radiation. However, the high costs, lengthy image acquisition, and low availability make CMR a good option mainly when stress echocardiography is nondiagnostic or not feasible. Computed tomography (CT) coronary angiography and coronary calcification scoring is the latest technique to enter the field of cardiac imaging. CT has the inherent limitations of radiation exposure, and more fundamentally, provides anatomic rather than functional information. Nevertheless, as with the other imaging techniques, its use has been advocated in patients with an intermediate pretest probability of CAD.

Contrast Echocardiography for Left Ventricular Opacification

Despite the advances in two-dimensional image quality with harmonic imaging, a significant minority of patients may have suboptimal images. This is particularly notable in patients with obesity, lung disease, or in the intensive care setting. Moreover, the need for very good endocardial definition is paramount in stress echocardiography. These concerns have prompted the development of ultrasound contrast agents to opacify the left ventricle. Since the 1990s, stabilized microbubble ultrasound contrast agents that are capable of transit through the pulmonary circulation have become available. These have been coupled with modifications in ultrasound technology to improve visualization of the microbubbles in the LV cavity and myocardium.[29–31]

Ultrasound Contrast Agents

Ultrasound contrast agents consist of acoustically active gas–filled microspheres designed to increase the signal strength of ultrasound waves. The microbubbles are smaller than the capillaries in the lungs allowing transit from the venous to the arterial side of the circulation. As they remain intravascular at all times, they act as red blood cell tracers. To prevent dissolution of the microbubble, a low-solubility, high-molecular-weight gas is used. The microbubbles are stabilized by the outer shell coated with a biocompatible surfactant to minimize reaction. The compressibility of the gas enables the microbubbles to be an efficient acoustic reflector. The microbubbles are eliminated from the body via the reticuloendothelial system with their gas escaping from the lungs.

Ultrasound Imaging of Contrast Agents

Myocardial tissue is capable of reflecting an equal and opposite frequency, and this is known as a *linear response*. Consequently, standard two-dimensional imaging originally involved the ultrasound receiver transmitting and receiving ultrasound impulses of the same frequency, known as *fundamental imaging*. However, ultrasound waves become distorted on passing through the body as they encounter tissues of differing composition and density. This may change the waveform and generate frequencies different from the incident frequency. The strongest harmonic signals are multiples of the fundamental frequency. A nonlinear response is one in which harmonic frequencies of the fundamental frequency can be produced. Because microbubbles have nonlinear scattering properties, harmonic imaging was originally introduced to enhance the detection of ultrasound contrast agents within the heart. Myocardial tissue has both

TABLE 11.1 Properties of Commercially Available Ultrasound Contrast Agents for Cardiac Imaging

	GAS	BUBBLE SIZE	SURFACE COATING
Sonovue	Sulphur hexafluoride	2–8 μm	Phospholipid
Optison	Perfluoropropane	3–4.5 μm	Albumin
Definity	Octafluoropropane	1.1–3.3 μm	Phospholipid

linear and nonlinear properties that have improved imaging of myocardial tissue using harmonic imaging, but microbubbles have greater nonlinearity and a number of techniques have been developed to help distinguish microbubbles from the surrounding tissue.

The mechanical index is a measure of the power generated by an ultrasound transducer within an acoustic field and gives an indication of the likelihood of bubble disruption. The mechanical index used during routine examinations destroys most contrast microbubbles. In order to image contrast within the LV cavity it is necessary to reduce the transmitted mechanical index, and using more contrast-specific imaging modalities this helps to remove the tissue signal and leave only the contrast. This type of imaging is very effective for LV endocardial border enhancement as it demonstrates a sharp demarcation between the contrast-enhanced cavity and the myocardium (see Fig. 11.4).

Administration and Indications for Use of Ultrasound Contrast Agents

Table 11.1 summarizes the characteristics of currently available ultrasound contrast agents. These ultrasound contrast agents are administered intravenously as a bolus or continuous infusion. Slow bolus injections (0.2–0.5 mL) are usually enough for the evaluation of the LV in the standard apical and parasternal views. A continuous infusion is sometimes preferred in more challenging cases to provide stable conditions for image acquisition from different views. The indications for the use of ultrasound contrast agents for LV opacification are broadly as follows:

- endocardial visualization and assessment of LV structure and function when two or more contiguous segments are not seen on noncontrast images;
- accurate and repeatable measurements of LV volumes and EF;
- to confirm or exclude apical pathology, LV thrombus, noncompaction, and ventricular pseudoaneurysm;
- to optimize images and diagnostic assessment of patients undergoing stress echocardiography.

By enhancing LV endocardial border definition, ultrasound contrast agents reduce the number of uninterpretable and technically difficult studies, increase the yield of definite apical pathology such as thrombus formation, and improve the quantification of LV volumes and EF.

Safety

Side effects have been noted with ultrasound contrast agents but these are usually mild and transient. Serious allergic reactions have been observed but are extremely rare, with an incidence of approximately 1 in 10,000 cases.[30–32] Absolute contraindications for the administration of contrast agents include bidirectional or right-to-left intracardiac shunting or known hypersensitivity to the agent.

Cost-Effectiveness

By improving image quality in patients with difficult acoustic windows, the use of contrast agents may shorten the time to diagnosis, enhance decision-making, and improve workflow through the echo lab by reducing the time needed to image challenging cases. A large prospective study in patients with technically difficult echocardiographic studies showed that the use of contrast echocardiography had a positive impact on diagnosis, resource utilization, and patient management.[33] Approximately one-third of patients had either a reduction in the number of additional diagnostic procedures, a significant alteration in medical management, or both. The impact of incorporating contrast agents was most pronounced in critically ill and hospitalized patients, those with the poorest quality images. Cost-effectiveness analysis showed a saving of $122 per patient.[33] In the setting of stress echocardiography, contrast agents have been shown to improve visualization of regional WMAs, thereby increasing reader confidence in study interpretation and improving diagnostic accuracy. Interobserver variability of interpretation of stress echocardiograms has also been shown to improve significantly with contrast administration, particularly in less experienced hands. It has been estimated that the use of contrast agents for suboptimal images during stress echocardiography may result in a saving of $238 per patient by reducing the need for further investigation.[30]

Myocardial Contrast Echocardiography

Ultrasound contrast agents may also be used to assess myocardial perfusion. After transit through the LV cavity, microbubbles enter the epicardial coronary arteries and the coronary microcirculation. The focus of myocardial contrast echocardiography is to use the best available imaging settings to visualize the microbubbles within the myocardium and hence assess myocardial perfusion. Continuous intravenous infusion of contrast agents is mandatory in order to provide a steady-state concentration of microbubbles and reduce the likelihood of artifacts. The technique relies on using imaging settings which initially destroy microbubbles and then observe the rate of microbubble replenishment within the myocardium.[29]

Real-Time Imaging

High mechanical index contrast imaging leads to early destruction of microbubbles and therefore does not allow continuous real-time imaging. Real-time imaging uses a mechanical index low enough to minimize microbubble destruction and thereby strengthen the signal from microbubbles while at the same time generating little harmonic signal from myocardial tissue. Microbubbles can be intentionally destroyed by a "flash" of high mechanical index ultrasound pulses, and contrast replenishment within the myocardium may then be observed by switching to a low mechanical index setting to allow qualitative and quantitative assessment of myocardial perfusion. This method allows the benefit of real-time assessment of both wall motion and perfusion (Video 11.6).

Intermittent Imaging

After microbubble destruction with flash imaging, a high mechanical index setting may be used to assess myocardial perfusion by intermittently imaging the myocardium at

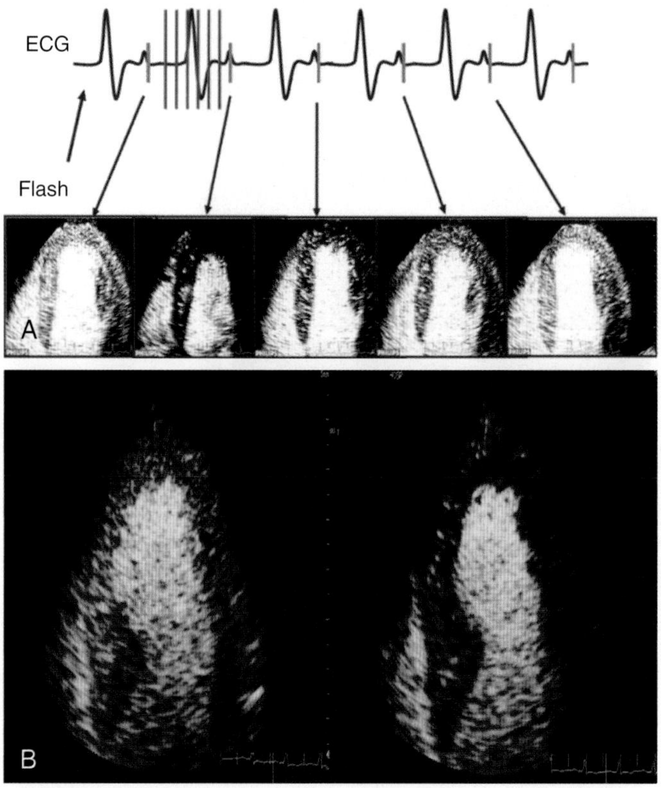

FIG. 11.5 **(A)** Myocardial contrast echocardiography by intermittent, high mechanical index imaging. After flash bubble destruction, replenishment of microbubbles in to the myocardium are imaged as snapshots in end-systole when the myocardium is at its thickest. (A, *Modified from Senior R, Becher H, Monaghan M, et al. Contrast echocardiography: evidence-based recommendations by European Association of Echocardiolgraphy. Eur J Echocardiogr. 2009;10:194-212).* **(B)** Apical 4-chamber view showing normal perfusion at rest (left) and perfusion defect in the septum, apex, and lateral wall with dipyridamole stress still present 3 seconds after microbubble destruction (right). This suggests significant disease in the LAD and LCx arteries, confirmed by coronary arteriography (B, *Modified from Senior R, Janardhanan, Jeetley P, Burden L. Myocardial contrast echocardiography for distinguishing ischemic from non-ischemic first-onset acute heart failure – insights into the mechanism of acute heart failure. Circulation 2005; 112: 1587-93).*

end-systole after every few cardiac cycles. Intermittent imaging avoids significant microbubble destruction and thereby allows replenishment of the microbubbles into the myocardium, imaged as snapshots in end-systole when the myocardium is at its thickest and easiest to discern (Fig. 11.5A). The main advantage of this technique is the high sensitivity, as the harmonic signals generated by bubble destruction at a high mechanical index are stronger than those emitted at a lower mechanical index. However, continuous imaging of wall motion and perfusion is not feasible (Video 11.7).

Quantification of Myocardial Perfusion

Approximately 90% of myocardial blood volume resides within the capillaries. When the entire myocardium is fully saturated with contrast during a continuous infusion of microbubbles, the signal intensity denotes the capillary blood volume. Any alteration of signal in such a situation must therefore occur predominantly as a result of change in capillary blood volume. As contrast agents are essentially red blood cell tracers, the rate at which contrast replenishment occurs after microbubble destruction represents red blood cell velocity. Myocardial blood flow is the product of myocardial blood volume and red blood cell velocity. If a graph is drawn plotting contrast video intensity against time,

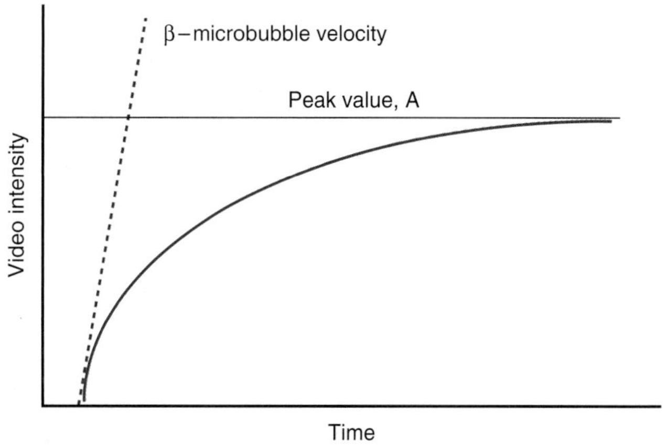

FIG. 11.6 **Quantification of myocardial perfusion.** The plateau represents the peak myocardial blood volume (denoted *A*) and the initial slope of the curve is the microbubble velocity (*β*). The product of A × β equals myocardial blood flow.

an exponential curve is obtained (Fig. 11.6). Mathematical analysis reveals that the plateau represents the peak myocardial blood volume (denoted A) and the initial slope of the curve is the microbubble velocity (denoted β). A × β then gives myocardial blood flow, and the ratio of myocardial blood flow at stress compared to rest then yields the CFR.

The capillary blood velocity is 1 mm/s with an ultrasound beam elevation of 5 mm. Thus, it takes 5 seconds for complete replenishment of the myocardium. Any decrease in myocardial blood flow prolongs replenishment time in proportion to the reduction in myocardial blood flow. Therefore, myocardial contrast echocardiography can detect capillary blood volume and, by virtue of its temporal resolution, can also assess myocardial blood flow.

Clinical Utility of Stress Myocardial Contrast Echocardiography

For the assessment of myocardial perfusion, vasodilator stress has been most commonly used, but dobutamine or exercise is just as accurate. As an alternative to dipyridamole and adenosine, a newer A_{2A} adenosine receptor agonist, regadenoson, may be given in conjunction with myocardial contrast echocardiography.[34] The latter agent is administered as a bolus injection and has a short half-life of only 2 to 3 min. This allows myocardial perfusion images to be acquired within 2 to 4 min of injection, permitting a rapid turnover of studies performed.

In the presence of a coronary stenosis, during stress, the perfusion pressure in the capillary bed supplied by the diseased artery falls significantly and these capillaries close. Consequently, there is a reduction in blood velocity and blood flow through the subtended myocardial segments, and this results in prolonged replenishment of microbubbles during destruction-replenishment imaging, indicating reduced perfusion (see Fig. 11.5B).

If wall thickening at rest is normal then, by definition, perfusion must also be normal. However, at intermediate stages of stress in a patient with flow limiting stenosis, there may be a reduction in myocardial perfusion before any change in wall motion. Therefore, perfusion assessment may be more sensitive than wall motion assessment, but with lower specificity. Numerous studies have shown good sensitivities and specificities of myocardial contrast echocardiography for the detection of CAD and myocardial viability.[29] A 2013 multicenter study found myocardial contrast echocardiography to be noninferior to single photon emission computed tomography

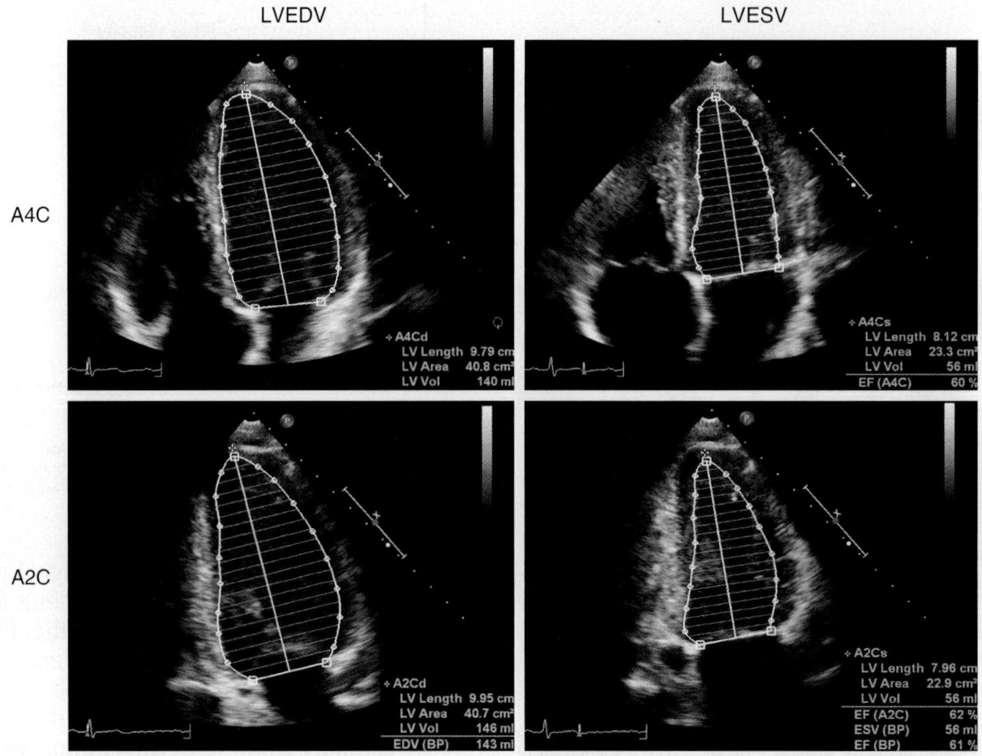

FIG. 11.7 Biplane method of disks for quantification of ejection fraction. *LVEDV*, Left ventricular end-diastolic volume; *LVESV*, left ventricular end-systolic volume; *A4C*, apical four-chamber; *A2C*, apical two-chamber.

(SPECT) imaging for the detection of CAD.[35] From the prognostic point of view, a negative stress myocardial contrast echocardiographic study is associated with a low event rate,[36] and in patients undergoing dobutamine stress echocardiography combined with myocardial contrast echocardiography, the assessment of myocardial perfusion provides incremental value in the prediction of 3-year event-free survival,[37] underlining the utility of combining myocardial contrast echocardiography with stress echocardiography.

Myocardial contrast echocardiography has good evidence to support its incorporation into clinical practice.[38,39] However, interobserver agreement is variable and the technique requires considerable expertise in order to avoid pitfalls associated with machine settings, perfusion imaging, contrast delivery, and patient anatomy. Ultrasound contrast agents are not currently licensed for perfusion imaging, and the technique has yet to gain momentum in the clinical arena.

ASSESSMENT OF LEFT VENTRICULAR DYSFUNCTION

Perhaps the most common indication for echocardiography is the assessment of LV systolic function. The data provide useful clinical, diagnostic, and prognostic information in virtually all types of organic heart disease.

Quantitative Assessment of Left Ventricular Systolic Function

Ejection Fraction

1. Two-Dimensional and Contrast Echocardiography

The recommended two-dimensional echocardiographic method for measurement of LV volumes and EF is the biplane method of disks. This method involves tracing the endocardial borders from the apical four-chamber and two-chamber views at end-diastole and end-systole[21] (Fig. 11.7). EF can then be derived from the end-diastolic volume (EDV) and end-systolic volume (ESV) as follows: EF = (EDV – ESV)/EDV. These measurements can be prone to error if image quality is suboptimal, but accuracy and reproducibility can be improved by the use of ultrasound contrast agents. LV volumes derived from contrast echocardiography are higher than those measured on standard tissue harmonic imaging, probably because contrast tracks the true endocardial surface better than noncontrast images. Consequently, LV volumes and EF measurements from contrast echocardiography have been shown to correlate better with CMR-derived measurements as the reference standard (e-Fig. 11.6). Interreader variability is also improved with contrast-enhanced versus unenhanced images.[40] This is clinically important because left ventricular ejection fraction (LVEF) after MI remains a major determinant of outcome and is pivotal for decision-making regarding the implantation of potentially life-saving but expensive device therapies.

2. Three-Dimensional Echocardiography

Importantly, the biplane method has the inherent limitation of using the geometric assumption that the LV is shaped like an ellipse. Another problem relates to potential foreshortening of the apex and therefore underestimation of cavity volumes. These limitations have been overcome by three-dimensional echocardiography that captures the entire volume of the LV during image acquisition.[41,42] Advances in computer and transducer technologies now allow real-time three-dimensional imaging of the heart without the need for intensive off-line postprocessing maneuvers. Three-dimensional echocardiographic images may be acquired in real time by the acquisition of multiple pyramidal datasets per second in a single cardiac cycle. Alternatively,

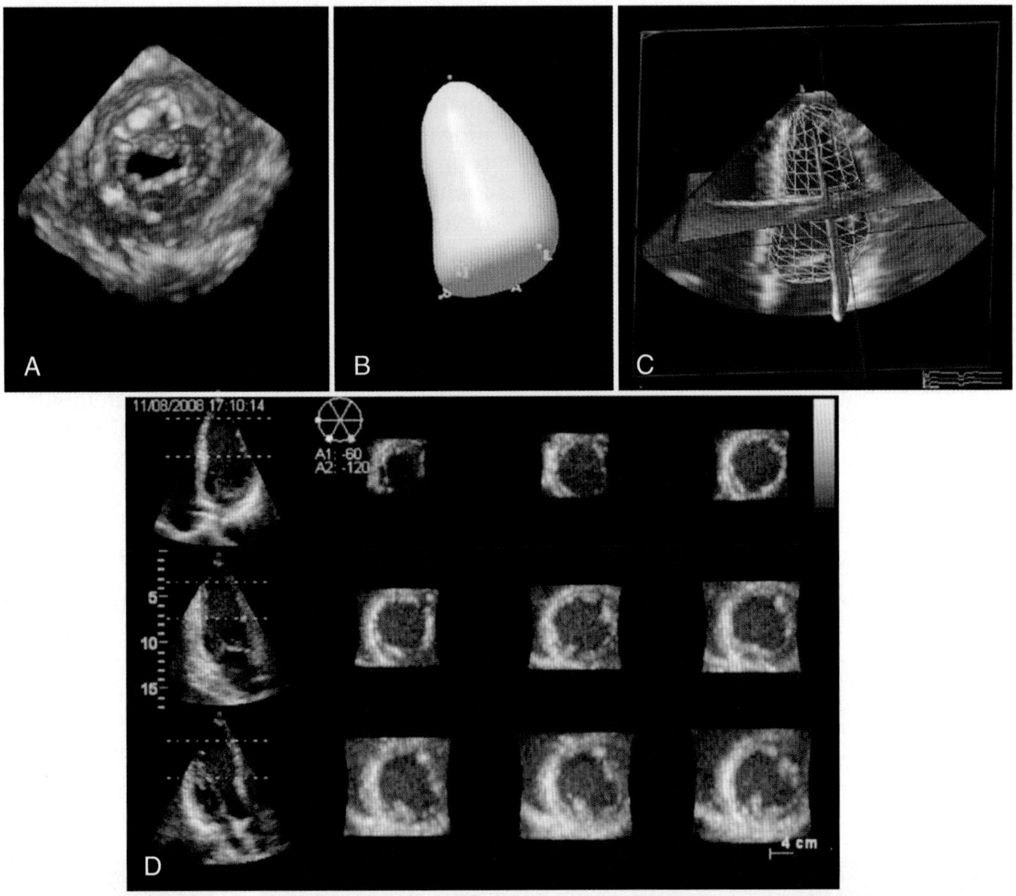

FIG. 11.8 **Three-dimensional echocardiographic images presented in four broad categories: (A) volume rendered, (B) surface rendered, (C) wire framed, and (D) two-dimensional tomographic slices.** *(From Mor-Avi V, Sugeng L, Lang RM. Real time 3-dimensional echocardiography: an integral component of the echocardiographic examination in adult patients?* Circulation *119:314-329, 2009.)*

ECG-gated multiple acquisitions of smaller volumes of data may be acquired that are then stitched together to create a full volume dataset (Video 11.8). The latter technique provides higher temporal resolution, but is prone to imaging artifacts created by movement or irregular cardiac rhythm. Three-dimensional images may be displayed as volume rendered, surface rendered, wire framed, or two-dimensional tomographic slices (Fig. 11.8).

Three-dimensional echocardiography is recommended for the evaluation of LV volumes and mass, anatomic presentation of the heart valves, and during transesophageal echocardiography–guided interventional procedures. LV volumes and EF measurements derived by three-dimensional echocardiography are more accurate and reproducible, and compare more favorably with CMR-derived measurements as the reference standard, compared to two-dimensional echocardiography[41] (e-Fig. 11.7). The use of ultrasound contrast agents in three-dimensional evaluation has not been shown to enhance the feasibility or accuracy of the technique, but may improve interreader variability.[40] Gender-specific normal values for LV volumes and EF using two-dimensional echocardiography and three-dimensional echocardiography were published in 2015.[21]

The feasibility of three-dimensional echocardiography is improving, but is limited by the need for high image quality and good operator experience. Further enhancements in temporal and spatial resolution, and in data manipulation, will be needed in the future to improve the utility of the technique.

Myocardial Mechanics

Because of its dynamic nature, echocardiography may be used to evaluate myocardial mechanics. Table 11.2 describes the main parameters of myocardial mechanics measured by echocardiography.[43] The LV myocardial architecture is such that the mid-myocardium consists of transverse fibers, the subendocardial layers have a right-handed helical arrangement, and the subepicardial layers have an opposite helical arrangement (e-Fig. 11.8). This structure broadly determines the components of myocardial deformation such that the subendocardial region contributes mainly to the longitudinal function of the LV, whereas the midwall and subepicardium contribute predominantly to rotational motion.

1. Myocardial Velocities

Tissue Doppler imaging (TDI) allows the measurement of high-amplitude, low-frequency Doppler signals arising from the myocardium and mitral annulus. A pulsed wave Doppler sample volume is placed within an area of the myocardium or the annulus, and the systolic and diastolic velocities at that point are then displayed (Fig. 11.9). Virtually any area of the myocardium can be interrogated in this manner allowing the quantitative assessment of regional systolic function by measuring the S wave peak velocity. Myocardial velocities in the longitudinal direction can be derived from apical views and in the radial direction from short-axis views. The technique may show changes in regional function that are not revealed by global LVEF measurements. However, velocity measurements are affected by translational movement and tethering, making it difficult to discriminate akinetic segments that are pulled, from actively contracting segments. In addition, velocities are not uniformly distributed across the myocardium, decreasing from base to apex, making it difficult to establish reference values.

TABLE 11.2 Measurable Indices of Myocardial Mechanics

PARAMETER	DEFINITION
Displacement	Distance moved by a cardiac structure between two consecutive frames.
Velocity	Displacement per unit time indicating the rate at which a cardiac structure changes location in a given direction.
Strain	Measure of myocardial deformation that describes the percentage change in length of a myocardial segment. Positive and negative values indicate lengthening or shortening, respectively.
Global strain	Average strain of all LV myocardial segments.
Strain rate	Rate of change in strain.
Rotation	Myocardial rotation around the long axis of the left ventricle.
Twist	Normally the base and apex rotate in opposite directions and the absolute difference in rotation is referred to as the net LV twist angle.
Torsion	Base-to-apex gradient normalized to the length of the left ventricle along the long axis.

LV, Left ventricular.

2. Myocardial Strain

Myocardial deformation imaging may overcome some of the limitations of velocity measurements. Strain measurements and strain rate measurements represent the magnitude and rate, respectively, of myocardial deformation, which is an energy-requiring process in both systole and diastole. Reductions in strain and strain rate are seen early in the development of many pathophysiologic states, including myocardial ischemia.

Color-coded TDI data allow simultaneous measurements of myocardial velocities from the entire myocardium. These data can be extrapolated to obtain displacement, strain, and strain rate measurements. Tissue Doppler data are readily available and allow online measurements of velocities and time intervals with high temporal resolution. However, the technique is limited by angle dependency, and strain and strain rate measurements with TDI require training and experience for proper interpretation and recognition of artifacts.

Two-dimensional speckle-tracking echocardiography is a new method for assessing myocardial deformation that may overcome some of the limitations of TDI. The technique allows myocardial motion to be analyzed through frame-by-frame tracking of natural acoustic markers (referred to as *speckles*) that are generated from interactions between ultrasound and myocardium within a defined region of interest. By analyzing and tracking the motion of speckles from standard apical and short-axis views, deformation may

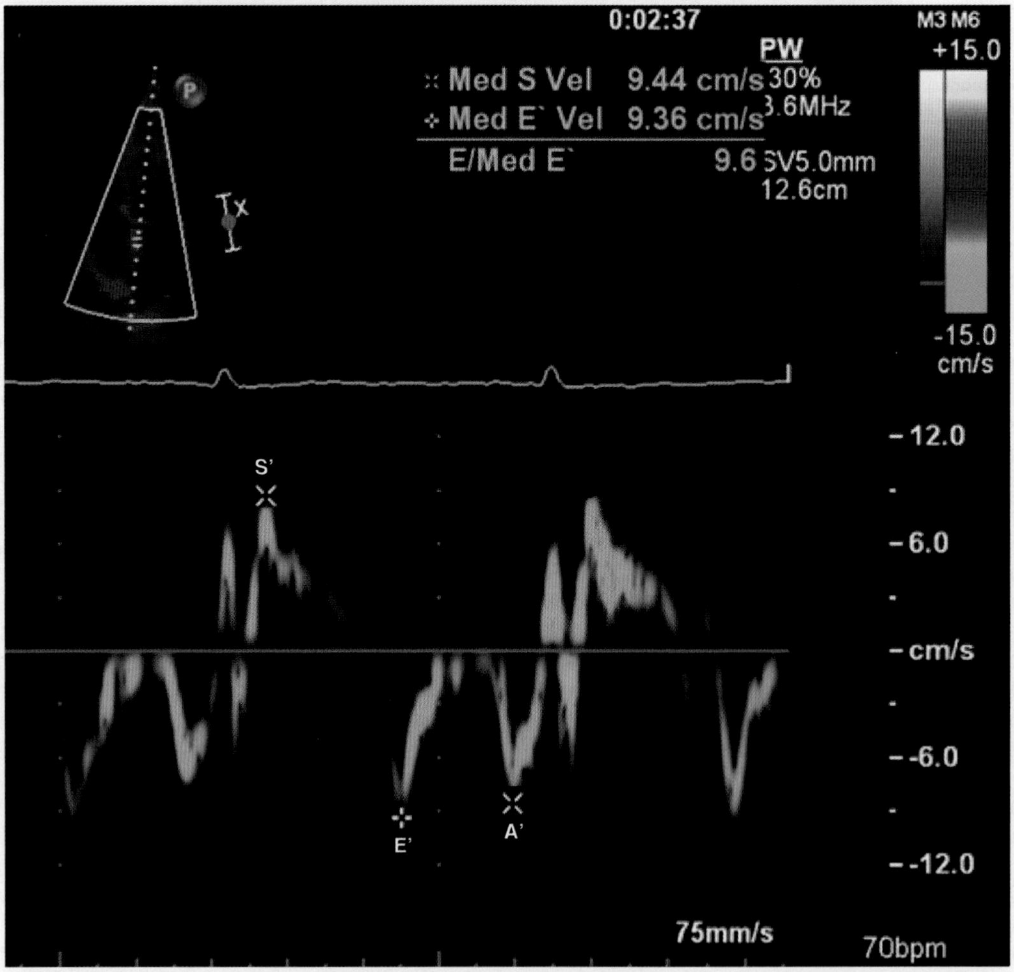

FIG. 11.9 Normal pattern of tissue Doppler–derived myocardial systolic (S′ wave), early diastolic (E′ wave), and late diastolic (A′ wave) velocities from the medial aspect of the mitral annulus.

be quantified along the longitudinal, radial, and circumferential axes independently from angulation. Moreover, the technique does not require high frame rate images and can be performed by dedicated software on normal two-dimensional pictures. The most commonly used strain-based measurement of LV systolic function is global longitudinal strain (GLS). Peak GLS describes the relative length change of the LV myocardium between end-diastole and end-systole such that GLS (%) = (MLs − MLd)/MLd, where ML is myocardial length at end-systole (MLs) and end-diastole (MLd). Because MLs is smaller than MLd, peak GLS is a negative number.

The data are analyzed off-line by manual definition of the region of interest and automated tracking of the myocardium. Strain and strain rate values can be obtained for a single myocardial segment or provide a global measure as the average of all segments of the LV (Fig. 11.10). The same segments may also be evaluated along the radial and circumferential axes. Reductions in myocardial strain have been shown to occur before any discernible change in EF in a variety of cardiac conditions. Measurements of longitudinal strain are more robust and reproducible than circumferential strain and radial strain. Normal ranges for GLS defined from a recent meta-analysis support the use of a normal cutoff exceeding −19%.[44] GLS measurements offer incremental predictive value in unselected patients undergoing echocardiography for the assessment of LV function.[45,46]

As the subendocardial layer mainly contributes to longitudinal function and is the most vulnerable to an ischemic insult, a reduced longitudinal strain may be noted in affected myocardial segments and areas of infarction. Reduced longitudinal strain in patients with normal EF and increased atherosclerotic risk has been related to increasing severity of coronary artery disease.[47] Longitudinal strain data have also been shown to provide incremental diagnostic and prognostic information in those undergoing dobutamine stress echocardiography. In patients with MI, GLS values seem to correlate with infarct size and EF and predict LV remodeling and cardiac events.[48] Reduced radial and circumferential strain have also been shown to differentiate viable from nonviable myocardium.[49,50]

Despite potentially useful applications,[51] strain measurements are not yet incorporated into clinical practice. Speckle-tracking echocardiography relies on good image quality and the assumption that a given speckle can be

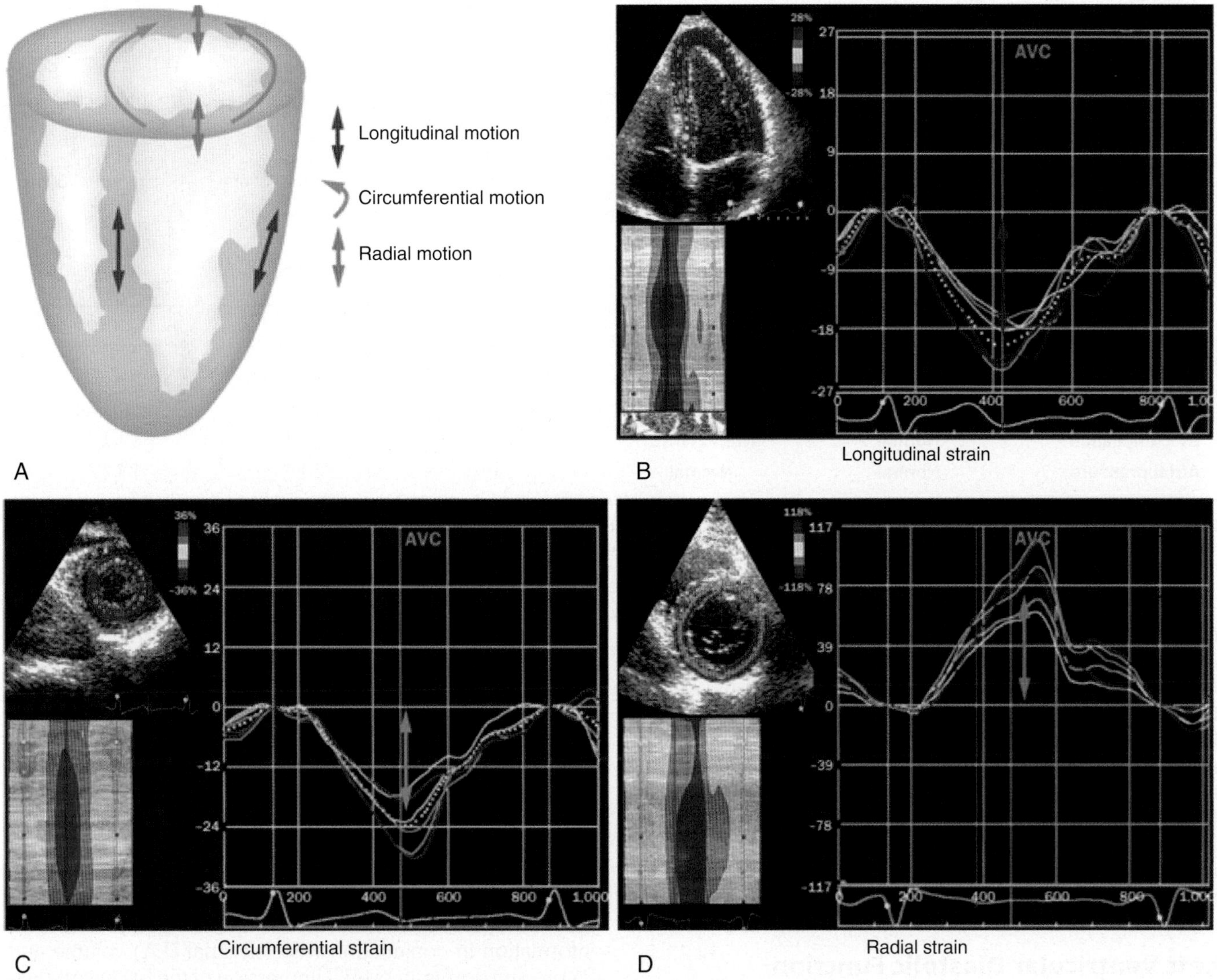

FIG. 11.10 Two-dimensional speckle tracking strain of the left ventricular myocardium. (A) *Arrows* denote the direction of movements. Myocardial fiber shortening in longitudinal **(B)** and circumferential directions **(C)** during systole represents negative strain, whereas thickening and lengthening in the radial direction **(D)** represents positive strain. *Arrows* in **B–D** represent mean strain values in these directions. *AVC*, Aortic valve closure. *(From Ozkan A, Kapadia S, Tuzcu M, Marwick TH.* Nat Rev Cardiol. *2011;8:494–501).*

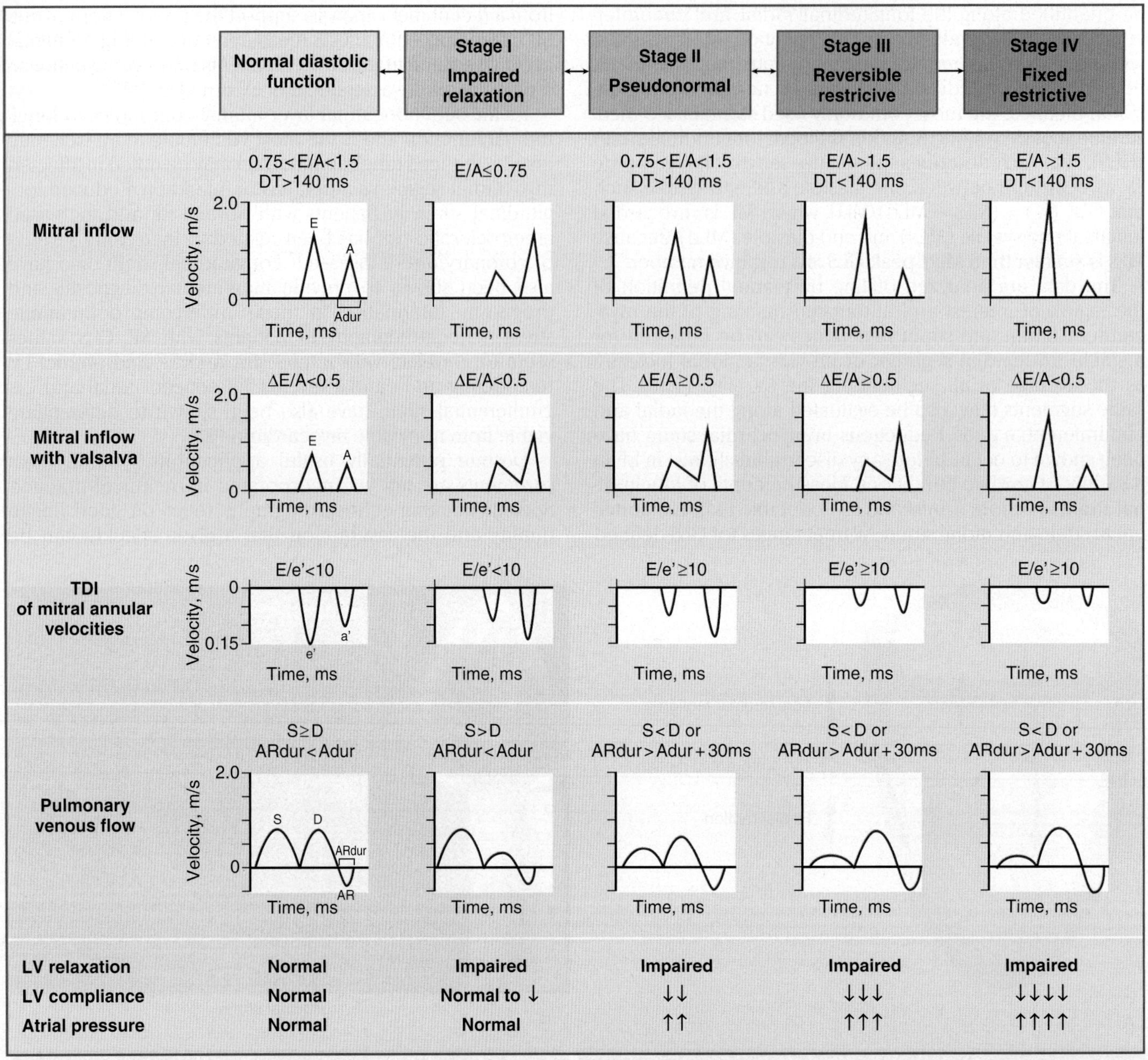

FIG. 11.11 **Grading of diastolic function from normal diastolic function to restrictive filling, based on pulsed wave trans-mitral inflow Doppler velocities, tissue Doppler myocardial diastolic velocities, and pulmonary venous flow velocities.** *(Modified from Daneshvar D, Wei J, Tolstrup K et al. Diastolic dysfunction: improved understanding from emerging imaging techniques.* Am Heart J *2010; 160: 394-404.)*

tracked from one frame to the next, which may not be the case when excessive cardiac motion occurs. Three-dimensional speckle-tracking echocardiography offers the advantages of overcoming foreshortening, the ability to measure a greater number of myocardial segments, and reduced examination time. However, three-dimensional techniques are highly dependent on image quality, use lower frame rates, and require rigorous validation. Most importantly, there are as yet unresolved differences in intervendor strain measurements that limit the widespread applicability of the technique.

Left Ventricular Diastolic Function

Virtually all forms of cardiac conditions including CAD are associated with abnormal diastolic function. Diastolic dysfunction is a significant contributor to the development of congestive heart failure. Diastole starts at aortic valve closure and includes LV pressure fall during isovolumic relaxation, rapid early passive LV filling immediately after mitral valve opening, diastasis, and late active filling during atrial contraction.

Echocardiography plays a central role in the assessment of LV diastolic function, and Doppler techniques evaluating mitral inflow, pulmonary venous flow, and tissue Doppler mitral annular velocities can be integrated to grade the severity of diastolic dysfunction[52] (Fig. 11.11). Moreover, Doppler-derived diastolic parameters can provide an estimate of left atrial pressure that may be useful in LV dysfunction due to CAD. This information in conjunction with left atrial (LA) volume and PA pressure forms an overall impression of the backward pressure due to LV systolic and diastolic dysfunction. Notably, the accuracy and validity of Doppler markers of diastolic function are greatest in the presence of systolic dysfunction.

Doppler Assessment of Diastolic Function

1. Mitral Inflow Velocities

Mitral inflow velocities are obtained in the apical four-chamber view with the pulsed wave Doppler sample volume positioned at the tips of the mitral valve. The main measurements of mitral inflow include the peak early filling velocity (E wave velocity), late diastolic filling velocity (A wave velocity), the E/A ratio, and deceleration time of early filling.

In a young, healthy individual the E/A ratio is greater than 1.0, but with advancing age, the natural increase in LV stiffness results in delayed relaxation with a progressive decrease in E wave velocity and an increase in A wave velocity such that there is E/A reversal with a ratio of less than 1.0. Pathologic changes in the myocardium lead to a hierarchy of changes in the mitral inflow pattern, from impaired relaxation to pseudonormal filling and, finally, restrictive filling (see Fig. 11.11). These patterns are dependent on intravascular volume and LV systolic function. The pseudonormal filling pattern may be hard to differentiate from normal LV filling. This mitral inflow pattern is caused by a mild-to-moderate increase in LA pressure in the setting of delayed myocardial relaxation. Because the Valsalva maneuver decreases preload during the strain phase, pseudonormal mitral inflow changes to a pattern of E/A reversal confirming impaired relaxation. A persistent restrictive filling pattern in the setting of LV systolic dysfunction following MI is associated with a poor prognosis.[53]

2. Pulmonary Venous Flow

Acquisition of pulmonary venous flow is performed in the apical four-chamber view with the pulsed wave Doppler sample volume placed in the right pulmonary vein. Normal pulmonary vein flow consists of a forward systolic and diastolic phase as well as a reversed atrial phase. Under normal circumstances, the systolic flow velocity exceeds the diastolic velocity and this is followed by a short, low-velocity reversed flow due to atrial contraction for those in sinus rhythm. With impaired LV systolic function and raised LA pressure, the pulmonary venous flow in systole is blunted and diastolic flow is increased because of greater emptying of the pulmonary veins into the LA following opening of the mitral valve. However, an increase in LA pressure leads to incomplete emptying and an increase in the reversed pulmonary A wave velocity and duration. If the pulmonary A wave duration exceeds the trans-mitral A wave duration, the LV end-diastolic pressure is usually elevated (see Fig. 11.11).

3. Tissue Doppler Mitral Annular Velocities

The acquisition of tissue Doppler mitral annular velocities is performed with the pulsed wave sample volume placed in the region of the septal and lateral insertion sites of the mitral leaflets. The early (e') and late (a') myocardial diastolic velocities are used as markers of global LV diastolic function in a manner similar to the trans-mitral inflow velocities. In normal conditions, e' is greater than a', but with diastolic dysfunction there is a reversal of this pattern. Importantly, unlike mitral inflow velocities, annular velocities are not load dependent and so the e' velocity remains depressed in the pseudonormal and restrictive trans-mitral filling patterns (see Fig. 11.11). In addition, the ratio of the trans-mitral E velocity and tissue Doppler annular e' velocity (E/e') has been shown to directly correlate with the pulmonary capillary wedge pressure. An elevated E/e' ratio is associated with an adverse outcome in both ischemic and nonischemic LV dysfunction. In the presence of regional LV systolic dysfunction as in CAD, use of the average of the septal and lateral e' velocities is recommended. An E/e' ratio of less than 8 is usually associated with normal LV filling pressure, whereas a ratio greater than 15 is associated with increased filling pressures. When the value is in the intermediate range, other echocardiographic indices should be integrated to gain an overall impression. Importantly, the E/e' ratio is not a reliable index of filling pressures in normal subjects, those with mitral valve disease, or those with constrictive pericarditis.

Left Atrial Volume

Whereas the previously mentioned parameters of diastolic function reflect LV filling pressures at the time of measurement, LA volume reflects the hemodynamic burden of elevated LV filling pressures over time. Left atrial volume should be measured in a similar fashion to LV volume, using the biplane method.[21] A left atrial volume index of less than 34 mL/m^2 is considered normal, as measurements above this cut-off level, in the absence of atrial fibrillation and significant valve disease, independently predict death, heart failure, atrial fibrillation, and ischemic stroke.[52]

Pulmonary Artery Pressure

In the absence of chronic pulmonary disease, a raised PA pressure in patients with LV dysfunction due to CAD usually implies increased LA and backward pressure causing secondary pulmonary hypertension. The peak velocity of the tricuspid regurgitation jet by continuous wave Doppler together with right atrial pressure (inferred by interrogation of the inferior vena cava) is used to derive PA systolic pressure. In addition, the end-diastolic velocity of the pulmonary regurgitation jet can be applied to derive PA diastolic pressure.[1] The latter correlates well with invasively measured pulmonary capillary wedge pressure.

Left Ventricular Dysfunction

In addition to the evaluation of LV function by echocardiography, information on cavity size, myocardial morphology, valvular involvement, and the regional or global nature of impaired LV systolic function may point to the etiology of the underlying disease process. Pathologic changes due to CAD result in regional rather than global abnormalities of LV systolic function that occur in well-defined territories (Video 11.9). Regional WMAs at rest may also occur in conditions such as myocarditis, Takotsubo cardiomyopathy, and sarcoidosis, but usually in patterns distinct from a specific coronary artery distribution. Septal abnormalities may arise from LBBB, from ventricular pacing, or following cardiac surgery and should therefore be interpreted in context. In some instances, it may be difficult to accurately separate ischemic from nonischemic causes of LV dysfunction, in which case direct assessment of the coronary arteries may be necessary. It should also be borne in mind that in rare circumstances a primary cardiomyopathy may coexist with CAD. The most common pattern under these circumstances is the presence of CAD that is milder than would be expected from the degree of LV dysfunction and dilatation.

1. Adverse Remodeling

In the presence of transmural infarction and depending on the size of infarction, the LV may undergo a series of changes in morphology and geometry known as *remodeling* (e-Fig. 11.9). Echocardiographically, there will be regional WMAs commonly associated with myocardial thinning and scar formation, highly suggestive of previous infarction in a typical coronary artery distribution and most commonly involving the septum and apex. Adverse LV remodeling leads to cavity dilatation and altered geometry with increased sphericity. There are usually varying degrees of mitral regurgitation either due to infarction involving the papillary muscle or as a result of the cavity dilatation leading to outward displacement of the papillary muscle, tethering of the mitral valve leaflets, and impaired coaptation. The LA may be dilated due to a combination of diastolic dysfunction, raised LV filling pressures, and mitral regurgitation. The PA pressures may be secondarily elevated and right ventricular function may be impaired, particularly if involved in previous inferior infarction.

2. Myocardial Viability

Myocardial walls that are akinetic at rest may either represent subendocardial or transmural infarction or demonstrate areas of myocardial viability due to stunning or hibernation. It is important to identify hibernating myocardium, as revascularization may lead to improved contractile function, reverse remodeling, and improved clinical outcome. Dobutamine stress echocardiography is the most widely used method for assessing myocardial viability. The varying patterns of contractile response to dobutamine of the akinetic myocardial region help to differentiate between infarcted, stunned, and hibernating myocardium. A low-dose dobutamine protocol is employed starting at a dose of 5 μg/kg per min, increasing at 5 minute intervals to 10 μg/kg per min and if necessary to 15 μg/kg per min, before resuming the standard protocol to the maximal dose of 40 μg/kg per min (see Fig. 11.2). At low doses, an inotropic effect is evoked with only a small increase in heart rate. In areas of myocardial viability, contractile proteins are recruited and wall thickening is observed on echocardiography. When dobutamine is then gradually increased to higher doses, the increase in myocardial oxygen consumption may provoke ischemia in the chronic, low blood flow state of hibernating myocardium, leading to severe hypokinesia or akinesia (Video 11.10). This biphasic response is a powerful predictor of recovery of LV function following revascularization. In stunned myocardium, higher doses of dobutamine lead to further improvement in contractile function in the previously akinetic area and therefore do not demonstrate a biphasic response. Truly infarcted myocardium fails to show any improvement in contractile function at low doses of dobutamine and remains akinetic throughout the test.

The detection of myocardial viability due to hibernating myocardium is based on the recovery of regional LV function following coronary revascularization.[54] The sensitivities and specificities of dobutamine stress echocardiography for detecting hibernating myocardium are approximately 80% to 85%. Retrospective data from a number of studies suggest that in patients with CAD and resting LV dysfunction the demonstration of myocardial viability in at least five myocardial segments is associated with better outcomes with coronary revascularization rather than medical therapy, whereas those without significant myocardial viability do not seem to derive any prognostic benefit from revascularization (e-Fig. 11.10). However, limited prospective data have not shown any clinical benefit of using viability testing to guide revascularization,[55,56] but the studies were relatively small and limited by methodological concerns.[54] Current guidelines endorse viability testing, stating that myocardial revascularization in patients with LV systolic dysfunction should be considered in the presence of viable myocardium.[57]

3. Left Ventricular Dyssynchrony

Progression of LV systolic dysfunction due to CAD may be accompanied by widening of the QRS duration, most commonly with an LBBB pattern. The prolonged interventricular and intraventricular conduction may cause dyssynchronous contraction within the LV leading to worsening systolic function. Modification of the electromechanical delay with cardiac resynchronization therapy (CRT) significantly improves morbidity and mortality.[58] CRT is mainly recommended in those with EF of less than 35% associated with a QRS duration of greater than or equal to 150 ms and New York Heart Association class II or III symptoms refractory to medical therapy. CRT may also be considered in subgroups with QRS duration of 120 to 149 ms, or in less symptomatic patients.

However, approximately one-third of patients fail to derive benefit from CRT using ECG criteria alone. Consequently, a number of echocardiographic parameters of mechanical dyssynchrony have been studied to predict the response to CRT[59] (e-Table 11.1). When assessed individually, these parameters have failed to demonstrate significant predictive value; it is likely that the mechanisms underlying dyssynchrony are more complex and varied than can be encompassed by a single measurement. Moreover, in LV dysfunction due to CAD, response to CRT is affected by other factors including location and extent of myocardial scar, LV lead position, right ventricular function, extent of cavity dilatation, and mitral regurgitation. At present, echocardiographic criteria for mechanical dyssynchrony are not integral to guidelines for CRT implantation.

Despite these limitations, a detailed echocardiographic assessment of multiple dyssynchrony parameters and myocardial viability may help to identify individual patients suitable for CRT.[60] In addition, strain imaging techniques and three-dimensional echocardiography may delineate the LV segments with the most delayed contraction in order to target LV lead placement in those particular regions if feasible. Using three-dimensional echocardiography, LV volumes can be divided into segments, and time to minimum volume in each segment can then be plotted. For speckle-tracking strain imaging, a similar principle can be applied by quantifying the time to peak systolic strain in individual LV segments.

Predischarge echocardiography following CRT implantation may be useful, as those with improved mechanical synchrony and contractile function are likely to benefit in the long term. A significant reduction in interventricular mechanical delay, normalized septal contraction pattern, reduction in mitral regurgitation, and improved LV synchronization by two-dimensional strain imaging or three-dimensional echocardiography have been associated with improved outcomes.[61–63] Echocardiography should also be performed at 3 or 6 months after implantation as improved LV function and reverse remodeling changes remain good prognostic signs.[64]

4. Mitral Regurgitation

Chronic CAD with LV dysfunction is usually accompanied by varying degrees of secondary mitral regurgitation (MR), most commonly due to progressive regional and global LV

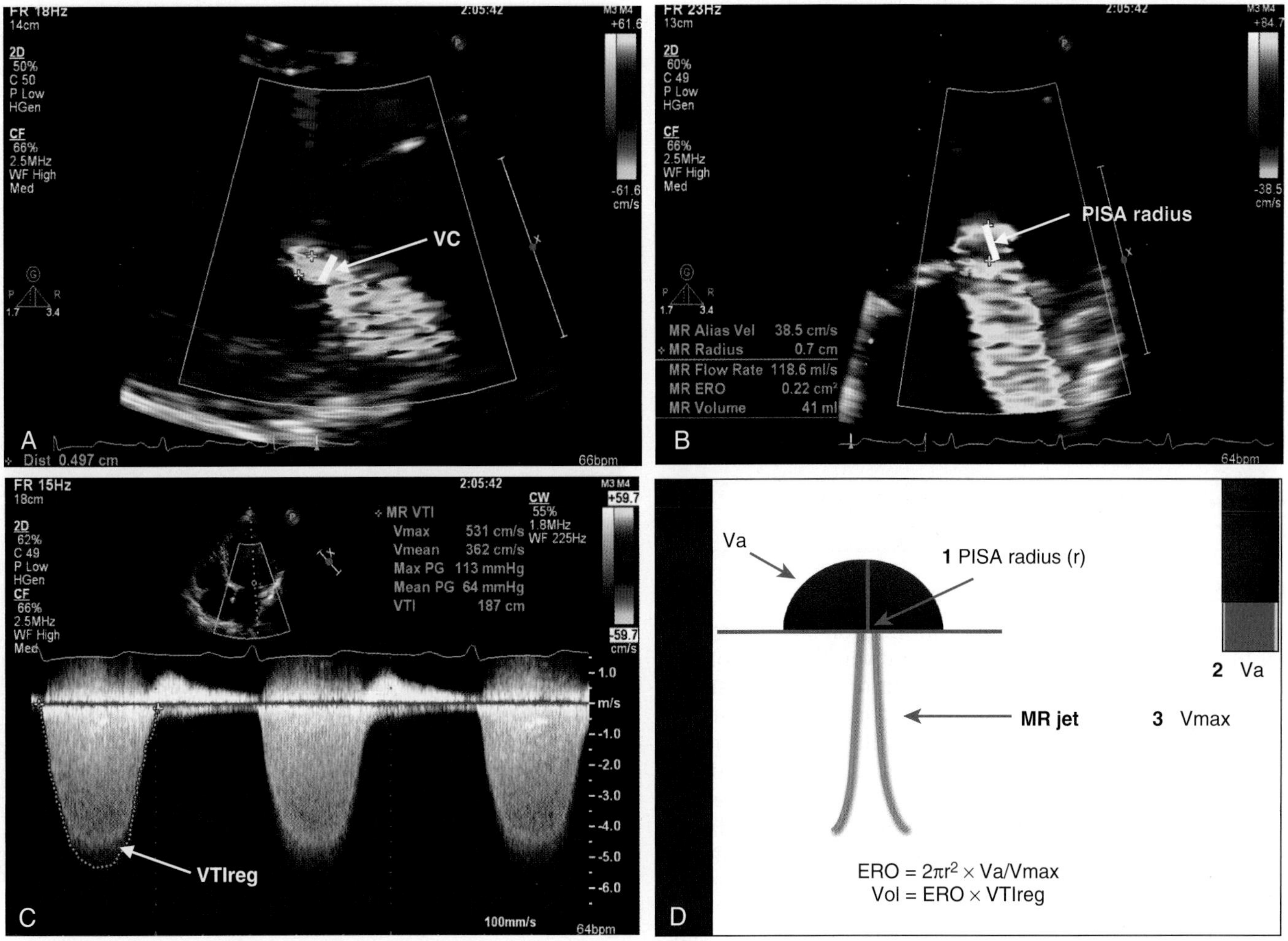

FIG. 11.12 Quantification of mitral regurgitation. (A) Magnified view of the mitral valve in the parasternal long-axis view showing measurement of vena contracta (*VC*) with color flow imaging. **(B)** Measurement of PISA radius in the apical four-chamber view. **(C)** Continuous wave spectral Doppler pattern of mitral regurgitation enabling measurement of peak velocity and velocity-time integral of the mitral regurgitation jet. **(D)** Calculation of effective regurgitant orifice area (*ERO*) and regurgitant volume (*Vol*), whereby *r* = PISA radius, *Va* = aliasing velocity, *Vmax* = peak velocity of mitral regurgitant jet, and *VTIreg* = velocity time integral of mitral regurgitation. *MR,* Mitral regurgitation; *PISA,* proximal isovelocity surface area.

remodeling rather than ongoing reversible ischemia. The chronic changes following inferolateral infarction or extensive anterior infarction lead to local LV remodeling contributing to varying degrees of apical, posterior, and lateral displacement of the posterior papillary muscle increased chordal tension and pulling of the valve leaflets leading to incomplete closure of the mitral valve in systole. At closure, the mitral valve has a tented appearance between the annular plane and displaced leaflets. In addition, the mitral annulus may become dilated in the remodeling process, further disrupting normal mitral valve closure leading to worsening MR.

Echocardiography is extremely valuable in characterizing the etiology, pathophysiology, and severity of the MR associated with CAD.[65] A number of quantitative parameters may be used to evaluate the severity of MR. The measurement of regurgitant jet area is no longer recommended because of numerous confounding factors and poor reproducibility. Vena contracta width is more reliable and robust, but guidelines favor the proximal isovelocity surface area (PISA) method as the most practical, allowing the measurement of effective regurgitant orifice area (EROA) and regurgitant volume (Fig. 11.12). However, there are many limitations to this approach. Firstly, the EROA changes during systole, tending to be higher in early and late systole and lower in mid-systole. Secondly, the shape of the PISA profile may be hemielliptic rather than truly hemispherical, and thirdly, the presence of multiple jets may lead to an underestimation of MR severity. Unlike organic MR in which severe MR is defined as an EROA of greater than 0.4 cm^2 and a regurgitant volume of greater than 60 mL, significant functional MR due to CAD is defined as an EROA of greater than 0.2 cm^2 and a regurgitant volume of greater than 30 mL because of an associated worse outcome and lower regurgitant volume in the presence of underlying impaired LV systolic function.

The severity of MR may vary with changes in loading conditions related to BP, level of hydration, physical activity, and appropriate medical therapy. The application of exercise echocardiography has shown that approximately 30% of patients develop significant MR and pulmonary hypertension with exercise, more often related to geometric and mechanical changes rather than to active reversible ischemia (Video 11.11). Serial measurements should include EROA, regurgitant volume, PA pressure, LV volumes, and EF. These can be combined with an assessment of regional wall motion to detect associated reversible ischemia. Exercise-induced worsening of MR severity by EROA of greater than 0.13 cm^2 of the resting EROA has been shown to indicate an increased risk of major adverse cardiac events.[66] Whether the MR is predominantly a marker of the LV remodeling and dysfunction or whether it independently contributes to the worse outcome is not clear.

Notably, there is no clear evidence to show that CRT, targeted percutaneous coronary revascularization, or surgical correction of the MR improves survival. Many percutaneous techniques for the treatment of MR are being investigated. In order to assess suitability of these techniques, several echo-based measurements such as leaflet length, tenting area, coaptation distance, and leaflet angles are needed. Transesophageal three-dimensional echocardiography may also be helpful in the measurement of tenting volume, better delineation of annular geometry and function,[41] and periprocedural guidance of mitral valve interventions.[67] At present, the management of ischemic MR should be tailored to the individual using an integrated approach that combines clinical information with the results of cardiac imaging data in which echocardiography plays an important role.

STRUCTURAL COMPLICATIONS DUE TO CORONARY ARTERY DISEASE

Left Ventricular Aneurysm

LV aneurysm formation is a complication of transmural MI that leads to a well-delineated outward bulging of the affected LV wall due to myocardial thinning and scar formation. Echocardiography can readily detect LV aneurysm formation (Fig. 11.13). The affected wall is either akinetic or dyskinetic, bulging outward in systole and sometimes associated with overlying laminar thrombus formation. The aneurysm has a wide neck communicating with the rest of the LV cavity. Aneurysms more commonly complicate anterior rather than inferior infarction, often involving the apex. Fortunately, with the advent of emergency reperfusion strategies for the treatment of acute coronary syndromes, the incidence of LV aneurysms has been reduced to approximately 10% to 15% following MI over the last few decades. Mechanically, the aneurysm does not contribute to LV ejection, but rather acts as a dead space for accommodating more blood in the LV cavity during systole and thereby compromising stroke volume. Surgical treatment of the LV aneurysm may be indicated in the setting of intractable heart failure or refractory ventricular arrhythmias. The aneurysm may be either resected and replaced with a Dacron graft or excluded by creating a partition between the normally functioning LV cavity walls and the aneurysm. Echocardiography may be helpful in determining the suitability for surgery and the approach used. In order for surgery to be feasible, the basal portions of the LV need to be normally functioning so that overall cardiac performance is preserved after surgery. Moreover, if the septum is involved in the aneurysmal dilatation, resection becomes less feasible and exclusion surgery may be the preferred choice.

Pseudoaneurysm

LV pseudoaneurysm occurs as a result of a contained rupture of the LV wall. Hemorrhage occurs into the pericardial space, which then becomes locally compressive preventing further leakage into the pericardium. The overlying thrombus then becomes organized within the pericardium creating a wall over the ruptured myocardium. In view of the limited structural integrity, pseudoaneurysms are prone to rupture, particularly within the first 3 months when the thrombus is relatively soft. However, incidental chronic pseudoaneurysms have been detected in part because of increasing use of imaging techniques and more effective postinfarction medical therapy. Other complications of pseudoaneurysms include thromboembolism and arrhythmias. Pseudoaneurysms tend to have a smaller opening than do true aneurysms. Echocardiography may identify the narrow opening with spontaneous contrast and swirling of blood within the cavity of the pseudoaneurysm, further delineated by the use of ultrasound contrast[68] (Fig. 11.14). However, the true size of the pseudoaneurysm—which incorporates the outer layer of pericardium, the inner layer of hematoma, and the cavity of the aneurysm—may be underestimated, as the thickness of the layer of hematoma cannot be determined. The size of the cavity may be modest compared to the full extent of the pericardial mass seen on CT or CMR imaging. In addition, pseudoaneurysm of the basal inferior wall may be difficult to distinguish from a true aneurysm, as the opening of the aneurysm may be wider than expected in this location.

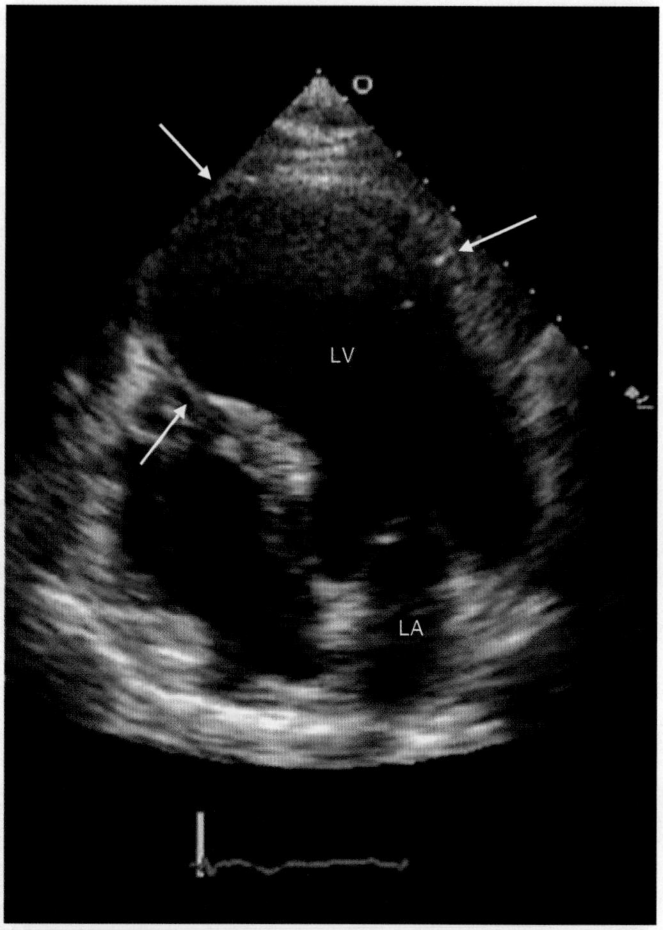

FIG. 11.13 **Large aneurysm of the left ventricular apex (*arrows*).** *LA*, left atrium; *LV*, left ventricle.

Thrombus Formation

LV thrombus formation is a well-recognized complication of MI, tending to occur more commonly after large anterior infarction and overlying the akinetic apex. Accurate detection of LV thrombus is of vital importance as anticoagulant therapy can be given to minimize the risk of embolic events leading to stroke or major organ loss. The likelihood of embolization is highest within the first 2 weeks of thrombus

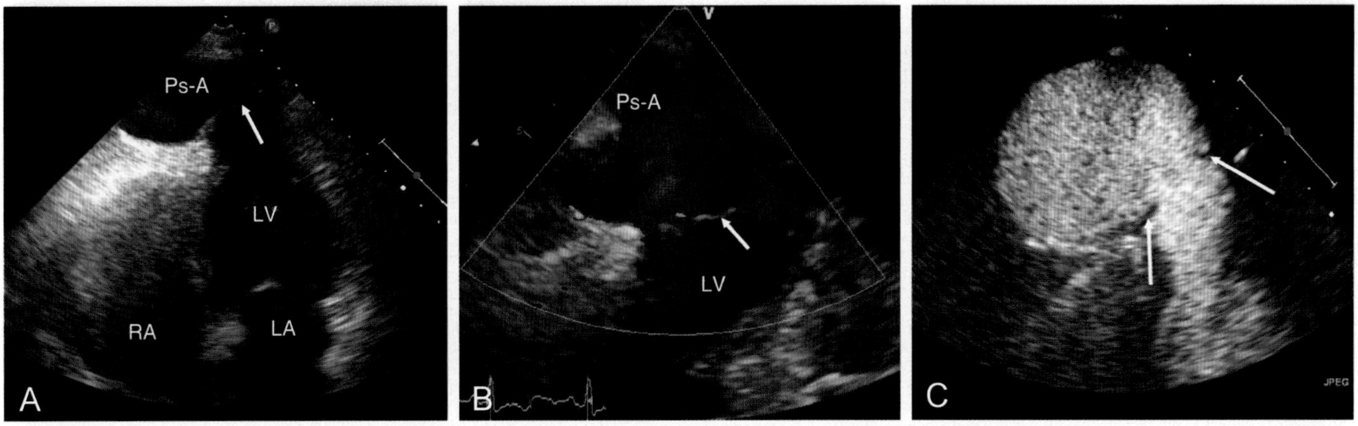

FIG. 11.14 Use of contrast echocardiography in delineating a left ventricular pseudoaneurysm. **(A)** Apical four-chamber view showing a pseudoaneurysm (*Ps-A*) adjacent to the apex and the ruptured myocardial flap (*arrow*). **(B)** Magnified view with color flow imaging showing bidirectional blood flow, due to swirling of blood within the aneurysmal cavity. **(C)** Contrast-enhanced echocardiography confirming site of rupture within the thinned apical wall of the left ventricle, measuring 15 mm in width, communicating freely with a large pseudoaneurysm (*Ps-A*). *LA*, Left atrium; *LV*, left ventricle; *Ps-A*, pseudoaneurysm; *RA*; right atrium.

formation, gradually reducing thereafter due to presumed organization and endothelialization of the thrombus.

Echocardiographically, thrombus is identified as a discrete echo dense mass with clear margins that are distinct from the endocardium and distinguishable from papillary muscles, chordae, trabeculations, and technical artifacts. Thrombus also tends to form over regional WMAs. Several characteristics of the thrombus should be noted, including size, shape, mobility, consistency, location, and presence of spontaneous echo contrast. Thrombus may be laminar in shape or protuberant and pedunculated. Laminar thrombus refers to a flattened or matted appearance of thrombus that is nonmobile and tends to imply a more chronic nature and lower potential for embolization. Pedunculated and mobile thrombi confer a greater likelihood of embolization. Fresh thrombi may have a softer appearance with an echolucent core giving them a more cystic appearance. The clinical setting and the appearance of associated regional WMA should distinguish them from cysts or tumors.

On occasion, there may be uncertainty as to whether thrombus is present over the apex, due to difficult echo windows or near-field artifacts. Under these circumstances, the use of ultrasound contrast agents is indicated to determine whether there is a true filling defect at the apex consistent with thrombus (Video 11.12). Use of contrast agents may yield a 90% reduction in the number of echoes interpreted as nondiagnostic for LV thrombus. Another scenario in which contrast agents may be helpful is when it is difficult on anatomic grounds to distinguish thrombus from surrounding myocardium and other cardiac masses such as neoplasms. Thrombus is intrinsically characterized by its avascular tissue properties, whereas neoplasm is reliant upon a vascular supply. Consequently, the use of myocardial contrast echocardiography may help to characterize the vascularity of a cardiac mass, thereby helping to differentiate between a possible tumor and thrombus[69,70] (Video 11.13).

SUMMARY

Echocardiography has become the first-line imaging modality for the assessment of cardiac structure and function in a variety of cardiac conditions. Advances in ultrasound technology now permit an accurate assessment of LV function by the introduction of ultrasound contrast agents and three-dimensional imaging. Ultrasound contrast agents may also be used to better delineate structural complications related to CAD. Speckle-tracking echocardiography allows a more detailed assessment of myocardial mechanics, beyond EF. Stress echocardiography has become a widely established technique for the detection of myocardial ischemia in patients with known or suspected cardiac chest pain, and for the assessment of myocardial viability in established chronic CAD and LV dysfunction. Consequently, the technique plays a central role in the broad range of pathophysiologic changes related to chronic CAD.

References

1. Armstrong WF, Ryan T: *Feigenbaum's Echocardiography*, ed. 7, Philadelphia, 2009, Lippincott, Williams & Wilkins.
2. Evangelista A, Flachskampf F, Lancellotti P, et al.: European Association of Echocardiography recommendations for standardization of performance, digital storage and reporting of echocardiographic studies, *Eur Heart J Cardiovasc Imaging* 9:438–448, 2008.
3. Douglas PS, Garcia MJ, Haines DE, et al.: ACCF/ASE/AHA/ASNC/HFSA/HRS/SCAI/SCCM/SCCT/SCMR 2011 appropriate use criteria for echocardiography, *J Am Coll Cardiol* 57:1126–1166, 2011.
4. *Journal of the American Society of Echocardiography*. Complete list of American Society of Echocardiography guidelines. *http://www.onlinejase.com/content/aseguidelines*.
5. European Society of Cardiology. Recommendations papers and consensus documents on echocardiography released by the European Association of Cardiovascular Imaging. *http://www.escardio.org/Guidelines-&-Education/Journals-and-publications/Consensus-and-position-documents/EACVI-position-papers/Echo*.
6. Cooper A, Calvert N, Skinner J, et al.: *Chest Pain of Recent Onset: Assessment and Diagnosis of Recent Onset Chest Pain or Discomfort of Suspected Cardiac Origin*, London, UK, 2010, National Clinical Guideline Centre for Acute and Chronic Conditions.
7. Montalescot G, Sechtem U, Achenbach S, et al.: 2013 ESC guidelines on the management of stable coronary artery disease, *Eur Heart J* 34:2949–3003, 2013.
8. Genders TSS, Steyerberg EW, Alkadhi H, et al.: A clinical prediction rule for the diagnosis of coronary artery disease: validation, updating, and extension, *Eur Heart J* 32:1316–1330, 2011.
9. Wolk MJ, Bailey SR, Doherty JU, et al.: ACCF/AHA/ASE/ASNC/HFSA/HRS/SCAI/SCCT/SCMR/STS 2013 multimodality appropriate use criteria for the detection and risk assessment of stable ischemic heart disease, *J Am Coll Cardiol* 63:380–406, 2014.
10. Sicari R, Nihoyannopoulos P, Evangelista A, et al.: Stress echocardiography expert consensus statement: European Association of Echocardiography, *Eur J Echocardiogr* 9:415–437, 2008.
11. Douglas PS, Kanderia B, Stainback RF, Weisssman NF: ACCF/ASE/ACEP/AHA/ASNC/SCAI/SCCT/SCMR 2008 appropriateness criteria for stress echocardiography: a report of the American College of Cardiology Foundation Appropriateness Criteria Task Force, American Society of Echocardiography, American College of Emergency Physicians, American Heart Association, American Society of Nuclear Cardiology, Society for Cardiovascular Angiography and Interventions, Society of Cardiovascular Computed Tomography, and Society for Cardiovascular Magnetic Resonance endorsed by the Heart Rhythm Society and the Society of Critical Care Medicine, *J Am Soc Echocardiogr* 51(11):1127–1147, 2008.
12. Pellikka PA, Nagueh SF, Elhendy AA, et al.: American Society of Echocardiography recommendations for performance, interpretation and clinical application of stress echocardiography, *J Am Soc Echocardiogr* 20(9):1021–1041, 2007.
13. Tweet MS, Arruda-Olson AM, Anavekar NS, Pellikka PA: Stress echocardiography: what is new and how does it compare with myocardial perfusion imaging and other modalities? *Curr Cardiol Rep* 17:43, 2015.
14. Fine NM, Pellikka PA, Scott CG, Gharacholou SM, McCully RB: Characteristics and outcomes of patients who achieve high workload (≥10 metabolic equivalents) during treadmill exercise echocardiography, *Mayo Clin Proc* 88:1408–1419, 2013.
15. Gilstrap LG, Bhatia RS, Weiner RB, Dudzinski D: Dobutamine stress echocardiography: a review and update, *Research Reports in Clinical Cardiology* 5:69–81, 2014.
16. Khattar RS: *WikiEcho*, Dobutamine stress echocardiography. *http://www.wikiecho.org/wiki/Dobutamine_Stress_Echo*.
17. Geleijnse ML, Krenning BJ, Nemes A, et al.: Incidence, pathophysiology, and treatment of complications during dobutamine-atropine stress echocardiography, *Circulation* 121:1756–1767, 2010.
18. *WikiEcho*. Dipyridamole stress echo. *http://www.wikiecho.org/wiki/Dipyridamole_Stress_Echo*.
19. Cortigiani L, Rigo F, Gherardi S, et al.: Coronary flow reserve during dipyridamole stress echocardiography predicts mortality, *JACC Cardiovasc Imaging* 5:1079–1085, 2012.

20. Gaibazzi N, Rigo F, Lorenzoni V, et al.: Comparative prediction of cardiac events by wall motion, wall motion plus coronary flow reserve, or myocardial perfusion analysis: a multicenter study of contrast stress echocardiography, *JACC Cardiovasc Imaging* 6:1–12, 2013.
21. Lang RM, Badano LP, Mor-Avi V, et al.: Recommendations for cardiac chamber quantification by echocardiography in adults. An update from the American Society of Echocardiography and the European Association of Cardiovascular Imaging, *Eur Heart J Cardiovasc Imaging* 16:233–271, 2015.
22. Shah BN, Zacharias K, Pabla JS, et al.: The clinical impact of contemporary stress echocardiography in morbid obesity for the assessment of coronary artery disease, *Heart* 102:370–375, 2016.
23. Shaw L, Vasey C, Sawada S, et al.: Impact of gender on risk stratification by exercise and dobutamine stress echocardiography: long-term mortality in 4234 women and 6898 men, *Eur Heart J* 26:447–456, 2005.
24. Metz LD, Beattie M, Hom R, et al.: The prognostic value of normal exercise myocardial perfusion imaging and exercise echocardiography: a meta-analysis, *J Am Coll Cardiol* 49:227–237, 2007.
25. From AM, Kane G, Bruce C, et al.: Characteristics and outcomes of patients with abnormal stress echocardiograms and angiographically mild coronary artery disease (< 50% stenoses) or normal coronary arteries, *J Am Soc Echocardiogr* 23:207–214, 2010.
26. Marwick TH1, Shaw L, Case C, Vasey C, Thomas JD: Clinical and economic impact of exercise electrocardiography and exercise echocardiography in clinical practice, *Eur Heart J* 24:1153–1163, 2003.
27. Zacharias K, Ahmed A, Shah BN, et al.: Relative clinical and economic impact of exercise echocardiography vs. exercise electrocardiography, as first line investigation in patients without known coronary artery disease and new stable angina: a randomized prospective study, *Eur Heart J Cardiovasc Imaging* 2016. [Epub ahead of print] *http://dx.doi.org/10.1093/ehjci/jew049.*
28. Jeetley P, Burden L, Stoykova B, Senior R: Clinical and economic impact of stress echocardiography compared with exercise electrocardiography in patients with suspected acute coronary syndrome but negative troponin: a prospective randomized controlled study, *Eur Heart J* 28:204–211, 2007.
29. European Society of Cardiology. Contrast echocardiography toolbox. *http://www.escardio.org/Guidelines-&-Education/Practice-tools/EACVI-toolboxes/Contrast-Echo/Contrast-Echocardiography-Box.*
30. Senior R, Becher H, Monaghan M, et al.: Contrast echocardiography: evidence-based recommendations by European Association of Echocardiography, *Eur J Echocardiogr* 10:194–212, 2009.
31. Porter TR, Abdelmoneim S, Belcik JT, et al.: Guidelines for the cardiac sonographer in the performance of contrast echocardiography: a focused update from the American Society of Echocardiography, *J Am Soc Echocardiogr* 27:797–810, 2014.
32. Dolan MS, Gala SS, Dodla S, et al.: Safety and efficacy of commercially available ultrasound contrast agents for rest and stress echocardiography: a multicenter experience, *J Am Coll Cardiol* 53:32–38, 2009.
33. Kurt M, Shaikh KA, Peterson L, et al.: Impact of contrast echocardiography on evaluation of ventricular function and clinical management in a large prospective cohort, *J Am Coll Cardiol* 53:802–810, 2009.
34. Porter TR, Adolphson M, High RR, et al.: Rapid detection of coronary artery stenosis with real-time myocardial perfusion echocardiography during regadenoson stress, *Circ Cardiovasc Imaging* 4:628–635, 2011.
35. Senior R, Moreo A, Gaibazzi N, et al.: Comparison of sulphur hexafluoride microbubble (SonoVue)-enhanced myocardial contrast echocardiography with gated single photon emission computed tomography for detection of significant coronary artery disease: a large European multicenter study, *J Am Coll Cardiol* 62:1353–1361, 2013.
36. Jeetley P, Burden L, Greaves K, Senior R: Prognostic value of myocardial contrast echocardiography in patients presenting to hospital with acute chest pain and negative troponin, *Am J Cardiol* 99:1369–1373, 2007.
37. Tsutsui JM, Elhendy A, Anderson JR, et al.: Prognostic value of dobutamine stress myocardial contrast perfusion echocardiography, *Circulation* 112:1444–1450, 2005.
38. Shah BN, Chahal NS, Bhattacharyya S, et al.: The feasibility and clinical utility of myocardial contrast echocardiography in clinical practice: results from the incorporation of myocardial perfusion assessment into clinical testing with stress echocardiography study, *J Am Soc Echocardiogr* 27:520–530, 2014.
39. Shah BN, Gonzalez-Gonzalez AM, Drakopoulou M, et al.: The incremental prognostic value of the incorporation of myocardial perfusion assessment into clinical testing with stress echocardiography study, *J Am Soc Echocardiogr* 28:1358–1365, 2015.
40. Hoffman R, Barletta G, von Bardeleben S, et al.: Analysis of left ventricular volumes and function: a multicentre comparison of cardiac magnetic resonance imaging, cine ventriculography, and unenhanced and contrast-enhanced two-dimensional and three-dimensional echocardiography, *J Am Soc Echocardiogr* 27:292–301, 2014.
41. Mor-Avi V, Sugeng L, Lang RM: Real time 3-dimensional echocardiography: an integral component of the echocardiographic examination in adult patients? *Circulation* 119:314–329, 2009.
42. Lang RM, Badano LP, Tsang W, et al.: EAE/ASE recommendations for image acquisition and display using three-dimensional echocardiography, *Eur Heart J Cardiovasc Imaging* 13:1–46, 2012.
43. Mor-Avi V, Lang RM, Badano LP, et al.: Current and evolving echocardiographic techniques for the quantitative evaluation of cardiac mechanics: ASE/EAE consensus statement on methodology and indications endorsed by the Japanese Society of Echocardiography, *Eur J Echocardiogr* 12:167–205, 2011.
44. Yingchoncharoen T, Agarwal S, Popović ZB, Marwick TH: Normal ranges of left ventricular strain: a meta-analysis, *J Am Soc Echocardiogr* 26:185–191, 2013.
45. Choi JO, Cho SW, Song YB, et al.: Longitudinal 2D strain at rest predicts the presence of left main and three-vessel coronary artery disease in patients without regional wall motion abnormality, *Eur J Echocardiogr* 10:695–701, 2009.
46. Nucifora G, Schuijf JD, Delgado V, et al.: Incremental value of subclinical left ventricular systolic dysfunction for the identification of patients with obstructive coronary artery disease, *Am Heart J* 159:148–157, 2010.
47. Ng ACT, Sitges M, Pham PN, et al.: Incremental value of 2-dimensional speckle tracking strain imaging to wall motion analysis for detection of coronary artery disease in patients undergoing dobutamine stress echocardiography, *Am Heart J* 158:836–844, 2009.
48. Hoit DB: Strain and strain rate echocardiography in coronary artery disease, *Circ Cardiovasc Imaging* 4:179–190, 2011.
49. Migrino RQ, Zhu X, Pajewski N, et al.: Assessment of segmental myocardial viability using regional 2-dimensional strain echocardiography, *J Am Soc Echocardiogr* 20:342–351, 2007.
50. Becker M, Lenzen A, Ocklenburg C, et al.: Myocardial deformation imaging based on ultrasonic pixel tracking to identify reversible myocardial dysfunction, *J Am Coll Cardiol* 51:1473–1481, 2008.
51. Smiseth OA, Torp H, Opdahl A, Haugaa KH, Urheim S: Myocardial strain imaging: how useful is it in clinical decision making? *Eur Heart J* 37:1196–1207, 2016.
52. Nagueh SF, Appleton CP, Gillebert TC, et al.: EAE/ASE recommendations for the evaluation of left ventricular diastolic function by echocardiography, *Eur J Echocardiogr* 10:165–193, 2009.
53. Meta-analysis Research Group in Echocardiography (MeRGE) AMI Collaborators, Møller JE, Whalley GA, et al.: Independent prognostic importance of a restrictive left ventricular filling pattern after myocardial infarction. An individual patient meta-analysis: Meta-analysis Research Group in Echocardiography acute myocardial infarction, *Circulation* 117:2591–2598, 2008.
54. Shah BN, Khattar RS, Senior R: The hibernating myocardium: current concepts, diagnostic dilemmas, and clinical challenges in the post-STICH era, *Eur Heart J* 34:1323–1336, 2013.
55. Bonow RO, Maurer G, Lee KL, et al.: Myocardial viability and survival in ischemic left ventricular dysfunction, *N Engl J Med* 364:1617–1625, 2011.
56. Cleland JG, Calvert M, Freemantle N, et al.: The Heart Failure Revascularisation Trial (HEART), *Eur J Heart Fail* 13:227–233, 2011.
57. Windecker S, Kolh P, Alfonoso F, et al.: 2014 ESC/EACTS guidelines on myocardial revascularization. The task force on myocardial revascularization of the European Society of Cardiology and the European Association for Cardiothoracic Surgery, *Eur Heart J* 35:2541–2619, 2014.
58. Daubert J-C, Saxon L, Adamson PB, et al.: 2012 EHRA/HRS expert consensus statement on cardiac resynchronisation therapy in heart failure: implant and follow-up recommendations and management, *Heart Rhythm* 9:1524–1576, 2012.
59. Chung ES, Leon AR, Tavazzi L, et al.: Results of the predictors of response to CRT (PROSPECT) trial, *Circulation* 117:2608–2616, 2008.
60. Lafitte S, Reant P, Zaroui A, et al.: Validation of an echocardiographic multiparametric strategy to increase responder patients after cardiac resynchronization: a multicentre study, *Eur Heart J* 30:2835–2837, 2009.
61. Pouleur AC, Knappe D, Shah AM, et al.: Relationship between improvement in left ventricular dyssynchrony and contractile function and clinical outcome with cardiac resynchronization therapy: the MADIT-CRT trial, *Eur Heart J* 32:1720–1729, 2011.
62. Parsai C, Bijnens B, Sutherland GR, et al.: Toward understanding response to cardiac resynchronization therapy: left ventricular dyssynchrony is only one of multiple mechanisms, *Eur Heart J* 30:940–949, 2009.
63. Di Biase L, Auricchio A, Mohanty P, et al.: Impact of cardiac resynchronization therapy on the severity of mitral regurgitation, *Europace* 13:829–838, 2011.
64. Goldenberg I, Moss AJ, Hall WJ, et al.: Predictors of response to cardiac resynchronization therapy in the Multicenter Automatic Defibrillator Implantation Trial with Cardiac Resynchronization Therapy (MADIT-CRT), *Circulation* 124:1527–1536, 2011.
65. Lancellotti P, Tribouilloy C, Hagendorff A, et al.: Recommendations for the echocardiographic assessment of native valvular regurgitation: an executive summary from the European Association of Cardiovascular Imaging, *Eur Heart J Cardiovasc Imaging* 14:611–644, 2013.
66. Pierard LA, Carabello BA: Ischaemic mitral regurgitation: pathophysiology, outcomes and the conundrum of treatment, *Eur Heart J* 31:2996–3005, 2010.
67. Lee AP, Lam Y, Yip GW, et al.: Role of real time three-dimensional transesophageal echocardiography in guidance of interventional procedures in cardiology, *Heart* 96:1485–1493, 2010.
68. Sehmi JS, Dungu J, Davies SW, et al.: Unsuspected large left ventricular pseudoaneurysm: rapid bedside diagnosis by contrast-enhanced echocardiography, *Oxf Med Case Reports* 11:358–359, 2015.
69. Mansencal N, Revault-d'Allonnes L, Pelage JP, et al.: Usefulness of contrast echocardiography for assessment of intracardiac masses, *Arch Cardiovasc Dis* 102:177–183, 2009.
70. Bhattacharyya S, Khattar RS, Gujral DM, Senior R: Cardiac tumors: the role of cardiovascular imaging, *Expert Rev Cardiovasc Ther* 12:37–43, 2014.

12 Nuclear Imaging and PET

Rory Hachamovitch and Marcelo F. Di Carli

FUNDAMENTALS OF RADIONUCLIDE IMAGING

Radionuclide imaging techniques are widely used in the evaluation of patients with known or suspected coronary artery disease (CAD). The basic principle underlying this approach is the use of radiolabeled agents or radiopharmaceuticals that are injected intravenously and enter viable cells (e.g., myocytes, autonomic neurons) or bind to cell receptors or other targets. These techniques use radiolabeled drugs or radiopharmaceuticals, which are injected intravenously and trapped in myocardial tissue or other cell types. This radioactivity within the heart decays by emitting gamma rays. The interaction between these gamma rays and the detectors in specialized scanners—single-photon emission computed tomography (SPECT) and positron emission tomography (PET)—creates a scintillation event or light output, which can be captured by digital recording equipment to form an image of the heart. Like computed tomography (CT) and magnetic resonance imaging (MRI), radionuclide images also generate tomographic (three-dimensional) views of the heart. Contemporary PET and SPECT scanners are frequently combined with a CT scanner (so-called hybrid PET/CT and SPECT/CT). CT is used primarily to guide patient positioning in the field of view and for correcting inhomogeneities in radiotracer distribution due to attenuation by soft tissues (so-called attenuation correction). However, the CT scanner is frequently used to obtain diagnostic data, including coronary artery calcium score and, occasionally, CT coronary angiography.

Protocols for Myocardial Perfusion and Viability Imaging

Imaging protocols are tailored to the individual patient based on clinical questions, patient's risk, ability to exercise, and body mass index, among other factors. Electrocardiogram (ECG)-triggered gated rest and stress images are acquired after the intravenous injection of the radiopharmaceutical and used to define the extent and severity of myocardial ischemia and scar, as well as regional and global cardiac function and remodeling.

Selecting a Stress Protocol

The choice of exercise versus pharmacologic stress has well-defined guidelines depending upon the patient's condition, clinical question, and safety considerations.[1] Exercise stress is always preferred over pharmacologic stress in patients who can exercise adequately due to the wealth of additional information that is provided—exercise capacity, hemodynamic response (maximal heart rate, heart rate recovery and reserve, peak blood pressure), stress-induced symptoms, exercise-induced arrhythmias, and ST-segment response. This approach permits coupling of clinical response and stress myocardial perfusion findings.

In patients unable to exercise adequately, pharmacologic stress with vasodilators (adenosine, dipyridamole, or regadenoson) or direct chronotropic/inotropic stimulation with dobutamine is used (Table 12.1). Pharmacologic stress is also preferred in patients with left bundle branch block (LBBB) or paced ventricular rhythm, as it reduces the frequency of false-positive tests related to mechanical dyssynchrony. Among the pharmacologic stress options, vasodilator stress is preferred primarily because it produces the greatest flow heterogeneity, thereby facilitating detection of regional perfusion defects. In patients with contraindications to vasodilator stress (e.g., asthma, AV block, etc.), dobutamine is a safe alternative. Finally, vasodilator stress is commonly used as an adjunct to exercise in patients unable to achieve a maximal exercise stress test.

TABLE 12.1 Pharmacologic Stress Agents in Nuclear Cardiology

	DIPYRIDAMOLE	ADENOSINE	REGADENOSON	DOBUTAMINE
Effect on coronary blood flow	× 3–4	× 3–5	× 2–3	× 2
Dose	0.56 mg/kg	140 u/kg per min	0.4 mg	Initial 3 minutes infusion of 5–10 μg/kg per min, incremental increases (2–3-minute intervals) to 20, 30, and 40 μg/kg per min. Atropine can be used to increase heart rate if target not achieved
Duration of action/half-life	30–45 minutes	< 10–15 seconds	Three phases: 1. Initial phase (maximal physiologic effect) 2–4 minutes 2. Intermediate phase (loss of pharmacologic effect) ~30 minutes 3. Final phase (decline in plasma concentration) ~2 hours	~2 minutes
Duration of infusion	4 minutes	4–6-minute infusion	~10 second	Depends on hemodynamic response
Maximal hyperemia	3–4 minutes after infusion	84 seconds (average)	1–4 minutes after injection	Peak infusion
Timing of radionuclide injection	3–5 minutes after infusion	At 3 minutes for a 6-minute infusion, at 2 minutes for a 4-minute infusion	~40 seconds after bolus injection	Goal of ≥ 85% age-predicted maximum heart rate
Reversal of effect	Aminophylline; used commonly	Aminophylline; used rarely	Aminophylline; used occasionally	β-blocker (preferably esmolol), used uncommonly

TABLE 12.2 Properties of Available SPECT Radiopharmaceuticals

	^{201}THALLIUM	^{99M}TECHNETIUM SESTAMIBI	^{99M}TECHNETIUM TETROFOSMIN
Source	Cyclotron	Generator	Generator
Physical half-life	73 hours	6 hours	6 hours
Clinical application	MPI and viability	MPI	MPI
Redistribution	Yes	No	No
Whole-body effective dose	~27 mSv per rest/stress study	~10 mSv per rest/stress study	~9 mSv per rest/stress study
Length of complete study (rest/stress imaging)	~4 hours	~2–3 hours	~2–3 hours

Imaging Protocols

A number of different protocols have been developed, validated, and tested for accuracy. Imaging protocols must be tailored to individual patients based on the clinical question, radiotracer used, and time constraints. For SPECT myocardial perfusion imaging (MPI) (Table 12.2), technetium 99m-labeled (^{99m}Tc-labeled) tracers are the most commonly used imaging agents because they are associated with the best image quality and the lowest radiation dose to the patient. After intravenous injection, myocardial uptake of ^{99m}Tc-labeled tracers is rapid (1–2 minutes). After uptake, these tracers become trapped intracellularly in mitochondria and show minimal change over time. Although used commonly in the past for perfusion imaging, ^{201}thallium protocols are now rarely used because they are associated with a higher radiation dose to the patient.

PET MPI is an alternative to SPECT and is associated with improved diagnostic accuracy and lower radiation dose to patients due to the fact that radiotracers are typically short-lived (Table 12.3). The ultra-short physical half-life of some PET radiopharmaceuticals in clinical use (e.g., ^{82}rubidium) is the primary reason that PET imaging is generally combined with pharmacologic stress, as opposed to exercise, as pharmacologic stress allows for faster imaging of these rapidly decaying radiopharmaceuticals. However, exercise is possible for relatively longer-lived radiotracers (e.g., ^{13}N-ammonia). For myocardial perfusion imaging, ^{82}rubidium does not require an onsite medical cyclotron (it is available from a ^{82}strontium/^{82}rubidium generator) and, thus, is the most commonly used radiopharmaceutical. ^{13}N-ammonia has better flow characteristics (higher myocardial extraction) and imaging properties than ^{82}rubidium but it does require access to a medical cyclotron in close proximity to the PET scanner. In comparison to SPECT, PET has improved spatial and contrast resolution and it provides absolute measures of myocardial perfusion (in mL/min per g of tissue), thereby providing a quantitative measure of regional and global coronary flow reserve that is unique.[2] Quantitative measures of myocardial blood flow and flow reserve help improve diagnostic accuracy and risk stratification.[2]

For the evaluation of myocardial viability in patients with severe left ventricular (LV) dysfunction, myocardial perfusion imaging (with SPECT or PET) is usually combined with metabolic imaging (i.e., ^{18}F-fluorodeoxyglucose [FDG] PET). In hospital settings lacking access to PET scanning, ^{201}thallium SPECT imaging is a useful alternative.[1]

TABLE 12.3 Properties of Commonly Used PET Radiopharmaceuticals

	^{13}N-AMMONIA	^{82}RUBIDIUM	^{18}F-FLUORODEOXYGLUCOSE	^{15}O-WATER*
Source	Cyclotron	Generator	Cyclotron	Cyclotron
Physical half-life	9.96 minutes	76 seconds	110 minutes	2.1 minutes
Clinical application	MPI	MPI	Myocardial viability	MPI
Exercise stress	Yes	No	NA	No
Myocardial blood flow measurement (mL/min per g)	Yes	Yes	NA	Yes
Whole-body effective dose	~2.96 mSv per rest/stress study	~3.72 mSv per rest/stress study	~7 mSv per study	~2.75 mSv per rest/stress study
Length of complete study (rest/stress imaging)	~70 minutes	~25 minutes	~2 hours	~25 minutes

*^{15}O-water is not FDA approved for clinical use and is only used in research studies.

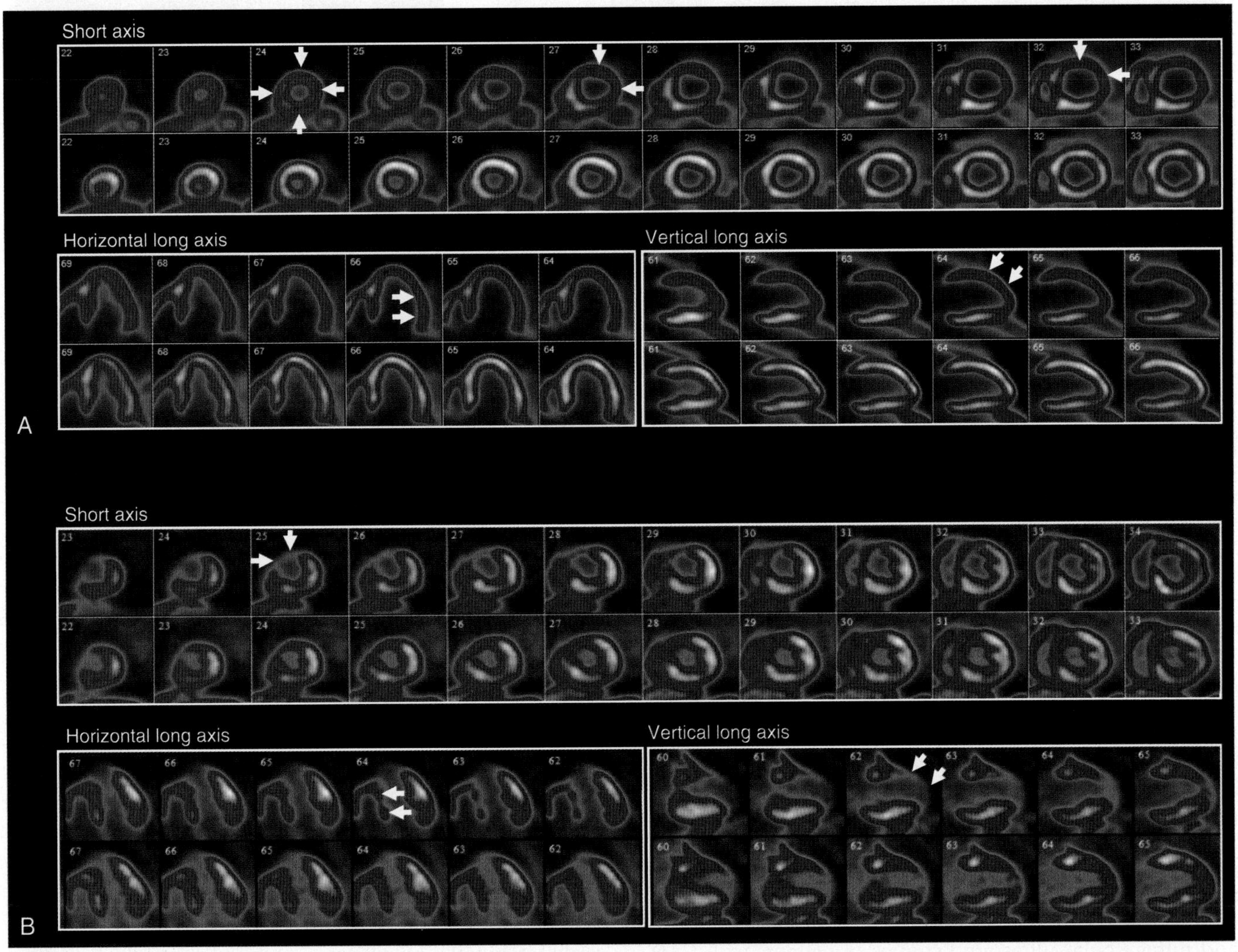

FIG. 12.1 Examples of reversible **(A)** and fixed **(B)** defects. In **(A)**, moderate- to severe-intensity reversible defects involving the basal and mid-anterior and lateral walls extending to the distal and apical ventricle are present. In **(B)**, there is a severe-intensity fixed defect involving the anteroseptal and anterior wall at the basal, mid, and distal LV extending to the apex with no clinically meaningful reversibility.

COMPREHENSIVE EVALUATION OF CORONARY ARTERY DISEASE

Detection of Coronary Artery Stenosis

The basic principle of radionuclide MPI for detecting CAD is based on the ability of a radiotracer to identify a transient regional perfusion deficit in a myocardial region subtended by a coronary artery with a flow-limiting stenosis. A reversible myocardial perfusion defect is indicative of ischemia (Fig. 12.1A), whereas a fixed perfusion defect generally reflects scarred myocardium from prior infarction (Fig. 12.1B). Generally, myocardial perfusion defects during stress develop downstream from epicardial stenosis with 50% to 70% luminal narrowing or greater and become progressively more severe with increasing degree of stenosis. It is noteworthy that coronary stenosis of intermediate severity (e.g., 50–90%) is associated with significant variability in

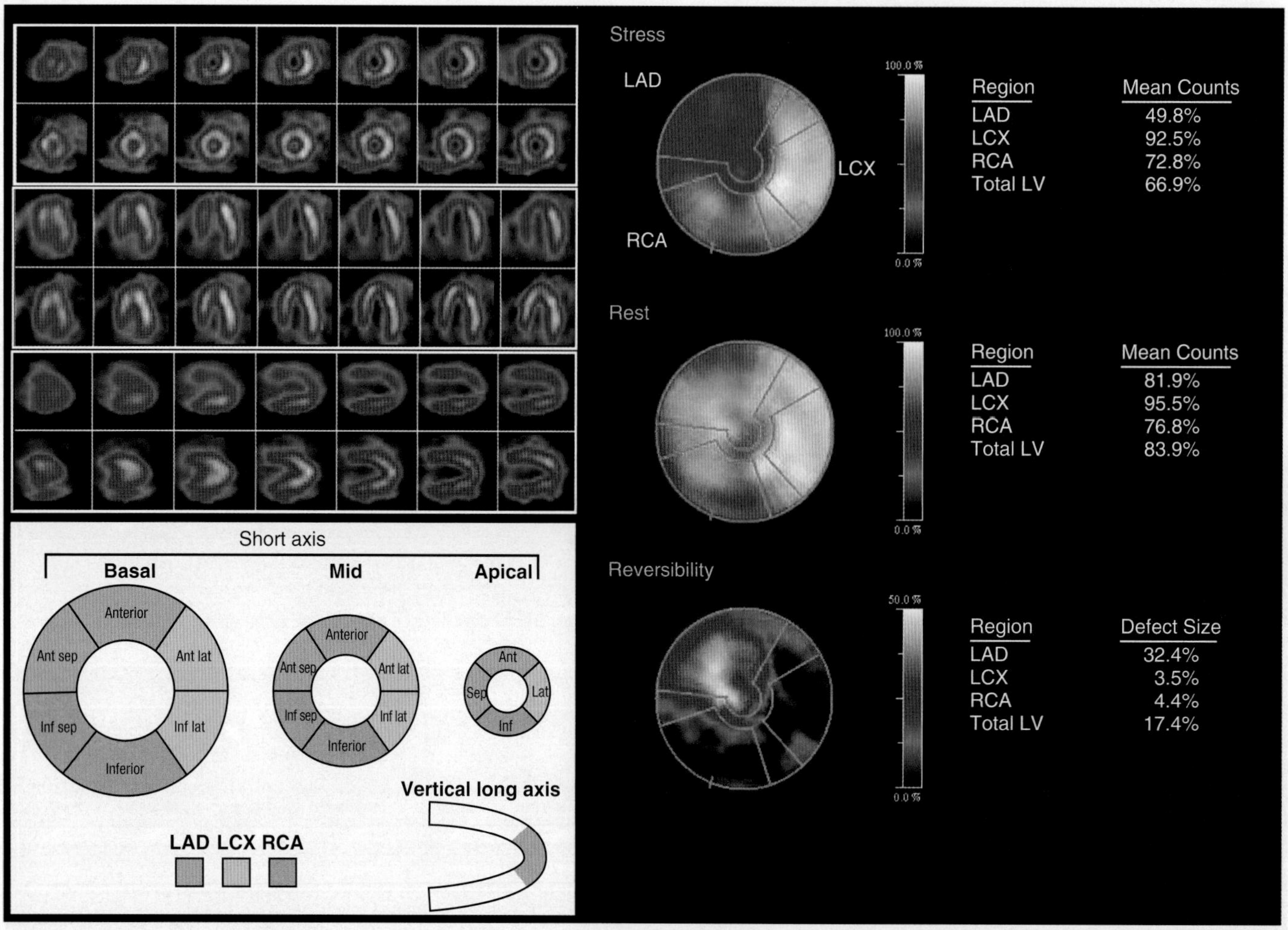

FIG. 12.2 Segmental scoring system used for interpretation and reporting of MPI. The perfusion images on the upper left reveal a severe-intensity reversible defect involving the basal, mid-, and distal anteroseptal region extending to the apex. The polar plot bullseye images on the upper right capture this defect as well. *LAD,* Left anterior descending artery; *LCX,* left circumflex artery; *LV,* left ventricle; *RCA,* right coronary artery.

the resulting maximal coronary blood flow, which in turns affects the presence and/or severity of regional perfusion defects. For any degree of intermediate luminal stenosis, the observed physiologic variability is multifactorial[3] and includes (1) geometric factors of coronary lesions not accounted for by a simple measure of minimal luminal diameter or percent stenosis, including shape, eccentricity, and length, as well as entrance and exit angles, all of which are known to modulate coronary resistance; (2) development of collateral blood flow; and (3) the presence of diffuse coronary atherosclerosis and microvascular dysfunction (combination of endothelial and smooth muscle cell dysfunction in resistive vessels, and microvascular rarefaction), all consistent findings in autopsy and intravascular ultrasound studies of patients with CAD. All these factors account for the frequent disagreements between angiographically defined CAD and its associated physiologic severity.

Quantification of Myocardial Ischemia

Regional myocardial perfusion is usually assessed by semi-quantitative visual analysis of the rest and stress images.[4] The segmental scores are then summed into global scores that reflect the total burden of ischemia and scar in the left ventricle (Fig. 12.2). Objective quantitative image analysis is a helpful tool for a more accurate and reproducible estimation of total defect size and severity and is generally used in combination with the semi-quantitative visual analysis. The semi-quantitative (visual) and quantitative scores of ischemia and scar are linearly related to the risk of adverse cardiovascular (CV) events and are useful in guiding patient management, especially the need for revascularization, and for assessing response to medical therapy. The presence of transient LV dilatation during stress imaging (so-called transient ischemic dilatation or TID) is an ancillary marker of risk that reflects extensive subendocardial ischemia and often accompanies radionuclide MPI studies with extensive and severe perfusion abnormalities (Fig. 12.3A). It is often an important finding, particularly when it occurs in patients with no or only mild perfusion abnormalities, suggesting the presence of more extensive balanced subendocardial ischemia. The presence of this abnormality has often been shown to be a harbinger of increased risk.[5–7] Similarly, the presence of transient pulmonary radiotracer retention and right ventricular uptake during stress along with a drop in left ventricular ejection fraction (LVEF) post-stress (a sign of post-ischemic stunning) are also markers of multivessel LV ischemia (Figs. 12.3B and C; Video 12.1).

Quantification of Myocardial Blood Flow and Coronary Flow Reserve

Myocardial blood flow (in mL/min per g of myocardium) and coronary flow reserve (CFR; defined as the ratio between peak

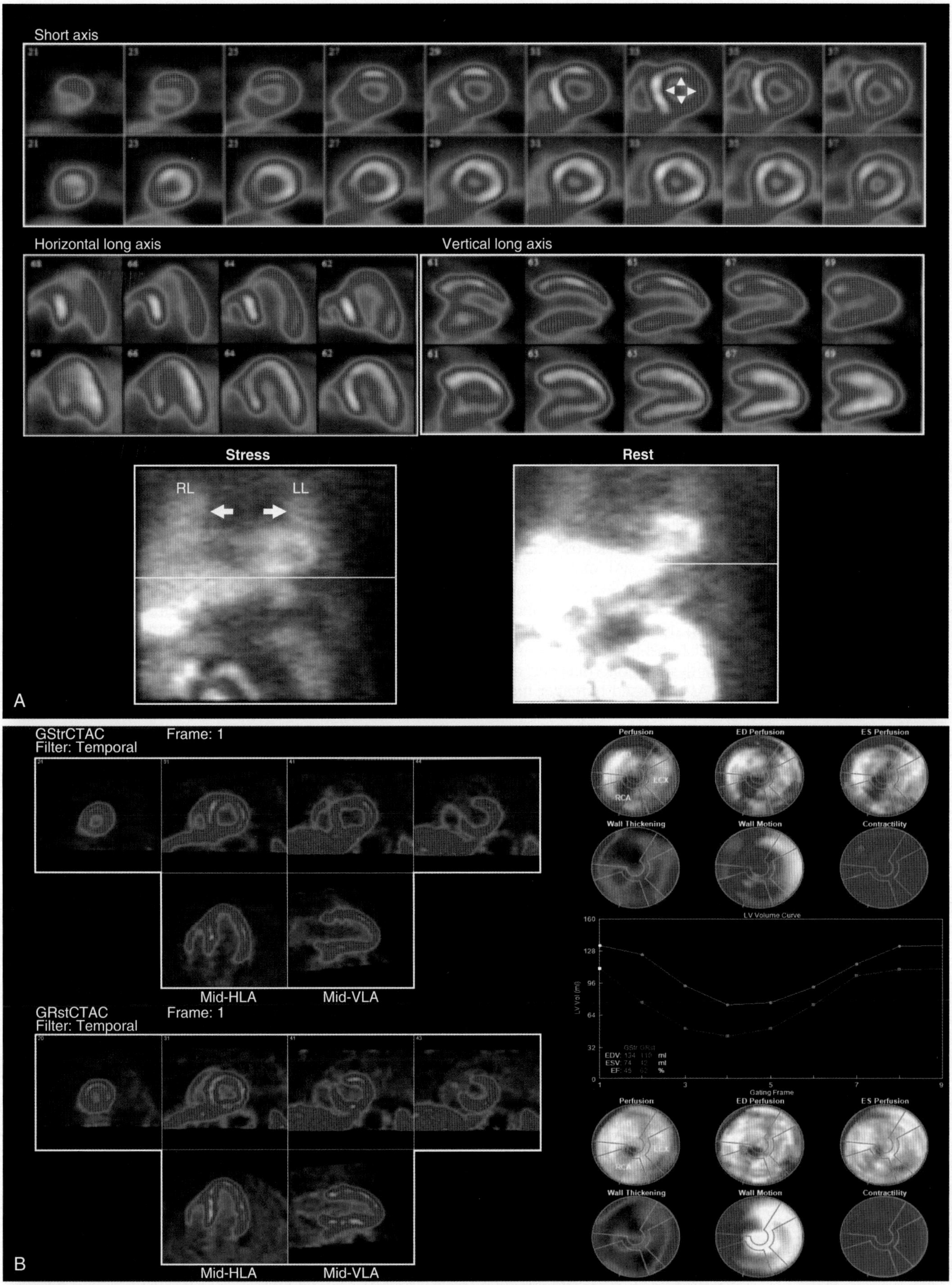

FIG. 12.3 Example of myocardial perfusion imaging (MPI) high-risk features (multivessel defects, transient ischemic dilatation [TID], pulmonary uptake, drop in left ventricular ejection fraction [LVEF] post stress). **(A)** Images reveal a moderate- to severe-intensity defect involving the mid to distal lateral and inferior walls extending to the apex and distal septum. Additionally, the projection images (*below*) reveal lung uptake of tracer on the stress views (*left*) not present on the rest view (*right*). **(B)** The decrease in LVEF is shown between the images on the upper and lower portions of the figure associated with these abnormalities. See corresponding Video 12.1.

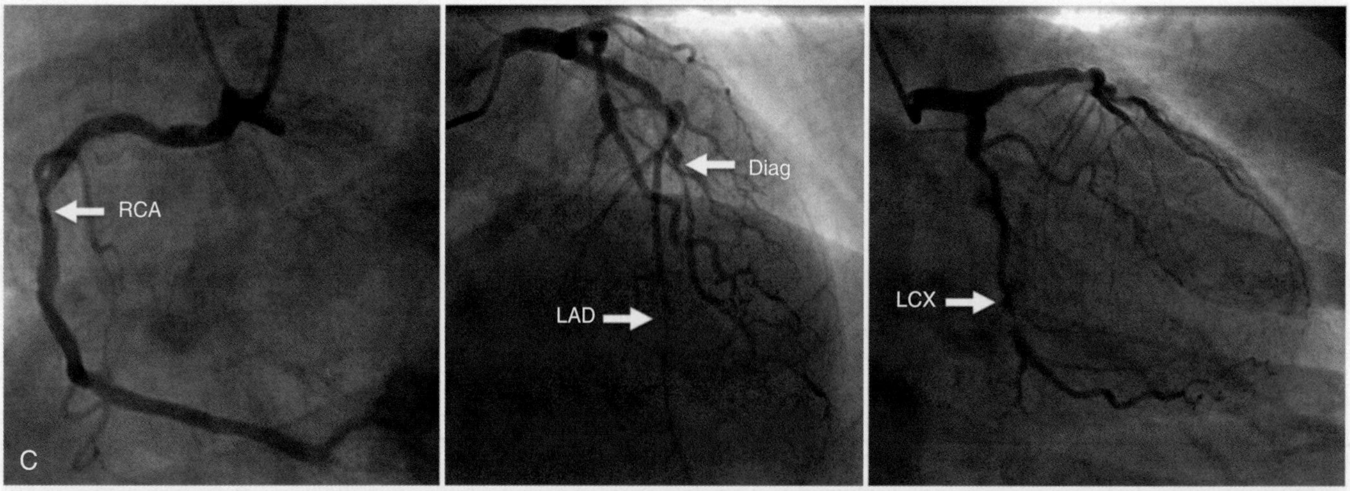

FIG. 12.3, cont'd (C) The catheterization correlate of the images (lesions in the distal left anterior descending artery (LAD), a diagonal artery (Diag), the left circumflex (LCX), and the right coronary artery (RCA) (*arrows*).

stress and rest myocardial blood flow) are important physiologic parameters that can be measured by routine post-processing of myocardial perfusion PET images.[2] These absolute measurements of tissue perfusion are accurate and reproducible. Pathophysiologically, CFR estimates provide a measure of the integrated effects of epicardial coronary stenoses, diffuse atherosclerosis and vessel remodeling, and microvascular dysfunction on myocardial perfusion, and, as such, the value obtained is a more sensitive measure of myocardial ischemia. In the setting of increased oxygen demand, a reduced CFR can upset the supply–demand relationship and lead to myocardial ischemia, subclinical LV dysfunction (diastolic and systolic), symptoms, and death. As discussed hereafter, these measurements of CFR have important diagnostic[8–12] and prognostic[13–19] implications in the evaluation and management[17] of patients with known or suspected CAD (Fig. 12.4).

Assessment of Myocardial Viability

Myocardial perfusion and metabolic imaging are commonly used to evaluate the patient with ischemic LV dysfunction, especially when the question of revascularization is being considered. Radionuclide imaging provides important quantitative information, including (1) myocardial infarct size; (2) extent of stunning and hibernating myocardium; (3) magnitude of inducible myocardial ischemia; and (4) LV function and volumes (see Fig. 12.3 and Fig. 12.5).

Both ^{201}thallium and, especially, ^{99m}Tc agents provide accurate and reproducible measurements of regional and global myocardial infarct size. The use of metabolic imaging with PET has been extensively validated and is commonly used for assessing myocardial viability. ^{18}FDG is used to assess regional myocardial glucose utilization (an index of tissue viability) and is compared with perfusion images to define metabolic abnormalities associated with infarction and hibernation.[20,21] Reduced perfusion and increased FDG uptake at rest (so-called perfusion–FDG mismatch) identifies areas of viable but hibernating myocardium, whereas regions showing both reduced perfusion and FDG uptake at rest (so-called perfusion–FDG match) are consistent with myocardial scar (Fig. 12.6). These metabolic patterns have important implications for selecting patients for revascularization.

Myocardial Neuronal Function

The use of imaging probes designed to evaluate presynaptic and postsynaptic targets of the cardiac autonomic nervous system allows quantification of autonomic function and offers insights into the pathophysiology of a variety of cardiovascular disorders, including CAD. For example, data suggest that quantitative imaging of the cardiac sympathetic nervous system may help identify patients with ischemic heart failure at risk for sudden cardiac death.[22,23] In experimental models of myocardial infarction (MI), the presence of functional sympathetic denervation within areas of viable myocardium identifies sites at higher risk of ventricular tachycardia inducibility.[24] There are emerging clinical trial data suggesting that this approach may provide a useful method for identification of patients at highest risk for sudden cardiac death.[22,23]

Quantification of Left Ventricular Function and Volumes

The acquisition of ECG-gated myocardial perfusion images allows quantification of regional and global systolic function and LV volumes. ECG-gated images are typically collected at rest and post-stress (SPECT) or rest and during stress (PET). Rest LVEF measurements are helpful to define the patient's risk after MI. A drop in LVEF post- or during stress testing can be helpful to identify high-risk patients with multivessel CAD[25] (see Fig. 12.3B).

PATIENT-CENTERED APPLICATIONS OF RADIONUCLIDE IMAGING IN CORONARY ARTERY DISEASE

To understand the efficacy and application of radionuclide MPI, it is important to first have a construct capturing its conceptual underpinnings. The use of noninvasive testing can be defined in the context of what is the underlying question to be addressed by the test. In general, this can be either defining whether obstructive CAD is present (anatomy-based endpoint) or what is the patient's downstream risk of adverse events (risk-based endpoint). The selection of patients for testing, the metrics and potential endpoints for assessing efficacy, and the post-test treatment strategies are determined by which of these are chosen.

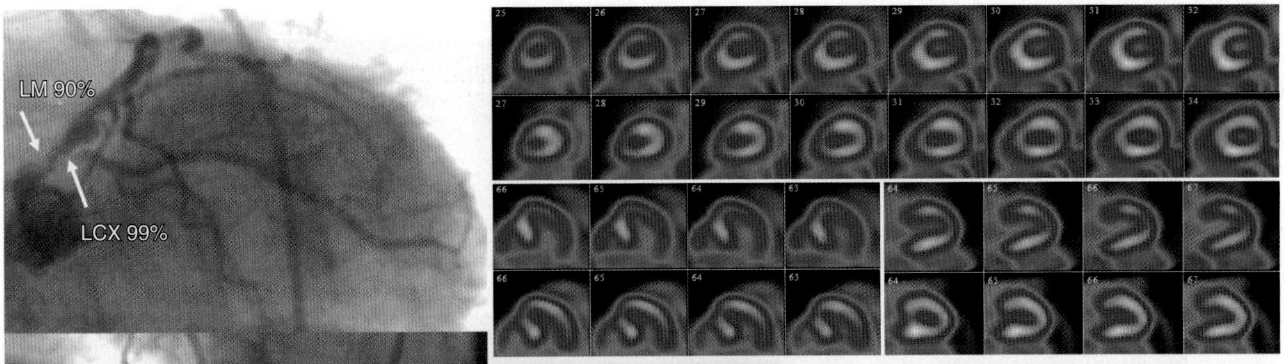

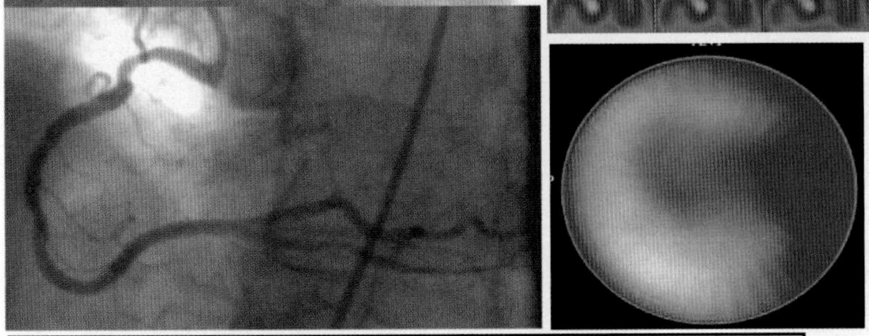

Quantitative myocardial blood flow and CFR

	Rest	Stress	CFR
LAD	1.21	1.19	0.99
LCX	1.16	0.82	0.71
RCA	1.30	1.73	1.33
Global LV	1.22	1.22	1.00

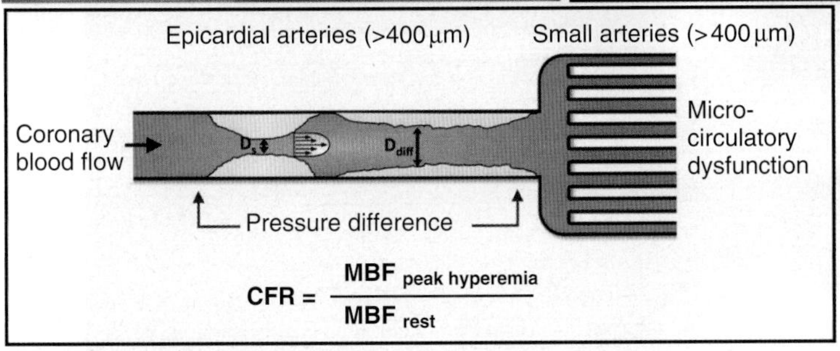

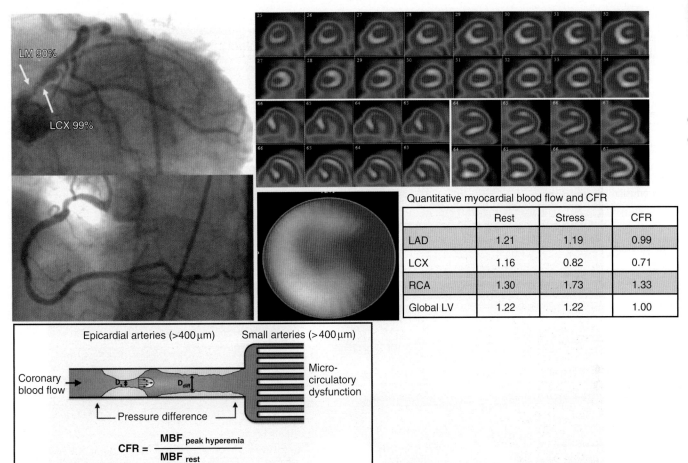

FIG. 12.4 Example of single vessel defect on PET MPI with diffuse abnormal coronary flow reserve (CFR) and left main (LM) disease. Perfusion images (*upper right*) reveal a severe-intensity reversible defect involving the lateral wall at the basal, mid, and distal LV. The CFR data (Table) reveal limitations of flow reserve both in the left circumflex (LCX) and left anterior descending artery (LAD) territories, the latter not evident on the PET MPI images. *Inset below*: Concept of coronary flow reserve. *MBF*, Myocardial blood flow. *(Adapted from Naya et al.[11])*

Appropriateness of MPI for Diagnosis of Angiographic CAD

Historically, the selection of patients for testing has been informed by determination of the patient's pretest likelihood of CAD. This estimate can be based on a variety of nomograms and models. For purposes of simplicity, rather than considering the entirety of the demographic, clinical, and historical information available, the estimates of pretest likelihood of CAD are based on a simplification of the Diamond and Forrester approach incorporating three data elements: patient age, sex, and symptoms. On the basis of these three elements, patients are classified as having low (< 10%), intermediate (10–90%), and high (> 90%) pretest likelihood of CAD. More accurate estimates of pretest likelihood based on more robust approaches would probably enhance the value of this assessment, and a number of other validated algorithms are available, albeit derived and validated in older studies.[26]

Given this estimate, a Bayesian approach, as first put forward by Diamond, is commonly used to identify the potential gain in diagnostic information from testing. This process considers the patient's pretest likelihood of CAD, the diagnostic accuracy of the test (defined by sensitivity and specificity), and the result of testing to yield a post-test likelihood of CAD. Although the greatest certainty with respect to the post-test likelihood of CAD occurs at the extremes of the spectrum (e.g., a negative test in a low pretest likelihood of CAD or a positive test in a high pretest likelihood of CAD patient), the greatest gain in information (magnitude of difference between pretest and post-test likelihood of CAD) occurs in the setting of intermediate pretest likelihood of CAD. For example, a patient with a pretest likelihood of 50% (intermediate) undergoing a test with a sensitivity and specificity of 90% will have a post-test likelihood of 90% (high) after an abnormal test result but a likelihood of 10% (low) after a normal test result. Thus, patients with a low pretest likelihood of CAD should not undergo radionuclide MPI testing because a positive test will increase their likelihood to intermediate and is more likely to be a false-positive than a true-positive result. Similarly, there is an unclear gain in diagnostic information from testing a high pretest likelihood of CAD patient. However, radionuclide MPI in high likelihood patients is sometimes performed to provide risk stratification and/or identification of the culprit vessel to guide revascularization. Hence, for the identification of anatomic endpoints, radionuclide MPI should be limited to those patients at intermediate pretest likelihood of CAD (based on demographic, clinical, historical, and exercise tolerance testing [ETT] data).

There has been a shift to appropriate use criteria (AUC) to define optimal patient selection for noninvasive testing. The recommendations from the 2013 multimodality AUC for the detection and risk assessment of stable ischemic heart disease indicate that in symptomatic patients with intermediate or high pretest likelihood of CAD, irrespective of resting ECG and ability to exercise, it is appropriate to use radionuclide MPI (Fig. 12.7). Additionally, radionuclide MPI is also appropriate in symptomatic patients with uninterpretable

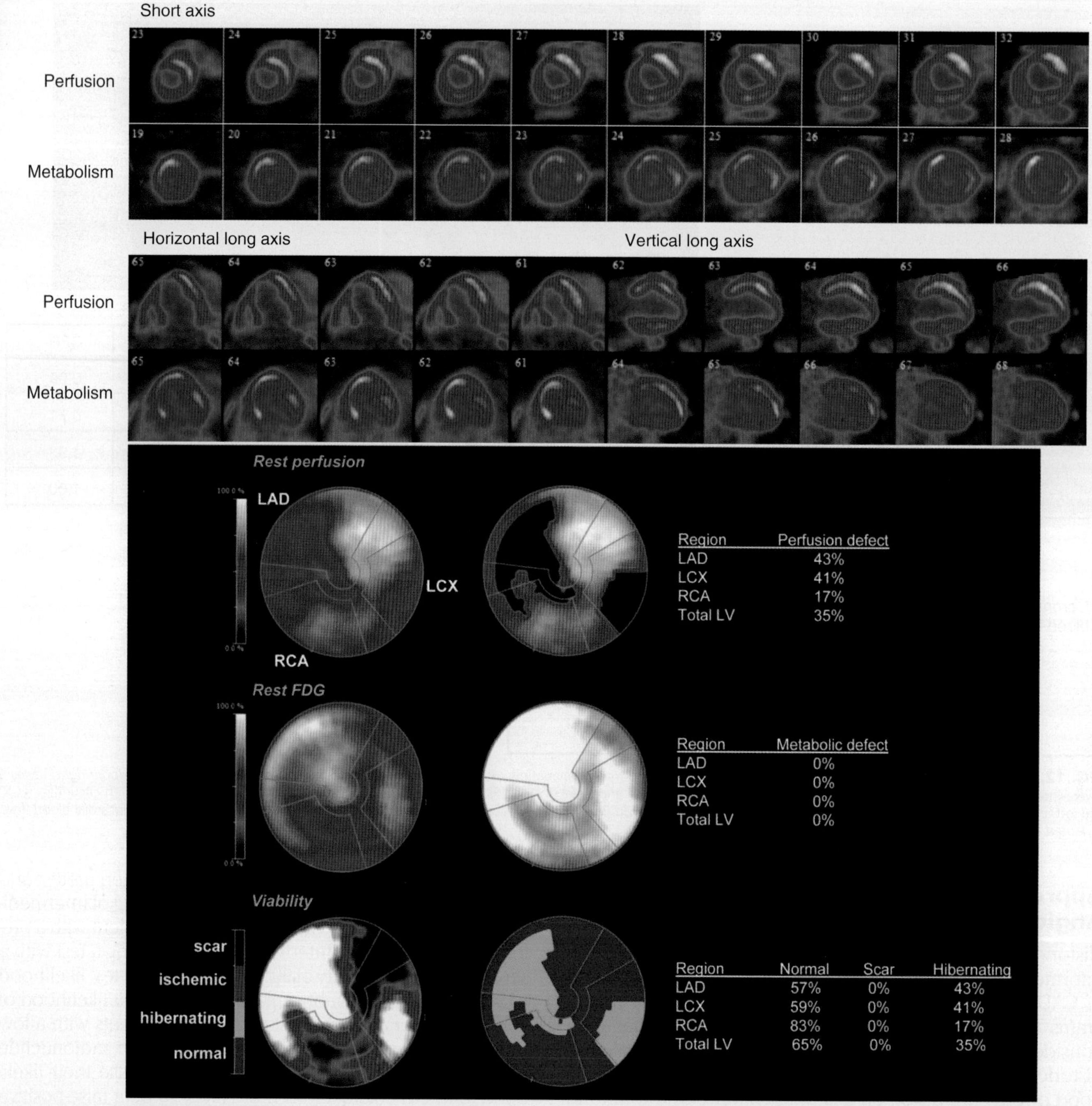

FIG. 12.5 Example of quantification of myocardial viability and scar in ischemic cardiomyopathy using PET MPI. A severe intensity perfusion defect involving the length of the septum to the apex is present on the rest images, with a small, basal inferolateral defect. The ^{18}F-fluorodeoxyglucose [FDG] (metabolism) images reveal uptake in the septal, but not the inferolateral, region, suggestive of hibernating myocardium in the former. *LAD,* Left anterior descending artery; *LCX,* left circumflex artery; *LV,* left ventricle; *RCA,* right coronary artery.

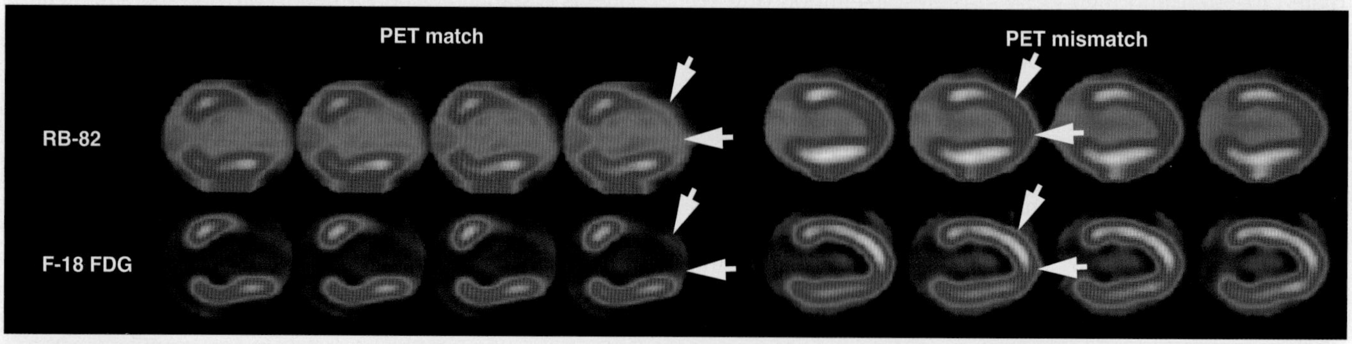

FIG. 12.6 Patterns of positron emission tomography (PET) viability; examples of PET myocardial perfusion imaging (MPI) match and mismatch. On the left, severe-intensity defects of the mid- to distal anterior wall and apex are present on perfusion and metabolism images (match). On the right, a mild resting abnormality in this same region is present with uptake of tracer on the metabolism images (mismatch). *FDG,* ^{18}F-fluorodeoxyglucose; *RB-82,* rubidium-82 chloride. *(From Di Carli MF and Hachamovitch R. New technology for noninvasive evaluation of coronary artery disease.* Circulation. *2007;115:1464-80.)*

resting ECG or who cannot exercise. Finally, in symptomatic patients able to exercise and with interpretable resting ECG, MPI is reported as rarely appropriate.[26]

In the asymptomatic patient, no symptoms or ischemic equivalent (Fig. 12.8), the AUC document considers patients in the context of global risk. Generally, this is defined as low (< 10% 10-year risk), intermediate (10–20% 10-year risk), or high (> 20% 10-year risk).[27] The thresholds for the former two categories are lowered in younger patients, and CAD equivalents can also define patients at high risk. In the setting of high risk (rest ECG interpretable or not, able to exercise or not) in the absence of symptoms, radionuclide MPI was only considered as "may be appropriate." Patients at intermediate risk with uninterpretable rest ECG or unable to exercise are given a similar "may be" rating. In patients at low risk or patients at intermediate risk who have interpretable ECG and can exercise, MPI is considered "rarely appropriate."[26] In patients with known CAD, radionuclide MPI is generally considered appropriate for the evaluation of new symptoms suspected of ischemia regardless of prior revascularization. Radionuclide MPI is considered rarely appropriate in patients with stable CAD without new symptoms.

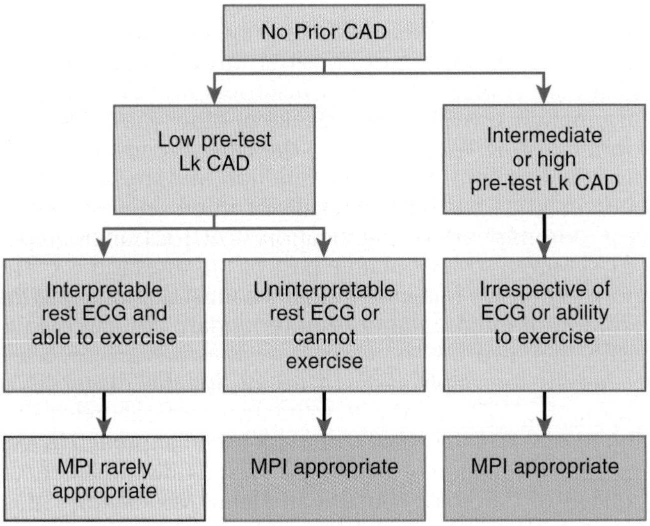

FIG. 12.7 Appropriate use criteria for MPI in symptomatic patients.

Accuracy of Radionuclide MPI for the Identification of Angiographic CAD

The accuracy of diagnostic testing for the identification of obstructive CAD is expressed in terms of sensitivity, specificity, and positive and negative predictive value. The threshold of abnormality on invasive angiographic results, the accepted gold standard, is either 50% or 70% in one or more coronary arteries. Left main (LM) coronary disease is usually defined on the basis of a 50% stenosis. An extensive literature exists defining the diagnostic accuracy of radionuclide MPI. This encompasses both SPECT and PET imaging, using different techniques, and for patients representing various subgroups.

A large meta-analysis examined the diagnostic accuracy of stress SPECT MPI for detecting obstructive CAD as defined by invasive coronary angiography.[28] This analysis examined 86 studies (10,870 patients) published between 2002 and 2009, with pooled accuracy estimates for various SPECT MPI subgroups. "Traditional" SPECT MPI (63 studies; performed without ECG gating or correction of soft tissue attenuation) had a sensitivity and specificity of 87% and 70%, respectively. The addition of ECG gating (19 studies) and attenuation correction (12 studies) increased specificity to 78% and 81%, respectively. Comparisons between ^{99m}Tc and ^{201}Tl, exercise versus pharmacologic stress, qualitative versus quantitative interpretation, 50% versus 70% thresholds, or history of prior MI were all nonsignificant.

Compared with SPECT MPI, meta-analyses[29,30] and a prospective European multicenter study (Evaluation of Integrated CAD Imaging in Ischemic Heart Disease—EVINCI)[31] suggest that PET MPI has higher sensitivity and overall accuracy for detecting obstructive angiographic stenosis. Furthermore, a 2015 meta-analysis using fractional flow reserve (FFR) rather than invasive angiography as a gold standard demonstrated higher sensitivity, specificity, and negative and positive predictive value for PET over SPECT MPI.[32] In this analysis, PET's performance at excluding abnormal FFR was comparable to cardiac MRI and CT and superior to both SPECT and echocardiography (Fig. 12.9). As discussed previously, one additional advantage of PET over SPECT is that it allows routine quantification of myocardial blood flow and coronary flow reserve. These quantitative measures of myocardial

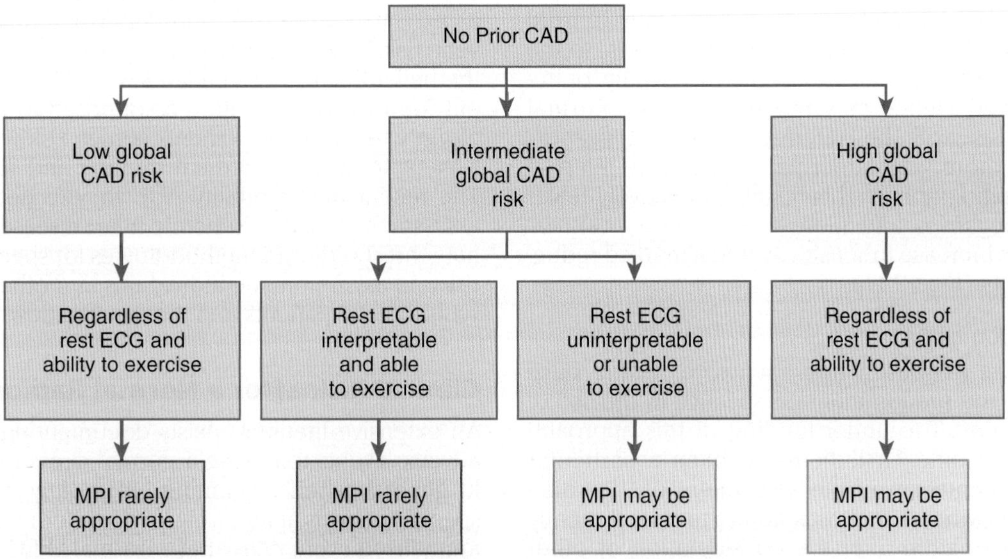

FIG. 12.8 Appropriate use criteria for MPI in asymptomatic patients.

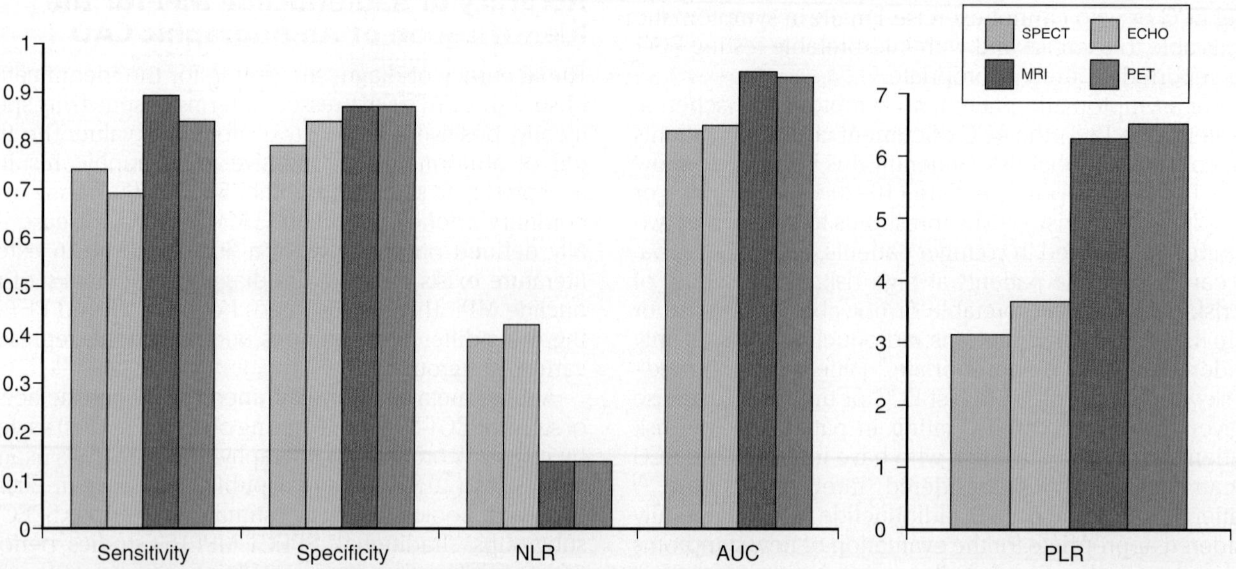

FIG. 12.9 Patient-level accuracy of noninvasive imaging methods for detection of fractional flow reserve (FFR)-positive CAD. *AUC*, Appropriate use criteria; *NLR*, neutrophil to lymphocyte ratio; *PLR*, platelet to lymphocyte ratio. *(Data from Takx RA, Blomberg BA, El Aidi H, et al. Diagnostic accuracy of stress myocardial perfusion imaging compared to invasive coronary angiography with fractional flow reserve meta-analysis.* Circ Cardiovasc Imaging. *2015;8.)*

perfusion improve the sensitivity and negative predictive value of PET for ruling out high-risk angiographic CAD[8–12] (Fig. 12.10). Although older studies reported superior accuracies for SPECT in men compared to women, the use of PET or SPECT with newer technology has largely eliminated this difference.[28,33] In general, the challenges to accurate SPECT MPI detection of ischemia occur with smaller hearts and the presence of increased tissue for photons to transverse (e.g., breast tissue in women, obese patients). In symptomatic patients without documentation of angiographic stenosis, PET MPI is helpful for identifying the presence and quantifying the severity of diffuse microvascular disease.[34]

Referral Bias and the Estimation of MPI Accuracy

The reported accuracies of noninvasive testing modalities are limited by the referral biases intrinsic to the design of most studies in this area, including the population from which patients were drawn, test selection, intersite variability in referral patterns, and especially partial verification bias. The latter refers to selective referral to the gold standard (catheterization) based on the results of the test being studied. Hence, very few patients with normal noninvasive tests will be referred to catheterization, whereas many more with abnormal tests will be referred for coronary angiography.[35] This results in relatively fewer true- or false-negatives and more true- or false-positives, yielding a slight increase in sensitivity and a marked reduction in specificity (Fig. 12.11).

Risk Stratification of CAD

Since the 1990s, risk-based approaches to testing have developed into the predominant perspective in the use of noninvasive testing. The understanding of this approach has evolved over time. First, there has been a particular focus on incrementalism in the assessment of the value of testing: that is, what is the test's ability to add clinically meaningful information after the consideration of other previously available information? Hence, the determination of whether radionuclide MPI has prognostic value in a specific patient cohort must consider this prognostic impact within the context of clinical, historical, and demographic information, as well as the results of other previously performed testing. With respect to the latter, the results of resting ECG, baseline LV size and function, and stress ETT have been emphasized, but the results of atherosclerosis testing (e.g., coronary artery calcification [CAC], CT angiography [CTA]) are also legitimately part of the question.[36,37] The more expensive imaging modalities must demonstrate the addition of unique rather than redundant clinical data to justify their use.

Just as the application of testing for the diagnosis of obstructive CAD begins with estimates of patient pretest likelihood of CAD, the first step of a risk-based approach to testing is the estimation of patient risk. Historically, the American College of Cardiology/American Heart Association (ACC/AHA) stable angina guidelines defined risk of hard cardiac events (cardiac death or nonfatal MI), with specific thresholds of low risk as less than 1%/year risk, intermediate risk as a 1% to 3%/year risk, and high risk as a greater than 3%/year risk.[38] Conceptually, these thresholds were based on the belief that low-risk patients would be least likely to benefit from revascularization as opposed to medical therapy alone, whereas those patients at high risk would most likely benefit from both medical therapy and revascularization. The recent multimodality AUC for the detection and risk assessment of stable ischemic heart disease[26] refers to alternate thresholds and methodologies for specific estimates of risk[27] in asymptomatic individuals and other approaches in symptomatic patients and those with known CAD.[39]

Clinical Risk after a Normal Radionuclide MPI

An extensive literature exists documenting the low risk of adverse events following a normal stress radionuclide MPI. In general, when examining either large patient series or specific cohorts at relatively low or intermediate overall risk, annualized event rates after a normal SPECT or PET MPI are very low, usually less than 1% annual risk of cardiac death

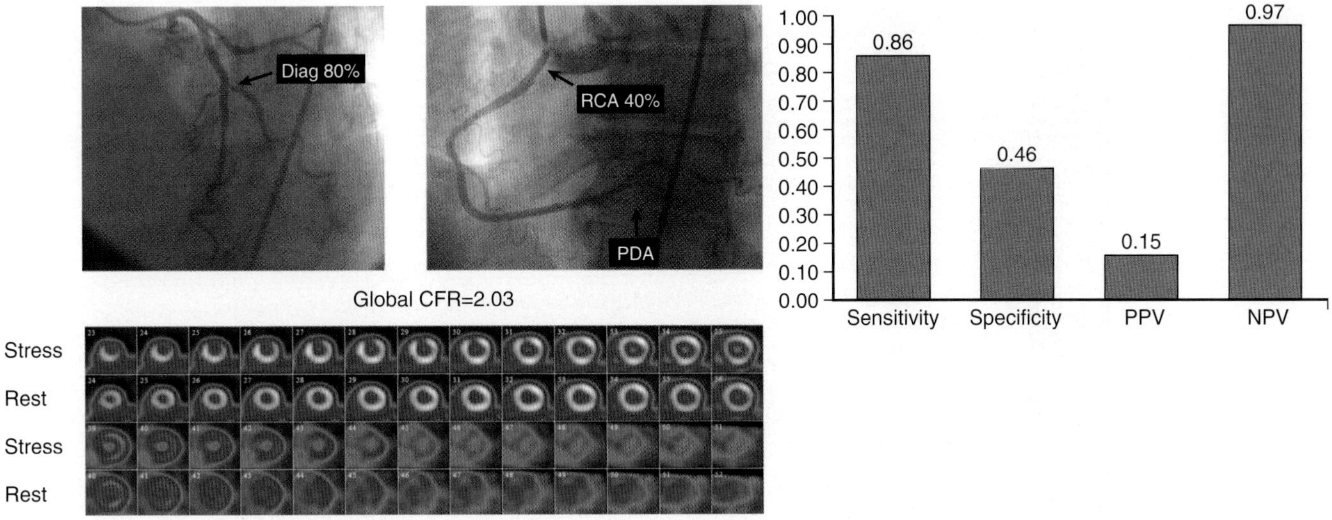

FIG. 12.10 Coronary flow reserve (CFR) measures increase the sensitivity and negative predictive value (NPV) of PET MPI. On the upper left are images from a 66-year-old female with high cholesterol and hypertension with atypical angina. On the perfusion images below is a small reversible defect in the diagonal artery distribution, with a normal global CFR (2.03). On the right, the outstanding NPV of this metric is shown. *PDA,* Posterior descending artery; *PPV,* positive predictive value; *RCA,* right coronary artery. *(Modified from Naya et al. Preserved coronary flow reserve effectively excludes high-risk coronary artery disease on angiography.* J Nucl Med. *2014;55:248–255.)*

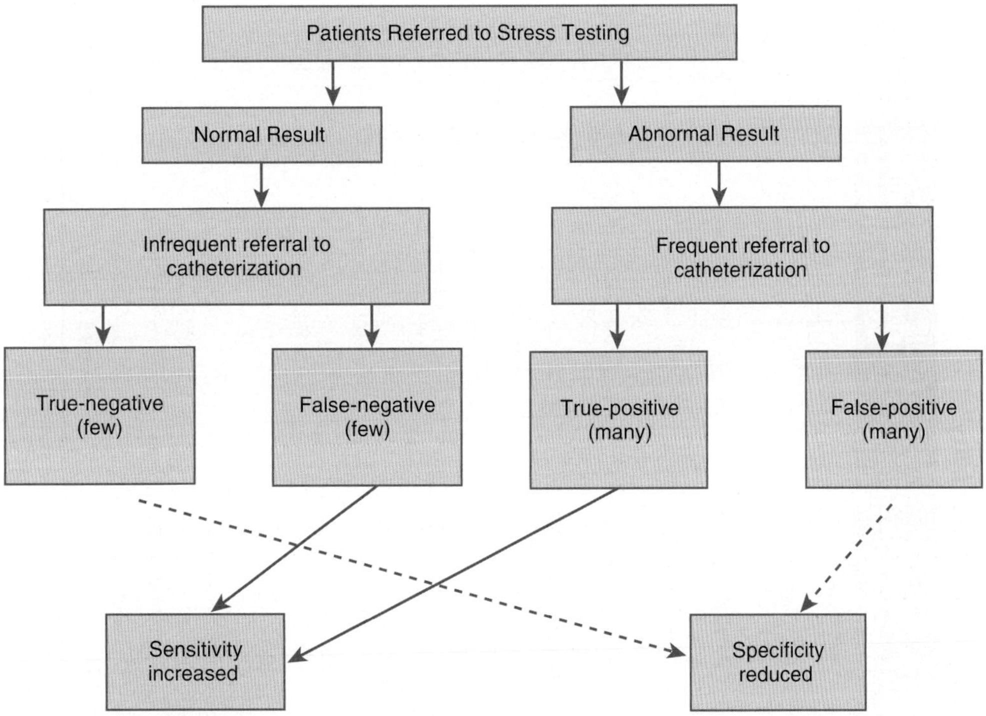

FIG. 12.11 Flow diagram demonstrating the etiology of post-verification bias. Patients with normal testing undergo few referrals to catheterization, resulting in few true- or false-negatives. Patients with abnormal testing results are referred to catheterization far more frequently, resulting in more true- and false-positives. The net result is an increased sensitivity and a reduced specificity.

and often less than 1% annual risk of the combined endpoint of cardiac death or nonfatal MI.[7] In a meta-analysis of almost 40,000 patients, a normal or low-risk rest/stress SPECT MPI was associated with an annual risk of major CV events of 0.6%.[40] Similar results have also been reported after a normal PET MPI.[16,19,25,41–43]

The low risk associated with normal SPECT MPI has been extended to the radiation-sparing, stress-only MPI protocols as well. All-cause mortality in 8034 patients followed for a median of 4.5 years after a normal stress-only SPECT was reported to be lower than in 8820 comparative patients undergoing stress-rest protocols.[44] These findings have been confirmed by other authors.[45–47]

Whereas the risk associated with a normal MPI is generally low, this is not necessarily the case in higher-risk cohorts (e.g., diabetes, chronic kidney impairment, elderly); that is, a normal scan is not always associated with low risk (Table 12.4).[6,7,39,48–50] This may be related in part to the presence of associated comorbidities that increase clinical risk, and that this increased hazard cannot be quantified by the results of the radionuclide MPI study. Another possibility is that notwithstanding the clinical utility of SPECT MPI, it is a somewhat insensitive test to uncover diffuse atherosclerosis and/or microvascular dysfunction associated with myocardial ischemia and increased risk of adverse events. For example, quantification of global coronary flow reserve by PET—an

TABLE 12.4 Risk after MPI by Degree of Perfusion Abnormality

STUDY	MODALITY	ENDPOINT	SUBGROUP	EVENT RATE AFTER NORMAL STUDY	EVENT RATE AFTER MILDLY ABNORMAL STUDY	EVENT RATE AFTER MODERATE TO SEVERELY ABNORMAL STUDY	FU (YEARS)
Hachamovitch et al.[49]	SPECT	CD	Age 75–84 yr	1.0%/yr (2332)	1.7%/yr (785)	4.9%/yr (1201)	2.8 ± 1.7
			Age ≥ 85 yr	3.3%/yr (443)	4.0%/yr (183)	11.1%/yr (256)	
			Pharmacologic stress; age ≥ 75 yr	1.9%/yr (1526)	2.7%/yr (609)	7.8%/yr (907)	
			Exercise stress; age ≥ 75 yr	0.7%/yr (1249)	1.0%/yr (359)	2.7%/yr (550)	
			Normal rest ECG	0.4%/yr (783)	0.9%/yr (169)	1.1%/yr (110)	
			Abnormal rest ECG	1.7%/yr (1992)	2.3%/yr (799)	6.3%/yr (1347)	
			Prior CAD; age ≥ 75 yr	1.8%/yr (682)	2.3%/yr (491)	6.6%/yr (1009)	
			No prior CAD; age ≥ 75 yr	1.2%/yr (1115)	1.8%/yr (477)	4.3%/yr (448)	
Kang et al.[119]	SPECT	CD	BMI < 25	0.8%/yr (605)	2.2%/yr (378)	4.0%/yr (882)	3.2 ± 2.0
			BMI 25–29.9	0.4%/yr (642)	0.8%/yr (405)	2.9%/yr (982)	
			BMI ≥ 30	0.4%/yr (272)	1.3%/yr (180)	2.2%/yr (374)	
Sood et al.[120]	SPECT	CD, NFMI, UA leading to hospitalization, or late revascularization	Low DTS in women	1.2%/yr (995)	1.5%/yr (55)	5.2%/yr (12)	2.4 ± 1.2
			Intermediate DTS in women	1.5%/yr (1012)	5.3%/yr (71)	10.8%/yr (23)	
Dorbala et al.[41]	PET	CD	Consecutive series	0.2% (664)	1.3% (381)	8.3% (387)	1.7 ± 0.7
		All cause death		3.5% (664)	6.1% (381)	16.5% (387)	

BMI, Body mass index; *CAD*, coronary artery disease; *CD*, cardiac death; *DTS*, Duke treadmill score; *NFMI*, nonfatal myocardial infarction; *PET*, positron emission tomography; *SPECT*, single photon emission computed tomography; *UA*, unstable angina.

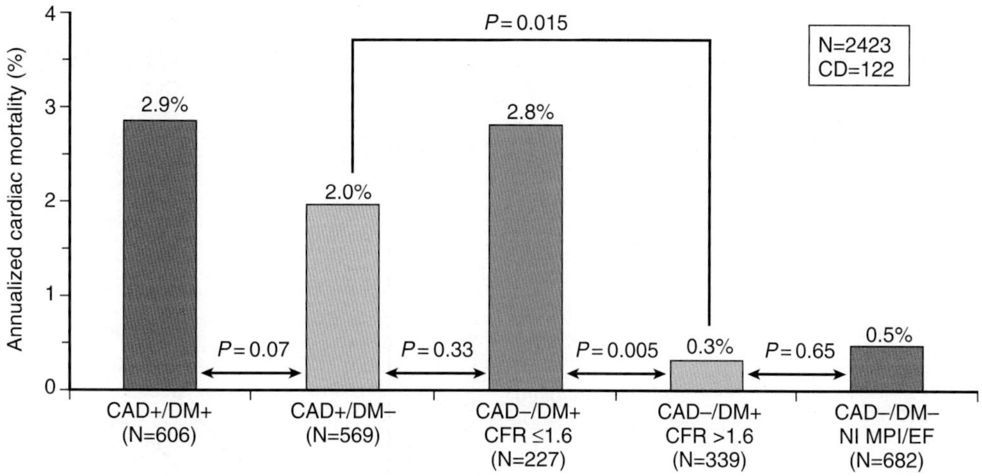

FIG. 12.12 Annualized cardiac mortality rates in patients (*N* = 2423) with diabetes mellitus (DM) or CAD (prior MI, PCI, or CABG). Results shown in patients with both CAD and DM (*purple*), patients with CAD but without DM (*yellow*), without CAD but with DM with abnormal CFR (*blue*), without CAD but with DM with normal CFR (*green*), and without CAD or DM with normal MPI perfusion and LVEF (*red*). *CAD,* Coronary artery disease; *CABG,* coronary artery bypass graft; *CFR,* coronary flow reserve; *LVEF,* left ventricular ejection fraction; *MI,* myocardial infarction; *MPI,* myocardial perfusion imaging; *PCI,* percutaneous coronary intervention. *(From Murthy VL, Naya M, Foster CR, et al. Association between coronary vascular dysfunction and cardiac mortality in patients with and without diabetes mellitus.* Circulation. *2012;126:1858–1868.)*

integrated marker of epicardial stenosis, diffuse atherosclerosis, and microvascular dysfunction—was able to identify truly low-risk individuals among patients with diabetes.[15] Indeed, diabetics without known CAD with abnormal CFR had a cardiac mortality risk similar to nondiabetics with known CAD, whereas those with relatively preserved CFR had an annual risk of less than 1% that was comparable to subjects without diabetes or CAD (Fig. 12.12). Similar findings have been shown by adding a coronary artery calcium score in patients with normal MPI.[36,51] Prognostic predictions in the elderly population also highlight the need for appropriate risk thresholds in formulating a risk estimate. For example, although the absolute risk after a normal SPECT MPI in a very elderly population was far greater than the conventionally accepted threshold of 1%/year, the risk of an elderly patient with a normal MPI was still lower than that of a similarly aged individual in the general US population.[49]

It is also important to note the *duration* of this low risk, the so-called "warranty period" of a normal scan. As initially described by Hachamovitch et al. in a general population, and later confirmed in a diabetic cohort, a patient history of prior CAD, sex, diabetes, the type of stress used (ability to walk on a treadmill), and age all influence this temporal component of risk.[6,48,52] These results suggest that patients at low clinical risk with little or no symptoms are at very low risk after a normal MPI, and this low risk persists for a number of years afterward.[53,54] However, it must also be noted that many of these patients were probably not candidates for MPI due to their low risk; thus, the "warranty" of a normal radionuclide MPI in clinically appropriate studies is unclear. Nonetheless, patients with normal radionuclide MPI without prior CAD, without significant symptoms, or able to exercise will be at very low risk for a number of years after initial testing, suggesting that retesting will have a low yield in the absence of a change in symptom status.

Clinical Risk after Abnormal Radionuclide MPI

The risk associated with an abnormal radionuclide MPI study is not only greater than that after a normal MPI but also increases as a function of the extent and severity of perfusion abnormalities (Fig. 12.13; see Table 12.4).[5,6,39,55] This concept is applicable to all radiotracers and scans (SPECT and PET), all forms of stress testing, as well as to a wide variety of patient cohorts. Similarly, numerous studies have shown the results of radionuclide MPI to yield incremental prognostic value over preimaging data. Thus, generally speaking, a mildly abnormal radionuclide MPI (defined as an abnormal study with < 10% of the myocardium abnormal) is associated with greater risk than that after a normal study, but the absolute risk of cardiac death tends to be low (< 1%/year), and the short- to intermediate-term risk is predominantly that of nonfatal MI and/or CV hospitalization. In the setting of moderately and severely abnormal radionuclide MPI results, the risk of cardiac death increases to intermediate and high levels. As previously outlined in the setting of normal test results, it is important to consider that the absolute risk associated with any level of abnormal radionuclide MPI result will be determined by the characteristics of the underlying population examined. Thus, whereas a mildly abnormal radionuclide MPI is generally considered low risk, in a cohort of patients with higher baseline clinical risk, the presence of increased age or need for pharmacologic stress is associated with a relatively high annual cardiac death (see Table 12.4). The further presence of abnormal rest ECG, prior CAD, or other high-risk scan findings (e.g., TID, resting or stress-induced LV dysfunction) further increases patient risk.

It must also be noted that not all radionuclide MPI findings carry similar prognostic implications. For example, fixed defects (and the presence of often-associated LV dilatation and reduced LV function) have been found to be associated with a greater risk of cardiac death than are reversible or ischemic defects, whereas the latter are more closely associated with the occurrence of nonfatal MI. The constellation of extensive myocardial scar, LV remodeling, and reduced ejection fraction represents the highest-risk subgroup.

A 2013 observational multicenter registry has also shown that the concept of progressive risk stratification demonstrated with SPECT MPI abnormalities is also applicable to PET studies.[42,43,56] In a study of 7061 patients with known or suspected CAD from four sites (median follow-up 2.2 years), stress PET results added incremental value over preimaging

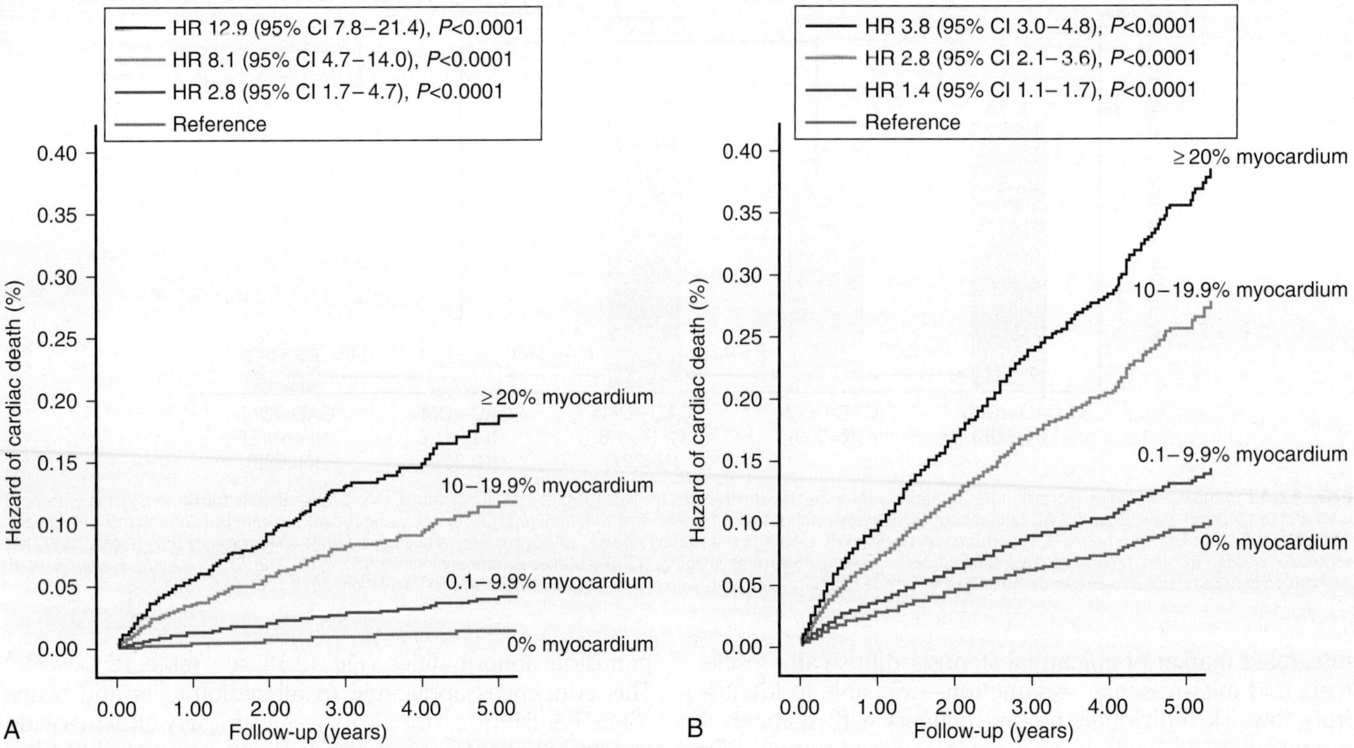

FIG. 12.13 Risk-adjusted hazard for cardiac death (**A**, 6037 patients) and all-cause death (**B**, 7061 patients). Risk was least in the setting of a normal PET MPI and increased progressively with worsening extent and severity of stress perfusion results. *(From Dorbala S, Di Carli MF, Beanlands RS, et al. Prognostic value of stress myocardial perfusion positron emission tomography: results from a multicenter observational registry.* J Am Coll Cardiol. *2013;61:176–184.)*

data for the prediction of cardiac death. Risk-adjusted analyses revealed that mild, moderately, and severely abnormal studies were associated with a stepwise increase in clinical risk (see Fig. 12.13). Furthermore, PET MPI results enhanced net reclassification improvement.[43] A subsequent study from this registry addressed the question of sex-related prognostic differences after stress PET and demonstrated that PET MPI yielded incremental prognostic value in both sexes, which, in turn, were associated with similar magnitudes of risk in men and women. A complementary study from this registry showed that a normal PET MPI was associated with an excellent prognosis with very low annual cardiac death rates in normal (0.38%), overweight (0.43%), and obese (0.15%) patients. As shown for other cohorts, risk increased with increasing degree of perfusion abnormalities in PET MPI.[56]

The use of ECG gating techniques has become an integral part of the radionuclide MPI examination, as this allows assessment of global and regional LV function. The presence of normal LVEF and wall motion has been shown to identify a lower-risk cohort even in the setting of perfusion abnormalities (Fig. 12.14).[41] Conversely, the presence of LV dilatation, wall motion abnormalities either at rest or post-stress, or reduced LVEF, have all been well described as markers of increased patient risk. Indeed, as high-risk markers, information on wall motion and LV function exceed perfusion data for the prediction of high-risk patients.[5,7,26]

The progressive increase in risk with worsening radionuclide MPI results generates progressive gradations in post-MPI patient risk, permitting relatively more detailed estimations of adverse outcomes. However, to achieve enhanced precision of these post-test risk estimates necessitates the incorporation of clinical, historical, and stress test information along with MPI results in formulating an estimate of risk. A prognostic score has been developed for patients undergoing vasodilator stress that incorporates clinical, historical, and stress test results as well as perfusion data to generate more precise estimates of short-term mortality risk (Table 12.5).[57] In distinction to SPECT MPI, post-PET MPI prognostic assessment also includes other risk markers, including a drop in LVEF during stress compared to rest and the presence of a globally reduced coronary flow reserve.[16,25,41,43]

As discussed previously, the other important quantitative component of stress PET MPI is the ability to accurately quantify regional and global myocardial blood flow at rest and during peak stress and estimate coronary flow reserve. A large 2011 study examined the incremental prognostic value of this measure in a large cohort of 2783 patients who underwent stress PET MPI and were followed up for a median of 1.4 years (interquartile range [IQR] 0.7–3.2 years) for cardiac death.[16] After adjusting for multiple factors, including rest LVEF, summed stress score, and LVEF reserve, CFR was prognostically important. Compared with the highest tertile of CFR, the lowest tertile had a hazard ratio of 5.6 (95% confidence interval [CI], 2.5–12.4; $p < 0.0001$) and the middle tertile had a hazard ratio of 3.4 (95% CI, 1.5–7.7; $p = 0.003$). These results were confirmed by a similar study in a smaller cohort followed for slightly more than 1 year.[19] As discussed, the noninvasive PET measure of CFR has been able to improve risk classification, especially among high-risk cohorts (e.g., diabetics, non-ST-elevation MI, in patients with chronic renal impairment, and in those with high coronary calcium scores).[58–60] Thus, the ability to assess CFR appears to permit a level of risk assessment beyond that achieved previously, with the potential to incorporate vascular/endothelial status into routine patient investigations.

This ability to quantify CFR extends the potential for evaluation of risk to those patients in the past not considered to be candidates for testing. Even in patients without CAD

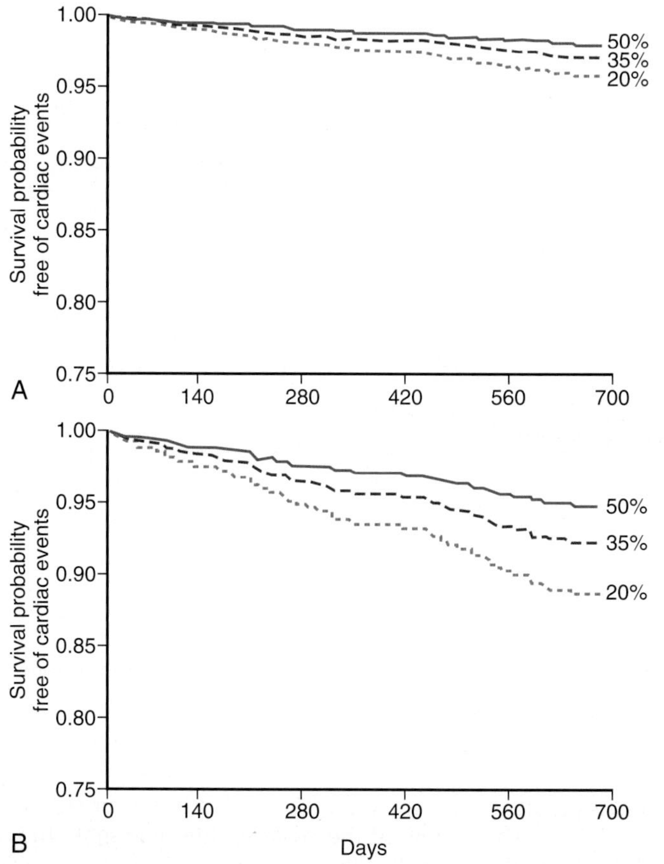

FIG. 12.14 Predicted survival free of cardiac events as a function of resting left ventricular ejection fraction (LVEF) and the extent and severity of ischemia on PET MPI. Survival predicted by multivariable modeling as a function of varying degrees of LVEF with **(A)** no ischemia and **(B)** severe ischemia. For any degree of ischemia, survival progressively worsened with decreasing LVEF and, conversely, improved with decreasing ischemia for any degree of LV function. *(From Dorbala S, Hachamovitch R, Curillova Z, et al. Incremental prognostic value of gated Rb-82 positron emission tomography myocardial perfusion imaging over clinical variables and rest LVEF.* JACC Cardiovasc Imaging. *2009;2:846–154.)*

and with normal LV function, after adjusting for multiple confounders, impaired CFR was associated with both the occurrence of a positive troponin and with major downstream adverse events.[59] Using PET-derived CFR, the prognostic impact of coronary microvascular dysfunction was assessed in 405 men and 813 women who were identified as having no prior CAD, as well as no perfusion abnormalities on their PET MPI studies.[34] Coronary microvascular dysfunction, defined as a CFR less than 2.0 mL/g/min in these patients, was a frequent finding in both men and women (51% and 54%, respectively) (Fig. 12.15). Patients were followed for a median of 1.3 years for the composite endpoint of cardiac death, nonfatal MI, late revascularization, and hospitalization for heart failure. In both men and women, CFR added incremental prognostic value (hazard ratio of 0.80 [95% CI 0.75–0.86] per 10% increase in CFR) and appropriately reclassified patients with respect to risk, as assessed by significant net reclassification improvement (NRI). These results suggest that coronary microvascular dysfunction is a widespread finding and that future work is needed to identify its putative role as a therapeutic target.

MANAGEMENT OF CAD

Ideally, the results of noninvasive testing should inform referring physicians as to which post-MPI treatment would

TABLE 12.5 Prognostic Adenosine Score

PARAMETER	MULTIPLIED BY
Age [decades]	5.19
Percent myocardium ischemic [per 10%]	4.66
Percent myocardium fixed [per 10%]	4.81
If diabetes mellitus present, value of 1	3.88
If patient treated with early revascularization, value of 1	4.51
If dyspnea was a presenting symptom, value of 1	5.47
Resting heart rate [per 10 beats]	2.88
Peak heart rate [per 10 beats]	−1.42
Resting ECG score*	1.95
If patient treated with early revascularization, percent myocardium ischemic [per 10%]	−4.47

*Resting ECG score = 0.628 (if "any block" was present) + 0.724 (if left ventricular hypertrophy with repolarization present) + 0.832 (if premature ventricular contraction[s] present) + 0.331 (if nonspecific ST-T wave changes).
The adenosine prognostic score is the sum of the products of the value of the parameters and the multipliers. Based on this score, patients can be categorized as:

- Low risk (< 1% cardiac death risk per year): score < 49 (observed cardiac mortality 0.9%/yr).
- Intermediate risk (1–3% cardiac death risk per year): score 49–57 (observed cardiac mortality 2.8%/yr).
- High risk (> 3% cardiac death risk per year): score > 57 (observed cardiac mortality 6.7%/yr).

Based on Hachamovitch et al.[57]

maximize health outcomes. To date, several avenues of clinical investigations have examined the question of whether the amount of inducible ischemia identified by radionuclide MPI can identify which patients may gain a relative survival benefit with revascularization versus medical therapy alone. Although studies to date have examined the potential to enhance patient survival, optimizing benefit may encompass improved patient perceived well-being, functional capacity, or symptom amelioration.[61]

An initial observational study utilizing survival modeling with a propensity score to adjust for nonrandomization of treatment in 10,627 patients without prior CAD revealed that patients in whom greater than 10% to 15% of the myocardium was ischemic experienced reduced incidence of cardiac death with revascularization compared to medical therapy alone.[5,7,26,62,63] On the other hand, patients with little or no ischemia had improved outcomes with medical therapy alone, although this treatment was not defined prospectively and its nature was unknown. The absolute survival benefit (e.g., lives saved per 100 patients treated) associated with early revascularization increased as the amount of ischemia present increased, as well as with increasing patient risk (increasing age, presence of diabetes, use of pharmacologic stress). These results were extended in a cohort of 5366 patients without prior revascularization in whom LVEF was also available.[63] Although LVEF was a more powerful predictor of cardiac death of any myocardial perfusion metric, only the extent and severity of ischemia on SPECT MPI identified patients in whom there was a potential benefit with revascularization compared to medical therapy. Indeed, in this analysis the use of revascularization eliminated the risk associated with ischemia.[62,63] The finding of enhanced survival with early revascularization versus medical therapy identified by SPECT MPI results was extended to asymptomatic diabetics with high-risk SPECT findings and to a large consecutive series of elderly patients.[49,62,63]

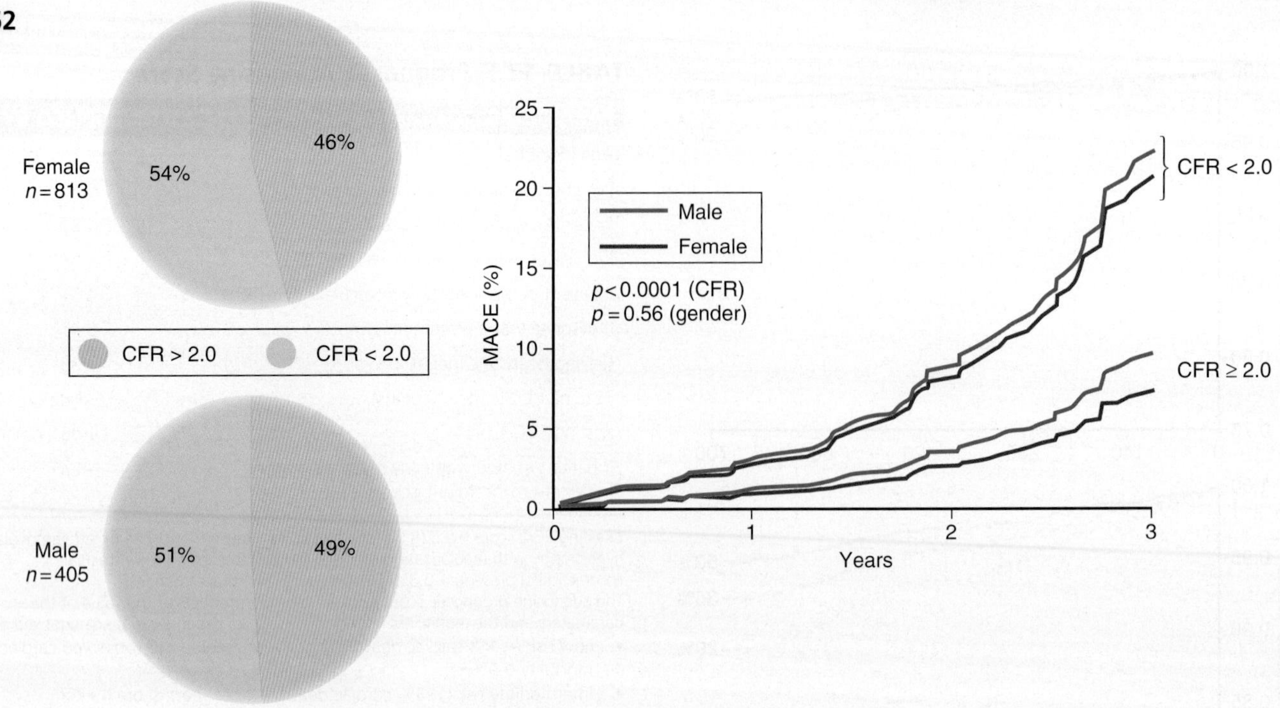

FIG. 12.15 Proportion of coronary microvascular dysfunction occurring in the setting of normal (CFR > 2.0) versus abnormal CFR (CFR < 2.0) as assessed by PET in symptomatic men and women without obstructive CAD. Rates of MACE over 3 years of follow-up in men and women with normal versus abnormal CFR. An abnormal CFR identified increased risk of MACE regardless of sex. *CAD*, Coronary artery disease; *CFR*, coronary flow reserve; *MACE*, major adverse coronary events. *(Modified from Murthy VL, Naya M, Taqueti VR, et al. Effects of sex on coronary microvascular dysfunction and cardiac outcomes.* Circulation. *2014;129:2518–27.)*

The generalizability of these results to patients with known CAD in whom significant amounts of fixed perfusion abnormality (suggestive of scar) is present was addressed by a large observational study of 13,969 patients followed for 8.7 years. The results confirmed the earlier finding of enhanced survival with revascularization over medical therapy in the setting of extensive ischemia in the subset of patients without prior CAD (n = 8791) and extended these findings to patients with prior CAD but without prior MI (n = 1542). Conversely, no such survival benefit with revascularization was found in patients with prior MI (Fig. 12.16).[62–64] However, when analyses excluded patients with fixed defect (scar) greater than 10% of the myocardium, revascularization was found to manifest a survival benefit in the setting of significant ischemia. Thus, it appears that the ability of MPI to identify revascularization candidates may not be impacted as much by prior CAD as it is by the presence of significant myocardial scar. LV volumes probably further confound this relationship, but they have not yet been fully evaluated.[63]

Data from randomized clinical trials have also examined this question. Whereas the overall Clinical Outcomes Utilizing Revascularization and Aggressive Drug Evaluation (COURAGE) trial identified no difference in death or nonfatal MI when patients were treated with medical therapy or percutaneous coronary intervention (PCI) plus medical therapy, the COURAGE nuclear substudy demonstrated a greater reduction in inducible ischemia with PCI combined with medical therapy compared to medical therapy alone in 314 patients.[65] Exploratory analysis of these data revealed that the magnitude of residual ischemia on follow-up radionuclide MPI was proportional to the risk of death, but this analysis was underpowered and risk-adjustment attenuated this finding. Similar results were described in the Bypass Angioplasty Revascularization Investigation 2 Diabetes (BARI 2D) nuclear substudy in that there were fewer perfusion abnormalities in patients assigned to revascularization versus medical management (3% versus 9% of myocardium, p = 0.01).[66] The results of the ongoing International Study of Comparative Health Effectiveness with Medical and Invasive Approaches (ISCHEMIA) trial examining outcomes with optimal medical therapy versus revascularization and optimal medical therapy will yield needed insight into these questions.

Influence of MPI Test Results on Patient Management

Little information is available describing how MPI results influence subsequent clinical decisions. Indeed, it appears that many physicians have presupposed assumptions regarding information provided by MPI that are not based on data.[67] If physicians follow a risk-based strategy, the primary drivers of therapeutic intervention should include the most powerful predictors of risk factors such as LVEF, LV volumes, and the degree of myocardial scar and/or ischemia. However, available data suggest that ischemia is the primary factor influencing referral patterns.

Beginning in the mid-1990s, a series of single-site studies identified a surprising pattern of post-MPI resource utilization as defined by early post-MPI referral rates to catheterization in patients without prior CAD.[62–64,68–70] Although the qualitative pattern of referrals for invasive angiography appeared reasonable—low referral rates after normal MPI, markedly increasing referral rates with worsening perfusion abnormalities—the absolute rates of referral were surprising. Even in the setting of moderate to severe ischemia in patients without prior CAD, referral rates to catheterization did not exceed 50% to 60%.[63,64,69,70] In fact, a recent multicenter prospective registry of patients with suspected CAD in the United States demonstrated that in the setting of the greatest testing abnormalities (and the greatest risk for adverse events), the referral rates to 90-day catheterization after

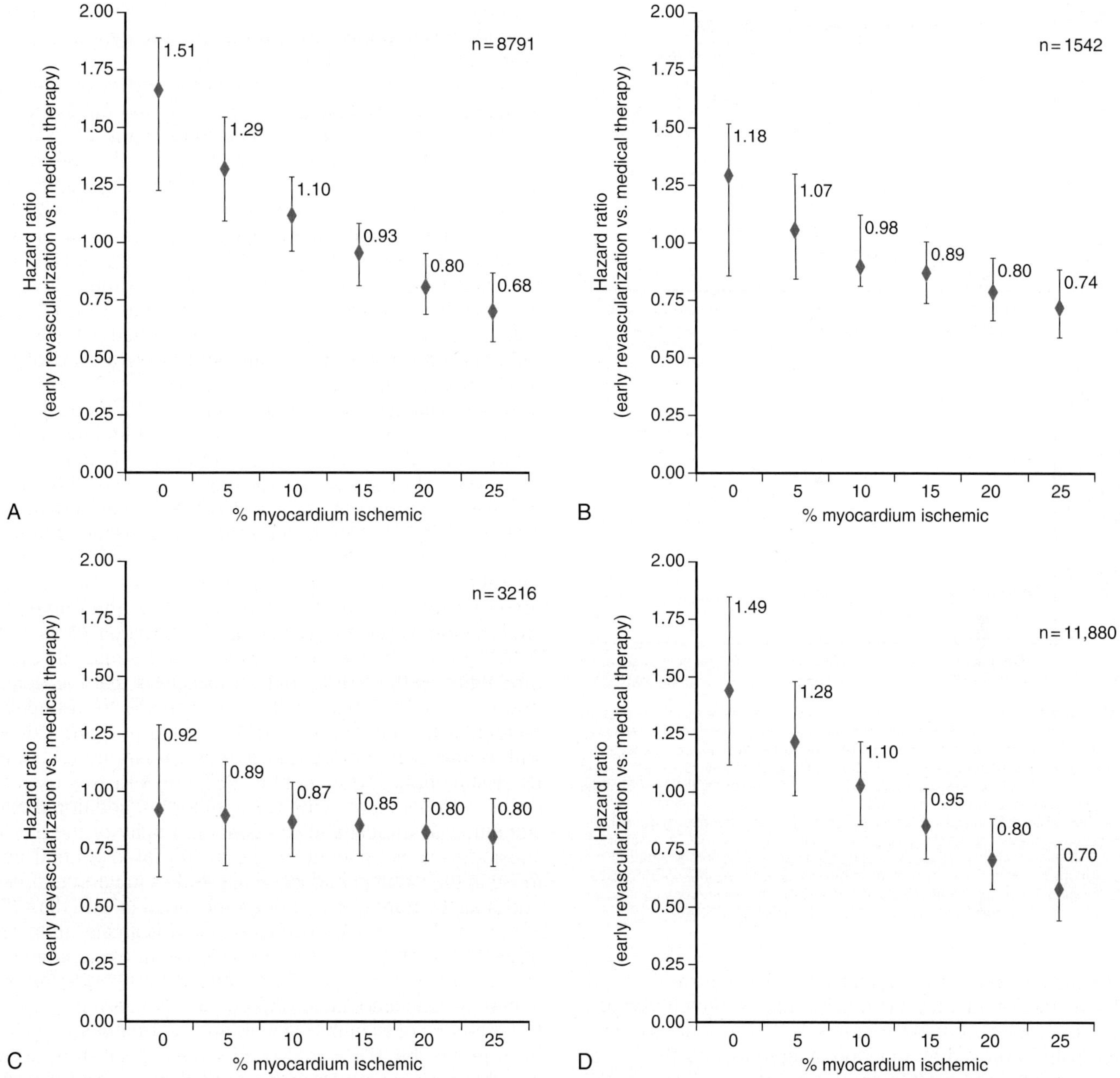

FIG. 12.16 Risk-adjusted hazard ratio based on Cox proportional hazards analysis associated with the use of early revascularization compared with medical therapy at specific values of percent myocardium ischemia: **(A)** in patients without prior CAD (MI or revascularization); **(B)** in patients with prior revascularization, but no prior MI; **(C)** in patients with prior MI; and **(D)** in patients with < 10% myocardium fixed. *(From Hachamovitch R, Rozanski A, Shaw LJ, et al. Impact of ischaemia and scar on the therapeutic benefit derived from myocardial revascularization vs. medical therapy among patients undergoing stress-rest myocardial perfusion scintigraphy.* Eur Heart J. *2011;32:1012–1024.)*

radionuclide MPI or coronary CTA only ranged from approximately 45% to 55% (Fig. 12.17).[69] Surprisingly, this study showed the results of testing did not influence post-test medical management, especially among patients with high-risk test results (Fig. 12.18). Indeed, only one in five patients with severe test abnormalities was receiving aspirin, lipid-lowering agents, and β-blockers 90 days post testing. A similar pattern of post-test management was observed in a recent ancillary analysis of the Prospective Multicenter Imaging Study for Evaluation of Chest Pain (PROMISE) trial.[71] This suggests that the evaluation of the relative prognostic utility of noninvasive imaging testing in patients with stable CAD must include a consideration of post-test change in management and that this may well serve as a quality metric for this previously unmonitored portion of the testing pathway.

MYOCARDIAL ISCHEMIA AND VIABILITY IMAGING TO GUIDE REVASCULARIZATION IN PATIENTS WITH ISCHEMIC LV DYSFUNCTION

Radionuclide imaging has an established role in the evaluation of myocardial ischemia and viability in patients with ischemic heart failure. Several studies using different radionuclide approaches have shown that the gain in global LVEF after revascularization is related to the magnitude of viable myocardium assessed preoperatively. These data demonstrate that clinically meaningful changes in global LV function can be expected after revascularization only in patients with relatively large areas of hibernating and/or stunned myocardium (approximately 20% of the LV mass).

More importantly, there is consistent data from single-center, observational studies demonstrating that the presence

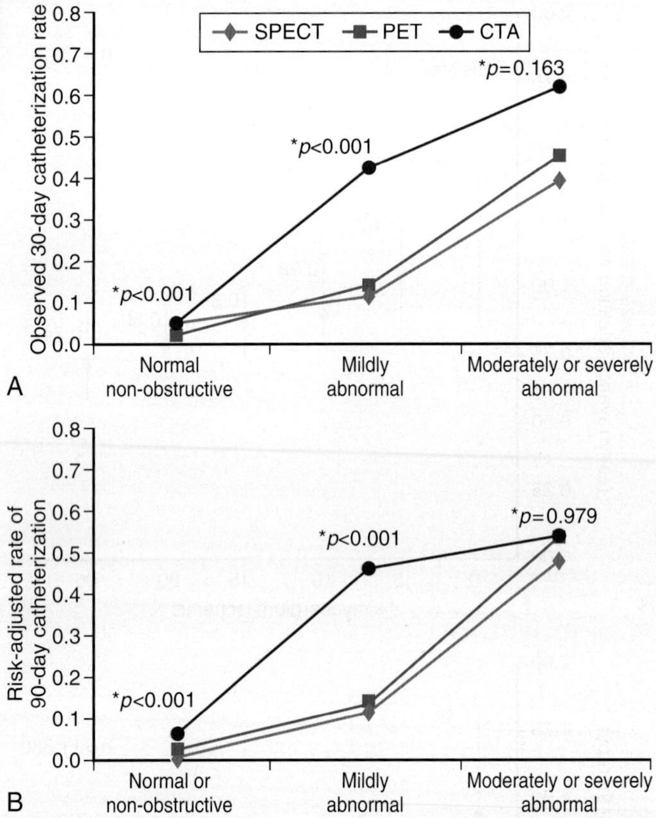

FIG. 12.17 Referral rates to catheterization after noninvasive testing in patients with suspected CAD from SPARC (Study of myocardial perfusion and coronary anatomy imaging roles in coronary artery disease). **(A)** Unadjusted frequency of 90-day catheterization referral after SPECT, PET, and CCTA as a function of test result. Results were significantly different across study results and between CCTA versus SPECT or PET in the setting of both abnormal test results. **(B)** Risk-adjusted 90-day catheterization referral rate after SPECT, PET, and CTA as a function of study result. After risk adjustment, differences were present across categories of test results and between CCTA versus SPECT or PET in the setting of normal and moderately to severely abnormal results. *(From Hachamovitch R, Nutter B, Hlatky MA, et al. Patient management after noninvasive cardiac imaging results from SPARC (Study of myocardial perfusion and coronary anatomy imaging roles in coronary artery disease). J Am Coll Cardiol. 2012;59:462–74.)*

of ischemic, viable myocardium among patients with severe LV dysfunction identifies patients at higher clinical risk and that prompt revascularization in selected patients is associated with improved LV function, symptoms, and survival as compared to medical therapy alone.[72] The randomized PET and Recovery Following Revascularization (PARR-2) clinical trial demonstrated that image-guided decisions regarding revascularization could also help improve clinical outcomes following revascularization if treatment decisions adhere to imaging recommendations.[73]

Nonetheless, the main criticism of those studies is that they were retrospective and medical therapy did not reflect current guideline-directed management of heart failure nor was it standardized in any way. The results of the Surgical Treatment for Ischemic Heart Failure (STICH) trial,[74] especially its ancillary viability,[75] and ischemia[76] substudies have challenged all prior data as they failed to demonstrate a significant interaction between ischemia or viability information, revascularization, and improved survival compared with optimal medical therapy. This casts significant uncertainty as to whether noninvasive characterization of ischemia, viability, and scar can actually provide useful information to guide revascularization decisions in patients with ischemic cardiomyopathy. This issue is currently undergoing intense debate in the medical community.[72,77] As we begin to incorporate the results of the STICH trial into practice, it is important to consider the strengths and weaknesses of the STICH substudies.

The STICH viability and ischemia substudies are the largest reports to date relating myocardial viability and ischemia to clinical outcomes of patients with CAD and LV dysfunction associated with heart failure. They are also the first to assess these relationships prospectively among patients who were all eligible for coronary artery bypass graft (CABG), as well as optimal medical management alone. As previously mentioned, medical therapy in the STICH trial was standardized and followed current published guidelines. However, these studies also have important limitations. First, viability data were only available in half of the enrolled patients, and ischemia information was available in only a third of the STICH trial population, which probably introduced selection bias. Patients in the STICH viability study had higher prevalence of prior MI, lower frequency of limiting angina symptoms, lower LVEF, and more advanced LV remodeling as compared to those who did not receive viability imaging before randomization. Secondly, the definition of viability in the STICH substudy was quite broad, resulting in 81% of the total study population being considered as having "viability" by study criteria. This number is notably higher than that reported in other studies such as the Carvedilol Hibernation Reversible Ischaemia Trial, Marker of Success (CHRISTMAS) trial (59%),[78] which used similar imaging modalities as the STICH trial, and suggests that the definition may not have been sufficiently specific to distinguish patients with ischemic but viable myocardium from those with primarily nontransmural scar or primary nonischemic LV dysfunction. Thirdly, neither PET nor MRI was used to evaluate ischemia or viability. An important additional consideration to understand the generalizability of the STICH substudies is that patients in the main trial in general, and those in the viability and ischemia studies in particular, had end-stage LV remodeling. Indeed, the mean LV end-diastolic volume index (to body surface area) was greater than 120 mL/m^2, and the LV end-systolic volume index approached 100 mL/m^2.[75] This degree of advanced LV remodeling has generally been associated with poor outcomes regardless of the presence of ischemia or viability and treatment applied. In summary, the STICH trial and its imaging substudies suggest that among patients with *heart failure* and *end-stage LV remodeling*, identification of moderate ischemia or viability is not associated with a significant survival advantage from revascularization. Whereas the benefits of optimal medical therapy in patients with ischemic cardiomyopathy are undeniable, we cannot and should not generalize the STICH findings to patients with heart failure, severe systolic dysfunction, but mild-to-moderate LV remodeling, as these patients were not studied in the STICH trial. Indeed, a contemporary observational study from the Cleveland Clinic in patients without advanced remodeling demonstrated that the extent of viability by PET had a significant interaction with revascularization, such that patients with extensive myocardial viability showed improved survival with revascularization compared to medical therapy.[79] As data from randomized clinical trials in such patients are limited, we should continue to carefully integrate clinical, anatomic, and functional information regarding ischemia and viability from noninvasive imaging and individualize these difficult management decisions based on the best available evidence and sound clinical judgment.

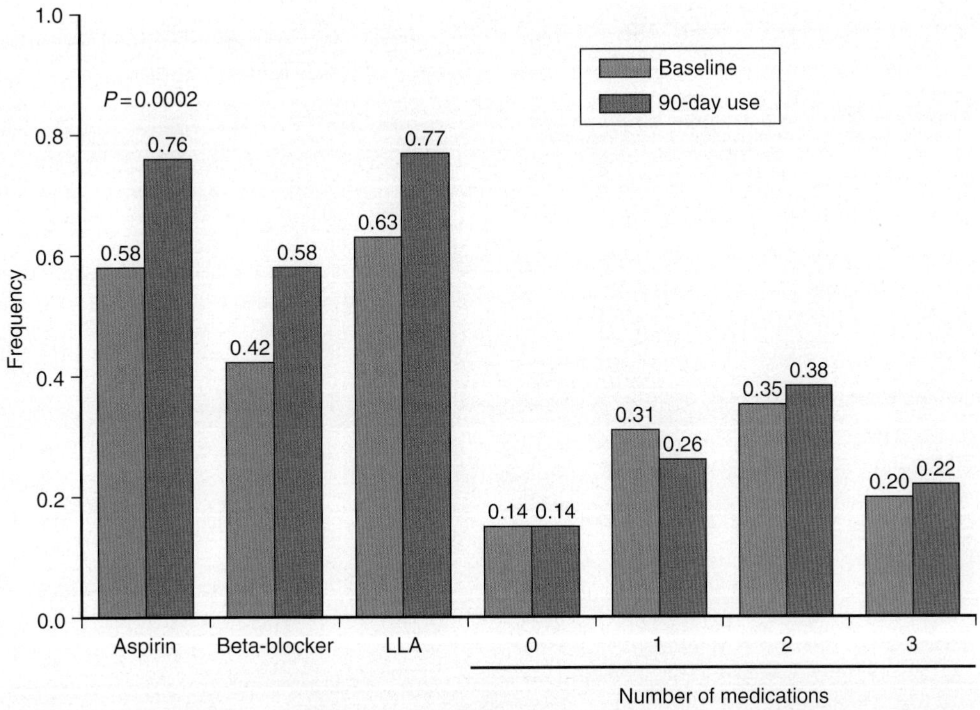

FIG. 12.18 Baseline and 90-day use of medications in SPARC in patients with suspected CAD with moderately or severely abnormal CCTA, SPECT, or PET results. Significant increases in the use of β-blockers and aspirin, but not lipid-lowering agents (LLA), were seen, but even at 90 days many patients were still not on these medications. No difference in the number of these medications used at 90 days was present, with few patients on all three medications. *(From Hachamovitch R, Nutter B, Hlatky MA, et al. Patient management after noninvasive cardiac imaging results from SPARC (Study of myocardial perfusion and coronary anatomy imaging roles in coronary artery disease).* J Am Coll Cardiol. *2012;59:462–474.)*

Estimating Post-MPI Likelihood, Risk, and Potential Benefit with Revascularization

The traditional approach to the assessment of patients after MPI focused on a post-MPI likelihood of CAD (in diagnostic patients) and likelihood of ischemia in patients with known CAD. The previously described shift toward a risk-based approach resulted in an attempt to estimate post-MPI risk of adverse events. Finally, as suggested by the studies already discussed, it may be possible to further extend this work and identify optimal treatment approaches on the basis of MPI results. A series of examples highlighting the potential inconsistencies between estimates of post-MPI likelihood, risk, and benefit with revascularization highlight these issues (Fig. 12.19A–G).

COST-EFFECTIVENESS OF RADIONUCLIDE IMAGING IN THE MANAGEMENT OF STABLE ISCHEMIC HEART DISEASE

With the increasing fiscal pressures brought to bear on the imaging community, the cost-effectiveness or cost implications of cardiac SPECT and PET are an important consideration. In the first multicenter study assessing the cost-effectiveness of radionuclide SPECT MPI, the Economics of Noninvasive Diagnosis (END) study examined cost and outcomes in 11,249 patients referred to SPECT or directly to cardiac catheterization.[80] A SPECT first strategy was found to have reduced costs (a 31–50% cost reduction) with comparative rates of cardiac and nonfatal MI at all levels of pretest clinical risk. The rates of cardiac catheterization, revascularization, and frequency of normal coronary angiographic findings were significantly reduced. These results suggested that compared to a direct strategy of referral to catheterization, initial use of cardiac SPECT was cost saving.

The Cost-Effectiveness of noninvasive Cardiac Testing (CECaT) trial compared the costs and outcomes of four noninvasive strategies (SPECT, cardiac magnetic resonance, stress echocardiography, and catheterization) in 898 patients with planned catheterization.[81] Overall, rates of catheterization were reduced by 20% to 25% by the use of noninvasive testing. Stress SPECT was found to be cost saving compared to cardiac MR and echocardiography with a greater than 70% probability of being cost-effective in bootstrap simulations. Compared to a strategy of direct catheterization, SPECT was more than $500 lower. This further confirmed the findings from END that the use of SPECT in a testing strategy was potentially cost saving.

The previously mentioned Study of myocardial perfusion and coronary anatomy imaging roles in coronary artery disease (SPARC) also reported economic data comparing cost-effectiveness of coronary computed tomography angiography (CCTA), SPECT, and PET.[82] Patients in the PET arm had the greatest downstream costs over the 2 years of follow-up ($6647 per patient), with CCTA having intermediate costs ($4909 per patient) and SPECT the least ($3695 per patient). In a decision analytic model comparing CCTA versus SPECT, the incremental cost-effectiveness ratio was $11,700 per life-year saved.

Finally, the PROMISE trial, a prospective comparison of outcomes in strategies of CCTA versus functional testing (exercise treadmill testing, stress echocardiography, SPECT), also compared the economic consequences of these strategies.[83] Despite the lower testing costs and enhanced efficiency of catheterization use after CCTA, there was no significant difference in overall costs of care after CCTA compared to functional testing. These results were due to the greater use of catheterization and revascularization after CCTA use compared to functional testing.

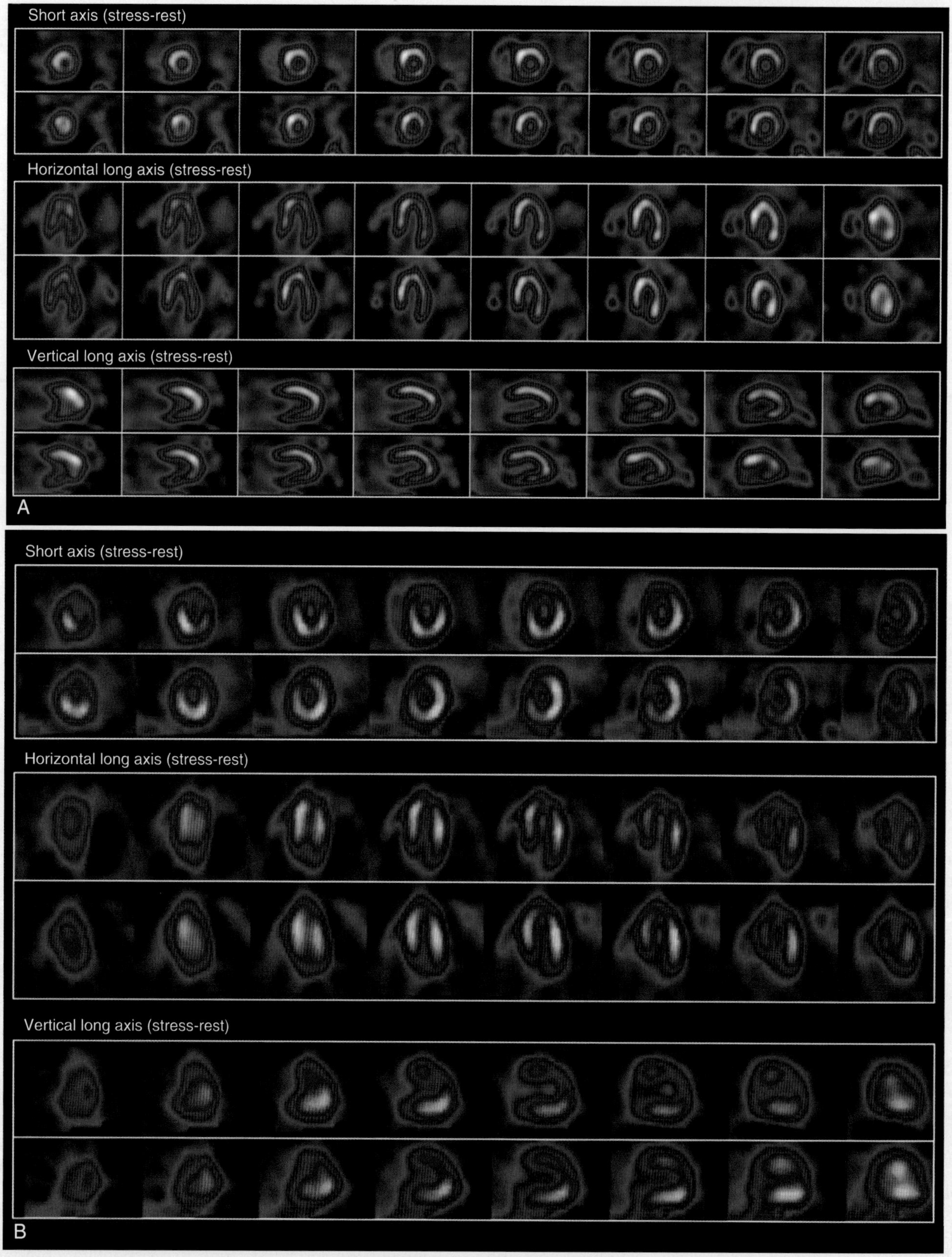

FIG. 12.19 **(A)** A 72-year-old male with hypertension and hypercholesterolemia, presenting with atypical angina, no prior CAD. Normal resting ECG. Exercise stress test (ETT) revealed excellent exercise tolerance without symptoms or ECG abnormalities. Stress perfusion images reveal no perfusion defects. Left ventricular ejection fraction was 65%.

- Pre-ETT likelihood of CAD: high.
- Post-ETT/pre-SPECT likelihood of CAD: intermediate.
- Post-SPECT likelihood of CAD: low.
- Post-SPECT risk of cardiac death: low.
- Potential benefit from revascularization: none, increased risk with revascularization.

(B) A 55-year-old female with diabetes mellitus and hypertension, presenting with atypical angina. Resting ECG showed mild ST-T wave abnormalities. ETT revealed fair exercise tolerance with dyspnea and nondiagnostic ST segment changes. Stress perfusion images demonstrate a medium-size, moderate-intensity reversible perfusion defect involving the mid- and apical anterior and apical lateral walls (9% myocardium ischemic). Left ventricular ejection fraction was 60%.

- Pre-ETT likelihood of CAD: intermediate.
- Post-ETT/pre-SPECT likelihood of CAD: intermediate.
- Post-SPECT likelihood of CAD: high.
- Post-SPECT risk of cardiac death: low.
- Potential benefit from revascularization: none, possibly increased risk with revascularization.

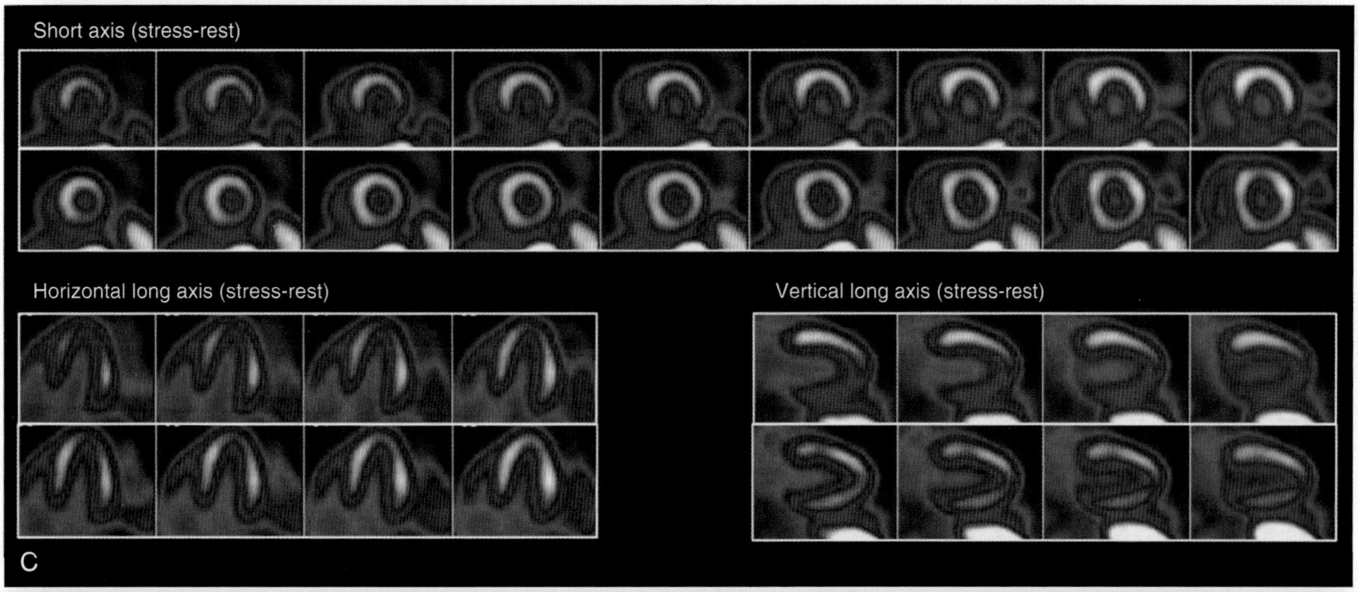

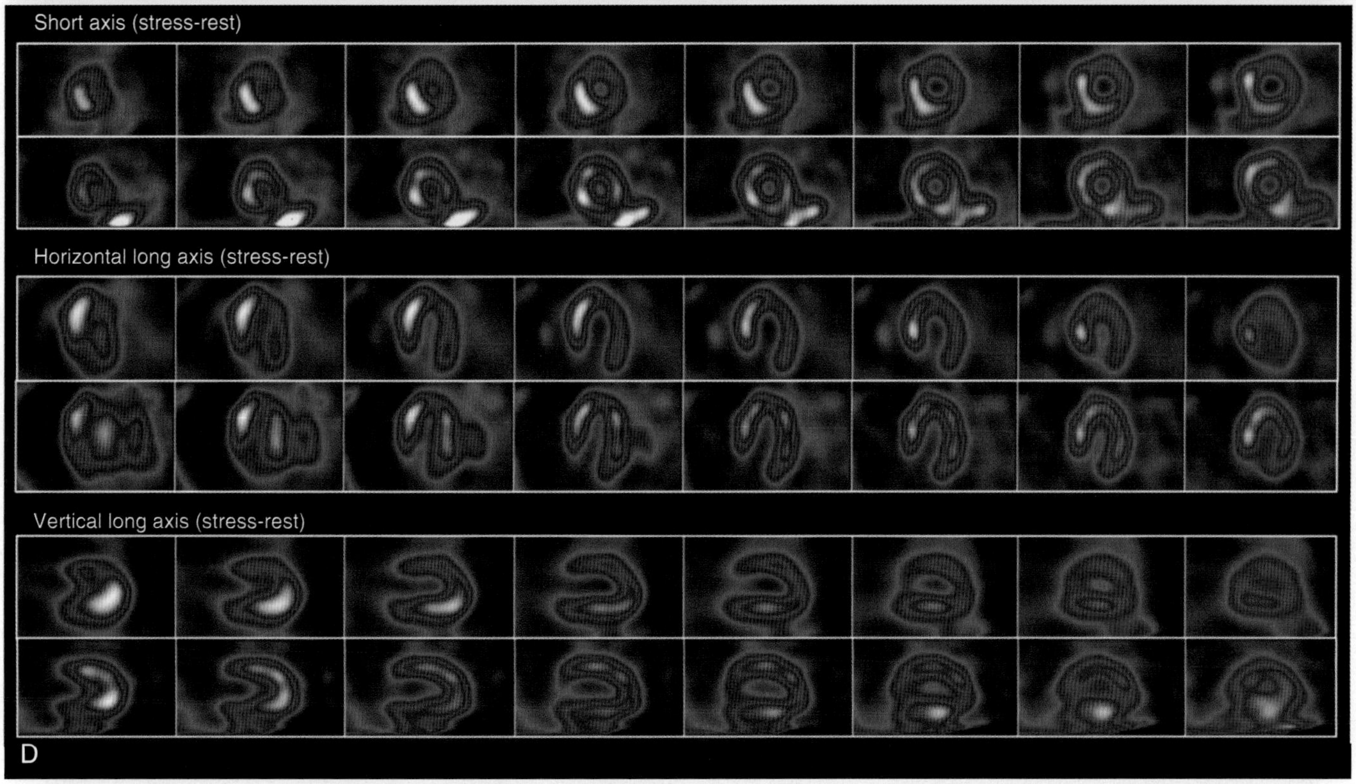

FIG. 12.19, cont'd **(C)** A 72-year-old female with hypertension and hypercholesterolemia, presenting with dyspnea. Resting ECG showed left bundle branch block. A vasodilator stress test revealed no symptoms or ECG changes. Stress perfusion images demonstrate a medium-size perfusion defect of severe intensity throughout the inferior and basal inferoseptal walls, showing complete reversibility (approximately 15% myocardium ischemic). Left ventricular ejection fraction was 72%.

- Pre-ETT likelihood of CAD: high.
- Post-ETT/pre-SPECT likelihood of CAD: high.
- Post-SPECT likelihood of CAD: high.
- Post-SPECT risk of cardiac death: intermediate to high.
- Potential benefit from revascularization: possibly reduced risk with revascularization.

(D) A 63-year-old male with a history of diabetes mellitus, hypertension, and prior coronary artery bypass graft (CABG) presenting with typical angina. Resting ECG showed mild ST-T wave abnormalities. ETT revealed good exercise tolerance with stress-induced angina and ischemic ECG changes. Stress perfusion images demonstrate a large perfusion defect of severe intensity throughout the anterior, anterolateral, and inferolateral walls, showing near complete reversibility (approximately 25% myocardium ischemic). Left ventricular ejection fraction was 57% at rest and drops to 52% post-stress.

- Pre-ETT likelihood of ischemia: intermediate.
- Post-ETT/pre-PET likelihood of ischemia: high.
- Post-PET likelihood of ischemia: high.
- Post-PET risk of cardiac death: high.
- Potential benefit from revascularization: probably reduced risk with revascularization.

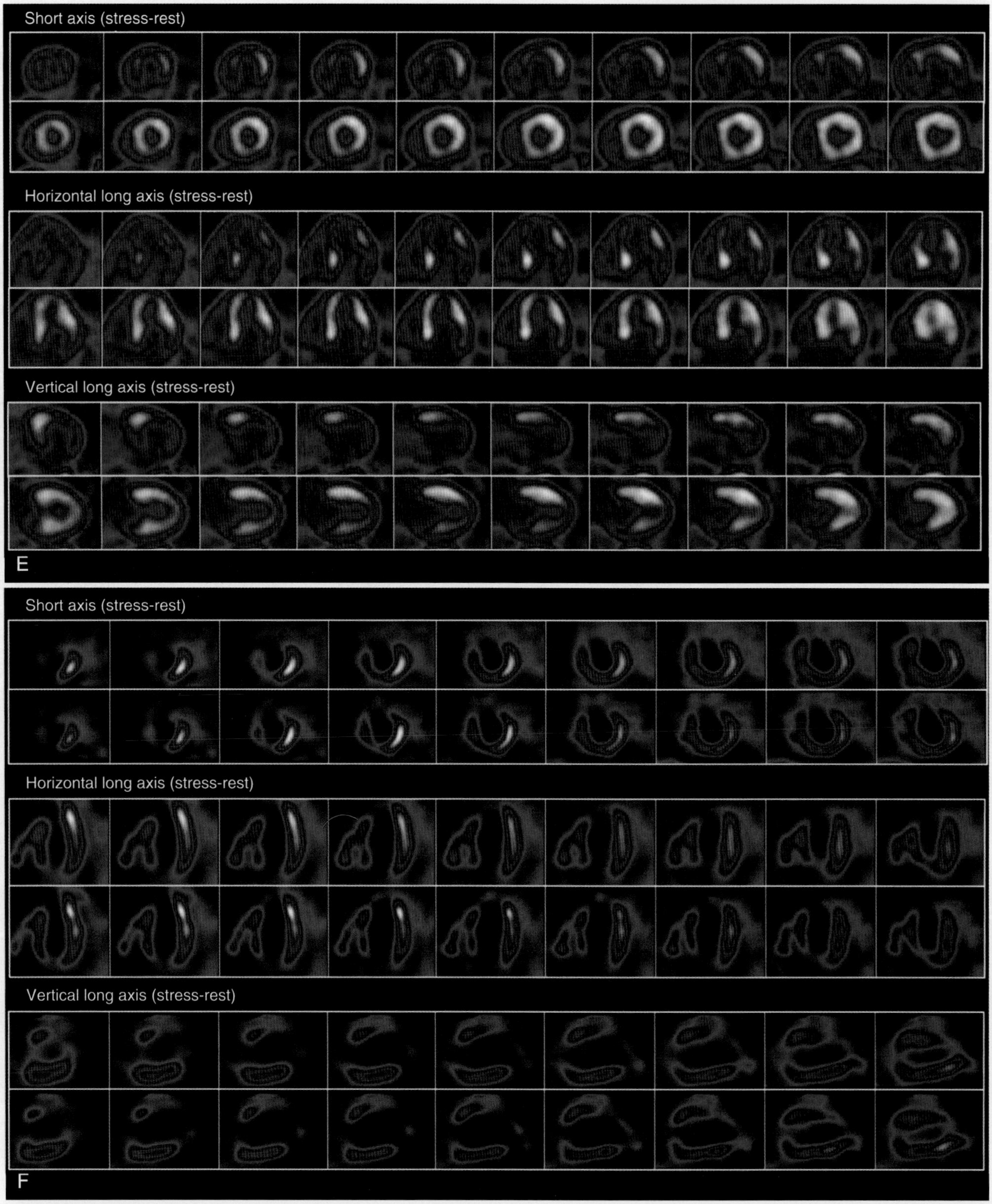

FIG. 12.19, cont'd **(E)** A 51-year-old male presenting with a history of hypertension, hypercholesterolemia, and prior percutaneous coronary intervention (PCI), presenting with dyspnea. Resting ECG showed right bundle branch block and ST-T wave abnormalities. A vasodilator stress test revealed dyspnea and was without ECG changes. Stress perfusion images demonstrate transient cavity dilatation and mildly increased radiotracer uptake during stress. There is a medium-sized perfusion defect of severe intensity throughout the inferior and inferoseptal walls, showing complete reversibility. In addition, there is a medium-size perfusion defect of moderate intensity involving the mid-anterior and anteroseptal walls, all the apical LV segments, and the LV apex, also showing near complete reversibility. Overall, there is > 30% myocardium ischemic. Left ventricular ejection fraction was 37% at rest and dropped to 26% post-stress.

- Pre-ETT likelihood of ischemia: high.
- Post-ETT/pre-SPECT likelihood of ischemia: high.
- Post-SPECT likelihood of ischemia: high.
- Post-SPECT risk of cardiac death: high.
- Potential benefit from revascularization: probably reduced risk with revascularization. Given the reduced LVEF, the absolute benefit associated with revascularization in this patient would be greater than in the patient shown in Fig. 12.19D.

(F) A 66-year-old male presenting with a history significant for prior CABG and multiple myocardial infarctions, presenting with symptoms of heart failure. Resting ECG showed left bundle branch block. A vasodilator stress test revealed dyspnea and without ECG changes. Stress perfusion images demonstrate severe LV dilatation on both stress and rest images. There is a large perfusion defect of severe intensity throughout the anterolateral, anterior, and septal walls, and the LV apex, which is fixed (> 30% scarred myocardium). LVEF was 22% post-stress.

- Pre-ETT likelihood of ischemia: intermediate.
- Post-ETT/pre-SPECT likelihood of ischemia: intermediate.
- Post-SPECT likelihood of ischemia: low.
- Post-SPECT risk of cardiac death: high.
- Potential benefit from revascularization: probably increased risk with revascularization.

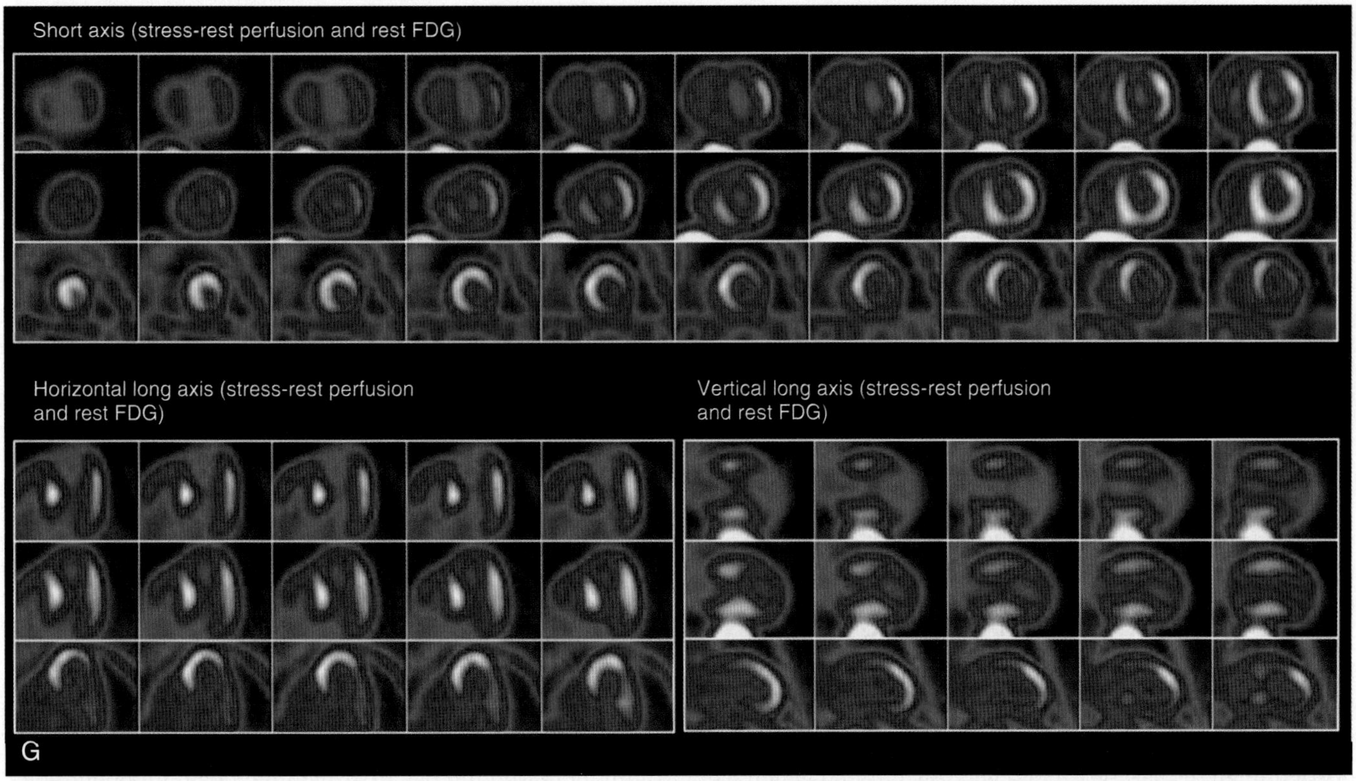

FIG. 12.19, cont'd (G) A 62-year-old female with a history of prior PCI and myocardial infarction, presenting with symptoms of heart failure and possible atypical angina. Resting ECG showed nonspecific intraventricular conduction delay and ST-T wave abnormalities. A vasodilator stress test revealed no symptoms or ECG changes. Images from a PET scan including stress-rest myocardial perfusion and metabolism (FDG) are shown. The stress perfusion images demonstrate a large perfusion defect of severe intensity throughout the mid-anterior and septal walls, the apical LV segments, and the LV apex, showing moderate partial reversibility. The FDG images demonstrate relatively preserved glucose uptake in all hypoperfused LV segments (perfusion–metabolism mismatch). Transient ischemic dilatation post stress is also present. Overall, the findings are consistent with a large territory of combined stress-induced ischemia and hibernating myocardium throughout the mid-LAD territory involving > 20% of the LV myocardium. LVEF was 46% at rest and dropped to 33% at peak stress.

- Pre-ETT likelihood of ischemia: intermediate.
- Post-ETT/pre-SPECT likelihood of ischemia: intermediate.
- Post-SPECT likelihood of ischemia: high.
- Post-SPECT risk of cardiac death: high.
- Potential benefit from revascularization: probably reduced risk with revascularization.

These results suggest that the use of functional testing is not intrinsically less cost- effective than anatomic imaging in patients with suspected CAD. The literature to date suggests that the use of stress radionuclide MPI is a cost-effective approach to the evaluation of the patient with known or suspected CAD.

MANAGING RADIATION EXPOSURE FROM RADIONUCLIDE IMAGING

Radionuclide imaging exposes patients to ionizing radiation. There is growing concern about the potential harmful effects of ionizing radiation associated with cardiac imaging. The "effective dose" is a measure used to estimate the absorbed radiation dose and is expressed in millisieverts (mSv). It is important to understand that measuring the radiation effective dose associated with diagnostic imaging studies is complex, imprecise, and often results in varying estimates, even among experts. The effective dose from a typical SPECT MPI scan ranges between approximately 4 mSv and 11 mSv, depending on the protocol and type of scanner that is used, whereas that for a typical PET MPI scan is lower, approximately 2.5 mSv to 4 mSv. By comparison, the average dose for invasive coronary angiography is approximately 7 mSv, and exposure to background radiation in the United States amounts to approximately 3 mSv annually. In epidemiologic studies, increased risk of cancer has not been observed consistently at "low" effective doses of less than 100 mSv delivered at low dose rates (i.e., over many years, as for most patients undergoing medical imaging). Because estimation of lifetime attributable cancer risk after low-dose radiation studies is difficult, measurements of activation of the DNA damage response pathways have emerged as a surrogate marker of DNA damage. Previous studies have found a strong correlation between the number of DNA double-stranded breaks and the degree of phosphorylation of proteins involved in the DNA damage response pathways after exposure of patients to high doses of radiation (> 100 mSv) in a dose-dependent manner. However, activation of the DNA damage response pathways has been more variable. Indeed, data from 2014 suggest most patients undergoing routine SPECT MPI do not have significant changes in phosphorylation of DNA damage-marker proteins, nor do they show significant changes in mRNA expression of DNA damage response genes in circulating T lymphocytes collected after injection of standard doses of ^{99m}Tc-labeled perfusion agents.[84] In contrast, most, if not all, patients undergoing cardiac catheterization show increased levels of protein markers of DNA damage.[84] This difference in biologic response may be related to the fact that patients undergoing radionuclide imaging receive fractionated radiation dosing with time intervals of 60 to 120 minutes between doses, as opposed to short continued bursts of radiation over a short period of time (typically < 30 minutes).

The introduction of new approaches and technologies to radionuclide MPI since 2014 has opened opportunities for significant dose reduction (i.e., > 50%) without compromising diagnostic information (Table 12.6).[85]

From a clinical viewpoint, the small but potential radiation risks from radionuclide imaging mandate an assessment of the risk versus benefit ratio in the individual patient. In this context, one must not fail to take into account the risks of missing important diagnostic information by not performing a test (which could potentially influence near-term management and outcomes) for a theoretical concern of long-term small risk of malignancy. Before ordering any test, especially one associated with ionizing radiation, we must ensure the appropriateness of the study and that the potential benefits outweigh the risks. The likelihood that the study being considered will affect clinical management of the patient should be addressed before testing is performed. It is also important that "routine" follow-up scans in asymptomatic individuals be avoided.

POTENTIAL OPPORTUNITIES FOR TARGETED MOLECULAR IMAGING

The use of imaging to study biology and uncover biomarkers of human disease provides a window through which we can phenotype disease in vivo, thereby offering an opportunity for early diagnosis of disease and assessing the potential value of novel therapies. Because the nuances of disease mechanisms and the subtleties of the responses to therapy are key to understanding and treating disease, molecular imaging is emerging as an essential tool for revealing pathogenic mechanisms and for developing therapeutic strategies. Importantly, many of these tools are slowly being integrated in the continuum of patient care, which offers a unique opportunity for clinical translation. The following is a brief description of potential applications of molecular imaging in the setting of stable ischemic heart disease.

Potential Applications of Neuronal Imaging in Patients with LV Dysfunction

There is experimental and clinical evidence supporting the concept that sympathetic activation plays an important role as a potential trigger of ventricular arrhythmias after MI.[86] Indeed, MI and ischemia can lead to sympathetic denervation in both the infarct and peri-infarct zone.[22] Viable but denervated myocardial regions show supersensitive shortening of effective refractory period in response to the infusion of norepinephrine and are more vulnerable to ventricular arrhythmias. These observations suggest that direct imaging of cardiac sympathetic innervation may have an important clinical role in risk stratification of patients after MI (Fig. 12.20).

The Prediction of ARrhythmic Events with Positron Emission Tomography (PAREPET) study was designed to test the hypothesis that the extent of inhomogeneity in myocardial sympathetic innervation and/or hibernating myocardium increased the risk of arrhythmic death independently of LV function in patients with ischemic cardiomyopathy (LVEF ≤ 35%).[22] The study included 204 patients who were eligible for primary prevention implantable cardiac defibrillator (ICDs). PET imaging was used to quantify myocardial sympathetic denervation (with ^{11}C-hydroxyephedrine [HED]), perfusion, and metabolism. The primary endpoint

TABLE 12.6 Radiation Reduction Techniques for SPECT MPI Using ^{99m}Tc Radiopharmaceuticals

TECHNIQUE	WHOLE-BODY EFFECTIVE DOSE	RELATIVE REDUCTION IN EFFECTIVE DOSE
Stress-only imaging with conventional gamma camera	~6–7 mSv	~30%
Half-dose stress-only imaging with new reconstruction techniques/collimators and a conventional gamma camera	~3–4 mSv	~60%
Half-dose rest-stress imaging with new reconstruction techniques/collimators and a conventional gamma camera	4–5 mSv	~50%
Low-dose stress-only imaging with CZT-equipped gamma cameras	~1–3 mSv	~80%
Low-dose rest-stress imaging with CZT-equipped gamma cameras	~4–5 mSv	~50%

CZT, Cadmium zinc telluride.

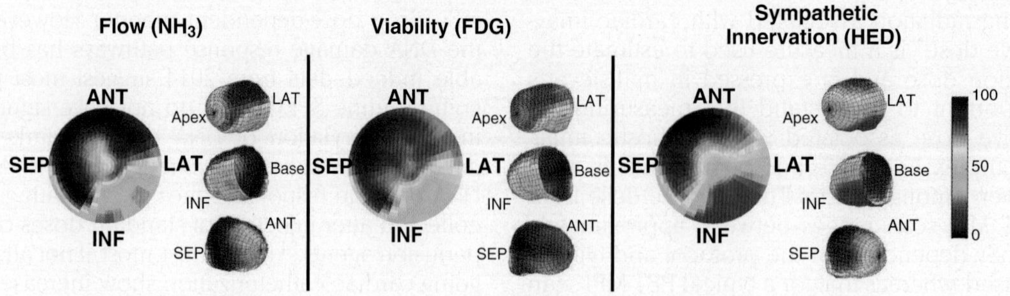

FIG. 12.20 Bullseye maps of myocardial perfusion (*left*), FDG viability (*middle*), and sympathetic innervation (*right*) in a patient who experienced sudden cardiac arrest (SCA). There is a large matched perfusion–metabolic defect involving the inferior and inferolateral walls, consistent with prior myocardial infarction. The ^{11}C-hydroxyephedrine (HED) images demonstrate a larger myocardial volume of sympathetic denervation (reduced HED uptake) compared to the scarred area. This mismatch between infarct size (reduced FDG) and the volume of sympathetic denervation (larger HED defect) has been identified as an imaging marker for ventricular arrhythmias. *ANT*, anterior; *INF*, inferior; *LAT*, lateral; *SEP*, septum. *(Courtesy of Dr. James A. Fallavollita, University of Buffalo, New York.)*

was sudden cardiac arrest defined as arrhythmic death or ICD discharge for ventricular fibrillation or ventricular tachycardia greater than 240 beats/min. Compared to patients in the lowest tertile of cardiac sympathetic denervation assessed by HED PET, patients in the highest tertile showed a greater than 6-fold increase in the risk of sudden cardiac arrest. In multivariable analysis, the extent of PET-defined sympathetic denervation, LV end-diastolic volume index, and creatinine were significantly associated with the risk of sudden cardiac arrest.

Similar findings were reported in the ADreView Myocardial Imaging for Risk Evaluation in Heart Failure (ADMIRE-HF) study using ^{123}I-*m*IBG imaging, in a more heterogeneous cohort of patients with ischemic and non-ischemic heart failure.[23] In this study, patients with a heart-to-mediastinum (H/M) count ratio greater than 1.6 had a relatively lower risk of death or ventricular arrhythmias. In a 2015 ancillary analysis of this trial, *m*IBG scores were able to reclassify risk in a significant number of patients regardless of whether it was used with a continuous or binary threshold.[87] Although *m*IBG-defined ICD candidates could not be identified in this analysis, the authors found that the number of lives saved per 100 patients receiving ICD (absolute benefit) varied across values of *m*IBG H/M results, thus identifying a potential role for this test in optimizing the cost-effectiveness of this intervention. The results of these clinical studies support the hypothesis that these techniques may be helpful in the identification of patients with sufficiently low risk of sudden cardiac death to guide subsequent therapy.

Atherosclerosis Imaging

Atherosclerosis is another area of great interest in the use of targeted molecular imaging biomarkers, especially in drug trials. Although anatomic (invasive and noninvasive) and functional imaging have traditionally been used in atherosclerosis trials, targeted imaging techniques have emerged as powerful markers of molecular and cellular processes directly involved in the pathobiology of this disease. Clinical imaging of plaque constituents is challenging because the plaque volume of interest in coronary and carotid arteries is small and the imaging signal is blurred by motion. However, imaging modalities with high sensitivity (PET) and high resolution (MRI) have demonstrated the greatest success for clinical translation, especially by using hybrid PET/CT and, potentially, PET/MRI.[88]

PET/CT is a highly sensitive and promising noninvasive approach for atherosclerosis imaging in humans.[89] The rationale behind the use of the glucose analog ^{18}F-FDG is that active inflammatory cells within human atheroma, especially monocyte/macrophages, show increased metabolic activity and avidity for glucose. Increased FDG uptake in human atherosclerotic plaques localizes primarily within macrophages[90] and correlates with macrophage density[88,91,92] and high-risk anatomic features of atherosclerotic plaque.[91,93,94] The FDG signal appears to be particularly enhanced in the setting of hypoxia[95] and increased plaque microvascularization.[88,96] In addition, the quantitative FDG PET signal correlates with clinical indices of cardiovascular risk[97] and circulating inflammatory biomarkers.[98–101] The quantitative vascular FDG PET signal has been widely used as a surrogate endpoint to test the effects of antiinflammatory drugs in clinical trials.[102–109] FDG PET is actively being used as a surrogate endpoint in many ongoing trials of atherosclerosis. More recently, other novel targeted imaging agents have been used with PET to characterize inflammation[110–115] and other aspects of plaque biology, including neoangiogenesis[116] and microcalcifications,[117] as well as complications from atherosclerosis[118] in experimental animals and humans.

SUMMARY

Radionuclide myocardial perfusion imaging, a long-practiced technique examining LV myocardial perfusion or viability, as well as LV function, has been extensively validated with respect to its diagnostic, prognostic, and cost-effectiveness characteristics. More recently, data have suggested that it may also have a role in predicting which patients may benefit from specific therapeutic approaches after testing. More widespread utilization of PET MPI with its enhanced performance characteristics will likely further augment the value of this modality. Its ability to accurately define CFR improves the accuracy of testing and may extend its potential applications. Ongoing developments in neuronal, molecular, and atherosclerosis imaging promise future avenues for this modality.

References

1. Henzlova MJ, Cerqueira MD, Hansen CL, et al.: ASNC imaging guidelines for nuclear cardiology procedures. Stress protocols and tracers. https://www.asnc.org/imageuploads/ImagingGuidelinesStressProtocols021109pdf, 2009.
2. Murthy VL, Di Carli MF: Non-invasive quantification of coronary vascular dysfunction for diagnosis and management of coronary artery disease, *J Nucl Cardiol* 19:1060–1072, 2012. quiz 1075.
3. Gould KL: Does coronary flow trump coronary anatomy? *JACC Cardiovasc Imaging* 2:1009–1023, 2009.
4. Tilkemeier PL, Cook CD, Grossman GB, et al.: ASNC imaging guidelines for nuclear cardiology procedures. Standardized reporting of radionuclide myocardial perfusion and function. https://www.asnc.org/imageuploads/ImagingGuidelinesReportingJuly2009pdf, 2009.
5. Beller GA, Heede RC: SPECT imaging for detecting coronary artery disease and determining prognosis by noninvasive assessment of myocardial perfusion and myocardial viability, *J Cardiovasc Transl Res* 4:416–424, 2011.
6. Task Force Members, Montalescot G, Sechtem U, et al.: 2013 ESC guidelines on the management of stable coronary artery disease: the Task Force on the management of stable coronary artery disease of the European Society of Cardiology, *Eur Heart J* 34:2949–3003, 2013.
7. Acampa W, Gaemperli O, Gimelli A, et al.: Document Reviewers. Role of risk stratification by SPECT, PET, and hybrid imaging in guiding management of stable patients with ischaemic heart disease: expert panel of the EANM cardiovascular committee and EACVI, *Eur Heart J Cardiovasc Imaging* 16:1289–1298, 2015.
8. Danad I, Uusitalo V, Kero T, et al.: Quantitative assessment of myocardial perfusion in the detection of significant coronary artery disease: cutoff values and diagnostic accuracy of quantitative [(15)O]H_2O PET imaging, *J Am Coll Cardiol* 64:1464–1475, 2014.
9. Johnson NP, Gould KL: Physiological basis for angina and ST-segment change PET-verified thresholds of quantitative stress myocardial perfusion and coronary flow reserve, *JACC Cardiovasc Imaging* 4:990–998, 2011.
10. Kajander S, Joutsiniemi E, Saraste M, et al.: Cardiac positron emission tomography/computed tomography imaging accurately detects anatomically and functionally significant coronary artery disease, *Circulation* 122:603–613, 2010.
11. Naya M, Murthy VL, Taqueti VR, et al.: Preserved coronary flow reserve effectively excludes high-risk coronary artery disease on angiography, *J Nucl Med* 55:248–255, 2014.
12. Ziadi MC, Dekemp RA, Williams K, et al.: Does quantification of myocardial flow reserve using rubidium-82 positron emission tomography facilitate detection of multivessel coronary artery disease? *J Nucl Cardiol* 19:670–680, 2012.
13. Fukushima K, Javadi MS, Higuchi T, et al.: Prediction of short-term cardiovascular events using quantification of global myocardial flow reserve in patients referred for clinical 82Rb PET perfusion imaging, *J Nucl Med* 52:726–732, 2011.
14. Herzog BA, Husmann L, Valenta I, et al.: Long-term prognostic value of ^{13}N-ammonia myocardial perfusion positron emission tomography added value of coronary flow reserve, *J Am Coll Cardiol* 54:150–156, 2009.
15. Murthy VL, Naya M, Foster CR, et al.: Association between coronary vascular dysfunction and cardiac mortality in patients with and without diabetes mellitus, *Circulation* 126:1858–1868, 2012.
16. Murthy VL, Naya M, Foster CR, et al.: Improved cardiac risk assessment with noninvasive measures of coronary flow reserve, *Circulation* 124:2215–2224, 2011.
17. Taqueti VR, Hachamovitch R, Murthy VL, et al.: Global coronary flow reserve is associated with adverse cardiovascular events independently of luminal angiographic severity and modifies the effect of early revascularization, *Circulation* 131:19–27, 2015.
18. Tio RA, Dabeshlim A, Siebelink HM, et al.: Comparison between the prognostic value of left ventricular function and myocardial perfusion reserve in patients with ischemic heart disease, *J Nucl Med* 50:214–219, 2009.
19. Ziadi MC, Dekemp RA, Williams KA, et al.: Impaired myocardial flow reserve on rubidium-82 positron emission tomography imaging predicts adverse outcomes in patients assessed for myocardial ischemia, *J Am Coll Cardiol* 58:740–748, 2011.
20. Bengel FM, Higuchi T, Javadi MS, Lautamaki R: Cardiac positron emission tomography, *J Am Coll Cardiol* 54:1–15, 2009.
21. Di Carli MF, Hachamovitch R: New technology for noninvasive evaluation of coronary artery disease, *Circulation* 115:1464–1480, 2007.
22. Fallavollita JA, Heavey BM, Luisi Jr AJ, et al.: Regional myocardial sympathetic denervation predicts the risk of sudden cardiac arrest in ischemic cardiomyopathy, *J Am Coll Cardiol* 63:141–149, 2014.

23. Jacobson AF, Senior R, Cerqueira MD, et al.: ADMIRE-HF Investigators. Myocardial iodine-123 meta-iodobenzylguanidine imaging and cardiac events in heart failure. Results of the prospective ADMIRE-HF (AdreView Myocardial Imaging for Risk Evaluation in Heart Failure) study, *J Am Coll Cardiol* 55:2212–2221, 2010.
24. Sasano T, Abraham MR, Chang KC, et al.: Abnormal sympathetic innervation of viable myocardium and the substrate of ventricular tachycardia after myocardial infarction, *J Am Coll Cardiol* 51:2266–2275, 2008.
25. Dorbala S, Di Carli MF: Cardiac PET perfusion: prognosis, risk stratification, and clinical management, *Semin Nucl Med* 44:344–357, 2014.
26. Wolk MJ, Bailey SR, Doherty JU, et al.: American College of Cardiology Foundation Appropriate Use Criteria Task F. ACCF/AHA/ASE/ASNC/HFSA/HRS/SCAI/SCCT/SCMR/STS 2013 multimodality appropriate use criteria for the detection and risk assessment of stable ischemic heart disease: a report of the American College of Cardiology Foundation Appropriate Use Criteria Task Force, American Heart Association, American Society of Echocardiography, American Society of Nuclear Cardiology, Heart Failure Society of America, Heart Rhythm Society, Society for Cardiovascular Angiography and Interventions, Society of Cardiovascular Computed Tomography, Society for Cardiovascular Magnetic Resonance, and Society of Thoracic Surgeons, *J Am Coll Cardiol* 63:380–406, 2014.
27. Goff Jr DC, Lloyd-Jones DM, Bennett G, et al.: American College of Cardiology/American Heart Association Task Force on Practice G. 2013 ACC/AHA guideline on the assessment of cardiovascular risk: a report of the American College of Cardiology/American Heart Association Task Force on Practice Guidelines, *Circulation* 129:S49–S73, 2014.
28. Secretariat MA: Single photon emission computed tomography for the diagnosis of coronary artery disease: an evidence-based analysis, *Ont Health Technol Assess Ser [internet]* 10:1–64, 2010.
29. McArdle BA, Dowsley TF, deKemp RA, et al.: Does rubidium-82 PET have superior accuracy to SPECT perfusion imaging for the diagnosis of obstructive coronary disease? A systematic review and meta-analysis, *J Am Coll Cardiol* 60:1828–1837, 2012.
30. Parker MW, Iskandar A, Limone B, et al.: Diagnostic accuracy of cardiac positron emission tomography versus single photon emission computed tomography for coronary artery disease: a bivariate meta-analysis, *Circ Cardiovasc Imaging* 5:700–707, 2012.
31. Neglia D, Rovai D, Caselli C, Pietila M, et al.: EVINCI Study Investigators. Detection of significant coronary artery disease by noninvasive anatomical and functional imaging, *Circ Cardiovasc Imaging* 8, 2015.
32. Takx RA, Blomberg BA, El Aidi H, et al.: Diagnostic accuracy of stress myocardial perfusion imaging compared to invasive coronary angiography with fractional flow reserve meta-analysis, *Circ Cardiovasc Imaging* 8, 2015.
33. Dolor RJ, Patel MR, Melloni C, et al.: *Noninvasive technologies for the diagnosis of coronary artery disease in women*, Rockville, MD, 2012.
34. Murthy VL, Naya M, Taqueti VR, et al.: Effects of sex on coronary microvascular dysfunction and cardiac outcomes, *Circulation* 129:2518–2527, 2014.
35. Hachamovitch R, Di Carli MF: Methods and limitations of assessing new noninvasive tests: part I: anatomy-based validation of noninvasive testing, *Circulation* 117:2684–2690, 2008.
36. Chang SM, Nabi F, Xu J, et al.: The coronary artery calcium score and stress myocardial perfusion imaging provide independent and complementary prediction of cardiac risk, *J Am Coll Cardiol* 54:1872–1882, 2009.
37. Uebleis C, Becker A, Griesshammer I, et al.: Stable coronary artery disease: prognostic value of myocardial perfusion SPECT in relation to coronary calcium scoring—long-term follow-up, *Radiology* 252:682–690, 2009.
38. Gibbons RJ, Chatterjee K, Daley J, et al.: ACC/AHA/ACP-ASIM guidelines for the management of patients with chronic stable angina: executive summary and recommendations. A report of the American College of Cardiology/American Heart Association Task Force on Practice Guidelines (Committee on Management of Patients with Chronic Stable Angina), *Circulation* 99:2829–2848, 1999.
39. Fihn SD, Gardin JM, Abrams J, et al.: American College of Cardiology. 2012 ACCF/AHA/ACP/AATS/PCNA/SCAI/STS guideline for the diagnosis and management of patients with stable ischemic heart disease: executive summary: a report of the American College of Cardiology Foundation/American Heart Association Task Force on Practice Guidelines, and the American College of Physicians, American Association for Thoracic Surgery, Preventive Cardiovascular Nurses Association, Society for Cardiovascular Angiography and Interventions, and Society of Thoracic Surgeons, *Circulation* 126:3097–3137, 2012.
40. Shaw LJ, Iskandrian AE: Prognostic value of gated myocardial perfusion SPECT, *J Nucl Cardiol* 11:171–185, 2004.
41. Dorbala S, Hachamovitch R, Curillova Z, et al.: Incremental prognostic value of gated Rb-82 positron emission tomography myocardial perfusion imaging over clinical variables and rest LVEF, *JACC Cardiovasc Imaging* 2:846–854, 2009.
42. Kay J, Dorbala S, Goyal A, et al.: Influence of sex on risk stratification with stress myocardial perfusion Rb-82 positron emission tomography: results from the PET (Positron Emission Tomography) Prognosis Multicenter Registry, *J Am Coll Cardiol* 62:1866–1876, 2013.
43. Dorbala S, Di Carli MF, Beanlands RS, et al.: Prognostic value of stress myocardial perfusion positron emission tomography: results from a multicenter observational registry, *J Am Coll Cardiol* 61:176–184, 2013.
44. Chang SM, Nabi F, Xu J, et al.: Normal stress-only versus standard stress/rest myocardial perfusion imaging: similar patient mortality with reduced radiation exposure, *J Am Coll Cardiol* 55:221–230, 2010.
45. Duvall WL, Hiensch RJ, Levine EJ, et al.: The prognosis of a normal Tl-201 stress-only SPECT MPI study, *J Nucl Cardiol* 19:914–921, 2012.
46. Edenbrandt L, Ohlsson M, Tragardh E: Prognosis of patients without perfusion defects with and without rest study in myocardial perfusion scintigraphy, *EJNMMI Res* 3:58, 2013.
47. Duvall WL, Wijetunga MN, Klein TM, et al.: The prognosis of a normal stress-only Tc-99m myocardial perfusion imaging study, *J Nucl Cardiol* 17:370–377, 2010.
48. Acampa W, Petretta M, Cuocolo R, et al.: Warranty period of normal stress myocardial perfusion imaging in diabetic patients: a propensity score analysis, *J Nucl Cardiol* 21:50–56, 2014.
49. Hachamovitch R, Kang X, Amanullah AM, et al.: Prognostic implications of myocardial perfusion single-photon emission computed tomography in the elderly, *Circulation* 120:2197–2206, 2009.
50. Johnson NP, Schimmel Jr DR, Dyer SP, et al.: Survival by stress modality in patients with a normal myocardial perfusion study, *Am J Cardiol* 107:986–989, 2011.
51. Schenker MP, Dorbala S, Hong EC, et al.: Interrelation of coronary calcification, myocardial ischemia, and outcomes in patients with intermediate likelihood of coronary artery disease: a combined positron emission tomography/computed tomography study, *Circulation* 117:1693–1700, 2008.
52. Romero-Farina G, Candell-Riera J, Aguade-Bruix S, et al.: Warranty periods for normal myocardial perfusion stress SPECT, *J Nucl Cardiol* 22:44–54, 2015.
53. Rozanski A, Gransar H, Min JK, et al.: Long-term mortality following normal exercise myocardial perfusion SPECT according to coronary disease risk factors, *J Nucl Cardiol* 21:341–350, 2014.
54. Schinkel AF, Boiten HJ, van der Sijde JN, et al.: 15-Year outcome after normal exercise ^{99m}Tc-sestamibi myocardial perfusion imaging: what is the duration of low risk after a normal scan? *J Nucl Cardiol* 19:901–906, 2012.
55. Taqueti VR, Di Carli MF: Radionuclide myocardial perfusion imaging for the evaluation of patients with known or suspected coronary artery disease in the era of multimodality cardiovascular imaging, *Prog Cardiovasc Dis* 57:644–653, 2015.
56. Chow BJ, Dorbala S, Di Carli MF, et al.: Prognostic value of PET myocardial perfusion imaging in obese patients, *JACC Cardiovasc Imaging* 7:278–287, 2014.
57. Hachamovitch R, Hayes SW, Friedman JD, et al.: A prognostic score for prediction of cardiac mortality risk after adenosine stress myocardial perfusion scintigraphy, *J Am Coll Cardiol* 45:722–729, 2005.
58. Murthy VL, Naya M, Foster CR, et al.: Coronary vascular dysfunction and prognosis in patients with chronic kidney disease, *JACC Cardiovasc Imaging* 5:1025–1034, 2012.
59. Taqueti VR, Everett BM, Murthy VL, et al.: Interaction of impaired coronary flow reserve and cardiomyocyte injury on adverse cardiovascular outcomes in patients without overt coronary artery disease, *Circulation* 131:528–535, 2015.
60. Naya M, Murthy VL, Foster CR, et al.: Prognostic interplay of coronary artery calcification and underlying vascular dysfunction in patients with suspected coronary artery disease, *J Am Coll Cardiol* 61:2098–2106, 2013.
61. Schulman-Marcus J, Boden WE: A PROMISE fulfilled that quality-of-life assessments afford incremental value to coronary artery disease management, *Circulation* 133:1989–1991, 2016.
62. Schoenhagen P, Hachamovitch R: Evaluating the clinical impact of cardiovascular imaging: is a risk-based stratification paradigm relevant? *J Am Coll Cardiol* 61:185–186, 2013.
63. Hachamovitch R: Does ischemia burden in stable coronary artery disease effectively identify revascularization candidates? Ischemia burden in stable coronary artery disease effectively identifies revascularization candidates, *Circ Cardiovasc Imaging* 8, 2015. discussion 8.
64. Hachamovitch R, Rozanski A, Shaw LJ, et al.: Impact of ischaemia and scar on the therapeutic benefit derived from myocardial revascularization vs. medical therapy among patients undergoing stress-rest myocardial perfusion scintigraphy, *Eur Heart J* 32:1012–1024, 2011.
65. Shaw LJ, Berman DS, Maron DJ, et al.: Investigators C. Optimal medical therapy with or without percutaneous coronary intervention to reduce ischemic burden: results from the Clinical Outcomes Utilizing Revascularization and Aggressive Drug Evaluation (COURAGE) trial nuclear substudy, *Circulation* 117:1283–1291, 2008.
66. Shaw LJ, Cerqueira MD, Brooks MM, et al.: Impact of left ventricular function and the extent of ischemia and scar by stress myocardial perfusion imaging on prognosis and therapeutic risk reduction in diabetic patients with coronary artery disease: results from the Bypass Angioplasty Revascularization Investigation 2 Diabetes (BARI 2D) trial, *J Nucl Cardiol* 19:658–669, 2012.
67. Maron DJ, Stone GW, Berman DS, et al.: Is cardiac catheterization necessary before initial management of patients with stable ischemic heart disease? Results from a web-based survey of cardiologists, *Am Heart J* 162:1034–1043, 2011. e13.
68. Nair SU, Ahlberg AW, Mathur S, et al.: The clinical value of single photon emission computed tomography myocardial perfusion imaging in cardiac risk stratification of very elderly patients (>/=80 years) with suspected coronary artery disease, *J Nucl Cardiol* 19:244–255, 2012.
69. Hachamovitch R, Nutter B, Hlatky MA, et al.: Patient management after noninvasive cardiac imaging results from SPARC (Study of myocardial perfusion and coronary anatomy imaging roles in coronary artery disease), *J Am Coll Cardiol* 59:462–474, 2012.
70. Hachamovitch R, Rozanski A, Hayes SW, et al.: Predicting therapeutic benefit from myocardial revascularization procedures: are measurements of both resting left ventricular ejection fraction and stress-induced myocardial ischemia necessary? *J Nucl Cardiol* 13:768–778, 2006.
71. Mark DB, Anstrom KJ, Sheng S, et al.: PROMISE Investigators. Quality-of-life outcomes with anatomic versus functional diagnostic testing strategies in symptomatic patients with suspected coronary artery disease: results from the PROMISE randomized trial, *Circulation* 133:1995–2007, 2016.
72. Mielniczuk LM, Beanlands RS: Does imaging-guided selection of patients with ischemic heart failure for high risk revascularization improve identification of those with the highest clinical benefit? Imaging-guided selection of patients with ischemic heart failure for high-risk revascularization improves identification of those with the highest clinical benefit, *Circ Cardiovasc Imaging* 5:262–270, 2012. discussion 270.
73. Beanlands RS, Nichol G, Huszti E, et al.: F-18-fluorodeoxyglucose positron emission tomography imaging-assisted management of patients with severe left ventricular dysfunction and suspected coronary disease: a randomized, controlled trial (PARR-2), *J Am Coll Cardiol* 50:2002–2012, 2007.
74. Velazquez EJ, Lee KL, Deja MA, et al.: Coronary-artery bypass surgery in patients with left ventricular dysfunction, *N Engl J Med* 364:1607–1616, 2011.
75. Bonow RO, Maurer G, Lee KL, et al.: Myocardial viability and survival in ischemic left ventricular dysfunction, *N Engl J Med* 364:1617–1625, 2011.
76. Panza JA, Holly TA, Asch FM, et al.: Inducible myocardial ischemia and outcomes in patients with coronary artery disease and left ventricular dysfunction, *J Am Coll Cardiol* 61:1860–1870, 2013.
77. Velazquez EJ: Does imaging-guided selection of patients with ischemic heart failure for high risk revascularization improve identification of those with the highest clinical benefit? Myocardial imaging should not exclude patients with ischemic heart failure from coronary revascularization, *Circ Cardiovasc Imaging* 5:271–279, 2012. discussion 279.
78. Cleland JG, Pennell DJ, Ray SG, et al.: Carvedilol hibernating reversible ischaemia trial. marker of success investigators. Myocardial viability as a determinant of the ejection fraction response to carvedilol in patients with heart failure (CHRISTMAS trial): randomised controlled trial, *Lancet* 362:14–21, 2003.
79. Ling LF, Marwick TH, Flores DR, et al.: Identification of therapeutic benefit from revascularization in patients with left ventricular systolic dysfunction: inducible ischemia versus hibernating myocardium, *Circ Cardiovasc Imaging* 6:363–372, 2013.
80. Des Prez RD, Shaw LJ, Gillespie RL, et al.: American Society of Nuclear Cardiology information statement: cost-effectiveness of myocardial perfusion imaging: a summary of the recent literature, 2011.
81. Thom H, West NE, Hughes V, CECaT study group, et al.: Cost-effectiveness of initial stress cardiovascular MR, stress SPECT or stress echocardiography as a gate-keeper test, compared with upfront invasive coronary angiography in the investigation and management of patients with stable chest pain: mid-term outcomes from the CECaT randomised controlled trial, *BMJ Open* 4:e003419, 2014.
82. Hlatky MA, Shilane D, Hachamovitch R, Dicarli MF, SPARC Investigators: Economic Outcomes in the Study of Myocardial Perfusion and Coronary Anatomy Imaging Roles in Coronary Artery Disease registry: the SPARC Study, *J Am Coll Cardiol* 63:1002–1008, 2014.
83. Mark_PROMISEecon.ppt. *clinical trialsorg*. 2016, 2016.
84. Lee WH, Nguyen P, Hu S, et al.: Variable activation of the DNA damage response pathways in patients undergoing single-photon emission computed tomography myocardial perfusion imaging, *Circ Cardiovasc Imaging* 8:e002851, 2015.
85. Dey D, Slomka PJ, Berman DS: Achieving very-low-dose radiation exposure in cardiac computed tomography, single-photon emission computed tomography, and positron emission tomography, *Circ Cardiovasc Imaging* 7:723–734, 2014.
86. Wellens HJ, Schwartz PJ, Lindemans FW, et al.: Risk stratification for sudden cardiac death: current status and challenges for the future, *Eur Heart J* 35:1642–1651, 2014.
87. Hachamovitch R, Nutter B, Menon V, Cerqueira MD: Predicting risk versus predicting potential survival benefit using 123I-*m*IBG imaging in patients with systolic dysfunction eligible for implantable cardiac defibrillator implantation: analysis of data from the prospective ADMIRE-HF study, *Circ Cardiovasc Imaging* 8, 2015.
88. Taqueti VR, Di Carli MF, Jerosch-Herold M, et al.: Increased microvascularization and vessel permeability associate with active inflammation in human atheromata, *Circ Cardiovasc Imaging* 7:920–929, 2014.

89. Tarkin JM, Joshi FR, Rudd JH: PET imaging of inflammation in atherosclerosis, *Nat Rev Cardiol* 11:443–457, 2014.
90. Rudd JH, Warburton EA, Fryer TD, et al.: Imaging atherosclerotic plaque inflammation with [18F]-fluorodeoxyglucose positron emission tomography, *Circulation* 105:2708–2711, 2002.
91. Figueroa AL, Subramanian SS, Cury RC, et al.: Distribution of inflammation within carotid atherosclerotic plaques with high-risk morphological features: a comparison between positron emission tomography activity, plaque morphology, and histopathology, *Circ Cardiovasc Imaging* 5:69–77, 2012.
92. Tawakol A, Migrino RQ, Bashian GG, et al.: In vivo 18F-fluorodeoxyglucose positron emission tomography imaging provides a noninvasive measure of carotid plaque inflammation in patients, *J Am Coll Cardiol* 48:1818–1824, 2006.
93. Graebe M, Pedersen SF, Hojgaard L, et al.: 18FDG PET and ultrasound echolucency in carotid artery plaques, *JACC Cardiovasc Imaging* 3:289–295, 2010.
94. Silvera SS, Aidi HE, Rudd JH, et al.: Multimodality imaging of atherosclerotic plaque activity and composition using FDG-PET/CT and MRI in carotid and femoral arteries, *Atherosclerosis* 207:139–143, 2009.
95. Folco EJ, Sheikine Y, Rocha VZ, et al.: Hypoxia but not inflammation augments glucose uptake in human macrophages: implications for imaging atherosclerosis with 18fluorine-labeled 2-deoxy-D-glucose positron emission tomography, *J Am Coll Cardiol* 58:603–614, 2011.
96. Pedersen SF, Graebe M, Hag AM, et al.: Microvessel density but not neoangiogenesis is associated with 18F-FDG uptake in human atherosclerotic carotid plaques, *Mol Imaging Biol* 14:384–392, 2012.
97. Noh TS, Moon SH, Cho YS, et al.: Relation of carotid artery 18F-FDG uptake to C-reactive protein and Framingham risk score in a large cohort of asymptomatic adults, *J Nucl Med* 54:2070–2076, 2013.
98. Choi HY, Kim S, Yang SJ, et al.: Association of adiponectin, resistin, and vascular inflammation: analysis with 18F-fluorodeoxyglucose positron emission tomography, *Arterioscler Thromb Vasc Biol* 31:944–949, 2011.
99. Rudd JH, Myers KS, Bansilal S, et al.: Relationships among regional arterial inflammation, calcification, risk factors, and biomarkers: a prospective fluorodeoxyglucose positron-emission tomography/computed tomography imaging study, *Circ Cardiovasc Imaging* 2:107–115, 2009.
100. Wu YW, Kao HL, Chen MF, et al.: Characterization of plaques using 18F-FDG PET/CT in patients with carotid atherosclerosis and correlation with matrix metalloproteinase-1, *J Nucl Med* 48:227–233, 2007.
101. Yoo HJ, Kim S, Park MS, et al.: Vascular inflammation stratified by C-reactive protein and low-density lipoprotein cholesterol levels: analysis with 18F-FDG PET, *J Nucl Med* 52:10–17, 2011.
102. Elkhawad M, Rudd JH, Sarov-Blat L, et al.: Effects of p38 mitogen-activated protein kinase inhibition on vascular and systemic inflammation in patients with atherosclerosis, *JACC Cardiovasc Imaging* 5:911–922, 2012.
103. Fayad ZA, Mani V, Woodward M, et al.: dal-PLAQUE Investigators. Safety and efficacy of dalcetrapib on atherosclerotic disease using novel non-invasive multimodality imaging (dal-PLAQUE): a randomised clinical trial, *Lancet* 378:1547–1559, 2011.
104. Maki-Petaja KM, Elkhawad M, Cheriyan J, et al.: Anti-tumor necrosis factor-alpha therapy reduces aortic inflammation and stiffness in patients with rheumatoid arthritis, *Circulation* 126:2473–2480, 2012.
105. Shaddinger BC, Xu Y, Roger JH, et al.: Platelet aggregation unchanged by lipoprotein-associated phospholipase A(2) inhibition: results from an in vitro study and two randomized phase I trials, *PLoS One* 9:e83094, 2014.
106. Tahara N, Kai H, Ishibashi M, et al.: Simvastatin attenuates plaque inflammation: evaluation by fluorodeoxyglucose positron emission tomography, *J Am Coll Cardiol* 48:1825–1831, 2006.
107. Tawakol A, Fayad ZA, Mogg R, et al.: Intensification of statin therapy results in a rapid reduction in atherosclerotic inflammation: results of a multicenter fluorodeoxyglucose-positron emission tomography/computed tomography feasibility study, *J Am Coll Cardiol* 62:909–917, 2013.
108. Tawakol A, Singh P, Rudd JH, et al.: Effect of treatment for 12 weeks with rilapladib, a lipoprotein-associated phospholipase A2 inhibitor, on arterial inflammation as assessed with 18F-fluorodeoxyglucose-positron emission tomography imaging, *J Am Coll Cardiol* 63:86–88, 2014.
109. Wu YW, Kao HL, Huang CL, et al.: The effects of 3-month atorvastatin therapy on arterial inflammation, calcification, abdominal adipose tissue and circulating biomarkers, *Eur J Nucl Med Mol Imaging* 39:399–407, 2012.
110. Bird JL, Izquierdo-Garcia D, Davies JR, et al.: Evaluation of translocator protein quantification as a tool for characterising macrophage burden in human carotid atherosclerosis, *Atherosclerosis* 210:388–391, 2010.
111. Li X, Samnick S, Lapa C, et al.: 68Ga-DOTATATE PET/CT for the detection of inflammation of large arteries: correlation with18F-FDG, calcium burden and risk factors, *EJNMMI Res* 2:52, 2012.
112. Pugliese F, Gaemperli O, Kinderlerer AR, et al.: Imaging of vascular inflammation with [11C]-PK11195 and positron emission tomography/computed tomography angiography, *J Am Coll Cardiol* 56:653–661, 2010.
113. Rominger A, Saam T, Vogl E, et al.: In vivo imaging of macrophage activity in the coronary arteries using 68Ga-DOTATATE PET/CT: correlation with coronary calcium burden and risk factors, *J Nucl Med* 51:193–197, 2010.
114. Weissleder R, Nahrendorf M, Pittet MJ: Imaging macrophages with nanoparticles, *Nat Mater* 13:125–138, 2014.
115. Majmudar MD, Yoo J, Keliher EJ, et al.: Polymeric nanoparticle PET/MR imaging allows macrophage detection in atherosclerotic plaques, *Circ Res* 112:755–761, 2013.
116. Beer AJ, Pelisek J, Heider P, et al.: PET/CT imaging of integrin αvβ3 expression in human carotid atherosclerosis, *JACC Cardiovasc Imaging* 7:178–187, 2014.
117. Joshi NV, Vesey AT, Williams MC, et al.: 18F-fluoride positron emission tomography for identification of ruptured and high-risk coronary atherosclerotic plaques: a prospective clinical trial, *Lancet* 383:705–713, 2014.
118. Ay I, Blasi F, Rietz TA, et al.: In vivo molecular imaging of thrombosis and thrombolysis using a fibrin-binding positron emission tomographic probe, *Circ Cardiovasc Imaging* 7:697–705, 2014.
119. Kang X, Shaw LJ, Hayes SW, et al.: Impact of body mass index on cardiac mortality in patients with known or suspected coronary artery disease undergoing myocardial perfusion single-photon emission computed tomography, *J Am Coll Cardiol* 47:1418–1426, 2006.
120. Sood N, Kazi FA, Lundbye JB, et al.: Risk stratification of CAD with SPECT-MPI in women with known estrogen status, *J Nucl Cardiol* 19:330–337, 2012.

13 CT and MRI

Stephan Achenbach and Gitsios Gitsioudis

INTRODUCTION

There are multiple aspects of imaging in the context of coronary artery disease. On the one hand, imaging is used to identify the presence of coronary artery stenoses, through two possible approaches. One approach is to visualize ischemia as the consequence of hemodynamically relevant coronary artery lesions. In clinical practice, this is most frequently done by stress echocardiography, stress cardiac magnetic resonance, or nuclear medicine techniques (*functional imaging*). The alternative approach is to directly visualize the coronary arteries and identify atherosclerotic lesions. Given the small dimensions and fast motion of the coronary vessels, this is technically challenging and requires a combination of high spatial resolution, high temporal resolution, and the ability to capture the entire complex course of the coronary artery tree. On the other hand, next to the mere identification of coronary artery disease, imaging fulfills other needs regarding management of patients, such as the assessment of left ventricular function or myocardial injury and viability.

Computed tomography (CT) and cardiac magnetic resonance (CMR) play an increasingly important role in the evaluation of patients with known or suspected coronary artery disease. The main application of CT in the context of chronic coronary artery disease is coronary CT angiography, that is, direct visualization of the coronary artery lumen to rule in or rule out coronary artery stenoses. Bypass grafts and stents can also be assessed but are significantly more challenging to evaluate than native coronary vessels. To some extent, CT can be used to characterize nonobstructive coronary atherosclerotic plaque. This may have applications in the context of risk stratification, but it is not yet a method with firmly established clinical applications. Other areas in which CT is used include the support of coronary interventions (in particular for chronic total coronary artery occlusions) and the identification of ischemia through myocardial perfusion imaging or simulation of the fractional flow reserve (FFR).

CMR is not used for visualization of the coronary arteries to the same extent as CT; rather, it is focused on imaging the myocardium. Late gadolinium enhancement imaging is a reliable, high-resolution technique to visualize and quantify myocardial scar and differentiate it from viable myocardial tissue, whereas stress CMR, typically after adenosine or dobutamine infusion, is an accurate method to identify myocardial ischemia.

Both methods complement each other regarding the assessment of patients with known or suspected chronic coronary artery disease. They have widespread clinical application and are firmly established in professional guidelines. Nevertheless, technical challenges exist that may impair image quality or lead to misinterpretation. Meticulous care in patient preparation and image acquisition, as well as sufficient expertise in interpretation, is therefore essential to maximize benefit to the patient.

CARDIAC COMPUTED TOMOGRAPHY

Imaging Protocols

Cardiac computed tomography is most frequently used to visualize the coronary artery lumen. The method is referred to as *coronary CT angiography* or *coronary CTA*. To achieve sufficient spatial and temporal resolution, high-end CT equipment and adequate imaging protocols must be used. Currently, 64-slice CT is considered the state of the art for coronary artery imaging.[1] Newer technology, such as dual source CT or volume scanners that have wide detectors with 256 or 320 detector rows, provides further improved and more robust image quality.

Typical datasets for coronary artery visualization by CT consist of approximately 200–300 transaxial slices with a thickness of 0.5 mm to 0.75 mm (Fig. 13.1). Data interpretation is based on interactive manipulation of these datasets using an image processing workstation, enhanced by post-processing tools such as maximum intensity projections and multiplanar reconstructions. Three-dimensional renderings, although impressive for visualization of the heart and coronary arteries, are not accurate for stenosis detection and play no role in data interpretation. Whereas many workstations provide prerendered reconstructions that are intended to show the coronary arteries over their entire course, readers should not rely on such automated post-processing tools alone. In fact, official recommendations mandate that the reader manipulate the original data and not rely on prerendered reconstructions of any kind.[2]

There are some conditions for patients to be suitable for coronary CT angiography (Box 13.1). Importantly, they include the ability to understand and follow breathhold commands, because even slight respiratory motion during data acquisition will cause substantial artifact. A regular and, preferably, low heart rate substantially improves image quality and reliability (optimally below 60 beats/min, even though this is not as strictly required for dual-source CT).[1]

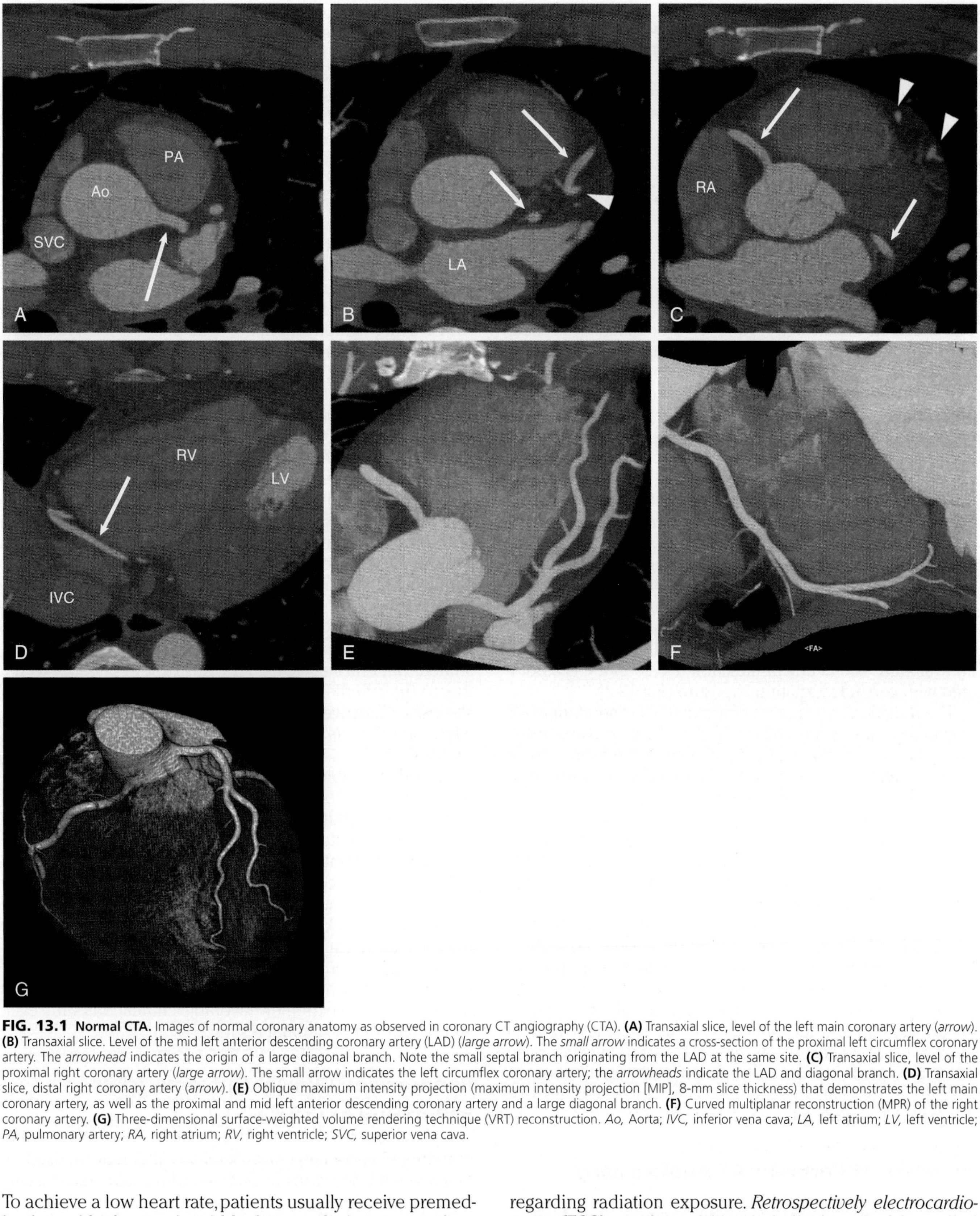

FIG. 13.1 Normal CTA. Images of normal coronary anatomy as observed in coronary CT angiography (CTA). **(A)** Transaxial slice, level of the left main coronary artery (*arrow*). **(B)** Transaxial slice. Level of the mid left anterior descending coronary artery (LAD) (*large arrow*). The *small arrow* indicates a cross-section of the proximal left circumflex coronary artery. The *arrowhead* indicates the origin of a large diagonal branch. Note the small septal branch originating from the LAD at the same site. **(C)** Transaxial slice, level of the proximal right coronary artery (*large arrow*). The small arrow indicates the left circumflex coronary artery; the *arrowheads* indicate the LAD and diagonal branch. **(D)** Transaxial slice, distal right coronary artery (*arrow*). **(E)** Oblique maximum intensity projection (maximum intensity projection [MIP], 8-mm slice thickness) that demonstrates the left main coronary artery, as well as the proximal and mid left anterior descending coronary artery and a large diagonal branch. **(F)** Curved multiplanar reconstruction (MPR) of the right coronary artery. **(G)** Three-dimensional surface-weighted volume rendering technique (VRT) reconstruction. *Ao,* Aorta; *IVC,* inferior vena cava; *LA,* left atrium; *LV,* left ventricle; *PA,* pulmonary artery; *RA,* right atrium; *RV,* right ventricle; *SVC,* superior vena cava.

To achieve a low heart rate, patients usually receive premedication with short-acting β-blockers, and nitrates are given to achieve coronary dilatation. For vascular enhancement during the scan, contrast agent is injected intravenously. Depending on scanner type and acquisition protocol, approximately 40 mL to 100 mL of iodinated contrast agent is used. Data acquisition can follow various principles,[1] and the mode of data acquisition has profound implications regarding radiation exposure. *Retrospectively electrocardiogram (ECG)-gated* acquisition in helical mode (also called *spiral mode*) provides for high and robust image quality and maximum flexibility to choose the cardiac phase during which images are reconstructed, including the ability to reconstruct functional datsasets throughout the entire cardiac cycle in order to assess wall motion (which, however, is not frequently necessary or clinically desired). *Prospectively*

BOX 13.1 Patient Characteristics for Optimal Image Quality in Cardiac CT and Coronary CT Angiography

- Ability to follow breathhold commands and perform a breathhold of approximately 10 seconds
- Regular heart rate (sinus rhythm) < 65 beats/min, optimally < 60 beats/min
- Lack of severe obesity
- Ability to establish a sufficiently large peripheral venous access (cubital vein preferred)
- Absence of contraindications to radiation exposure and iodinated contrast media

ECG-triggered axial acquisition is associated with substantially lower radiation exposure. Image quality is high, especially in patients with stable and low heart rates. Less flexibility to reconstruct data at different time instants in the cardiac cycle, as well as greater susceptibility to artifacts caused by arrhythmia, can be downsides of this acquisition mode but rarely affect individuals if they are well prepared. Overall, prospectively ECG-triggered axial acquisition is the preferred image acquisition mode in many experienced centers. Finally, *prospectively ECG-triggered high-pitch* helical or spiral acquisition, often referred to as *flash* acquisition, is an imaging mode that combines aspects of the former two techniques but can only be used on single source or dual-source CT systems with very wide detectors and only in patients with low and truly regular heart rates. It allows coverage of the volume of the heart within a very short time and maximizes efficacy of radiation use, so that it is associated with very low radiation exposure (Fig. 13.2).

The radiation exposure of coronary CTA (and cardiac CT in general) varies widely. When CT of the heart was first developed, use of radiation was not efficient and effective doses up to 25 mSv were not uncommon for standard acquisition protocols. With the use of improved data acquisition protocols, complemented by image reconstruction techniques that compensate for image noise, radiation exposure in the context of coronary CT angiography has been substantially reduced and typical values for effective radiation dose of contemporary CT protocols range between 1 and 5 mSv. In very strictly selected patient cohorts, it has even been reported that doses below 0.5 mSv and even below 0.1 mSv are possible,[3,4] but image quality at this extreme end of the spectrum is not robust enough for routine clinical practice. Without going to the extreme and by using measures that are widely available, do not require special training, and are straightforward to implement, Chinnaiyan et al. reported a mean effective dose of 6.4 mSv across 15 centers routinely performing coronary CTA.[5] In a 2014 multicenter trial, the average effective dose for coronary CT angiography was 3.2 mSv.[6]

Accuracy of Coronary CT Angiography

Coronary CT angiography has high accuracy for the detection of coronary artery stenoses (Figs. 13.3 and 13.4). Three multicenter trials assessed the accuracy of coronary CT angiography for the identification of coronary artery stenosis in comparison with invasive coronary angiography. Two trials performed in patients with suspected coronary artery disease using 64-slice CT have demonstrated sensitivities of 95% to 99% and specificities of 64% to 83%, as well as negative predictive values of 97% to 99% for the identification of individuals with at least one coronary artery stenosis.[7,8] The positive predictive values were 64% and 86% in these two trials, which is due to a tendency to overestimate stenosis degree in coronary CTA, as well as the fact that image artifacts often result in false-positive interpretations. In a third multicenter study of 291 patients with 56% prevalence of coronary artery stenoses, as well as 20% of patients with previous myocardial infarction and 10% with prior revascularization, specificity was high (90%) and the resulting positive predictive value was 91%.[9] However, this came at the cost of decreased sensitivity (85%) and negative predictive value (83%).

A 2016 meta-analysis summarized 30 clinical trials that evaluated the accuracy of coronary CTA performed with systems composed of 64 slices or greater in comparison with invasive angiography. A total of 3722 patients were included. The authors determined that, on average, 6.6% of studies were unevaluable. They also reported a pooled sensitivity of 95.6% and a specificity of 81.5% for systems with at least 64 detector rows.[10] Of particular importance, the negative likelihood ratio was 0.022, rendering coronary artery stenoses extremely unlikely if coronary CTA is normal.

Accuracy values are not uniform across all patients. High heart rates, obesity, and extensive calcification negatively influence accuracy. Degraded images will lead to false-positive rather than false-negative findings. Specificity and positive predictive value will therefore be most affected. Along with patient factors that influence image quality, the accuracy of coronary CTA depends on pretest likelihood of disease.[11] In an analysis of 254 patients referred to invasive angiography and also studied by CT, it was demonstrated that coronary CTA performs best in patients with a low to intermediate clinical likelihood of coronary artery stenoses (negative predictive value: 100% in both groups), while accuracy is substantially lower in high-risk patients (Table 13.1).[11]

Overall, the ability of coronary CTA to reliably rule out the presence of coronary artery stenoses and the fact that it performs best in situations of low to intermediate likelihood of disease indicate that coronary CTA is a clinically useful tool in symptomatic patients who do not have a high pretest likelihood of coronary artery disease but require further work-up to rule out significant coronary stenoses. A negative coronary CTA scan, if of high quality, will obviate the need for further testing. Indeed, several observational trials and registry reports with up to 35,000 patients clearly demonstrated that symptomatic patients, when coronary CTA is negative, have an extremely favorable clinical outcome even without further additional testing.[12–16]

Randomized Clinical Outcome Trials Evaluating Coronary CTA

Two pivotal randomized clinical trials emphasize the fact that coronary CTA is a clinically useful tool that may be used for management decisions in patients with suspected chronic coronary artery disease.[17,18] In the multicenter Prospective Multicenter Imaging Study for Evaluation of Chest Pain (PROMISE) trial, published in 2015,[17] 10,003 patients with suspected coronary artery disease were randomized to either ischemia testing or coronary CTA as the initial test. After 2 years, outcome in terms of major cardiovascular adverse events or complications associated with testing was equal between the two groups. The rate of invasive coronary

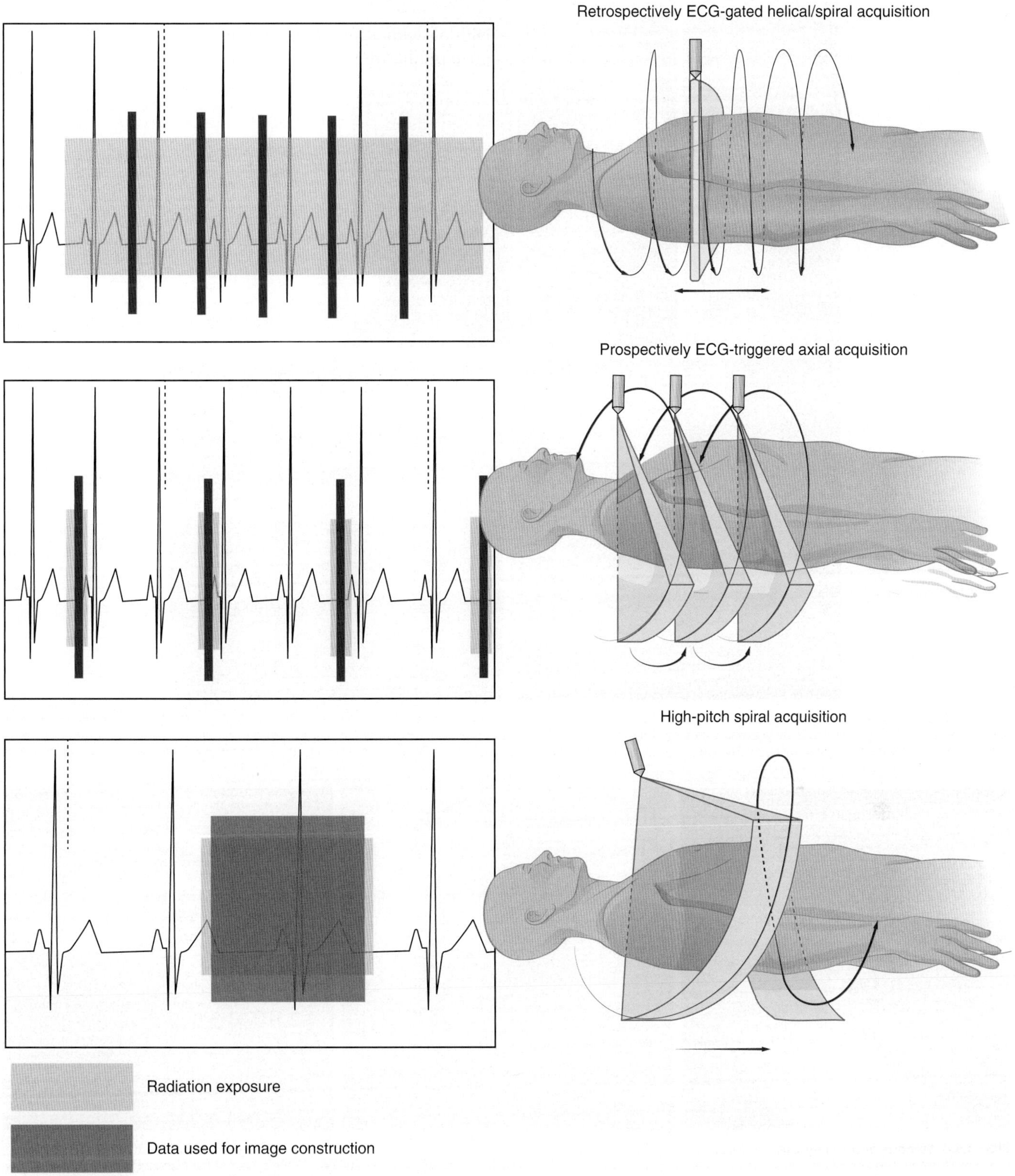

FIG. 13.2 Modes of data acquisition in cardiac CT. Currently, there are three data acquisition modes for coronary CT angiography. **(Top)** Retrospectively ECG-gated helical or spiral acquisition encompasses continuous rotation of the x-ray tube, combined with slow and continuous table motion. Wide x-ray detectors provide oversampling to an extent that every anatomic level is covered during each time point of a cardiac cycle. Hence, the continuously recorded ECG signal can be used to retrospectively select the time instant during the cardiac cycle (gating), during which the cross-sectional images are to be reconstructed. **(Middle)** Prospectively ECG-triggered axial acquisition refers to a data acquisition mode in which the table remains stationary during data acquisition. x-ray exposure is prospectively triggered by the ECG to fit into the desired segment of the cardiac cycle. Additional levels are acquired in subsequent cardiac cycles until the entire anatomy of the heart is covered. **(Bottom)** High-pitch spiral acquisition is a hybrid of the two previously mentioned techniques. Radiation exposure is prospectively triggered by the ECG, but data acquisition is combined with very rapid table motion so that each level of the heart is covered at a slightly different time instant of the cardiac cycle. Because the temporal offset between consecutive levels is very small, and overall acquisition time can be limited to less than 200 ms with very wide detectors and dual-source systems, resulting image quality is high.

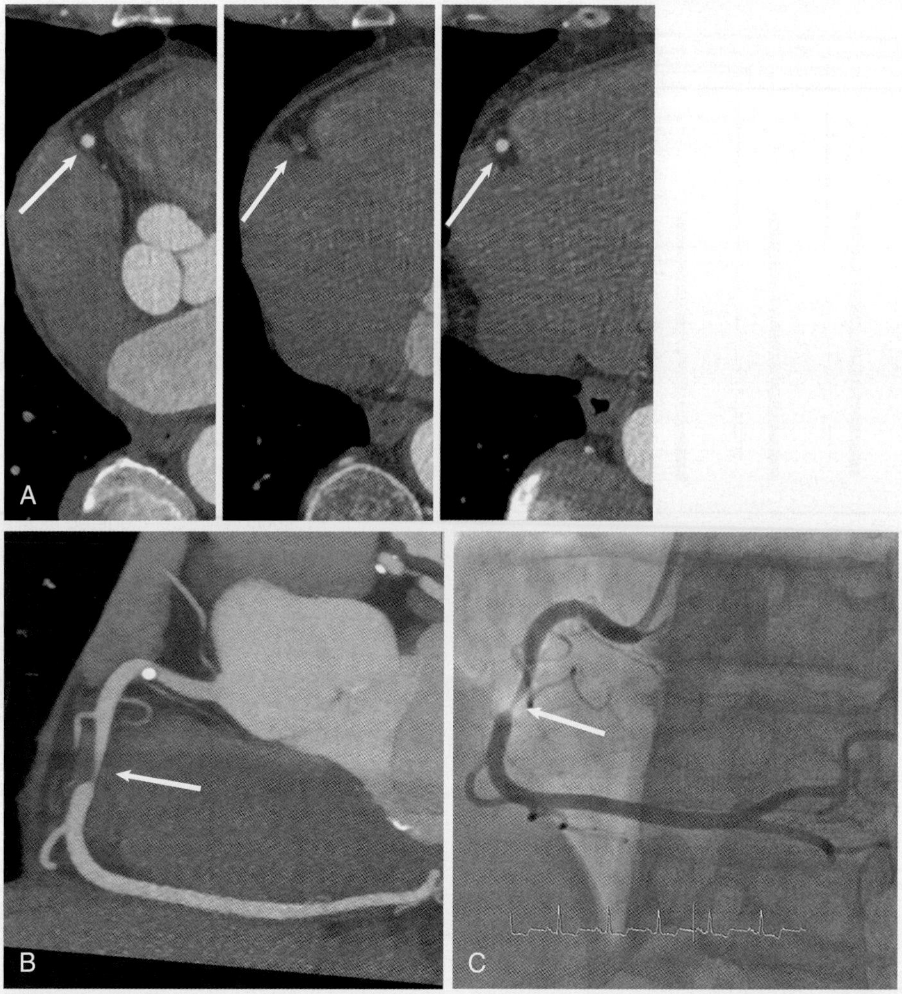

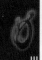

FIG. 13.3 Stenosis in coronary CTA. Visualization of a stenosis of the right coronary artery in coronary CTA **(A, B)** and invasive angiography **(C)**. **(A)** Cross-section of the right coronary artery (*arrow*) in three consecutive levels. A stenosis of the mid right coronary artery is present. **(B)** Maximum intensity projection (MIP) in a plane that corresponds to the spatial orientation of the right coronary artery. The stenosis is detectable in the mid segment (*arrow*). **(C)** Invasive coronary angiogram (*arrow* = stenosis). *CTA,* CT angiography.

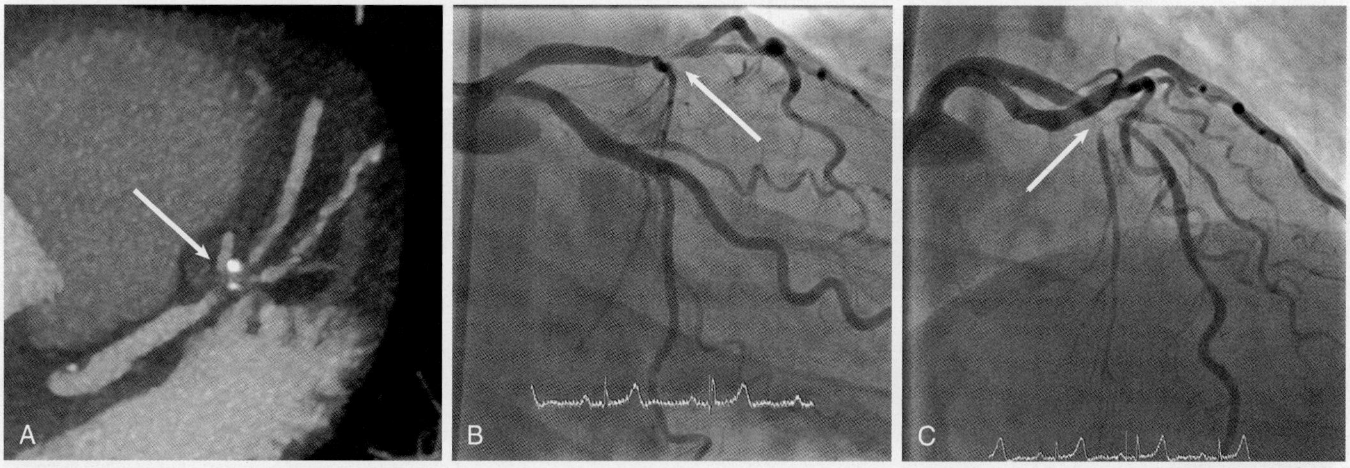

FIG. 13.4 Stenosis in coronary CTA. Visualization of a stenosis of the left anterior coronary artery in coronary CTA. **(A)** Oblique maximum-intensity projection showing a complex bifurcation stenosis of the mid left anterior descending coronary artery (Medina 1/1/1, *arrow*). Note the stenoses in the course of the diagonal branch. **(B and C)** Corresponding invasive coronary angiograms (*arrow* = stenosis). *CTA,* CT angiography.

TABLE 13.1 Diagnostic Performance of 64-slice CT Depending on the Clinical Pretest Likelihood of Coronary Artery Disease in 254 Patients

PRETEST PROBABILITY*	*n*	SENSITIVITY	SPECIFICITY	POSITIVE PRED. VALUE	NEGATIVE PRED. VALUE
High	105	98%	74%	93%	89%
Intermediate	83	100%	84%	80%	100%
Low	66	100%	93%	75%	100%

*Estimated with the Duke Clinical Risk Score.

Meijboom WB, van Mieghem CA, Mollet NR, et al. 64-slice computed tomography coronary angiography in patients with high, intermediate, or low pretest probability of significant coronary artery disease. J Am Coll Cardiol. *2007;50:1469–1475.*

TABLE 13.2 Overview of the Design and the Main Findings of the Multicenter Randomized Trials PROMISE and the SCOT-HEART

	PROMISE	SCOT-HEART
Patients	*n* = 10,003 patients	*n* = 4146 patients
Inclusion criteria	– Suspicion for significant CAD – New/worsening chest pain syndrome or equivalent symptoms – Planned noninvasive testing – Men/women age ≥ 45/50 years	– Attendance at a chest pain unit – Age: > 18 years, but ≤ 75 years
Methods	Functional stress testing* versus coronary CTA	Usual care (ECG stress testing) versus usual care *plus* coronary CTA
Study endpoints	Death, nonfatal MI Hospitalization for unstable angina, Major procedural complications†	Certainty of diagnosis Angina due to CAD
Management	– Increased rate of ICA and increased rate of revascularizations when coronary CTA was initially applied – Less frequently ICA showing no obstructive lesions when coronary CTA was initially applied	Increased preventive prescription
Outcome	No difference	– No difference for overall event rates – Trend for reduced cardiac death and MI in the coronary CTA group after 20 months

*Exercise treadmill, nuclear stress, or stress echocardiography.
†Major procedural complications: anaphylaxis, stroke, major bleeding, renal failure.
CAD, Coronary artery disease; *CTA*, computed tomography angiography; *ICA*, invasive coronary angiography; *MI*, myocardial infarction.
Data from Douglas PS, Hoffmann U, Patel MR, et al. Outcomes of anatomical versus functional testing for coronary artery disease. Engl J Med. *2015;372(14):1291–1230; SCOT-HEART Investigators. CT coronary angiography in patients with suspected angina due to coronary heart disease (SCOT-HEART): an open-label, parallel-group, multicentre trial.* Lancet. *2015;385(9985):2383–2391.*

angiograms (12.2% vs 8.1%) and the rate of revascularizations (6.2% vs 3.2%, $p < 0.001$) were significantly higher if coronary CTA was used as the initial test. On the other hand, catheterization showing no obstructive lesions occurred significantly less frequently if coronary CTA had been used as the initial test (3.4% vs 4.3% of the population, $p < 0.02$). In summary, the trial demonstrated that there is no clinical risk to using coronary CTA as an anatomic test, as opposed to functional imaging, as a first diagnostic method in patients with suspected coronary artery disease.

The Scottish Computed Tomography of the Heart (SCOT-HEART) multicenter trial randomized 4146 patients with stable chest pain to receiving only functional testing or functional testing plus coronary CTA in the setting of suspected coronary artery disease. The additional information from coronary CTA to standard care changed planned management (15% vs 1%, $p < 0.001$) and treatment (23% vs 5%, $p < 0.001$) but did not affect 6-week symptom status ($p = 0.22$) or the frequency of initial admissions ($p = 0.21$) or subsequent hospital admissions for chest pain (11.9% vs 12.7%, $p = 0.40$) as compared to standard care alone. However, after 1.7 years of follow-up, the trial demonstrated that there was a trend toward lower event rates of fatal and nonfatal myocardial infarction by 38% ($p = 0.05$) if ischemia testing was complemented by coronary CTA.[18]

These two pivotal randomized imaging clinical outcome trials (PROMISE and SCOT-HEART) and several smaller trials[19,20] demonstrated coronary CTA to have a proven role in management of patients with suspected chronic coronary artery disease. An overview of the PROMISE and SCOT-HEART trials is presented in Table 13.2.

Imaging of Patients With Bypass Grafts and Stent

The follow-up of patients after previous revascularization is a frequent question in clinical cardiology. It needs to be taken into account that coronary CTA has relevant limitations in patients with previous coronary revascularization. Assessment of coronary artery stents (Fig. 13.5) is often unreliable because the dense metal of the stents can cause artifacts that render the stent lumen unevaluable or create false-positive findings of stenosis. The ability to assess stents concerning in-stent restenosis depends on many factors. They include stent type and diameter, as well as the overall image quality. The analysis of large stents (eg, stents implanted in the left main coronary artery) may be possible by CT in most cases. In general, however, there is uncertainty about the accuracy of coronary CTA to detect and rule out in-stent stenosis. A meta-analysis reported that 20% of stents were unevaluable by CT, and sensitivity for stenosis detection was only 82% in evaluable stents.[21] With the exception of large stents (≥ 3.0-mm diameter) in locations very amenable to CT imaging (eg, left main coronary artery), and if invasive coronary angiography is to be avoided, imaging of patients with previously implanted stents by coronary CTA should therefore not be routinely considered. Bioresorbable vascular scaffolds, on the other hand, are typically made of material that does not have the high attenuation of metal in CT imaging. No systematic evaluations have been performed, but imaging of the coronary lumen should not be impaired by these devices. CT may therefore be a useful method for the follow-up after percutaneous coronary intervention (PCI) performed with bioresorbable scaffolds (Fig. 13.6).[22]

Regarding the follow-up after bypass surgery, the accuracy of coronary CTA for the detection of bypass graft stenosis and occlusion is very high (Fig. 13.7).[23,24] However, assessing the native coronary arteries in patients after bypass surgery is typically difficult. The native vessels frequently have a small diameter and substantial calcification (Fig. 13.8). Consequently, accuracy for detecting and ruling out stenoses in nongrafted and run-off vessels is relatively low, false-positive findings are frequent, and unevaluable segments impair the clinical utility of the test.

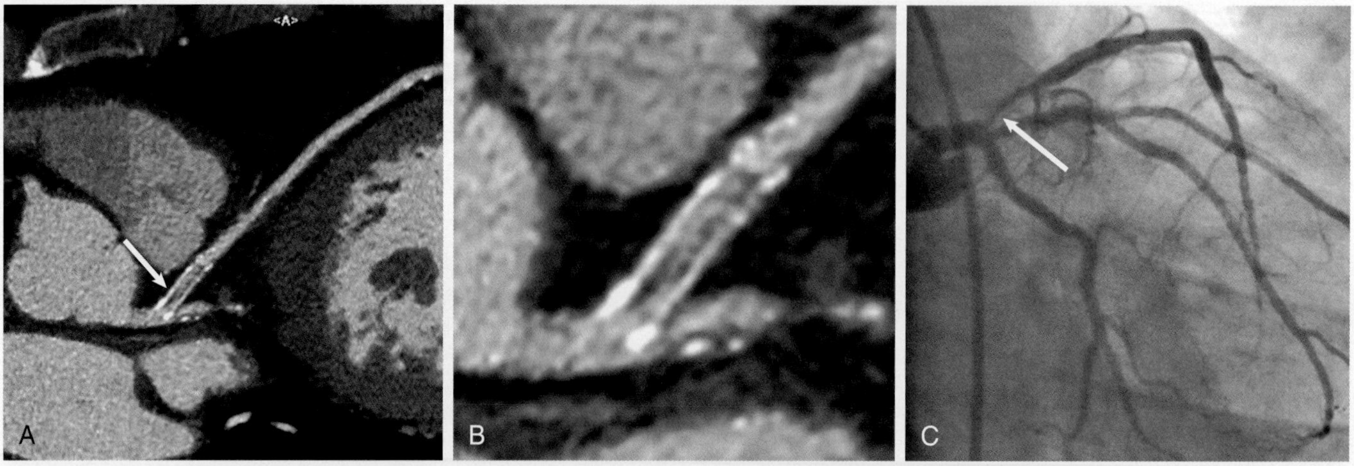

FIG. 13.5 Imaging of stents in coronary CTA. (A) In-stent stenosis of a drug-eluting stent placed in the ostium of the left anterior descending coronary artery (*arrow*). **(B)** Enlarged image of the stent. **(C)** Corresponding invasive coronary angiogram (*arrow* = ostial in-stent stenosis). *CTA,* CT angiography.

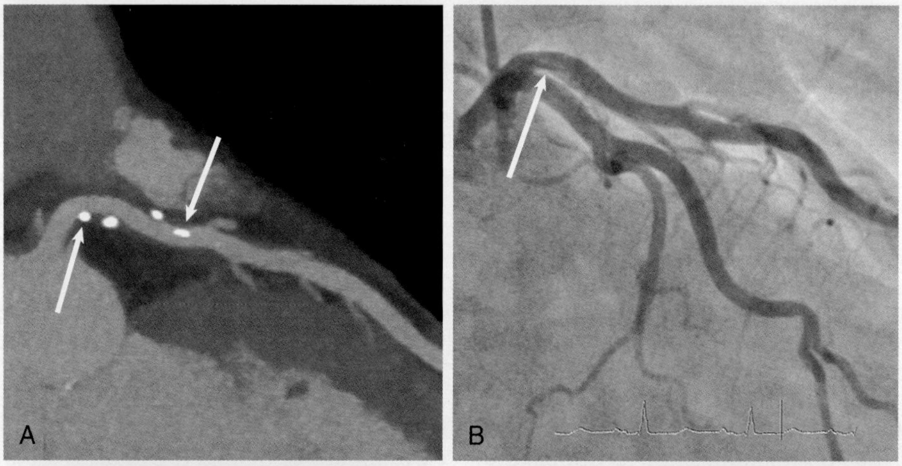

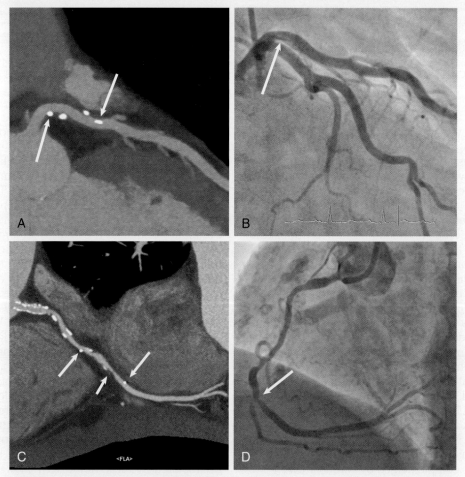

FIG. 13.6 Imaging of bioresorbable vascular scaffolds in coronary CTA. The material of the bioresorbable scaffold itself shows no attenuation in CT and is therefore not depicted. Two platinum markers at either end of the scaffold indicate the position of the device. **(A)** Coronary CT angiography, curved multiplanar reconstruction. The *arrows* indicate the platinum pellets at the distal and proximal end of a bioresorbable vascular scaffold placed in the very proximal left anterior descending coronary artery. The scaffold material itself is not visible. Two calcifications are seen in the course of the scaffold. **(B)** Invasive coronary angiogram (*arrow* = scaffold position). No restenosis is present. **(C)** Different patient. Curved multiplanar reconstruction of a patient with a bioresorbable vascular scaffold placed in a right coronary artery. The *large arrows* point at the platinum markers that indicate the proximal and distal margins of the scaffold. The *small arrow* indicates a focal in-scaffold stenosis. A conventional metal stent is placed in the ostium of the right coronary artery. **(D)** Invasive coronary angiogram. The *arrow* points at the focal in-scaffold stenosis. *CTA,* CT angiography.

Coronary CTA and Ischemia

Coronary CTA, like invasive coronary angiography, is a purely morphologic imaging modality and cannot demonstrate the functional relevance of stenoses (ie, resulting ischemia). In fact, the correlation of CT results with the presence of ischemia is poor.[25] Not surprisingly, coronary CTA is a better predictor of angiographic findings than of findings on nuclear perfusion imaging.[25] A negative coronary CTA result is a reliable predictor to rule out the presence of coronary artery stenoses and the need for revascularization, and CT may therefore be used as a gatekeeper to avoid invasive coronary angiograms.[26] Nevertheless, presence of a stenosis

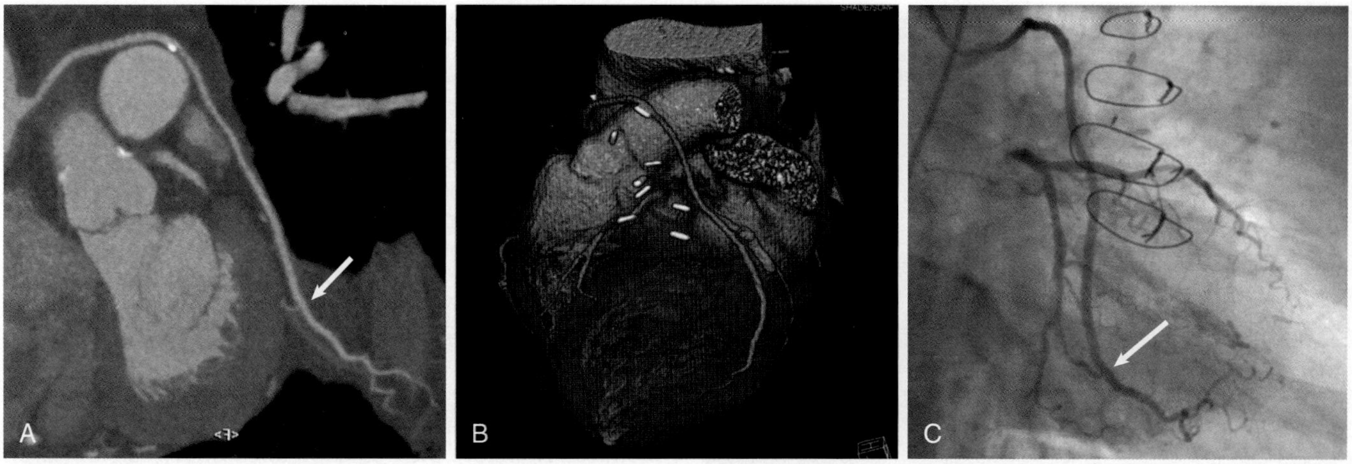

FIG. 13.7 Bypass graft in coronary CTA. (A) Curved multiplanar reconstruction of a vein graft to the left circumflex territory. The *arrow* indicates the site of the coronary anastomosis. **(B)** Three-dimensional reconstruction of the bypass graft. **(C)** Invasive coronary angiogram of the bypass graft (*arrow* = site of coronary anastomosis). *CTA,* CT angiography.

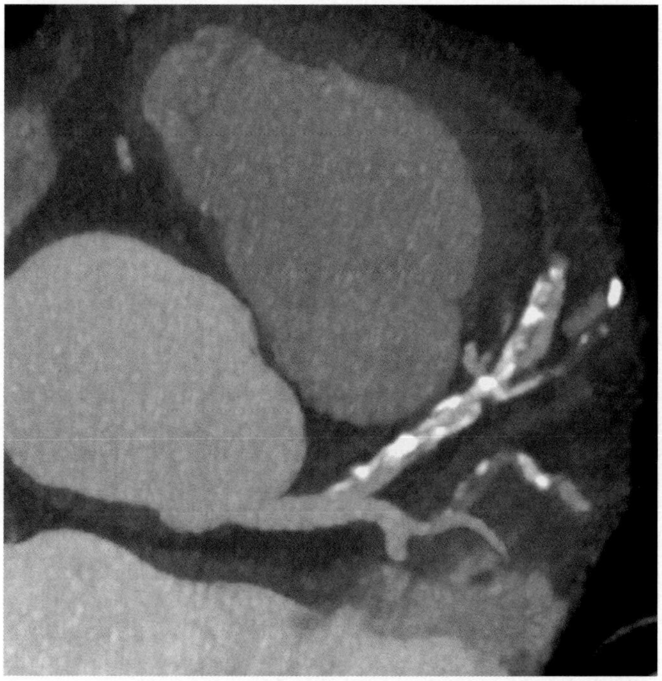

FIG. 13.8 Severe native coronary artery calcification in coronary CTA of a bypass patient. Transaxial cross-sectional contrast-enhanced CT image of a post-bypass surgery patient. There is severe calcification of the proximal and mid left anterior descending coronary artery. This severe calcification is frequently seen in patients after bypass surgery and limits the ability of coronary CTA to evaluate native coronary vessels in post-bypass patients. *CTA,* CT angiography.

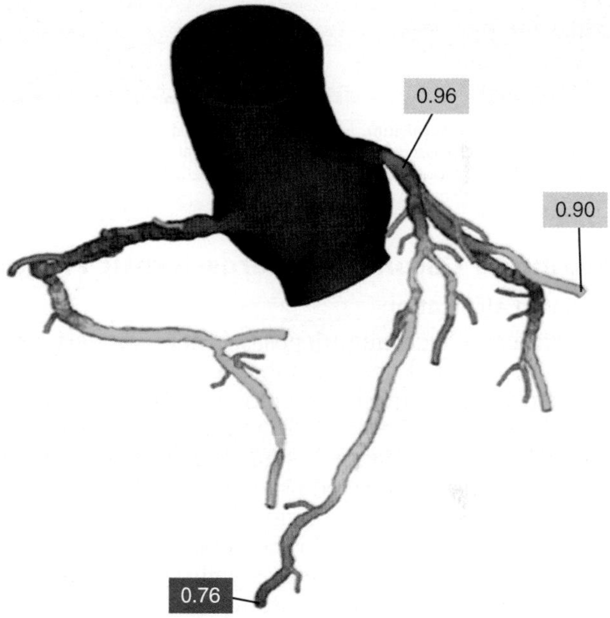

FIG. 13.9 FFR-CT. Determination of CT-based fractional flow reserve (FFR-CT) by fluid dynamic modeling. FFR values are derived from coronary anatomy as depicted by CT, using standard values for microvascular resistance. Local FFR values are color-coded.

on coronary CTA does not mean that a hemodynamically relevant stenosis is present and revascularization should unconditionally be performed. Ischemia testing, whether noninvasive or as an FFR measurement in the context of invasive angiography, will typically be required before revascularization of a stenosis first detected in coronary CTA.

Several methods are under evaluation to improve the ability of coronary CTA to predict ischemia. To this effect, specific analysis methods, such as the transluminal attenuation gradient or CT-based determination of the fractional flow reserve (FFR-CT),[27,28] are used. In particular, the latter receives widespread interest. Based on the anatomic CT dataset, computational fluid dynamics is applied to model the flow and resistance pattern under adenosine stress and to obtain the FFR value for all segments of the coronary artery tree (Fig. 13.9). Initial publications show that FFR-CT is feasible as long as image quality is sufficient and that FFR-CT values correlate rather closely to invasively measured reference values.[28] A large prospective cohort study (Prospective LongitudinAl Trial of FFR-CT: Outcome and Resource Impacts [PLATFORM]) including a total of 584 patients suggests that coronary CTA with FFR-CT may be an effective gatekeeper to invasive coronary angiography. In patients planned for invasive angiography as a work-up for chest pain, adding coronary CTA with FFR-CT before the planned angiogram resulted in a significantly lower rate of invasive coronary angiograms without obstructive coronary artery disease (direct angiography: 73.3% vs FFR-CT first: 12.4%, $p < 0.0001$).[29] Patients were followed for 90 days, and the CT-based strategy was demonstrated to be safe, with low clinical event rates in both groups.

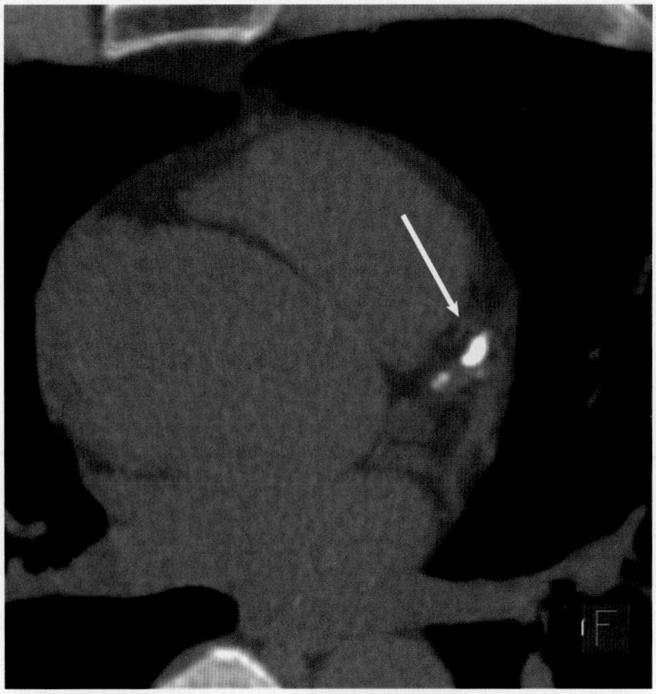

FIG. 13.10 Coronary calcium. Non–contrast-enhanced CT image (3-mm slice thickness) showing a localized calcification in the proximal left anterior descending coronary artery (*arrow*). The Agatston score of this calcified plaque is 179.

Imaging of Coronary Atherosclerotic Plaque

Coronary Calcification

Using cardiac CT, calcium deposits in the coronary arteries can be detected and quantified in low-radiation, nonenhanced image acquisition protocols (Fig. 13.10). Tissue within the vessel wall with a CT number of 130 Hounsfield units (HU) or more is defined as *calcified*, and the amount of calcium is typically classified using the so-called "Agatston score," which takes into account the area and the peak density of calcified lesions. In the general population, the coronary calcium score increases with age and, on average, is higher in men than in women.[30] For the Agatston score, age- and gender-specific percentiles exist for various populations.[30–32]

Coronary calcifications are always due to coronary atherosclerotic plaque, with the possible exception of medial coronary artery calcification seen in patients in renal failure. The amount of calcium roughly correlates to the overall plaque volume.[33] Because coronary artery disease events are typically caused by plaque rupture and erosion, the amount of coronary calcium is associated with individual coronary artery disease risk. Coronary calcium allows for improved risk stratification in primary prevention and is more robust than other markers of risk, such as C-reactive protein or intima-media thickness.[34] In asymptomatic individuals, the absence of coronary calcium is associated with very low (< 1% per year) risk of major cardiovascular events over the next 3 to 5 years, whereas an up to 11-fold relative risk increase of major cardiac events has been reported in asymptomatic subjects with extensive coronary calcification. Prospective large-scale studies, including the Multiethnic Study of Atherosclerosis (MESA)[35] and the Heinz Nixdorf Recall Study,[36] have convincingly demonstrated that coronary calcium measurement by CT has incremental prognostic information beyond assessment of traditional risk factors. The presence of coronary calcium will reclassify individuals who seem to be at low or intermediate risk based on traditional risk factors to a high-risk category, and that this may mandate more intense risk factor modification.

The correlation between calcium and stenosis is poor. Atherosclerotic lesions, and even stenosis, may be present even in the absence of calcium, especially in younger patients with recent onset of symptoms.[37] The lack of calcium therefore does not reliably eliminate the possibility of coronary artery stenoses, particularly in young individuals and those with suspected acute coronary syndromes. Nevertheless, even substantial amounts of coronary calcium are not necessarily associated with the presence of hemodynamically relevant luminal narrowing. Frequently, very high calcium scores can be found in the absence of coronary stenoses. Therefore, the detection of coronary calcium, even in large amounts, should not prompt invasive coronary angiography in otherwise asymptomatic individuals.

In summary, the predictive value of coronary calcium concerning the occurrence of future cardiovascular disease events in asymptomatic individuals is widely accepted. A potential clinical role of coronary calcium for further risk stratification exists for individuals who are at intermediate risk as assessed by traditional risk factors. In patients at high or very low risk, coronary calcium imaging will usually not be indicated, because the result is unlikely to influence treatment decisions.[38,39] Unselected screening or patient self-referral is not recommended.[38,39]

Atherosclerotic Plaque in Coronary CTA

Next to the identification of stenoses, coronary CTA allows us to visualize—and, to a certain extent, to quantify and characterize—nonobstructive coronary atherosclerotic plaque (Fig. 13.11). For risk stratification purposes, the analysis not only of calcified but also of noncalcified plaque components is a promising tool for refined assessment of individual event risk. In comparison to intravascular ultrasound (IVUS), accuracy for detecting noncalcified plaque has been reported to be approximately 80% to 90%, albeit in selected patients within small studies. Several trials and large registries have been able to demonstrate prognostic value of atherosclerotic lesions detected by coronary CT angiography both in symptomatic and asymptomatic individuals. In a landmark publication, Min et al.[40] demonstrated increased overall mortality in patients with atherosclerotic lesions in more than five coronary artery segments. Ostrom et al.[41] demonstrated increased mortality during long-term follow-up in patients with nonobstructive lesions in all three coronary arteries, or in patients who had obstructive lesions. An analysis of a clinical registry comprising more than 23,000 patients confirmed the prognostic value of coronary CTA, where the presence of coronary stenoses, but also the presence of nonobstructive plaque, was associated with an increased risk of mortality.[42] However, the hazard ratio (HR) for nonobstructive plaque was relatively low (HR = 1.6; 95% confidence interval [CI] 1.2–2.2). Also, another analysis of the same registry was unable to demonstrate, for this mostly symptomatic patient group, an incremental prognostic value of contrast-enhanced coronary CTA over coronary calcium measurements.[43]

For further characterization of plaque, assessment of features that are associated with plaque vulnerability has been suggested. The two most important features are positive remodeling and low CT attenuation (< 30 HU) within

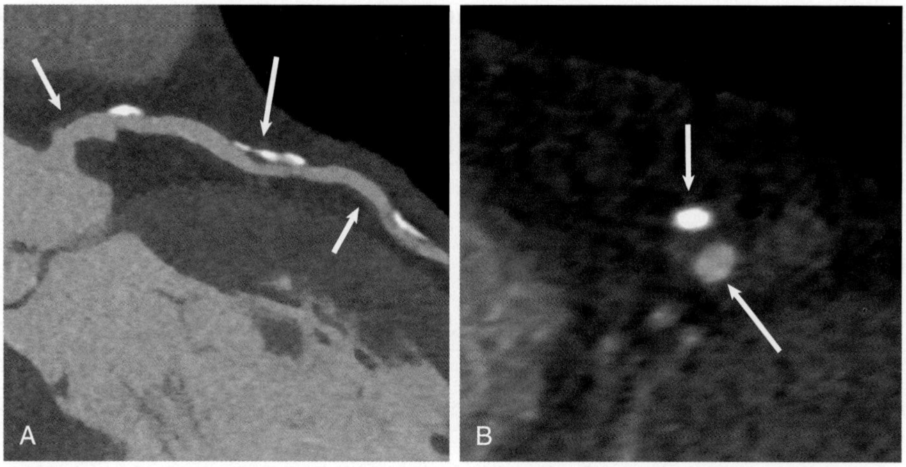

FIG. 13.11 Plaque in coronary CTA. (A) Curved multiplanar reconstruction of the left main and proximal left anterior descending coronary artery showing areas of completely noncalcified plaque (*small arrows*), as well as a large partially calcified plaque (*large arrow*). Furthermore, there are two small entirely calcified plaques. **(B)** Cross-sectional view of the partially calcified plaque (calcification [*small arrow*]; coronary lumen [*large arrow*]). *CTA,* CT angiography.

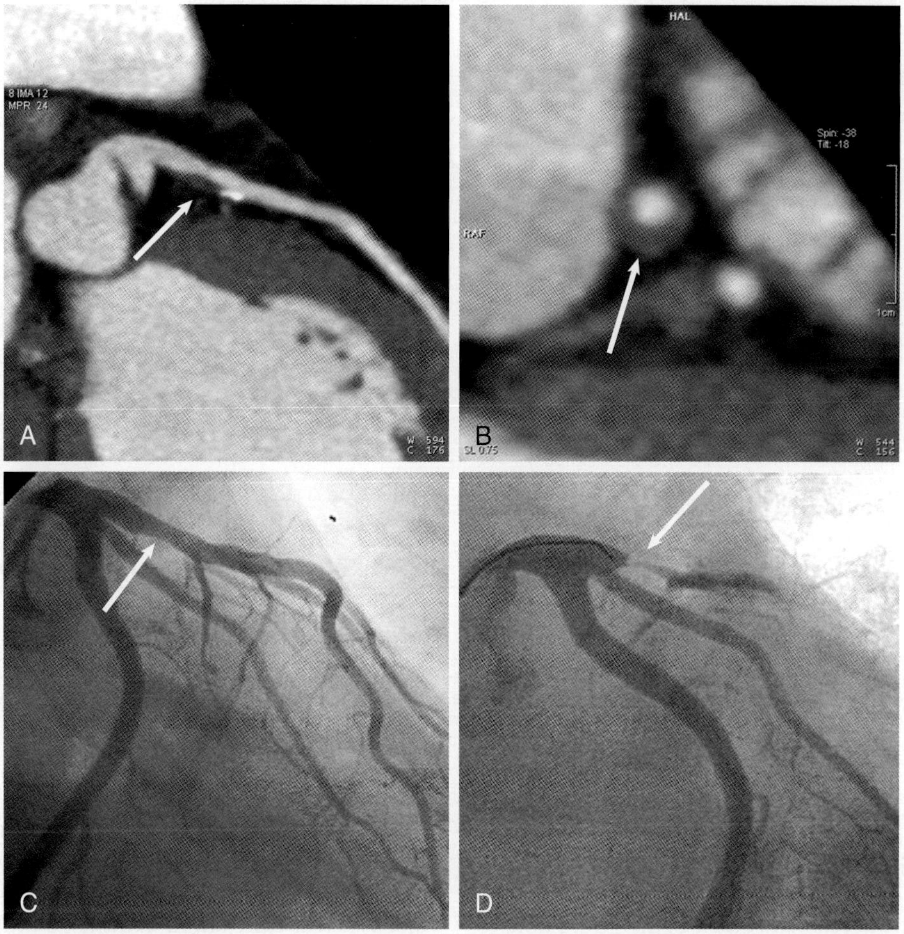

FIG. 13.12 Vulnerable plaque in coronary CTA. (A) Longitudinal reconstruction of the left main and proximal left anterior descending coronary artery. A partly calcified plaque has low CT attenuation and positive remodeling, signs of plaque vulnerability in coronary CTA (*arrow*). **(B)** Cross-sectional view of the plaque (*arrow*). **(C)** Corresponding invasive angiogram showing a mild luminal stenosis at the site of the plaque (*arrow*). **(D)** Seven years later, the patient experienced ST-elevation myocardial infarction of the anterior wall as a consequence of plaque rupture (*arrow*). *CTA,* CT angiography.

coronary atherosclerotic plaque (Fig. 13.12). It has been shown that these characteristics are associated with the occurrence of future acute coronary syndromes[44] (Table 13.3). It is very interesting to note that features associated with vulnerability of coronary atherosclerotic plaque are also predictors of the hemodynamic relevance of a given lesion. In several trials that compared coronary CTA to invasively measured FFR, plaque characteristics such as aggregate plaque volume, positive remodeling, and low CT attenuation were incremental to stenosis degree in predicting whether a lesion was associated with a pathologic FFR result (≤ 0.80)[45,46] (Fig. 13.13).

TABLE 13.3 Results of a Prospective Study That Followed 1059 Patients Who Had Undergone Coronary CTA for an Average Duration of 27 Months

FINDING AT BASELINE	TOTAL NUMBER OF PATIENTS	ACS DURING FOLLOW-UP	NO ACS DURING FOLLOW-UP
Plaques with positive remodeling **AND** CT attenuation < 30 HU	45	10 (22%)	35 (78%)
Plaques with positive remodeling **OR** CT attenuation < 30 HU	27	1 (4%)	26 (96%)
Plaques with **Neither** positive remodeling **NOR** CT attenuation < 30 HU	822	4 (0.5%)	816 (99%)
No plaque	167	0 (0%)	167 (100%)

The rate of acute coronary syndromes (ACS) during follow-up was substantially higher in patients with plaques that demonstrated positive remodeling and low CT attenuation (< 30 HU) as compared to patients with plaque of another type or without plaque.
Data from Motoyama S, Sarai M, Harigaya H, et al. Computed tomographic angiography characteristics of atherosclerotic plaques subsequently resulting in acute coronary syndrome. J Am Coll Cardiol. *2009;54:49–57.*

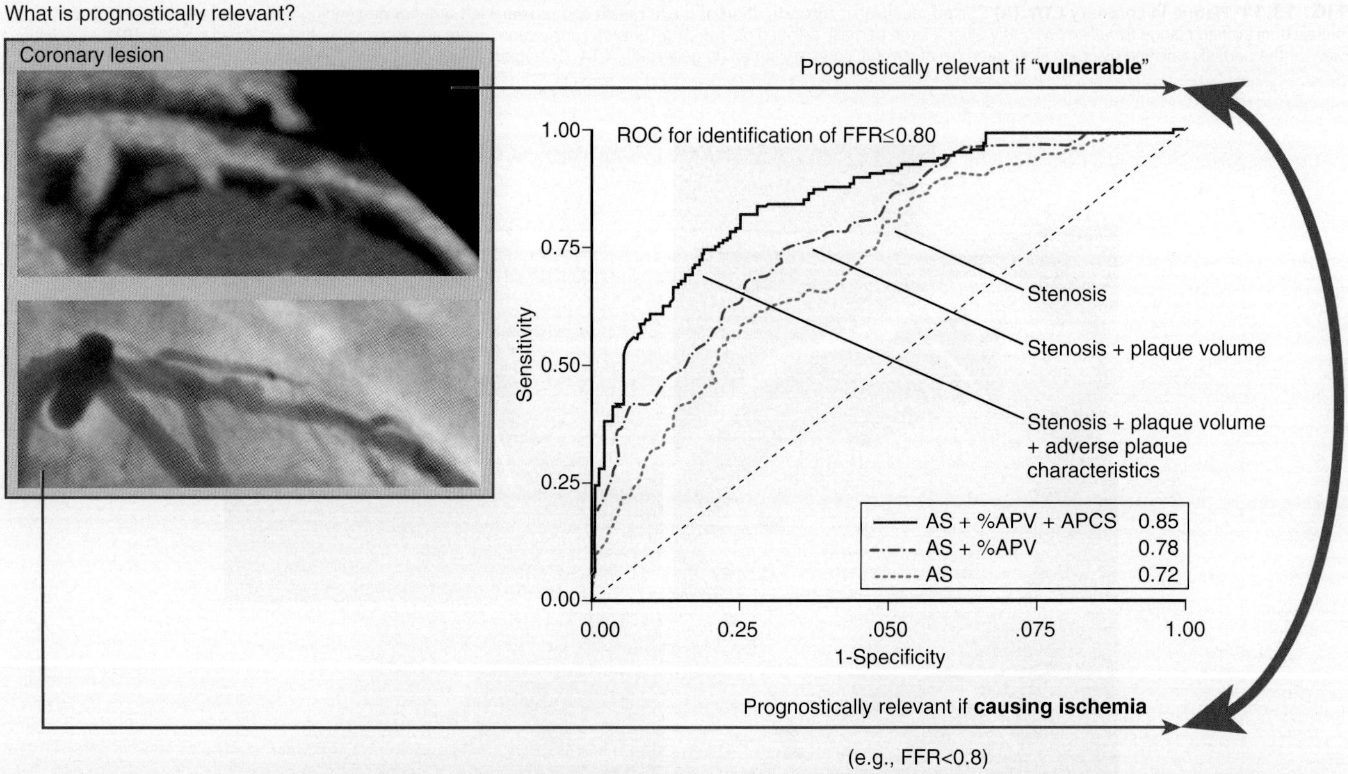

FIG. 13.13 Plaque vulnerability and FFR. Both the hemodynamic effect and the presence of "vulnerable" characteristics are associated with the prognostic relevance of a given coronary lesion. CT-based studies demonstrate that there is a relationship between both aspects: parameters associated with plaque vulnerability (referred to as *adverse plaque characteristics*) are predictive regarding the presence of hemodynamic relevance (FFR < 0.80) beyond the degree of stenosis. This was shown in several studies.[45] *APCs,* Atherosclerotic plaque characteristics; *APV,* aggregate plaque volume; *AS,* lumen area stenosis; *FFR,* fractional flow reserve; *ROC,* receiver operating characteristic. *(Graph from Park HB, Heo R, ó Hartaigh B, et al. Atherosclerotic plaque characteristics by CT angiography identify coronary lesions that cause ischemia: a direct comparison to fractional flow reserve.* JACC Cardiovasc Imaging. *2015;8(1):1–1.)*

Clinical consequences of plaque imaging by coronary CTA are unclear (Fig. 13.14), and plaque analysis has not been incorporated into guidelines and recommendations for risk modification. Interestingly, Chow et al.[47] were able to show in a large registry (10,418 individuals without obstructive coronary stenoses, followed for 4 years) that the use of statin medication in primary prevention was only associated with lower event rates if plaque was present in coronary CTA. In the absence of detectable plaque, event rates between individuals with and without statin therapy were not different.

CT Myocardial Perfusion Imaging

After intravenous injection of contrast agent, CT imaging permits visualization of myocardial enhancement. Myocardial perfusion defects at rest have been shown to be associated with myocardial infarction in patients with acute chest pain (Fig. 13.15).[48] In patients with suspected chronic coronary disease, rest and stress contrast-enhanced images of the myocardium can be acquired before and after adenosine injection. It has not yet been clarified whether rest-stress protocols (rest acquisition first, followed by stress perfusion imaging) or stress-rest protocols (in opposite order) provide better results. Neither has it been clarified whether static protocols that acquire images only at one time point or dynamic protocols with repeated image acquisition to establish time–density curves and potentially calculate myocardial blood flow are the optimal approach.[49] The average estimated effective radiation dose for static protocols is 5.9 mSv, whereas the average dose for dynamic

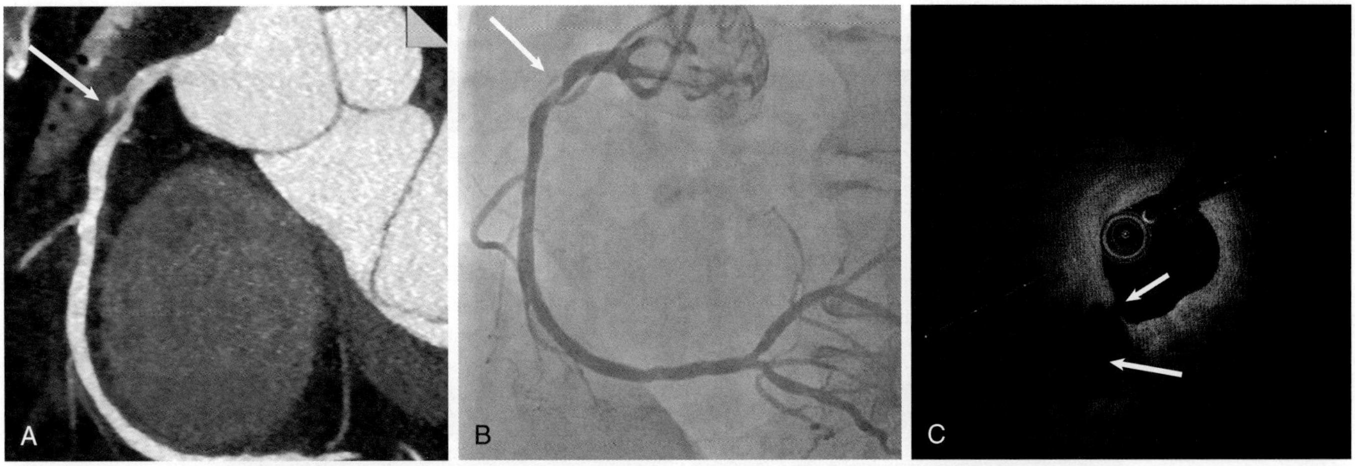

FIG. 13.14 Plaque rupture in coronary CT angiography, invasive coronary angiography, and optical coherence tomography. (A) Plaque rupture ("ulcerated plaque") with contrast density within noncalcified plaque (*arrow*) of the proximal right coronary artery. **(B)** Invasive coronary angiography showing a mild stenosis in the proximal right coronary artery. Some gray density at the site of the stenosis indicates contrast agent that has penetrated into the plaque as a sign of plaque rupture (*arrow*). **(C)** Optical coherence tomography showing the ruptured fibrous cap (*small arrow*) and washed-out cavity within the plaque (*large arrow*).

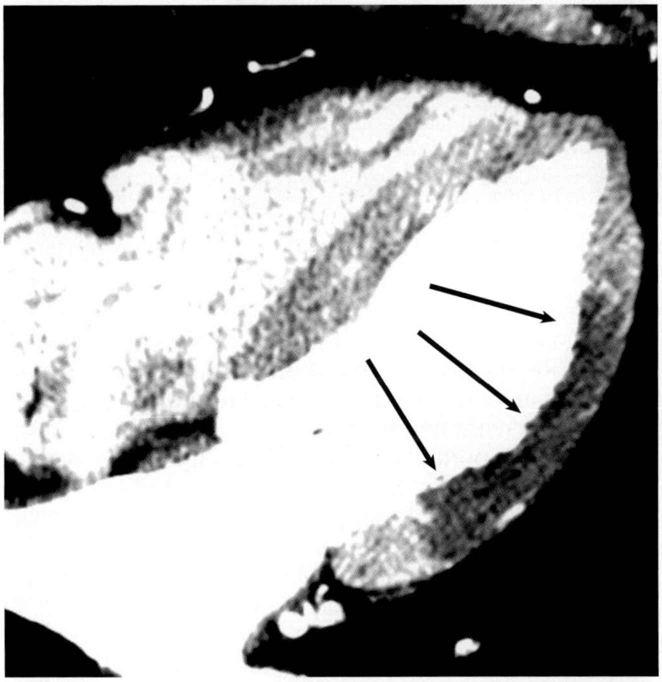

FIG. 13.15 Myocardial perfusion defect in contrast-enhanced cardiac CT. Shown here (*arrows*) in a patient with NSTEMI (non-ST-elevation myocardial infarction).

protocols is 9.2 mSv.[49] So far, the method is not used widely in clinical practice, even though, according to published studies, diagnostic accuracy is high. In a meta-analysis of 22 articles with 1507 subjects, Pelgrim et al.[50] reported a mean per-patient sensitivity of 89% and specificity of 88% for CT myocardial perfusion compared to single-photon emission computed tomography (SPECT), whereas in a smaller meta-analysis that summarized 316 patients with comparisons between CT perfusion and invasive FFR the sensitivity of CT was 88% and the specificity was 80%[51] (Table 13.4). Obviously, CT myocardial perfusion imaging would rarely be a stand-alone test. Typically, its combination with CT assessment of coronary morphology would enhance the diagnostic value. In a multicenter approach, the combined use of CT angiography and CT perfusion in 381 patients (Coronary Artery Evaluation Using 320-Row Multidetector CT Angiography [CORE320] study) yielded a sensitivity of 80% and specificity of 74% against the combined reference standard of a stenosis greater than 50% in invasive angiography with a perfusion defect in SPECT.[6]

In summary, the field of CT myocardial perfusion imaging is still evolving. Results of initial accuracy trials are encouraging, but the optimal methodology has not yet been identified. There is room for further improvement of acquisition and image processing through, for example, dual energy imaging, monochromatic imaging, iterative reconstruction, or specific algorithms to remove artifacts.[49] CT myocardial perfusion imaging will, on the other hand, never exhibit the same elegant ease that makes coronary CTA so compellingly attractive. Hence, the future clinical role of CT myocardial perfusion imaging is currently unclear.

MAGNETIC RESONANCE IMAGING

Magnetic resonance imaging (MRI)—in the context of heart disease often referred to as *cardiovascular magnetic resonance* or *cardiac magnetic resonance* (CMR)—has the capability to assess, with high accuracy, various aspects of cardiac morphology and function. As far as coronary artery disease is concerned, they include left ventricular global and regional function and characterization of myocardial tissue (thickness, fibrosis, and edema) and viability, as well as myocardial perfusion and, with some limitations, visualization of the coronary artery lumen and coronary atherosclerotic plaque.

Whereas, previously, the limited availability of suitable MR systems, long examination times, and small bore sizes prevented a more widespread application of MRI in the context of coronary artery disease, new technical developments have made MRI much more accessible and widely used. Mainly, they include imaging techniques that provide for shorter examination times, such as parallel imaging techniques, k–t undersampling strategies, and compressed sensing, so that the examination time for a comprehensive MR examination is less than 45 minutes.[52]

Sequences and Image Acquisition in Cardiac MRI

For MRI, a high-strength constant external magnetic field is applied (typically 0.5–3.0 tesla). This aligns the spins of

TABLE 13.4 Accuracy of Myocardial Perfusion Techniques for the Identification of Hemodynamically Relevant Coronary Artery Disease, Validated Against the Gold Standard of Invasive FFR (meta-analysis)

METHOD	SENSITIVITY	SPECIFICITY	POSITIVE LIKELIHOOD RATIO	NEGATIVE LIKELIHOOD RATIO	DIAGNOSTIC ODDS RATIO
SPECT	61%	84%	3.76	0.47	8.17
MRI	87%	91%	8.26	0.16	66.86
CT*	78%	86%	5.74	0.22	28.90
PET	83%	89%	7.43	0.15	48.53

*CT myocardial perfusion.

Data was derived from a total of 37 studies, with 2048 patients and 4721 vessels compared to invasive FFR.[65]

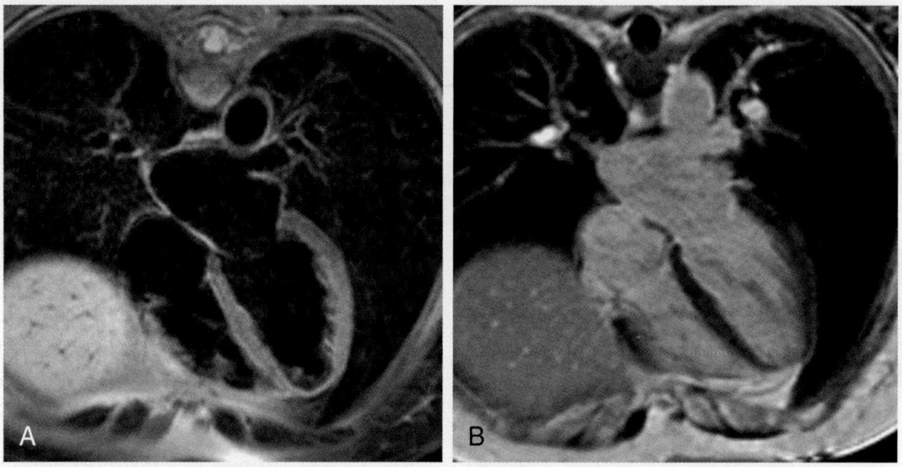

FIG. 13.16 Dark-blood and bright-blood images in CMR. Four-chamber view of the heart using dark-blood **(A)** and bright-blood **(B)** sequences. *CMR,* Cardiac magnetic resonance.

protons (nuclei of hydrogen atoms, for example within water) within the patient's body with the direction of the external magnetic field. Radiofrequency pulses are then emitted that deflect the spins from their aligned direction, and as they gradually realign after the end of the external radiofrequency pulse, the protons emit radiofrequency signals themselves. These signals are detected by antennae and form the basis for creating magnetic resonance images. The magnitude of the radiofrequency signals that the protons emit depends on the density of protons (eg, the water content of tissue), the movement of protons (eg, blood flow), and two so-called "relaxation times" (T1 and T2). T1 is the time constant that describes the return of longitudinal magnetization to baseline (after the external radio frequency [RF] pulse has deflected proton spin), and T2 describes the return of transverse magnetization to baseline. T1 and T2 are independent from each other and depend on the type of tissue the proton is embedded in. Water, for example, has long T1 and T2 times, whereas fat has short T1 and T2 times. T1-weighted images are images that exploit the difference of T1 relaxation times of various tissues. For instance, in T1-weighted images, fat is bright, water is dark, and myocardium is gray. On the other hand, in T2-weighted images, blood is bright whereas fat is dark (Fig. 13.16).

Both T1- and T2-weighted images (and also so-called "proton-density weighted images") can be acquired using spin-echo techniques or gradient-echo techniques. Spin-echo techniques are slower to acquire but provide very good contrast and are robust regarding the occurrence of artifacts, whereas gradient-echo techniques are more rapid to acquire, but have higher susceptibility to artifacts. Parallel imaging is a technique that requires specific coils to detect emitted RF signals and enables us to increase sampling speed: it can therefore either be used to shorten scan duration or to increase image resolution.

A further important aspect of CMR is the suppression of motion. To this effect, ECG gating is used to eliminate cardiac motion. In order to suppress respiratory motion, image acquisition can be performed in repeated breathholds (requiring good patient cooperation) or with navigator techniques that monitor respiratory movement of, for example, the diaphragm. Finally, real-time MRI is possible to some extent and can be used when other techniques to suppress motion fail.

For some aspects of CMR, intravenous contrast agent is required. For example, this concerns late enhancement and myocardial perfusion, whereas cardiac morphology and function can be assessed without contrast agent injection. The most commonly used contrast agents are chelates of the metal gadolinium (eg, gadolinium (Gd)-DTPA), where the chelation is required to avoid toxic effects of gadolinium itself. The contrast agents are eliminated renally in an unchanged form. Side effects are rare, but some concern exists when renal function is impaired. Because of observed associations with nephrogenic systemic fibrosis,[53] it is typically recommended to avoid Gd-based contrast agents when the glomerular filtration rate (GFR) is less than 30 mL/min per $1.73m^2$. First-pass imaging of the contrast-enhanced myocardium, usually at rest and with vasodilator stress, is used to determine myocardial perfusion. Late gadolinium enhancement (or delayed enhancement) images are acquired at least 10 minutes after contrast injection and display areas of

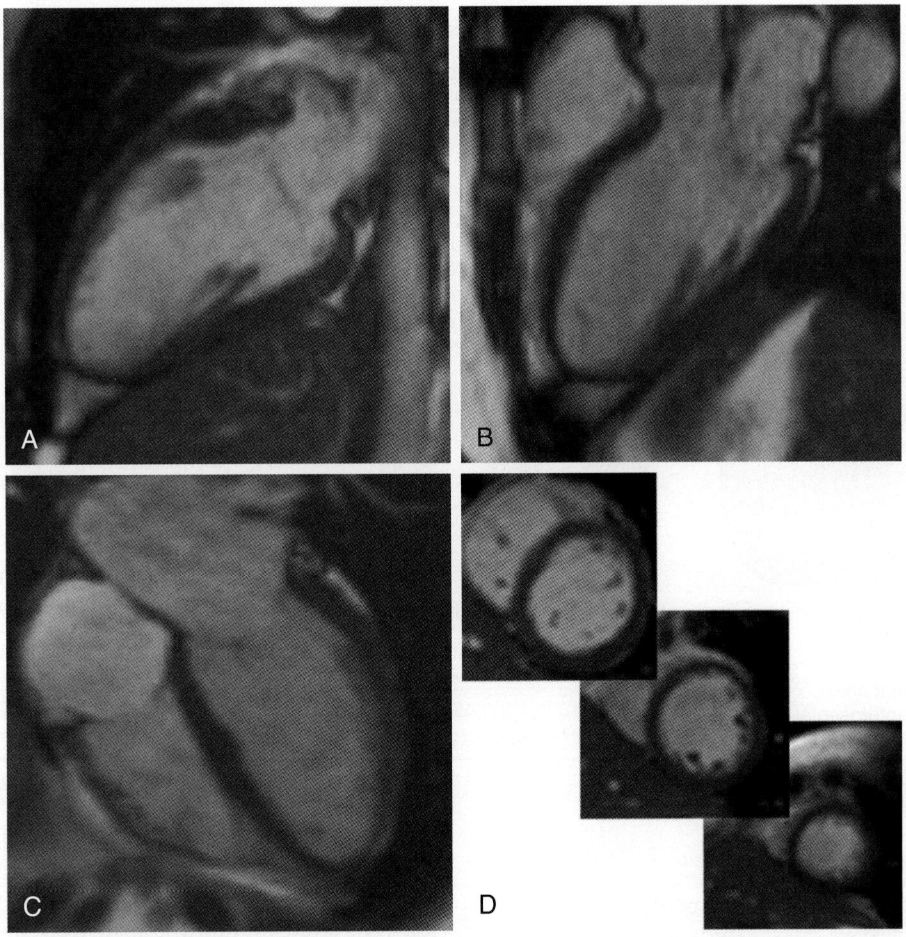

FIG. 13.17 CMR images in various standard anatomic planes. (A) Two-chamber long-axis view; **(B)** three-chamber view; **(C)** four-chamber view; and **(D)** short-axis views at the basal, mid-ventricular, and apical level. *CMR,* Cardiac magnetic resonance.

increased extracellular space where Gd is trapped and not washed out. In this way, ischemic myocardial scars retain Gd and appear bright in the resulting images. However, other areas of scar and increased fibrosis equally appear bright, and the differentiation between ischemic scar (myocardial infarction) and nonischemic causes of scar and fibrosis (eg, myocarditis, hypertrophic cardiomyopathy) has to be made based on the morphology and localization of the scar.

A typical CMR examination in the context of coronary artery disease will first assess cardiac morphology and function. Axial, two-, and four-chamber views, as well as stacks of short-axis images, are used for morphology assessment (Fig. 13.17). Stacks of 10 to 12 contiguous short-axis images, acquired at approximately 20 to 30 phases of the cardiac cycle and displayed in continuous loops, are used to visually and quantitatively assess left ventricular global and regional function. This basic assessment is then followed by further acquisition sequences that are tailored to the specific clinical question. Specifically, in patients with known or suspected chronic coronary artery disease, they will often include myocardial perfusion at rest and stress, as well as delayed enhancement images to identify ischemic scar. To identify the localization of detected pathology, and to assign areas of impaired function, perfusion, or scar to specific coronary arteries, the 17-segment model proposed by the American Society of Echocardiography is typically used[54] (Fig. 13.18).

Ischemia Detection

In clinical practice, the two basic methods to identify ischemia in CMR are (1) MR perfusion imaging during hyperemia using vasodilators (typically adenosine) and (2) dobutamine stress MR to identify stress-induced wall motion abnormalities. Both methods have high diagnostic accuracy and proven prognostic value (event rates in the order of 1% per year if the examination is normal).[55,56] In clinical practice, adenosine stress CMR is used approximately four times more frequently than dobutamine stress CMR.[57]

Dobutamine Stress CMR Imaging

In dobutamine stress CMR, ischemic myocardial segments are identified by assessing local left ventricular wall motion in four standard cine MRI sequences (two-chamber, three-chamber, four-chamber, and short-axis view) at rest and under stepwise increasing doses of dobutamine from 10 to 40 μg/kg per min (plus up to 2 mg atropine if required). The medication protocol of dobutamine stress CMR is equal to that of stress echocardiography.[58] However, because delineation of endocardial borders in CMR is better than in echocardiography, diagnostic accuracy is higher if echocardiographic image quality is suboptimal.[59] In head-to-head comparisons between dobutamine stress and adenosine perfusion CMR, accuracy was equal.[60] However, side effects are not infrequent and require close monitoring of the patients, as well as the infrastructure, to handle arrhythmic events. The reported event rate is 1.6% for atrial fibrillation,

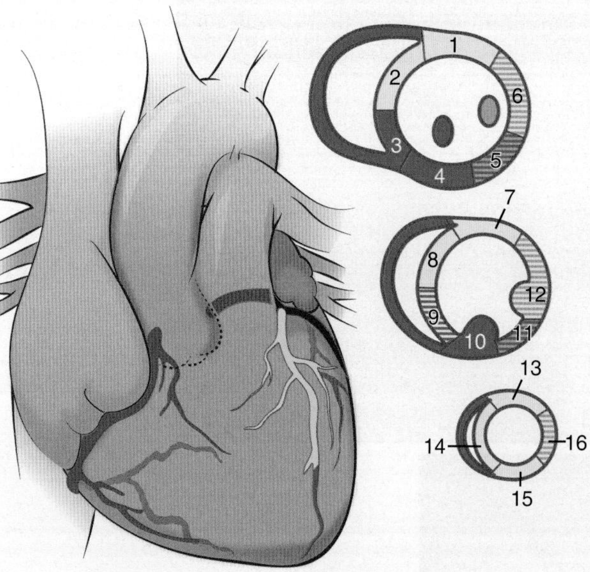

Segment	Typical coronary territory
1 basal anterior	LAD
2 basal anteroseptal	LAD
3 basal inferoseptal	RCA
4 basal inferior	RCA
5 basal inferolateral	LCX or RCA
6 basal anterolateral	LCX or LAC
7 mid anterior	LAD
8 mid anteroseptal	LAD
9 mid inferoseptal	LAD or RCA
10 mid inferior	RCA
11 mid inferolateral	LCX or RCA
12 mid anterolateral	LCX or LAD
13 apical anterior	LAD
14 apical septal	LAD
15 apical inferior	LAD
16 apical lateral	LCX or LAD
17 apical (not depicted)	LAD

FIG. 13.18 Myocardial segments and coronary territories in CMR. *CMR,* Cardiac magnetic resonance; *LAC,* left anterior cardinal vein; *LAD,* left anterior descending artery; *LCX,* left circumflex artery; *RCA,* right coronary artery.

0.4% for nonsustained ventricular tachycardia (VT), and 0.1% for sustained VT.[61] Contraindications for dobutamine stress MRI include acute coronary syndromes, severe aortic stenosis, hypertrophic obstructive cardiomyopathy, and glaucoma. Interestingly, it has been shown that the addition of myocardial stress perfusion imaging can increase the sensitivity of a dobutamine stress CMR, particularly in the presence of left ventricular hypertrophy and/or resting segmental wall motion abnormalities.[62]

Vasodilator Stress CMR

The more frequently used myocardial perfusion test in CMR is vasodilator stress myocardial perfusion with intravenous injection of gadolinium-based contrast agent. Because gadolinium is a positive contrast agent that appears bright in T1-weighted images, normally perfused myocardial segments appear bright in T1-weighted image sequences performed at rest or under pharmacologically induced hyperemia. Coronary arteries with significant stenoses cannot adequately respond to vasodilating stimuli, so the influx of contrast in the dependent segments is delayed and ischemic territories appear darker than the normally perfused segments of the myocardium (Figs. 13.19 and 13.20).

Most frequently, adenosine is used to induce hyperemia (140–210 μg/kg per min for 3 minutes). The typical contrast dose is 0.05–0.1 mmol/kg body weight administered as a bolus. Adenosine has an extremely short half-life of 12 to 20 seconds. Side effects include bronchospasm and atrioventricular (AV) block but are transient in nature given the very short half-life of adenosine. Nevertheless, conduction disturbances and severe chronic obstructive pulmonary disease (COPD)/asthma are considered contraindications. Regadenoson may be an alternative in patients who cannot receive adenosine.[63]

For imaging of myocardial perfusion, T1-weighted sequences with a minimal spatial resolution of 2 mm to 3 mm should be used. In most cases, three short-axis slices are acquired (basal, mid-ventricular, and apical). Typical perfusion sequences are performed in breathhold, because the first pass of injected contrast agent lasts approximately 10 seconds. Although quantitative approaches are available, images are typically interpreted visually. Comparison between rest and stress can be useful to avoid false-positive findings (or between stress perfusion CMR and late enhancement, see following).

The diagnostic accuracy of adenosine stress myocardial perfusion CMR imaging is high. Validated against the presence of coronary artery stenosis in invasive angiography, sensitivity in the multicenter Clinical Evaluation of Magnetic Resonance Imaging in Coronary Heart Disease (CE-MARC) trial was 87% and specificity was 83%.[64] A better reference standard is invasively measured FFR (which serves as the gold standard for ischemia detection). A 2015 meta-analysis that summarized the diagnostic accuracy of various techniques as compared to the gold standard invasive FFR summarized, for stress perfusion CMR imaging, 15 studies and 1830 vessels. Sensitivity (as compared to FFR ≤ 0.80) of CMR perfusion was 87%, specificity was 91%, for a diagnostic odds ratio of 67, making it the noninvasive test that best discriminates between the presence and absence of ischemia (see Table 13.4).[65] Given the high diagnostic performance of CMR stress perfusion, it would be appropriate to use it more frequently for ischemia detection, both in patients with suspected and known coronary artery disease.

Myocardial Viability and Scar

The identification of viable myocardium that is dysfunctional but may recover function after revascularization is of crucial importance in the work-up of patients with chronic coronary artery disease. According to a meta-analysis, revascularization of viable segments reduces mortality by 78%,[66] whereas revascularization of nonviable segments does not change mortality. Mechanisms that can lead to impaired contractility of viable myocardium are stunning and hibernation. Stunning refers to myocardium that displays prolonged dysfunction after ischemia, or chronic dysfunction due to repetitive ischemia and that can regain function after perfusion is normalized. Hibernation refers to myocardium that exhibits chronic dysfunction due to persistently reduced coronary flow and that has the potential to regain function after revascularization. Late gadolinium enhancement imaging can discriminate these two dysfunctional but viable states with the potential for recovery from

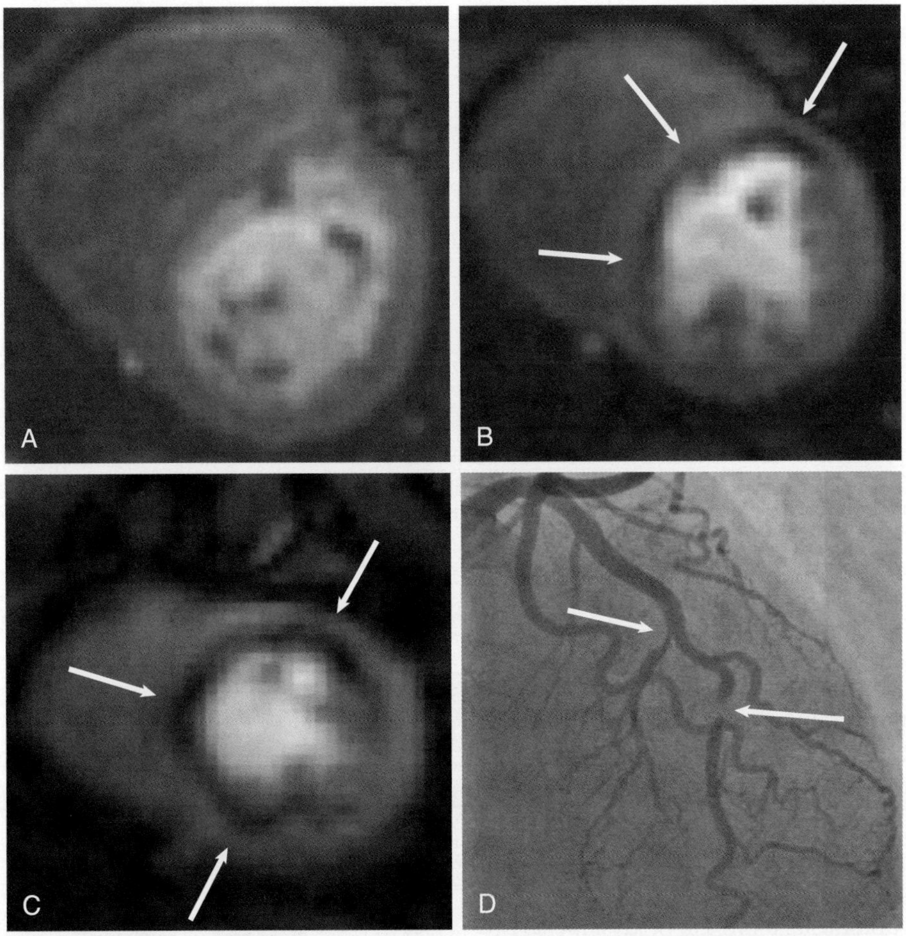

FIG. 13.19 Large myocardial perfusion defect in adenosine stress CMR. (A) Short-axis view, basal level: no perfusion defect. **(B)** Short-axis view, mid-ventricular level: stress-induced hypoenhancement in the mid-inferoseptal, mid-anteroseptal, and mid-anterior segment (*arrows*). **(C)** Short-axis view, apical level: hypoenhancement in the apical inferior, apical septal, and apical anterior segment (*arrows*). **(D)** Corresponding invasive coronary angiogram with a subtotal mid-LAD stenosis and stenosis of a septal branch (*arrows*). *CMR,* Cardiac magnetic resonance.

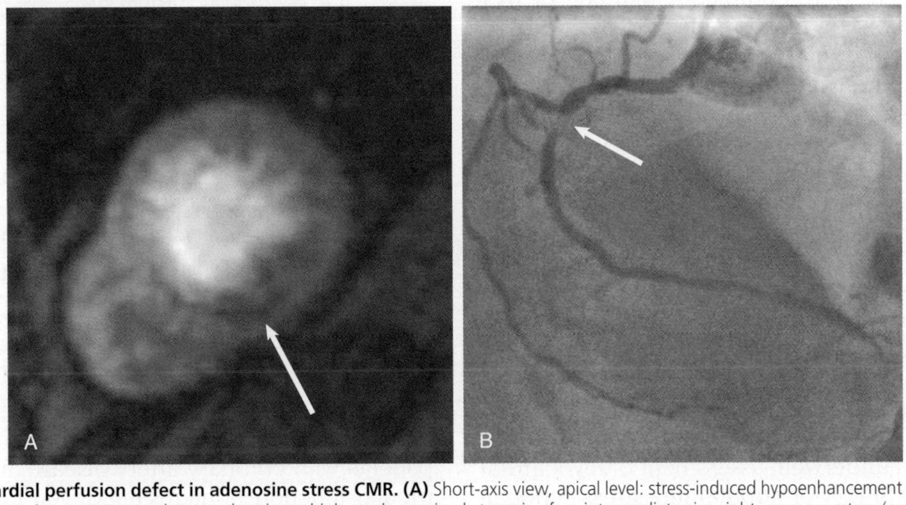

FIG. 13.20 Small myocardial perfusion defect in adenosine stress CMR. (A) Short-axis view, apical level: stress-induced hypoenhancement in the apical inferior segment (*arrow*). **(B)** Corresponding invasive coronary angiogram showing a high-grade proximal stenosis of an intermediate-size right coronary artery (*arrow*). *CMR,* Cardiac magnetic resonance.

irreversibly damaged myocardium in chronic infarction. In vital myocardium, there is little extracellular space and the extravascular gadolinium contrast agents do not accumulate because intact membranes keep them from penetrating into the viable cells. In acute infarction, on the other hand, gadolinium-based contrast agents penetrate into the enlarged extracellular space and are retained to display hyperenhancement in T1-weighted images. In chronic scar tissue, gadolinium-based contrast agents also accumulate (through mechanisms not completely understood). It is assumed that the increased extracellular space plays a relevant role.[67]

For late gadolinium enhancement imaging, T1-weighted sequences, preferably with high resolution between 1.5×1.5

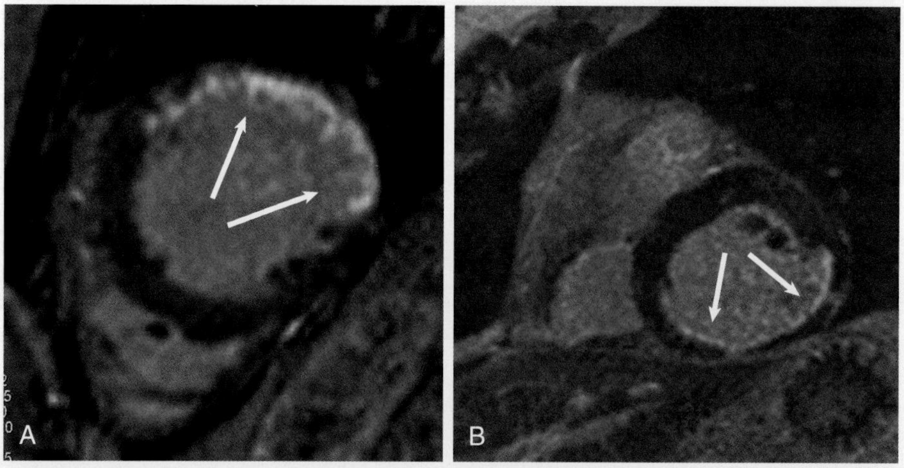

FIG. 13.21 Transmurality of scar in CMR (transmural vs nontransmural < 50%). (A) Transmural late enhancement of the lateral wall (*arrows*: anterolateral and inferolateral segment). **(B)** Late enhancement of the inferolateral wall, with transmurality in small areas and nontransmurality (< 50%) in the majority of the infarct territory (*arrows*: inferior and inferolateral segment). *CMR,* Cardiac magnetic resonance.

mm and 1.0 × 1.0 mm, are used. They are run in standard two-chamber, three-chamber, four-chamber, and short-axis orientations.

The extent of transmurality determines the likelihood of a myocardial segment to regain improved contractility after revascularization (Figs. 13.21 and 13.22). Importantly, it is not a "yes/no" issue, but rather a question of probability. This was first demonstrated by Kim et al.[68] in a landmark paper published in 2000, examining 41 patients with 806 dysfunctional segments. The likelihood of dysfunctional segments (hypokinesia, akinesia, or dyskinesia) to improve contractility after revascularization ranged from 80%, if there was complete absence of late enhancement, to 2%, if late enhancement was transmural (see Fig. 13.21). Importantly, in segments without transmural late gadolinium enhancement that were completely akinetic or dyskinetic at baseline, revascularization resulted in improved contractility in 100% of cases (12 of 12).[68] A meta-analysis confirmed these findings, demonstrating that late gadolinium enhancement had a sensitivity of 95% and specificity of 51% to predict recovery of function after revascularization, using a cut-off of 50% transmurality for viability.[69] This threshold is typically used in clinical practice, labeling myocardial segments with less than 50% transmurality of late enhancement as "viable" and those with more than 50% late enhancement as "nonviable." Potentially, adding low-dose dobutamine may increase the diagnostic accuracy of cardiac MRI for viability assessment, but this is rarely done in clinical practice. In a substudy of the multicenter, nonblinded, randomized Surgical Treatment for Ischemic Heart Failure (STICH) trial that enrolled a total of 1212 patients, 601 patients underwent assessment of myocardial viability using either SPECT or dobutamine stress echocardiography.[70] This study failed to show that the assessment of myocardial viability would identify patients with a survival benefit after coronary artery bypass grafting. However, several limitations make the study results difficult to generalize: (1) viability testing was not randomized; (2) significant differences in baseline characteristics of the patient groups were present; (3) there was a relatively small group of patients without viability; and (4) a binary classification of viability was used with controversial thresholds for extent and uptake.

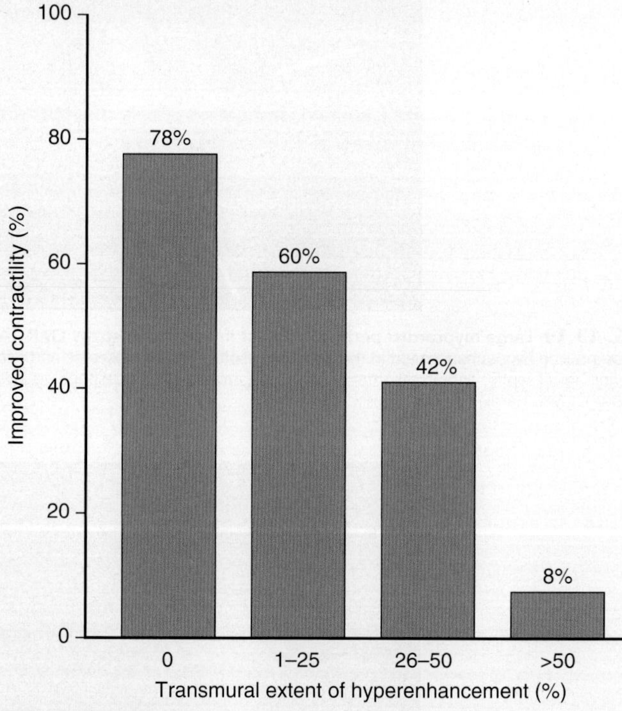

FIG. 13.22 Relationship between transmurality of scar and likelihood for functional improvement. *(Kim RJ, Wu E, Rafael A, et al. The use of contrast-enhanced magnetic resonance imaging to identify reversible myocardial dysfunction.* N Engl J Med. *2000;343:1445–1453.)*

On the other hand, the presence of late gadolinium enhancement identified by CMR has prognostic relevance in patients with coronary artery disease and impaired left ventricular function.[71] Interestingly, even the incidental identification of small ischemic scars in asymptomatic individuals, for example, with diabetes, has substantial prognostic relevance.[72] In a study of 107 diabetic individuals who were free of symptoms and known coronary artery disease, delayed enhancement consistent with ischemic myocardial scar was observed in 30 patients. Their odds ratios for major adverse cardiac events (MACE) and death were 3.7 and 3.6, respectively, as compared to individuals without scar. Currently, however, there are no recommendations for screening of asymptomatic individuals with delayed enhancement CMR.

Magnetic Resonance Angiography

Magnetic resonance imaging is able to visualize the coronary artery lumen and to identify coronary atherosclerotic plaque.[73] However, the limited spatial resolution of MR and the very small dimensions of the coronary vessels, along with the rapid motion, make MR coronary angiography extremely challenging. In a meta-analysis, the sensitivity for stenosis detection was 89%, with a specificity of 78%; 3-tesla equipment, whole-heart examinations, and contrast injection improved diagnostic accuracy.[74] However, coronary imaging by CMR is too difficult and unstable to play a relevant clinical role and, for the foreseeable future, CT imaging will remain superior to MR regarding the direct visualization of the coronary arteries. Only for visualization of coronary anomalies is the use of coronary MRI angiography considered fully appropriate.[73]

CT AND MRI: GUIDELINES

With the technical improvements over the past years and the vast amount of clinical data that have accumulated and confirm the clinical, diagnostic, and prognostic value of cardiac CT and cardiac MR, the two diagnostic techniques have been incorporated into numerous clinical practice guidelines issued by professional societies. Understandably, guideline writers are reluctant to include new techniques and applications, given the often overly positive study results of early technology validation.

For suspected stable coronary artery disease, the American College of Cardiology/American Heart Association assign, in their 2012 guidelines, a class IIa recommendation ("should be considered") to stress perfusion CMR imaging if patients have an intermediate to high pretest likelihood of coronary artery disease and are unable to exercise (or if they are able to exercise but have an uninterpretable ECG).[75] A class IIa recommendation is issued to coronary CTA if patients are unable to exercise and have a low to intermediate pretest likelihood of disease. A class IIb recommendation ("may be considered") is given to coronary CTA in patients who can exercise and have an intermediate pretest likelihood of disease. Coronary CTA is also endorsed with a class IIa recommendation if patients have an intermediate pretest likelihood of disease and an inconclusive exercise test, ongoing symptoms in spite of a normal exercise test, or are unable to undergo stress testing by myocardial perfusion imaging or stress echocardiography. Furthermore, stress CMR carries a class I recommendation (along with other perfusion tests) to determine the hemodynamic relevance and need for revascularization of stenoses that are already known.

Guidelines on stable coronary artery disease issued by the European Society of Cardiology (ESC) in 2013 differentiate between stress ECG and imaging-based stress tests, but do not differentiate between the various available imaging-based ischemia tests.[76] They assign a class I recommendation to stress imaging (rather than stress ECG) tests if pretest likelihood in suspected coronary artery disease is greater than 50% or if there is impaired left ventricular function. They also assign a class IIa recommendation to stress imaging tests in symptomatic patients with prior revascularization and to assessing the functional severity of intermediate lesions on invasive coronary angiography.[76]

Interestingly, the ESC acknowledges a potential role of stress imaging (class IIb recommendation)—for example, myocardial stress perfusion CMR imaging—in asymptomatic, high-risk individuals, stating that "In asymptomatic adults with diabetes or asymptomatic adults with a strong family history of CAD or when previous risk assessment testing suggests high risk of CAD, such as a coronary artery calcium score of 400 or greater stress imaging tests (myocardial perfusion imaging [MPI], stress echocardiography, perfusion CMR) may be considered for advanced cardiovascular risk assessment."

For coronary CTA, the ESC acknowledges a role (class IIa recommendation) in patients with suspected coronary artery disease, a pretest likelihood between 15% and 50%, and suitable patient characteristics for high-quality CT with low radiation dose.

It is likely that future guidelines will strengthen the recommendations supporting coronary CTA in symptomatic patients, based on the results from PROMISE and SCOT-HEART that demonstrated comparable or even improved outcomes for a CTA-based approach as compared with a functional testing approach.

CONCLUSIONS

Both cardiac CT (mainly in the form of coronary CTA) and cardiac MR play an increasingly important role in the management of patients with suspected or known coronary artery disease. Coronary CTA has its major application in ruling out stenoses in patients with a relatively low pretest likelihood of disease. CMR, on the other hand, has a role that extends to the more advanced stages of disease and includes ischemia detection in patients with known intermediate coronary artery stenoses or returning symptoms after revascularization, and the assessment of viability in the context of complex revascularization decisions in patients with regional wall motion abnormalities. Both technologies require expertise in image acquisition and interpretation, and image quality is not constant across all patient subsets. Therefore, their utilization depends on regional and patient-specific circumstances.

Technology progresses both in CT and MRI, and new applications are constantly being developed and evaluated. It can be expected that the role of both techniques in patients with chronic coronary artery disease will continue to expand in the future.

References

1. Abbara S, Arbab-Zadeh A, Callister TQ, et al.: SCCT guidelines for performance of coronary computed tomographic angiography: a report of the Society of Cardiovascular Computed Tomography Guidelines Committee, *J Cardiovasc Comput Tomogr* 3:190–204, 2009.
2. Leipsic J, Abbara S, Achenbach S, et al.: SCCT guidelines for the interpretation and reporting of coronary CT angiography: a report of the Society of Cardiovascular Computed Tomography Guidelines Committee, *J Cardiovasc Comput Tomogr* 8(5):342–358, 2014.
3. Schuhbaeck A, Achenbach S, Layritz C, et al.: Image quality of ultra-low radiation exposure coronary CT angiography with an effective dose < 0.1 mSv using high-pitch spiral acquisition and raw data-based iterative reconstruction, *Eur Radiol* 23(3):597–606, 2013.
4. Hell MM, Bittner D, Schuhbaeck A, et al.: Prospectively ECG-triggered high-pitch coronary angiography with third-generation dual-source CT at 70 kVp tube voltage: feasibility, image quality, radiation dose, and effect of iterative reconstruction, *J Cardiovasc Comput Tomogr* 8:418–425, 2014.
5. Chinnaiyan KM, Boura JA, DePetris A, et al.: Advanced Cardiovascular Imaging Consortium Coinvestigators. Progressive radiation dose reduction from coronary computed tomography angiography in a statewide collaborative quality improvement program: results from the Advanced Cardiovascular Imaging Consortium, *Circ Cardiovasc Imaging* 6:646–654, 2013.
6. Rochitte CE, George RT, Chen MY, et al.: Computed tomography angiography and perfusion to assess coronary artery stenosis causing perfusion defects by single photon emission computed tomography: the CORE320 study, *Eur Heart J* 35:1120–1130, 2014.
7. Budoff MJ, Dowe D, Jollis JG, et al.: Diagnostic performance of 64-multidetector-row coronary computed tomographic angiography for evaluation of coronary artery stenosis in individuals without known coronary artery disease, *J Am Coll Cardiol* 52:1724–1732, 2008.
8. Meijboom WB, Meijs MF, Schuijf JD, et al.: Diagnostic accuracy of 64-slice computed tomography coronary angiography: a prospective, multicenter, multivendor study, *J Am Coll Cardiol* 52: 2135–2144, 2008.

9. Miller JM, Rochitte CE, Dewey M, et al.: Diagnostic performance of coronary angiography by 64-row CT, *N Engl J Med* 359:2324–2336, 2008.
10. Menke J, Kowalski J: Diagnostic accuracy and utility of coronary CT angiography with consideration of unevaluable results: a systematic review and multivariate Bayesian random-effects meta-analysis with intention to diagnose, *Eur Radiol* 26(2):451–458, 2016.
11. Meijboom WB, van Mieghem CA, Mollet NR, et al.: 64-slice computed tomography coronary angiography in patients with high, intermediate, or low pretest probability of significant coronary artery disease, *J Am Coll Cardiol* 50:1469–1475, 2007.
12. Hadamitzky M, Freissmuth B, Meyer T, et al.: Prognostic value of coronary computed tomographic angiography for prediction of cardiac events in patients with suspected coronary artery disease, *JACC Cardiovasc Imaging* 2:404–411, 2009.
13. Ostrom MP, Gopal A, Ahmadi N, et al.: Mortality incidence and the severity of coronary atherosclerosis assessed by computed tomography angiography, *J Am Coll Cardiol* 52:1335–1343, 2008.
14. Otaki Y, Arsanjani R, Gransar H, et al.: What have we learned from CONFIRM? Prognostic implications from a prospective multicenter international observational cohort study of consecutive patients undergoing coronary computed tomographic angiography, *J Nucl Cardiol* 19:787–795, 2012.
15. Min JK, Dunning A, Lin FY, et al.: CONFIRM Investigators. Age- and sex-related differences in all-cause mortality risk based on coronary computed tomography angiography findings results from the International Multicenter CONFIRM (Coronary CT Angiography Evaluation for Clinical Outcomes: An International Multicenter Registry) of 23,854 patients without known coronary artery disease, *J Am Coll Cardiol* 58(8):849–860, 2011.
16. Shaw LJ, Hausleiter J, Achenbach S, et al.: CONFIRM Registry Investigators. Coronary computed tomographic angiography as a gatekeeper to invasive diagnostic and surgical procedures: results from the multicenter CONFIRM (Coronary CT Angiography Evaluation for Clinical Outcomes: an International Multicenter) registry, *J Am Coll Cardiol* 60(20):2103–2114, 2012.
17. Douglas PS, Hoffmann U, Patel MR, et al.: PROMISE Investigators. Outcomes of anatomical versus functional testing for coronary artery disease, *N Engl J Med* 372(14):1291–1300, 2015.
18. SCOT-HEART Investigators: CT coronary angiography in patients with suspected angina due to coronary heart disease (SCOT-HEART): an open-label, parallel-group, multicentre trial, *Lancet* 385(9985):2383–2391, 2015.
19. Linde JJ, Hove JD, Sorgaard M, et al.: Long-term clinical impact of coronary CT angiography in patients with recent acute-onset chest pain: the randomized controlled CATCH trial, *J Am Coll Cardiol* 8:1404–1413, 2015.
20. McKavanagh P, Lusk L, Ball PA, et al.: A comparison of cardiac computerized tomography and exercise stress electrocardiogram test for the investigation of stable chest pain: the clinical results of the CAPP randomized prospective trial, *Eur Heart J Cardiovasc Imaging* 16:441–448, 2015.
21. Vanhoenacker PK, Decramer I, Bladt O, et al.: Multidetector computed tomography angiography for assessment of in-stent restenosis: meta-analysis of diagnostic performance, *BMC Med Imaging* 8:14, 2008.
22. Onuma Y, Dudek D, Thuesen L, et al.: Five-year clinical and functional multislice computed tomography angiographic results after coronary implantation of the fully resorbable polymeric everolimus-eluting scaffold in patients with de novo coronary artery disease: the ABSORB cohort A trial, *JACC Cardiovasc Interv* 6(10):999–1009, 2013.
23. Barbero U, Iannaccone M, d'Ascenzo F, et al.: 64 slice-coronary computed tomography sensitivity and specificity in the evaluation of coronary artery bypass graft stenosis: a meta-analysis, *Int J Cardiol* 216:52–57, 2016.
24. Heye T, Kauczor HU, Szabo G, Hosch W: Computed tomography angiography of coronary artery bypass grafts: robustness in emergency and clinical routine settings, *Acta Radiol* 55(2):161–170, 2014.
25. Schuijf JD, Wijns W, Jukema JW, et al.: Relationship between noninvasive coronary angiography with multi-slice computed tomography and myocardial perfusion imaging, *J Am Coll Cardiol* 48:2508–2514, 2006.
26. Shaw LJ, Hausleiter J, Achenbach S, et al.: CONFIRM Registry Investigators. Coronary computed tomographic angiography as a gatekeeper to invasive diagnostic and surgical procedures: results from the multicenter CONFIRM (Coronary CT Angiography Evaluation for Clinical Outcomes: an International Multicenter) registry, *J Am Coll Cardiol* 60(20):2103–2114, 2012.
27. Min JK, Taylor CA, Achenbach S, et al.: Noninvasive fractional flow reserve derived from coronary CT angiography: clinical data and scientific principles, *JACC Cardiovasc Imaging* 8(10):1209–1222, 2015.
28. Nørgaard BL, Leipsic J, Gaur S, et al.: NXT Trial Study Group. Diagnostic performance of noninvasive fractional flow reserve derived from coronary computed tomography angiography in suspected coronary artery disease: the NXT trial (Analysis of Coronary Blood Flow Using CT Angiography: Next Steps), *J Am Coll Cardiol* 63(12):1145–1155, 2014.
29. Douglas PS, Pontone G, Hlatky MA, et al.: PLATFORM Investigators. Clinical outcomes of fractional flow reserve by computed tomographic angiography-guided diagnostic strategies vs. usual care in patients with suspected coronary artery disease: the prospective longitudinal trial of FFR(CT): outcome and resource impacts study, *Eur Heart J* 36(47):3359–3367, 2015.
30. Hoff JA, Chomka EV, Krainik AJ, et al.: Age and gender distribution of coronary artery calcium detected by electron beam tomography, *Am J Cardiol* 87:1335–1339, 2001.
31. McClelland RL, Chung H, Detrano R, et al.: Distribution of coronary artery calcium by race, gender, and age: results from the Multi-Ethnic Study of Atherosclerosis (MESA), *Circulation* 113:30–37, 2006.
32. Schmermund A, Mohlenkamp S, Berenbein S, et al.: Population-based assessment of subclinical coronary atherosclerosis using electro-beam computed tomography, *Atherosclerosis* 185:117–182, 2006.
33. Rumberger JA, Simons DB, Fitzpatrick LA, et al.: Coronary artery calcium area by electron-beam computed tomography and coronary atherosclerotic plaque area. A histopathologic correlative study, *Circulation* 92:2157–2162, 1995.
34. Folsom AR, Kronmal RA, Detrano RC, et al.: Coronary artery calcification compared with carotid intima-media thickness in the prediction of cardiovascular disease incidence: the Multi-Ethnic Study of Atherosclerosis (MESA), *Arch Intern Med* 168(12):1333–1339, 2008.
35. Detrano R, Guerci AD, Carr JJ, et al.: Coronary calcium as a predictor of coronary events in four racial or ethnic groups, *N Engl J Med* 358:1336–1345, 2008.
36. Erbel R, Möhlenkamp S, Moebus S, et al.: Heinz Nixdorf Recall Study Investigative Group. Coronary risk stratification, discrimination, and reclassification improvement based on quantification of subclinical coronary atherosclerosis: the Heinz Nixdorf Recall study, *J Am Coll Cardiol* 56(17):1397–1406, 2010.
37. Marwan M, Ropers D, Pflederer T, et al.: Clinical characteristics of patients with obstructive coronary lesions in the absence of coronary calcification: an evaluation by coronary CT angiography, *Heart* 95:1056–1060, 2009.
38. Greenland P, Bonow RO, Brundage BH, et al.: ACCF/AHA 2007 clinical expert consensus document on coronary artery calcium scoring by computed tomography in global cardiovascular risk assessment and in evaluation of patients with chest pain: a report of the American College of Cardiology Foundation Clinical Expert Consensus Task Force (ACCF/AHA Writing Committee to Update the 2000 Expert Consensus Document on Electron Beam Computed Tomography), *Circulation* 115:402–426, 2007.
39. Taylor AJ, Cerqueira M, Hodgson JM, et al.: American College of Cardiology Foundation Appropriate Use Criteria Task Force; Society of Cardiovascular Computed Tomography; American College of Radiology; American Heart Association; American Society of Echocardiography; American Society of Nuclear Cardiology; North American Society for Cardiovascular Imaging; Society for Cardiovascular Angiography and Interventions; Society for Cardiovascular Magnetic Resonance. ACCF/SCCT/ACR/AHA/ASE/ASNC/NASCI/SCAI/SCMR 2010 appropriate use criteria for cardiac computed tomography. A report of the American College of Cardiology Foundation Appropriate Use Criteria Task Force, the Society of Cardiovascular Computed Tomography, the American College of Radiology, the American Heart Association, the American Society of Echocardiography, the American Society of Nuclear Cardiology, the North American Society for Cardiovascular Imaging, the Society for Cardiovascular Angiography and Interventions, and the Society for Cardiovascular Magnetic Resonance, *J Am Coll Cardiol* 56(22):1864–1894, 2010.
40. Min JK, Shaw LJ, Devereux RB, et al.: Prognostic value of multidetector coronary computed tomographic angiography for prediction of all-cause mortality, *J Am Coll Cardiol* 50:1161–1170, 2007.
41. Ostrom MP, Gopal A, Ahmadi N, et al.: Mortality incidence and the severity of coronary atherosclerosis assessed by computed tomography angiography, *J Am Coll Cardiol* 52:1335–1343, 2008.
42. Min JK, Dunning A, Lin FY, et al.: CONFIRM Investigators. Age- and sex-related differences in all-cause mortality risk based on coronary computed tomography angiography findings results from the International Multicenter CONFIRM (Coronary CT Angiography Evaluation for Clinical Outcomes: An International Multicenter Registry) of 23,854 patients without known coronary artery disease, *J Am Coll Cardiol* 58(8):849–860, 2011.
43. Al-Mallah MH, Qureshi W, Lin FY, et al.: Does coronary CT angiography improve risk stratification over coronary calcium scoring in symptomatic patients with suspected coronary artery disease? Results from the prospective multicenter international CONFIRM registry, *Eur Heart J Cardiovasc Imaging* 15(3): 267–267, 2014.
44. Motoyama S, Sarai M, Harigaya H, et al.: Computed tomographic angiography characteristics of atherosclerotic plaques subsequently resulting in acute coronary syndrome, *J Am Coll Cardiol* 54:49–57, 2009.
45. Park HB, Heo R, ó Hartaigh B, et al.: Atherosclerotic plaque characteristics by CT angiography identify coronary lesions that cause ischemia: a direct comparison to fractional flow reserve, *JACC Cardiovasc Imaging* 8(1): 1–1, 2015.
46. Diaz-Zamudio M, Dey D, Schuhbaeck A, et al.: Automated quantitative plaque burden from coronary CT angiography noninvasively predicts hemodynamic significance by using fractional flow reserve in intermediate coronary lesions, *Radiology* 276(2):408–415, 2015.
47. Chow BJ, Small G, Yam Y, et al.: CONFIRM Investigators. Prognostic and therapeutic implications of statin and aspirin therapy in individuals with nonobstructive coronary artery disease: results from the CONFIRM (COronary CT Angiography EvaluatioN For Clinical Outcomes: An InteRnational Multicenter registry) registry, *Arterioscler Thromb Vasc Biol.* 35:981–989, 2015.
48. Schepis T, Achenbach S, Marwan M, et al.: Prevalence of first-pass myocardial perfusion defects detected by contrast-enhanced dual-source CT in patients with non-ST segment elevation acute coronary syndromes, *Eur Radiol* 20(7):1607–1614, 2010.
49. Danad I, Szymonifka J, Schulman-Marcus J, Min JK: Static and dynamic assessment of myocardial perfusion by computed tomography, *Eur Heart J Cardiovasc Imaging* 17(8):836–844, 2016. pii: jew044.
50. Pelgrim GJ, Dorrius M, Xie X, et al.: The dream of a one-stop-shop: meta-analysis on myocardial perfusion CT, *Eur J Radiol* 84(12):2411–2420, 2015.
51. Takx RA, Blomberg BA, El Aidi H, et al.: Diagnostic accuracy of stress myocardial perfusion imaging compared to invasive coronary angiography with fractional flow reserve meta-analysis, *Circ Cardiovasc Imaging* 8(1), pii: e002666, 2015.
52. Gotschy A, Niemann M, Kozerke S, et al.: Cardiovascular magnetic resonance for the assessment of coronary artery disease, *Int J Cardiol* 193:84–92, 2015.
53. Morcos SK: Nephrogenic systemic fibrosis following the administration of extracellular gadolinium based contrast agents: is the stability of the contrast agent molecule an important factor in the pathogenesis of this condition? *Br J Radiol* 80:73–76, 2007.
54. Lang RM, Badano LP, Mor-Avi V, et al.: Recommendations for cardiac chamber quantification by echocardiography in adults: an update from the American Society of Echocardiography and the European Association of Cardiovascular Imaging, *J Am Soc Echocardiogr* 28(1):1–39. e14, 2015.
55. Lipinski MJ, McVey CM, Berger JS, et al.: Prognostic value of stress cardiac magnetic resonance imaging in patients with known or suspected coronary artery disease: a systematic review and meta-analysis, *J Am Coll Cardiol* 62:826–838, 2013.
56. Gargiulo P, Dellegrottaglie S, Bruzzese D, et al.: The prognostic value of normal stress cardiac magnetic resonance in patients with known or suspected coronary artery disease: a meta-analysis, *Circ Cardiovasc Imaging* 6:574–582, 2013.
57. Bruder O, Wagner A, Lombardi M, et al.: European Cardiovascular Magnetic Resonance (EuroCMR) registry—multinational results from 57 centers in 15 countries, *J Cardiovasc Magn Reson* 15:9, 2013.
58. Schwitter J, Arai AE: Assessment of cardiac ischaemia and viability: role of cardiovascular magnetic resonance, *Eur Heart J* 32:799–809, 2011.
59. Nagel E, Lehmkuhl HB, Boksch C, et al.: Noninvasive diagnosis of ischemia-induced wall motion abnormalities with the use of high-dose dobutamine stress MRI: comparison with dobutamine stress echocardiography, *Circulation* 99:763–770, 1999.
60. Manka R, Jahnke C, Gebker R, et al.: Head-to-head comparison of first-pass MR perfusion imaging during adenosine and high-dose dobutamine/atropine stress, *Int J Cardiovasc Imaging* 27: 995–1002, 2011.
61. Wahl A, Paetsch I, Gollesch A, et al.: Safety and feasibility of high-dose dobutamine-atropine stress cardiovascular magnetic resonance for diagnosis of myocardial ischaemia: experience in 1000 consecutive cases, *Eur Heart J* 25:1230–1236, 2004.
62. Gebker R, Jahnke C, Manka R, et al.: Additional value of myocardial perfusion imaging during dobutamine stress magnetic resonance for the assessment of coronary artery disease, *Circ Cardiovasc Imaging* 1:122–130, 2008.
63. Vasu S, Bandettini WP, Hsu LY, et al.: Regadenoson and adenosine are equivalent vasodilators and are superior than dipyridamole—a study of first pass quantitative perfusion cardiovascular magnetic resonance, *J Cardiovasc Magnet Reson* 15:85, 2013.
64. Greenwood JP, Maredia N, Younger JF, et al.: Cardiovascular magnetic resonance and single-photon emission computed tomography for diagnosis of coronary heart disease (CE-MARC): a prospective trial, *Lancet* 379:453–460, 2012.
65. Takx RA, Blomberg BA, El Aidi H, et al.: Diagnostic accuracy of stress myocardial perfusion imaging compared to invasive coronary angiography with fractional flow reserve meta-analysis, *Circ Cardiovasc Imaging* 8, 2015, http://dx.doi.org/10.1161/CIRCIMAGING.114.00266.
66. Allman KC, Shaw LJ, Hachamovitch R, Udelson JE: Myocardial viability testing and impact of revascularization on prognosis in patients with coronary artery disease and left ventricular dysfunction: a meta-analysis, *J Am Coll Cardiol* 39:1151–1158, 2002.
67. Van Assche LM, Kim HW, Kim RJ: Cardiac MR for the assessment of myocardial viability, *Methodist DeBakey Cardiovasc J* 9:163–168, 2013.
68. Kim RJ, Wu E, Rafael A, et al.: The use of contrast-enhanced magnetic resonance imaging to identify reversible myocardial dysfunction, *N Engl J Med* 343:1445–1453, 2000.
69. Romero J, Xue X, Gonzalez W, Garcia MJ: CMR imaging assessing viability in patients with chronic ventricular dysfunction due to coronary artery disease: a meta-analysis of prospective trials, *JACC Cardiovasc Imaging* 5:494–508, 2012.
70. Bonow RO, Maurer G, Lee KL, et al.: STICH Trial Investigators. Myocardial viability and survival in ischemic left ventricular dysfunction, *N Engl J Med* 364:1617–1625, 2011.
71. Gerber BL, Rousseau MF, Ahn SA, et al.: Prognostic value of myocardial viability by delayed-enhanced magnetic resonance in patients with coronary artery disease and low ejection fraction: impact of revascularization therapy, *J Am Coll Cardiol* 59:825–833, 2012.
72. Kwong RY, Sattar H, Wu H, et al.: Incidence and prognostic implication of unrecognized myocardial scar characterized by cardiac magnetic resonance in diabetic patients without clinical evidence of myocardial infarction, *Circulation* 118:1011–1020, 2008.

73. Dweck MR, Puntman V, Vesey AT, et al.: MR imaging of coronary arteries and plaques, *JACC Cardiovasc Imaging* 9:306–316, 2016.
74. Di Leo G, Fisci E, Secchi F, et al.: Diagnostic accuracy of magnetic resonance angiography for detection of coronary artery disease: a systematic review and meta-analysis, *Eur Radiol* 26:3706–3718, 2016.
75. Fihn SD, Gardin JM, Abrams J, et al.: American College of Cardiology Foundation/American Heart Association Task Force. 2012 ACCF/AHA/ACP/AATS/PCNA/SCAI/STS guideline for the diagnosis and management of patients with stable ischemic heart disease: a report of the American College of Cardiology Foundation/American Heart Association Task Force on Practice Guidelines, and the American College of Physicians, American Association for Thoracic Surgery, Preventive Cardiovascular Nurses Association, Society for Cardiovascular Angiography and Interventions, and Society of Thoracic Surgeons, *Circulation* 126:e354–e471, 2012.
76. Task Force Members, Montalescot G, Sechtem U, Achenbach S, et al.: ESC Committee for Practice Guidelines, Zamorano JL, Achenbach S, Baumgartner H, et al.; Document Reviewers, Knuuti J, Valgimigli M, Bueno H, et al. 2013 ESC guidelines on the management of stable coronary artery disease: the Task Force on the management of stable coronary artery disease of the European Society of Cardiology, *Eur Heart J* 34:2949–3003, 2013.

14 Invasive Testing

William F. Fearon

When noninvasive testing for coronary artery disease (CAD) is inconclusive or suggests significant pathology, invasive testing is necessary. X-ray coronary angiography provides an overview of the coronary circulation and in particular helps to identify obstructive epicardial CAD. However, the coronary angiogram is often misleading. Significant-appearing CAD may not be responsible for myocardial ischemia and symptoms, whereas occult diffuse epicardial disease not apparent on the angiogram can be. Moreover, the coronary angiogram focuses on fixed obstructive epicardial disease, but it does not provide information regarding endothelial dysfunction or vasospasm, nor does it identify coronary microvascular dysfunction. A number of adjunctive techniques including both coronary wire-based measures and catheter-based systems allow for further interrogation of the coronary circulation at the time of coronary angiography. This chapter will focus on the main methods for assessing coronary physiology, namely coronary flow reserve, fractional flow reserve, and the index of microcirculatory resistance, as well as the two main methods for invasively imaging the epicardial coronary anatomy, namely intravascular ultrasound and optical coherence tomography.

CORONARY ANGIOGRAPHY

Coronary angiography is defined as the visualization of the coronary arteries after injection of contrast media. Typically, the angiographic diagnosis of CAD is made subjectively by the cardiologist who performed the procedure. In general, a visual estimation of the severity of a coronary narrowing is reported, for which a 50% stenosis is considered as obstructive coronary disease and greater than 70% stenosis as significant coronary disease. Classification systems aimed at standardizing the interpretation of an angiogram have been created that incorporate lesion characteristics such as degree of calcification, length, eccentricity, tortuosity, and location at a bifurcation. These techniques, however, are inherently limited by interobserver variability.[1]

Quantitative coronary angiography is a computer-assisted method of measuring lesion length and stenosis severity. By using an object of known size, such as the catheter, to calibrate the system, quantitative coronary angiography ideally is less subjective and more accurate than other methods. Unfortunately, it too is prone to error and subjectivity due to operator technique. Despite these issues, the presence and severity of coronary disease as assessed by coronary angiography are predictors of long-term adverse outcome.

A number of limitations to angiography hamper its ability to accurately diagnose coronary disease, especially in the setting of moderate narrowing or diffuse disease. First, because the angiogram is a two-dimensional representation of a three-dimensional object, an eccentric narrowing can be missed if the correct angle is not used to image the vessel.[2] Second, because a diseased area of a coronary artery is generally compared with an adjacent "normal" area, patients with diffuse disease without any focal component can be incorrectly classified as having normal coronary arteries. Finally, the angiogram highlights the lumen of the coronary artery but provides no information about the wall of the vessel. Positive remodeling of the artery at the site of atherosclerotic plaque development can result in preservation of the lumen and a near normal angiogram, which hide the atherosclerosis from the angiographer. Because of these limitations a number of adjunctive techniques have been developed to improve the invasive diagnosis of ischemic heart disease.

CORONARY FLOW RESERVE

Coronary flow reserve (CFR) is defined as the ratio of the maximal or hyperemic flow down a coronary vessel to the resting flow.[3] It can be measured invasively with a Doppler-tipped coronary guidewire that determines coronary velocity at rest and during hyperemia, typically induced with intracoronary or intravenous adenosine.[4] Because velocity is proportional to flow, the coronary flow velocity reserve is a reflection of the CFR. If in addition to the velocity the area of the coronary vessel is known, the absolute CFR can be calculated. CFR also can be measured invasively by using a wire-based thermodilution technique.[5] On one of the commercially available coronary pressure wires (St. Jude Medical, MIN), the pressure sensor also can act as a thermistor. With the commercially available software, the shaft of the wire acts as a proximal thermistor. Room temperature saline can be injected into the coronary artery and this system will calculate the transit time, which is inversely proportional to coronary flow. After three injections at rest, the resting mean transit time is calculated. Hyperemia is then induced with intravenous adenosine, and three injections are performed to determine the hyperemic mean transit time. CFR is measured in this situation by dividing the resting mean transit time by the hyperemic mean transit time. The thermodilution-derived CFR has been validated in animal and human models and has been compared in an animal model to a reference standard of absolute flow.[5–7] It appears to correlate more closely to the standard than does Doppler-derived CFR.

A normal CFR is considered to be greater than 2.0 and in most patients should be somewhere between 3 and 5. Initially, invasive CFR was performed to interrogate the functional significance of an intermediate coronary stenosis with studies showing a correlation between CFR and noninvasive tests for ischemia.[8] However, a number of limitations of invasively measured CFR impaired its broad clinical utility. First, it can be difficult to measure with a Doppler wire because of the challenge in obtaining a suitable Doppler signal. Second, because CFR relies on resting flow for its calculation, the repeatability of measurements is less than optimal. Any hemodynamic perturbation such as a change in heart rate, blood pressure, or left ventricular contractility will significantly change the CFR value as a result of the change in resting flow.[9] The lack of a clear cut-off between a normal and abnormal CFR makes it difficult to use for clinical decisions. Because there is a range of normal CFR values between approximately 2.5 and 6, in one patient a value of 3.0 might be normal whereas in another patient normal CFR may be 5.0 and therefore a recorded value of 3.0 could be quite abnormal. Finally, by definition CFR is a measure of the entire coronary circulation. It interrogates the epicardial vessel as well as the coronary microvasculature (Fig. 14.1). Therefore, a low CFR value may be a result of significant epicardial CAD, microvascular dysfunction, or both.[10] For all of these reasons, invasively measured CFR has largely been abandoned as a method for interrogating intermediate coronary lesions. However, in patients with normal appearing epicardial coronary vessels, invasively measured CFR can be used to assess microvascular function. However, because of the previously mentioned limitations and the availability of other methods for assessing the microvasculature independently of the epicardial system (for example, the index of microcirculatory resistance, which will be discussed later), invasively measured CFR is not performed routinely on a clinical basis.

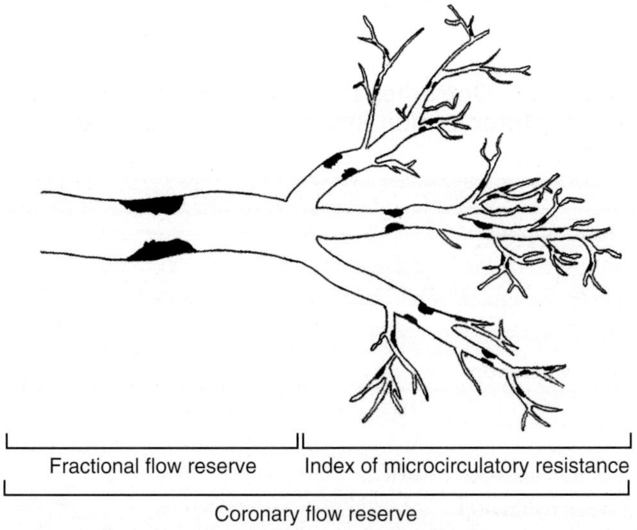

FIG. 14.1 Diagram depicting the coronary circulation. Fractional flow reserve is a specific of the epicardial coronary artery resistance, index of microcirculatory resistance interrogates the microvascular resistance independent of the epicardial system, and coronary flow reserve assesses the entire coronary circulation, both the epicardial artery and the microcirculation. *(Reproduced with permission from Yong AS, Fearon WF. Coronary microvascular dysfunction after ST-segment-elevation myocardial infarction: local or global phenomenon?* Circ Cardiovasc Interv. *2013;6:201–203.)*

FRACTIONAL FLOW RESERVE

Because of the issues surrounding CFR mentioned earlier, in the early 1990s Pijls, De Bruyne, et al. introduced fractional flow reserve (FFR) as a method for assessing the functional significance of epicardial CAD.[11,12] FFR is defined as the maximum myocardial blood flow in the presence of an epicardial stenosis compared with the maximum flow in the hypothetical absence of the stenosis. During maximal hyperemia microvascular resistance is minimized and assumed to be similar in the presence and absence of an epicardial stenosis. Therefore, flow becomes proportional to pressure, and the definition for FFR can be stated as the distal pressure in the presence of a stenosis compared with the distal pressure in the theoretical absence of the stenosis. In a normal epicardial vessel, distal coronary pressure is similar to proximal coronary pressure. Therefore, in a diseased epicardial vessel, what the distal coronary pressure would be in the absence of the disease can be approximated by measuring the proximal coronary pressure. This concept allows for measurement of FFR invasively by using a coronary pressure wire to measure mean distal pressure during maximal hyperemia and dividing that by the mean proximal coronary or aortic pressure measured simultaneously with the guiding catheter (Fig. 14.2).

FFR has a number of unique attributes that makes it more attractive than CFR for assessing epicardial CAD (Box 14.1).[13] First, it has a normal value of 1.0 in every patient and every vessel. Second, it has a well-defined cut-off value of 0.75, with a "gray" zone extending to 0.80. If the FFR value is above 0.80, then it can be assumed that the epicardial vessel being interrogated is not responsible for significant ischemia. FFR values below 0.75 indicate that epicardial vessel disease is responsible for ischemia, whereas values

Derivation of Fractional Flow Reserve

$$\text{FFR} = \frac{\text{Myocardial Flow (Stenosis)}}{\text{Myocardial Flow (Normal)}}$$

$$\text{Myocardial Flow} = \frac{\Delta\ \text{Pressure}}{\text{Resistance}}$$

$$\text{FFR} = \frac{(P_d - P_v)\ /\ \cancel{\text{Resistance}}}{(P_a - P_v)\ /\ \cancel{\text{Resistance}}} \quad \textit{at maximal hyperemia}$$

$$\text{FFR} = \frac{P_d - P_v}{P_a - P_v}$$

$$\text{FFR} = \frac{P_d}{P_a}$$

FIG. 14.2 Derivation of fractional flow reserve (FFR). P_a indicates proximal coronary or aortic pressure; P_d indicates distal coronary pressure; P_v indicates venous pressure. *(Reproduced with permission from Fearon WF. Percutaneous coronary intervention should be guided by fractional flow reserve measurement.* Circulation. *2014;129:1860–1870.)*

BOX 14.1 Unique Attributes of Fractional Flow Reserve

1. Normal value of 1.0 in every patient and every vessel
2. Well-defined ischemic cut-off value
3. Independent of hemodynamic perturbations
4. Extremely reproducible
5. Relatively easy to measure
6. Specific for the epicardial vessel
7. Independent of the microvasculature

in the gray zone require clinical judgment. It is important to remember that FFR is not a dichotomous variable, but a continuous one. In the same vessel, the lower the FFR value, the greater the degree of myocardial ischemia present, and the greater the benefit of revascularization compared with medical therapy.[14]

A third attribute of FFR is that, because it is measured during maximal hyperemia, it is independent of changes in resting flow and other hemodynamic perturbations.[7] For this reason, FFR has excellent reproducibility. Fourth, FFR is relatively easy to measure, at least in comparison to Doppler-derived CFR. Finally, FFR is a specific measure of the contribution of the epicardial CAD to myocardial ischemia. It is independent of microvascular dysfunction. This is an important advantage during invasive assessment because it provides information regarding the expected improvement in myocardial flow should a stent be placed across an epicardial stenosis. For example, in a vessel that subtends previously infarcted myocardium, the maximum flow down the vessel will be less than expected, leading to a lower gradient and a higher FFR across a given upstream epicardial stenosis.[15] However, this does not mean that the FFR is inaccurate, it simply means that the epicardial stenosis does not have a significant effect on myocardial flow and is not responsible for myocardial ischemia.

Data Supporting the Clinical Utility of FFR Measurement

FFR was first validated in a landmark study by Pijls, De Bruyne, et al. in which FFR was compared with three different noninvasive stress tests for the assessment of ischemia in patients with intermediate coronary narrowings.[16] If any one of the stress tests was positive for ischemia, the patient was defined as having ischemia. By using composite information from all three stress tests, the authors were able to increase the accuracy of the noninvasive diagnosis of ischemia. Using a cut-off point of 0.75, they found that 100% of the 21 patients with an FFR below 0.75 had ischemia and 88% of the 24 patients with an FFR of 0.75 or greater did not have ischemia. Importantly, revascularization was not performed in these 24 patients and at an average of 14-month follow-up there were no cardiac events in this group. The overall accuracy of FFR for identifying ischemia-producing lesions in patients with single-vessel intermediate disease was 93%.

The clinical utility of FFR has been documented in three large randomized trials and multiple registries and observational studies. The first important randomized study validating FFR was the deferral of percutaneous coronary intervention (DEFER) trial.[17] In this study, 325 patients with chest pain and moderate coronary lesions who were scheduled for percutaneous coronary intervention (PCI) had FFR measured. If the FFR was less than 0.75, the patient was thought to have a functionally significant coronary stenosis and underwent PCI. If the FFR was greater than or equal to 0.75, the patient was randomized to performance of PCI anyway or to deferral of PCI with medical treatment. At 2-year follow-up, the major adverse cardiac event rate was 11% in the 91 patients randomized to deferral of PCI compared with 17% (p = 0.27) in the 90 patients randomized to performance of PCI. This initial report was important because it was the first large-scale study to demonstrate the safety of *deferring* PCI for lesions that appeared to be associated with significant epicardial obstruction but that were not functionally significant based on FFR.

Subsequently, this same group of patients was followed up to 5 years, at which point in time the cardiac death and myocardial infarction rate was 3.3% in the deferral group versus 7.9% in the performance group (p = 0.21), further documenting safety of medical treatment of coronary lesions that are not hemodynamically significant.[18] Most recently, the 15-year follow-up of this cohort was published.[19] At 15 years, the mortality rate was no different between the two groups, but the myocardial infarction rate was significantly lower in the deferral group compared with the performance group (2.2% vs 10%, p = 0.03). During follow-up this benefit came without any significant difference in revascularization between the two groups (44% vs 34%, respectively, p = 0.25). This report reinforced the safety of medically managing CAD that is not functionally significant based on FFR (Table 14.1).

The next important multicenter, randomized study, the Fractional Flow Reserve Versus Angiography for Multivessel Evaluation (FAME) trial, established the role of FFR in guiding PCI in patients with multivessel CAD.[20] FAME included 1005 stable and unstable patients (not including those with acute ST elevation myocardial infarction [STEMI]) who had 50% or greater stenoses in at least two of the major epicardial arteries and were thought to require PCI based on the angiographic appearance and the clinical scenario. After the identification of which lesions required PCI, the patients were randomized to either angiography-guided PCI, in which case PCI was performed in the usual fashion, or to FFR-guided PCI, in which case first FFR was measured across each lesion and then only if the FFR was less than or equal to 0.80 was PCI performed. The primary endpoint was the 1-year rate of death, myocardial infarction, or repeat revascularization.

Significantly fewer drug-eluting stents were placed in the group randomized to FFR-guidance than in those receiving usual care (1.9 vs 2.7 stents per patient, $p < 0.001$) despite a similar number of lesions identified in both groups. Importantly, the procedure time was similar between both groups; although measurement of FFR adds some time, avoiding unnecessary stents saves time. Most importantly,

TABLE 14.1 Outcomes after Deferring Percutaneous Coronary Intervention Based on Fractional Flow Reserve

ADVERSE EVENT	DEFERRAL (n = 91)	PCI (n = 90)
2-Year Follow-Up		
Death (%)	4.4	2.2
MI (%)	0	3.3
Revascularization (%)	5.6	7.8
5-Year Follow-Up		
Death (%)	6.6	5.7
MI (%)	0	5.6
Revascularization (%)	10.0	15.9
15-Year Follow-Up		
Death (%)	33.0	31.1
MI (%)	2.2	10.0[a]
Revascularization (%)	36.3	27.8

[a]p = 0.04; other comparisons are nonsignificant.
MI, Myocardial infarction; *PCI*, percutaneous coronary intervention.

outcomes were improved in the FFR-guided group at 1 year with a significantly lower rate of the primary endpoint (13% vs 18%, $p = 0.02$). In addition, the rate of death or myocardial infarction was also significantly reduced in the FFR-guided patients (7% vs 11%, $p = 0.04$). Both 2-year and 5-year follow-up confirmed the durability of these results.[21,22] Additionally, a cost-effectiveness study found that FFR-guided PCI was unique in that it not only improved outcomes but also saved resources (Fig. 14.3).[23]

The FAME trial was important because it highlighted the benefit of a new concept, functional revascularization, which involves performing PCI on only those lesions responsible for myocardial ischemia, as directed by an abnormal FFR, and treating medically those lesions that are not functionally significant, despite their angiographic appearance. In this manner the benefits of PCI are maximized while its risks are minimized.

An angiographic substudy of the FAME trial further emphasized the discordance between the coronary angiogram and the functional significance of lesions based on FFR.[24] Of the lesions that were graded between 50% and 70% by the operator, 35% had an ischemic FFR, whereas for those between 70% and 90%, 20% were not significant based on FFR. This discrepancy is especially relevant in patients with three-vessel CAD for whom coronary artery bypass graft surgery is being considered. Guidelines suggest calculating the SYNTAX score and favor bypass surgery if the SYNTAX score is in the intermediate or highest tertile. However, the SYNTAX score is inherently limited by the fact that it is based on the angiographic appearance of the CAD and does not take into account the functional significance. To address this limitation, a so-called Functional SYNTAX Score has been proposed and evaluated in the cohort assigned to FFR-guided PCI in the FAME trial.[25]

The Functional SYNTAX Score takes into account only those lesions that are significant based on FFR. It was shown to be a better discriminator of the risk for death and myocardial infarction as compared with the SYNTAX score (Fig. 14.4). This concept is being tested prospectively in the FAME 3 trial, comparing FFR-guided PCI with current generation drug-eluting stents to coronary artery bypass graft surgery in a multicenter, randomized trial.[26]

The FAME 2 trial is the most recent large, multicenter randomized FFR study. This study compared FFR-guided PCI plus optimal medical therapy with optimal medical therapy alone in patients with stable angina who had at least one major epicardial vessel with a proximal or mid stenosis of greater than 50%.[27] The primary endpoint was the rate of death, myocardial infarction, or hospitalization with urgent revascularization at 2 years. The difference between FAME 2 and prior studies comparing PCI with medical therapy in stable patients is that FFR was performed across all lesions, and only if the FFR was less than or equal to 0.80 was the patient randomized either to PCI with current generation drug-eluting stents plus optimal medical therapy or to optimal medical therapy alone. In this manner, it was ensured

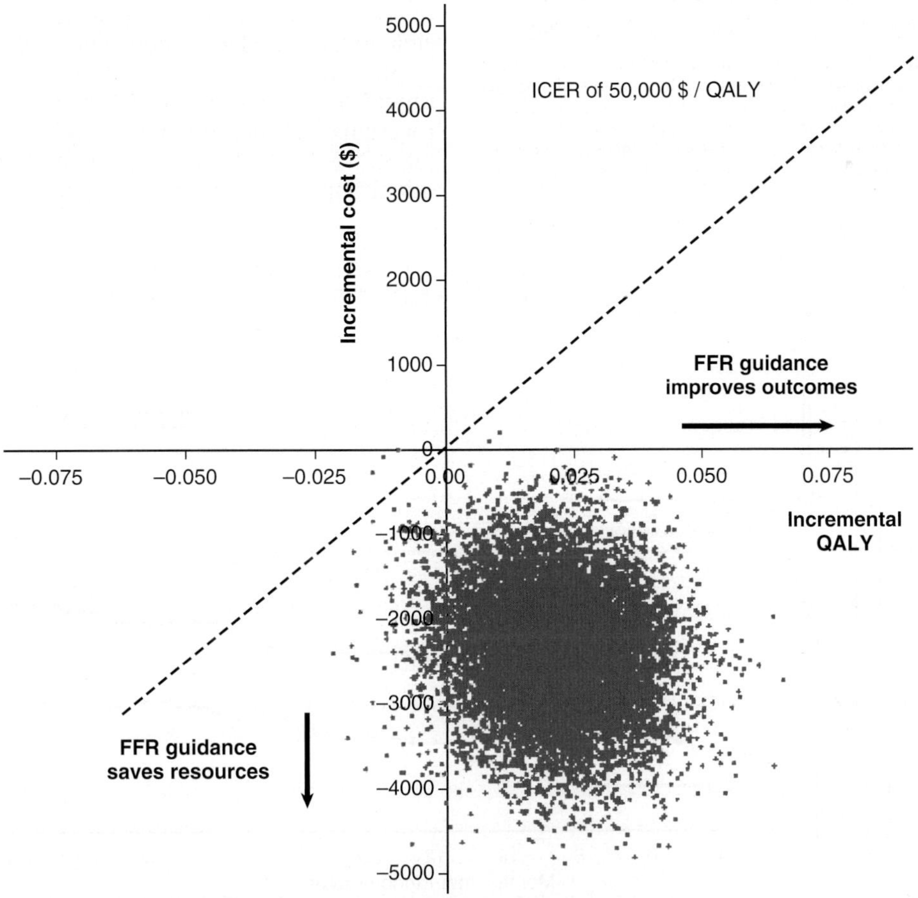

FIG. 14.3 Bootstrap simulation of incremental costs and effects from the FAME 1 trial. Fractional flow reserve (FFR)-guided percutaneous coronary intervention (PCI) not only improved outcomes but also saved resources. ICER indicates incremental cost-effectiveness ration and QALY indicates quality-adjusted life-years. *(With permission from Fearon WF, Bornschein B, Tonino PAL, et al. Economic evaluation of fractional flow reserve-guided percutaneous coronary intervention in patients with multivessel disease.* Circulation. *2010;122:2545–2550.)*

that patients with significant myocardial ischemia were included in the randomized portion of the study. Those patients with angiographic disease that was not significant based on FFR were also treated with optimal medical therapy and were followed in a registry.

The goal of FAME 2 was to evaluate the benefit of PCI in patients with stable CAD and abnormal FFR or, alternatively, the potential hazard of medical therapy alone for patients with lesions responsible for myocardial ischemia. After inclusion of 1220 patients (randomization of 888), enrollment was discontinued on the advice of the data safety monitoring board because of a highly significant difference in the primary endpoint between the two groups and because of concern regarding future adverse events in the medically treated patients. At a mean follow-up of roughly 7 months, the primary endpoint occurred in 4.3% of the PCI group and 12.7% of the medical therapy group ($p < 0.001$). This difference was due primarily to a difference in hospitalization with the need for urgent revascularization. A second report of the complete 2-year follow-up in all patients continued to show a significantly lower rate of the primary endpoint in the PCI group (8.1% vs 19.5%, $p < 0.001$), again driven primarily by a higher rate of urgent revascularization in the medically treated patients.[28] Of interest was a landmark analysis looking at the death and myocardial infarction rate more than 7 days after randomization. In this manner, periprocedural myocardial infarctions occurring in the PCI group were ignored. The rate of death and myocardial infarction after 7 days was significantly higher in the medically treated patients compared with the PCI arm (8.0% vs 4.6%, $p = 0.04$) (Fig. 14.5). Equally important are the results from the registry component of the study, which demonstrated that outcomes were excellent in those patients without ischemia in whom all lesions had an FFR greater than 0.80 and were managed medically. The rate of the primary endpoint in these patients was similar to that in the PCI patients and significantly lower than in the patients with abnormal FFR values who received medical therapy alone (Table 14.2).

Other important aspects of treating patients with stable coronary disease based on FFR-guided PCI are quality of life and cost-effectiveness. The FAME 2 trial demonstrated a significant improvement in angina and quality of life in the PCI patients and an attractive cost-effectiveness ratio of $36,000 per quality-adjusted life-years.[29] Thus the FAME 2 trial reinforced the advantage of identifying CAD responsible for ischemia based on FFR measurement and performing PCI to relieve ischemia, while safely managing CAD not responsible for ischemia with medications alone.

Some have criticized the FAME 2 trial because it included urgent revascularization in the primary endpoint. Urgent revascularization is not traditionally considered a hard endpoint, like death or myocardial infarction. They argue that an initial approach with medical management is reasonable.

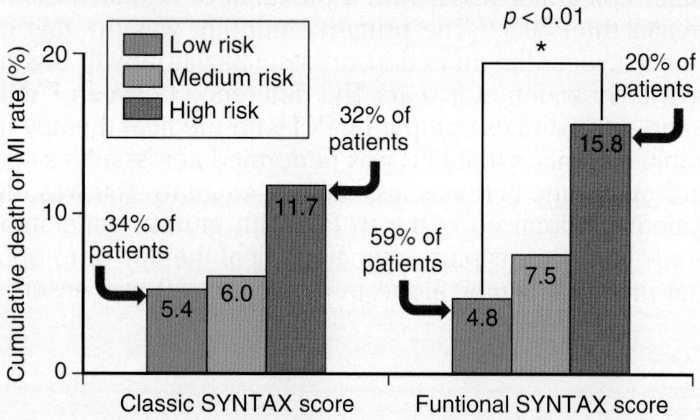

FIG. 14.4 The functional SYNTAX score outperforms the classic SYNTAX score by being a better predictor of subsequent death or myocardial infarction (MI). Additionally, the percentage of patients in the highest risk group is lower after calculation of the functional SYNTAX score, and the percentage in the lowest risk group increases. *(Adapted from Nam CW, Mangiacapra F, Entjes R, et al. Functional SYNTAX score for risk assessment in multivessel coronary artery disease.* J Am Coll Cardiol. *2011;58:1211–1218.)*

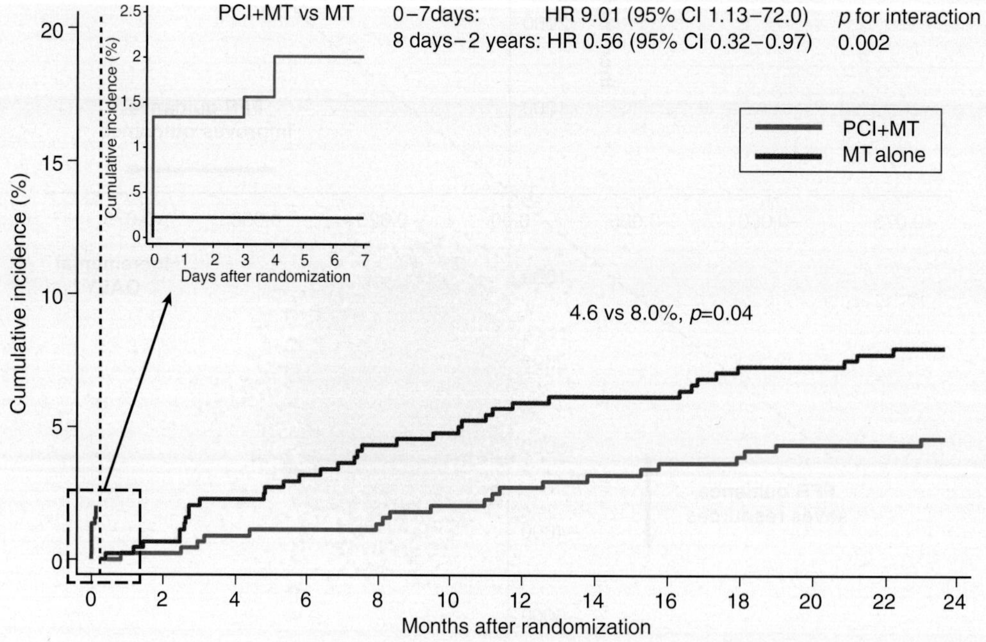

FIG. 14.5 Landmark analysis from the FAME 2 trial. Comparison of medical therapy with fractional flow reserve–guided percutaneous coronary intervention in patients with stable coronary disease and demonstrating lower rates of subsequent death or myocardial infarction in the PCI patients greater than 7 days after randomization. *CI*, Confidence interval; *HR*, hazard ratio; *MT*, medical therapy; *PCI*, percutaneous coronary intervention. *(Adapted from De Bruyne B, Fearon WF, Pijls NH, et al. Fractional flow reserve-guided PCI for stable coronary artery disease.* N Engl J Med. *2014;371:1208-1217.)*

However, those who support the results of the FAME 2 trial believe that the improved angina relief and quality of life at an acceptable cost-effectiveness ratio make FFR-guided PCI the preferred approach for stable angina patients.

The findings from the FAME 2 trial and the other randomized studies have been reinforced by a number of observational studies, registries, and meta-analyses. For example, FFR measurement has been shown to be a valuable method for interrogating intermediate left main CAD,[30] jailed sidebranches[31] (a branching vessel with a main vessel stent covering its ostium), diffuse CAD,[32] residual disease in previously infarcted vessels,[33] and nonculprit vessels in patients with acute coronary syndromes.[34] However, in the culprit vessel of patients presenting with STEMI, FFR measurement is not recommended because of the transient microvascular dysfunction that can occur in this setting, which may result in a higher FFR acutely and a lower FFR days to weeks later, once the microvascular stunning has resolved. Specifically, an important observational study and a meta-analysis both highlighted the concept that FFR is not a dichotomous variable but represents a continuum of risk.[12] The lower the FFR, the greater the risk for major adverse cardiac events with medical therapy and the greater the benefit of revascularization, whereas when the FFR is above 0.80 the risks of revascularization are not outweighed by any benefit and, in general, medical therapy is recommended.

INTRAVASCULAR IMAGING

Ultrasound

In some situations, the anatomic characteristics of CAD are more important than the physiologic effects. In these scenarios, intravascular imaging with either intravascular ultrasound (IVUS) or optical coherence tomography (OCT) can be useful. Intravascular ultrasound is performed by passing an approximately 3-French monorail catheter, which houses the miniaturized ultrasound probe, over a coronary guidewire in the coronary artery. The ultrasound transducer can then be pulled back manually or automatically and the vessel can be imaged. IVUS has an axial resolution of approximately 100 μm and imaging depth of 4–10 mm. Multiple studies have demonstrated its superior resolution compared with coronary angiography.[35]

The primary indications for IVUS can be divided into diagnostic purposes and optimization of PCI. From the diagnostic standpoint FFR has supplanted IVUS as the preferred method for determining whether or not an intermediate lesion is responsible for ischemia. This is because routine IVUS interrogation provides information about lesion severity and length of the lesion but does not provide information regarding effect of the stenosis on coronary flow. A stenosis in the proximal left anterior descending coronary artery (LAD) typically will be of greater functional significance than an identical stenosis in an obtuse marginal branch of the circumflex. This is because the amount of myocardium subtended by the LAD is much greater and therefore the greater maximum flow across the stenosis will result in a lower FFR. However, the IVUS image will be identical. Many do still advocate using IVUS for interrogating intermediate left main coronary disease, especially if one will be performing PCI, as IVUS optimization may improve outcomes in this setting.[36] The guidelines provide a class IIa indication for using IVUS in the assessment of intermediate left main disease.[37]

The other main role for IVUS is in planning and optimizing PCI. IVUS allows determination of lesion composition, especially the degree and depth of calcification, which can affect the operator's approach to lesion preparation prior to stenting. It can also be helpful for determining lesion length and the involvement of a coronary bifurcation. After stenting has been performed, IVUS allows assessment of stent expansion, stent apposition, and evidence for edge dissection or residual uncovered disease. Multiple randomized studies have compared IVUS-guided stenting with angiography-guided stenting in the bare-metal stent era with variable results.[38,39] Many observational studies and meta-analyses have suggested that IVUS guidance improves outcomes after PCI.[40,41] One large randomized study has compared IVUS-guided PCI to angiography-guided PCI in 1400 patients with long coronary lesions (≥28 mm).[42] The primary endpoint was the composite of cardiac death, target lesion–related myocardial infarction, or ischemia-driven target lesion revascularization at 1 year; this occurred significantly less often in the 700 IVUS-guided PCI patients than in the 700 angiography-guided PCI patients (2.9% vs 5.8%, $p = 0.007$). This difference was explained by the 2.5% difference in target lesion revascularization. It is not clear that this benefit alone will be enough to increase IVUS utilization during PCI.

A final rationale for performing IVUS is to investigate angiographic findings of unclear significance such as spontaneous dissection, thrombus, and vulnerable/ruptured plaque. The use of IVUS for identification of vulnerable plaque (coronary lesions more likely to progress and cause a cardiac event) has been especially disappointing,[43] likely because multiple factors beyond lesion morphology determine which lesions will ultimately be responsible for myocardial infarction. Moreover, because of its enhanced resolution, OCT has supplanted IVUS for some of these indications.

TABLE 14.2 Adverse Events at 2 Years in the FAME 2 Trial

ADVERSE EVENT	PCI (n = 447)	MEDICAL THERAPY (n = 441)	REGISTRY (n = 166)
Primary endpoint (%)	8.1	19.5*	9.0
Death (%)	1.3	1.8	1.2
MI (%)	5.8	6.8	5.4
Death or MI (%)	6.5	8.2	6.0
Urgent revascularization (%)	4.0	16.3**	5.4

*$p < 0.001$ compared with PCI and $p = 0.002$ compared with the Registry.
**$p < 0.001$ compared with PCI and $p = 0.001$ compared with the Registry.
MI, Myocardial infarction; *PCI*, percutaneous coronary intervention.

Optical Coherence Tomography

OCT is analogous to IVUS in that it is a catheter-based method for imaging within the coronary vessel, but it uses light instead of ultrasound. OCT has a number of advantages over IVUS and a few disadvantages. On the one hand, because OCT uses light, the entire coronary vessel can be imaged in a few seconds as compared with a few minutes with IVUS. The axial resolution of OCT is on the order of 10–15 μm, as compared with 100–150 μm with IVUS. This allows OCT to provide detailed vascular information regarding, for example, fibroatheroma cap thickness (a marker

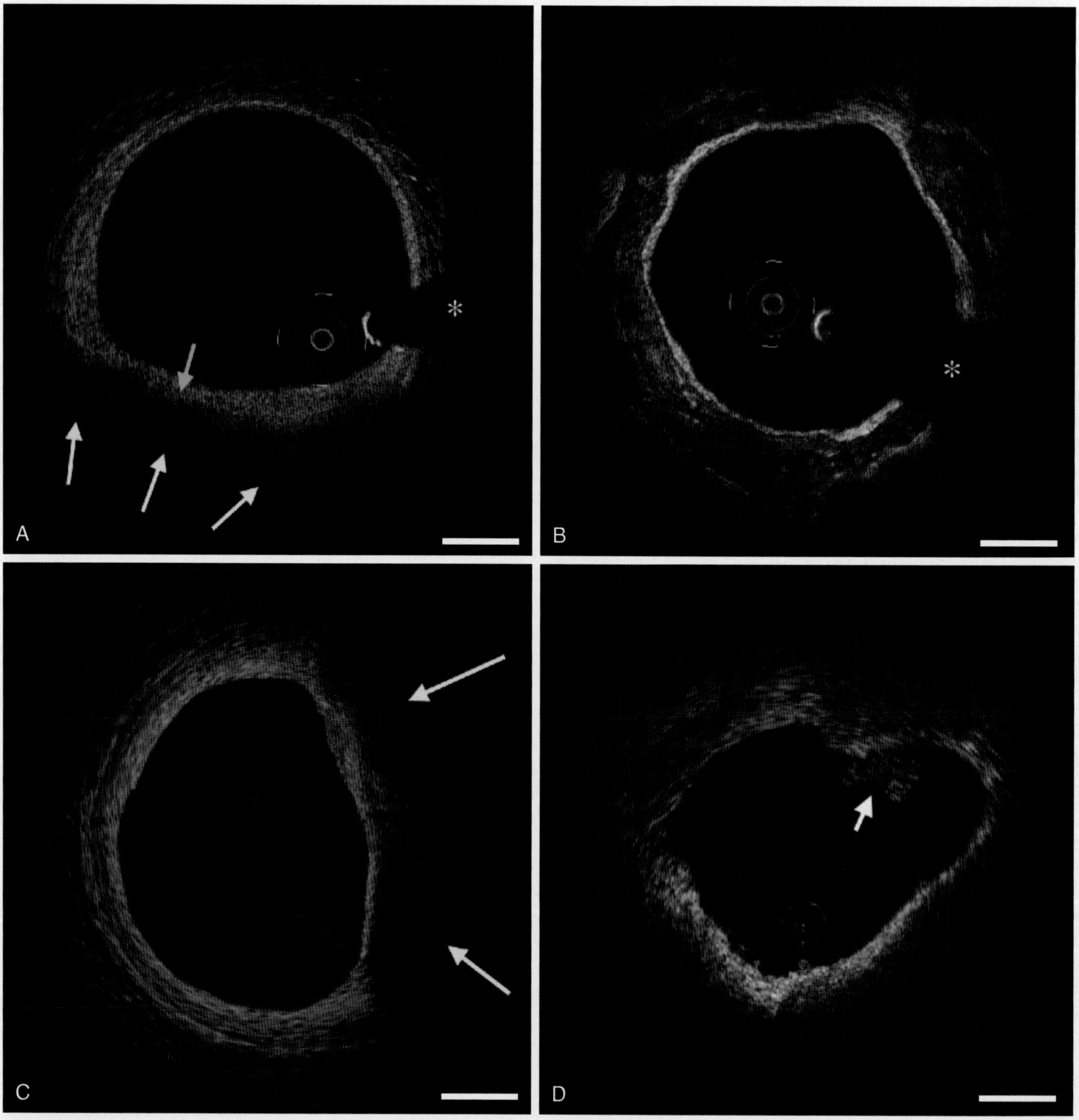

FIG. 14.6 Still frames from optical coherence tomographic images. Demonstration of **(A)** Fibroatheroma *(green arrow)*, **(B)** fibrocalcific lesion, **(C)** thin-capped fibroatheroma *(red arrow)*, **(D)** thrombus *(white arrow)*. *Guidewire artifact. *(Adapted from Tearney GJ, Regar E, Akasaka T, et al. Consensus standards for acquisition, measurement, and reporting of intravascular optical coherence tomography studies: a report from the International Working Group for Intravascular Optical Coherence Tomography Standardization and Validation.* J Am Coll Cardiol. *2012;59:1058–1072.)*

of plaque instability), coronary dissection, stent malapposition, and endothelialization of stent struts (Fig. 14.6). On the other hand, because OCT uses light, which cannot penetrate blood, in order to obtain optimal images the blood is typically replaced with contrast injection. If multiple OCT imaging pullbacks are performed, contrast media use can be a limitation, especially in patients with kidney disease. Another potential disadvantage of OCT is the fact that its imaging depth into the vessel wall ranges from only 1 to 3 μm. Therefore, it is not possible to quantify plaque burden or assess vessel remodeling with OCT, as can be done with IVUS (Box 14.2).

BOX 14.2 Important Differences Between Intravascular Ultrasound (IVUS) and Optical Coherence Tomography (OCT)

1. OCT is light based, whereas IVUS is ultrasound based.
2. OCT imaging can be performed more quickly than IVUS imaging.
3. OCT imaging requires replacement of blood, generally with contrast media injection.
4. OCT has greater axial resolution than IVUS, allowing more detailed vascular information.
5. IVUS has greater imaging depth than IVUS, allowing assessment of plaque burden and vessel remodeling.

$$\text{Resistance} = \Delta\,\text{Pressure} / \text{Flow}$$

$$\Delta\,\text{Pressure} = P_d - P_v \qquad \text{Flow} = 1 / T_{mn}$$

$$\text{IMR} = P_d - P_v / (1 / T_{mn})$$

$$\text{IMR} = P_d \times T_{mn} \textit{ measured during maximal hyperemia}$$

FIG. 14.7 Derivation of the index of microcirculatory resistance (IMR). P_d indicates distal coronary pressure; P_v indicates coronary venous pressure; T_{mn} indicates mean transit time.

Large-scale randomized outcomes trials comparing OCT with angiography-guided or IVUS-guided PCI have not been performed to date. In an observational study, OCT-guided PCI was compared in 335 patients with angiography-guided PCI in another 335 matched patients and was associated with significantly lower rates of cardiac death or myocardial infarction at 1 year (6.6% vs 13.0%, $p = 0.006$).[44] These data should be interpreted with caution given the observational study design, which introduces selection biases and confounding. For widespread routine use of OCT or IVUS to be recommended, large-scale randomized studies demonstrating clinical benefit will be necessary.

INDEX OF MICROCIRCULATORY RESISTANCE

As mentioned previously, one of the limitations of measuring CFR in the cardiac catheterization laboratory is that it interrogates the entire coronary circulation, both the epicardial vessel and the microvasculature. FFR is an index specific for the epicardial vessel. The index of microcirculatory resistance (IMR) is a relatively newer index that specifically interrogates the coronary microcirculation, independent of epicardial stenosis.[45] It is defined as the change in pressure across the microvasculature (distal coronary artery pressure minus coronary venous pressure) divided by flow during maximal hyperemia, and it is a reflection of the minimum achievable microvascular resistance. It can be calculated using a coronary pressure/thermistor–tipped wire and measuring the distal coronary pressure and mean transit time of room temperature saline during maximal hyperemia (Fig. 14.7). IMR was first validated in an animal model and subsequently tested extensively in humans.[46] A normal value for IMR has been found to be less than 25.[47–49]

The advantages of IMR include that it is relatively easy to measure and can be performed simultaneously while measuring FFR without any extra equipment; it has been shown to have a low inter- and intraobserver variability; it is independent of hemodynamic variability; it is specific for the microvasculature; and it is predictive of outcomes.

The prognostic role of IMR has been studied in stable patients undergoing PCI, in which case elevated levels of IMR measured before PCI can predict periprocedural myocardial infarction.[50] However, IMR has been most extensively evaluated in patients undergoing primary PCI for STEMI. In this situation an elevated IMR immediately after primary PCI correlates with the size of the myocardial infarction and predicts recovery of left ventricular function.[51] In a large series of patients with STEMI, IMR was an independent predictor of long-term mortality.[52] In stable patients without obstructive CAD but with chest pain, IMR is elevated in roughly 20% of patients, a finding suggesting microvascular dysfunction as a cause for the chest pain.[53] The prognostic value of IMR in this setting has not been reported.

EVALUATION OF CHEST PAIN AND NO OBSTRUCTIVE CORONARY ARTERY DISEASE

Because as many as 20% of patients presenting to the catheterization laboratory are found to have no obstructive epicardial CAD (NOCAD), there has been growing interest in the invasive evaluation of these patients. In many cases, these patients undergo multiple noninvasive tests with variable results and often multiple coronary angiograms and are told everything is normal and/or their symptoms are psychosomatic. It is now possible to perform safely and reasonably quickly a more thorough evaluation in the catheterization laboratory.

A patient with chest pain in whom NOCAD is suspected and who is scheduled for an invasive angiogram should stop any vasoactive medications for 48 hours before the procedure. After a baseline coronary angiogram is performed, endothelial function can be assessed by administering intracoronary acetylcholine. This can be performed through an infusion catheter in the proximal vessel with a gradual increase in the dose, or more commonly, by an intracoronary bolus given over 30 seconds, starting at 20–50 μg and increasing to as high as 200 μg. An angiogram is performed after each dose and can be subjectively evaluated for changes in vessel size. A final angiogram is performed after administering 100–200 μg of intracoronary nitroglycerin to assess endothelial-independent vasodilatation. Off-line quantitative coronary angiography allows more accurate comparison of changes in vessel dimensions and of the presence of endothelial dysfunction, typically defined as a greater than 20% decrease in vessel diameter after acetylcholine administration. A coronary pressure/thermistor-tipped wire is then advanced down the vessel of interest and simultaneous FFR and IMR can be measured to assess the epicardial and microvascular compartments independently. Finally, IVUS is performed to evaluate further for diffuse epicardial CAD and for myocardial bridging (Fig. 14.8).

This series of tests was performed in 139 patients without complication, and 77% of patients had at least one abnormality (occult epicardial disease, endothelial dysfunction, microvascular dysfunction, or myocardial bridging).[50] Importantly, almost one-quarter of patients did not have any detectable epicardial or microvascular coronary cause for their chest pain and therefore could be reassured and hopefully avoid further unnecessary coronary testing and treatment (Fig. 14.9). For those patients who do have an occult abnormality, guideline-directed therapy can be instituted and individualized based on the abnormality found. In the case of microvascular dysfunction, the most effective therapy remains unclear and further studies are warranted (see Chapters 5 and 25).

CONCLUSION

Cardiologists now have a number of invasive techniques beyond x-ray coronary angiography to obtain more detailed information regarding a patient's coronary circulation. FFR allows the specific assessment of the functional significance of epicardial CAD to guide decisions regarding the need for revascularization, whereas IMR independently interrogates the microvasculature. IVUS and OCT provide anatomic information that can help to optimize PCI. In patients with chest pain and no obstructive CAD, these methods allow more accurate diagnosis of the etiology of the patient's symptoms.

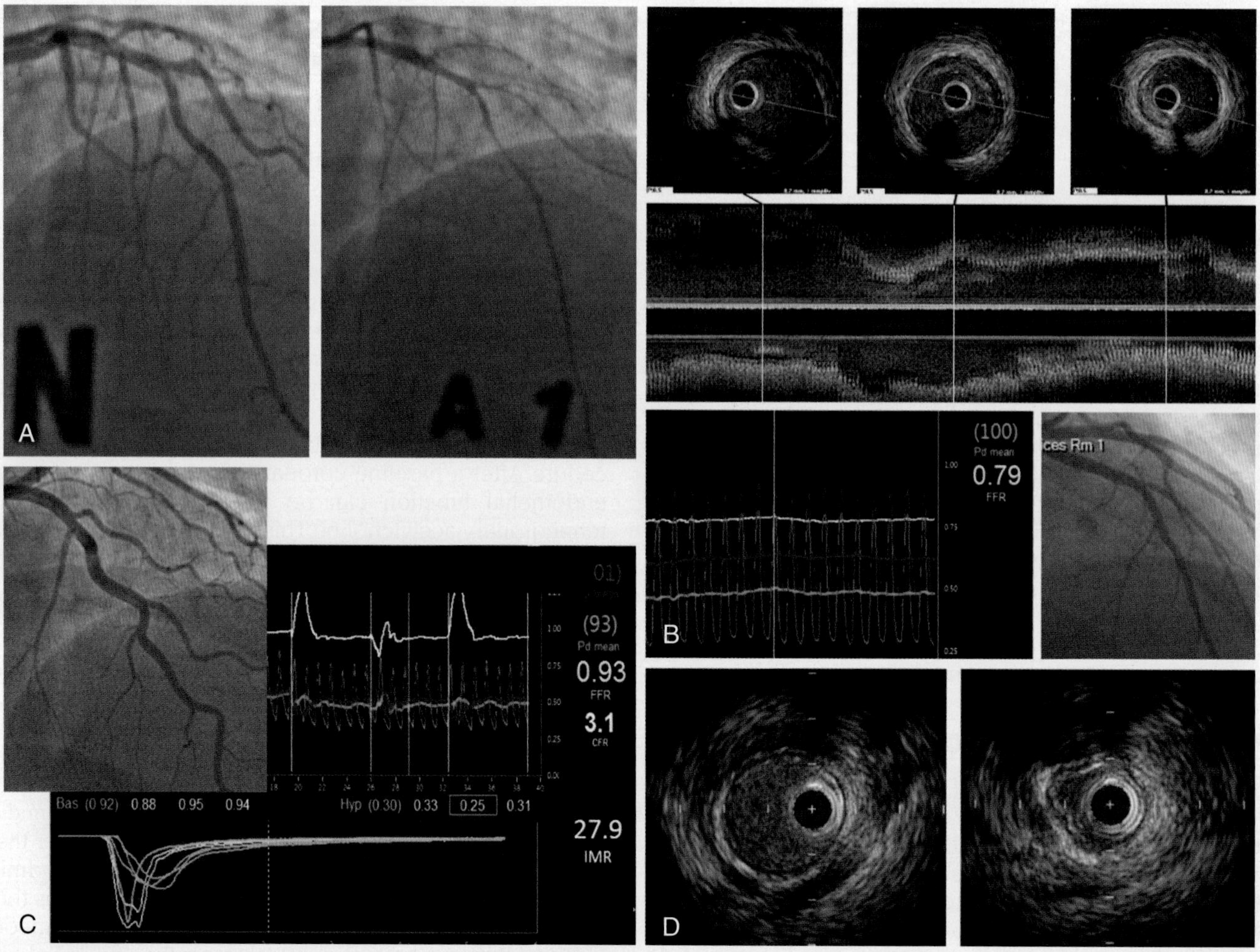

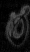

FIG. 14.8 (A) Baseline coronary angiogram and subsequent angiogram after intracoronary acetylcholine demonstrating diffuse endothelial dysfunction with vasoconstriction. (B) Cross-sectional and longitudinal intravascular ultrasound images demonstrating diffuse atherosclerosis and coronary pressure tracing revealing an abnormal fractional flow reserve in a normal appearing left anterior descending coronary artery on angiography. (C) Coronary angiogram revealing a normal left anterior descending coronary artery with a pressure tracing showing an abnormal index of microcirculatory resistance. (D) Cross-sectional intravascular ultrasound images of a myocardial bridge segment. *(With permission from Lee BK, Lim HS, Fearon WF, et al. Invasive evaluation of patients with angina in the absence of obstructive coronary artery disease.* Circulation. *2015;131:1054–1060.)*

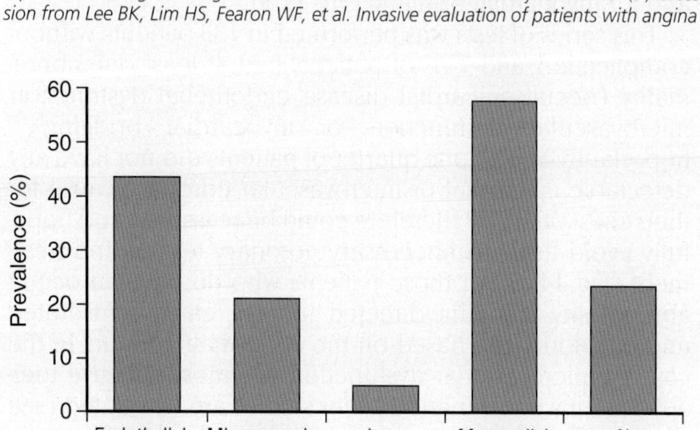

FIG. 14.9 Potential causes for chest pain in patients with no obstructive coronary artery disease. *FFR,* Fractional flow reserve. *(With permission from Lee BK, Lim HS, Fearon WF, et al. Invasive evaluation of patients with angina in the absence of obstructive coronary artery disease.* Circulation. *2015;131:1054–1060.)*

References

1. Kini AS: Coronary angiography, lesion classification and severity assessment, *Cardiol Clin* 24: 153–162, 2006.
2. Topol EJ, Nissen SE: Our preoccupation with coronary luminology. The dissociation between clinical and angiographic findings in ischemic heart disease, *Circulation* 92:2333–2342, 1995.
3. Kern MJ, Lerman A, Bech JW, et al.: Physiological assessment of coronary artery disease in the cardiac catheterization laboratory: a scientific statement from the American Heart Association Committee on Diagnostic and Interventional Cardiac Catheterization, Council on Clinical Cardiology, *Circulation* 114:1321–1341, 2006.
4. Doucette JW, Corl PD, Payne HM, et al.: Validation of a Doppler guide wire for intravascular measurement of coronary artery flow velocity, *Circulation* 85:1899–1911, 1992.
5. De Bruyne B, Pijls NH, Smith L, et al.: Coronary thermodilution to assess flow reserve: experimental validation, *Circulation* 104:2003–2006, 2001.
6. Pijls NH, De Bruyne B, Smith L, et al.: Coronary thermodilution to assess flow reserve: validation in humans, *Circulation* 105:2482–2486, 2002.
7. Fearon WF, Farouque HM, Balsam LB, et al.: Comparison of coronary thermodilution and Doppler velocity for assessing coronary flow reserve, *Circulation* 108:2198–2200, 2003.
8. Joye JD, Schulman DS, Lasorda D, et al.: Intracoronary Doppler guide wire versus stress single-photon emission computed tomographic thallium-201 imaging in assessment of intermediate coronary stenoses, *J Am Coll Cardiol* 24:940–947, 1994.
9. De Bruyne B, Bartunek J, Sys SU, et al.: Simultaneous coronary pressure and flow velocity measurements in humans. Feasibility, reproducibility, and hemodynamic dependence of coronary flow velocity reserve, hyperemic flow versus pressure slope index, and fractional flow reserve, *Circulation* 94:1842–1849, 1996.
10. Fearon WF: Invasive coronary physiology for assessing intermediate lesions, *Circ Cardiovasc Interv* 8:e001942, 2015.
11. Pijls NHJ, van Son JAM, Kirkeeide RL, et al.: Experimental basis of determining maximum coronary, myocardial and collateral blood flow by pressure measurements for assessing functional stenosis severity before and after percutaneous transluminal coronary angioplasty, *Circulation* 86:1354–1367, 1993.
12. De Bruyne B, Baudhuin T, Melin JA, et al.: Coronary flow reserve calculated from pressure measurements in humans. Validation with positron emission tomography, *Circulation* 89:1013–1022, 1994.
13. Fearon WF: Percutaneous coronary intervention should be guided by fractional flow reserve measurement, *Circulation* 129:1860–1870, 2014.
14. Johnson NP, Tóth GG, Lai D, et al.: Prognostic value of fractional flow reserve: linking physiologic severity to clinical outcomes, *J Am Coll Cardiol* 64:1641–1654, 2014.
15. De Bruyne B, Pijls NH, Bartunek J, et al.: Fractional flow reserve in patients with prior myocardial infarction, *Circulation* 104:157–162, 2001.
16. Pijls NH, De Bruyne B, Peels K, et al.: Measurement of fractional flow reserve to assess the functional severity of coronary-artery stenoses, *N Engl J Med* 334:1703–1708, 1996.
17. Bech GJ, De Bruyne B, Pijls NH, et al.: Fractional flow reserve to determine the appropriateness of angioplasty in moderate coronary stenosis: a randomized trial, *Circulation* 103:2928–2934, 2001.
18. Pijls NH, van Schaardenburgh P, Manoharan G, et al.: Percutaneous coronary intervention of functionally nonsignificant stenosis: 5-year follow-up of the DEFER Study, *J Am Coll Cardiol* 49:2105–2111, 2007.
19. Zimmermann FM, Ferrara A, Johnson NP, et al.: Deferral vs. performance of percutaneous coronary intervention of functionally non-significant coronary stenosis: 15-year follow-up of the DEFER trial, *Eur Heart J* 36:3182–3188, 2015.
20. Tonino PAL, De Bruyne B, Pijls NHJ, et al.: Fractional flow reserve versus angiography for guiding percutaneous coronary intervention in patients with multivessel coronary artery disease, *N Engl J Med* 360:213–224, 2009.

21. Pijls NH, Fearon WF, Tonino PA, et al.: FAME Study Investigators. Fractional flow reserve versus angiography for guiding percutaneous coronary intervention in patients with multivessel coronary artery disease: 2-year follow-up of the FAME (Fractional Flow Reserve Versus Angiography for Multivessel Evaluation) study, *J Am Coll Cardiol* 56:177–184, 2010.
22. van Nunen LX, Zimmermann FM, Tonino PA, et al.: FAME Study Investigators. Fractional flow reserve versus angiography for guidance of PCI in patients with multivessel coronary artery disease (FAME): 5-year follow-up of a randomised controlled trial, *Lancet* 386:1853–1860, 2015.
23. Fearon WF, Bornschein B, Tonino PAL, et al.: Economic evaluation of fractional flow reserve-guided percutaneous coronary intervention in patients with multivessel disease, *Circulation* 122:2545–2550, 2010.
24. Tonino PA, Fearon WF, De Bruyne B, et al.: Angiographic versus functional severity of coronary artery stenoses in the FAME study fractional flow reserve versus angiography in multivessel evaluation, *J Am Coll Cardiol* 55:2816–2821, 2010.
25. Nam CW, Mangiacapra F, Entjes R, et al.: FAME Study Investigators. Functional SYNTAX score for risk assessment in multivessel coronary artery disease, *J Am Coll Cardiol* 58:1211–1218, 2011.
26. Zimmermann FM, De Bruyne B, Pijls NH, et al.: Rationale and design of the Fractional Flow Reserve versus Angiography for Multivessel Evaluation (FAME) 3 Trial: a comparison of fractional flow reserve-guided percutaneous coronary intervention and coronary artery bypass graft surgery in patients with multivessel coronary artery disease, *Am Heart J* 170:619–626, 2015.
27. De Bruyne B, Pijls NH, Kalesan B, et al.: FAME 2 Trial Investigators. Fractional flow reserve-guided PCI versus medical therapy in stable coronary disease, *N Engl J Med* 367:991–1001, 2012.
28. De Bruyne B, Fearon WF, Pijls NH, et al.: FAME 2 Trial Investigators. Fractional flow reserve-guided PCI for stable coronary artery disease, *N Engl J Med* 371:1208–1217, 2014.
29. Fearon WF, Shilane D, Pijls NHJ, et al.: Cost-effectiveness of percutaneous coronary intervention in patients with stable coronary disease and abnormal fractional flow reserve, *Circulation* 128:1335–1340, 2013.
30. Hamilos M, Muller O, Cuisset T, et al.: Long-term clinical outcome after fractional flow reserve-guided treatment in patients with angiographically equivocal left main coronary artery stenosis, *Circulation* 120:1505–1512, 2009.
31. Koo BK, Kang HJ, Youn TJ, et al.: Physiologic assessment of jailed side branch lesions using fractional flow reserve, *J Am Coll Cardiol* 46:633–637, 2005.
32. De Bruyne B, Hersbach F, Pijls NH, et al.: Abnormal epicardial coronary resistance in patients with diffuse atherosclerosis but "normal" coronary angiography, *Circulation* 104:2401–2406, 2001.
33. De Bruyne B, Pijls NH, Bartunek J, et al.: Fractional flow reserve in patients with prior myocardial infarction, *Circulation* 104:157–162, 2001.
34. Ntalianis A, Sels JW, Davidavicius G, et al.: Fractional flow reserve for the assessment of nonculprit coronary artery stenoses in patients with acute myocardial infarction, *JACC Cardiovasc Interv* 3:1274–1281, 2010.
35. Nissen SE, Gurley JC, Booth DC, DeMaria AN: Intravascular ultrasound of the coronary arteries: current applications and future directions, *Am J Cardiol* 69:18H–29H, 1992.
36. Park SJ, Kim YH, Park DW, et al.: MAIN-COMPARE Investigators. Impact of intravascular ultrasound guidance on long-term mortality in stenting for unprotected left main coronary artery stenosis, *Circ Cardiovasc Interv* 2:167–177, 2009.
37. Levine GN, Bates ER, Blankenship JC, et al.: 2011 ACCF/AHA/SCAI Guideline for Percutaneous Coronary Intervention: executive summary: a report of the American College of Cardiology Foundation/American Heart Association Task Force on Practice Guidelines and the Society for Cardiovascular Angiography and Interventions, *Circulation* 124:2574–2609, 2011.
38. Schiele F, Meneveau N, Vuillemenot A, et al.: Impact of intravascular ultrasound guidance in stent deployment on 6-month restenosis rate: a multicenter, randomized study comparing two strategies—with and without intravascular ultrasound guidance. RESIST Study Group. REStenosis after Ivus guided Stenting, *J Am Coll Cardiol* 32:320–328, 1998.
39. Fitzgerald PJ, Oshima A, Hayase M, et al.: Final results of the Can Routine Ultrasound Influence Stent Expansion (CRUISE) study, *Circulation* 102:523–530, 2000.
40. Zhang Y, Farooq V, Garcia-Garcia HM, et al.: Comparison of intravascular ultrasound versus angiography-guided drug-eluting stent implantation: a meta-analysis of one randomised trial and ten observational studies involving 19,619 patients, *EuroIntervention* 8:855–865, 2012.
41. Witzenbichler B, Maehara A, Weisz G, et al.: Relationship between intravascular ultrasound guidance and clinical outcomes after drug-eluting stents: the assessment of dual antiplatelet therapy with drug-eluting stents (ADAPT-DES) study, *Circulation* 129:463–470, 2014.
42. Hong SJ, Kim BK, Shin DH, et al.: IVUS-XPL Investigators. Effect of intravascular ultrasound-guided vs angiography-guided everolimus-eluting stent implantation: The IVUS-XPL randomized clinical trial, *JAMA* 314:2155–2156, 2015.
43. Stone GW, Maehara A, Lansky AJ, et al.: PROSPECT Investigators. A prospective natural-history study of coronary atherosclerosis, *N Engl J Med* 364:226–235, 2011.
44. Prati F, Di Vito L, Biondi-Zoccai G, et al.: Angiography alone versus angiography plus optical coherence tomography to guide decision-making during percutaneous coronary intervention: the Centro per la Lotta contro l'Infarto-Optimisation of Percutaneous Coronary Intervention (CLI-OPCI) study, *EuroIntervention* 8:823–829, 2012.
45. Fearon WF, Balsam LB, Farouque HMO, et al.: Novel index for invasively assessing the coronary microcirculation, *Circulation* 107:3129–3132, 2003.
46. Ng MK, Yeung AC, Fearon WF: Invasive assessment of the coronary microcirculation: superior reproducibility and less hemodynamic dependence of index of microcirculatory resistance compared with coronary flow reserve, *Circulation* 113:2054–2061, 2006.
47. Melikian N, Vercauteren S, Fearon WF, et al.: Quantitative assessment of coronary microvascular function in patients with and without epicardial atherosclerosis, *EuroIntervention* 5:939–945, 2010.
48. Luo C, Long M, Hu X, et al.: Thermodilution-derived coronary microvascular resistance and flow reserve in patients with cardiac syndrome X, *Circ Cardiovasc Interv* 7:43–48, 2014.
49. Solberg OG, Ragnarsson A, Kvarsnes A, et al.: Reference interval for the index of coronary microvascular resistance, *EuroIntervention* 9:1069–1075, 2014.
50. Ng MK, Yong AS, Ho M, et al.: The index of microcirculatory resistance predicts myocardial infarction related to percutaneous coronary intervention, *Circ Cardiovasc Interv* 5:515–522, 2012.
51. Fearon WF, Shah M, Ng M, et al.: Predictive value of the index of microcirculatory resistance in patients with ST segment elevation myocardial infarction, *J Am Coll Cardiol* 51:560–565, 2008.
52. Fearon WF, Low AF, Yong AC, et al.: Prognostic value of the Index of Microcirculatory Resistance measured after primary percutaneous coronary intervention, *Circulation* 127:2436–2441, 2013.
53. Lee BK, Lim HS, Fearon WF, et al.: Invasive evaluation of patients with angina in the absence of obstructive coronary artery disease, *Circulation* 131:1054–1060, 2015.

15 Putting It All Together: Which Test for Which Patient?

Christopher B. Fordyce and Pamela S. Douglas

THE CHALLENGE OF NONINVASIVE TEST SELECTION FOR STABLE CHEST PAIN

The prevalence of angina is high in the general population and increases with age in both sexes, from approximately 3% to 4% in patients aged 40–59 years to 10% to 11% in those older than 80 years old.[1] New-onset stable chest pain among patients without known coronary artery disease (CAD) is a common clinical problem that results in approximately 4 million outpatient stress tests annually in the United States.[2] An initial evaluation always includes a full history and physical examination as well as basic ancillary studies, which should be sufficient for the physician to generate a hypothesis regarding the etiology of the chest pain (including cardiac vs. noncardiac). As described in more detail later, this initial evaluation should determine the patient's risk factors for atherosclerotic coronary disease and classify symptoms as typical, atypical, or noncardiac chest pain, which, in combination with age, can be used to quantify the pretest probability of underlying coronary disease. Important ancillary studies include fasting lipids, a resting 12-lead electrocardiogram, and possibly a chest x-ray. In addition to implementing any needed risk factor modification, empiric treatment with aspirin, β-blockers, and/or nitroglycerin may be considered in a patient who has an intermediate-to-high likelihood of obstructive coronary artery disease while awaiting an outpatient diagnostic test. Decisions then need to be made regarding testing, i.e.:

1. who to test (and who should not be tested)
2. if testing is chosen, which initial test to perform, including the type of noninvasive test or an invasive strategy.

Goals of Testing for the Diagnosis of CAD

While test selection for the diagnosis of CAD has the immediate goal of trying to determine if obstructive CAD accounts for the patient's symptoms, there are many other potential and salient goals that are both patient specific and system specific (Fig. 15.1). Related short-term patient-centric goals include determining the presence, severity, and extent of CAD, lifestyle and medical treatment optimization, risk stratification, and referral for invasive angiography or possible revascularization, if necessary. The overall long-term goal is to improve clinical outcomes for both individual patients and the overall population. Additional longer-term

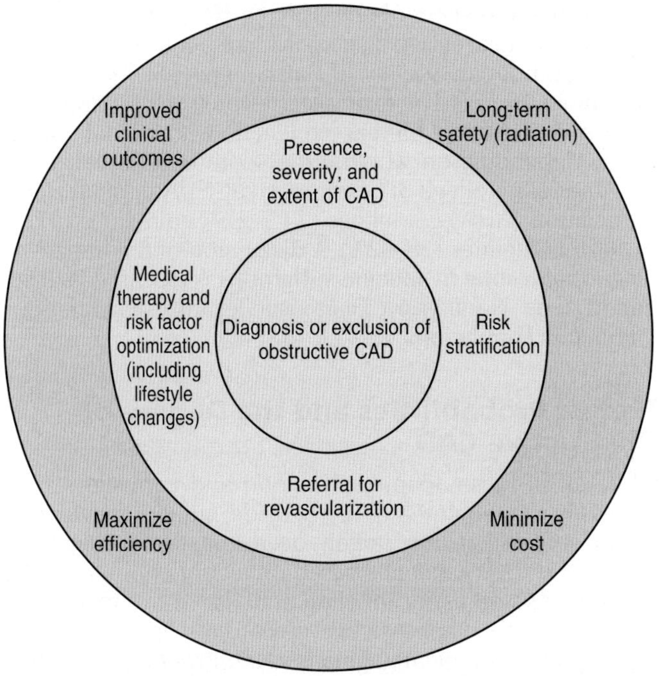

FIG. 15.1 Immediate *(beige)*, short-term *(green)*, and long-term *(blue)* goals of noninvasive cardiac testing for the diagnosis of obstructive coronary artery disease among patients with chest pain.

patient-centric goals include safety, such as reducing radiation exposure to prevent adverse sequelae, while goals for the healthcare system include maximizing efficiency and minimizing cost.

However, selection of patients for testing and selecting initial tests for the diagnosis of CAD are not always straightforward. Major US and European guidelines differ fairly substantially in their basic approaches to determining both the pretest probability of CAD in symptomatic patients and how to proceed with test selection. This may be related to a variation in features at presentation and regional preferences for diagnostic strategies and may be influenced by differences in healthcare systems, access to testing technologies, and risk tolerance.[2–4] Importantly, limited information on health-related outcomes exists in this stable as-yet-undiagnosed population, and there is little consensus about which test is preferable or even when one is required.[5–7] The discrepancies between guidelines differ significantly from other areas in cardiology (i.e., therapy for acute coronary syndromes or chronic heart failure), in which general consensus exists largely based on the availability of randomized clinical trial data. To date, current guidelines for imaging stable chest pain of suspected cardiac etiology have not yet incorporated the results of recent, large, randomized trials comparing functional versus anatomic testing strategies.[8,9]

Complicating the uncertainty are several potential adverse downstream consequences associated with noninvasive tests. These include patient-centered outcomes of false-positive testing such as discomfort during cardiac catheterization, procedural complications,[10] and the effects of radiation,[11] as well as the impact of changes in medical therapy after test result findings[12–14] and cost.[4] Recent reports of high rates of finding nonobstructive CAD on angiography[15] may speak to the quality of clinical assessment, including the crucial step of patient selection for noninvasive testing.[16] The majority of studies on outpatients with a clinical syndrome of possible ischemia show that, in contrast to past data, at present up to 90% of such tests are normal and approximately 99% of those patients will not experience an untoward clinical event.[17–20] The risks of false-negative testing include those of a missed diagnosis and failure to treat CAD or risk factors properly. The high incidence of normal noninvasive testing and weak correlations between noninvasive testing results and the presence of obstructive CAD provide further impetus to improve patient selection for noninvasive testing. These issues have important implications for healthcare utilization as well as for the individual patient.

In addition, the fundamental concepts about how we define "significant" CAD have been recently evolving, contributing to the uncertainty of how to best evaluate specific patient populations with chest pain. Recent evidence has found that the association between angiographically defined coronary stenosis and ischemia is variable, as many patients have no ischemia despite the presence of significant stenosis and others may have ischemia with no severe stenosis.[21] Furthermore, the extent to which routine revascularization to treat ischemia reduces death or myocardial infarction (MI), or improves quality of life in patients with stable ischemic heart disease, remains one of the most fundamental uncertainties in cardiology today.[22]

Therefore, decisions regarding noninvasive test use and selection remain common but challenging for many clinicians and a controversial topic for practice guidelines. This chapter reviews important patient characteristics that influence noninvasive test selection for the diagnosis of CAD, including an emphasis on comparing major guideline recommendations and evaluating very recent data, including promising technologies. We review contemporary considerations in cardiovascular imaging, such as how best to evaluate special populations, and appropriate use, including the consequences of noninvasive testing that are sometimes overlooked, such as radiation and cost. Finally, we present a step-by-step practical proposal for a unified approach, incorporating the latest trial evidence, to optimize test selection for both functional and anatomic strategies.

OVERVIEW: PATIENT SELECTION FOR NONINVASIVE TESTING

The current discussion applies specifically to stable, symptomatic patients with suspected ischemic heart disease on the basis of a thorough history, physical examination, and laboratory data. First, angina is both a continuum and a collection of disparate symptoms, ranging from atypical pain or angina equivalent to typical angina to low-risk unstable angina; delineating these categories can be difficult but the implications for testing and prognosis are significant. While new-onset angina is generally regarded as unstable angina, if the chest pain first occurs with heavy exertion—such as prolonged or fast running (Canadian Cardiovascular Society I)—the patient with new-onset angina may instead fall under the definition of stable, rather than unstable, angina.[23] Further confusing the issue is the fact that research is often conducted on the basis of location of care (e.g., office, rapid access chest pain center, or emergency department) rather than solely on symptom type, such that differences in healthcare systems or access to care may obscure differences in clinical presentation. Second, the physical examination, while often normal, should help to exclude other causes

TABLE 15.1 Traditional Clinical Classification of Chest Pain

Typical angina (definite)	Meets all three of the following characteristics: 1. Substernal chest discomfort of characteristic quality and duration 2. Provoked by exertion or emotional stress 3. Relieved by rest and/or nitrates within minutes
Atypical angina (probable)	Meets two of these characteristics
Nonanginal chest pain	Lacks or meets only one or none of the characteristics

From Diamond GA, Forrester JS, Hirsch M, et al. Application of conditional probability analysis to the clinical diagnosis of coronary artery disease. J Clin Invest. *1980;65:1210–1221.*

of chest pain (e.g., chest wall tenderness or pericarditis), including life-threatening causes (e.g., aortic stenosis, aortic dissection, or pulmonary embolism). The resting 12-lead electrocardiogram (ECG) is also usually normal or has only minor abnormalities, and patients undergoing assessment should have negative or minimally abnormal cardiac biomarkers, if measured. Thus, in addition to patient-specific considerations such as suitability for revascularization, the next critical step for consideration of noninvasive testing is determination of the pretest probability of obstructive CAD.

Clinical Classification of Chest Pain and the Pretest Probability of Obstructive CAD

Classically, chest pain symptoms are categorized as typical, atypical, or noncardiac chest, which in combination with age can be used to quantify the pretest probability of underlying coronary disease (Table 15.1).[24] This must be distinguished from other tools such as the Framingham Risk Score[25] or newer atherosclerotic cardiovascular disease (ASCVD) score,[26] which are helpful in evaluating overall risk burden and prognosis using baseline clinical characteristics, but are not designed to evaluate the likelihood of obstructive CAD in the presence of symptoms. While the Coronary CT Angiography Evaluation for Clinical Outcomes: An International Multicenter (CONFIRM) registry risk score[27] provides incremental prognostic information from plaque burden and stenosis found on coronary computed tomographic angiography (CCTA), it was derived in a mixed population of patients (asymptomatic and symptomatic) and requires noninvasive testing by definition, and thus does not aid in the decision to test or in test selection itself.

The Diamond and Forrester algorithms represent the gold standard for prediction of obstructive CAD in symptomatic patients. However, calculation of pretest probability using this score differs depending on which guideline is followed, as each country or region has adopted a different modification. In the United States, current guidelines recommend use of a Diamond and Forrester likelihood score combined with data from the Coronary Artery Surgery Study risk score (Table 15.2).[6] The UK National Institute for Health and Care Excellence (NICE) guidelines advocate calculating CAD likelihood using another modified Diamond and Forrester clinical prediction rule by Pryor et al.[5,28] This score incorporates the additional high-risk features of diabetes, smoking, hyperlipidemia, and resting ECG changes. More recently, a clinical prediction rule by Genders et al., which aimed to validate, update, and extend the Diamond and Forrester model to a more contemporary population and especially women, had the effect of reclassifying 16% of men and 64% of females. This revised risk score has been incorporated into the European Society of Cardiology (ESC) guidelines (see Table 15.2).[29] For example, the pretest probability of obstructive CAD in a 55-year-old female with typical angina differs depending on whether the score used is based on the American College of Cardiology (ACC)/American Heart Association (AHA) guidelines (73%), ESC guidelines (47%), or NICE guidelines (38–92%). A discussion of the impact of diagnostic testing in specific subgroups is discussed subsequently (see "Noninvasive Diagnostic Testing Considerations for Special Populations").

Pretest Probabilities and the Degree of Obstructive CAD

While all of these adapted Diamond and Forrester scores are easily implemented at the bedside, mounting evidence demonstrates that they largely overestimate the degree of obstructive CAD. Estimates based on a contemporary CCTA registry,[30] as well as recent clinical trials,[8,9] have found that the prevalence of obstructive epicardial CAD in patients with typical or atypical angina is much lower than that predicted by Diamond and Forrester in 1979, or any subsequent modification.[24] There are also increasing questions about the need to predict other coronary abnormalities besides severe stenoses. Several studies have found that high rates of nonobstructive CAD are routinely identified during elective coronary angiography, with a significant variation in the rate of nonobstructive CAD between centers.[15,16,31–33] Plaque burden and location each carries incremental prognostic value above traditional obstructive stenosis.[27] Therefore, while we continue to rely on likelihood scores to predict pretest probability of CAD based mainly on age and symptoms alone, improved strategies for likelihood of CAD, risk stratification, and subsequent test selection are warranted and have been proposed or are in development (see "Noninvasive Imaging Integrating Functional and Anatomical Strategies"). Validation in other populations may encourage future adoption.

Quantifying "Intermediate" Pretest Probability of CAD

Determination of pretest probability also impacts the performance of the available diagnostic methods (the likelihood that this patient has obstructive disease if the test is positive, or does not have disease if the test is negative).[7] Diagnostic testing is most valuable when the pretest probability of ischemic heart disease (IHD) is intermediate, since the application of a test result using Bayesian analysis drives the posttest probability sufficiently lower (negative test) or higher (positive test) to inform future decision-making—usually whether or not the patient should proceed to cardiac catheterization.[34]

Nevertheless, there remains no universal definition of intermediate pretest probability. The definition of 10% to 90%, first advocated in 1980,[35] has been applied in several studies and is the current definition used in the ACC/AHA guidelines for stable IHD (Table 15.3).[36,37] Low and high pretest probabilities are thus less than 10% and greater than 90%, respectively. This risk stratification scheme is also used by the most recent ACC/AHA Appropriate Use Criteria Task Force.[38] In contrast, the current ESC guidelines using the

TABLE 15.2 Calculation of Patient Pretest Probabilities of CAD Used to Determine Eligibility for Noninvasive Test Selection in the 2012 ACC/AHA, 2013 ESC, and 2010 UK NICE Guidelines in Males and Females[156]

	MALES								
	NONANGINAL CHEST PAIN			ATYPICAL ANGINA			TYPICAL ANGINA		
Guideline	**ACC/AHA**[A]	**ESC**[B]	**Nice**[C]	**ACC/AHA**	**ESC**	**Nice**	**ACC/AHA**	**ESC**	**Nice**
Age									
30–39	4	18	3–35	34	29	8–59	76	59	30–88
40–49	13	25	9–47	51	38	21–70	87	69	51–92
50–59	20	34	23–59	65	49	45–79	93	77	80–95
60–69	27	44	49–69	72	59	71–86	94	84	93–97
70–79		54			69			89	
> 80		65			78			93	
	FEMALES								
	NONANGINAL CHEST PAIN			**ATYPICAL ANGINA**			**TYPICAL ANGINA**		
Guideline	**ACC/AHA**	**ESC**	**Nice**	**ACC/AHA**	**ESC**	**Nice**	**ACC/AHA**	**ESC**	**Nice**
Age									
30–39	2	5	1–19	12	10	2–39	26	28	10–78
40–49	3	8	2–22	22	14	5–43	55	37	20–79
50–59	7	12	4–25	31	20	10–47	73	47	38–92
60–69	14	17	9–29	51	28	20–51	86	58	56–84
70–79		24			37			68	
> 80		32			47			76	

ACC, American College of Cardiology; *AHA,* American Heart Association; *CAD,* coronary artery disease; *ESC,* European Society of Cardiology; *NICE,* National Institute for Health and Care Excellence.

[a]ACC/AHA uses combined Diamond and Forrester and Coronary Artery Surgery Study risk score. Each value represents the percent with obstructive CAD on catheterization. *Modified from Fihn SD, Gardin JM, Abrams J, et al. 2012 ACCF/AHA/ACP/AATS/PCNA/SCAI/STS guideline for the diagnosis and management of patients with stable ischemic heart disease: a report of the American College of Cardiology Foundation/American Heart Association Task Force on Practice Guidelines, and the American College of Physicians, American Association for Thoracic Surgery, Preventive Cardiovascular Nurses Association, Society for Cardiovascular Angiography and Interventions, and Society of Thoracic Surgeons.* J Am Coll Cardiol. *2012;60:e44–e164.*

[b]ESC uses updated Diamond and Forrester prediction score. *Modified from Genders TS, Steyerberg EW, Alkadhi H, et al. A clinical prediction rule for the diagnosis of coronary artery disease: validation, updating, and extension.* Eur Heart J. *2011;32:1316–1330.*

[c]NICE uses modified Diamond and Forrester prediction score. *Modified from Pryor DB, Shaw L, McCants CB, et al. Value of the history and physical in identifying patients at increased risk for coronary artery disease.* Ann Intern Med. *1993;118:81–90.* A range is provided for each estimate from "Low" to "High" risk depending on the presence of the additional factors of diabetes, smoking, and hyperlipidemia (total cholesterol > 6.4 mmol/L).

TABLE 15.3 Selected Sensitivities and Specificities of Noninvasive Tests for the Detection of CAD as Reported in the ACC/AHA 2012 and ESC 2013 Guidelines

	SENSITIVITY		SPECIFICITY	
	ACC/AHA 2012	ESC 2013	ACC/AHA 2012	ESC 2013
Exercise ECG	0.68	0.45–0.50	0.77	0.85–0.90
ECHO				
Exercise or pharm	0.76		0.88	
Exercise		0.80–0.85		0.80–0.88
Pharm		0.79–0.83		0.82–0.86
SPECT				
Exercise or pharm	0.88		0.77	
Exercise		0.73–0.92		0.63–0.87
Pharm		0.90–0.91		0.75–0.84
PET				
Exercise or pharm	0.91		0.82	
Pharm PET		0.81–0.97		0.74–0.91
CMR				
Dobutamine		0.79–0.88		0.82–0.86
Vasodilator		0.67–0.94		0.61–0.85
CCTA		0.95–0.99		0.64–0.93

ACC, American College of Cardiology; *AHA,* American Heart Association; *CCTA,* coronary computed tomographic angiography; *CMR,* cardiac magnetic resonance; *ECG,* electrocardiogram; *ECHO,* echocardiography; *ESC,* European Society of Cardiology; *NICE,* National Institute for Health and Care Excellence; *PET,* positron emission tomography; *SPECT,* single photon emission computed tomography.

ACC/AHA 2012 estimates were modified from Garber AM, Solomon NA. Cost-effectiveness of alternative test strategies for the diagnosis of coronary artery disease. *Ann Intern Med.* 1999;130:719–728.

ESC 2013 estimates were collated from multiple studies and modified from Montalescot G, Sechtem U, Achenbach S, et al. 2013 ESC guidelines on the management of stable coronary artery disease. *Eur Heart J.* 2013;34:2949–3003.

Genders et al.–modified Diamond and Forrester clinical prediction rule stratifies patients into four groups: less than 15%, 15–65%, 66–85%, and greater than 85%. In comparison to the US guidelines, the intermediate group is defined by a pretest probability of 15% to 85% by combining the two mid-risk groups. Based on these four groups, the ESC guidelines recommend specific test strategies (see later). Finally, the UK NICE guidelines differ compared to both the ACC/AHA and ESC guidelines, identifying an intermediate pretest probability as 30% to 60%.[5]

Is There a Role for Watchful Waiting in Patients with Stable Chest Pain?

Due to low event rates in stable chest pain populations undergoing imaging or ECG testing,[8,9,39] and the similar outcomes with medical treatment and coronary revascularization in trials such as Clinical Outcomes Utilizing Revascularization and Aggressive Drug Evaluation (COURAGE),[40,41] some have recommended that a strategy of deferred testing may be preferable to performing any test at all. In this scenario, a patient with a sufficiently low pretest probability of obstructive CAD as the cause of their stable chest pain would not undergo any initial noninvasive cardiac testing, would be monitored clinically, and would be treated according to primary prevention strategies. This is on a background of the explosive growth in cardiac imaging in the United States, which has become central to discussions surrounding the high cost of healthcare, including a rapid escalation of costs for testing (twice that of other physician services).[4] However, there is as yet no direct clinical trial evidence to support a deferred testing strategy. This is in contrast to the robust evidence now available that supports a testing strategy with either functional testing or CCTA as being safe and effective (see "A New Standard for Pragmatic, Imaging Trials: PROMISE and SCOT-HEART").[8,9]

Another important aspect in the decision regarding whether to defer testing is first considering whether the patient would benefit from revascularization. If the patient has significant comorbidities or their quality of life is not expected to benefit from revascularization, then optimizing medical therapy may be a more reasonable approach than testing.

GENERAL APPROACH TO CHOOSING A NONINVASIVE TEST

Following identification of a symptomatic patient with no prior history of CAD and an intermediate pretest probability of CAD, the clinician is generally advised to consider a functional or, more rarely, an anatomic strategy. The NICE guidelines are an exception to this rule; they recommend an anatomic strategy for lower pretest probabilities (<30%).[5]

Approach to Choosing a Functional Test

For functional testing, the choice of stress must first be considered (exercise vs. pharmacologic) and, if exercise is employed, consideration must also be given to whether or not additional imaging should be performed. Several stress imaging modalities currently exist, each with their advantages and disadvantages (Table 15.4). These include radionuclide stress myocardial perfusion imaging (MPI) using single photon emission computed tomography (SPECT) or positron emission tomography (PET), stress echocardiography, and stress cardiac magnetic resonance (CMR). SPECT,

TABLE 15.4 Advantages and Disadvantages of Stress Imaging Techniques and CCTA

TECHNIQUE	ADVANTAGES	DISADVANTAGES
Echocardiography	• wide access • portability • no radiation • low cost	• echo contrast needed in patients with poor ultrasound windows • dependent on operator skills
SPECT	• wide access • extensive data	• radiation
PET	• flow quantitation	• radiation • limited access • high cost
CMR	• high soft tissue contrast • precise imaging of myocardial scar • no ionizing radiation	• limited access in cardiology • contra-indications • functional analysis limited in arrhythmias • limited 3D quantification of ischemia • high cost
CCTA	• high NPV in patients with lower pretest probability	• limited availability • radiation • assessment limited with extensive coronary calcium • image quality limited with arrhythmias or higher heart rates that cannot be lowered • low NPV in higher pretest probability

3D, Three-dimensional; *CMR,* cardiac magnetic resonance; *CCTA,* coronary computed tomographic angiography; *NPV,* negative predictive value; *PET,* positron emission tomography; *SPECT,* single photon emission computed tomography.
From Montalescot G, Sechtem U, Achenbach S, et al. 2013 ESC guidelines on the management of stable coronary artery disease. Eur Heart J. *2013;34:2949–3003.*

PET, and echocardiography may be coupled to either exercise or pharmacologic stress, whereas stress CMR is only performed with pharmacologic stress.

In the absence of contraindications,[33,34] symptom-limited exercise with an exercise treadmill test (ETT) or bicycle ergometer is the preferred stress-testing modality (over pharmacologic stress) since it provides information concerning reproducibility of symptoms, cardiovascular function, exercise capacity, ECG changes, and the hemodynamic response during usual forms of activity. Exercise capacity alone is a powerful predictor of mortality. Furthermore, a score such as the Duke Treadmill Score when applied to data generated by the ETT can improve diagnostic certainty in addition to its prognostic implications.[42] However, a patient may be unable to exercise due to one or more noncardiac reasons. These include obesity, orthopedic limitations, balance issues, pulmonary limitations, frailty, or limb dysfunction as a result of paraplegia from a prior cerebrovascular event. A detailed discussion on the various forms of exercise modalities (treadmill, or upright or supine bicycle) and protocols (Bruce, Modified Bruce, Naughton) is presented elsewhere (see Chapter 10).[43] If absolute contraindications exist, then pharmacologic stress should be used; if relative contraindications exist, pharmacologic stress should be considered.

In addition to considering exercise capacity, several conditions interfere with the ability to make an ECG diagnosis of ischemia (e.g., left bundle branch block, right ventricular pacing, resting ST depression > 1 mm) and may result in an uninterpretable exercise ECG. When such conditions are present, imaging should be used regardless of the stress modality.[44]

If the patient is unable to exercise to sufficient workload, then pharmacologic stress is required. The decision regarding which imaging modality to use will depend on patient factors including suitability of the stress agents for that purpose as well as patient tolerance; ischemic endpoints may vary accordingly.[45] If MPI is used, vasodilators are the preferred pharmacologic stress agents, and perfusion is assessed. If echocardiography is performed, inotropic agents are the most commonly used (although this can vary by country), and wall motion is assessed. For CMR, either inotropes or vasodilators can be used with corresponding endpoints. However, as for exercise testing, contraindications to vasodilator stress agents (adenosine, dipyridamole, and the selective A2A receptor agonists, including regadenoson, binodenoson, and apadenoson)[46–49] or inotropic agents (typically dobutamine)[50] should be taken into account in selecting the test modality.

If the patient is not a candidate for exercise or pharmacologic stress testing, an anatomic strategy with coronary artery calcium (CAC) scoring or CCTA should be considered. Moreover, based on recently published trial data, an anatomic-first strategy may be a reasonable alternative in selected patients (see "A New Standard for Pragmatic Imaging Trials: PROMISE and SCOT-HEART") as discussed later.

Diagnostic Accuracy of Functional Testing Strategies

There are distinct strengths and weaknesses associated with each imaging modality (see Table 15.4), and test selection ultimately depends on many factors, including local availability, local expertise, existence and relevance of prior imaging data, cost, the patient's body habitus (e.g., morbid obesity), radiation exposure, and the need for concomitant assessment of hemodynamic function or valvular disease. Diagnostic performance should be considered when multiple options exist, ideally based on local laboratory performance rather than the literature. Since such detailed data are often not available, a cost-effectiveness meta-analysis by Garber and Solomon may be used. This analysis includes information on diagnostic accuracy of individual tests and is cited by the ACC/AHA guidelines as evidence for differing diagnostic accuracy between modalities (see Table 15.3).[51] PET is the most sensitive noninvasive functional test, and exercise ECG is the least sensitive. SPECT is nearly as sensitive as and somewhat less specific than PET (specificity, 0.77 [range in individual studies: 0.53–0.96] for SPECT and 0.82 [0.73–0.88] for PET). Echocardiography is more specific than PET (0.88 [0.80–0.95] compared with 0.82 [0.73–0.88]) but less sensitive (0.76 [0.40–1.00] compared with 0.91 [0.69–1.00]). The Clinical Evaluation of Magnetic Resonance Imaging in Coronary Heart Disease (CE-MARC) study directly and prospectively compared CMR to SPECT.[52] Compared to SPECT, CMR had greater sensitivity (0.87 [95% CI 0.82–0.90] compared with 0.67 [0.60–0.72]) and similar specificity (0.83 [0.80–0.87 for CMR]; 0.83 [0.79–0.86 for SPECT]). CE-MARC2 is a three-arm trial that is ongoing and will provide valuable insights by comparing outcomes following CMR-guided care, positron emission tomography–computed tomography (PET-CT)-guided care (according to ACC/AHA appropriate-use criteria), and NICE guideline-based management.[53]

TABLE 15.5 Summary of Multimodality Appropriate Use Criteria for the Detection of Ischemic Heart Disease in Symptomatic Patients

TARGET POPULATION	EXERCISE ECG	STRESS RNI	STRESS ECHO	STRESS CMR	CAC	CCTA
Low pretest probability of CAD ECG interpretable AND able to exercise	A	R	M	R	R	R
Low pretest probability of CAD ECG uninterpretable OR unable to exercise		A	A	M	R	M
Intermediate pretest probability of CAD ECG interpretable AND able to exercise	A	A	A	M	R	M
Intermediate pretest probability of CAD ECG uninterpretable OR unable to exercise		A	A	A	R	A
High pretest probability of CAD ECG interpretable AND able to exercise	M	A	A	A	R	M
High pretest probability of CAD ECG uninterpretable OR unable to exercise		A	A	A	R	M

Appropriate Use Key: *A,* appropriate; *M,* may be appropriate; *R,* rarely appropriate.
CAC, Coronary artery calcium; *CAD,* coronary artery disease; *CCTA,* coronary computed tomographic angiography; *CMR,* cardiac magnetic resonance; *ECG,* electrocardiogram; *ECHO,* echocardiography; *RNI,* radionuclide imaging.
Modified from Wolk MJ, Bailey SR, Doherty JU, et al. ACCF/AHA/ASE/ASNC/HFSA/HRS/SCAI/SCCT/SCMR/STS 2013 multimodality appropriate use criteria for the detection and risk assessment of stable ischemic heart disease: a report of the American College of Cardiology Foundation Appropriate Use Criteria Task Force, American Heart Association, American Society of Echocardiography, American Society of Nuclear Cardiology, Heart Failure Society of America, Heart Rhythm Society, Society for Cardiovascular Angiography and Interventions, Society of Cardiovascular Computed Tomography, Society for Cardiovascular Magnetic Resonance, and Society of Thoracic Surgeons. J Am Coll Cardiol. *2014;63:380–406.*

The ESC guidelines use multiple primary studies to summarize test performance.[7] A major difference between the reference data used by each guideline is the lower sensitivity of the exercise ECG reported in the ESC guidelines—only 50% (despite an excellent specificity of 90%). The marked differences in these values are at least partially, if not fully, explained by the ESC's use of data obtained from studies avoiding verification bias;[54] ACC/AHA guidelines do not restrict data to studies avoiding verification bias. Because this lower sensitivity means that the number of incorrect test results will become higher than the number of correct test results in populations with a pretest probability of greater than 65%,[55] the ESC does not recommend employing the exercise stress test without imaging in such higher-risk populations for diagnostic purposes. In general, it may be more appropriate to employ more specific testing for patients with a low-intermediate pretest probability of CAD and reserve more sensitive testing for those with high-intermediate pretest probabilities. Therefore the precision of pretest probability estimates to impact the choice the optimal noninvasive test is important even within the intermediate ranges.

Guideline Recommendations for Choosing a Functional Test

ACC/AHA 2012 Guideline

Among patients who can exercise, there are strong recommendations for nonimaging ETT for patients with an intermediate pretest probability of CAD, and exercise stress with nuclear MPI or echocardiography for those with an intermediate-to-high pretest probability of CAD who have an uninterpretable ECG (Class I).[6] The remaining Class I recommendation is for pharmacologic stress with nuclear MPI or echocardiography for patients who are unable to exercise. The guideline recommends against the use of pharmacologic stress with nuclear MPI, echocardiography, or CMR for patients who can exercise with interpretable ECGs, or amongst patients who can exercise with an interpretable ECG and who have only a low pretest probability of IHD (< 10%; Class III). The other testing strategies fall within the IIa or IIb classes of recommendations. While no specific recommendations are provided for patients with a pretest probability greater than 90%, it is reasonable to consider cardiac catheterization as the initial test, which is supported by the ACC/AHA 2012 diagnostic angiography appropriate use criteria.[56]

ACC Multimodality Appropriate Use Criteria 2014

The ACC Appropriate Use Criteria (AUC) document development process uses an independent technical panel to rate each testing modality as either appropriate, may be appropriate, or rarely appropriate for given symptomatic target populations.[38] The following appropriate functional testing situations are summarized here and in further detail in Table 15.5:

- Exercise ECG
  - Patients who are able to exercise with a low-to-intermediate pretest probability of CAD and an interpretable ECG
- Stress radionuclide imaging or stress echocardiography
  - All patient groups are appropriate, with the exception of those with a low pretest probability of CAD who are able to exercise and have an interpretable ECG, for whom stress echocardiography may be appropriate but stress MPI is rarely appropriate
- Stress CMR
  - Patients with an intermediate pretest probability of CAD who are unable to exercise or have an uninterpretable ECG
  - Patients with a high pretest probability of CAD, irrespective of their ability to exercise or whether their ECG is interpretable

Notably, in this most recent AUC guidance document, ratings for stress CMR were more often in accord with the ratings for stress radionuclide imaging (RNI), stress echo, and exercise treadmill testing. This may reflect the simultaneous rating of modalities, the growing body of evidence supporting the utility and accuracy of stress CMR,[38] and its increasing use in the community.

Despite guidance that exercise treadmill testing without imaging may be routinely used in many patients, the practice of stress imaging still dominates the US testing landscape for both symptomatic and asymptomatic patients. Among intermediate-risk patients with chest pain assigned to the functional arm of the Prospective Multicenter Imaging Study for Evaluation of Chest Pain (PROMISE) trial, only 10.2% of patients received exercise testing without imaging as a prespecified test.[9] Furthermore, in 2012, the *Choosing Wisely* campaign (http://www.choosingwisely.org) brought together nine leading medical organizations (including the ACC and the American Society of Nuclear Cardiology [ASNC]) to each pick five tests which they viewed as overused.[57] The cardiac tests felt to be most overused by both the ACC and ASNC for the testing of CAD were all imaging-based modalities in patients with few symptoms: stress imaging in patients without symptoms or high-risk markers for diabetes, regular stress cardiac imaging in asymptomatic patients during routine follow-up after treatment, and stress cardiac imaging during preoperative assessment. Therefore, the practice of US providers does not appear to reflect current US guideline recommendations.

ESC 2013 Guideline

In patients able to exercise and who have an evaluable ECG, exercise treadmill testing is recommended as the initial test for establishing a diagnosis of CAD in patients with symptoms of angina and intermediate pretest probability of CAD of 15% to 65% (Class I).[7] Furthermore, stress imaging (echocardiography, CMR, SPECT, or PET) is strongly recommended as the initial option if local expertise and availability permit (Class I). Exercise ECG without imaging in patients with an ST depression greater than or equal to 0.1 mV on resting ECG or taking digitalis is not recommended for diagnostic purposes (Class III). An imaging stress test is recommended as the initial test for diagnosing CAD with a high-intermediate pretest probability between 66% and 85% or if the left ventricular ejection fraction is less than 50% in patients without typical angina (Class I). While there are no specific recommendations for pharmacologic stress, exercise is recommended over pharmacologic testing whenever possible (Class I). A pretest probability of greater than 85% establishes a presumptive diagnosis of CAD, at which point risk stratification should be performed. In patients with severe symptoms or a clinical constellation suggesting high-risk coronary anatomy, clinicians are advised to initiate guideline-directed medical therapy and consider invasive catheterization as the initial test. In patients who have mild symptoms, noninvasive testing for risk stratification should be considered only if there is agreement to proceed to revascularization in the event of high-risk test findings.

UK 2010 NICE Guideline

For patients with chest pain and an estimated pretest probability of 30% to 60% the clinician is advised to offer noninvasive functional imaging for myocardial ischemia as the first-line test.[5] In contrast to the other guidelines, NICE incorporates an anatomic strategy as the front-line test for patients with a low-intermediate pretest probability. If the pretest probability is 10% to 29%, a "rule out" CAD strategy was felt to be best achieved with initial CAC scoring (and then CCTA if the CAC score is 1–400) and is justified based on cost-effectiveness and low radiation doses.[58–61] Alternatively, patients with a high CAC score may be investigated by functional assessment, depending on the score and patient factors (see next section), or invasive angiography. If the estimated pretest probability is 61% to 90%, the clinician should offer invasive coronary angiography as the first-line diagnostic investigation. Notably, exercise testing without imaging is never recommended in the investigative pathway for patients with no prior history of established CAD, representing a significant change to current practice and in contrast with other major guidelines.[61] This is based on the evidence of poorer diagnostic accuracy of exercise testing compared to the other tests and supported by a cost-effectiveness model derived specifically for these guidelines.[58]

Approach to Choosing an Anatomic Test Using CAC or CCTA

Until recently, the use of an anatomic strategy using CAC or CCTA has not generally been considered first-line in the diagnosis of CAD in intermediate pretest probability patients with stable chest pain (apart from the NICE guidelines for low-intermediate pretest probability patients, discussed previously), and receives weak, if any, recommendations in current ACC/AHA and ESC guidelines as well as the AUC (see later section). However, two recent randomized controlled trials (PROMISE and Scottish Computed Tomography of the Heart [SCOT-HEART]) directly comparing anatomic and functional testing in the setting of low-risk chest pain provide potential support for its inclusion as a reasonable choice in selected patients (see later discussion).

Patient Selection for CAC

While CAC imaging has been mostly used for risk stratification in asymptomatic individuals, some studies have evaluated the use of CAC in the diagnostic work-up of patients with suspected CAD (by excluding CAD). Data from a high-risk symptomatic population suggest a non-negligible rate of obstructive CAD (i.e., 20% of patients with a high pretest probability of CAD) in the absence of detectable calcium.[62] In contrast, data from lower-risk cohorts have demonstrated that among patients with a negative calcium scan, severe CAD requiring percutaneous coronary intervention (PCI) or coronary artery bypass grafting (CABG) occurs in less than or equal to 1% of patients.[63,64] The Computed Tomography vs. Exercise Testing in Suspected Coronary Artery Disease (CRESCENT) randomized controlled trial assessed the effectiveness and safety of a tiered cardiac CT protocol, consisting of a calcium scan and selective performance of CCTA if CAC was present. It found that this tiered approach offered an effective and safe alternative to functional testing while lowering diagnostic expenses and radiation exposure.[65] Patients in the CRESCENT trial had a pretest probability of approximately 45% per Diamond–Forrester criteria. Therefore, incorporation of CAC into stepwise CCTA imaging protocols may be beneficial in symptomatic patients, provided they have a low-to-intermediate pretest probability of CAD, although further studies are required for confirmation. One caveat is that this could lead to a higher false-negative rate in younger patients, who may have CAD without detectable CAC, since atherosclerotic calcification increases with age.[66,67] This may also be seen in women and ethnic minorities.[68–70]

Patient Selection for CCTA

As with functional testing, the clinician must first consider whether the patient is a good candidate for CCTA. According to a report from the 2014 Society of Cardiovascular Computed Tomography Guidelines Committee,[71] only patients with adequate breath-holding capabilities, without severe obesity (body mass index [BMI] >39 kg/m^2), with sinus rhythm and with a heart rate less than or equal to 60 beats per minute (BPM), and with normal or near-normal renal function should be considered for CCTA. If necessary, the patient should be able to tolerate use of short-acting β-blockers or other heart rate–lowering medication to achieve target heart rates. State-of-the-art multidetector scanners reduce radiation exposure and may obviate the need for adjunctive medications in many patients, as they allow accurate imaging with higher heart rates. Absolute contraindications must also be ruled out and include definite acute coronary syndromes, glomerular filtration rate (GFR) of less than 30 mL/min per 1.73m^2 unless on chronic dialysis, previous anaphylaxis after iodinated contrast administration, previous episode of contrast allergy after adequate steroid/antihistamine preparation, inability to cooperate (including inability to raise arms), or pregnancy or uncertain pregnancy status in premenopausal women.[71] Finally, one constraint is that CCTA accuracy may be limited with a high CAC score (Agatston score > 400 U), which can only be determined once the image acquisition has started.

Diagnostic Accuracy of CCTA

Multicenter studies evaluating the diagnostic accuracy of 64-slice multidetector CCTA for detection of significant (at least 50% stenosis) CAD on quantitative invasive coronary angiography have found sensitivities of between 85% and 99% and specificities between 64% and 90%,[72–74] although newer equipment and scan protocols may improve the diagnostic accuracy.[75] The Assessment by Coronary Computed Tomographic Angiography of Individuals Undergoing Invasive Coronary Angiography (ACCURACY) trial found that specificity was reduced significantly in the presence of coronary artery calcium.[72] In contrast, negative predictive values for CCTA have generally been high (95–100%).[72,73,76] This has garnered significant interest in using CCTA in scenarios to "rule out" coronary artery stenosis, or patients with lower pretest probability. Three randomized controlled trials have found a CCTA strategy to provide superior efficiency in the emergency department for low- to intermediate-risk chest pain to "rule out" acute coronary syndromes while providing excellent event-free survival similar to usual care, with no increase in costs or radiation exposure[77–79] (see Chapter 13).

Guideline Recommendations for Choosing an Anatomic Test with CAC and CCTA

ACC/AHA 2012 Guideline

There are currently no strong (Class I) recommendations for CAC or CCTA as the initial test.[6] CCTA may be considered for patients who cannot exercise or for those patients who have a prior normal functional test but ongoing symptoms, have an inconclusive functional test, or are unable to undergo stress MPI or echocardiography (all Class IIa).

ACC Multimodality Appropriate Use Criteria 2014

As in the preceding section, the document rated each testing modality as either appropriate, may be appropriate, or rarely appropriate for given symptomatic target populations.[38] The following anatomic testing situations are summarized here and in further detail in Table 15.4:

- CAC
  - Rarely appropriate for a symptomatic population of patients with chest pain
- CCTA
  - Appropriate only for symptomatic patients with an intermediate pretest probability of CAD and an uninterpretable ECG or unable to exercise

ESC 2013 Guideline

Similar to the ACC/AHA 2012 guideline, there are no strong recommendations (Class I) for CAC or CCTA as the initial test.[7] It is a Class IIa recommendation that CCTA should be considered as an alternative to stress imaging techniques for ruling out CAD in patients with a low-intermediate pretest probability (15–65%) who have an inconclusive exercise ECG or stress imaging test or who have contraindications to stress testing. This recommendation includes patients who can exercise, but excludes the highest range of pretest probability to improve accuracy by selecting patients less likely to have significant coronary calcium, which decreases diagnostic accuracy (discussed previously). Class III recommendations include using CCTA for patients with prior coronary revascularization (not applicable to this population) or as a "screening" test in asymptomatic individuals.

UK 2010 NICE Guideline

In contrast to the ESC guidelines, NICE recommends CAC scoring as the first-line test in patients with an estimated pretest probability of CAD of 10% to 29%.[5] Further management depends on the calcium score: if 0, consider other causes of chest pain; if 1–400, offer 64-slice (or greater) CCTA or imaging stress testing; and if higher than 400, offer invasive coronary angiography. If this is not clinically appropriate or acceptable to the person and/or revascularization is not being considered, offer noninvasive functional imaging.

Major differences between guideline recommendations for the diagnosis of CAD in patients with stable chest pain have several notable differences and are summarized in Table 15.6.

A NEW STANDARD FOR PRAGMATIC IMAGING TRIALS: PROMISE AND SCOT-HEART

The first two large randomized trials to directly compare noninvasive anatomic and functional imaging modalities in the setting of stable chest pain were published in early 2015. A comparison of the characteristics of each trial is shown in Table 15.7, and the overall trial results are compared in Fig. 15.2. The PROMISE trial randomly assigned 10,003 symptomatic stable outpatients requiring evaluation for suspected CAD to either CCTA or functional stress testing (ETT, nuclear stress testing, or stress echocardiography, at the discretion of the clinician caring for the patient) with a median follow-up of 25 months.[9] The composite primary endpoint (death, MI, hospitalization for unstable angina, or major cardiovascular procedural complication) occurred at similar rates in the CCTA and functional testing groups (3.3% and 3.0%, respectively; adjusted hazard ratio, 1.04), which was lower than previously established historical rates (Fig. 15.3). More patients in the CCTA group underwent cardiac catheterization within 90 days after randomization (12.2% vs. 8.1%), but the frequency of catheterization showing no obstructive CAD (a prespecified secondary endpoint) was lower in the CCTA group (27.9% vs. 52.5%).

TABLE 15.6 Selected Guideline Recommendations for the Use of Noninvasive Testing for the Diagnosis of Ischemic Heart Disease

	AHA/ACC (2012)	ESC (2013)	NICE (2010)
Patient Selection			
Risk score to calculate pretest probability	Combined Diamond Forrester - CASS	Genders et al. (2011)	Pryor et al. (1993)
Intermediate pretest probability	10–90%	15–85%	10–60%
Functional Test Selection			
Exercise treadmill test alone if pretest probability 15–65%*	Class I	Class I	Not recommended
Stress imaging if local expertise and availability	Class IIa	Class I	First line if pretest probability 30–60%
Stress imaging if pretest probability 66–85%**	Class IIa	Class I	Invasive angiography if pretest probability 60–90%
Stress imaging if nonevaluable ECG	Class I	Class I	Not specified
Anatomic (CTA) Test Selection			
"Rule out" if pretest probability 15–65%	Not specified	Class IIa	CAC scoring first line if pretest probability 10–29%; proceed to other testing depending on score
Nonconclusive functional test or contraindications	Class IIa	Class IIa	Not specified

ACC, American College of Cardiology; *AHA,* American Heart Association; *CAC,* coronary artery calcium; *CASS,* Coronary Artery Surgery Study; *CTA,* computed tomographic angiography; *ESC,* European Society of Cardiology; *NICE,* National Institute for Health and Care Excellence.
*Able to exercise with an evaluable ECG.
**ACC/AHA quantify risk as "intermediate to high."
Modified from Fordyce CB, Douglas PS. Optimal non-invasive imaging test selection for the diagnosis of ischaemic heart disease. Heart. *2016;102(7):555–564.*

TABLE 15.7 SCOT-HEART and PROMISE: Trial Characteristics

	SCOT-HEART	PROMISE
Country	United Kingdom	United States and Canada
Comparators	CCTA + standard of care vs. standard of care	CCTA vs. functional stress test
Trial design	Open-label	Open-label
Recruiting centers	12	193
Length of follow-up	20 months	25 months
Sample size	4146	10,003
Primary endpoint	Certainty of diagnosis of angina due to coronary heart disease	Death, nonfatal MI, hospitalization for unstable angina, major procedural complications (anaphylaxis, stroke, major bleeding, and renal failure)
Follow-up	National Health Record systems	Mail and telephone

CCTA, Coronary computed tomographic angiography; *MI,* myocardial infarction.
Modified from Fordyce CB, Newby DE, Douglas PS. Diagnostic strategies for the evaluation of chest pain: clinical implications from SCOT-HEART and PROMISE. J Am Coll Cardiol. *2016;67(7):843–852.*

The SCOT-HEART trial randomized 4146 patients with stable chest pain to CCTA in addition to usual care (which generally included stress testing) or to usual care alone.[8] The trial's primary endpoint, certainty of the attribution of symptoms to CAD, showed an increase in the CCTA group (relative risk 1.79, 95% CI 1.62–1.96), as did the secondary endpoint of certainty of diagnosis of coronary artery disease (2.56, 95% CI 2.33–2.79). There was also a nonsignificant reduction in some long-term clinical outcomes, including the rate of death or MI in the CCTA group at 1.7 years, although event rates were low in both arms (Fig. 15.4). While the trials were of different design, event rates were comparable, and there was a consistent finding that obstructive coronary disease was more frequently detected using an anatomic strategy of CCTA. Moreover, these top-line results provide support for consideration of an anatomic strategy as a viable option for initial noninvasive test selection. This notion is further supported by other smaller, but contemporary studies favoring a role for CCTA over functional imaging to improve both diagnostic accuracy[80] and patient outcomes.[81,82] This may be particularly important in the future, as patient selection for CCTA may become less restricted (i.e., due to arrhythmias, or high CAC) as a result of newer technologies and software algorithms.[83] Finally, it is anticipated that a number of secondary analyses will be performed in both PROMISE and SCOT-HEART, providing important additional details such as test performance, cost efficiency, and differences between special populations.

Clinical Implications from PROMISE and SCOT-HEART

PROMISE and SCOT-HEART extend findings from prior observational studies that contemporary patients with stable chest pain are at lower risk for subsequent clinical events than previously believed, despite a calculated intermediate pretest probability of obstructive disease according to traditional scoring systems. They also confirm findings of high rates of nonobstructive CAD on invasive angiography in prior observational studies, which may speak to the difficulty of clinical assessment, including the crucial step of patient selection for invasive testing.[16] The studies also

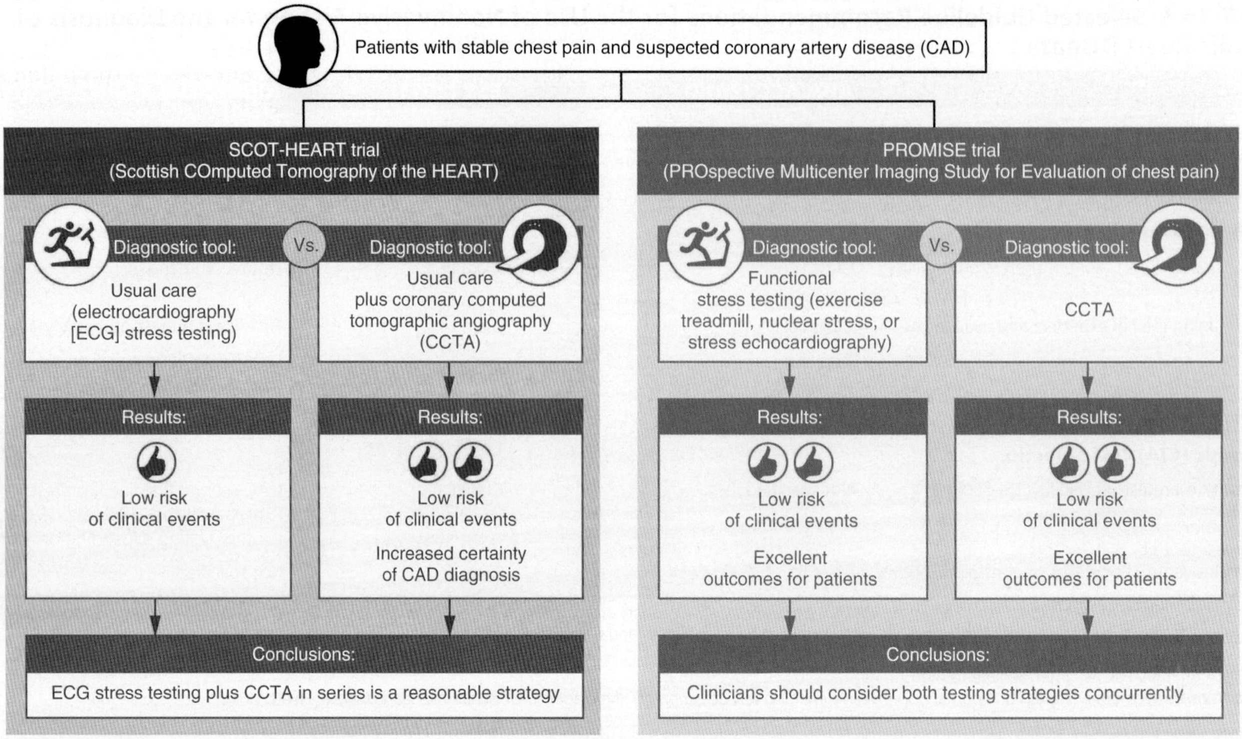

FIG. 15.2 Comparison of diagnostic tools, main results, and conclusions from the SCOT-HEART and PROMISE trials. *(Modified with permission from Fordyce CB, Newby DE, Douglas PS. Diagnostic strategies for the evaluation of chest pain: clinical implications from SCOT-HEART and PROMISE.* J Am Coll Cardiol. *2016:843–852.)*

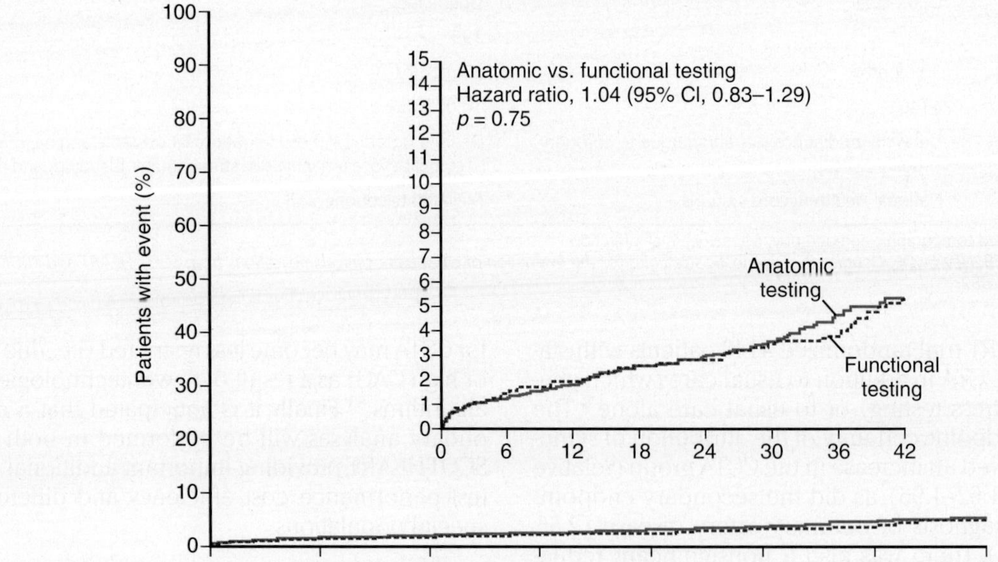

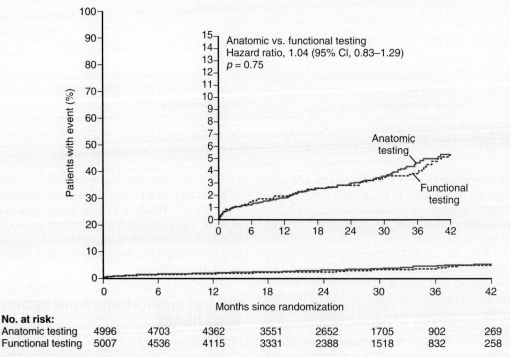

FIG. 15.3 PROMISE trial composite primary endpoint. The graph shows the unadjusted Kaplan–Meier estimates of the primary composite endpoint (death from any cause, nonfatal myocardial infarction, hospitalization for unstable angina, or major procedural complication). The adjusted hazard ratio for a computed tomographic angiography (CTA) strategy, as compared with a usual-care strategy of functional testing, was 1.04 (95% CI, 0.83–1.29), with adjustment for age, sex, risk equivalent of coronary artery disease (history of diabetes, peripheral arterial disease, or cerebrovascular disease), and the prespecification of the intended functional test if the patient were to be randomly assigned to the functional-testing group. The inset shows the same data on an enlarged *y* axis. *(Reproduced with permission from Douglas PS, Hoffmann U, Patel MR, et al. Outcomes of anatomical versus functional testing for coronary artery disease.* N Engl J Med. *2015;372:1291–1300.)*

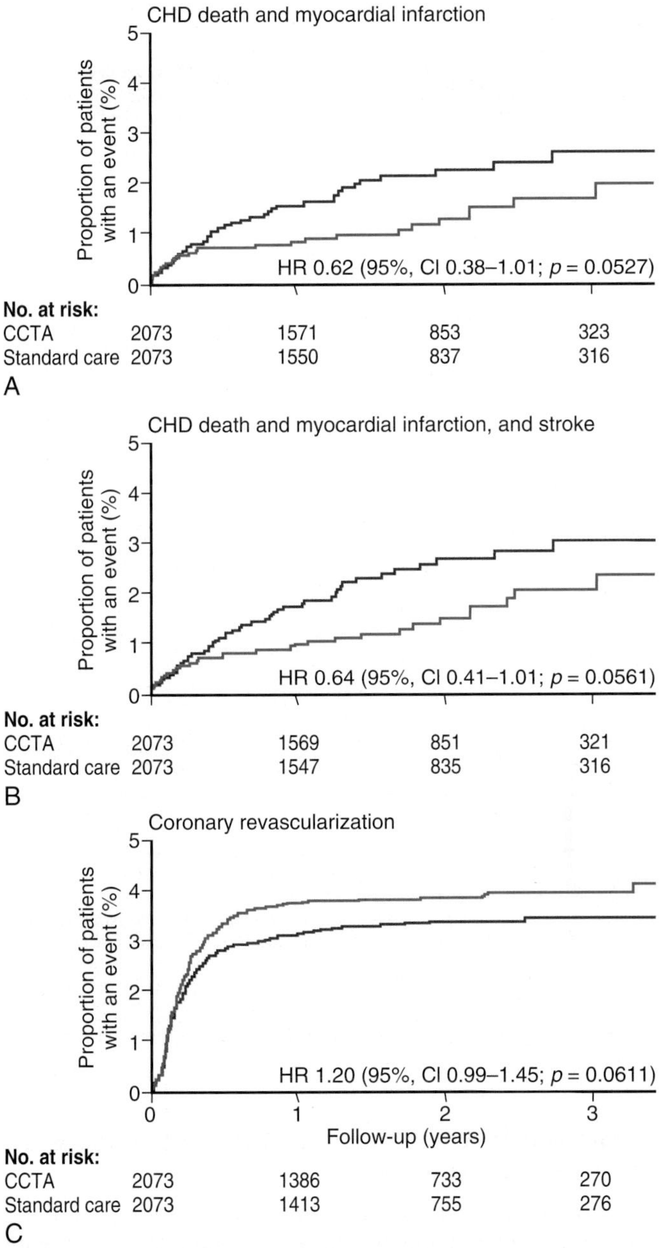

FIG. 15.4 SCOT-HEART trial long-term clinical outcomes. Kaplan–Meier curves for coronary heart disease (CHD) death and myocardial infarction (MI) **(A)**, CHD death, MI, and stroke **(B)**, and coronary revascularization **(C)** in patients assigned to coronary computed tomographic angiography *(blue)* and standard care *(red)*. *CCTA,* Coronary computed tomographic angiography. *(Modified with permission from Newby D, Williams M, Hunter A, et al. CT coronary angiography in patients with suspected angina due to coronary heart disease (SCOT-HEART): an open-label, parallel-group, multicentre trial.* Lancet. *2015;385:2383–2391.)*

corroborate several reports showing that the results of up to 90% of noninvasive tests performed in patients with stable chest pain of suspected ischemic etiology are normal or signify nonobstructive CAD disease and that many of these patients will not experience an untoward clinical event.[17–20] However, only an anatomic approach can identify nonobstructive disease, which is associated with event rates similar to obstructive single-vessel disease.[84] Both trials demonstrate that both anatomic and functional strategies resulted in few safety endpoints related to testing in either arm or downstream events such as cardiac catheterization, and relatively low levels of radiation exposure. However, despite this high degree of safety, testing should be judiciously performed, given recent calls for reducing inappropriate cardiac testing to prevent unnecessary risk to patients.[2,38,56]

PROMISE and SCOT-HEART also demonstrate that stress testing will continue to play an important and highly appropriate front-line role in our assessment of stable, symptomatic patients for risk stratification and diagnosis. However, it should be acknowledged that despite widespread adaptation into practice, stress testing had not previously undergone the same rigorous assessment for determining the impact of a diagnostic test on downstream clinical endpoints that both stress testing and CCTA have now undergone with these two trials. For PROMISE, there was a head-to-head comparison of stress versus anatomic testing in which CCTA did not improve outcomes compared to functional testing. Both strategies resulted in acceptable if not excellent outcomes for patients. For SCOT-HEART, stress testing and CCTA were performed sequentially and were therefore integrated as part of a care pathway. Some have since advocated routinely using exercise stress testing and CCTA in a serial manner to evaluate patients with stable chest pain.[85] This trial's findings suggest that stress testing alone will provide a somewhat different diagnostic formulation than using both tests. Overall, event rates were low and, while not directly addressed by either trial, the incremental benefit of performing *any* testing in the lowest risk patients may reasonably be questioned. For example, if CCTA is used indiscriminately, SCOT-HEART would suggest that approximately 100 CCTAs would need to be performed to prevent one MI.

Finally, the totality of the evidence generated from PROMISE and SCOT-HEART demonstrates that CCTA is a reasonable first-choice alternative in the routine assessment of patients with stable chest pain. When stress imaging and CCTA are compared head-to-head, the PROMISE trial demonstrated similar clinical outcomes compared to usual care but better selection of patients for invasive coronary angiography. Compared to standard of care, SCOT-HEART demonstrated that using exercise ECG and CCTA in series clarified the diagnosis of angina due to coronary heart disease and altered patient management (selection of invasive coronary angiography and preventative therapies). Both trials demonstrated that CCTA can be performed safely at acceptable or low radiation doses (see later). Although not statistically significant, trends for reductions in clinical events may be plausibly related to changes in medical and revascularization therapies, although further analysis is required. It should also be remembered that, for the patient, discontinuation of unnecessary investigations and treatments is greatly valued even if there is limited impact on clinical outcomes.

IMPORTANT DOWNSTREAM SEQUELAE OF NONINVASIVE TESTING

Radiation

As a result of increases in procedure volumes, total magnitude of radiation dose received by some patients as a consequence of cardiac testing, and the association of radiation exposure with malignancy, radiation is a topic of immense interest.[11,86] Differences in radiation exposure between imaging modalities (Table 15.8) may be an important secondary consideration when deciding upon test selection.[87] Notably, radiation doses for CCTA continue to be reduced, particularly with newer technologies, including a

TABLE 15.8 Representative Values and Ranges of Effective Dose Estimates Reported for Selected Cardiac Imaging Studies

EXAMINATION	REPRESENTATIVE EFFECTIVE DOSE VALUE (mSv)	RANGE OF REPORTED DOSE VALUES (mSv)	ADMINISTERED ACTIVITY (MBq)
Chest x-ray PA and lateral	0.1	0.05–0.24	NA
CT chest	7	4–18	NA
CT abdominal	8	4–25	NA
CT pelvis	6	3–10	NA
Coronary calcium CT*	3	1–12	NA
Coronary CT angiogram	16	5–32	NA
64-Slice CCTA‡			
Without tube current modulation	15	12–18	NA
With tube current modulation[21]	9	8–18	NA
Dual-source CCTA‡			
With tube current modulation	13	6–17	NA
Prospectively triggered CCTA‡ [22]	3	2–4	NA
Diagnostic invasive coronary angiogram	7	2–16	NA
Percutaneous coronary intervention or radiofrequency ablation	15	7–57	NA
Myocardial perfusion study			
Sestamibi (1-day) stress/rest	9	—	1100
Thallium stress/rest	41	—	185
F-18 FDG	14	—	740
Rubidium-82	5	—	1480

CT, Computed tomography; *CCTA*, coronary computed tomographic angiography; *FDG*, fluorodeoxyglucose; *mSv*, millisieverts; *MBq*, megabecquerels; *NA*, not applicable; *PA*, posteroanterior.
*Data combine prospectively triggered and retrospectively gated protocols. The Writing Group estimates the representative effective dose estimate to be approximately 1 mSv for prospectively triggered coronary calcium CT scans and 3 mSv for retrospectively gated scans.
‡64-Slice multidetector-row CT and dual-source CT studies published since 2005 only; data include a survey of the literature by the Writing Group.
Modified from Gerber TC, Carr JJ, Arai AE, et al. Ionizing radiation in cardiac imaging: a science advisory from the American Heart Association Committee on Cardiac Imaging of the Council on Clinical Cardiology and Committee on Cardiovascular Imaging and Intervention of the Council on Cardiovascular Radiology and Intervention. Circulation. *2009;119:1056–1065.*

320–Detector Row CT scanner enabling submillisievert radiation exposures,[88] as well as the implementation of novel software algorithms such as iterative reconstruction.[89] In a setting of chest pain in the emergency department, the use of CCTA did not increase radiation exposure and was found to provide superior efficiency to "rule out" acute coronary syndromes while providing excellent event-free survival, compared to usual care.[77–79] Mean cumulative radiation exposure in the PROMISE trial, amongst those patients randomized in an intended nuclear test strata, was lower in the CCTA group compared to that in the functional testing group (12.0 vs. 14.1 mSv).[9] This included all downstream radiation within 90 days, including that associated with cardiac catheterization, and is particularly intriguing given that a greater proportion of CCTA patients received cardiac catheterization. Radiation doses were even lower in the CCTA arms of SCOT-HEART (4.1 mSv, using mainly 320 Detector Row CT scanners), as well as in the recent PLATFORM trial (5.2 mSv, using ≥ 64 Detector Row CT scanners). Similarly, newer nuclear scanner technology, image-reconstruction software, and strategies employing low-dose and ultra-low-dose radiotracers are also expected to yield lower radiation doses in the future,[90] including targeting doses of 9 mSv or less in 50% of patients referred for SPECT or PET MPI studies.[91] The comparative effectiveness of newer scanners and scan protocols on reducing both CCTA and nuclear radiation exposure is unknown at this time. Importantly, both the Society of Computer Cardiovascular Tomography and the ASNC are undertaking national quality control initiatives to routinely minimize exposure while preserving diagnostic image quality.[91,92]

A Growing Awareness of the Importance of Nonobstructive CAD

The potential benefit of modifying medical therapy and lifestyle to reduce clinical events among patients with recently diagnosed nonobstructive CAD on imaging is a compelling concept, but is as yet unproven by prospective intervention trials. As discussed previously, only an anatomic approach can identify nonobstructive CAD.[84] An analysis from the CONFIRM registry found that baseline statin use was associated with reduced mortality, but only among patients with CCTA-identified nonobstructive CAD and not those with normal coronary arteries.[93] Recent studies have found increased rates of medical therapy intensification once CCTA results showed nonobstructive CAD,[12–14] but not consistently for functional testing.[94,95] In the SCOT-HEART trial, 27% of participants randomized to CCTA had a change in pharmacologic therapy, including the implementation of therapies associated with improved outcomes, as compared with 5% in the usual care arm.[8,85] Similarly, in the PROMISE trial, a CCTA strategy was associated with a higher proportion of patients initiating therapies following testing compared to a functional strategy, including aspirin (11.6% vs. 7.6%), statin (12.7% vs. 6.2%), and β-blockers (8.2% vs. 5.4%) ($p < 0.0001$ for each).[96] Taken together, mounting evidence suggests that the identification of nonobstructive CAD on

CCTA leads to greater intensification of therapy, with the potential to improve outcomes. However, future analyses are required to determine whether this hypothesis holds true.

Appropriate Use and Cost-Effectiveness of the Various Imaging Modalities

Concerns regarding overuse of both noninvasive and invasive diagnostic testing are long-standing, based on growth in use. In addition, the vast majority of noninvasive stress tests on outpatients with a clinical syndrome of possible ischemia show that, increasingly, the results of up to 90% of such tests are normal, and approximately 99% of those patients will not experience an untoward clinical event.[17–20] Furthermore, typically half of the patients referred for coronary angiography are found not to have obstructive CAD.[15,30,97-99] The overuse of cardiac testing has significant healthcare system and cost implications.

In order to provide guidance for cardiac testing and procedures, and reduce both over- and under-use testing, the Appropriate Use Criteria Task Force was developed for both multimodality imaging[38] and coronary angiography.[56] The AUC stipulate that clinical benefits should always be considered first, and costs should be considered relative to these benefits in order to better convey net value. Because event and complication rates are so low, cost-effectiveness of the various imaging modalities become a more relevant concern. However, this varies according to payer and site of service, making true estimates challenging.[38] This is especially true as healthcare reimbursement in the United States transitions to shared risk and quality-based models. Quality of care and access should also be paramount when considering appropriate use of the various imaging modalities.[100] A recent finding that rates of appropriate test ordering varied between provider types (cardiologists vs. primary care physicians) speaks not only to the complexity of the issue, but suggests that provider-specific interventions may be helpful in mitigating unnecessary testing in the future.[101] The AUC for the various testing modalities for specific patient populations was discussed previously (see "Guideline Recommendations for Choosing a Functional / Anatomic Test with CCTA").

The AUC appear to have had a modest impact on at least some practice patterns. A recent systematic review involving 103,567 tests from 2000 to 2012 found that rates of reported appropriate use in imaging show improvements for transthoracic echocardiography and computed tomographic angiography but not for stress MPO or either stress or transesophageal echocardiography.[102] Similarly, despite the fact that inappropriate MPI studies were less likely to yield abnormal results or demonstrate myocardial ischemia, a second systematic review with over 23,443 patients found that rates of inappropriate MPI have not decreased over time.[103] Finally, a systematic review of studies evaluating quality improvement initiatives aimed at reducing inappropriate cardiac imaging found that interventions using physician audit and feedback are associated with lower rates of inappropriate cardiac testing.[104]

As the gaps between the costs of various modalities have narrowed, most contemporary analyses have suggested that CCTA is comparable to functional testing from a cost-effectiveness standpoint. A recent study using both US and European data found CCTA to be as cost-effective as MPI and CMR.[105] The final PROMISE cost analyses showed similar true costs (vs. reimbursement) in the anatomic and functional arms.[106] Furthermore, when compared to functional testing alone, a decision analysis found that a two-step diagnostic strategy of CCTA followed by SPECT for intermediate lesions is likely to be less costly and more effective than functional testing alone for the diagnosis of symptomatic patients at low risk of an acute coronary syndrome.[107] In contrast, Medicare beneficiaries who underwent CCTA in a nonacute setting were more likely to undergo subsequent invasive cardiac procedures and have higher CAD-related spending than patients who underwent stress testing.[108] However, the generalizability of this study may be limited, since it was based on administrative data, included only traditional fee-for-service Medicare beneficiaries, and had no information on the diagnostic performance of the various noninvasive tests or the appropriateness of the invasive cardiac procedures performed. A possible role for use of newer genomic approaches such as the Corus CAD gene expression score in selecting patients for testing is as yet unknown; such a strategy may be more cost-efficient as well as effective.[109,110] Taken together, the evidence to date suggests that cost-effectiveness alone does not favor any imaging test over another for routine practice.

NONINVASIVE DIAGNOSTIC TESTING CONSIDERATIONS FOR SPECIAL POPULATIONS

Sex

Until recently, there has been a dearth of evidence supporting specific noninvasive diagnostic testing strategies in important subgroups such as those categorized by sex, race, and age. It is clear that prevalence of coronary disease is a function of sex, as is prevalence of angina.[111] Experts have long advocated that diagnostic imaging tests are generally not optimized for—and hence are less accurate for—females.[68–70] The reasons for this are multifactorial, but females are thought to present with more atypical symptoms and at an older age.[112] Moreover, the diagnostic accuracy of exercise treadmill testing is lower in women, with pooled sensitivities and specificities of 61% and 70%, respectively, compared with corresponding values of 68% and 77% in men.[113] The decreased specificity of ST-segment depression in women is thought to be partially due to poorer exercise capacity, a digoxin-like estrogen effect, lower ECG voltage, and an increased prevalence of baseline ST-T changes.[113] Differences in diagnostic accuracy using various imaging modalities have also been observed between males and females, but these have been based on relatively small and underpowered studies, none of which studied CCTA.[114–116] Fortunately, over 50% of patients enrolled in the PROMISE trial were female,[9] while 44% of patients in the SCOT-HEART trial were female,[8] so the contemporary clinical trial data very much apply to both sexes, and we can anticipate several important secondary analyses to help refine the optimal testing strategy for each sex.

Race

The relative performances of diagnostic testing in racial minorities are not well understood, but disparities in care delivery likely exist. A study of Medicare beneficiaries found that, compared to patients who did not receive testing, patients receiving noninvasive testing were younger, less likely to be female or black, but more likely to live in high-income, highly educated, and urban areas.[117] A recent analysis found no evidence of a lower likelihood of black patients receiving a cardiac stress test, but there was some evidence of disparity between Hispanic patients and other groups.[2]

Age

Advancing age and associated comorbidities have the potential to impact both functional and anatomic test performance characteristics. Older patients may experience several challenges with exercise treadmill testing, including decreased exercise tolerance, higher incidence of comorbidities, and mobility issues. A recent meta-analysis of 17 studies in 13,304 patients aged 65 years or older undergoing either MPI, stress echocardiography, or exercise treadmill testing found effective risk stratification by the two imaging techniques but not by exercise treadmill testing alone.[118] A separate study found that dobutamine stress echocardiography was predictive of cardiac events among all age groups and of death in patients 60 years of age or above.[119] However, among patients below 60 years of age, stress-induced echocardiographic abnormalities were not independently associated with mortality. Furthermore, while increasing age is also associated with a higher burden of coronary artery calcium (CAC),[66] compared to younger patients, the ability of CAC to provide long-term risk stratification may be lower, due principally to an increased all-cause mortality rate in patients with lower CAC scores in the older age group.[97] However, a CAC score of 0 confers a 15-year warranty period against mortality in individuals at low to intermediate risk that is unaffected by age.[120] Additionally, age may impact the presentation of potential ischemic symptoms with various comorbidities including congestive heart failure, contributing to symptoms.

EMERGING CONCEPTS: BEYOND THE SILOED CHOICE OF A FUNCTIONAL OR ANATOMIC STRATEGY

Presence of Ischemia with no Significant Stenosis and No Ischemia in the Presence of Significant Stenosis

Mounting evidence demonstrates that the association between coronary stenosis and ischemia is variable, as patients can have no ischemia in the presence of significant stenosis (NIPSS) and presence of ischemia with no severe stenosis (PINNS).[21] The nuclear substudy of the COURAGE trial found that 40% of patients who had stenotic lesions with over 70% stenosis had either no myocardial ischemia or only a mild degree of myocardial ischemia.[121] Even among severe lesions with 71% to 90% stenosis by visual assessment in the FAME (Fractional Flow Reserve Versus Angiography in Multivessel Evaluation) trial, 20% were found not to be functionally significant, with a fractional flow reserve (FFR) greater than 0.8.[98] In contrast, 35% of lesions with 50% to 70% stenosis in the FAME trial demonstrated an FFR of less than 0.8.[98] Other studies have found that plaque features found on CCTA (i.e., positive remodeling or low attenuation plaque) better predicted ischemia compared to severity of stenosis by visual assessment alone.[99,122,123] This has led to the addition of the concepts of NIPSS and PINSS, which extends from the conventional formulations of significant stenosis plus ischemia and no stenosis without ischemia. In part, these seeming incongruities may be explained by non-obstructive atherosclerosis leading to endothelial dysfunction through local inflammation and oxidative stress, resulting in a decrease in bioavailability of nitric oxide and inhibition of vasodilatation.[21] Regardless of mechanism, the recognition of a not-infrequent disconnect between anatomic and functional significance is an important consideration in test selection and interpretation of noninvasive imaging data.

Noninvasive Imaging Integrating Functional and Anatomic Strategies

As a result of these merging concepts, imaging modalities that combine both anatomic and functional strategies are highly appealing. Fractional flow reserve computed tomography (FFR CT) is a noninvasive means of estimating coronary ischemia using principles of fluid dynamics to create three-dimensional mathematic modeling of coronary flow, pressure, and resistance under varying hemodynamic conditions. It is intended to provide similar information to invasive FFR performed via traditional coronary angiography, which is considered the gold standard to measure severity of ischemia. Analysis is performed centrally following secure data upload from the site to HeartFlow as previously described.[124–126] Briefly, simulation of three-dimensional coronary blood flow (under conditions modeling intravenous adenosine) is performed using proprietary software, with quantitative image quality analysis, image segmentation, and physiologic modeling using computational fluid dynamics. Data are then provided to the clinical site consisting of the lowest FFR CT numeric value in each coronary distribution, and color-scale representations of the coronary tree showing FFR CT values in all vessels greater than 1.8 mm in diameter. A concise review by Min et al. includes a detailed description of the applied computational fluid dynamics used to calculate "three-vessel" FFR from conventionally acquired coronary CCTA images with no need for additional imaging or vasodilators (Fig. 15.5).[127] Use of FFR to guide revascularization in randomized trials (vs. anatomic guided revascularization only) has resulted in improved event-free survival[128,129] and reduced costs.[130] Diagnostic performance of the addition of FFR CT to anatomic CCTA has been validated in three prospective multicenter studies assessing FFR CT performance against the reference standard of invasive FFR for the identification of lesion-specific ischemia.[122,124,131]

To determine the "real world" impact of integrating FFR CT into practice, the Prospective Longitudinal Trial of FFR CT: Outcome and Resource Impacts (PLATFORM) trial was performed. In this study of 584 patients, the rate of coronary angiography showing no stenosis greater than or equal to 50% in a vessel larger than 2 mm by quantitative coronary angiography at 90 days was 12% in the FFR CT guided arm, versus 73% with usual care ($p < 0.0001$), among those patients who had this test performed before a planned invasive catheterization.[132] Indeed, 61% of patients had their scheduled invasive coronary angiography canceled as a result in the FFR CT guided arm. Secondary endpoints of major adverse cardiac events occurred in only two patients, and mean cumulative radiation exposure was similar in the FFR CT guided planned invasive arm (9.9 + 8.7 mSv) versus usual care arm (9.4 + 4.9 mSv; $p = 0.20$). In a prespecified substudy, FFR CT was associated with less resource use and lower costs within 90 days

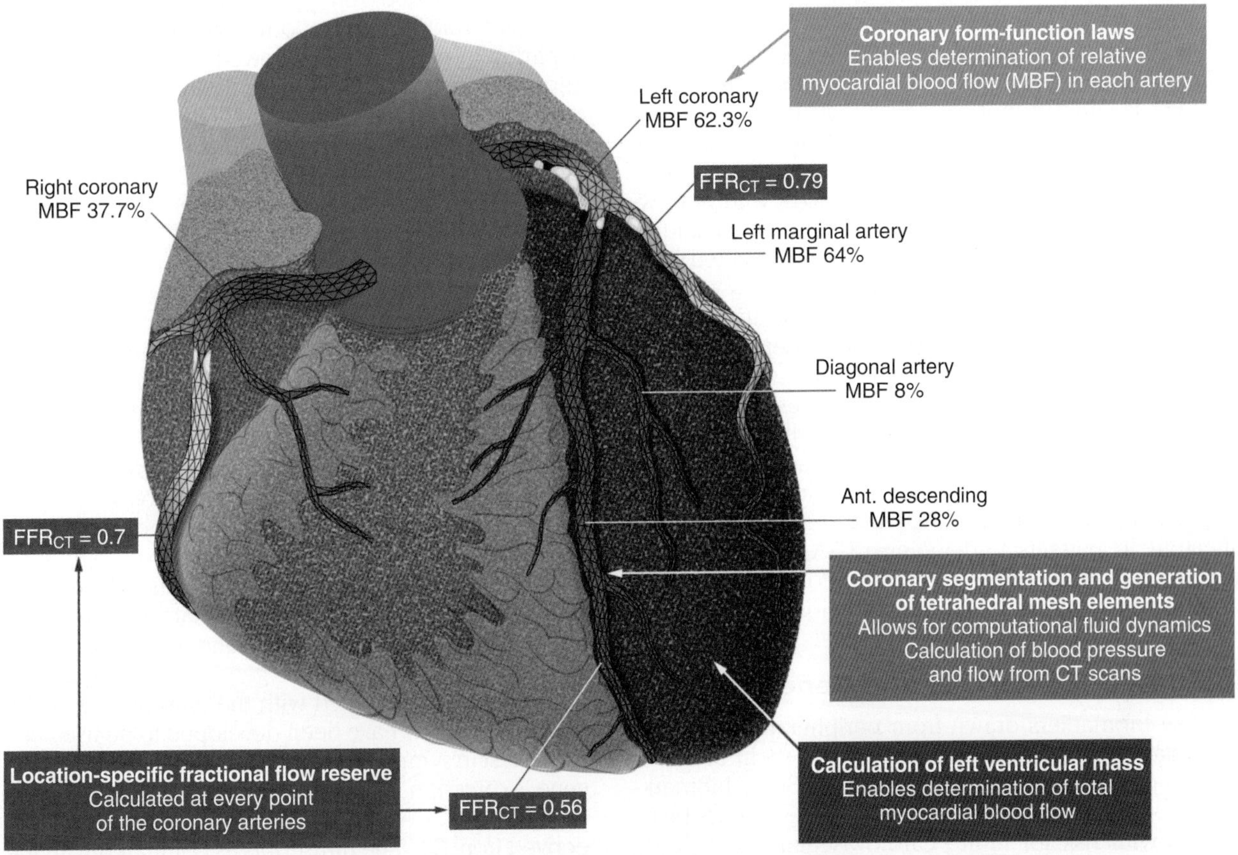

FIG. 15.5 Important components for calculation of fractional flow reserve from fractional flow reserve computed tomography (FFR CT). This figure demonstrates several of the important components of FFR CT. Patient-specific geometry from computed tomography allows for accurate segmentation of coronary artery geometry. Each of these coronary artery segments undergoes mesh segmentation, and the governing equations of fluid dynamics are solved for each of these meshes to calculate FFR CT within the entire vascular bed. Coupling arterial form with myocardial mass enables calculation of relative myocardial blood flow. *MBF*, Myocardial blood flow. *(Reproduced with permission from Min JK, Taylor CA, Achenbach S, et al. Noninvasive fractional flow reserve derived from coronary CT angiography: clinical data and scientific principles.* JACC Cardiovasc Imaging. *2015;8:1209–1222.)*

than evaluation with invasive coronary angiography, as well as being associated with greater improvement in quality of life than evaluation with usual noninvasive testing.[133]

Imaging Strategies to Improve the Yield of Obstructive CAD on Subsequent Coronary Angiography

Importantly, PLATFORM builds on SCOT-HEART's finding of increased diagnostic certainty with CCTA by finding that FFR CT resulted in the cancelation of planned invasive coronary angiography in 61% of patients, without adverse consequences, and resulted in a dramatically higher rate of finding obstructive CAD on coronary angiography. To put this in perspective, the yield of obstructive CAD (≥50% stenosis) at elective cardiac catheterization was higher in the FFR CT arm of PLATFORM (76%), compared to the CCTA arm in PROMISE (72%) or the usual care arms in PLATFORM (43%) or PROMISE (48%), as well as prior large observational analyses from US registries (38–52%) (Fig. 15.6).[9,15,32,132,134] This suggests that FFR CT may be a meaningful diagnostic strategy to guide care, improve efficiency, and reduce costs in those with planned invasive catheterization, with substantial practical and clinical implications. Ongoing trials comparing the diagnostic performance of FFR CT versus stress imaging methods will further inform its most appropriate use in clinical practice.[127]

While FFR CT appears to be the most promising modality combining functional and anatomic imaging, other strategies are being developed. Other modifications of CT technology including CT perfusion are of particular interest. Although prospective evidence supporting this modality is limited to date, it may also be a promising future strategy to combine anatomic and functional imaging in patients with stable chest pain.[135] Hybrid SPECT/CCTA imaging results in improved specificity and positive predictive value to detect hemodynamically significant coronary lesions in patients with chest pain.[136] However, there is some concern that radiation doses may be prohibitive. Other hybrid imaging modalities remain an area of increasing interest and research.[137] Finally, while data for CMR perfusion detection of ischemia are excellent (see earlier), data are not sufficient to support clinical CMR for the routine anatomic identification of CAD.[138] However, there may be a role for CMR in the assessment of congenital coronary anomalies and coronary artery aneurysms.

FUTURE HORIZONS FOR NONINVASIVE IMAGING AND CAD

Plaque Morphology and Burden

As discussed in the previous section, an emerging concept is the notion that the relationship between stenosis and ischemia, and potentially that of symptom burden, is variable (PINNS and NIPPS).[21] In a recent secondary analysis from the Determination of Fractional Flow Reserve by Anatomic

Computed Tomographic Angiography (DEFACTO) study, both plaque volume and plaque characteristics (positive remodeling, low attenuation plaque, and spotty calcification) by CCTA improved identification of coronary lesions that cause ischemia.[99] Positive remodeling was associated with all ischemia-causing lesions regardless of degree of stenosis, whereas plaque volume and low attenuation plaque were only associated with ischemia-causing lesions with narrowing of greater than or equal to 50%. This follows other studies that found that plaque characteristics better predicted ischemia compared to severity of stenosis by visual assessment alone.[122,123] Although untested, these lesion-specific features could putatively help to guide therapy. Such recent studies are additive to our understanding of the prognostic value of both the distribution and degree of plaque as assessed via CCTA (i.e., number of diseased vessels, including whether obstructive or nonobstructive), which is now well established.[139–141] Quantitative analysis of plaque burden predicts future events among patients with stable CAD and may improve risk stratification in patients undergoing CCTA.[142] Other novel approaches gain incremental prognostic information through the combined use of plaque burden and biomarkers.[143]

Blood-Based Biomarkers and Gene Scores

Only a few biomarkers drawn from peripheral blood have been validated for diagnosing obstructive CAD in the nonacute setting in patients without known CAD. Some biomarkers, such as high sensitivity C-reactive protein, have been associated with risk for future cardiovascular events.[144,145] Similarly, troponin T and I levels carry incremental prognostic value in both patients with stable CAD and apparently healthy subjects in the general population.[146–148] While biomarkers currently have no established role in the assessment of symptoms that suggest CAD in stable patients, several potential strategies are in development and could aid clinicians with test selection, e.g., high-sensitivity troponin (hs-troponin). A Rule Out Myocardial Infarction/Ischemia using Computer Assisted Tomography II (ROMICAT II) trial subanalysis found that hs-troponin I at the time of emergency department presentation, followed by early advanced CCTA, improved risk stratification and diagnostic accuracy for acute coronary syndromes compared to conventional troponin and traditional CCTA assessment. In contrast, the Better Evaluation of Acute Chest Pain with Computed Tomography Angiography (BEACON) trial assessed whether a diagnostic strategy supplemented by early CCTA improved clinical effectiveness compared with contemporary standard of care that included high-sensitivity troponin in patients presenting to the emergency department with chest pain.[149] CCTA did not identify more patients with significant CAD requiring coronary revascularization, shorten hospital stay, or allow for more direct discharge from the emergency department. Furthermore, in a more stable population of CAD, an analysis from the Bypass Angioplasty Revascularization Investigation in Type 2 Diabetes (BARI 2D) trial, hs-troponin T predicted adverse cardiovascular events, but did not seem to identify a subgroup of patients who benefited from random assignment to prompt coronary revascularization.[150] Although not specifically evaluated, this suggests that this biomarker would not be additive to information found in noninvasive testing.

While a number of genetic, genomic, and metabolic markers have been associated with the presence of CAD and/or future events, few have been developed to be used as a diagnostic test in symptomatic patients.[151] However, the CardioDx gene expression score modestly improved the prediction of obstructive CAD using a sex- and age-specific algorithm derived from 23 gene transcripts as compared with the traditional Diamond and Forrester method among patients receiving coronary angiography,[152] and was subsequently found to outperform clinical factors and nuclear stress imaging in symptomatic patients referred for noninvasive imaging.[110] It is also associated with plaque burden and stenosis by CCTA.[153] Future outcomes studies will be required to determine if this score incremental predicts adverse outcomes as well as obstructive CAD in a symptomatic population.

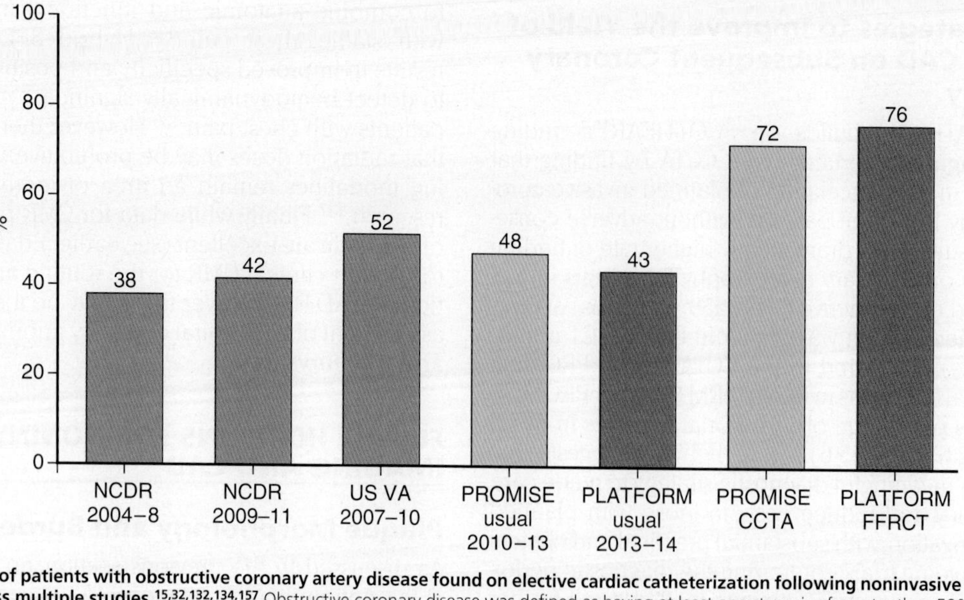

FIG. 15.6 Proportion of patients with obstructive coronary artery disease found on elective cardiac catheterization following noninvasive testing for suspected cardiac chest pain across multiple studies.[15,32,132,134,157] Obstructive coronary disease was defined as having at least one stenosis of greater than 50% of an epicardial coronary artery measuring at least 2 mm in diameter. Dates represent the timeframe during which patient data were accrued. *CCTA*, Coronary computed tomographic angiography; *FFRCT*, fractional flow reserve computed tomography; *NCDR*, National Cardiovascular Data Registry; *PLATFORM*, Prospective Longitudinal Trial of FFR CT: Outcome and Resource Impacts; *PROMISE*, Prospective Multicenter Imaging Study for Evaluation of Chest Pain trial; *US VA*, United States Veterans Affairs. *(Modified with permission from Fordyce CB, Newby DE, Douglas PS. Diagnostic strategies for the evaluation of chest pain: clinical implications from SCOT-HEART and PROMISE.* J Am Coll Cardiol. *2016;67(7):843–852.)*

Future Trials Involving Noninvasive Imaging and Clinical Outcomes as Endpoints

The International Study of Comparative Health Effectiveness with Medical and Invasive Approaches (ISCHEMIA) trial (NCT01471522) will determine whether an initial invasive strategy of cardiac catheterization and revascularization (with PCI or CABG) plus optimal medical therapy (OMT) will reduce the primary composite endpoint of cardiovascular death or nonfatal MI in stable ischemic heart disease (SIHD) patients with moderate or severe ischemia compared with an initial conservative strategy of OMT alone, and cardiac catheterization if OMT fails. The trial design is shown in Fig. 15.7. The trial involves over 30 countries and 300 sites, with an expected enrollment of 8000 patients and a 3-year follow-up. Patients will have either absent or medically controlled symptoms. Blinded CCTA will be performed before randomization in participants with normal renal function to exclude those with significant left main disease or no obstructive CAD. With enrollment expected to finish in 2017, ISCHEMIA is expected to address the following limitations of prior studies:[22]

- enrolling patients before catheterization, so that anatomically high-risk patients are not excluded
- enrolling a higher-risk group with at least moderate ischemia
- minimizing crossovers
- using contemporary drug eluting stents and physiologically guided decision-making (FFR) to achieve complete ischemic (rather than anatomic) revascularization
- being adequately powered to demonstrate whether routine revascularization reduces cardiovascular death or nonfatal MI in patients with SIHD and at least moderate ischemia

While ISCHEMIA uses noninvasive test information to select a population of patients with high-risk functional imaging features but whose symptoms are otherwise well controlled (or asymptomatic), other smaller trials enrolling patients with stable chest pain are currently underway. They mainly compare the effectiveness of various imaging strategies, but with the key common goal (like PROMISE and SCOT-HEART) of evaluating clinical outcomes and not only test performance (Table 15.9).

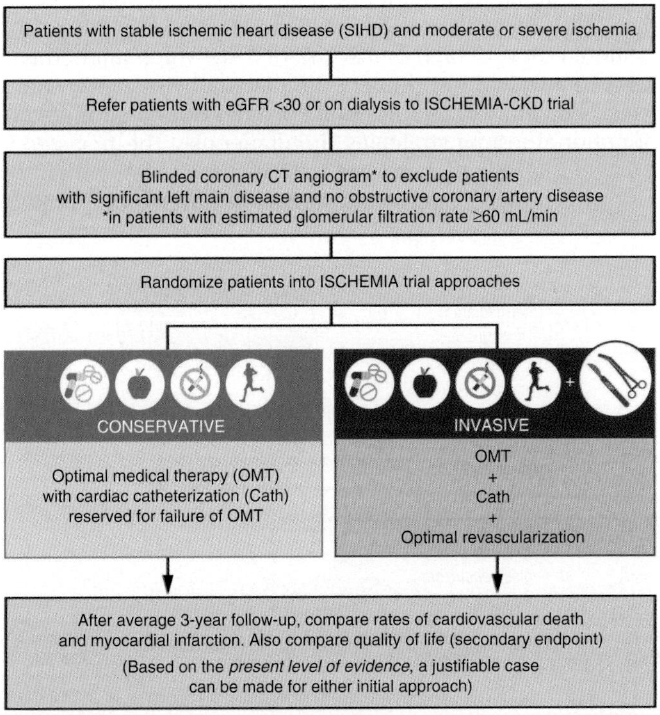

FIG. 15.7 ISCHEMIA trial design. Patients are excluded with an estimated glomerular filtration rate less than 60 mL/min or if the coronary computer tomographic angiography shows significant left main disease (≥ 50% stenosis) or no obstructive disease. *Cath,* Catheterization; *CCTA,* coronary computed tomographic angiography; *CKD,* chronic kidney disease; *eGFR,* estimated glomerular filtration rate; *OMT,* optimal medical therapy; *SIHD,* stable ischemic heart disease. *(Modified with permission from Stone GW, Hochman JS, Williams DO, et al. Medical therapy with versus without revascularization in stable patients with moderate and severe ischemia: the case for community equipoise.* J Am Coll Cardiol. *2016;67:81–99.)*

TABLE 15.9 Ongoing Selected Prospective Noninvasive Imaging Outcomes Studies for the Evaluation of Stable Chest Pain Patients

TRIAL	*N*	COUNTRY	STUDY POPULATION	RANDOMIZATION ARMS	PRIMARY OUTCOME ENDPOINT(S)	STUDY COMPLETION*
Gurunathan et al. (NCT02346565)	450	United Kingdom	Female; ≥ 30 years; no known CAD	Exercise stress testing vs. stress echo	CV death or nonfatal MI (at 2 years)	June 2018
CRESCENT2 (NCT02291484)	250	Netherlands	≥18 years; >10% pretest probability of CAD	Comprehensive cardiac CT (CAC, CCTA, CT perfusion) vs. standard care	Rate of negative invasive angiograms (at 6 months)	December 2015
DISCHARGE (NCT02400229)	3546	Europe	≥30 years; 10–60% pretest probability of CAD referred for angiography	CCTA vs. coronary angiography	CV death, nonfatal MI, and nonfatal stroke (at 1 year)	September 2019
MR-INFORM[159] (NCT01236807)	918	United Kingdom	≥18 years; ≥ two cardiac risk factors or positive exercise treadmill test	MR perfusion vs. coronary angiography with FFR	All-cause death, MI and repeat revascularization (at 1 year)	June 2016

CAC, Coronary artery calcium; *CAD,* coronary artery disease; *CCTA,* coronary computed tomographic angiography; *CT,* computed tomography; *CV,* cardiovascular; *FFR,* fractional flow reserve; *MI,* myocardial infraction; *MR,* magnetic resonance.

*http://ClinicalTrials.gov. Included only open trials evaluating patients with stable chest pain with a clinical outcome as the primary endpoint. Excluded trials with unknown status or ACS, including those studies requiring a positive cardiac biomarker for study inclusion, and those including admitted patients or those in the emergency department. Search terms were chest pain AND stress test, imaging, CT, nuclear, echo, or cardiac magnetic resonance imaging. CRESCENT2, Comprehensive Cardiac CT Versus Exercise Testing in Suspected Coronary Artery Disease (2); DISCHARGE, Diagnostic Imaging Strategies for Patients with Stable Chest Pain and Intermediate Risk of Coronary Artery Disease; MR-INFORM, MR Perfusion Imaging to Guide Management of Patients with Stable Coronary Artery Disease

A PROPOSED APPROACH FOR SELECTING THE OPTIMAL NONINVASIVE TEST FOR CAD DIAGNOSIS

The approach to selection of noninvasive testing for the diagnosis of suspected CAD in patients with stable chest pain must take into account the goals of testing in tandem with patient and test characteristics, cost, as well as local availability, and expertise. For example, access to CMR is greater in some parts of Europe[154] compared to the rest the world, including the United States. However, as data from pragmatic clinical trials emerge, other salient features should also be considered. These include imaging of other possible abnormalities or causes for chest pain that could be captured with a given imaging modality, as well as radiation exposure. The PROMISE and SCOT-HEART trials demonstrate that an initial anatomic strategy with CCTA could be considered a reasonable alternative to functional testing. While FFR CT remains promising, additional randomized trials are warranted to properly position this new technology into practice.[127] This proposed contemporary approach, integrating the latest clinical trial data, is outlined in Fig. 15.8.

After deciding whether the patient is a potential revascularization candidate, the next step is to assess whether the patient is at very high or low risk of CAD, which might direct care to a watchful waiting or direct to catheterization strategies. The clinician should then consider both anatomic and functional testing strategies simultaneously. The first step is to exclude tests that are not suitable for a given patient by asking a series of simple questions relevant to each strategy.

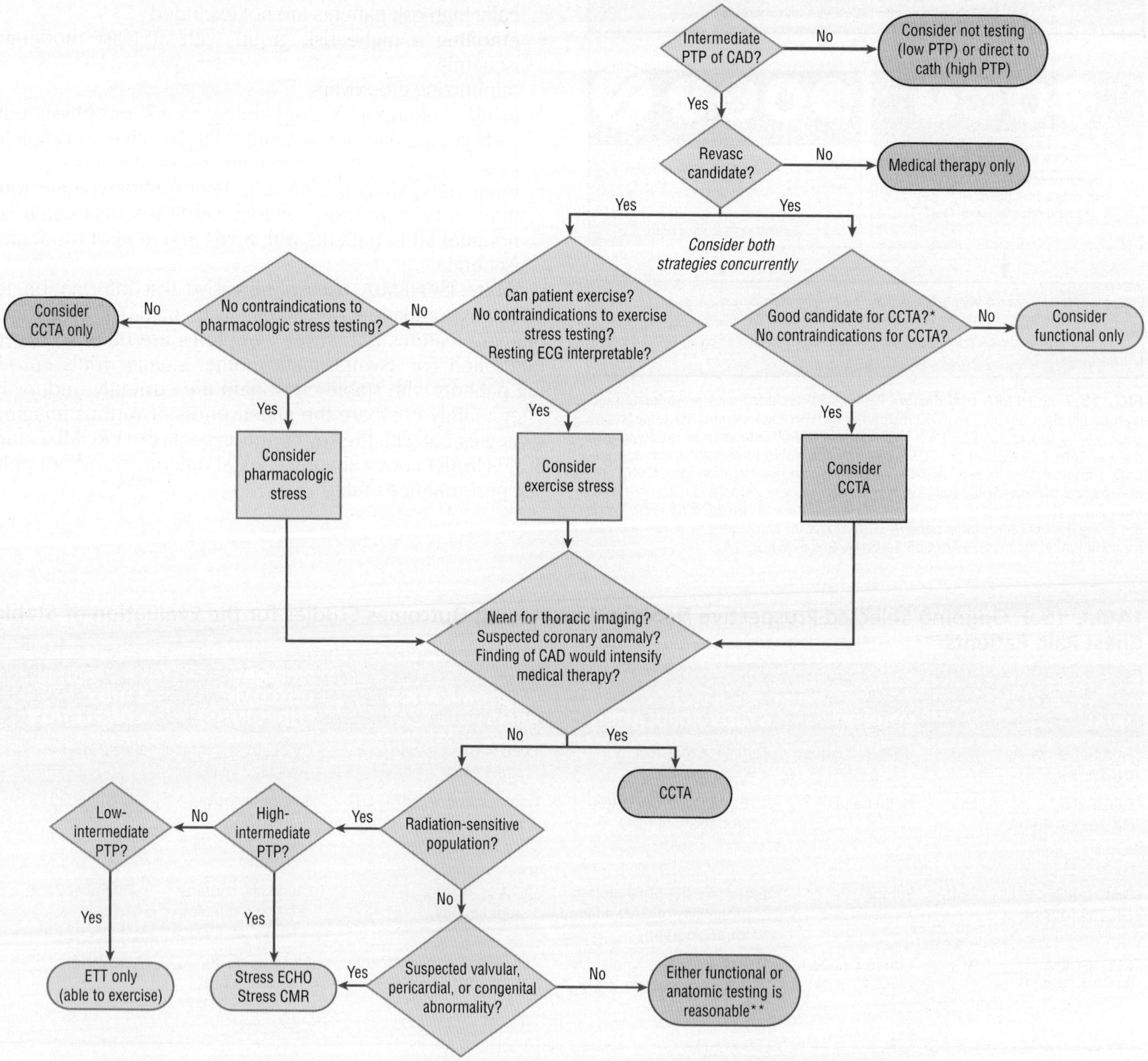

FIG. 15.8 Proposed integrated approach to initial noninvasive test selection using both functional and anatomic approaches for the diagnosis of ischemic heart disease in stable chest pain patients. *See text. **Consider exercise treadmill test or coronary computed tomographic angiography for low-intermediate pretest probability; consider stress echocardiography, myocardial perfusion imaging, or cardiac magnetic resonance for high-intermediate pretest probability. *CAD,* Coronary artery disease; *CCTA,* coronary computed tomographic angiography; *CMR,* cardiac magnetic resonance; *ECHO,* echocardiograph; *ECG,* electrocardiogram; *ETT,* exercise treadmill test; *PTP,* pretest probability. *(Modified with permission from Fordyce CB, Douglas PS. Optimal non-invasive imaging test selection for the diagnosis of ischaemic heart disease.* Heart. *2016;102(7):555–564.)*

The second step is to ask whether additional considerations exist that would warrant use of a given test over another. Such important imaging-specific considerations include:

- Consider CCTA
  - if needed for additional thoracic CT imaging, e.g., a triple or double rule out in suspected pulmonary embolism (D-dimer positive) and aortic dissection or if an intra-thoracic pathology is suspected, such as pericardial disease[71]
  - if there is a suspected coronary anomaly[155]
  - if diagnosis of nonobstructive or obstructive CAD alone would result in a change in medical therapy[12–14]
- Consider stress echocardiography or CMR
  - if evaluation of radiation-sensitive population is required, e.g., female and younger age or previous radiation exposure history[71]
  - if suspected valvular, pericardial, or congenital abnormality is concomitantly suspected
- Consider ETT
  - if evaluation of radiation-sensitive population is required, e.g., female and younger age or previous radiation exposure history[71]
  - to mitigate cost

Other considerations include preference for ETT and CCTA in patients with low-intermediate pretest probability versus preference for use of other imaging modalities for high-intermediate pretest probability. If the patient is somehow not eligible for any form of invasive testing, the diagnosis of CAD could then be obtained through invasive coronary angiography.

SUMMARY

The prevalence of angina is high in the general population and increases with age. Little consensus exists about which initial test is preferable when one is required for diagnosis; there are significant differences between the current US and European guidelines. However, the recent PROMISE and SCOT-HEART trials incorporating the use of CCTA have demonstrated that an anatomic strategy is a reasonable alternative initial approach in intermediate-risk patients with stable chest pain for the diagnosis of IHD. Other features must also be considered when employing noninvasive testing, including radiation, impact of testing on subsequent medical therapy, and cost-effectiveness. FFR CT and hybrid imaging represent promising new techniques with the potential to revolutionize noninvasive cardiac testing. Further understanding of the true relationships between coronary ischemia and stenosis, the ability to better characterize and utilize the diagnostic power of potentially important coronary plaque features, and novel biomarkers may help to refine the diagnostic yield of noninvasive imaging. Taken together, contemporary approaches should consider both functional and anatomic strategies, while taking into account important patient factors, in an integrated decision-making model.

References

1. Mozaffarian D, Benjamin EJ, Go AS, et al.: Heart disease and stroke statistics—2015 update: a report from the American Heart Association, *Circulation* 131:e29–e322, 2015.
2. Ladapo JA, Blecker S, Douglas PS: Physician decision making and trends in the use of cardiac stress testing in the United States: an analysis of repeated cross-sectional data, *Ann Intern Med* 161:482–490, 2014.
3. Daly CA, Clemens F, Sendon JLL, et al.: The clinical characteristics and investigations planned in patients with stable angina presenting to cardiologists in Europe: from the Euro Heart Survey of Stable Angina, *Eur Heart J* 26:996–1010, 2005.
4. Shaw LJ, Min JK, Hachamovitch R, et al.: Cardiovascular imaging research at the crossroads, *JACC Cardiovasc Imaging* 3:316–324, 2010.
5. *Chest pain of recent onset: assessment and diagnosis of recent onset chest pain or discomfort of suspected cardiac origin*. NICE Guidelines [CG95]. http://www.nice.org.uk/guidance/CG95.
6. Fihn SD, Gardin JM, Abrams J, et al.: 2012 ACCF/AHA/ACP/AATS/PCNA/SCAI/STS guideline for the diagnosis and management of patients with stable ischemic heart disease: a report of the American College of Cardiology Foundation/American Heart Association Task Force on Practice Guidelines, and the American College of Physicians, American Association for Thoracic Surgery, Preventive Cardiovascular Nurses Association, Society for Cardiovascular Angiography and Interventions, and Society of Thoracic Surgeons, *J Am Coll Cardiol* 60:e44–e164, 2012.
7. Montalescot G, Sechtem U, Achenbach S, et al.: 2013 ESC guidelines on the management of stable coronary artery disease, *Eur Heart J* 34:2949–3003, 2013.
8. CT coronary angiography in patients with suspected angina due to coronary heart disease (SCOT-HEART): an open-label, parallel-group, multicentre trial, *Lancet* 385:2383–2391, 2015.
9. Douglas PS, Hoffmann U, Patel MR, et al.: Outcomes of anatomical versus functional testing for coronary artery disease, *N Engl J Med* 372:1291–1300, 2015.
10. Wagener JF, Rao SV: A comparison of radial and femoral access for cardiac catheterization, *Trends Cardiovasc Med* 25:707–713, 2015.
11. Eisenberg MJ, Afilalo J, Lawler PR, et al.: Cancer risk related to low-dose ionizing radiation from cardiac imaging in patients after acute myocardial infarction, *CMAJ* 183:430–436, 2011.
12. Cheezum MK, Hulten EA, Smith RM, et al.: Changes in preventive medical therapies and CV risk factors after CT angiography, *JACC Cardiovasc Imaging* 6:574–581, 2013.
13. Hulten E, Bittencourt MS, Singh A, et al.: Coronary artery disease detected by coronary computed tomographic angiography is associated with intensification of preventive medical therapy and lower low-density lipoprotein cholesterol, *Circ Cardiovasc Imaging* 7:629–638, 2014.
14. Pursnani A, Schlett CL, Mayrhofer T, et al.: Potential for coronary CT angiography to tailor medical therapy beyond preventive guideline-based recommendations: insights from the ROMICAT I trial, *J Cardiovasc Comput Tomogr* 9:193–201, 2015.
15. Patel MR, Peterson ED, Dai D, et al.: Low diagnostic yield of elective coronary angiography, *N Engl J Med* 362:886–895, 2010.
16. Douglas PS, Patel MR, Bailey SR, et al.: Hospital variability in the rate of finding obstructive coronary artery disease at elective, diagnostic coronary angiography, *J Am Coll Cardiol* 58:801–809, 2011.
17. Hachamovitch R, Berman DS, Kiat H, et al.: Exercise myocardial perfusion SPECT in patients without known coronary artery disease incremental prognostic value and use in risk stratification, *Circulation* 93:905–914, 1996.
18. Bangalore S, Gopinath D, Yao S-S, Chaudhry FA: Risk stratification using stress echocardiography: incremental prognostic value over historic, clinical, and stress electrocardiographic variables across a wide spectrum of bayesian pretest probabilities for coronary artery disease, *J Am Soc Echocardiogr* 20:244–252, 2007.
19. Mudrick DW, Cowper PA, Shah BR, et al.: Downstream procedures and outcomes after stress testing for chest pain without known coronary artery disease in the United States, *Am Heart J* 163:454–461, 2012.
20. Rozanski A, Gransar H, Hayes SW, et al.: Temporal trends in the frequency of inducible myocardial ischemia during cardiac stress testing: 1991 to 2009, *J Am Coll Cardiol* 61:1054–1065, 2013.
21. Ahmadi A, Kini A, Narula J: Discordance between ischemia and stenosis, or PINSS and NIPSS: are we ready for new vocabulary? *JACC Cardiovasc Imaging* 8:111–114, 2015.
22. Stone GW, Hochman JS, Williams DO, et al.: Medical therapy with versus without revascularization in stable patients with moderate and severe ischemia: the case for community equipoise, *J Am Coll Cardiol* 67:81–99, 2016.
23. Hamm CW, Bassand JP, Agewall S, et al.: ESC guidelines for the management of acute coronary syndromes in patients presenting without persistent ST-segment elevation: the Task Force for the management of acute coronary syndromes (ACS) in patients presenting without persistent ST-segment elevation of the European Society of Cardiology (ESC), *Eur Heart J* 32:2999–3054, 2011.
24. Diamond GA: A clinically relevant classification of chest discomfort, *J Am Coll Cardiol* 1:574–575, 1983.
25. D'Agostino Sr RB, Vasan RS, Pencina MJ, et al.: General cardiovascular risk profile for use in primary care: the Framingham Heart Study, *Circulation* 117:743–753, 2008.
26. Goff Jr DC, Lloyd-Jones DM, Bennett G, et al.: 2013 ACC/AHA guideline on the assessment of cardiovascular risk: a report of the American College of Cardiology/American Heart Association Task Force on Practice Guidelines, *Circulation* 129(25 Suppl 2):S49–S73, 2014.
27. Hadamitzky M, Achenbach S, Al-Mallah M, et al.: Optimized prognostic score for coronary computed tomographic angiography: results from the CONFIRM registry (COronary CT Angiography EvaluatioN For Clinical Outcomes: an InteRnational Multicenter Registry), *J Am Coll Cardiol* 62:468–476, 2013.
28. Pryor DB, Shaw L, McCants CB, et al.: Value of the history and physical in identifying patients at increased risk for coronary artery disease, *Ann Intern Med* 118:81–90, 1993.
29. Genders TS, Steyerberg EW, Alkadhi H, et al.: A clinical prediction rule for the diagnosis of coronary artery disease: validation, updating, and extension, *Eur Heart J* 32:1316–1330, 2011.
30. Cheng VY, Berman DS, Rozanski A, et al.: Performance of the traditional age, sex, and angina typicality-based approach for estimating pretest probability of angiographically significant coronary artery disease in patients undergoing coronary computed tomographic angiography: results from the multinational coronary CT angiography evaluation for clinical outcomes: an international multicenter registry (CONFIRM), *Circulation* 124:2423–2432, 2011. 1–8.
31. Ko DT, Tu JV, Austin PC, et al.: Prevalence and extent of obstructive coronary artery disease among patients undergoing elective coronary catheterization in New York State and Ontario, *JAMA* 310:163–169, 2013.
32. Bradley SM, Maddox TM, Stanislawski MA, et al.: Normal coronary rates for elective angiography in the Veterans Affairs Healthcare System: insights from the VA CART program (Veterans Affairs clinical assessment reporting and tracking), *J Am Coll Cardiol* 63:417–426, 2014.
33. Christman MP, Bittencourt MS, Hulten E, et al.: Yield of downstream tests after exercise treadmill testing: a prospective cohort study, *J Am Coll Cardiol* 63:1264–1274, 2014.
34. Rifkin RD, Hood Jr WB: Bayesian analysis of electrocardiographic exercise stress testing, *N Engl J Med* 297:681–686, 1977.
35. Diamond GA, Forrester JS, Hirsch M, et al.: Application of conditional probability analysis to the clinical diagnosis of coronary artery disease, *J Clin Invest* 65:1210–1221, 1980.
36. Goldman L, Cook EF, Mitchell N, et al.: Incremental value of the exercise test for diagnosing the presence or absence of coronary artery disease, *Circulation* 66:945–953, 1982.
37. Melin JA, Wijns W, Vanbutsele RJ, et al.: Alternative diagnostic strategies for coronary artery disease in women: demonstration of the usefulness and efficiency of probability analysis, *Circulation* 71:535–542, 1985.
38. Wolk MJ, Bailey SR, Doherty JU, et al.: ACCF/AHA/ASE/ASNC/HFSA/HRS/SCAI/SCCT/SCMR/STS 2013 multimodality appropriate use criteria for the detection and risk assessment of stable ischemic heart disease: a report of the American College of Cardiology Foundation Appropriate Use Criteria Task Force, American Heart Association, American Society of Echocardiography, American Society of Nuclear Cardiology, Heart Failure Society of America, Heart Rhythm Society, Society for Cardiovascular Angiography and Interventions, Society of Cardiovascular Computed Tomography, Society for Cardiovascular Magnetic Resonance, and Society of Thoracic Surgeons, *J Am Coll Cardiol* 63:380–406, 2014.

39. Muhlestein JB, Lappe DL, Lima JA, et al.: Effect of screening for coronary artery disease using CT angiography on mortality and cardiac events in high-risk patients with diabetes: the FACTOR-64 randomized clinical trial, *JAMA* 312:2234–2243, 2014.
40. Sedlis SP, Hartigan PM, Teo KK, et al.: Effect of PCI on long-term survival in patients with stable ischemic heart disease, *N Engl J Med* 373:1937–1946, 2015.
41. Boden WE, O'Rourke RA, Teo KK, et al.: Optimal medical therapy with or without PCI for stable coronary disease, *N Engl J Med* 356:1503–1516, 2007.
42. Shaw LJ, Peterson ED, Shaw LK, et al.: Use of a prognostic treadmill score in identifying diagnostic coronary disease subgroups, *Circulation* 98:1622–1630, 1998.
43. Fletcher GF, Balady GJ, Amsterdam EA, et al.: Exercise standards for testing and training a statement for healthcare professionals from the American Heart Association, *Circulation* 104:1694–1740, 2001.
44. Gibbons RJ, Balady GJ, Bricker JT, et al.: ACC/AHA 2002 guideline update for exercise testing: summary article: a report of the American College of Cardiology/American Heart Association Task Force on Practice Guidelines (Committee to Update the 1997 Exercise Testing Guidelines), *J Am Coll Cardiol* 40:1531–1540, 2002.
45. Shaw LJ, Berman DS, Picard MH, et al.: Comparative definitions for moderate-severe ischemia in stress nuclear, echocardiography, and magnetic resonance imaging, *JACC Cardiovasc Imaging* 7:593–604, 2014.
46. Chan SY, Brunken RC, Czernin J, et al.: Comparison of maximal myocardial blood flow during adenosine infusion with that of intravenous dipyridamole in normal men, *J Am Coll Cardiol* 20:979–985, 1992.
47. Trochu JN, Zhao G, Post H, et al.: Selective A2A adenosine receptor agonist as a coronary vasodilator in conscious dogs: potential for use in myocardial perfusion imaging, *J Cardiovasc Pharmacol* 41:132–139, 2003.
48. Wilson RF, Wyche K, Christensen BV, Zimmer S, Laxson DD: Effects of adenosine on human coronary arterial circulation, *Circulation* 82:1595–1606, 1990.
49. Sunderland JJ, Pan XB, Declerck J, Menda Y: Dependency of cardiac rubidium-82 imaging quantitative measures on age, gender, vascular territory, and software in a cardiovascular normal population, *J Nucl Cardiol* 22:72–84, 2015.
50. Geleijnse ML, Elhendy A, Fioretti PM, Roelandt JR: Dobutamine stress myocardial perfusion imaging, *J Am Coll Cardiol* 36:2017–2027, 2000.
51. Garber AM, Solomon NA: Cost-effectiveness of alternative test strategies for the diagnosis of coronary artery disease, *Ann Intern Med* 130:719–728, 1999.
52. Greenwood JP, Maredia N, Younger JF, et al.: Cardiovascular magnetic resonance and single-photon emission computed tomography for diagnosis of coronary heart disease (CE-MARC): a prospective trial, *Lancet* 379:453–460, 2012.
53. Ripley DP, Brown JM, Everett CC, et al.: Rationale and design of the Clinical Evaluation of Magnetic Resonance Imaging in Coronary heart disease 2 trial (CE-MARC 2): a prospective, multicenter, randomized trial of diagnostic strategies in suspected coronary heart disease, *Am Heart J* 169:17–24.e1, 2015.
54. Gibbons RJ, Abrams J, Chatterjee K, et al.: ACC/AHA 2002 guideline update for the management of patients with chronic stable angina—summary article: a report of the American College of Cardiology/American Heart Association Task Force on Practice Guidelines (Committee on the Management of Patients with Chronic Stable Angina), *J Am Coll Cardiol* 41:159–168, 2003.
55. Diamond GA, Kaul S: Gone fishing!: on the "real-world" accuracy of computed tomographic coronary angiography: comment on the "Ontario multidetector computed tomographic coronary angiography study, *Arch Intern Med* 171:1029–1031, 2011.
56. Patel MR, Bailey SR, Bonow RO, et al.: ACCF/SCAI/AATS/AHA/ASE/ASNC/HFSA/HRS/SCCM/SCCT/SCMR/STS 2012 appropriate use criteria for diagnostic catheterization: a report of the American College of Cardiology Foundation Appropriate Use Criteria Task Force, Society for Cardiovascular Angiography and Interventions, American Association for Thoracic Surgery, American Heart Association, American Society of Echocardiography, American Society of Nuclear Cardiology, Heart Failure Society of America, Heart Rhythm Society, Society of Critical Care Medicine, Society of Cardiovascular Computed Tomography, Society for Cardiovascular Magnetic Resonance, and Society of Thoracic Surgeons, *J Am Coll Cardiol* 59:1995–2027, 2012.
57. Rao VM, Levin DC: The overuse of diagnostic imaging and the Choosing Wisely initiative, *Ann Intern Med* 157:574–576, 2012.
58. Cooper A, Calvert N, Skinner J, et al.: *Chest Pain of Recent Onset: assessment and Diagnosis of Recent Onset Chest Pain or Discomfort of Suspected Cardiac Origin*, London, 2010, National Clinical Guideline Centre for Acute and Chronic Conditions.
59. Mowatt G, Cummins E, Waugh N, et al.: Systematic review of the clinical effectiveness and cost-effectiveness of 64-slice or higher computed tomography angiography as an alternative to invasive coronary angiography in the investigation of coronary artery disease, *Health Technol Assess* 12:iii–iv, 2008. ix–143.
60. Gosling O, Loader R, Venables P, et al.: A comparison of radiation doses between state-of-the-art multislice CT coronary angiography with iterative reconstruction, multislice CT coronary angiography with standard filtered back-projection and invasive diagnostic coronary angiography, *Heart* 96:922–926, 2010.
61. Skinner JS, Smeeth L, Kendall JM, Adams PC, Timmis A: NICE guidance. Chest pain of recent onset: assessment and diagnosis of recent onset chest pain or discomfort of suspected cardiac origin, *Heart* 96:974–978, 2010.
62. Gottlieb I, Miller JM, Arbab-Zadeh A, et al.: The absence of coronary calcification does not exclude obstructive coronary artery disease or the need for revascularization in patients referred for conventional coronary angiography, *J Am Coll Cardiol* 55:627–634, 2010.
63. Mouden M, Timmer JR, Reiffers S, et al.: Coronary artery calcium scoring to exclude flow-limiting coronary artery disease in symptomatic stable patients at low or intermediate risk, *Radiology* 269:77–83, 2013.
64. Al-Mallah MH, Qureshi W, Lin FY, et al.: Does coronary CT angiography improve risk stratification over coronary calcium scoring in symptomatic patients with suspected coronary artery disease? Results from the prospective multicenter international CONFIRM registry, *Eur Heart J Cardiovasc Imaging* 15:267–274, 2014.
65. Lubbers M, Dedic A, Coenen A, et al.: Calcium imaging and selective computed tomography angiography in comparison to functional testing for suspected coronary artery disease: the multicentre, randomized CRESCENT trial, *Eur Heart J* 37:1232–1243, 2016.
66. Kronmal RA, McClelland RL, Detrano R, et al.: Risk factors for the progression of coronary artery calcification in asymptomatic subjects: results from the Multi-Ethnic Study of Atherosclerosis (MESA), *Circulation* 115:2722–2730, 2007.
67. Tota-Maharaj R, Blaha MJ, Rivera JJ, et al.: Differences in coronary plaque composition with aging measured by coronary computed tomography angiography, *Int J Cardiol* 158:240–245, 2012.
68. Clarke JL, Ladapo JL, Monane M, et al.: The Diagnosis of CAD in Women: addressing the Unmet Need—A Report from the National Expert Roundtable Meeting, *Popul Health Manag* 18:86–92, 2015.
69. Mieres JH, Shaw LJ, Arai A, et al.: Role of noninvasive testing in the clinical evaluation of women with suspected coronary artery disease: consensus statement from the Cardiac Imaging Committee, Council on Clinical Cardiology, and the Cardiovascular Imaging and Intervention Committee, Council on Cardiovascular Radiology and Intervention, American Heart Association, *Circulation* 111:682–696, 2005.
70. Dolor RJ, Patel MR, Melloni C, et al.: *AHRQ Comparative Effectiveness Reviews. Noninvasive Technologies for the Diagnosis of Coronary Artery Disease in Women*, Rockville (MD), 2012, Agency for Healthcare Research and Quality (US).
71. Raff GL, Chinnaiyan KM, Cury RC, et al.: SCCT guidelines on the use of coronary computed tomographic angiography for patients presenting with acute chest pain to the emergency department: a report of the Society of Cardiovascular Computed Tomography Guidelines Committee, *J Cardiovasc Comput Tomogr* 8:254–271, 2014.
72. Budoff MJ, Dowe D, Jollis JG, et al.: Diagnostic performance of 64-multidetector row coronary computed tomographic angiography for evaluation of coronary artery stenosis in individuals without known coronary artery disease: results from the prospective multicenter ACCURACY (Assessment by Coronary Computed Tomographic Angiography of Individuals Undergoing Invasive Coronary Angiography) trial, *J Am Coll Cardiol* 52:1724–1732, 2008.
73. Meijboom WB, Meijs MF, Schuijf JD, et al.: Diagnostic accuracy of 64-slice computed tomography coronary angiography: a prospective, multicenter, multivendor study, *J Am Coll Cardiol* 52:2135–2144, 2008.
74. Miller JM, Rochitte CE, Dewey M, et al.: Diagnostic performance of coronary angiography by 64-row CT, *N Engl J Med* 359:2324–2336, 2008.
75. Meinel FG, Bayer 2nd RR, Zwerner PL, et al.: Coronary computed tomographic angiography in clinical practice: state of the art, *Radiol Clin North Am* 53:287–296, 2015.
76. Stein PD, Yaekoub AY, Matta F, Sostman HD: 64-slice CT for diagnosis of coronary artery disease: a systematic review, *Am J Med* 121:715–725, 2008.
77. Hoffmann U, Bamberg F, Chae CU, et al.: Coronary computed tomography angiography for early triage of patients with acute chest pain: the ROMICAT (Rule Out Myocardial Infarction using Computer Assisted Tomography) trial, *J Am Coll Cardiol* 53:1642–1650, 2009.
78. Hoffmann U, Truong QA, Schoenfeld DA, et al.: Coronary CT angiography versus standard evaluation in acute chest pain, *N Engl J Med* 367:299–308, 2012.
79. Litt HI, Gatsonis C, Snyder B, et al.: CT angiography for safe discharge of patients with possible acute coronary syndromes, *N Engl J Med* 366:1393–1403, 2012.
80. Neglia D, Rovai D, Caselli C, et al.: Detection of significant coronary artery disease by noninvasive anatomical and functional imaging, *Circ Cardiovasc Imaging* 8, 2015.
81. Levsky JM, Spevack DM, Travin MI, et al.: Coronary computed tomography angiography versus radionuclide myocardial perfusion imaging in patients with chest pain admitted to telemetry: a randomized trial, *Ann Intern Med* 163:174–183, 2015.
82. McKavanagh P, Lusk L, Ball PA, et al.: A comparison of cardiac computerized tomography and exercise stress electrocardiogram test for the investigation of stable chest pain: the clinical results of the CAPP randomized prospective trial, *Eur Heart J Cardiovasc Imaging* 16:441–448, 2015.
83. Rubin GD, Leipsic J, Joseph Schoepf U, Fleischmann D, Napel S: CT angiography after 20 years: a transformation in cardiovascular disease characterization continues to advance, *Radiology* 271:633–652, 2014.
84. Cho I, Chang HJ, Sung JM, et al.: Coronary computed tomographic angiography and risk of all-cause mortality and nonfatal myocardial infarction in subjects without chest pain syndrome from the CONFIRM Registry (coronary CT angiography evaluation for clinical outcomes: an international multicenter registry), *Circulation* 126:304–313, 2012.
85. Moss AJ, Newby DE: CT coronary angiographic evaluation of suspected anginal chest pain, *Heart* 102:263–268, 2016.
86. Einstein AJ: Effects of radiation exposure from cardiac imaging: how good are the data? *J Am Coll Cardiol* 59:553–565, 2012.
87. Gerber TC, Carr JJ, Arai AE, et al.: Ionizing radiation in cardiac imaging: a science advisory from the American Heart Association Committee on Cardiac Imaging of the Council on Clinical Cardiology and Committee on Cardiovascular Imaging and Intervention of the Council on Cardiovascular Radiology and Intervention, *Circulation* 119:1056–1065, 2009.
88. Chen MY, Shanbhag SM, Arai AE: Submillisievert median radiation dose for coronary angiography with a second-generation 320-detector row CT scanner in 107 consecutive patients, *Radiology* 267:76–85, 2013.
89. Leipsic J, Heilbron BG, Hague C: Iterative reconstruction for coronary CT angiography: finding its way, *Int J Cardiovasc Imaging* 28:613–620, 2012.
90. Dorbala S, Blankstein R, Skali H, et al.: Approaches to reducing radiation dose from radionuclide myocardial perfusion imaging, *Journal Nucl Med* 56:592–599, 2015.
91. Cerqueira MD, Allman KC, Ficaro EP, et al.: Recommendations for reducing radiation exposure in myocardial perfusion imaging, *J Nucl Cardiol* 17:709–718, 2010.
92. Halliburton SS, Abbara S, Chen MY, et al.: SCCT guidelines on radiation dose and dose-optimization strategies in cardiovascular CT, *J Cardiovasc Comput Tomogr* 5:198–224, 2011.
93. Chow BJ, Small G, Yam Y, et al.: Prognostic and therapeutic implications of statin and aspirin therapy in individuals with nonobstructive coronary artery disease: results from the CONFIRM (COronary CT Angiography EvaluatioN For Clinical Outcomes: an InteRnational Multicenter registry) registry, *Arterioscler Thromb Vasc Biol* 35:981–989, 2015.
94. Young LH, Wackers FJ, Chyun DA, et al.: Cardiac outcomes after screening for asymptomatic coronary artery disease in patients with type 2 diabetes: the DIAD study: a randomized controlled trial, *JAMA* 301:1547–1555, 2009.
95. Hachamovitch R, Nutter B, Hlatky MA, et al.: Patient management after noninvasive cardiac imaging results from SPARC (Study of myocardial perfusion and coronary anatomy imaging roles in coronary artery disease), *J Am Coll Cardiol* 59:462–474, 2012.
96. Ladapo JA, Hoffmann U, Lee KL, et al.: Changes in medical therapy and lifestyle after anatomical versus functional testing for coronary artery disease: the PROMISE trial (PROspective Multicenter Imaging Study for Evaluation of Chest Pain), *Circulation* 132, 2015.A14051–A.
97. Nakanishi R, Li D, Blaha MJ, et al.: All-cause mortality by age and gender based on coronary artery calcium scores, *Eur Heart J Cardiovasc Imaging*, 2015.
98. Tonino PA, Fearon WF, De Bruyne B, et al.: Angiographic versus functional severity of coronary artery stenoses in the FAME study fractional flow reserve versus angiography in multivessel evaluation, *J Am Coll Cardiol* 55:2816–2821, 2010.
99. Park HB, Heo R, Ó Hartaigh B, et al.: Atherosclerotic plaque characteristics by CT angiography identify coronary lesions that cause ischemia: a direct comparison to fractional flow reserve, *JACC Cardiovasc Imaging* 8:1–10, 2015.
100. Douglas PS, Picard MH: Healthcare reform for imagers: finding a way forward now, *JACC Cardiovasc Imaging* 6:385–391, 2013.
101. Ladapo JA, Blecker S, Douglas PS: Appropriateness of cardiac stress test use among primary care physicians and cardiologists in the United States, *Int J Cardiol* 203:584–586, 2016.
102. Fonseca R, Negishi K, Otahal P, Marwick TH: Temporal changes in appropriateness of cardiac imaging, *J Am Coll Cardiol* 65:763–773, 2015.
103. Elgendy IY, Mahmoud A, Shuster JJ, Doukky R, Winchester DE: Outcomes after inappropriate nuclear myocardial perfusion imaging: a meta-analysis, *J Nucl Cardiol*, 2015.
104. Chaudhuri D, Montgomery A, Gulenchyn K, Mitchell M, Joseph P: Effectiveness of quality improvement interventions at reducing inappropriate cardiac imaging: a systematic review and meta-analysis, *Circ Cardiovasc Qual Outcomes*, 2016.
105. Genders TS, Petersen SE, Pugliese F, et al.: The optimal imaging strategy for patients with stable chest pain: a cost-effectiveness analysis, *Ann Intern Med* 162:474–484, 2015.
106. Mark DB: The PROspective Multicenter Imaging Study for Evaluation of Chest Pain (PROMISE) Trial: economic outcomes, *American College of Cardiology Scientific Sessions*, 2015, San Diego.

107. Priest VL, Scuffham PA, Hachamovitch R, Marwick TH: Cost-effectiveness of coronary computed tomography and cardiac stress imaging in the emergency department: a decision analytic model comparing diagnostic strategies for chest pain in patients at low risk of acute coronary syndromes, *JACC Cardiovasc Imaging* 4:549–556, 2011.
108. Shreibati JB, Baker LC, Hlatky MA: Association of coronary CT angiography or stress testing with subsequent utilization and spending among Medicare beneficiaries, *JAMA* 306:2128–2136, 2011.
109. Phelps CE, O'Sullivan AK, Ladapo JA, et al.: Cost effectiveness of a gene expression score and myocardial perfusion imaging for diagnosis of coronary artery disease, *Am Heart J* 167:697–706. e2, 2014.
110. Thomas GS, Voros S, McPherson JA, et al.: A blood-based gene expression test for obstructive coronary artery disease tested in symptomatic nondiabetic patients referred for myocardial perfusion imaging the COMPASS study, *Circ Cardiovasc Genet* 6:154–162, 2013.
111. Hemingway H, Langenberg C, Damant J, et al.: Prevalence of angina in women versus men: a systematic review and meta-analysis of international variations across 31 countries, *Circulation* 117:1526–1536, 2008.
112. Kohli P, Gulati M: Exercise stress testing in women: going back to the basics, *Circulation* 122:2570–2580, 2010.
113. Bourque JM, Beller GA: Value of exercise ECG for risk stratification in suspected or known CAD in the era of advanced imaging technologies, *JACC Cardiovasc Imaging* 8:1309–1321, 2015.
114. Dodi C, Cortigiani L, Masini M, et al.: The incremental prognostic value of pharmacological stress echo over exercise electrocardiography in women with chest pain of unknown origin, *Eur Heart J* 22:145–152, 2001.
115. Raman SV, Donnally MR, McCarthy B: Dobutamine stress cardiac magnetic resonance imaging to detect myocardial ischemia in women, *Prev Cardiol* 11:135–140, 2008.
116. Shaw LJ, Mieres JH, Hendel RH, et al.: Comparative effectiveness of exercise electrocardiography with or without myocardial perfusion single photon emission computed tomography in women with suspected coronary artery disease: results from the What Is the Optimal Method for Ischemia Evaluation in Women (WOMEN) trial, *Circulation* 124:1239–1249, 2011.
117. Lucas FL, Siewers AE, DeLorenzo MA, Wennberg DE: Differences in cardiac stress testing by sex and race among Medicare beneficiaries, *Am Heart J* 154:502–509, 2007.
118. Rai M, Baker WL, Parker MW, Heller GV: Meta-analysis of optimal risk stratification in patients >65 years of age, *Am J Cardiol* 110:1092–1099, 2012.
119. Bernheim AM, Kittipovanonth M, Takahashi PY, et al.: Does the prognostic value of dobutamine stress echocardiography differ among different age groups? *Am Heart J* 161:740–745, 2011.
120. Valenti V, Ó Hartaigh B, Heo R, et al.: A 15-year warranty period for asymptomatic individuals without coronary artery calcium: a prospective follow-up of 9,715 individuals, *JACC Cardiovasc Imaging* 8:900–909, 2015.
121. Shaw LJ, Berman DS, Maron DJ, et al.: Optimal medical therapy with or without percutaneous coronary intervention to reduce ischemic burden: results from the Clinical Outcomes Utilizing Revascularization and Aggressive Drug Evaluation (COURAGE) trial nuclear substudy, *Circulation* 117:1283–1291, 2008.
122. Nakazato R, Park HB, Berman DS, et al.: Noninvasive fractional flow reserve derived from computed tomography angiography for coronary lesions of intermediate stenosis severity: results from the DeFACTO study, *Circ Cardiovasc Imaging* 6:881–889, 2013.
123. Shmilovich H, Cheng VY, Tamarappoo BK, et al.: Vulnerable plaque features on coronary CT angiography as markers of inducible regional myocardial hypoperfusion from severe coronary artery stenoses, *Atherosclerosis* 219:588–595, 2011.
124. Min JK, Leipsic J, Pencina MJ, et al.: Diagnostic accuracy of fractional flow reserve from anatomic CT angiography, *JAMA* 308:1237–1245, 2012.
125. Koo BK, Erglis A, Doh JH, et al.: Diagnosis of ischemia-causing coronary stenoses by noninvasive fractional flow reserve computed from coronary computed tomographic angiograms. Results from the prospective multicenter DISCOVER-FLOW (Diagnosis of Ischemia-Causing Stenoses Obtained Via Noninvasive Fractional Flow Reserve) study, *J Am Coll Cardiol* 58:1989–1997, 2011.
126. Taylor CA, Fonte TA, Min JK: Computational fluid dynamics applied to cardiac computed tomography for noninvasive quantification of fractional flow reserve: scientific basis, *J Am Coll Cardiol* 61:2233–2241, 2013.
127. Min JK, Taylor CA, Achenbach S, et al.: Noninvasive fractional flow reserve derived from coronary CT angiography: clinical data and scientific principles, *JACC Cardiovasc Imaging* 8:1209–1222, 2015.
128. Pijls NH, De Bruyne B, Peels K, et al.: Measurement of fractional flow reserve to assess the functional severity of coronary-artery stenoses, *N Engl J Med* 334:1703–1708, 1996.
129. Pijls NH, Van Gelder B, Van der Voort P, et al.: Fractional flow reserve. A useful index to evaluate the influence of an epicardial coronary stenosis on myocardial blood flow, *Circulation* 92:3183–3193, 1995.
130. Fearon WF, Bornschein B, Tonino PA, et al.: Economic evaluation of fractional flow reserve-guided percutaneous coronary intervention in patients with multivessel disease, *Circulation* 122:2545–2550, 2010.
131. Norgaard BL, Leipsic J, Gaur S, et al.: Diagnostic performance of noninvasive fractional flow reserve derived from coronary computed tomography angiography in suspected coronary artery disease: the NXT trial (Analysis of Coronary Blood Flow Using CT Angiography: next Steps), *J Am Coll Cardiol* 63:1145–1155, 2014.
132. Douglas PS, Pontone G, Hlatky MA, et al.: Clinical outcomes of fractional flow reserve by computed tomographic angiography-guided diagnostic strategies vs. usual care in patients with suspected coronary artery disease: the prospective longitudinal trial of FFRct: outcome and resource impacts study, *Eur Heart J* 36:3359–3367, 2015.
133. Hlatky MA, De Bruyne B, Pontone G, et al.: Quality-of-life and economic outcomes of assessing fractional flow reserve with computed tomography angiography: PLATFORM, *J Am Coll Cardiol* 66:2315–2323, 2015.
134. Patel MR, Dai D, Hernandez AF, et al.: Prevalence and predictors of nonobstructive coronary artery disease identified with coronary angiography in contemporary clinical practice, *Am Heart J* 167:846–852.e2, 2014.
135. Techasith T, Cury RC: Stress myocardial CT perfusion: an update and future perspective, *JACC Cardiovasc Imaging* 4:905–916, 2011.
136. Rispler S, Keidar Z, Ghersin E, et al.: Integrated single-photon emission computed tomography and computed tomography coronary angiography for the assessment of hemodynamically significant coronary artery lesions, *J Am Coll Cardiol* 49:1059–1067, 2007.
137. Acampa W, Gaemperli O, Gimelli A, et al.: Role of risk stratification by SPECT, PET, and hybrid imaging in guiding management of stable patients with ischaemic heart disease: expert panel of the EANM cardiovascular committee and EACVI, *Eur Heart J Cardiovasc Imaging*, 2015.
138. Hundley WG, Bluemke DA, Finn JP, et al.: ACCF/ACR/AHA/NASCI/SCMR 2010 expert consensus document on cardiovascular magnetic resonance: a report of the American College of Cardiology Foundation Task Force on Expert Consensus Documents, *Circulation* 121:2462–2508, 2010.
139. Bamberg F, Sommer WH, Hoffmann V, et al.: Meta-analysis and systematic review of the long-term predictive value of assessment of coronary atherosclerosis by contrast-enhanced coronary computed tomography angiography, *J Am Coll Cardiol* 57:2426–2436, 2011.
140. Min JK, Dunning A, Lin FY, et al.: Age- and sex-related differences in all-cause mortality risk based on coronary computed tomography angiography findings results from the International Multicenter CONFIRM (Coronary CT Angiography Evaluation for Clinical Outcomes: an International Multicenter Registry) of 23,854 patients without known coronary artery disease, *J Am Coll Cardiol* 58:849–860, 2011.
141. Puchner SB, Liu T, Mayrhofer T, et al.: High-risk plaque detected on coronary CT angiography predicts acute coronary syndromes independent of significant stenosis in acute chest pain: results from the ROMICAT-II trial, *J Am Coll Cardiol* 64:684–692, 2014.
142. Versteylen MO, Kietselaer BL, Dagnelie PC, et al.: Additive value of semiautomated quantification of coronary artery disease using cardiac computed tomographic angiography to predict future acute coronary syndrome, *J Am Coll Cardiol* 61:2296–2305, 2013.
143. Gitsioudis G, Schussler A, Nagy E, et al.: Combined assessment of high-sensitivity troponin T and noninvasive coronary plaque composition for the prediction of cardiac outcomes, *Radiology* 276:73–81, 2015.
144. Melander O, Newton-Cheh C, Almgren P, et al.: Novel and conventional biomarkers for prediction of incident cardiovascular events in the community, *JAMA* 302:49–57, 2009.
145. Ridker PM, Paynter NP, Rifai N, Gaziano JM, Cook NR: C-reactive protein and parental history improve global cardiovascular risk prediction: the Reynolds Risk Score for men, *Circulation* 118:2243–2251, 2008. 4p following 2251.
146. Wallace TW, Abdullah SM, Drazner MH, et al.: Prevalence and determinants of troponin T elevation in the general population, *Circulation* 113:1958–1965, 2006.
147. Zethelius B, Johnston N, Venge P: Troponin I as a predictor of coronary heart disease and mortality in 70-year-old men: a community-based cohort study, *Circulation* 113:1071–1078, 2006.
148. Omland T, Pfeffer MA, Solomon SD, et al.: Prognostic value of cardiac troponin I measured with a highly sensitive assay in patients with stable coronary artery disease, *J Am Coll Cardiol* 61:1240–1249, 2013.
149. Dedic A, Lubbers MM, Schaap J, et al.: Coronary CT angiography for suspected ACS in the era of high-sensitivity troponins: randomized multicenter study, *J Am Coll Cardiol* 67:16–26, 2016.
150. Everett BM, Brooks MM, Vlachos HE, et al.: Troponin and cardiac events in stable ischemic heart disease and diabetes, *N Engl J Med* 373:610–620, 2015.
151. Bjorkegren JL, Kovacic JC, Dudley JT, Schadt EE: Genome-wide significant loci: how important are they? Systems genetics to understand heritability of coronary artery disease and other common complex disorders, *J Am Coll Cardiol* 65:830–845, 2015.
152. Rosenberg S, Elashoff MR, Beineke P, et al.: Multicenter validation of the diagnostic accuracy of a blood-based gene expression test for assessing obstructive coronary artery disease in nondiabetic patients, *Ann Intern Med* 153:425–434, 2010.
153. Voros S, Elashoff MR, Wingrove JA, et al.: A peripheral blood gene expression score is associated with atherosclerotic plaque burden and stenosis by cardiovascular CT-angiography: results from the PREDICT and COMPASS studies, *Atherosclerosis* 233:284–290, 2014.
154. Bruder O, Wagner A, Lombardi M, et al.: European Cardiovascular Magnetic Resonance (EuroCMR) registry—multi national results from 57 centers in 15 countries, *J Cardiovasc Magn Reson* 15:9, 2013.
155. Roberts WT, Bax JJ, Davies LC: Cardiac CT and CT coronary angiography: technology and application, *Heart* 94:781–792, 2008.
156. Fordyce CB, Newby DE, Douglas PS: Diagnostic strategies for the evaluation of chest pain: clinical implications from SCOT-HEART and PROMISE, *J Am Coll Cardiol* 843–852, 2016.
157. Douglas PS, Hoffmann U, Lee KL, et al.: PROspective Multicenter Imaging Study for Evaluation of chest pain: rationale and design of the PROMISE trial, *Am Heart J* 167:796–803.e1, 2014.
158. Fordyce CB, Douglas PS: Optimal non-invasive imaging test selection for the diagnosis of ischaemic heart disease, *Heart* 555–564, 2016.
159. Hussain ST, Paul M, Plein S, et al.: Design and rationale of the MR-INFORM study: stress perfusion cardiovascular magnetic resonance imaging to guide the management of patients with stable coronary artery disease, *J Cardiovasc Magn Reson* 14:65, 2012.

SECTION IV

MANAGEMENT

16 Goals of Therapy

Mikhail Kosiborod and Suzanne V. Arnold

By its definition, chronic stable coronary artery disease (CAD) refers predominantly to patients who have a prior history of or current demonstrable obstructive atherosclerotic disease of the epicardial coronary arteries and who are either asymptomatic, or have stable symptoms, with no evidence of recent symptomatic, hemodynamic, or electrical decompensation. Because the process of atherosclerosis usually evolves over several decades, the natural history of CAD typically involves long periods during which patients are asymptomatic, minimally symptomatic, or have stable symptoms that can be effectively managed; however, these periods of clinical stability can rapidly transition to acute coronary syndromes (ACSs), resulting in serious, and sometimes fatal, adverse cardiac events. The major goals of treating patients with chronic stable CAD are, therefore, 2-fold. One is to prolong life and prevent or reduce major adverse cardiovascular events. The second, and equally important, goal is to control symptoms of CAD—primarily angina—with the purpose of improving symptoms, functional status, and quality of life, as well as reducing hospitalizations. These goals are achieved, in part, by administering evidence-based medical therapies that have been proven to provide prognostic benefit, improve symptoms of angina, or achieve both goals; and by identifying (through appropriate testing) a subgroup of patients that may derive a prognostic benefit from coronary revascularization. This section will summarize the key therapeutic approaches to achieving these goals and direct the reader to additional details for each of the treatment strategies in other chapters.

IMPROVING SURVIVAL AND PREVENTION OF MAJOR ADVERSE CARDIAC EVENTS

Lifestyle Interventions

Numerous prior studies have documented the positive impact of dietary interventions and physical activity on surrogate markers of cardiovascular risk (such as blood pressure, lipids, blood glucose, and weight), and meta-analyses suggest that an intensive lifestyle intervention program may have a modest beneficial effect on cardiovascular mortality and prevention of myocardial infarction (MI). Multiple beneficial effects of cardiac rehabilitation programs have also been demonstrated in several prior studies, and they are endorsed by professional guidelines in patients who have sustained an ACS or have had a revascularization procedure. See Chapter 18 for more on this topic.

Medical Therapy

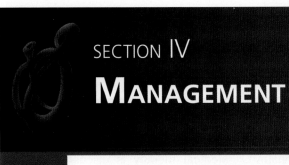

Few treatment approaches have been definitively shown to reduce mortality and prevent Major Adverse Cardiac Events (MACE) in patients with chronic stable CAD. Although β-blockers are a mainstay of therapy in chronic stable CAD, little evidence exists that their prolonged use results in improved survival or lower MACE rate. A meta-analysis of older clinical trials[1] demonstrated an overall 23% relative risk reduction in mortality in patients following acute MI; however, this meta-analysis primarily included studies performed before the modern era of coronary revascularization/reperfusion and medical therapy and did not examine truly long-term treatment (median duration of follow-up was 1.4 years). Data from the REduction of Atherothrombosis for Continued Health (REACH) registry, which included over 20,000 propensity-matched patients that were and were not treated with β-blockers,[2] demonstrated no statistically significant difference in the rates of MACE between patients with established CAD and no prior MI during a median follow up of nearly 4 years.[2] Among patients with previous history of MI, the outcomes were numerically favorable in patients with versus without β-blocker use, but this difference was not statistically significant. Other large observational studies also suggest a modest benefit in patients with a recent MI, but not in those without prior acute MI.[3] As a result, current guidelines for chronic stable CAD management give a strong recommendation for the use of β-blockers in patients with prior MI or history of heart failure, but not in other patients with chronic stable CAD.[4]

Other medical therapies used for treating symptoms of CAD, such as calcium-channel blockers, nitrates, and ranolazine, have not been shown to have an effect on survival or MACE events. In randomized clinical trials, neither nifedipine nor amlodipine was shown to reduce the rates of cardiovascular death or MI.[5–7] In the Metabolic Efficiency with Ranolazine for Less Ischemia in Non–ST-Elevation Acute Coronary Syndromes (MERLIN-TIMI36) trial, which was performed in patients stabilized after an ACS event, ranolazine did not significantly reduce the primary endpoint of cardiovascular death, MI, or recurrent ischemia compared with placebo.[8] No cardiovascular outcomes trials have ever been performed with long- or short-acting nitrates in this patient population.

Antiplatelet therapy has been proven to improve outcomes in patients with established CAD and is endorsed by practice guidelines. The Antithrombotic Trialists' Collaboration meta-analysis of over 135,000 patients, which included those with prior vascular events but also patients with previous coronary revascularization procedures and/or stable angina, demonstrated a significant reduction in MACE (nonfatal MI, nonfatal stroke, or vascular death) with antiplatelet therapy, primarily aspirin There was no difference in efficacy or safety between low-dose (75 to 150 mg daily) and higher-dose aspirin. The use of thienopyridines, such as clopidogrel, instead of aspirin may provide an additional modest benefit,[9] but is not recommended unless patients are unable to tolerate aspirin. The use of dual antiplatelet therapy (aspirin plus P2Y12 receptor blocker) in patients with chronic stable CAD (and without another indication, such as recent coronary stent implantation) is more controversial; an in-depth discussion of antiplatelet therapy, as well as anticoagulants, is provided in Chapter 21.

Lowering of low-density lipoprotein cholesterol (LDL-C) with statin therapy is a mainstay of chronic stable CAD management. Numerous clinical trials and multiple meta-analyses have demonstrated the benefits of LDL-C lowering—specifically with statins—on cardiovascular outcomes. Specifically, both in trials of statins versus placebo, and in trials of more intensive versus less intensive statin regimens, a consistent benefit of intensive statin therapy is observed in patients with established CAD, including reductions in cardiovascular and all-cause mortality, and MI,[10] and, therefore, clinical guidelines strongly endorse high-intensity statin treatment for all eligible patients with established CAD.[11] For patients with established CAD that require additional LDL lowering despite maximally tolerated statin therapy, several options for nonstatin LDL-C lowering exist; however, only ezetimibe has been shown to provide additional, modest clinical benefit in combination with a statin.[12] Of note, the modest benefit with ezetimibe was observed in patients in whom treatment was initiated following an ACS event and was predominantly seen in the subgroup of patients with type 2 diabetes;[13] whether these data can be extrapolated to patients with chronic stable CAD without prior ACS is unclear. Therapies aimed at raising high-density lipoprotein (HDL) and/or lowering triglycerides have so far failed to provide additional clinical benefit in recent clinical trials. The effects of LDL cholesterol lowering therapies in patients with established CAD are discussed in detail elsewhere (Chapter 30).

In the broad population of patients with stable CAD, angiotensin-converting enzyme inhibitor (ACE-I), angiotensin receptor blocker (ARB), and mineralocorticoid receptor antagonists have not been consistently demonstrated to improve outcomes above and beyond blood pressure lowering; however, these agents have important benefits (including reduction in total mortality, MI, stroke, and heart failure) in several key subgroups of patients, such as those after acute MI with reduced left ventricular ejection fraction (LVEF), symptomatic heart failure, and high-risk diabetes, and may also improve renal outcomes in patients with chronic kidney disease (CKD) (particularly diabetic nephropathy).[14] Medical therapy is discussed in more detail in Chapter 20.

Coronary Revascularization

A benefit of coronary revascularization (Chapter 23) on death and MI has been difficult to demonstrate in patients with stable CAD, except in select patient populations (high-grade left main disease, multivessel disease with reduced LVEF and/or large ischemic burden, etc.) in whom coronary artery bypass graft (CABG) surgery is indicated. Percutaneous coronary intervention (PCI), even with the latest generation drug-eluting stents, has not been shown to improve the natural history of stable CAD. This contrasts with evidence in patients with ACS, where routine use of PCI lowers the risk of recurrent ischemic events.

An important goal of management is to identify the minority of patients with stable ischemic heart disease (IHD) who have clear indications for coronary revascularization. Multiple noninvasive testing options are available for risk stratification, including standard stress electrocardiography (Chapter 10), echocardiography and stress echocardiography (Chapter 11), nuclear and positron emission tomography (PET) imaging (Chapter 12) and cardiac computed tomography (CT), and magnetic resonance imaging (MRI) (Chapter 13). Selection among the different testing options should be based on individual patient factors, local expertise, and cost considerations. (Chapter 15). When high-risk findings are found on noninvasive testing, coronary angiography is generally indicated. Incorporation of functional assessment of the impact of coronary stenoses using hemodynamic assessments such as fractional flow reserve (Chapter 14) improves decision-making regarding coronary revascularization, allowing deferral of revascularization for lesions with minimal hemodynamic significance.

IMPROVING SYMPTOMS AND QUALITY OF LIFE

Importance of Angina as Outcome in Patients with Chronic Stable CAD

Whereas prolonging survival and reducing the risk of recurrent adverse cardiac events are important, many of the treatments used for chronic CAD are used for the explicit purpose of reducing angina and improving quality of life. Despite improvements in interventional techniques and medications to reduce the burden of atherosclerosis, angina continues to be a substantial issue for many patients with chronic CAD. Understanding the burden and impact of angina on our patients and working to reduce that burden remain important goals of treatment of chronic CAD. Among patients with CAD, those with more frequent angina and more physical limitations due to angina are more likely to be hospitalized for an ACS and are more likely to die, as compared with those with minimal angina,[15] even after adjusting for demographic and clinical factors. Among 5558 patients with CAD, nearly 20% of those who reported severe functional limitations due to angina died by 2 years versus less than 5% of those who reported minimal limitations from angina (Fig. 16.1).

Importantly, treatment of angina in patients with chronic CAD, either with medications or revascularization, has not been shown to improve prognosis except in rare circumstances (e.g., large ischemic burden, disease in the proximal left anterior descending coronary artery). As such, the association of burden of angina with increased risk of mortality is likely more of a marker of a higher risk patient, as opposed to a mediator of poor outcomes that can be modulated. However, there are other benefits of aggressively treating angina, namely in improving quality of life and reducing healthcare utilization. Angina is not only associated with substantial impairment in disease-specific and generic quality of life, but relief of angina after revascularization has been shown to be the primary determinant of improvement in quality of life.[16]

Beyond its impact on quality of life, angina is also related to healthcare utilization. In a study of 5460 patients after a hospitalization for an ACS, residual angina was associated with a graded risk for both cardiovascular hospitalizations and increased resource utilization (Fig. 16.2).[17]

Patients with angina had incremental costs of approximately \$125 (monthly angina) to \$500 (daily angina) per month of follow-up over the monthly costs of those without residual angina, which were primarily driven by hospitalizations for recurrent acute coronary events or coronary revascularization. Whereas treatment of angina has not specifically been shown to reduce healthcare utilization, in an era of increasing capitation and reimbursement based on quality of care, interventions that effectively reduce the burden of angina, including disease management programs, could potentially reduce both morbidity and healthcare costs.

Measuring Angina Burden

A unique feature of angina is that there is no biologic or imaging assay that can quantify it. In research studies, semi-quantitative methods of treadmill testing with time to chest pain or ST-segment depression have been used as a means of quantifying the patient's burden of angina and response to antianginal medications. However, these methods, although reasonably assessing ischemia, are artificial in their assessment of angina, as they do not represent patients' daily lives nor are they practical to serially assess in clinical practice. Instead, the physician/patient interaction is the primary means by which physicians assess patients' responses to therapy and the need for further testing or treatment. As such, the evaluation of angina is subject to all the limitations inherent in history taking, including physical and psychosocial barriers to the proper conveyance of information, pre-existing biases on the part of both physicians and patients, and the inherent inter-rater variability across physicians. Studies have shown that both cardiologists and primary care doctors often underestimate the burden of angina of their patients when they rely on free-form interviews.[18,19] In a multicenter, cross-sectional sample of patients with coronary artery disease, 42% of patients who reported chest pain in the prior month had their angina underrecognized by the treating physician. Few patient factors were associated with underrecognition; instead, it was explained by variation in the quality of physician assessment, with some physicians being quite good at angina recognition while others were poor (range of underrecognition rates of 0–86%). These data underscore that a more systematic approach is needed for assessing angina in patients with CAD.

Many physicians rely on Canadian Cardiovascular Society (CCS) grading of angina, which asks the physician to grade the level of activity that brings on chest pain, ranging from a score of 0 to 4 (Table 16.1).

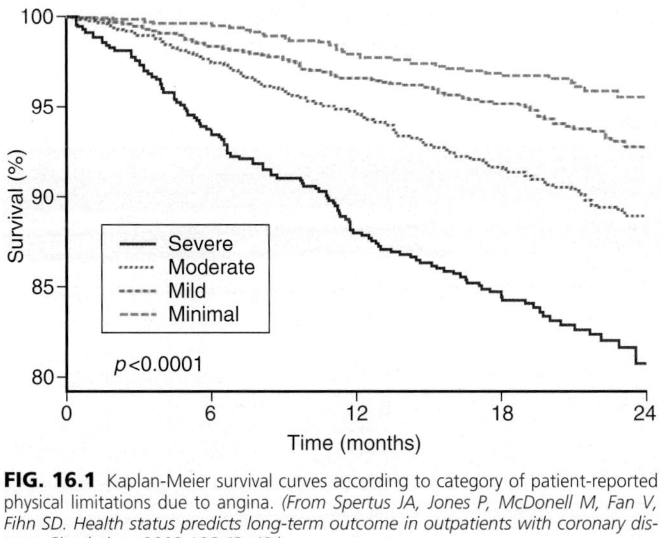

FIG. 16.1 Kaplan-Meier survival curves according to category of patient-reported physical limitations due to angina. *(From Spertus JA, Jones P, McDonell M, Fan V, Fihn SD. Health status predicts long-term outcome in outpatients with coronary disease.* Circulation. *2002;106:43–49.)*

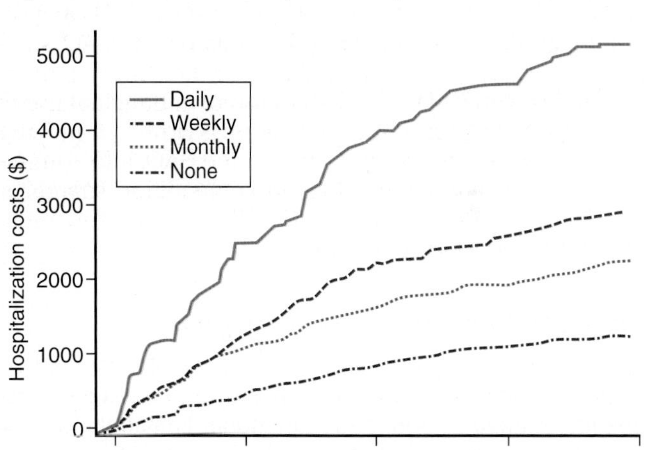

FIG. 16.2 Cumulative healthcare costs according to patient-reported angina at 4 months after hospitalization for acute coronary syndrome. *(From Arnold SV, Morrow DA, Lei Y, et al. Economic impact of angina after an acute coronary syndrome: insights from the MERLIN-TIMI 36 trial.* Circ Cardiovasc Qual Outcomes. *2009;2:344–353.)*

TABLE 16.1 Canadian Cardiovascular Society Grading of Angina

Class 0	Asymptomatic
Class I	Angina during strenuous or prolonged physical activity only
Class II	Angina with moderate physical activity, such as walking or climbing stairs briskly
Class III	Angina with ordinary physical activity, such as walking on level ground at normal pace
Class IV	Angina at rest or with minimal activity, such as dressing or showering

This grading scale is used in the Appropriateness Criteria for coronary revascularization and is easy to calculate, as it arises simply from the information gathered in the physician/patient interview. However, similar to New York Heart Association functional class in heart failure, it does not provide any standardized assessment directly from the patient and, therefore, is susceptible to biases and errors. For example, in a clinical trial of patients undergoing revascularization, physicians tended to overestimate the burden of angina of their patients using CCS class when compared to a patient-reported measure prior to revascularization and underestimate residual angina after revascularization.[20]

Assessing symptoms directly from patients with a validated instrument, such as the Seattle Angina Questionnaire (SAQ),[21] provides more reliable and reproducible results than physician-derived scales. The SAQ has been used to document angina burden and disease-specific quality of life in patients with CAD in numerous clinical trials and registries and has been shown to correlate closely with daily angina and sublingual nitroglycerin diaries.[22] Despite its established validity, its widespread use in research studies, and its promotion for clinical use by major societies, the routine clinical use of the SAQ (along with other similar health status measures for conditions such as heart failure and peripheral artery disease) has been hindered by logistic barriers. A shorter, seven-item version of the SAQ has been developed, which was designed to simplify this transition from being a research instrument to an effective clinical tool. The SAQ-7 is a reliable and valid measure of the burden of angina from the patient's perspective and changes in scores over time (≥ 10 points on the SAQ angina frequency domain score or ≥ 5 points on the SAQ summary score) can support clinicians in their management of patients with CAD (e.g., up-titration of antianginal medications, referral for revascularization). However, moving patient-reported outcomes, such as the SAQ, into routine clinical care requires creative implementation strategies, including novel mechanisms to collect, score, and interpret these data, work that is on-going.

Medical Therapy to Treat Angina

Pharmacologic treatment is the mainstay of treatment of angina (Chapter 20) and has been shown to reduce the frequency of angina, reduce the functional limitations due to angina, and improve quality of life. Medications to treat angina are generally grouped into those that decrease myocardial demand (e.g., β-blockers, calcium-channel blockers, ranolazine) and those that improve myocardial oxygen supply (e.g., calcium-channel blockers, long-acting nitrates) (Table 16.2).

β-Blockers are the recommended first-line therapy for treatment of chronic exertional angina and work by reducing heart rate, contractility, and left ventricular wall stress, which results in decreased myocardial oxygen demand. β-Blockers improve exercise capacity, reduce exercise-induced ischemia, and decrease the frequency of angina and the requirement for sublingual nitroglycerin. Ideally, β-blockers can be titrated up to a resting heart rate in the 50 to 60 beats/min range, recognizing that bradycardia is often the limiting step in up-titration of these medications.

Calcium-channel blockers are also effective antianginal medications, doing so through both increasing oxygen supply (via coronary vasodilatation) and reducing oxygen demand (via reduction in wall stress from peripheral vasodilation and reduction in myocardial contractility). Both long-acting nondihydropyridines (e.g., diltiazem or verapamil) and second generation dihydropyridines (e.g., amlodipine or felodipine) are typically safe and effective antianginal medications and are the first-line medications for vasospastic angina. Whereas short-acting dihydropyridines also reduce angina, there is evidence of increased mortality with these agents when used after an MI, and so their general use is discouraged. The addition of nondihydropyridines to maximally tolerated β-blockers is often limited by bradycardia and so dihydropyridines may be preferred. In a meta-analysis in patients with stable CAD, patients with stable CAD treated with a calcium-channel blocker had 0.11 fewer episodes of angina a week as compared with those treated with a β-blocker.[23] In addition, there was no difference in morbidity or mortality between the two treatment groups, indicating that both β-blockers and calcium-channel blockers are effective and safe antianginal medications.

Short-acting nitrates are recommended for immediate relief of acute episodes of angina. Nitroglycerin causes coronary vasodilation, augments collateral flow, and reduces preload, thereby reducing myocardial wall tension and myocardial oxygen demand. However, this benefit of reduced wall tension is countered by an increase in sympathetic activity that results in increased heart rate and myocardial contractility. Long-acting nitrates have been shown to improve time to angina and ischemia with exercise in short-term studies. Prolonged benefit of long-acting nitrates is limited due to tolerance and can also result in increases in oxidative stress and endothelial dysfunction.

TABLE 16.2 Effects of Antianginal Medications on Myocardium

	OXYGEN DEMAND					OXYGEN SUPPLY	
	HEART RATE	ARTERIAL PRESSURE/ AFTERLOAD	VENOUS RETURN/ PRELOAD	MYOCARDIAL CONTRACTILITY	OVERALL EFFECT	CORONARY FLOW	OVERALL EFFECT
β-Blockers	↓↓	↓	--	↓↓	↓↓	--	--
Calcium-channel blockers							
Dihydropyridine	↑/--	↓↓	--	↓	↓	↑↑	↑↑
Nondihydropyridine	↓↓	↓	--	↓↓	↓↓	↑↑	↑↑
Long-acting nitrates	--	↓	↓↓	--	↓	↑	↑
Ranolazine	--	--	--	--	↓↓*	--	--

*Reduces ischemia/demand at the cellular level.
↓, Decrease; ↑, increase; --, no change.

Ranolazine is a selective inhibitor of the late sodium current (late I_{Na}) and reduces ischemia at the cellular level; it is therefore unique among the antianginal medications available as it has no hemodynamic effects. Because of this, it is particularly useful for patients in whom titration of β-blockers or calcium antagonists is limited by low heart rate or blood pressure. It reduces chronic angina both as a monotherapy and in combination with other commonly prescribed antianginal medications. Similar to other medications for stable angina, it has not been shown to impact mortality. Due to its mechanism of action, ranolazine can be particularly effective in patients with concomitant diabetes—it is both a more effective antianginal medication in the setting of hyperglycemia and can also improve blood glucose control.[24] It is currently recommended as add-on therapy or as a first-line medication for angina when β-blockers cannot be used.

The choice of antianginal medications for individual patients, both as classes of medications and particular medications within classes, often depends on hemodynamics, comorbidities, and side effects. It is also important to note that combinations of two different classes of medications generally provide superior angina relief and better tolerability. Typically, this is a β-blocker combined with a long-acting dihydropyridine, nitrate, or ranolazine, although ranolazine has also been tested in combination with calcium-channel blockers. Despite the prevalence of revascularization (the role of which is discussed separately), angina remains a substantial burden in the lives of many patients with chronic CAD. As such, the appropriate medical management of angina continues to be important to study and understand, as this has potential to greatly improve patients' quality of life, as well as reduce healthcare utilization.

Exercise

Beyond the available pharmacologic therapies, exercise (Chapter 18) has the potential to increase exercise tolerance and reduce symptoms of ischemia. Low-impact aerobic exercises such as walking or cycling, which involve large, lower-body muscles groups, are generally safe and well-tolerated in patients with stable angina. Exercise reduces endothelial dysfunction and systemic inflammation, which can improve microvascular function and progression of atherosclerosis. In addition, exercise can be markedly effective in the management of cardiovascular risk factors, such as hypertension, diabetes, and obesity. Patients should be instructed to avoid extreme weather conditions, to work up to regular exercise, and to stop exercising if angina occurs. Patients who develop angina during exercise should have a goal heart rate 10 bpm lower than the heart rate that results in angina.

Coronary Revascularization

Although the role of coronary revascularization (Chapter 23) in improving mortality in stable CAD is limited to subgroups of patients with coronary anatomy suitable for CABG (see previous discussion), both PCI and CABG are highly effective strategies for relief of angina. The best evidence comparing medical therapy with medical therapy plus PCI in patients with stable angina comes from the Clinical Outcomes Utilizing Revascularization and Aggressive Drug Evaluation (COURAGE) trial. In this trial, which (importantly) allowed for cross-over from medical therapy to PCI, showed that PCI improved angina more quickly than medical therapy. At 1 year after randomization, 52% of patients randomized to PCI had a clinically significant improvement in angina frequency (assessed with the SAQ) versus 46% of patients randomized to medical therapy, which translates to a number needed to treat of 17. As a result, revascularization for stable angina (in the absence of select cases where revascularization may have improved survival) is generally recommended after an initial trial of medical therapy with at least two antianginal medications.

Treating Refractory Angina

Enhanced external counterpulsation is the most commonly used mechanical therapy for stable angina and has evidence from multiple registries demonstrating benefit in angina reduction. The mechanism of action is largely unknown, and importantly, it has not been (and probably cannot be) tested in a blinded manner, suggesting that the results of these studies potentially may be due to a placebo effect. Other mechanical therapies, such as spinal cord stimulation, transmyocardial laser revascularization, ethylenediamine tetra-acetic acid (EDTA) chelation, and coronary sinus reducers, also have limited favorable data to support their use in reducing angina but have not yet gained much popularity in use. Despite the prevalence of revascularization, angina remains a substantial burden in the lives of many patients with chronic CAD. As such, the appropriate noninterventional management of angina continues to be important to study and understand, as this has the potential to greatly improve patients' quality of life, as well as reduce healthcare utilization. For more on treating refractory angina, see Chapter 27.

SPECIAL POPULATIONS

Women

Women are more likely to present with symptomatic CAD at an older age than are men and more typically present with stable angina, as opposed to ACS. The traditional teaching is that women present with atypical symptoms, such as dyspnea and fatigue, and not typical exertional chest pain or tightness. Whereas it is true that atypical angina is more often reported in women than in men, the majority of women still present with typical symptoms.[25] In addition, women are more likely to have microvascular disease, as opposed to obstructive CAD that is amenable to revascularization. There have not been any substantial differences in response to medical therapy for angina between men and women, either in general (e.g., COURAGE trial) or in specific trials of antianginal medications. However, women are more likely than men to have complications[26] and worse long-term outcomes after revascularization.[27,28]

Elderly

Older adults often present with more diffuse CAD than younger patients, which can be difficult to treat with revascularization. As such, medical therapy of CAD has a more prominent role in older adults. Older patients generally have higher event rates (morbidity and mortality), and therefore, medications that reduce cardiovascular risk (e.g., statins) have larger absolute risk reductions in these patients. However, they also tend to be more susceptible to adverse events with both revascularization (e.g., more periprocedural complications) and medications (e.g., bleeding with dual antiplatelet therapy). In addition, due to the relatively larger number of medications that they often take, older adults are at greater risk of medication interactions and polypharmacy. Older patients are more prone to side effects of medications, such as orthostasis and myalgias. As such, care must be taken to try to consolidate medications (e.g., choose one medication instead of two), simplify medication regimens (e.g., choose once daily medications), and select medications with lower risk of side effects. Older patients are more likely than younger patients to curtail their activities to avoid angina, and thus they may not complain as much about chest pain. In addition, for the same degree of angina, older patients report better quality of life, indicating that they have differing expectations about their symptoms and functional status than do younger patients. As such, a careful history about activity level and avoidance of activities is needed to avoid undertreatment of angina, as medical management can still substantially improve older patients' symptoms and quality of life.

Diabetes

Patients with diabetes (Chapter 24) represent a substantial and growing proportion of those with established CAD. Among those presenting with ACS, less than 30% of patients have normal glucose metabolism, with the rest having either known or newly diagnosed diabetes, or prediabetes;[29] these findings are similar in patients with stable CAD. Because of the high prevalence of glucose abnormalities, screening for diabetes with glycated hemoglobin (HbA1c) assay is recommended in patients with CAD.[30]

There are several important considerations in the management of this high-risk group for several reasons: first, the presence of diabetes may impact the management of CAD itself (risk stratification strategies, medical management and revascularization options); and second, treatment choices for the management of diabetes may impact cardiovascular events.

Patients with diabetes mellitus (DM) do have more extensive and severe CAD[31] than their nondiabetic counterparts, and, therefore, revascularization strategies are of importance in this patient group. Despite more extensive and severe CAD, prior clinical trials have demonstrated no impact on mortality or MACE with either percutaneous or surgical revascularization versus optimal medical therapy in patients with DM and stable CAD.[32] Therefore, the decisions regarding appropriate patient selection for revascularization should be guided by similar considerations in patients with and without DM (i.e., left main disease, multivessel disease, large ischemic burden, reduced LVEF, etc.). However, if revascularization is being pursued, the presence of DM may significantly impact the choice of revascularization strategy. Specifically, large clinical trials have definitively demonstrated superiority of CABG over PCI (even with drug-eluting stents [DES]) in patients with type 2 diabetes and multivessel stable CAD, both in terms of clinical outcomes (including survival) and cost-effectiveness.[33,34]

Whereas patients with DM have more extensive coronary disease, the data on whether they experience more angina are conflicting. Although a few older studies suggested that patients with DM are more likely to have asymptomatic (or "silent") ischemia, with diabetic autonomic neuropathy posited as one potential explanation,[35,36] data from more up-to-date clinical trials and large observational registries indicate that there is little difference in the degree of silent ischemia between diabetic and nondiabetic patients with CAD[37–39] and that the burden of angina may actually be greater in patients with diabetes.[40] Therefore, more aggressive screening for asymptomatic CAD in patients with DM (vs no diabetes) with advanced imaging techniques is not currently recommended and has not been shown to meaningfully impact outcomes in clinical trials.[41] Furthermore, aggressive management of angina is at least as important in this patient group. To this end, there are additional considerations in terms of the choice of antianginal medications in patients with diabetes. As one example, vasodilating β-blockers, such as carvedilol, may be preferable in patients with DM, as they have similar antianginal properties as nonvasodilating β-blockers but a more favorable effect on glycemia.[42]

Finally, the choice of glucose-lowering medications may have an important impact on cardiovascular events in patients with type 2 diabetes and stable CAD. The general strategy of aggressive HbA1C lowering has generally produced modest (if any) benefit for cardiovascular events, which emerged after more than 10 years of follow-up, and no demonstrable reduction in cardiovascular or all-cause mortality.[43–45] However, in large randomized clinical trials from 2015 and 2016, several type 2 diabetes compounds have been shown to substantially reduce cardiovascular complications, including in some cases cardiovascular and total mortality.[46–48] Importantly, these effects were observed within a relatively short time period (3–4 years), and were almost certainly mediated by mechanisms other than glucose-lowering. These findings have not yet been incorporated into most practice guidelines, and the data from future trials are needed to determine whether these benefits represent class effects. Nevertheless, because cardiovascular disease is the leading cause of death and disability in patients with type 2 diabetes, it is reasonable to prioritize type 2 diabetes treatments that have been proven to reduce cardiovascular and all-cause mortality, and prevent cardiovascular complications of type 2 diabetes within a short time frame, irrespective of their "efficacy" as it relates to glucose lowering.

CONCLUSIONS: DEVELOPING AN INDIVIDUALIZED PLAN OF CARE

By its definition, the stable nature of chronic stable CAD indicates absence of recent deterioration and therefore affords time for collecting appropriate clinical data for thoughtful consideration, meaningful discussion of treatment options with patients, and shared decision-making. As previously noted, the dual goals of management are to prolong life/prevent major cardiovascular events and to improve symptoms, functional status, and quality of life. Guideline-directed optimal medical therapy is the foundation for achieving both of these goals. Careful risk stratification, using appropriate noninvasive modalities and/or coronary angiography, can help identify subgroups of patients that may benefit from percutaneous or surgical coronary revascularization for prognostic reasons. In addition, careful and accurate assessment of angina frequency and severity, and an individualized approach to symptom management that incorporates, among other important factors, patient-reported angina burden and treatment preferences, is most likely to produce the optimal outcomes in patients with chronic stable CAD.

References

1. Freemantle N, Cleland J, Young P, Mason J, Harrison J: β-Blockade after myocardial infarction: systematic review and meta regression analysis, *BMJ* 318:1730–1737, 1999.
2. Bangalore S, Steg G, Deedwania P, et al.: β-Blocker use and clinical outcomes in stable outpatients with and without coronary artery disease, *JAMA* 308:1340–1349, 2012.
3. Andersson C, Shilane D, Go AS, et al.: β-Blocker therapy and cardiac events among patients with newly diagnosed coronary heart disease, *J Am Coll Cardiol* 64:247–252, 2014.
4. Fihn SD, Gardin JM, Abrams J, et al.: 2012 ACCF/AHA/ACP/AATS/PCNA/SCAI/STS Guideline for the diagnosis and management of patients with stable ischemic heart disease: a report of the American College of Cardiology Foundation/American Heart Association Task Force on Practice Guidelines, and the American College of Physicians, American Association for Thoracic Surgery, Preventive Cardiovascular Nurses Association, Society for Cardiovascular Angiography and Interventions, and Society of Thoracic Surgeons, *J Am Coll Cardiol* 60:e44–e164, 2012.
5. Dargie HJ, Ford I, Fox KM: Total Ischaemic Burden European Trial (TIBET). Effects of ischaemia and treatment with atenolol, nifedipine SR and their combination on outcome in patients with chronic stable angina. The TIBET Study Group, *Eur Heart J* 17:104–112, 1996.
6. Nissen SE, Tuzcu EM, Libby P, et al.: Effect of antihypertensive agents on cardiovascular events in patients with coronary disease and normal blood pressure: the CAMELOT study: a randomized controlled trial, *JAMA* 292:2217–2225, 2004.
7. Poole-Wilson PA, Lubsen J, Kirwan BA, et al.: Effect of long-acting nifedipine on mortality and cardiovascular morbidity in patients with stable angina requiring treatment (ACTION trial): randomised controlled trial, *Lancet* 364:849–857, 2004.
8. Morrow DA, Scirica BM, Karwatowska-Prokopczuk E, et al.: Effects of ranolazine on recurrent cardiovascular events in patients with non-ST-elevation acute coronary syndromes: the MERLIN-TIMI 36 randomized trial, *JAMA* 297:1775–1783, 2007.
9. A randomised, blinded, trial of clopidogrel versus aspirin in patients at risk of ischaemic events (CAPRIE). CAPRIE Steering Committee, *Lancet* 348:1329–1339, 1996.
10. Baigent C, Blackwell L, Emberson J, et al.: Efficacy and safety of more intensive lowering of LDL cholesterol: a meta-analysis of data from 170,000 participants in 26 randomised trials, *Lancet* 376:1670–1681, 2010.
11. Stone NJ, Robinson J, Lichtenstein AH, et al.: 2013 ACC/AHA Guideline on the treatment of blood cholesterol to reduce atherosclerotic cardiovascular risk in adults: a report of the American College of Cardiology/American Heart Association Task Force on Practice Guidelines, *J Am Coll Cardiol* 63(25 Pt B):2889–2934, 2014.
12. Cannon CP, Blazing MA, Giugliano RP, et al.: Ezetimibe added to statin therapy after acute coronary syndromes, *N Engl J Med* 372:2387–2397, 2015.
13. Exetimibe Reduces Cardiovascular Events in Diabetics with Recent Acute Coronary Syndrome [article online]. Available at http://www.medscape.com/viewarticle/850261. Accessed 2016.
14. Yusuf S, Sleight P, Pogue J, Bosch J, Davies R, Dagenais G: Effects of an angiotensin-converting-enzyme inhibitor, ramipril, on cardiovascular events in high-risk patients. The Heart Outcomes Prevention Evaluation Study Investigators, *N Engl J Med* 342:145–153, 2000.
15. Spertus JA, Jones P, McDonell M, Fan V, Fihn SD: Health status predicts long-term outcome in outpatients with coronary disease, *Circulation* 106:43–49, 2002.
16. Spertus JA, Salisbury AC, Jones PG, Conaway DG, Thompson RC: Predictors of quality-of-life benefit after percutaneous coronary intervention, *Circulation* 110:3789–3794, 2004.
17. Arnold SV, Morrow DA, Lei Y, et al.: Economic impact of angina after an acute coronary syndrome: insights from the MERLIN-TIMI 36 trial, *Circ Cardiovasc Qual Outcomes* 2:344–353, 2009.
18. Beltrame JF, Weekes AJ, Morgan C, Tavella R, Spertus JA: The prevalence of weekly angina among patients with chronic stable angina in primary care practices: the Coronary Artery Disease in General Practice (CADENCE) Study, *Arch Intern Med* 169:1491–1499, 2009.
19. Arnold SV, Grodzinsky A, Gosch KL, et al.: Predictors of Physician Under-recognition of Angina in Outpatients with Stable Coronary Artery Disease, *Circ Cardiovasc Qual Outcomes*, 9:554–559, 2016.
20. Nassif ME, Cohen DJ, Arnold SV, et al.: Comparison of Patient Reported Angina with Provider Assigned Canadian Cardiovascular Society Angina Class Before and After Revascularization, *Circ Cardiovasc Qual Outcomes* 9:A11, 2016.
21. Spertus JA, Winder JA, Dewhurst TA, et al.: Development and evaluation of the Seattle Angina Questionnaire: a new functional status measure for coronary artery disease, *J Am Coll Cardiol* 25:333–341, 1995.
22. Arnold SV, Kosiborod M, Li Y, et al.: Comparison of the Seattle Angina Questionnaire with daily angina diary in the TERISA clinical trial, *Circ Cardiovasc Qual Outcomes* 7:844–850, 2014.
23. National Institute for Health and Care Excellence: Stable angina: management. https://www.nice.org.uk/guidance/cg126. *NICE guidelines*, 2011.
24. Arnold SV, McGuire DK, Spertus JA, et al.: Effectiveness of ranolazine in patients with type 2 diabetes mellitus and chronic stable angina according to baseline hemoglobin A1c, *Am Heart J* 168:457–465, 2014. e452.
25. Canto JG, Goldberg RJ, Hand MM, et al.: Symptom presentation of women with acute coronary syndromes: myth vs reality, *Arch Intern Med* 167:2405–2413, 2007.
26. Singh M, Lennon RJ, Holmes Jr DR, Bell MR, Rihal CS: Correlates of procedural complications and a simple integer risk score for percutaneous coronary intervention, *J Am Coll Cardiol* 40:387–393, 2002.
27. Holubkov R, Laskey WK, Haviland A, et al.: Angina 1 year after percutaneous coronary intervention: a report from the NHLBI Dynamic Registry, *Am Heart J* 144:826–833, 2002.
28. Dey S, Flather MD, Devlin G, et al.: Global Registry of Acute Coronary Events i. Sex-related differences in the presentation, treatment and outcomes among patients with acute coronary syndromes: the Global Registry of Acute Coronary Events, *Heart* 95:20–26, 2009.
29. Arnold SV, Lipska KJ, Li Y, et al.: Prevalence of glucose abnormalities among patients presenting with an acute myocardial infarction, *Am Heart J* 168:466–470, 2014. e461.
30. Ryden L, Grant PJ, Anker SD, et al.: ESC Guidelines on diabetes, pre-diabetes, and cardiovascular diseases developed in collaboration with the EASD: the Task Force on diabetes, pre-diabetes, and cardiovascular diseases of the European Society of Cardiology (ESC) and developed in collaboration with the European Association for the Study of Diabetes (EASD), *Eur Heart J* 34:3035–3087, 2013.
31. Duarte R, Castela S, Reis RP, et al.: Acute coronary syndrome in a diabetic population—risk factors and clinical and angiographic characteristics, *Rev Port Cardiol* 22:1077–1088, 2003.
32. Frye RL, August P, Brooks MM, et al.: A randomized trial of therapies for type 2 diabetes and coronary artery disease, *N Engl J Med* 360:2503–2515, 2009.
33. Influence of diabetes on 5-year mortality and morbidity in a randomized trial comparing CABG and PTCA in patients with multivessel disease: the Bypass Angioplasty Revascularization Investigation (BARI), *Circulation* 96:1761–1769, 1997.
34. Farkouh ME, Domanski M, Sleeper LA, et al.: Strategies for multivessel revascularization in patients with diabetes, *N Engl J Med* 367:2375–2384, 2012.
35. Murray DP, O'Brien T, Mulrooney R, O'Sullivan DJ: Autonomic dysfunction and silent myocardial ischaemia on exercise testing in diabetes mellitus, *Diabet Med* 7:580–584, 1990.
36. Marchant B, Umachandran V, Stevenson R, Kopelman PG, Timmis AD: Silent myocardial ischemia: role of subclinical neuropathy in patients with and without diabetes, *J Am Coll Cardiol* 22:1433–1437, 1993.
37. Caracciolo EA, Chaitman BR, Forman SA, et al.: Diabetics with coronary disease have a prevalence of asymptomatic ischemia during exercise treadmill testing and ambulatory ischemia monitoring similar to that of nondiabetic patients. An ACIP database study. ACIP Investigators. Asymptomatic Cardiac Ischemia Pilot Investigators, *Circulation* 93:2097–2105, 1996.
38. Peterson PN, Spertus JA, Magid DJ, et al.: The impact of diabetes on one-year health status outcomes following acute coronary syndromes, *BMC Cardiovasc Disord* 6:41, 2006.
39. Morrow DA, Scirica BM, Chaitman BR, et al.: Evaluation of the glycometabolic effects of ranolazine in patients with and without diabetes mellitus in the MERLIN-TIMI 36 randomized controlled trial, *Circulation* 119:2032–2039, 2009.
40. Arnold SV, Spertus JA, Lipska KJ, et al.: Association between diabetes mellitus and angina after acute myocardial infarction: analysis of the TRIUMPH prospective cohort study, *Eur J Prev Cardiol*, 2014.
41. Young LH, Wackers FJ, Chyun DA, et al.: Cardiac outcomes after screening for asymptomatic coronary artery disease in patients with type 2 diabetes: the DIAD study: a randomized controlled trial, *JAMA* 301:1547–1555, 2009.
42. Arnold SV, Spertus JA, Lipska KJ, et al.: Type of beta-blocker use among patients with versus without diabetes after myocardial infarction, *Am Heart J* 168:273–279, 2014. e271.
43. Action to Control Cardiovascular Risk in Diabetes Study G, Gerstein HC, Miller ME, et al.: Effects of intensive glucose lowering in type 2 diabetes, *N Engl J Med* 358:2545–2559, 2008.
44. Duckworth W, Abraira C, Moritz T, et al.: Glucose control and vascular complications in veterans with type 2 diabetes, *N Engl J Med* 360:129–139, 2009.
45. Hayward RA, Reaven PD, Emanuele NV: Follow-up of glycemic control and cardiovascular outcomes in type 2 diabetes, *N Engl J Med* 373:978, 2015.
46. Zinman B, Wanner C, Lachin JM, et al.: Empagliflozin, cardiovascular outcomes, and mortality in type 2 diabetes, *N Engl J Med* 373:2117–2128, 2015.
47. Kernan WN, Viscoli CM, Furie KL, et al.: Pioglitazone after ischemic stroke or transient ischemic attack, *N Engl J Med* 374:1321–1331, 2016.
48. Marso SP, Daniels GH, Brown-Frandsen K, et al.: Liraglutide and cardiovascular outcomes in type 2 diabetes, *N Engl J Med* 375:311–322, 2016.

17 Global Risk Assessment

Jesper K. Jensen, Amit V. Khera, and Connor A. Emdin

INTRODUCTION

This chapter is focused on tools for risk assessment in patients with stable coronary heart disease. In general, patients with stable ischemic heart disease have a good prognosis. However, these data summarize the population average, and the clinician is able to significantly refine the estimate of risk for the individual using methods described in this chapter. The central goal of risk assessment is to guide therapeutic decision-making and, in some cases, additional diagnostic evaluation. These diagnostic and prognostic assessments, although overlapping, are not identical. The prognostic assessment is valuable because the risk of recurrent events is strongly linked to the potential absolute and relative benefits of specific therapeutic interventions. In patients with stable coronary heart disease, an estimate of risk is similarly pivotal in management such as in identifying candidates for coronary angiography and revascularization. In this chapter we will review individual prognostic markers that are associated with adverse outcomes in stable coronary artery disease (CAD). We will also review multivariable models that incorporate multiple markers to quantitatively estimate risk and examine current approaches to match therapies to individual risk of an adverse outcome.

PROGNOSIS OVERALL AND IN SUBGROUPS

The assessment of cardiovascular disease risk and the prevention of recurrent events in patients with established CAD represent an opportunity for major public health gain.[1] Aligning diagnostic studies and therapeutic interventions with clinical risk is a cornerstone of secondary prevention. Previous epidemiologic studies have demonstrated that established CAD is a major risk factor for incident events. For example, data from the Framingham Study, obtained before the widespread use of aggressive medication and modification of risk factors, revealed an average annual mortality rate of 4% in patients with stable CAD. Current therapies and management have improved the prognosis of the disease substantially, with an annual mortality rate of 1% to 3% and a rate of major ischemic events of 1% to 2%. In contemporary clinical trials, patients with stable CAD have an annual rate of major cardiovascular events of 1.2–2.4% per annum.[2–4]

However, substantial heterogeneity in overall risk exists amongst patients with stable CAD with baseline cardiovascular risk factors, functional characteristics, and coronary anatomy each playing an important role. For example, in the international Reduction for Continued Health (REACH) Registry—which included asymptomatic adults with risk factors, patients with stable atherosclerosis, and individuals with prior ischemic events—large variations in cardiovascular risk between subgroups of patients were observed.[5] Patients with a prior history of ischemic events at baseline had the highest rate of subsequent ischemic events (18.3%); patients with stable coronary, cerebrovascular, or peripheral artery disease had a lower risk (12.2%); and patients without established atherothrombosis but with risk factors only had the lowest risk (9.1%) during 4-year follow-up.[5]

As might be expected, conventional risk factors for the development of CAD[6,7]—hypertension,[8] diabetes,[9] smoking,[10] hypercholesterolemia,[11] obesity,[12] and family history[13]—each retain their prognostic value in the context of established CAD. The prognosis for patients with stable CAD is also worsened in patients with reduced left ventricular ejection fraction,[14] by the severity and intensity of angina pectoris, with the presence of dyspnea,[15] and by the presence of three-vessel disease or left main disease.[16,17] The estimation of the long-term risk of adverse outcomes is crucial to effectively apply measures of secondary prevention and prevent overtreatment of patients at low risk of an adverse outcome, or under-treatment of patients at high risk of an adverse outcome.

Individual prognostic markers that are associated with adverse outcomes in stable CAD are summarized in Box 17.1.

PROGNOSIS IN SUBGROUPS

Coronary Artery Spasm

Although the pathophysiology is incompletely understood, known triggers for coronary vasospasm include smoking, electrolyte disturbances (potassium, magnesium), cocaine use, cold stimulation, autoimmune diseases, hyperventilation, or insulin resistance. The symptoms vary from silent myocardial ischemia to angina and even myocardial infarction. Long-term survival is usually good as long as patients

BOX 17.1 Risk Stratification Based on Noninvasive Testing

High Risk (> 3% Annual Risk for Death or Myocardial Infarction)

1. Severe resting left ventricular dysfunction (LVEF < 35%) not readily explained by noncoronary causes
2. Resting perfusion abnormalities involving ≥ 10% of the myocardium without previous known MI
3. High-risk stress findings on the ECG, including
   - ≥ 2 mm ST-segment depression at low workload or persisting into recovery
   - Exercise-induced ST-segment elevation
   - Exercise-induced VT/VF
4. Severe stress-induced LV dysfunction (peak exercise LVEF < 45% or drop in LVEF with stress ≥ 10%)
5. Stress-induced perfusion abnormalities encumbering ≥ 10% myocardium or stress segmental scores indicating multiple vascular territories with abnormalities
6. Stress-induced LV dilation
7. Inducible wall motion abnormality (involving more than two segments or two coronary beds)
8. Wall motion abnormality developing at low dose of dobutamine (≤ 10 mg/kg per min) or at a low heart rate (< 120 beats/min)
9. Multivessel obstructive CAD (≥ 70% stenosis) or left main stenosis (≥ 50% stenosis) on CCTA

Intermediate Risk (1–3% Annual Risk for Death or Myocardial Infarction)

1. Mild to moderate resting LV dysfunction (LVEF of 35–49%) not readily explained by noncoronary causes
2. Resting perfusion abnormalities involving 5–9.9% of the myocardium in patients without a history or previous evidence of MI
3. ST-segment depression of ≥ 1 mm occurring with exertional symptoms
4. Stress-induced perfusion abnormalities encumbering 5–9.9% of the myocardium or stress segmental scores (in multiple segments) indicating one vascular territory with abnormalities but without LV dilation
5. Small wall motion abnormality involving one to two segments and only one coronary bed
6. One-vessel CAD with ≥ 70% stenosis or moderate CAD stenosis (50–69% stenosis) in two or more arteries on CCTA

Low Risk (< 1% Annual Risk for Death or Myocardial Infarction)

1. Low-risk treadmill score (score ≥ 5) or no new ST-segment changes or exercise-induced chest pain symptoms when achieving maximal levels of exercise
2. Normal or small myocardial perfusion defect at rest or with stress encumbering < 5% of the myocardium*
3. Normal stress or no change in limited resting wall motion abnormalities during stress
4. No coronary stenosis > 50% on CCTA

*Although the published data are limited, patients with these findings will probably not be at low risk in the presence of either a high-risk treadmill score or severe resting LV dysfunction (LVEF < 35%).

CAC, Coronary artery calcium; *CAD*, coronary artery disease; *CCTA*, coronary computed tomography angiography; *ECG*, electrocardiogram; *LV*, left ventricular; *LVEF*, left ventricular ejection fraction; *MI*, myocardial infarction; *VF*, ventricular fibrillation; *VT*, ventricular tachycardia.

Modified from Fihn SD, et al. 2012 ACCF/AHA/ACP/AATS/PCNA/SCAI/STS Guideline for the diagnosis and management of patients with stable ischemic heart disease: a report of the American College of Cardiology Foundation/American Heart Association Task Force on Practice Guidelines, and the American College of Physicians, American Association for Thoracic Surgery, Preventive Cardiovascular Nurses Association, Society for Cardiovascular Angiography and Interventions, and Society of Thoracic Surgeons. *Circulation*. 2012;e354–471.

are on calcium antagonists and avoid smoking.[18,19] The incidence of cardiac death among patients with coronary artery spasm is up to 10% during 3 years of follow-up.[19] The prognosis of vasospastic angina depends on the extent of underlying CAD and on disease activity (frequency and duration of spastic episodes), the amount of myocardium at risk, and the presence of severe ventricular tachyarrhythmias or advanced atrioventricular block during ischemia.[20] The prognosis of vasospasm may be better in Japanese patients than patients of European ancestry, potentially due to differences in baseline characteristics, ascertainment of individuals of less severe disease, and fewer patients of Japanese ancestry having multivessel coronary spasm and/or reduced left ventricular function.[20a]

Women

Cardiovascular disease remains the leading cause of death in women and is responsible for 42% of premature deaths in women under the age of 75 years.[21] Although coronary heart disease develops 5–10 years later in women than in men and women have historically been at lower risk for CAD, more recent data indicate that the prevalence of cardiac events in men is decreasing, whereas women are experiencing an increase in cardiac events, including myocardial infarction.[22] Women have been underrepresented in cardiovascular clinical trials to date, representing 30% of participants in trials conducted since 2006, thus diminishing the quality of the evidence base available to guide therapy. The increasing recognition of heart disease in women is likely to stimulate key additional research in coming years.[23] The considerable decline in mortality from CAD is mainly caused by population-level improvements in risk factors and by improvements in primary and secondary prevention.[24–26]

Although the risk factors for CAD in women and men are similar, their distribution differs over time and between regions. Smoking seems to be associated with a higher relative risk of CAD in women than men,[27] and the prevalence of hypertension increases more with age in women than men, resulting in higher rates of stroke, hypertrophy of the left ventricle, and diastolic heart failure.[28] Diabetes is associated with a higher risk of CAD in women than in men.[29] Previously, circulating estrogens were believed to have a beneficial effect on the risk of CAD, but exogenous hormone administration has not led to a similar effect.[30]

Women and men of every age presenting with stable angina have increased coronary mortality relative to the general population, and several studies have indicated gender-related bias in care of both acute and chronic CAD.[31] However, in a large international prospective population (CLARIFY) of outpatients with stable CAD, the rates for cardiovascular clinical outcomes were similar between men and women at 1-year follow-up.[32]

Diabetes Mellitus (See Chapter 24)

Diabetes mellitus doubles the risk of major cardiovascular complications in patients with and in patients without established cardiovascular disease,[5,33] such that the majority of patients with diabetes die of cardiovascular diseases.[34] Patients with angina and concomitant type 2 diabetes mellitus often have more diffuse and extensive CAD compared with those without type 2 diabetes mellitus.[35] Furthermore, patients with CAD and type 2 diabetes may also have a greater burden of angina leading to a worsening prognosis.[35] If diabetes mellitus is accompanied by other coronary risk factors or target organ damage, the patient is considered to be at very high risk and maximal preventive efforts are warranted.[36] The control of risk factors appears to be efficacious in preventing future major adverse cardiovascular events in patients with stable CAD and diabetes mellitus.[37] The clinical manifestations of cardiovascular disease in diabetic patients are similar to those in nondiabetic patients. In particular, angina, myocardial infarction, and heart failure are the most prominent clinical manifestations in patients with diabetes and tend to occur at an earlier age. The cardiac assessment of symptomatic ischemia in diabetic patients should follow the same indications as for patients without diabetes. The Bypass Angioplasty Revascularization Investigation 2 Diabetes trial showed that patients with CAD and diabetes had the same risk of cardiovascular events and mortality regardless of whether or not they had angina symptoms.[38] Therefore, the management of CAD in these patients should not be predicated solely on the presence or absence of angina symptoms. However, routine screening for cardiovascular disease in asymptomatic patients is not currently recommended.[36] The greater degree of plaque burden together with comorbidity (e.g., renal failure) and smaller distal vessels in patients with diabetes influence the prognosis and may guide the choice of coronary revascularization strategy.[39,40]

Chronic Renal Failure

Chronic kidney disease is a risk factor for CAD and has a major impact on outcomes and therapeutic decisions within stable CAD. There are several risk factors in patients with chronic kidney disease that interact with the medical and diagnostic management of stable CAD and accelerate the development of CAD. Cardiovascular disease mortality is increased in patients with end-stage renal disease, therefore these patients should be monitored for symptoms suggestive of CAD. In CAD patients, the risk of sudden cardiac death is increased by 11% for every 10 mL/min decline in glomerular filtration rate.[41] Myocardial perfusion imaging carries prognostic value in end-stage renal disease patients who are asymptomatic for CAD, although the screening for asymptomatic patients is not currently in routine clinical use.[42,43] The work-up of suspected CAD in symptomatic patients with renal disease follows the same patterns as in patients with normal renal function. However, the presence of impaired renal function increases the pretest probability of CAD in patients who report chest pain, and noninvasive test results need to be interpreted accordingly. In addition, the use of iodinated contrast agent should be minimized in patients with preterminal renal failure and in dialysis patients with preserved urine production, in order to prevent contrast-induced nephropathy. Similarly, special attention should be paid to the drugs that are renally cleared and may need dose down-adjustment or substitution.

The same treatment options should be initiated in patients with CAD with or without renal insufficiency. Thus, treatment for risk modification should be initiated.[44] However, mortality rates and the risk of complications are high in this type of patient compared to those without impaired renal function.[45] In general, coronary bypass surgery is associated with higher procedural mortality and a greater likelihood of hemodialysis in nonhemodialysis-dependent patients after revascularization, while available studies suggest a trend toward better long-term survival, as compared with percutaneous coronary intervention (PCI).[46,47]

TOOLS FOR RISK ASSESSMENT

Medical History (See Chapter 7)

The approach to the patient with stable CAD starts with the medical history, in which several variables can provide important prognostic information and serve as an effective gatekeeper. Additional findings of heart failure or atherosclerosis in noncoronary vascular beds are associated with a poorer prognosis. Traditional models have estimated the likelihood of obstructive CAD rather than the risk of clinical events.[48] The pattern and duration of chest pain, and the frequency of chest pain, in addition to traditional risk factors for atherosclerosis, confer prognostic information.[49–51] In a study published in 2015, a model based on medical history–taking alone was able to identify a majority of patients with low risk (1%) of future clinical events (myocardial infarction and death) during 3 years of follow-up.[50]

Resting Electrocardiogram (See Chapter 10)

A normal resting electrocardiogram (ECG) is common in patients with stable CAD and may assist the clinician in differential diagnosis and defining the mechanisms of chest pain. Stable angina pectoris patients with an abnormal ECG are at greater risk of adverse outcomes than those with a normal ECG. A normal resting ECG suggests underlying normal left ventricular function whereas presence of a left bundle branch block on an ECG is associated with multivessel disease, impaired left ventricular function, and a poorer prognosis. ECG evidence of left ventricular dysfunction (left bundle branch block, nonspecific intraventricular conduction delays) is also a well-characterized indicator of adverse prognosis and increases the likelihood of future cardiac events almost twofold to fourfold.[52]

Exercise Testing (Treadmill Test) (See Chapter 10)

Exercise ECG is an important tool for risk stratification in patients with stable CAD. The exercise capacity is measured by maximum exercise duration, workload, and metabolic equivalent level. Maximum exercise capacity is one of the strongest prognostic markers and there are no major differences between the specific variables used to measure exercise capacity. The prognostic information is incorporated in the Duke treadmill score, which is well validated, and patients with a normal treadmill test have an excellent prognosis.[53] The Duke treadmill score classifies patients into three risk groups: low, moderate, and high. Mean annual mortality is 0.25% in the low-risk group and 5% in the high-risk group.[53] Cycle ergometry is an alternative to treadmill testing and is widely used in Europe. The work intensity can be adjusted by variations in resistance and cycling rate and is typically calculated in watts.

Echocardiography (See Chapter 11)

Echocardiography has a range of uses in ischemic heart disease including diagnosis, risk stratification, and clinical decision-making. Quantitative indices of global and regional systolic function are also valuable in describing left ventricular function, determining prognosis, and evaluating treatment outcome. Measurement of left ventricular ejection fraction is useful for risk stratification and is a strong predictor of adverse outcomes. Reduced left ventricular ejection fraction is associated with a high risk of cardiovascular death.[54] Echocardiography is also important for excluding other conditions such as significant valvular heart disease, pulmonary hypertension, or hypertrophic cardiomyopathy. The introduction of global longitudinal strain measurement may complement the traditional measurement of ejection fraction in the future, as the prognostic value of global longitudinal strain appears to be superior to that of ejection fraction for predicting major adverse cardiac events.[55]

The sensitivity of stress echocardiography averages approximately 88% (range, 76–94%), and its specificity is 83% for detecting myocardial ischemia in patients with stable CAD and carries prognostic information.[48,56] However, the diagnostic performance is dependent on the operator skills to obtain good image quality (adequate images can normally be obtained in more than 85% of patients, and the test is highly reproducible). The accuracy of stress echocardiography is in line with stress myocardial radionuclide perfusion imaging.[48] A normal result portends a good prognosis, whereas an abnormal result indicates an increased risk of cardiac events.[57]

Stress Perfusion Scintigraphy and Cardiac Magnetic Resonance Imaging (See Chapters 12 and 13)

Myocardial perfusion imaging using single photon emission computed tomography (SPECT) is a useful tool in risk stratification of patients with stable CAD.[58] On the one hand, among individuals with stable CAD and a normal stress imaging result, the annual cardiac mortality and myocardial infarction rate is similar to the general population.[31] On the other hand, stress-induced reversible perfusion defects of greater than 10% of the total myocardium are associated with a poor prognosis.[59,60] However, myocardial perfusion imaging has limited sensitivity for the detection of high-risk CAD, but a normal global coronary flow reserve (CFR) seems to be helpful in excluding the presence of high-risk CAD on angiography.[61,62] A growing body of evidence supports the prognostic ability of absolute flow when quantified by cardiac positron emission tomography (PET) showing that intact CFR is associated with a favorable prognosis during follow-up of up to 5 years.[63] Mechanistically, a reduced CFR leads to a worse prognosis either through a severe, focal defect and its future risk of plaque rupture with an acute coronary syndrome, or through a global flow reduction that serves as a marker for diffuse disease and overall CAD burden.[63]

Evidence of the prognostic value of stress cardiac magnetic resonance and outcome is more limited but, in general, the same principles as for SPECT are shared. Thus, stress-induced reversible wall abnormalities of greater than 10% of the left ventricle are associated with a high-risk situation (Fig. 17.1).[64]

Coronary Computed Tomography Angiography (See Chapter 13)

Noninvasive coronary computed tomography angiography (CTA) is very sensitive in detecting obstructive CAD, but is limited in its positive predictive value. Therefore, at present, the strength of CTA is its ability to exclude significant CAD with a high negative predictive value. In addition, CTA does not assess the functional significance of visualized lesions and often leads to further evaluation with either stress testing or invasive angiography, or both.[65] However, new technologies with CTA are now available to estimate the functional significance of individual coronary lesion flow (fractional flow reserve).[66,67]

Risk stratification using CTA is well established and large prospective international multicenter studies have demonstrated that the extent and severity of CAD is associated with all-cause mortality and demonstrated the independent prognostic value of both obstructive as well as nonobstructive CAD by CTA.[68] However, the clinical event rate is very low in the absence of any coronary plaque or with plaque, but without stenosis (Fig. 17.2).[65,68–71]

Coronary Angiography (See Chapter 14)

Coronary angiography provides important information both in the diagnosis of CAD and in assessing the risk of cardiovascular events. In the stable angina setting, coronary angiography provides information on the number of vessels involved.[72] The severity is assessed by the overall number of lesions, lesion location, severity, and the extent of involvement of branch vessels.[31]

The classification of disease into single-, double-, or triple-vessel or left main CAD is the most widely used and can be translated into prognostic information (Fig. 17.3). The SYNTAX (Synergy Between Percutaneous Coronary Intervention with Taxus and Cardiac Surgery) score extends this simple classification, provides a detailed risk assessment of the severity of epicardial CAD, and has been validated.[16,17]

The angiogram is not always sufficient to characterize the coronary atheroma, and therefore advanced invasive imaging techniques, such as intravascular ultrasound and optical coherence tomography, are evolving as additional tools, but so far have not translated into prognostic information in patients with stable CAD.[72,73]

The functional significance of a stenosis can be measured by fractional flow reserve (FFR). FFR is calculated as the ratio of distal coronary pressure to aortic pressure measured during maximal hyperemia. A normal value for FFR (> 0.80) indicates that a stenosis is not flow limiting and the prognosis is therefore excellent (< 1% risk of cardiovascular event).[74]

Genetic Testing (See Chapter 3)

Long known to be a heritable condition, genetic analyses have validated more than 50 loci across the genome that are independently related to risk of coronary disease.[75] A genetic risk score based on a combination of 27 such variants was recently shown to predict risk of recurrent coronary events in participants from the CARE (Cholesterol and Recurrent Events) and PROVE-IT TIMI 22 (Pravastatin or Atorvastatin Evaluation and Infection Therapy–Thrombolysis in Myocardial Infarction 22) clinical trials.[76] For example, those in the top quintile of the genetic risk score had a hazard ratio of 1.81 (95% confidence interval [CI] 1.22–2.67) for incident events. Furthermore, enhanced relative and absolute risk reduction was noted with statin/higher-intensity statin therapy within this subgroup. This finding has led to the hypothesis that identification of patients at increased genetic risk may allow for tailored therapy.

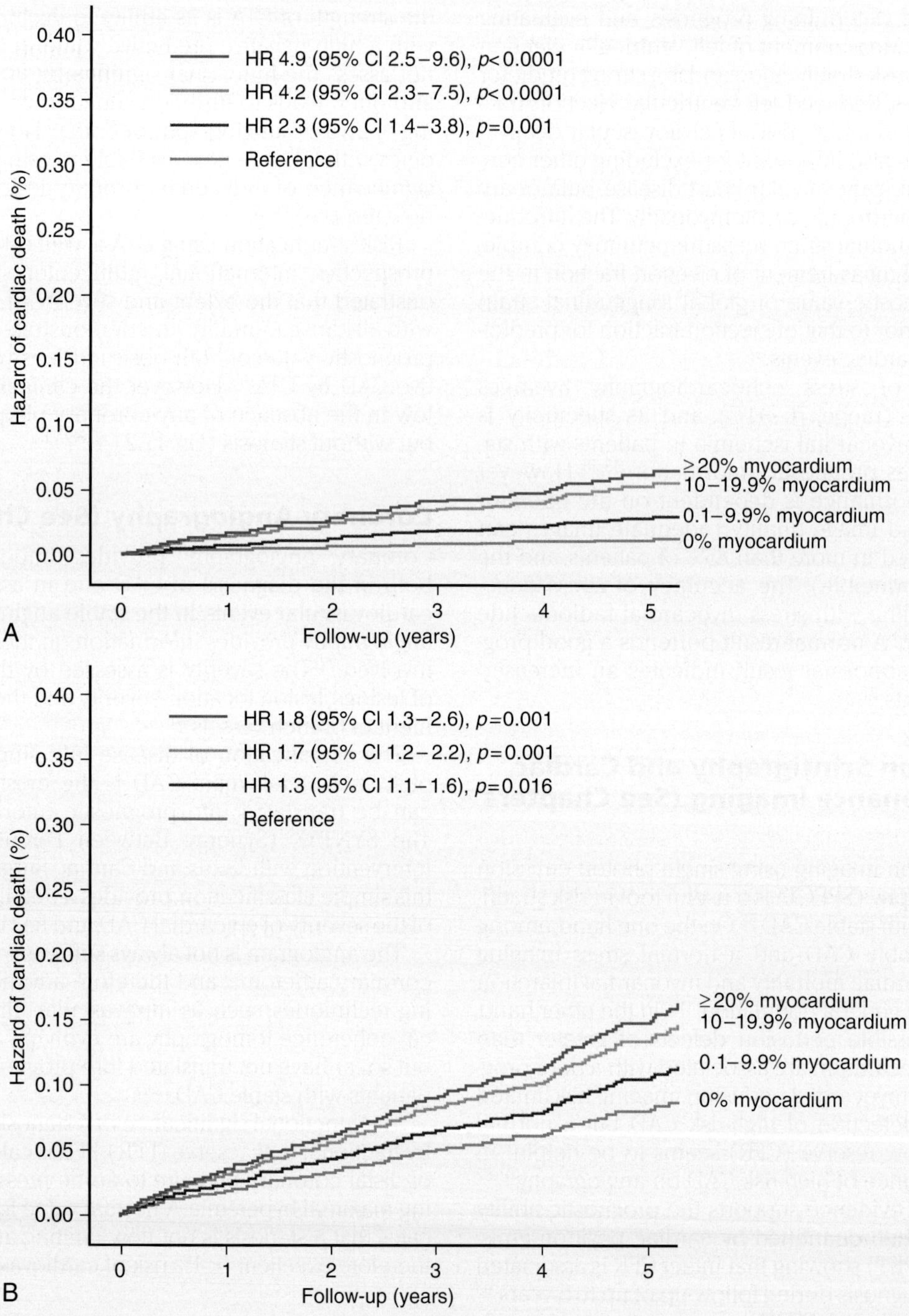

FIG. 17.1 Risk-adjusted hazard of events by percent myocardium abnormal on vasodilator stress Rb-82 PET. Hazard of (A) cardiac death (6037 patients, 169 cardiac deaths) and (B) all-cause death (7061 patients, 570 all-cause deaths) was lowest in patients with normal PET myocardial perfusion imaging and increased gradually in patients with minimal, mild, moderate, and severe degrees of scan abnormality. *CI,* Confidence interval; *HR,* hazard ration; *PET,* positron emission tomography. *(Modified from Dorbala S, Di Carli MF, Beanlands RS, et al. Prognostic value of stress myocardial perfusion positron emission tomography: results from a multicenter observational registry.* J Am Coll Cardiol. *2013;61:176.)*

MULTIVARIABLE RISK PREDICTION MODELS IN CHRONIC CORONARY ARTERY DISEASE

Informal methods of risk prediction, such as identification of clinical signs, symptoms, or biomarkers associated with adverse outcomes, have long been applied in the treatment of chronic CAD to identify individuals who may benefit from more intensive therapy.[15] However, informal methods of risk stratification or use of single markers to predict risk have significant disadvantages. First, observed rates of adverse outcomes may vary substantially among individuals who have a prognostic marker associated with adverse outcomes due to the presence of other observed and unobserved risk factors. For example, both age and the presence of comorbidities such as diabetes and heart failure influence the prognosis of patients with chronic CAD.[77] Second, the ability of clinicians to estimate the likelihood of patients' outcomes using clinical signs and symptoms may be poorly related to patients' observed risk of adverse outcomes.[78]

Global risk scores that quantitatively estimate patients' absolute risk of outcomes using multiple variables can avoid these disadvantages. Quantitative risk scores can allow physicians to predict patients' absolute risk of adverse outcomes using greater information and with greater consistency than

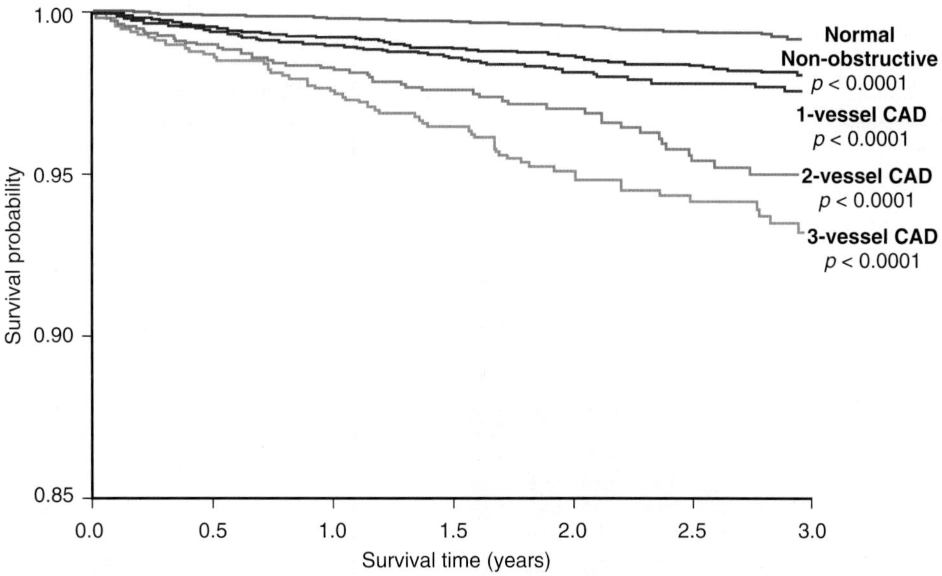

At risk	Year 0	Year 1	Year 2	Year 3
Normal	10,146	9357	5800	2907
Non-obstructive	8114	7437	4081	1930
1-vessel	3118	2873	1747	782
2-vessel	1346	1228	742	324
3-vessel/left main	1130	1034	664	324

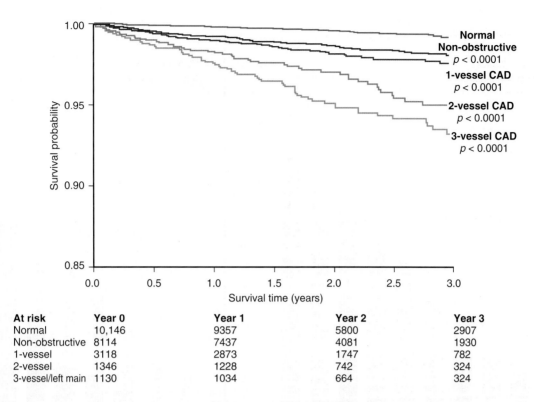

FIG. 17.2 Unadjusted all-cause 3-year Kaplan-Meier survival by the presence, extent, and severity of CAD by CCTA. Note the dose-response relationship of mortality to increasing numbers of vessels with obstructive CAD. *CAD*, Coronary artery disease; *CCTA*, coronary computed tomography angiography. *(Modified from Min JK, Dunning A, Lin FY, et al. Age- and sex-related differences in all-cause mortality risk based on coronary computed tomography angiography findings results from the International Multicenter CONFIRM (Coronary CT Angiography Evaluation for Clinical Outcomes: An International Multicenter Registry) of 23,854 patients without known coronary artery disease.* J Am Coll Cardiol. *2011;58:849.)*

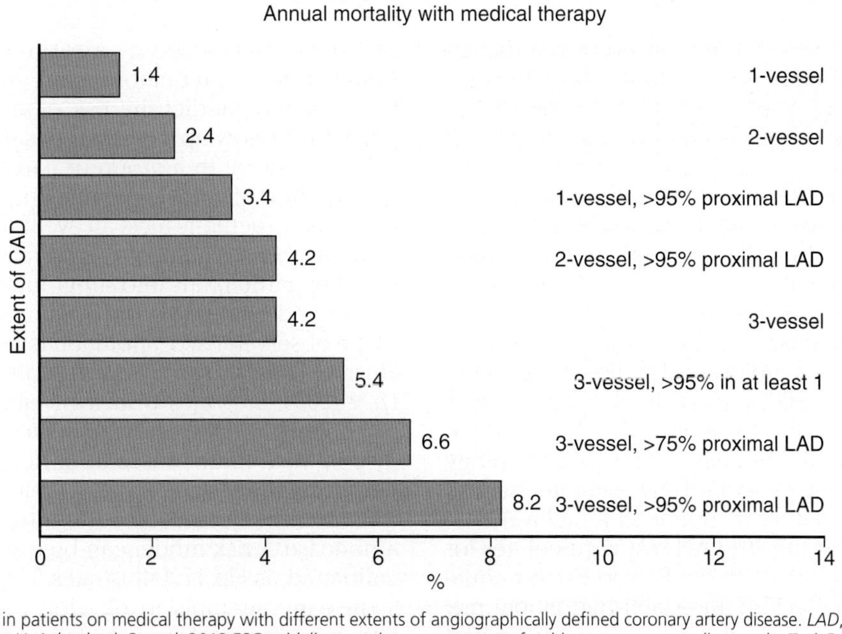

FIG. 17.3 Cardiac death rates in patients on medical therapy with different extents of angiographically defined coronary artery disease. *LAD*, Left anterior descending. *(Modified from Montalescot G, Sechtem U, Achenbach S, et al. 2013 ESC guidelines on the management of stable coronary artery disease: the Task Force on the management of stable coronary artery disease of the European Society of Cardiology.* Eur Heart J. *2013;34:2949–3003; and Mark DB, Nelson CL, Califf RM, et al. Continuing evolution of therapy for coronary artery disease. Initial results from the era of coronary angioplasty.* Circulation. *1994;89:2015–2025.)*

a single sign or symptom.[15] Indeed, use of multivariable risk prediction models to guide therapy for the primary prevention of cardiovascular disease has become common and has been the focus of intensive research over the past two decades.[79]

The Framingham Coronary Heart Disease risk model has been widely applied to predict risk of coronary heart disease among individuals without cardiovascular disease[79] and has been recently extended to prediction of cardiovascular events including stroke.[80] For the 2013 American Heart Association/American College of Cardiology (AHA/ACC) guidelines on the initiation of statin therapy, the Pooled Cohort equations were developed to predict cardiovascular risk and identify individuals at greater than 7.5% risk

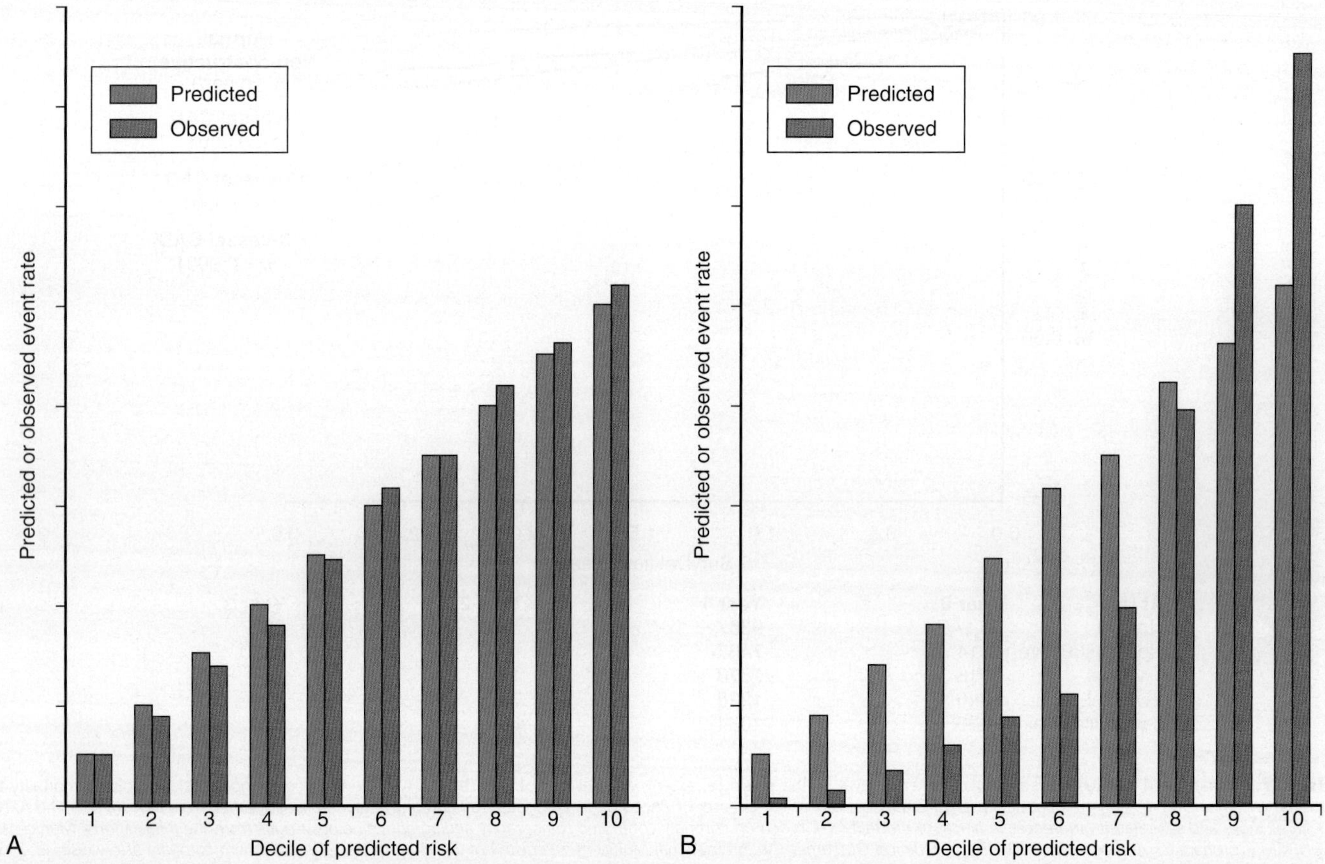

FIG. 17.4 Examples of models which are (A) well calibrated and discriminatory and (B) discriminatory but not well calibrated. *(Modified from Lloyd-Jones DM. Cardiovascular risk prediction: basic concepts, current status, and future directions.* Circulation. *2010;121:1768–1777.)*

of a hard atherosclerotic cardiovascular event (cardiovascular death, myocardial infarction, or stroke) over 10 years for potential initiation of statin therapy.[11,81] In the United Kingdom, the QRISK2 score has been developed to predict risk of a cardiovascular event and has also been incorporated into National Institute for Health and Care Excellence guidelines for the initiation of statin therapy.[82] A 2011 systematic review on cardiovascular risk prediction identified more than one hundred different risk models aiming to predict incident cardiovascular disease.[83]

In contrast to the intensive research into risk models for primary prevention of cardiovascular disease, research into risk prediction of cardiovascular disease among individuals with chronic CAD has been limited.[15] Although the 2014 AHA/ACC[48] and 2013 European Society of Cardiology guidelines[31] on treatment of stable CAD recommend risk assessment of patients, neither recommend a multivariable risk assessment model, as the 2013 AHA/ACC guidelines for initiation of statin therapy do with the Pooled Cohort equations,[11] likely due to the lack of an established global risk score. This section will review the comparatively limited research on multivariable risk prediction models in chronic CAD, including current multivariable risk models that use traditional risk factors, research into novel markers to improve risk prediction, and limitations of current models for risk prediction in chronic CAD.

Risk Prediction Using Multivariable Models

Although numerous statistical methods have been developed to characterize risk prediction models, they can be broadly characterized by measures of calibration and discrimination.[79] Calibration refers to the ability of models to accurately predict the risk of an event observed over a period of follow-up. For example, if a model estimates the risk of an event in a group of participants to be 7% over a given period of follow-up, while only 3.5% of participants are observed to actually have an event, the model would be considered poorly calibrated. Calibration can be assessed by dividing participants into subgroups (often tenths of participants) and comparing the predicted risk in each subgroup to the observed risk. Calibration is often quantified using the Hosmer-Lemeshow chi-square statistic, which, if significant ($p < 0.05$), indicates a lack of calibration. Discrimination, in contrast to calibration, refers to the ability of models to discriminate future cases from noncases. It is often quantified using the C-statistic, which refers to the probability that a randomly selected case has a higher predicted risk than a noncase. A risk model can be discriminatory, but not well calibrated, as Fig. 17.4 illustrates.[79]

In early attempts to develop multivariable risk prediction models in CAD, quantitative measures of discrimination and calibration were inconsistently reported (Table 17.1).[15,31,39,77,84–88] For example, one of the first multivariable models to be developed for patients with CAD, published in 1988, was a risk score developed from a database of all patients undergoing cardiac catheterization at Duke.[31] Stepwise selection was used to identify significant predictors of risk of death or myocardial infarction over a median 22 months of follow-up, with ejection fraction, number of diseased vessels, left main stenosis, angina score, age, and sex included in the final model. The dataset was divided into

TABLE 17.1 Multivariable Risk Prediction Models Using Traditional Risk Factors Developed for Predicting Events in Stable CAD

NAME OF MODEL (AUTHOR)	YEAR OF PUBLICATION	ENDPOINT(S)	POPULATION	PREDICTOR VARIABLES	DISCRIMINATION	CALIBRATION	VALIDATED IN AN EXTERNAL COHORT?	VALIDATED BY EXTERNAL RESEARCHERS?	OTHER LIMITATIONS
Duke (Califf et al.)	1988	Death and nonfatal MI	5886 participants with CAD	Demographic and clinical characteristics	Not assessed	Visually assessed through KM curves	No	No	Single center, baseline 1971
LIPID (Marschner et al.)	2001	CHD death and nonfatal MI	8557 participants with stable CAD and a history of myocardial infarction	Demographic and clinical characteristics	Visually assessed	Visually assessed	No	Yes, C-statistic = 0.61[25]	Baseline 1990
TIBET (Daly et al.)	2003	Cardiac death, nonfatal MI, unstable angina	682 participants with stable angina	Demographic, clinical, and noninvasive test variables	Not assessed	Not assessed	No	No	Baseline before 1995
ACTION (Clayton et al.)	2005	Death, MI or stroke	1063 participants with stable angina	Demographic, clinical, and noninvasive test variables	Visually assessed	Visually assessed	No	No	Baseline 1996
Olmsted County (Miller et al.)	2005	1.Death 2.Cardiac death 3.Cardiac death or nonfatal MI	3546 participants undergoing stress testing for CAD	Demographic and clinical variables	Not assessed	Not assessed	No	No	Baseline 1987
Euro Heart Angina (Daly et al.)	2006	1. Death and nonfatal MI 2. Cardiovascular event	3031 participants with stable angina	Clinical and test variables	C-statistic = 0.74	Not assessed	No	No	
PEACE (Hsia et al.)	2008	Sudden cardiac death	8290 participants with stable CAD	Demographic, clinical, and test variables	C-statistic = 0.71	Not assessed	No	No	
Duke SCD (Atwater et al.)	2009	Sudden cardiac death	37,258 participants with angiographic CAD	Demographic, clinical, and test variables	C-statistic = 0.75	Visually assessed	Yes, C-statistic = 0.64	No	Baseline 1985
VILCAD (Goliasch et al.)	2012	Death	547 participants with stable CAD	Demographic, clinical, and test variables	C-statistic = 0.77	Not assessed	Yes, C-statistic = 0.73	No	
EUROASPIRE (De Bacquer et al.)	2013	Cardiovascular death	5216 participants with CAD	Demographic, clinical, and test variables	No	No	No	No	Baseline 1995
EUROPA (Battes et al.)	2013	1. Cardiovascular death 2. Cardiovascular death, nonfatal MI, and cardiac arrest Other endpoints	12,218 participants with stable CAD	Demographic and clinical variables	C-statistic = 0.70	Visually assessed	No	No	
CALIBER (Rapsomaniki et al.)	2014	1. Death 2. CAD death or nonfatal MI	102,023 participants with CAD	Demographic and clinical variables	C-statistic = 0.81	Visually assessed	Yes, C-statistic = 0.74	No	

CAD, coronary artery disease; *CHD*, coronary heart disease; *KM*, Kaplan-Meier; *MI*, myocardial infarction.

NOTE: Prakash et al. risk score was excluded as it examined individuals referred for exercise testing (not known CAD). Framingham Secondary Model was *excluded* as it included participants after ischemic stroke. Acampa et al. risk score was excluded as it was restricted to post CABG.

a training set, used to develop the model, and validation set, which was used to roughly examine the calibration of the final model. Kaplan-Meier curves for the model in the training set and the validation set overlapped, suggesting that the model was reasonably calibrated. However, quantitative measures of discrimination and calibration, such as the C-statistic or predicted versus observed event rate, were not reported.

In contrast to the modest attempt to visually evaluate the calibration of the Duke model, measures of calibration and discrimination were not reported at all for the Total Ischaemic Burden European Trial (TIBET) model.[31] Published in 2003, this model was developed to predict risk of coronary heart disease events (cardiac death, myocardial infarction, or unstable angina) at 2-year follow-up from 612 participants. Four variables were selected for inclusion in the model after stepwise regression: coronary artery bypass grafting (yes or no), left ventricular hypertrophy (yes or no), end-diastolic dimension, and time to 1-mm ST depression on exercise. Two-year probability of coronary heart disease ranged from a minimum of 3% to a maximum of 79%. No effort was made to compare predicted risks to observed risks (calibration) or the ability of the model to discriminate between cases and noncases (discrimination). The performance of the model is thus unknown and it should not be used in clinical practice.

The A Coronary disease Trial Investigating Outcome with Nifedipine GITS (ACTION) trial model, published 2 years later in 2005 and available as an online calculator (http://www.anginarisk.org/), was developed to predict risk of all-cause death, myocardial infarction, and stroke in a cohort of 7311 participants with stable angina over 5 years of follow-up. Forward stepwise selection was used to choose variables, with significant variables ($p < 0.001$) included in the model. The strongest predictor of risk was age, followed by mean ejection fraction, current smoking, and white blood cell count. Model calibration was assessed visually by comparing observed risk in tenths of participants to predicted risk. Risk in the bottom tenth was 4% whereas risk in the top tenth was 36% (Fig. 17.5). The model appeared well calibrated, with similar levels of observed and predicted risk across tenths, although quantitative methods of assessing calibration and discrimination were again not reported.

A 2014 publication of a risk prediction model for stable CAD from the CArdiovascular disease research using Linked Bespoke studies and Electronic health Records (CALIBER) cohort represented a methodological advancement over these prior reports.[77] This model used variables from routinely collected electronic health records in United Kingdom general practices to predict risk of all-cause death and risk of myocardial infarction/coronary death over a mean of 4.4 years. These variables included age, sex, deprivation (socioeconomic status), CAD subtype, history of myocardial infarction, traditional cardiovascular risk factors (smoking, hypertension, diabetes, cholesterol), cardiovascular and noncardiovascular morbidities, depression, anxiety, and biomarkers (heart rate, creatinine, white cell count, and hemoglobin). Among the 102,023 patients for whom the model was developed, the C-index was 0.81 (95% CI 0.81–0.82) for all-cause mortality and 0.78 (CI 0.77–0.79) for nonfatal myocardial infarction or cardiovascular death, suggesting excellent discrimination. The model also appeared well calibrated when visually assessed, although a Hosmer-Lemeshow chi-square statistic was not reported. When the model was tested on a new cohort (the Appropriateness of Coronary Revascularization study), discrimination was moderate (C-statistic 0.74, CI 0.72–0.76, for all-cause mortality and C-statistic 0.72, CI 0.70–0.74, for nonfatal myocardial infarction/cardiovascular death) although the model appeared well calibrated. In addition to examining measures

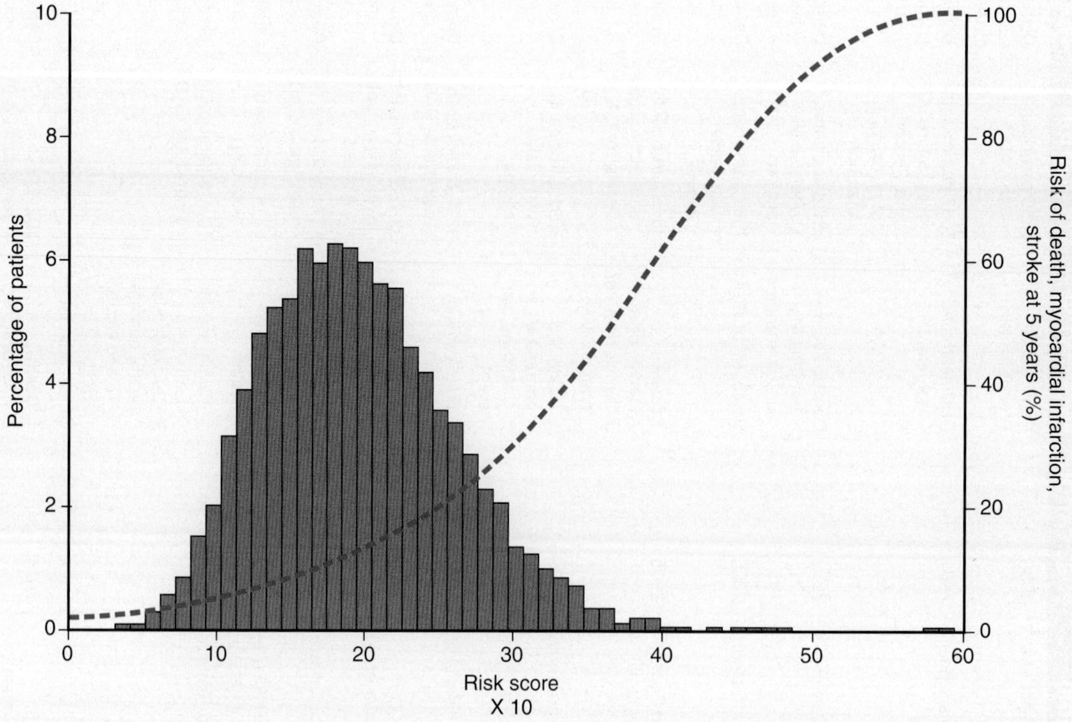

FIG. 17.5 Distribution of ACTION risk score and risk of death, myocardial infarction, or disabling stroke at 5 years. *ACTION*, A Coronary disease Trial Investigating Outcome with Nifedipine GITS. *(Adapted from Clayton TC, Lubsen J, Pocock SJ, et al. Risk score for predicting death, myocardial infarction, and stroke in patients with stable angina, based on a large randomised trial cohort of patients.* BMJ. *2005;331(7521):869.)*

of discrimination and calibration, the authors also modeled the clinical impact of use of the model, assuming that high-risk patients could be more intensively treated to reduce their risk of all-cause death or coronary heart disease by 20%. They estimated that screening 1000 participants with their model would lead to 15 life-years relative to a model that used only demographic characteristics (Fig. 17.6). The methodological approach of the authors, including evaluating the performance of the model in both a derivation cohort and a validation cohort, and estimating the clinical impact of their model, is an improvement over prior reports of risk prediction models in chronic CAD and should be adopted in future research into risk prediction in chronic coronary disease.

Table 17.1 summarizes reported multivariable risk prediction models for use in patients with chronic CAD. The majority of the models predict death or cardiovascular death as the outcome, although two models (Duke SCD and Prevention of Events with Angiotensin-Converting Enzyme Inhibition [PEACE]) predict sudden cardiac death. Eleven of the 12 models included demographic variables such as age and sex as predictors, whereas all of the models included clinical variables, such as the presence of comorbidities, as predictors. Seven of the 11 models included test variables, such as measures of ejection fraction, as predictors.

Almost all of the models reported in Table 17.1 are not suitable for clinical use for two reasons. First, many of the models do not report measures of discrimination or calibration, preventing their performance from being compared to other risk prediction models or evaluated by clinicians. Without metrics of calibration and discrimination, it is unclear how the models can be expected to stratify patients' risks of events. Second, the majority of the models do not report an attempt to validate the model in an external cohort. Validation of models in a new cohort is important, as a model will typically show overly optimistic results on the cohort from which the model was developed.[89] To estimate how the models would perform in a novel setting, they must be applied to external cohorts.

The CALIBER,[77] VILCAD,[90] LIPID,[15] and Duke SCD[86] models are the exceptions to these limitations, as calibration and discrimination were assessed and these models were validated in an external cohort (see Table 17.1). It would therefore seem reasonable to use these models for prediction of risk in chronic CAD in similar populations from which they were derived (European populations for CALIBER and VILCAD, Australian populations for LIPID, and American populations for Duke SCD). However, only the LIPID model has been validated by external investigators. In addition, the discrimination and calibration of predictive models can vary substantially by geographic region,[89] so without further validation studies, use of these models in different geographic settings may not be prudent. The Duke SCD model was also derived in patients presenting from as early as 1987, making it unclear if it would be well calibrated in current populations.

Novel Markers to Improve Risk Prediction

Numerous risk markers have been shown to be associated with cardiovascular events in the primary and secondary prevention setting. Inflammatory markers such as C-reactive protein and interleukin-6, and cardiovascular function markers such as B-type natriuretic peptide and high-sensitivity cardiac troponin T, among other markers, have been demonstrated to be associated with secondary cardiovascular events in CAD.[91–93] However, demonstration of a significant association with cardiovascular events, after controlling for traditional risk factors, is not sufficient to demonstrate that a marker improves risk prediction. Traditional risk factors may be easier and less costly to capture, and addition of a novel marker may not add clinically important information to traditional risk factors, even if it is significantly associated.[94] To evaluate whether novel markers improve risk prediction,

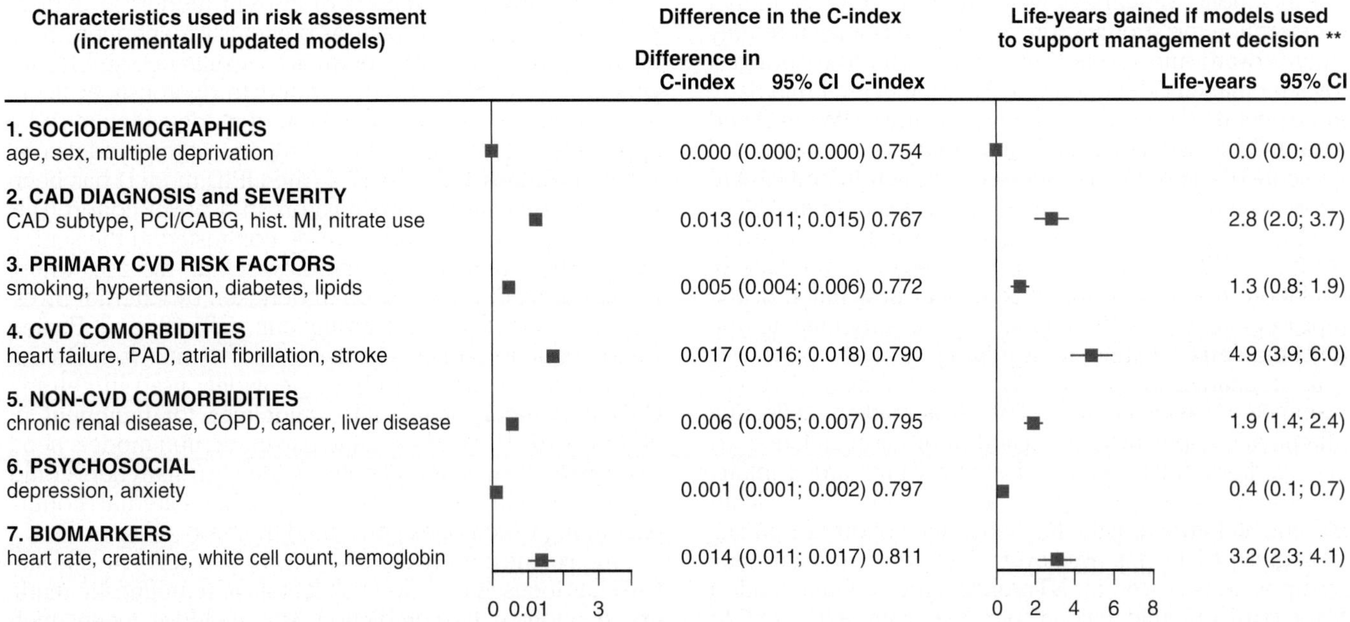

Characteristics used in risk assessment (incrementally updated models)
Difference in the C-index
Difference in C-index
95% CI
C-index
Life-years gained if models used to support management decision **
Life-years
95% CI
1. SOCIODEMOGRAPHICS
age, sex, multiple deprivation
0.000 (0.000; 0.000) 0.754
0.0 (0.0; 0.0)
2. CAD DIAGNOSIS and SEVERITY
CAD subtype, PCI/CABG, hist. MI, nitrate use
0.013 (0.011; 0.015) 0.767
2.8 (2.0; 3.7)
3. PRIMARY CVD RISK FACTORS
smoking, hypertension, diabetes, lipids
0.005 (0.004; 0.006) 0.772
1.3 (0.8; 1.9)
4. CVD COMORBIDITIES
heart failure, PAD, atrial fibrillation, stroke
0.017 (0.016; 0.018) 0.790
4.9 (3.9; 6.0)
5. NON-CVD COMORBIDITIES
chronic renal disease, COPD, cancer, liver disease
0.006 (0.005; 0.007) 0.795
1.9 (1.4; 2.4)
6. PSYCHOSOCIAL
depression, anxiety
0.001 (0.001; 0.002) 0.797
0.4 (0.1; 0.7)
7. BIOMARKERS
heart rate, creatinine, white cell count, hemoglobin
0.014 (0.011; 0.017) 0.811
3.2 (2.3; 4.1)
0 0.01 3
0 2 4 6 8

FIG. 17.6 Progressive addition of variables to model and changes in C-index as well as life-years used if models used to support management decision. *CABG,* Coronary artery bypass grafting; *CAD,* coronary artery disease; *CI,* confidence interval; *COPD,* chronic obstructive pulmonary disease; *CVD,* cardiovascular disease; *MI,* myocardial infarction; *PAD,* peripheral arterial disease; *PCI,* percutaneous coronary intervention. *(Modified from Rapsomaniki E, Shah A, Perel P, et al. Prognostic models for stable coronary artery disease based on electronic health record cohort of 102 023 patients.* Eur Heart J. *2014;35(13):844–852.)*

they must be added into models and changes in model performance evaluated.

Comprehensive reviews of individual risk factors that have been suggested to improve risk prediction in chronic CAD are provided elsewhere.[79,95] Among the best studied risk factors, however, have been markers of cardiovascular function, particularly B-type natriuretic peptides[93] and cardiac troponins T and I.[32,96] In a systematic review of B-type natriuretic peptides that included seven studies conducted in populations with stable cardiovascular disease, inclusion of B-type natriuretic peptides led to modest improvements in discrimination, with increases in C-statistics increasing from 0.02 to 0.1.[93] In an analysis of the PEACE trial, inclusion of cardiac troponin T measured using a highly sensitive assay led to an increase in the C-statistic by approximately 0.02 and high-sensitivity cardiac troponin I led to an increase by 0.015 relative to a model with traditional risk factors.[96] In an analysis of the Dallas Heart Study, inclusion of high-sensitivity cardiac troponin T led to reclassification of participants and improved model fit.[32] Inflammatory markers, such as C-reactive protein, and markers of kidney function, such as cystatin C, have also been suggested to improve risk prediction in stable coronary heart disease.[15]

Whereas these analyses have examined whether introduction of a single variable improves risk prediction over a model containing traditional risk factors, a single binary risk factor, in isolation, requires an odds ratio of 9 or greater to achieve excellent discrimination.[79] As a single novel risk marker (or, indeed, any risk factor) is unlikely to have such a strong association with an outcome of interest, inclusion of multiple novel markers, each of which is modestly associated with the outcome of interest, may be more likely to substantially improve model performance in a clinically relevant manner.

Over the past 5 years, several studies have attempted to undertake such a multimarker approach to improve risk prediction and generate multivariable risk models containing novel markers (Table 17.2).[97–101] In the BIO-VILCAD study of 1275 patients with stable CAD, 135 novel biochemical and metabolic biomarkers were added into a Cox model to determine the strongest predictors of all-cause mortality using forward and reverse selection.[100] The four strongest novel biomarkers identified were N-terminal pro-brain natriuretic peptide (NT-proBNP), renin, 25-hydroxy vitamin D, and cystatin C. Inclusion of these four biomarkers in a traditional risk score of age, sex, heart rate, ejection fraction, and HbA1c led to a significant improvement in C-statistic from 0.73 to 0.78. However, when considering the very high likelihood of overfitting (135 different variables tested) and the lack of validation in a new cohort, it is unclear how much of the improvement in discrimination can be attributed to the novel biomarkers relative to overfitting.

In an analysis of the AtheroGene study, Schnabel et al.[97] examined the association of 12 novel biomarkers (reflecting inflammation, lipid metabolism, and cardiovascular function) with cardiovascular death and nonfatal myocardial infarction. The strongest associations with cardiovascular death and nonfatal myocardial infarction in the cohort of 1781 stable angina patients, followed over a median of 3.6 years of follow-up, were observed for NT-proBNP, growth-differentiation factor (GDF)-15, mid-regional pro-atrial natriuretic peptide, cystatin C, and mid-regional pro-adrenomedullin. When these five biomarkers were included in a model containing traditional risk factors, the C-statistic improved from 0.656 to 0.690 with improvements in classification of participants across clinically relevant risk categories. However, inclusion of the five biomarkers did not improve discrimination or reclassification relative to including the single strongest biomarker (NT-proBNP).

In a recent analysis of the Heart and Soul study,[101] six novel biomarkers were evaluated along with traditional risk factors for prediction of secondary events among individuals with stable CAD (912 participants with 202 cardiovascular events). The four strongest risk factors were NT-proBNP, high-sensitivity cardiac troponin T, urinary albumin:creatinine ratio, and smoking. Traditional risk factors, including age, sex, and ejection fraction, did not meaningfully improve discrimination and calibration. This four-predictor model with novel biomarkers was well calibrated and discriminating, with a C-statistic of 0.73 and similar rates of predicted and observed events. Importantly, the authors then validated their model in a separate cohort (the PEACE trial). Although the overall C-statistic was reduced in the validation cohort, addition of the novel risk factors to the model with traditional risk factors improved the C-statistic from 0.57 to 0.65.

Overall, these results suggest that use of novel biomarkers, particularly natriuretic peptides and high sensitivity cardiac troponins, has the potential to improve risk prediction in chronic CAD. Combining multiple markers in a multimarker approach appears to result in larger increases in model performance than use of a single marker.

Limitations of Current Models and Future Directions

Whereas development of models for risk prediction in chronic CAD has been limited relative to prediction of incident cardiovascular disease, there have been more than 10 models developed for risk prediction in chronic CAD that use either traditional risk factors or novel markers (see Tables 17.1 and 17.2). The major limitation to the use of global risk prediction models in chronic CAD is therefore not that risk prediction models have not been developed but is that the performance of current models in clinical practice is largely unknown. As previously mentioned, models typically show overly optimistic results on samples for which development was performed; to rigorously evaluate the calibration and discrimination of models, they must be applied to external cohorts.[89] Only one of the models presented in Tables 17.1 and 17.2 (the LIPID model) has been validated by external investigators in a novel cohort. This lack of external validation can be contrasted to the setting of primary prevention of cardiovascular disease, where numerous studies have been undertaken by external investigators validating the Framingham, QRisk2, and Pooled Cohort equations in novel cohorts.[102,103] If multivariable risk prediction models are to become widely used in chronic CAD, and incorporated into guidelines for treatment of chronic CAD,[48,56] multivariable risk prediction models need to be assessed in external cohorts. Ideally, researchers could compare multiple models in the same external cohort, examining which ones performed the best.

Much of the current research on risk prediction in chronic CAD has focused on novel risk factors and prognostic markers to improve risk prediction. This includes recent high profile analyses of the predictive value of natriuretic peptides, cardiac troponins, and inflammatory markers.[32,96,97] However, without well-validated models that clinicians can

TABLE 17.2 Multivariable Risk Prediction Models Using Multiple Novel Markers and Traditional Risk Factors Developed for Predicting Events in Stable CAD

NAME OF MODEL (AUTHOR)	YEAR OF PUBLICATION	ENDPOINT(S)	POPULATION	PREDICTOR VARIABLES	NOVEL BIOMARKERS INCLUDED IN FINAL MARKER	DISCRIMINATION	CALIBRATION	VALIDATED IN A NEW COHORT?	VALIDATED BY EXTERNAL RESEARCHERS?	OTHER LIMITATIONS
AtheroGene (Schnabel et al.)	2010	Cardiovascular death and nonfatal MI	1781 participants	Demographic, clinical, and noninvasive test variables	NT-proBNP, MR-proADM, MR-proANP, cystatin C, GDF-15	C-statistic = 0.69	Not assessed	No	No	Full model not reported in publication
TNT (Mora et al.)	2012	Major cardiovascular events	9251 participants with stable CAD	Demographic, clinical, and noninvasive test variables	Apolipoprotein A1, apolipoprotein B, blood urea nitrogen	C-statistic = 0.68	Not assessed	No	No	Full model not reported in publication
PEACE (Sabatine et al.)	2012	Cardiovascular death or heart failure	3717 participants with stable CAD	Demographic, clinical, and noninvasive test variables	MR-proANP, MR-proADM, CT-proET-1, copeptin	C-statistic = 0.81	Not assessed	No	No	
BIO-VILCAD (Kleber et al.)	2014	Death	1275 participants with stable CAD	Demographic, clinical, and noninvasive test variables	Pro-BNP, renin, 25-hydroxy vitamin D, cyastatin C	C-statistic = 0.78	Not assessed	No	No	
Heart and Soul (Beatty et al.)	2015	Cardiovascular death, MI, or stroke	912 participants with stable CAD	Demographic, clinical, and noninvasive test variables	NT-proBNP, Cardiac troponin T, albumin:creatinine	C-statistic = 0.73	*p*-value = 0.07, also visually assessed	Yes, C-statistic = 0.65	No	

CAD, coronary artery disease; *CT-proET-1*, C-terminal pro-endothelin-1; *GDF*, growth-differentiation factor; *KM*, Kaplan-Meier; *MI*, myocardial infarction; *MR-proADM*, midregional pro-adrenomedullin; *MR-proANP*, midregional pro-atrial natriuretic peptide; *NT-proBNP*, N-terminal pro-B-type natriuretic peptide.

TABLE 17.3 Current Examples of Therapies Tailored to Clinical Risk

DISEASE SUBTYPE	HIGH RISK DEFINITION	THERAPY	AUTHOR AND YEAR
Sudden cardiac death	Ischemic-cardiomyopathy and EF ≤ 30%	Implantable cardioverter defibrillator	Moss AJ et al. 2002
In-stent thrombosis	Drug-eluting stent implantation Prior MI	Dual antiplatelet therapy ≥12 months	Levine GN et al. 2011
Recurrent ischemic events vs. bleeding	Multivariable DAPT score	Dual antiplatelet therapy continuation beyond 12 months	Yeh RW et al. 2015
Multivessel disease in context of diabetes	High anatomic complexity (three-vessel disease or high SYNTAX score)	CABG preferred over PCI	Fihn SD et al. 2014

CABG, coronary artery bypass grafting; *DAPT*, dual antiplatelet therapy; *EF*, ejection fraction; *MI*, myocardial infarction; *PCI*, percutaneous coronary intervention; *SYNTAX*, Synergy Between Percutaneous Coronary Intervention with Taxus and Cardiac Surgery.

apply in practice and that novel models can be compared to, the value of such research is uncertain. Hopefully, in the future, risk prediction research in chronic CAD will consistently include evaluation and validation of current models in different settings, in addition to developing new models and examining new risk factors.

Aligning Therapy with Risk in Stable Coronary Heart Disease

The alignment of therapies according to individual patient risk is a key component of the widely endorsed "precision medicine" concept. Applied optimally, this strategy enables those at highest risk to gain benefit while protecting lower risk subgroups from the costs and potential side effects of a given therapeutic.

However, despite the conceptual appeal, this notion has proven difficult to apply to clinical medicine with only a few examples that are in current widespread use (Table 17.3). For example, observational evidence describing an increased risk of sudden cardiac death amongst those with an ischemic cardiomyopathy provided the foundation for the pivotal Multicenter Automatic Defibrillator Implantation Trial II (MADIT II trial), in which implantation of an implantable cardioverter defibrillator led to a 31% decrease in all-cause mortality.[104] The identification of an increased rate of in-stent thrombosis following drug-eluting stent implantation related to delayed endothelialization has led to a recommendation of dual antiplatelet therapy for at least 12 months.[105] Finally, the SYNTAX (Synergy Between Percutaneous Coronary Intervention with TAXUS and Cardiac Surgery) trial randomized 1800 patients with multivessel coronary disease to revascularization with either drug eluting stents or coronary artery bypass surgery. Post hoc analyses noted substantial decrements in cardiovascular events in those with intermediate to high anatomic CAD complexity but similar event rates in those with more straightforward anatomy.[106] This has led to a preference for coronary artery bypass grafting in those with complex/diffuse CAD, particularly in those with diabetes.[48]

The development of individualized therapy paradigms has proven challenging largely because it requires well-conceived identification of those at highest risk and subsequent application of an appropriate intervention. A recent *post hoc* analysis from the Bypass Angioplasty Revascularization in Type 2 Diabetes trial (BARI-2D) illustrated these challenges by successfully demonstrating a strong relationship between abnormal troponin T concentrations at baseline and incident cardiovascular events (hazard ratio [HR] 1.85, 95% CI 1.48–2.32).[107] However, random assignment of these high-risk individuals to revascularization, as compared to optimal medical therapy, did not lead to a reduction in cardiovascular events (HR 0.96 in both subgroups of those with normal and abnormal baseline troponin T). Similarly, although levels of LDL-cholesterol are predictive of incident cardiovascular events, the clinical benefit of statin therapy is largely uniform across a broad range of baseline LDL-C levels.[108]

Furthermore, cardiovascular therapeutics for ischemic heart disease often confers both benefits and potential side effects. Few efforts to date have sought to combine these endpoints into subpopulations that receive net clinical benefit. A recent example sought to guide clinicians deciding whether or not to continue dual antiplatelet therapy beyond the 12 months currently stipulated in ACC/AHA guidelines. The Dual Antiplatelet Therapy (DAPT) study investigators used multivariate models to predict both benefit (reduction in recurrent myocardial infarction or stent thrombosis) and risk (moderate/severe bleeding).[109] Although the overall discriminative ability for both endpoints was modest, the resulting score combines clinical characteristics to predict overall net clinical utility of drug continuation. The DAPT score awaits replication in similar clinical trial datasets prior to widespread clinical implementation.

Moving forward, the identification and combination of risk factors into scores that are appropriately calibrated and provide adequate discrimination will pave the way for confirmatory studies of their utility. Two conceptual frameworks exist to build this evidence base (Fig. 17.7). The traditional approach has been to conduct a trial in a broad population with subsequent subgroup analyses to assess for heterogeneity of effect (i.e., stratification of SYNTAX trial participants into subgroups based on anatomic complexity as previously discussed). This strategy increases efficiency in allowing investigators to test multiple subgroup hypotheses in a *post hoc* fashion. However, the multiple testing burden and power limitations of subgroup analyses often preclude definitive conclusions. An alternate approach involves the *a priori* definition of a high-risk patient population for a clinical trial, as in the restriction of the MADIT-II trial to participants with ischemic cardiomyopathy and a depressed ejection fraction. Although this allows for the most formal validation of the risk criteria, it requires an individual study to test each hypothesis and a successful intervention may lead some to wonder whether the findings are generalizable to the lower risk strata as well.

SUMMARY

Risk assessment is essential to effective medical decision-making for prevention in CAD (Fig. 17.8). A variety of clinical tools, including the most basic elements of the clinical history

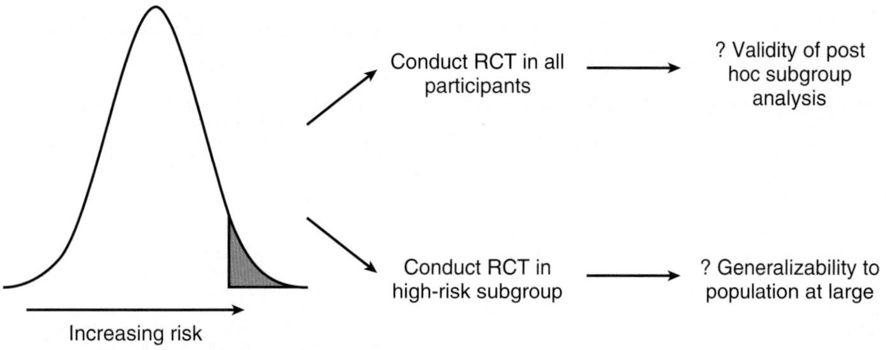

FIG. 17.7 Building the evidence base for precision medicine. *RTC*, Randomized controlled trial.

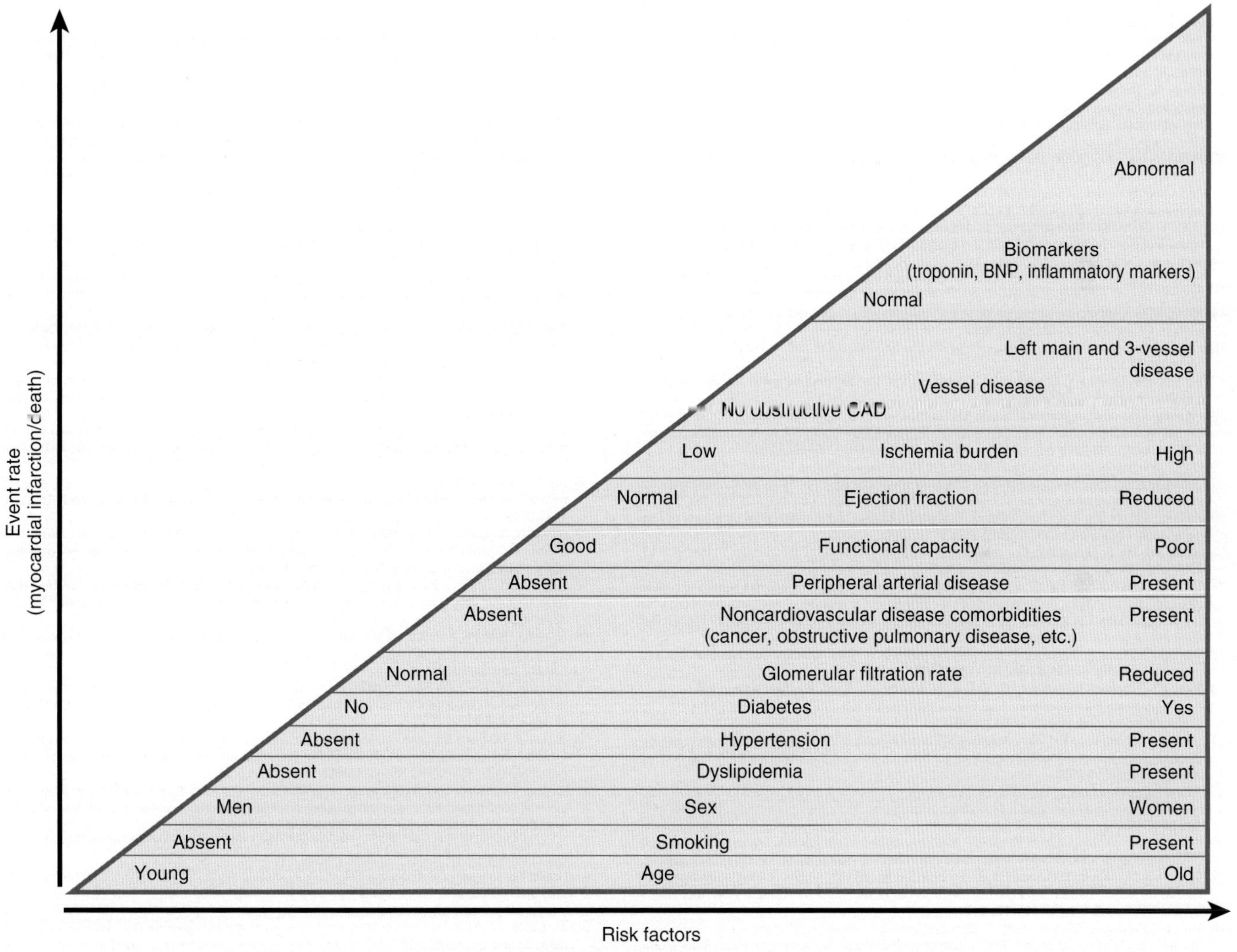

FIG. 17.8 Summary.

and the physical examination, provide valuable information on prognosis. In addition, data from the ECG, laboratory testing, and noninvasive and invasive imaging are complementary with respect to prognosis and can aid in informing patients and their families, directing triage, and guiding medical therapy. An integrated approach to risk assessment is optimal, and simple clinical risk scores can assist the clinician in assimilating the diverse sources of data on prognosis. Several multivariable risk models using traditional risk factors with and without multibiomarker approaches, have been developed for prediction of cardiovascular events in patients with stable CAD, but unfortunately they have not been assessed in external cohorts.

The alignment of therapy according to individual patient risk is a strategy that enables those at highest risk to benefit while protecting lower risk subgroups from the costs and potential side effects of a given therapy. This notion has proven difficult to apply to clinical medicine and indeed in patients with stable ischemic heart disease. This is an area for future research that may advance the extent to which the promise of personalized medicine can be realized in our routine care of patients with cardiovascular disease.

References

1. Lloyd-Jones D, Adams RJ, Brown TM, et al.: Heart disease and stroke statistics—2010 update: a report from the American Heart Association, *Circulation* 121:e46–e215, 2010.
2. Chung SC, Hlatky MA, Faxon D, et al.: The effect of age on clinical outcomes and health status BARI 2D (Bypass Angioplasty Revascularization Investigation in Type 2 Diabetes), *J Am Coll Cardiol* 58:810–819, 2011.
3. Frye RL, August P, Brooks MM, et al.: A randomized trial of therapies for type 2 diabetes and coronary artery disease, *N Engl J Med* 360:2503–2515, 2009.
4. Steg PG, Greenlaw N, Tardif JC, et al.: Women and men with stable coronary artery disease have similar clinical outcomes: insights from the international prospective CLARIFY registry, *Eur Heart J* 33:2831–2840, 2012.
5. Bhatt DL, Eagle KA, Ohman EM, et al.: Comparative determinants of 4-year cardiovascular event rates in stable outpatients at risk of or with atherothrombosis, *JAMA* 304:1350–1357, 2010.
6. Bayturan O, Kapadia S, Nicholls SJ, et al.: Clinical predictors of plaque progression despite very low levels of low-density lipoprotein cholesterol, *J Am Coll Cardiol* 55:2736–2742, 2010.
7. Chhatriwalla AK, Nicholls SJ, Wang TH, et al.: Low levels of low-density lipoprotein cholesterol and blood pressure and progression of coronary atherosclerosis, *J Am Coll Cardiol* 53: 1110–1115, 2009.
8. Nicholls SJ, Hsu A, Wolski K, et al.: Intravascular ultrasound-derived measures of coronary atherosclerotic plaque burden and clinical outcome, *J Am Coll Cardiol* 55:2399–2407, 2010.
9. Bayturan O, Tuzcu EM, Uno K, et al.: Comparison of rates of progression of coronary atherosclerosis in patients with diabetes mellitus versus those with the metabolic syndrome, *Am J Cardiol* 105:1735–1739, 2010.
10. Frey P, Waters DD, DeMicco DA, et al.: Impact of smoking on cardiovascular events in patients with coronary disease receiving contemporary medical therapy (from the Treating to New Targets [TNT] and the Incremental Decrease in End Points Through Aggressive Lipid Lowering [IDEAL] trials), *Am J Cardiol* 107:145–150, 2011.
11. Stone NJ, Robinson JG, Lichtenstein AH, et al.: 2013 ACC/AHA guideline on the treatment of blood cholesterol to reduce atherosclerotic cardiovascular risk in adults: a report of the American College of Cardiology/American Heart Association Task Force on Practice Guidelines, *Circulation* 129:S1–S45, 2014.
12. Perk J, De Backer G, Gohlke H, et al.: European Guidelines on cardiovascular disease prevention in clinical practice (version 2012). The Fifth Joint Task Force of the European Society of Cardiology and Other Societies on Cardiovascular Disease Prevention in Clinical Practice (constituted by representatives of nine societies and by invited experts), *Eur Heart J* 33:1635–1701, 2012.
13. Otaki Y, Gransar H, Berman DS, et al.: Impact of family history of coronary artery disease in young individuals (from the CONFIRM registry), *Am J Cardiol* 111:1081–1086, 2013.
14. Mentz RJ, Fiuzat M, Shaw LK, et al.: Comparison of clinical characteristics and long-term outcomes of patients with ischemic cardiomyopathy with versus without angina pectoris (from the Duke Databank for Cardiovascular Disease), *Am J Cardiol* 109:1272–1277, 2012.
15. Morrow DA: Cardiovascular risk prediction in patients with stable and unstable coronary heart disease, *Circulation* 121:2681–2691, 2010.
16. Head SJ, Farooq V, Serruys PW, Kappetein AP: The SYNTAX score and its clinical implications, *Heart* 100:169–177, 2014.
17. Serruys PW, Onuma Y, Garg S, et al.: Assessment of the SYNTAX score in the Syntax study, *EuroIntervention* 5:50–56, 2009.
18. Figueras J, Domingo E, Ferreira I, Lidon RM, Garcia-Dorado D: Persistent angina pectoris, cardiac mortality and myocardial infarction during a 12 year follow-up in 273 variant angina patients without significant fixed coronary stenosis, *Am J Cardiol* 110:1249–1255, 2012.
19. Ong P, Athanasiadis A, Borgulya G, Voehringer M, Sechtem U: 3-year follow-up of patients with coronary artery spasm as cause of acute coronary syndrome: the CASPAR (coronary artery spasm in patients with acute coronary syndrome) study follow-up, *J Am Coll Cardiol* 57:147–152, 2011.
20. Kusniec J, Iakobishvili Z, Haim M, et al.: Prinzmetal angina in the differential diagnosis of syncope, *Acute Card Care* 14:45–47, 2012.

20a. Hung MJ, Hu P, Hung MY: Coronary artery spasm: review and update, *Int J Med Sci* 11: 1161–1171, 2014.

21. Maas AH, van der Schouw YT, Regitz-Zagrosek V, et al.: Red alert for women's heart: the urgent need for more research and knowledge on cardiovascular disease in women: proceedings of the workshop held in Brussels on gender differences in cardiovascular disease, 29 September 2010, *Eur Heart J* 32:1362–1368, 2011.
22. Towfighi A, Zheng L, Ovbiagele B: Sex-specific trends in midlife coronary heart disease risk and prevalence, *Arch Intern Med* 169:1762–1766, 2009.
23. Mosca L, Mochari-Greenberger H, Dolor RJ, Newby LK, Robb KJ: Twelve-year follow-up of American women's awareness of cardiovascular disease risk and barriers to heart health, *Circ Cardiovasc Qual Outcomes* 3:120–127, 2010.
24. Hardoon SL, Whincup PH, Wannamethee SG, et al.: Assessing the impact of medication use on trends in major coronary risk factors in older British men: a cohort study, *Eur J Cardiovasc Prev Rehabil* 17:502–508, 2010.
25. Young F, Capewell S, Ford ES, Critchley JA: Coronary mortality declines in the U.S. between 1980 and 2000 quantifying the contributions from primary and secondary prevention, *Am J Prev Med* 39:228–234, 2010.
26. Wijeysundera HC, Machado M, Farahati F, et al.: Association of temporal trends in risk factors and treatment uptake with coronary heart disease mortality, 1994–2005, *JAMA* 303:1841–1847, 2010.
27. Grundtvig M, Hagen TP, German M, Reikvam A: Sex-based differences in premature first myocardial infarction caused by smoking: twice as many years lost by women as by men, *Eur J Cardiovasc Prev Rehabil* 16:174–179, 2009.
28. Mosca L, Benjamin EJ, Berra K, et al.: Effectiveness-based guidelines for the prevention of cardiovascular disease in women—2011 update: a guideline from the American Heart Association, *Circulation* 123:1243–1262, 2011.
29. Lee C, Joseph L, Colosimo A, Dasgupta K: Mortality in diabetes compared with previous cardiovascular disease: a gender-specific meta-analysis, *Diabetes Metab* 38:420–427, 2012.
30. Wild RA, Wu C, Curb JD, et al.: Coronary heart disease events in the Women's Health Initiative hormone trials: effect modification by metabolic syndrome: a nested case-control study within the Women's Health Initiative randomized clinical trials, *Menopause* 20:254–260, 2013.
31. Montalescot G, Sechtem U, Achenbach S, et al.: 2013 ESC guidelines on the management of stable coronary artery disease: the Task Force on the management of stable coronary artery disease of the European Society of Cardiology, *Eur Heart J* 34:2949–3003, 2013.
32. de Lemos JA, Drazner MH, Omland T, et al.: Association of troponin T detected with a highly sensitive assay and cardiac structure and mortality risk in the general population, *JAMA* 304: 2503–2512, 2010.
33. Preis SR, Hwang SJ, Coady S, et al.: Trends in all-cause and cardiovascular disease mortality among women and men with and without diabetes mellitus in the Framingham Heart Study, 1950 to 2005, *Circulation* 119:1728–1735, 2009.
34. Go AS, Mozaffarian D, Roger VL, et al.: Heart disease and stroke statistics—2013 update: a report from the American Heart Association, *Circulation* 127:e6–e245, 2013.
35. Deedwania PC: Management of patients with stable angina and type 2 diabetes, *Rev Cardiovasc Med* 16:105–113, 2015.
36. American Diabetes Association: Standards of medical care in diabetes—2013, *Diabetes Care* 36(Suppl 1):S11–S66, 2013.
37. Li S, Zhang Y, Guo YL, et al.: Effect of glycemic and lipid achievements on clinical outcomes type 2 diabetic, Chinese patients with stable coronary artery disease, *J Diabetes Complications* 30:115–120, 2015.
38. Dagenais GR, Lu J, Faxon DP, et al.: Prognostic impact of the presence and absence of angina on mortality and cardiovascular outcomes in patients with type 2 diabetes and stable coronary artery disease: results from the BARI 2D (Bypass Angioplasty Revascularization Investigation 2 Diabetes) trial, *J Am Coll Cardiol* 61:702–711, 2013.
39. Park DW, Kim YH, Song HG, et al.: Long-term outcome of stents versus bypass surgery in diabetic and nondiabetic patients with multivessel or left main coronary artery disease: a pooled analysis of 5775 individual patient data, *Circ Cardiovasc Interv* 5:467–475, 2012.
40. Farkouh ME, Domanski M, Sleeper LA, et al.: Strategies for multivessel revascularization in patients with diabetes, *N Engl J Med* 367:2375–2384, 2012.
41. Cai Q, Mukku VK, Ahmad M: Coronary artery disease in patients with chronic kidney disease: a clinical update, *Curr Cardiol Rev* 9:331–339, 2013.
42. De Vriese AS, De Bacquer DA, Verbeke FH, et al.: Comparison of the prognostic value of dipyridamole and dobutamine myocardial perfusion scintigraphy in hemodialysis patients, *Kidney Int* 76:428–436, 2009.
43. De Vriese AS, Vandecasteele SJ, Van den Bergh B, De Geeter FW: Should we screen for coronary artery disease in asymptomatic chronic dialysis patients? *Kidney Int* 81:143–151, 2012.
44. Baigent C, Landray MJ, Reith C, et al.: The effects of lowering LDL cholesterol with simvastatin plus ezetimibe in patients with chronic kidney disease (Study of Heart and Renal Protection): a randomised placebo-controlled trial, *Lancet* 377:2181–2192, 2011.
45. Zheng H, Xue S, Lian F, et al.: Meta-analysis of clinical studies comparing coronary artery bypass grafting with percutaneous coronary intervention in patients with end-stage renal disease, *Eur J Cardiothorac Surg* 43:459–467, 2013.
46. Ashrith G, Lee VV, Elayda MA, Reul RM, Wilson JM: Short- and long-term outcomes of coronary artery bypass grafting or drug-eluting stent implantation for multivessel coronary artery disease in patients with chronic kidney disease, *Am J Cardiol* 106:348–353, 2010.
47. Ashrith G, Elayda MA, Wilson JM: Revascularization options in patients with chronic kidney disease, *Tex Heart Inst J* 37:9–18, 2010.
48. Fihn SD, Blankenship JC, Alexander KP, et al.: 2014 ACC/AHA/AATS/PCNA/SCAI/STS focused update of the guideline for the diagnosis and management of patients with stable ischemic heart disease: a report of the American College of Cardiology/American Heart Association Task Force on Practice Guidelines, and the American Association for Thoracic Surgery, Preventive Cardiovascular Nurses Association, Society for Cardiovascular Angiography and Interventions, and Society of Thoracic Surgeons, *Circulation* 130:1749–1767, 2014.
49. Wilson PW, D'Agostino Sr R, Bhatt DL, et al.: An international model to predict recurrent cardiovascular disease, *Am J Med* 125:695–703 e1, 2012.
50. Min JK, Dunning A, Gransar H, et al.: Medical history for prognostic risk assessment and diagnosis of stable patients with suspected coronary artery disease, *Am J Med* 128:871–878, 2015.
51. Steg PG, Greenlaw N, Tendera M, et al.: Prevalence of anginal symptoms and myocardial ischemia and their effect on clinical outcomes in outpatients with stable coronary artery disease: data from the International Observational CLARIFY Registry, *JAMA Intern Med* 174:1651–1659, 2014.
52. Haataja P, Anttila I, Nikus K, et al.: Prognostic implications of intraventricular conduction delays in a general population: the Health 2000 Survey, *Ann Med* 47:74–80, 2015.
53. Cheezum MK, Subramaniyam PS, Bittencourt MS, et al.: Prognostic value of coronary CTA vs. exercise treadmill testing: results from the Partners registry, *Eur Heart J Cardiovasc Imaging* 16:1338–1346, 2015.
54. Yancy CW, Jessup M, Bozkurt B, et al.: 2013 ACCF/AHA guideline for the management of heart failure: a report of the American College of Cardiology Foundation/American Heart Association Task Force on Practice Guidelines, *Circulation* 128:e240–e327, 2013.
55. Kalam K, Otahal P, Marwick TH: Prognostic implications of global LV dysfunction: a systematic review and meta-analysis of global longitudinal strain and ejection fraction, *Heart* 100:1673–1680, 2014.
56. Shah BN, Gonzalez-Gonzalez AM, Drakopoulou M, et al.: The incremental prognostic value of the incorporation of myocardial perfusion assessment into clinical testing with stress echocardiography study, *J Am Soc Echocardiogr* 28:1358–1365, 2015.
57. Gaibazzi N, Reverberi C, Lorenzoni V, Molinaro S, Porter TR: Prognostic value of high-dose dipyridamole stress myocardial contrast perfusion echocardiography, *Circulation* 126:1217–1224, 2012.
58. Shaw LJ, Hage FG, Berman DS, Hachamovitch R, Iskandrian A: Prognosis in the era of comparative effectiveness research: where is nuclear cardiology now and where should it be? *J Nucl Cardiol* 19:1026–1043, 2012.
59. Dorbala S, Di Carli MF, Beanlands RS, et al.: Prognostic value of stress myocardial perfusion positron emission tomography: results from a multicenter observational registry, *J Am Coll Cardiol* 61:176–184, 2013.
60. Williams BA, Dorn JM, LaMonte MJ, et al.: Evaluating the prognostic value of positron-emission tomography myocardial perfusion imaging using automated software to calculate perfusion defect size, *Clin Cardiol* 35:E14–E21, 2012.
61. Taqueti VR, Hachamovitch R, Murthy VL, et al.: Global coronary flow reserve is associated with adverse cardiovascular events independently of luminal angiographic severity and modifies the effect of early revascularization, *Circulation* 131:19–27, 2015.
62. Naya M, Murthy VL, Taqueti VR, et al.: Preserved coronary flow reserve effectively excludes high-risk coronary artery disease on angiography, *J Nucl Med* 55:248–255, 2014.
63. Gould KL, Johnson NP, Bateman TM, et al.: Anatomic versus physiologic assessment of coronary artery disease. Role of coronary flow reserve, fractional flow reserve, and positron emission tomography imaging in revascularization decision-making, *J Am Coll Cardiol* 62:1639–1653, 2013.
64. Korosoglou G, Elhmidi Y, Steen H, et al.: Prognostic value of high-dose dobutamine stress magnetic resonance imaging in 1,493 consecutive patients: assessment of myocardial wall motion and perfusion, *J Am Coll Cardiol* 56:1225–1234, 2010.
65. Douglas PS, Hoffmann U, Patel MR, et al.: Outcomes of anatomical versus functional testing for coronary artery disease, *N Engl J Med* 372:1291–1300, 2015.
66. Douglas PS, Pontone G, Hlatky MA, et al.: Clinical outcomes of fractional flow reserve by computed tomographic angiography-guided diagnostic strategies vs. usual care in patients with suspected coronary artery disease: the prospective longitudinal trial of FFRct: outcome and resource impacts study, *Eur Heart J* 36:3359–3367, 2015.
67. Hlatky MA, De Bruyne B, Pontone G, et al.: Quality of life and economic outcomes of assessing fractional flow reserve with computed tomography angiography: the PLATFORM study, *J Am Coll Cardiol* 66:2315–2323, 2015.
68. Min JK, Dunning A, Lin FY, et al.: Age- and sex-related differences in all-cause mortality risk based on coronary computed tomography angiography findings results from the International Multicenter CONFIRM (Coronary CT Angiography Evaluation for Clinical Outcomes: an International Multicenter Registry) of 23,854 patients without known coronary artery disease, *J Am Coll Cardiol* 58:849–860, 2011.
69. The SCOT-HEART Investigators. CT coronary angiography in patients with suspected angina due to coronary heart disease (SCOT-HEART): an open-label, parallel-group, multicentre trial, *Lancet* 385:2383–2391, 2015.
70. Motoyama S, Sarai M, Harigaya H, et al.: Computed tomographic angiography characteristics of atherosclerotic plaques subsequently resulting in acute coronary syndrome, *J Am Coll Cardiol* 54:49–57, 2009.

71. Hulten EA, Carbonaro S, Petrillo SP, Mitchell JD, Villines TC: Prognostic value of cardiac computed tomography angiography: a systematic review and meta-analysis, *J Am Coll Cardiol* 57:1237–1247, 2011.
72. Iannaccone M, Quadri G, Taha S, et al.: Prevalence and predictors of culprit plaque rupture at OCT in patients with coronary artery disease: a meta-analysis, *Eur Heart J Cardiovasc Imaging* 16:2–8, 2015.
73. Dong L, Mintz GS, Witzenbichler B, et al.: Comparison of plaque characteristics in narrowings with ST-elevation myocardial infarction (STEMI), non-STEMI/unstable angina pectoris and stable coronary artery disease (from the ADAPT-DES IVUS Substudy), *Am J Cardiol* 115:860–866, 2015.
74. Pijls NH, Sels JW: Functional measurement of coronary stenosis, *J Am Coll Cardiol* 59:1045–1057, 2012.
75. Nikpay M, Goel A, Won H-H: A comprehensive 1000 genomes-based genome-wide association meta-analysis of coronary artery disease, *Nat Genet* 47:1121–1130, 2015.
76. Mega JL, Stitziel NO, Smith JG, et al.: Genetic risk, coronary heart disease events, and the clinical benefit of statin therapy: an analysis of primary and secondary prevention trials, *Lancet* 385:2264–2271, 2015.
77. Rapsomaniki E, Shah A, Perel P, et al.: Prognostic models for stable coronary artery disease based on electronic health record cohort of 102 023 patients, *Eur Heart J* 35:844–852, 2014.
78. Yan AT, Yan RT, Huynh T, et al.: Understanding physicians' risk stratification of acute coronary syndromes: insights from the Canadian ACS 2 Registry, *Arch Intern Med* 169:372–378, 2009.
79. Lloyd-Jones DM: Cardiovascular risk prediction: basic concepts, current status, and future directions, *Circulation* 121:1768–1777, 2010.
80. D'Agostino Sr RB, Vasan RS, Pencina MJ, et al.: General cardiovascular risk profile for use in primary care: the Framingham Heart Study, *Circulation* 117:743–753, 2008.
81. Goff Jr DC, Lloyd-Jones DM, Bennett G, et al.: 2013 ACC/AHA guideline on the assessment of cardiovascular risk: a report of the American College of Cardiology/American Heart Association Task Force on Practice Guidelines, *J Am Coll Cardiol* 63:2935–2959, 2014.
82. Rabar S, Harker M, O'Flynn N, Wierzbicki AS: Lipid modification and cardiovascular risk assessment for the primary and secondary prevention of cardiovascular disease: summary of updated NICE guidance, *BMJ* 349:g4356, 2014.
83. Matheny M, McPheeters ML, Glasser A, et al.: Systematic review of cardiovascular disease risk assessment tools, *Evidence Synthesis/Technology Assessment No* 85, 2011.
84. Fihn SD, Gardin JM, Abrams J, et al.: 2012 ACCF/AHA/ACP/AATS/PCNA/SCAI/STS guideline for the diagnosis and management of patients with stable ischemic heart disease: a report of the American College of Cardiology Foundation/American Heart Association Task Force on Practice Guidelines, and the American College of Physicians, American Association for Thoracic Surgery, Preventive Cardiovascular Nurses Association, Society for Cardiovascular Angiography and Interventions, and Society of Thoracic Surgeons, *Circulation* 126:e354–e471, 2012.
85. Hsia J, Jablonski KA, Rice MM, et al.: Sudden cardiac death in patients with stable coronary artery disease and preserved left ventricular systolic function, *Am J Cardiol* 101:457–461, 2008.
86. Atwater BD, Thompson VP, Vest 3rd RN, et al.: Usefulness of the Duke Sudden Cardiac Death risk score for predicting sudden cardiac death in patients with angiographic (>75% narrowing) coronary artery disease, *Am J Cardiol* 104:1624–1630, 2009.
87. De Bacquer D, Dallongeville J, Kotseva K, et al.: Residual risk of cardiovascular mortality in patients with coronary heart disease: the EUROASPIRE risk categories, *Int J Cardiol* 168:910–914, 2013.
88. Battes L, Barendse R, Steyerberg EW, et al.: Development and validation of a cardiovascular risk assessment model in patients with established coronary artery disease, *Am J Cardiol* 112:27–33, 2013.
89. Moons KG, Kengne AP, Grobbee DE, et al.: Risk prediction models: II. External validation, model updating, and impact assessment, *Heart* 98:691–698, 2012.
90. Goliasch G, Kleber ME, Richter B, et al.: Routinely available biomarkers improve prediction of long-term mortality in stable coronary artery disease: the Vienna and Ludwigshafen Coronary Artery Disease (VILCAD) risk score, *Eur Heart J* 33:2282–2289, 2012.
91. Omland T, de Lemos JA, Sabatine MS, et al.: A sensitive cardiac troponin T assay in stable coronary artery disease, *N Engl J Med* 361:2538–2547, 2009.
92. Zakynthinos E, Pappa N: Inflammatory biomarkers in coronary artery disease, *J Cardiol* 53:317–333, 2009.
93. Di Angelantonio E, Chowdhury R, Sarwar N, et al.: B-type natriuretic peptides and cardiovascular risk: systematic review and meta-analysis of 40 prospective studies, *Circulation* 120:2177–2187, 2009.
94. Moons KG, Kengne AP, Woodward M, et al.: Risk prediction models: I. Development, internal validation, and assessing the incremental value of a new (bio)marker, *Heart* 98:683–690, 2012.
95. Cassar A, Holmes Jr DR, Rihal CS, Gersh BJ: Chronic coronary artery disease: diagnosis and management, *Mayo Clin Proc* 84:1130–1146, 2009.
96. Omland T, Pfeffer MA, Solomon SD, et al.: Prognostic value of cardiac troponin I measured with a highly sensitive assay in patients with stable coronary artery disease, *J Am Coll Cardiol* 61:1240–1249, 2013.
97. Schnabel RB, Schulz A, Messow CM, et al.: Multiple marker approach to risk stratification in patients with stable coronary artery disease, *Eur Heart J* 31:3024–3031, 2010.
98. Mora S, Wenger NK, Demicco DA, et al.: Determinants of residual risk in secondary prevention patients treated with high- versus low-dose statin therapy: the Treating to New Targets (TNT) study, *Circulation* 125:1979–1987, 2012.
99. Sabatine MS, Morrow DA, de Lemos JA, et al.: Evaluation of multiple biomarkers of cardiovascular stress for risk prediction and guiding medical therapy in patients with stable coronary disease, *Circulation* 125:233–240, 2012.
100. Kleber ME, Goliasch G, Grammer TB, et al.: Evolving biomarkers improve prediction of long-term mortality in patients with stable coronary artery disease: the BIO-VILCAD score, *J Intern Med* 276:184–194, 2014.
101. Beatty AL, Ku IA, Bibbins-Domingo K, et al.: Traditional risk factors versus biomarkers for prediction of secondary events in patients with stable coronary heart disease: from the Heart and Soul Study, *J Am Heart Assoc* 4, 2015.
102. DeFilippis AP, Young R, Carrubba CJ, et al.: An analysis of calibration and discrimination among multiple cardiovascular risk scores in a modern multiethnic cohort, *Ann Intern Med* 162:266–275, 2015.
103. Collins GS, Altman DG: An independent and external validation of QRISK2 cardiovascular disease risk score: a prospective open cohort study, *BMJ* 340:c2442, 2010.
104. Moss AJ, Zareba W, Hall WJ, et al.: Prophylactic implantation of a defibrillator in patients with myocardial infarction and reduced ejection fraction, *N Engl J Med* 346:877–883, 2002.
105. Levine GN, Bates ER, Blankenship JC, et al.: 2011 ACCF/AHA/SCAI Guideline for Percutaneous Coronary Intervention: a report of the American College of Cardiology Foundation/American Heart Association Task Force on Practice Guidelines and the Society for Cardiovascular Angiography and Interventions, *Circulation* 124:e574–e651, 2011.
106. Serruys PW, Morice MC, Kappetein AP, et al.: Percutaneous coronary intervention versus coronary-artery bypass grafting for severe coronary artery disease, *N Engl J Med* 360:961–972, 2009.
107. Everett BM, Brooks MM, Vlachos HE, et al.: Troponin and cardiac events in stable ischemic heart disease and diabetes, *N Engl J Med* 373:610–620, 2015.
108. Baigent C, Blackwell L, Emberson J, et al.: Efficacy and safety of more intensive lowering of LDL cholesterol: a meta-analysis of data from 170,000 participants in 26 randomised trials, *Lancet* 376:1670–1681, 2010.
109. Yeh RW: Individualizing treatment duration of dual antiplatelet therapy after percutaneous coronary intervention: an analysis from the DAPT study. Presented at, Orlando, FL, 2015, *American Heart Association Scientific Sessions November 7–11, 2015.*

18 Lifestyle Interventions

Eva Prescott

More than 90% of all cardiovascular disease (CVD) deaths are thought to be preventable through lifestyle changes. In the INTERHEART study, a case-control study of myocardial infarction (MI) in 52 countries worldwide, nine lifestyle-related risk factors accounted for 90% of the risk in men and 94% of the risk in women.[1] The nine risk factors were: (1) abnormal lipids, (2) smoking, (3) hypertension, (4) diabetes, (5) abdominal obesity, (6) psychosocial factors, (7) low consumption of fruit and vegetables, (8) alcohol consumption, and (9) lack of regular physical activity. Western countries have seen a decline in mortality from CVD in recent decades with mortality dropping to less than a third of previous levels in some countries. Half of this impressive decline in coronary heart disease mortality in the last three to four decades is generally ascribed to effects of population-level lifestyle changes, mainly reductions in smoking and cholesterol through improved diet, and the remaining decline is ascribed to improved treatments, including medical therapy for cardiovascular risk factors.[2]

Revascularization through percutaneous coronary intervention (PCI) or coronary artery bypass grafting (CABG), whether in the acute or elective setting, addresses the need for improved oxygen supply to the affected area of myocardium but does not address the underlying atherosclerotic process. For this, secondary prevention comprising lifestyle adaptation and medical treatment are necessary, and the effects of these adaptations have a rapid onset. In the Organization to Assess Strategies in Acute Ischemic Syndromes (OASIS) 5 study, a multicenter trial of 18,809 patients from 41 countries, patients were assessed for adherence to the lifestyle factors diet, exercise and smoking one month after their MI and subsequently followed for a total of 6 months for cardiovascular events. Patients who reported to be persistent smokers and nonadherent to diet and exercise recommendations had a 3.8-fold increased risk of MI, stroke, or death compared with never-smokers who modified their diet and exercise.[3] Smoking cessation alone was associated with a 43% reduction in risk of recurrent MI within the following 5 months, and adherence to diet and exercise was associated with a 48% reduction. Although this was an observational study and effects may be overestimated, data illustrate that the potential effects of lifestyle changes in cardiac patients are considerable even in the short term.

Despite decades of recommending lifestyle changes in patients with CVD, uptake remains suboptimal at best. In the EUROASPIRE IV survey, a cross-sectional study of secondary prevention in 8000 patients with coronary artery disease in 78 centers in 24 European countries, lifestyle changes were not widely adopted: little or no physical activity was reported by 59.9%, 48.6% of those smoking at the time of their event were still smoking, 37.6% were obese, 42.7% did not reach the blood pressure target of less than 140/90 mm Hg, 80.5% had low-density lipoprotein cholesterol (LDL-C) above the 1.8 mmol/L goal, and 26.8% reported to have diabetes. Half the patients (50.7%) had been offered cardiac rehabilitation and 81.3% of these had only attended half the program. Somewhat better adherence was seen for the main cardioprotective medications, antiplatelet agents and statins. These had been widely prescribed and were used by 85% to 94% of the population. These figures are likely to give an optimistic view of the status of secondary prevention because of selection mechanisms regarding both participating centers and patients.[4] Thus the implementation of lifestyle adaptations in patients with coronary heart disease continues to present a challenge.

In the following chapter, the lifestyle factors of smoking, physical activity, and nutrition will be covered, as will cardiac rehabilitation issues of adherence, whereas lipids, weight management, and psychosocial factors (stress and depression) are covered in other chapters.

SMOKING

Epidemiology

Smoking is a strong risk factor for coronary heart disease and, due to a persistently high use of tobacco products, remains responsible for a large proportion of coronary heart disease cases. In the INTERHEART study the population attributable fraction for smoking in causing MI was 35.7%.[1] Smoking has declined in the Western world in recent decades, and this decline has been an important contribution to the observed decline in mortality from coronary heart disease. Nonetheless, it is estimated that active and passive smoking remains responsible for more than 480,000 annual deaths in the United States, equivalent to one in five deaths, almost half of these from CVD.[5]

The decline in smoking has been greatest among light smokers, men, and the socioeconomically privileged, leading to increased disparities in smoking-attributable disease. Even in smokers with established coronary heart disease many continue to smoke. European survey data indicate that 16% of patients with coronary heart disease are smokers more than one year after their event, and only half of smokers have quit smoking. The survey also found that smoking cessation tools were underused.[4]

Types, Dosage, and Passive Smoking

Smoking is a strong and independent risk factor for all CVD. Smokers on average reduce their life span by 10 years, and their risk of developing CVD is increased two- to threefold.[6] In younger smokers the excess risk is five times higher than in nonsmokers of similar age.[7] All types of tobacco are deleterious, whether low-tar ("mild" or "light"), filter cigarettes, pipe, or cigar. Moreover, significantly increased risk is still seen in smokers that have limited inhalation of smoke, such as habitual pipe or cigar smokers. There is no lower limit below which smoking is safe. Passive smoking or environmental tobacco smoke also increases the risk of smoking-related diseases. For example, work-related exposure to environmental tobacco smoke has been reported to increase the risk of MI by approximately 20% to 30%.[8,9] The deleterious effect of environmental tobacco smoke is corroborated by animal and mechanistic studies showing measurable levels of tobacco and nicotine degradation substances in blood and urine of passive smokers and a measurable effect on endothelial function and platelet aggregation in study subjects exposed to passive smoking.[6] Correspondingly, since legislation on passive smoking has been implemented in various settings, the rate of MI has dropped by an estimated 17%.[10] This decline in incidence of MI was seen mainly among nonsmokers. These data indicate that patients at increased risk of CVD, including post-MI patients, should be advised to avoid exposure to environmental tobacco smoke.[11] Smokeless tobacco, which is popular in some subgroups as, for example, "snus" (a moist powder tobacco placed under the upper lip), is also associated with a small but significantly increased risk of MI and stroke.[12]

Mechanism

The effects of smoking on cardiovascular pathogenesis are several. When tobacco is burned, thousands of chemical compounds are developed and inhaled. These chemical compounds have numerous effects on the cardiovascular system. Smoking acts chronically by accelerating the atherosclerotic process and acutely by increasing the risk of plaque rupture and thrombus formation. Central to the effects of smoking is increased oxidative stress and endothelial dysfunction and injury (Fig. 18.1). The atherosclerotic plaques of smokers are more vulnerable with unfavorable plaque lipid composition, more inflammatory activity, degradation of extracellular matrix proteins, and thinner fibrous caps through inappropriate activation of matrix metalloproteinases and higher risk of intraplaque hemorrhage. Smoking exposure affects the balance of procoagulant and anticoagulant factors leading to a prothrombotic state with increased platelet activation, activation of coagulation pathways, and downregulation of fibrinolytic pathways. These mechanisms also lead to higher risk of in-stent thrombosis in smokers, and prothrombotic effects are amplified by concomitant oral contraceptive use. Further effects include changes in vasomotor function through impairment of endothelial function, increased leucocyte count, and lowering of high-density lipoprotein cholesterol (HDL-C).[6,13]

Corresponding to these effects, after smoking cessation cardiovascular risk decreases in a biphasic manner with rapid onset of reduction through decreased propensity to thrombus formation and increased plaque stability, followed by more long-term effects in reduced atherosclerosis disease progression. The first beneficial cardiovascular effects of smoking cessation are also seen very soon after quitting: within hours, heart rate (HR) drops and carbon monoxide returns to normal; within days to weeks, effects on platelet and endothelial function are reversed. Correspondingly, the risk of recurrent events after quitting immediately drops. In a study of smoking cessation after MI, smokers who had quit within the first month had a 43% reduced risk of recurrent events within the next 5 months in comparison with continuing smokers.[3] This first risk reduction is followed by a more prolonged effect, and epidemiologic studies have shown that the risk of recurrent events in ex-smokers approaches that of never-smokers asymptotically by 15 to 20 years.[14,13] Although the atherosclerotic plaque is not dissolved after smoking cessation, plaque stability is increased and plaques are less prone to rupture and erosion causing MI.[13]

Smoking Cessation Benefits

Evidence of effects of quitting smoking are based on observational studies of smoking cessation among the general population as well as cardiac patients. Smokers who give up smoking in the context of a cardiovascular event differ from smokers who continue smoking with regard to other aspects associated with cardiovascular risk: they are, for instance, also more likely to adhere to other lifestyle changes and to medication. Therefore, these studies have the inherent risk of overestimating the benefits of smoking cessation. However, given the strong evidence of the effects of smoking from basic science, animal studies, and observational studies, as well as short-term mechanistic intervention trials, the evidence supporting cardiovascular benefits and general health benefits of smoking cessation is overwhelming.

In a smoker, smoking cessation is potentially the lifestyle change with greatest impact on risk of recurrent events. Because smoking has such profound effects on overall health status, the benefits of cessation are multiple. Quitting smoking in patients with coronary heart disease was associated with a 36% reduced mortality risk and a 32% reduced risk of fatal MI when compared with continued smokers in a large meta-analysis (Fig. 18.2).[16] This benefit was consistent across gender, age, and duration of follow-up. Due to the relatively small effect of the intervention on smoking prevalence, large-scale randomized smoking cessation trials are generally required. The few existing randomized controlled trials of smoking cessation with mortality or morbidity

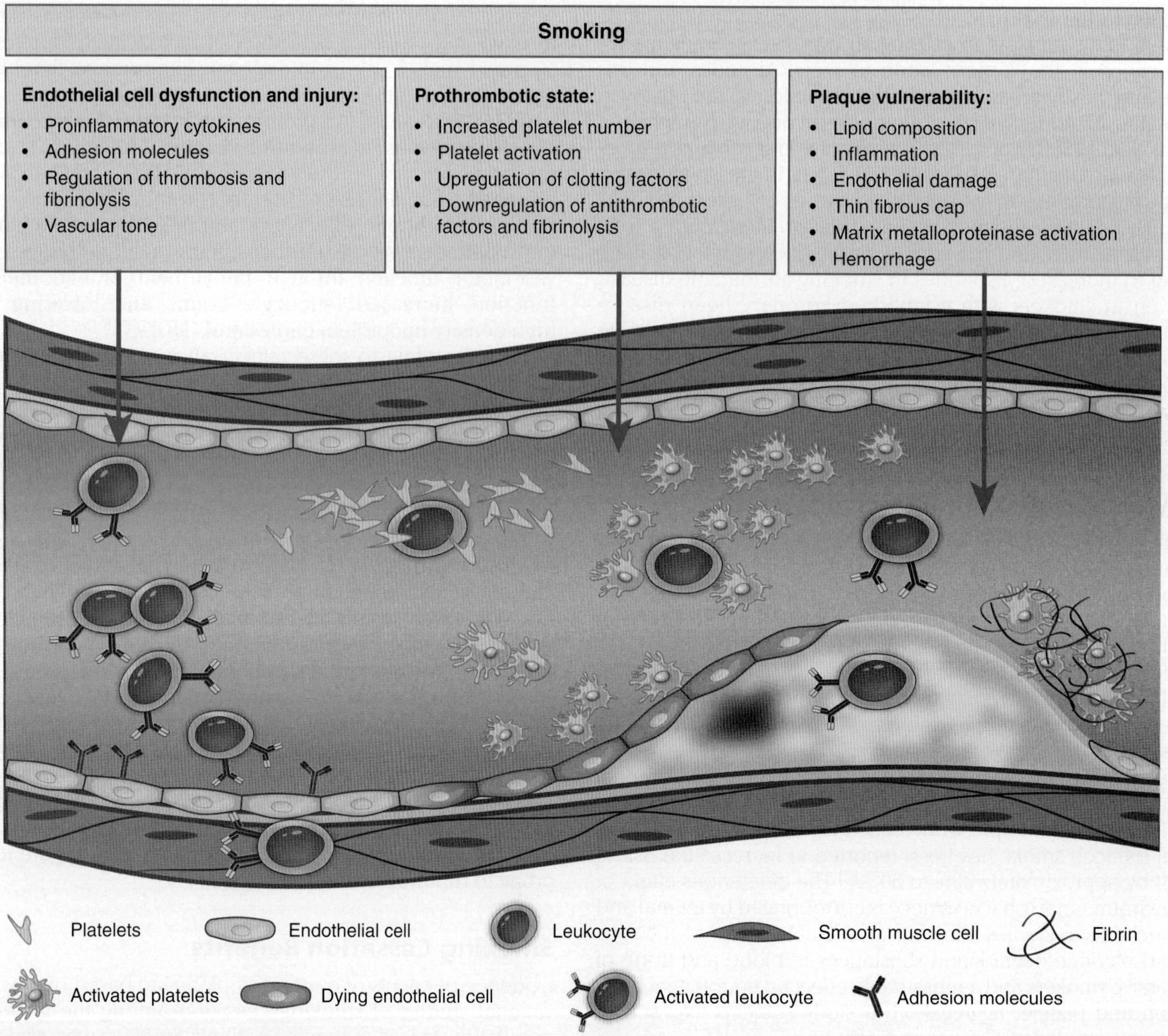

FIG. 18.1 Overview of atherothrombotic effects of smoking exposure. *(Modified from Csordas A, Bernhard D. The biology behind the atherothrombotic effects of cigarette smoke.* Nat Rev Cardiol. *2013;10(4):219–230.)*

outcomes indicate effects similar to those reported in the observational meta-analyses.[17,18]

Smoking Cessation Aid

Smoking cessation is difficult to achieve because the habit is strongly addictive pharmacologically and psychologically and is enforced by smoking habits in the family and social environment of the patient. The most important predictor of successful smoking cessation is patient motivation. Studies have shown that other factors also affect the likelihood of quitting smoking; women, the socioeconomically deprived, and patients with depressive symptoms are less likely to achieve their goal. As with other lifestyle changes, support from the surrounding environment, including through antitobacco legislation and policy changes, is important for sustainable effects.

To achieve smoking cessation, health professionals should give a strong, clear, and consistent message to the patient. Smoking habits should be addressed in all contact with patients with CVD and smokers should be encouraged to quit, regardless of age.[11,19] Contacts with the patient during hospital admission for a cardiovascular event or for revascularization are moments of opportunity to reinforce the message. Notably, brief advice from health physicians, nurses, and other health professionals are evidence-based interventions that increase the likelihood of quitting by 60% to 70%.[20,21] Allied health professionals should assess nicotine addiction[22] and degree of patient motivation, set a quit date, and arrange follow-up (see the five As in Table 18.1). Smokers should be informed that smoking cessation is accompanied by a mean weight increase of 5 kg but that the health benefits of smoking cessation far outweigh the effects of potential weight gain.

The majority of smokers who quit do so unaided. Individual, group, and telephone counseling increase quit rates, whereas smoking reduction, nicotine fading, relaxation techniques, hypnosis, and acupuncture are methods that have not been proven successful in trials. Quitting rates can be increased by use of pharmacologic agents diminishing withdrawal symptoms in addicted smokers (Table 18.2). Nicotine replacement therapy, the mild antidepressant bupropion, and the

Review: Smoking cessation for the secondary prevention of coronary heart disease
Comparison: Ceased vs. continued smoking
Outcome: Total deaths

Study or subgroup	Ceased smoking n/N	Continued smoking n/N	Weight	Risk ratio M-H, Random, 95% CI
Aberg 1983	110/542	142/443	8.3%	0.63 (0.51, 0.79)
Baughman 1982	9/45	14/32	1.8%	0.46 (0.23, 0.92)
Bednarzewski 1984	136/455	205/555	9.3%	0.81 (0.68, 0.67)
Burr 1992	27/665	41/521	3.5%	0.52 (0.32, 0.83)
Daly 1983	80/217	129/157	9.0%	0.45 (0.37, 0.54)
Greenwood 1995	64/396	29/136	4.5%	0.76 (0.51, 1.12)
Gupta 1993	56/173	24/52	4.9%	0.70 (0.49, 1.01)
Hallstrom 1986	34/91	104/219	6.1%	0.79 (0.58, 1.06)
Johansson 1985	14/81	27/75	2.6%	0.48 (0.27, 0.84)
Perkins 1985	9/52	30/67	2.1%	0.39 (0.20,0.74)
Salonen 1980	26/221	60/302	4.0%	0.59 (0.39, 0.91)
Sato 1992	5/59	7/28	0.9%	0.34 (0.12, 0.97)
Sparrow 1978	10/56	40/139	2.3%	0.62 (0.33, 1.15)
Tofler 1993	14/173	37/220	2.5%	0.48 (0.27, 0.86)
Van Domburg 2000	109/238	202/318	9.8%	0.72 (0.61, 0.85)
Vliestra 1986	223/1490	588/2675	10.4%	0.68 (0.59, 0.78)
Voors 1996	26/72	37/95	4.4%	0.93 (0.62, 1.38)
Total (95% CI)	**5659**	**6944**	**100.0%**	**0.64 (0.58, 0.71)**

Total events: 1044 (ceased smoking), 1884 (continued smoking)
Heterogeneity: $Tau^2 = 0.002$; $Chi^2 = 36.74$, $df = 19$ ($p = 0.001$); $I^2 = 45\%$
Test of overall effect: $Z = 8.42$ ($P < 0.00001$)

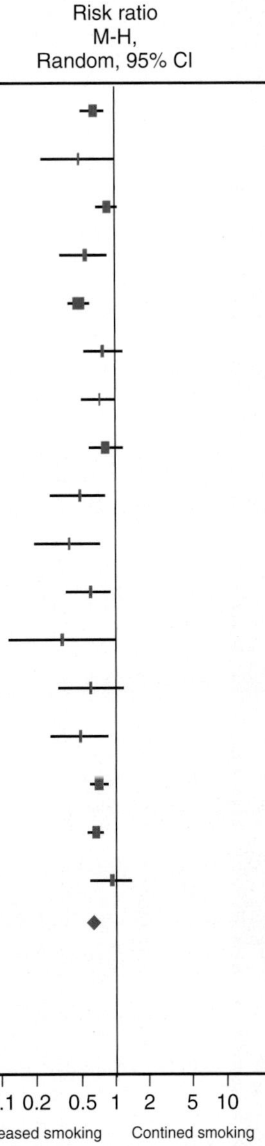

FIG. 18.2 Cochrane review smoking cessation after coronary heart disease. *CI*, Confidence interval; *df*, degrees of freedom; *M-H*, Mantel-Haenzsel; *n/N*, number of deaths/total number of study subjects in group. *(Based on Critchley J, Capewell S. Smoking cessation for the secondary prevention of coronary heart disease.* Cochrane Database Syst Rev. *2003;(1):DOI 10.1002/14651858.CD003041.)*

TABLE 18.1 The Five As of Smoking Cessation

A-Ask:	Systematically inquire about smoking status at every opportunity.
A-Advise:	Unequivocally urge all smokers to quit.
A-Assess:	Determine the person's degree of addiction and readiness to quit.
A-Assist:	Agree on a smoking-cessation strategy, including setting a quit date, behavioral counseling, and pharmacologic support.
A-Arrange:	Arrange a schedule of follow-up.

partial nicotine agonists varenicline and cytisine have all been shown to increase quit rates.[23] Nicotine replacement therapy, whether delivered as gum, transdermal patch, nasal spray, lozenge, or inhaler, increased the success rate by 84%.[24,25] Bupropion had similar effects (quit rate increased by 82%), confirmed by head-to-head comparison studies. Varenicline has mainly been tested against singular nicotine replacement therapy and shown to result in an approximately 50% higher success rate. However, combination therapies of nicotine replacement therapy are more efficient than singular use.[24] A combination of varenicline and nicotine replacement therapy may be superior to either used alone.[26] Cytisine, although less studied, has been found to increase quit rates and may be more clinically effective and cost-effective than varenicline, although they have not been compared head to head.[23,27] Cytisine is not approved for smoking cessation aid by regulatory authorities outside Eastern Europe. There was initial concern regarding possible minor adverse effects of varenicline on CVD outcomes, but these adverse effects have not been confirmed[23] and nicotine replacement therapy, bupropion, and varenicline are currently all considered safe agents to use, including in cardiac patients.

TABLE 18.2 Smoking Cessation Aid

	TREATMENT DURATION	MODE OF USE	MECHANISM	EFFECTIVENESS RELATIVE TO PLACEBO	COMMON SIDE-EFFECTS (1–10%)	RELATIVE EFFICACY	NOTE
NR	Dosage adjusted to level of addiction and gradually reduced. Up to 3 months, prolonged treatment not associated with better effect but preferable to smoking reuptake	Patch, gum, lozenge, inhaler, nasal spray	Stimulates nicotinic acetylcholine receptors in CNS and reduces withdrawal symptoms	OR 1.6 vs. control, combination of several NR products increased effectivity	Local irritation, pain and paresthesia, headache, nausea, dizziness, hiccups, upset stomach	+ as monotherapy, ++ in combination	
Bupropion	150 mg daily for 3–4 d followed by 150 mg bid for 7–12 wk, up to 6 months	Smoking cessation planned after 1 week of treatment	Antidepressant, inhibits noradrenaline and dopamine reuptake	OR 1.9 vs. control	Insomnia, dry mouth, abdominal pain, nausea, oral dryness, obstipation	+	Caution in patients with risk of seizure. Patients should be monitored for mood changes.
Varenicline	0.5 mg daily for 1–3 d, 0.5 mg bid for 4–7 d, then 1 mg bid for 12 wk	Smoking cessation planned after 1 week of treatment	Partial nicotine receptor agonist with agonist and antagonist effects	OR 1.8 vs. bupropion, not documented more efficient than combination of NR	Nausea, rhinitis, sleep disturbance, vomiting, obstipation, flatulence, headache, changed appetite, dyspnea, chest pain, myalgias, dizziness	++	Reduced dosage in renal failure (GFR < 30 mL/min) Caution in patients with a history of psychiatric disorder, including depression, anxiety or previous attempted suicide

CNS, Central nervous system; *GFR,* glomerular filtration rate; *NR,* nicotine replacement; *OR,* odds ratio.

E-Cigarettes

Electronic cigarettes (e-cigarettes) have been recently introduced and have achieved increasing popularity. The e-cigarette is an electronic vaporizer for delivery of nicotine. Because nicotine is addictive, e-cigarettes can be regarded as either a smoking cessation pharmaceutical and treated under pharmaceutical legislation, or as a tobacco product covered by regulations for tobacco products. Long-term nicotine addiction and usefulness of e-cigarettes as a smoking cessation tool have not yet been clarified. Currently, there is insufficient evidence that e-cigarettes are efficient in supporting smoking cessation.[28] Concerns have been voiced of an increasing likelihood of nicotine addiction in youth if e-cigarettes are perceived as socially acceptable. However, e-cigarettes have been used as a means of reducing deleterious effects of smoking for smokers who are unable or unwilling to quit. Whereas there is little doubt that e-cigarettes are less harmful than smoking cigarettes, the long-term consequences are not known, and, at the time of writing, guidelines on both sides of the Atlantic recommend care. However, short-time use has not been associated with health risks.

NUTRITION

A healthy diet is recognized as a cornerstone in maintaining cardiovascular health. Dietary habits influence not only CVD but also other chronic diseases including cancer. Effects of diet on cardiovascular health are through a number of known and unknown factors, including effects on lipoproteins. A number of food constituents have been identified and tested in randomized controlled trials but all have been disappointing. In general, when following the recommendations for a healthy dietary pattern, no dietary supplements are needed. In addition to the diet pattern, energy intake should be limited to what is necessary to maintain, or obtain, a healthy bodyweight, i.e., a body mass index (BMI) of 20 to 25 kg/m^2. Several studies have reported that coronary heart disease patients who are overweight have lower mortality rates than normal weight coronary heart disease patients. This has been termed the obesity paradox and is also seen in chronic heart failure, chronic obstructive pulmonary disease (COPD), and other chronic disease conditions. Whether this association is causal or caused by bias in the observational studies remains unclear. No randomized large-scale trial of substantial weight loss in coronary heart disease patients with CVD endpoints has been undertaken. In the Look AHEAD (Action for Health in Diabetes) trial, a randomized trial of weight loss and physical activity in overweight and obese patients with type 2 diabetes, there was no benefit of a modest weight loss (2.5%) on the primary combined outcome over a 9-year follow-up period (hazard ratio 0.95, $p = 0.51$).[29] However, the Swedish Obesity Study, a nonrandomized, controlled study comparing the outcome of bariatric surgery with usual care in obese subjects, found a 33% (0.54–0.83) reduced incidence of fatal and nonfatal CVD events in patients who underwent surgery.[30] Weight loss in overweight patients is associated with multiple beneficial effects on cardiovascular risk factors such as dyslipidemia, hypertension, and hyperglycemia, and maintenance of a normal body weight remains an objective in secondary prevention of coronary heart disease.[11,31]

Mediterranean and Other Diets

The Mediterranean diet is a diet similar to the traditional dietary patterns in Greece, Italy, and Spain. The diet was first described as beneficial in the seven countries study in which the diet in the Greek island of Crete was studied.[32] The Mediterranean diet is defined as a diet rich in olive oils, fruit, vegetables, legumes, unrefined cereals, and fish; a moderate consumption of wine and dairy products (cheese and yogurt); and a relatively low consumption of meat. Mediterranean dietary patterns tend to be moderate in total fat, low in saturated fat, and high in fiber and polyunsaturated fatty acids, including n-3 (omega 3) fatty acids from fish consumption.[19] The Mediterranean diet has been declared by UNESCO to be on the Representative List of the Intangible Cultural Heritage of Humanity of the Mediterranean countries Portugal, Spain, Italy, Croatia, Greece, and Morocco.

The evidence for the beneficial effect of the Mediterranean diet comes from multicenter observational studies and meta-analyses and also from randomized controlled trials. Meta-analyses of observational studies of the Mediterranean diet in primary prevention have found reduced incidence of diabetes, lower triglyceride concentrations, lower blood sugar levels, and lower blood pressure.[33] Recent meta-analyses comprising data from more than 4 million individuals found significant reductions of overall mortality of 8% and of CVD morbidity of 10%.[34,35] It should be noted, however, that two Cochrane reviews in 2013 found only limited evidence to date in randomized trials that the Mediterranean diet or increased fruit and vegetables consumption had a beneficial effect on CVD risk.[36,37]

The two main trials showing a benefit of the Mediterranean diet on cardiovascular outcomes are the Lyon Diet Heart study and the Prevención con Dieta Mediterránea (PREDIMED) trial. Based on these trials, the plausibility through mechanistic studies, and the overwhelming evidence from observational studies, 2016 guidelines for secondary prevention recommend a diet that is close to the Mediterranean diet[11,19] (Box 18.1).

The PREDIMED trial was a Spanish multicenter trial comparing three diets: two arms with a Mediterranean diet supplemented with either extra virgin olive oil or mixed nuts, and one arm with a low-fat diet, in 7447 persons without CVD but at high risk of developing CVD. The Mediterranean diet recommended was rich in olive oil, nuts, fruit, vegetables, legumes, fish, and wine and low in soda drinks, bakery items, red meat, and spread fats. The low-fat diet arm also recommended fruit, vegetables, and fish/seafood in addition to low-fat dairy products and potatoes, pasta, and rice, whereas fatty fish, olive oil, and nuts were discouraged. The study was halted after 4.8 years after an interim analysis finding the Mediterranean diet superior. There was an overall 30% reduction in the primary major adverse cardiac event (MACE) outcome of MI, stroke, or death from CVD causes with similar risk reduction in the nut group and in the extra virgin olive oil group.[38] The absolute risk in the PREDIMED study, although based on individuals with risk factors for CVD, was low, with overall CVD event rate in the range of 4% per year. The main event driving differences between groups was stroke. The reductions achieved were reported to be consistent with that calculated based on the PREDIMED population applying risk reductions achieved from observational studies on individual dietary components.

BOX 18.1 Example of Recommended Dietary Pattern for Secondary Prevention of Cardiovascular Disease

Choose a dietary pattern that emphasizes intake of vegetables, fruit, whole grains, low-fat dairy products, poultry, fish, legumes, nontropical vegetable oils, and nuts and limits the intake of sugar-sweetened beverages and red meats:

- Saturated FAs should account for < 5–10% of total energy intake, through replacement by PUFAs.
- Trans unsaturated FAs intake should be as little as possible, preferably no intake from processed food and < 1% of total energy intake from natural origin.
- Lower sodium intake to < 5 g per day; in patients with hypertension aim at 2.4 g or less.
- 30–45 g of fiber per day, preferably from whole-grain products
- 200 g of fruit per day (2–3 servings)
- 200 g of vegetables per day (2–3 servings)
- Fish at least twice a week, one of which to be oily fish
- Consumption of alcoholic beverages should be limited to 2 glasses per day (20 g/d of alcohol) in men and 1 glass per day (10 g/d of alcohol) for women.
- Sugar-sweetened soft drinks and alcoholic beverages consumption must be discouraged.

FAs, Fatty acids; *PUFAs*, poly-unsaturated fatty acids.
Modified from Eckel RH, Jakicic JM, Ard JD, et al. 2013 AHA/ACC guideline on lifestyle management to reduce cardiovascular risk: a report of the American College of Cardiology/American Heart Association Task Force on Practice Guidelines. *Circulation* 129(25 Suppl 2):S76-S99, 2014; Perk J, De BG, Gohlke H, et al. European Guidelines on cardiovascular disease prevention in clinical practice (version 2012). The Fifth Joint Task Force of the European Society of Cardiology and Other Societies on Cardiovascular Disease Prevention in Clinical Practice (constituted by representatives of nine societies and by invited experts). *Eur Heart J.* 2012;33(13):1635–1701.

The PREDIMED trial has also been criticized. These criticisms include that it was halted early and that effects were seen in the beginning of the trial only and were exclusively mediated by reduction in stroke. Also, critics have suggested that the control diet was not only low in fat but also high in carbohydrates, or that the control diet was not low enough in fat.[39] Finally, the absolute risk reduction was limited and the overall strong conclusions are based on a relatively low number of events.

The PREDIMED study was a primary prevention study in high-risk individuals. The only secondary prevention study powered for CVD events was the Lyon Diet Heart Study in which 605 patients with MI were randomized to a recommendation of Mediterranean diet versus no specific study-based recommendation. This study was also halted early. The study found a risk reduction for the main outcome of cardiac death or MI of 73% after 27 months, and the effect was maintained after 4 years' follow-up.[40,41]

The effect of diet on CVD risk seems to be rapid with significant differences seen within one year, which is also consistent with observational population studies[42] and with effect on intermediary outcomes in controlled feeding studies. As previously mentioned the potential mechanisms are multiple: the Mediterranean diet has been shown to reduce the prevalence of the metabolic syndrome and, in patients with diabetes, to improve glycemic control. This diet has also been shown to reduce intima media progression, reduce blood pressure, reduce low-grade inflammation, improve insulin sensitivity, and reduce use of antihyperglycemic medication.[43–47] Importantly, although the Mediterranean diet also leads to improved weight control, the beneficial effects are not mediated via weight loss but primarily through dietary composition.

Other dietary patterns deemed beneficial are the Dietary Approaches to Stop Hypertension (DASH), also recommended by the American Heart Association (AHA).[19] The DASH diet is high in vegetables, fruit, low-fat dairy products, whole grains, poultry, fish, and nuts and is low in sweets, sugar-sweetened beverages, and red meats. The DASH diet is rich in potassium, magnesium, and calcium, as well as protein and fiber, but lower in total fat than the Mediterranean diet. Vegetarian diets, which are also very low in total fat, have also been shown to be somewhat beneficial to CVD endpoints in observational studies and smaller trials.[48] One problem with diets that are very low in fat is less enjoyment, and thus in some patient groups lower adherence to the diet.

Based on the totality of the evidence from observational studies and intervention studies on individual nutrients, as well as from the PREDIMED and DASH trials, there is worldwide consensus that healthy dietary patterns are of greater importance than single nutrients for the prevention of CVD.

Fatty Acids, Including Trans-Fat

Fatty acids (FAs) are available as saturated FAs, monounsaturated fatty acids (MUFAs), and polyunsaturated fatty acids (PUFAs). A higher intake of saturated FAs comes mainly from animal products, including meats and dairy products, and is associated with higher LDL-C, lower HDL-C, and higher risk of CVD. Conversely, a higher intake of PUFAs, in particular, is associated with a lower risk of CVD. Substitution of MUFAs for saturated FAs lowers LDL-C and, to some extent, HDL-C, but the evidence of a beneficial effect on CVD outcome is limited. Substitution of PUFAs for saturated FAs is associated with reduced risk, whereas substitution with carbohydrates is associated with a more diabetogenic risk profile, higher triglycerides, lower HDL-C, and a higher CVD risk.

A 2014 meta-analysis has questioned the harmful effect of saturated FAs intake and has led to considerable discussion.[49] However, the key point is what the saturated FAs are replaced with, as previously described. Thus saturated animal fat should be replaced mainly by unsaturated fat, i.e., plant oils. These are key constituents in the Mediterranean diet. Prevailing dietary recommendations include consumption of food low in saturated fat, with saturated fat constituting a maximum of 10% of the total energy intake, or preferably less.[11,19]

Dietary intake of cholesterol has a limited effect on serum lipoproteins, in comparison with the effect of FAs and carbohydrates, and most guidelines do not give a specific recommendation on cholesterol consumption.

Trans FAs are industrially developed products to stiffen liquid fats for spread. A higher trans FAs intake leads to higher LDL-C, lower HDL-C, and a higher risk of CVD. The association has been proven beyond doubt. Prevailing guidelines recommend no consumption of industrially produced trans FAs. Several countries have introduced legislation banning the use of trans FAs, and this ban may be associated with the steep decline in CVD mortality seen in some countries. In the United States, trans FAs have been classified as not safe by the Food and Drug Administration (FDA) and are being phased out from food production.

Polyunsaturated Fatty Acids, Fish, and Fish Oils

PUFAs include n-6 (omega 6) FAs, derived mainly from plant foods, and n-3 (omega 3) FAs, derived mainly from fish oils and fats. The n-3 FAs eicosapentaenoic acid and docosahexaenoic acid (EPA/DHA) are particularly important subclasses of n-3 FAs. Dietary intake of fish is associated with lower risk of CVD. The association is not linear, with the highest risk seen for no fish consumption. The beneficial effect is thought to be mediated via the content of n-3 FAs. Several randomized trials in secondary prevention of CVD have tested the effect of supplementation with EPA/DHA in the form of fish oil capsules. These have not consistently shown a beneficial effect, and a lack of effect on CVD outcomes has been confirmed in a meta-analysis that included 20 secondary prevention trials with more than 60,000 patients.[50] Overall, n-3 supplementation was not associated with a lower risk of all-cause mortality, cardiac death, sudden death, MI, or stroke. The recommendation is thus to eat fish twice weekly or more, with one of the meals containing fatty fish,[11] whereas fish oils may be used for reduction of triglycerides.

Vitamins

Observational and case-control studies have indicated that low levels of vitamin A and E are associated with increased risk of CVD. However, randomized controlled trials have not shown beneficial effects of vitamin supplementation. The same is true for vitamin C and B, including folic acid. In addition, low levels of vitamin D are associated with a higher incidence of CVD in observational cohort studies,[51] but results may be confounded by smoking, less physical activity (and thus less exposure to the sun), diet, and other lifestyle factors. Most intervention trials have been small and not aimed at CVD outcomes. A recent meta-analysis of 22 randomized controlled trials with a total of approximately 30,000 individuals randomized to vitamin D supplementation or control/placebo has given limited support for a beneficial effect: vitamin D3 (cholecalciferol) supplementation was associated with an 11% reduced all-cause mortality risk (0.80–0.98), and vitamin D2 (ergocalciferol) supplementation was not associated with mortality risk reduction (Hazard ratio 1.04).[51] Vitamin D supplementation (mainly cholecalciferol) did not significantly reduce risk of MI or stroke in a meta-analysis of 21 randomized trials including 13,033 patients.[52] Results of several large ongoing trials of vitamin D3 supplementation with CVD outcomes expected in 2017 must be awaited before supplementation can be recommended for prevention of CVD.[53]

Fiber

Diets with a higher content of fibers inhibit or delay gastric emptying and are associated with lower postprandial glucose and reduction in total cholesterol and LDL-C. Soluble fiber may also improve insulin sensitivity and endothelial function and may lower inflammation, body weight, and blood pressure. In observational studies, higher fiber content in food has been linked to reduced risk of coronary heart disease, stroke, and diabetes. Another beneficial effect of dietary fiber is lower risk of gastrointestinal cancer. High fiber content is a key constituent of both the Mediterranean and DASH diets.

Minerals—Sodium and Potassium

Higher sodium consumption is associated with higher blood pressure, higher risk of coronary heart disease, and stroke. The effect of sodium on blood pressure is well established. It has been estimated that for every gram per day increase in sodium consumption, systolic blood pressure increases by 3.1 mm Hg in hypertensive patients and by 1.6 mm Hg in normotensive patients.[11] Little sodium is found naturally in food; the majority of sodium consumption is through added salt, in particular in prefabricated and processed food. Sodium consumption varies between countries but is as high as 8–12 g/day in many countries. Sodium consumption is recommended to be under 5 g/day in general, and the optimal intake is even lower. It has been estimated that a reduction in sodium intake in the United States to 3 g/day would result in a 5.9% to 9.6% reduction in the incidence of coronary heart disease and a 2.6% to 4.1% reduction in all-cause mortality.[19] In the United Kingdom a reduction from the current 8.5 g/day to 3 g/day would reduce the population average blood pressure by 2.5 mm Hg and reduce annual deaths from CVD by 4450.[54] Patients who would benefit from blood pressure lowering are advised to reduce their sodium consumption to 2.4 g/day, and further reduction to 1.5 g/day can result in greater blood pressure reduction.[19] Conversely, higher potassium intake is associated with lower blood pressure. The main source of potassium is intake of fruit and vegetables. Indeed, diets rich in potassium such as the Mediterranean diet and the DASH diet have been shown to reduce blood pressure.

Alcohol

Alcohol consumption is associated with higher blood pressure, higher BMI, and higher triglyceride and HDL-C. However, since the mid1980s observational studies have consistently found that moderate alcohol consumption is associated with a lower risk of CVD, with the relationship being J-shaped. The lowest risk is observed in persons consuming one to two drinks per day. The higher risk in teetotalers does not seem to be explained by residual confounding. Earlier studies indicated a beneficial effect of wine particularly, perhaps because of the content of flavonoids and resveratrol. However, wine drinkers, beer drinkers, and drinkers of other types of alcohol may differ in other aspects related to cardiovascular risk and the more beneficial association seen for wine in some studies may be caused by residual confounding.

The beneficial effect of alcohol consumption on cardiovascular risk has been questioned, however, in particular after a Mendelian randomization study was not able to confirm this J-shaped relationship. This study was based on the pooling of 56 cohort studies comprising more than 260,000 individuals and 20,000 outcomes. Participants in the study with a genetic variation associated with side effects of drinking alcohol [a single nucleotide polymorphism in the coding for alcohol dehydrogenase (rs1229984 ADH1B)] were observed to consume less alcohol. Contrary to the expectation, carriers of the polymorphism were less likely to develop coronary heart disease, indicating that reduced alcohol exposure is beneficial for CVD health.[55] Conversely, a moderate consumption of alcohol mainly as wine has traditionally been part of the Mediterranean diet and was also part of the recommended diet in the PREDIMED trial. Observational studies of patients with established coronary heart disease have also indicated reduced risk with a moderate alcohol consumption.[56] Controlled trials with alcohol supplementation are not ethically feasible and accepted recommendations are therefore prudent: in patients with coronary heart disease who already have a moderate alcohol consumption (7–14 units per week in men, less in women), no recommendation for change is given.[11,57] Recommendations may be more restrictive in conditions such as hypertension and hypertriglyceridemia. Any recommendations regarding alcohol should be cautious due to the effects beyond cardiovascular health and the wide social implications of alcohol consumption. Thus, CVD patients who do not consume alcohol should not be encouraged to become regular drinkers.[56]

PHYSICAL ACTIVITY

Epidemiologic Evidence of Benefits of Exercise

Plato (400 BC) stated that "In order for man to succeed in life, God provided two means, education and physical activity. Lack of activity destroys the good condition of every human being, whereas movement and methodical physical exercise can save it and preserve it." The beneficial effects of exercise have been recognized since the beginning of medicine. Hippocrates has been quoted for being of the opinion that exercise is necessary to keep a man well.[58] In modern times the first rigorously performed epidemiologic studies to observe a protective effect of exercise on risk of coronary heart disease were the seminal studies by Morris observing that conductors in the London double-decker buses, being physically active climbing the stairs of the bus all day, had a lower risk of coronary heart disease than the less active but otherwise socioeconomically similar bus drivers.[59] Since the 1950s the amount of physical activity during working hours has declined, as the nature of work has changed with less aerobic conditioning physical activity. Furthermore, occupational physical activity is strongly confounded by socioeconomic factors. The strongest evidence supporting the role of physical inactivity in the pathogenesis of CVD relates to leisure time aerobic physical activity.

Physical activity has multiple beneficial effects on a variety of health outcomes and is a cornerstone of a healthy life. There is abundant evidence from epidemiology, basic science, and mechanistic studies supporting the causal role of exercise on prevention of CVD. Multiple large population studies have confirmed the association between physical activity and cardiorespiratory fitness, CVD, and mortality.[60–63] Exercise is associated with an estimated reduction in development of coronary heart disease of 30% to 50%, and physical inactivity is now considered the fourth leading cause of death worldwide.[64] The beneficial effects of physical activity apply to healthy individuals, individuals with cardiovascular risk factors, and patients who have already developed CVD. There is a strong and clear association between exercise and cardiovascular fitness on the one hand and development and progression of CVD on the other hand. Accordingly, physical activity and exercise training are considered important nonpharmacologic tools for primary and secondary CVD prevention in all contemporary prevention guidelines.[11,65]

Definitions of Physical Activity, Exercise, and Fitness

Physical activity is defined as any bodily movement produced by skeletal muscles that requires energy expenditure. One type of physical activity is exercise, which can be defined as a planned and structured physical activity involving increased muscular activity, HR, cardiac output, and energy expenditure. For most persons the activities of daily living will constitute the majority of their energy expenditure, although activities may be at low intensity levels and may not necessarily lead to higher degrees of cardiorespiratory fitness. Cardiorespiratory fitness is the ability of the cardiovascular and respiratory system to supply oxygen to the musculature. Cardiorespiratory fitness is usually expressed as peak VO_2, i.e., the oxygen uptake during maximum exercise standardized to body weight and measured during a cardiopulmonary exercise test. Expected cardiorespiratory fitness is often measured in metabolic equivalents (METs), which is the ratio of energy expenditure during exercise to baseline energy expenditure. The baseline energy expenditure of one MET is equivalent to 3.5 mL oxygen consumption/kg per min. Expected cardiorespiratory fitness depends on age and gender and ranges from 10.5 METs in a 40-year-old male and 9.5 in a 40-year-old female to 6 and 4.5 METS, respectively, in their 80-year-old correlates.[66]

Measuring Physical Activity

Physical activity can be characterized by the duration (the time spent doing the exercise), intensity (the energy expenditure associated with the activity), and frequency (the number of times the physical activity is performed, e.g., per week). Aerobic exercise may be further characterized as continuous aerobic exercise or interval training. Physical activity is often quantified by a summary measure, either as MET-hours, i.e., intensity in METs multiplied by hours of exercise, or as energy expenditure in calories. In studies based on self-reported exercise, METs and MET-hours are calculated from assumed energy expenditure for categories of exercise. None of the measures, however, capture all the important characteristics of physical activity.

Activities of less than 3 METs are characterized as light, e.g., walking at leisure speed (Table 18.3). However, METs is an absolute measure and does not take into account that a younger person can deliver more METs than an older person, a heavier person can deliver more METs than a slim person, and a man can deliver more METs than a woman. For instance, an 80-year-old man working at 6 METs may be close to his physiologic limit, whereas this is very light work for a 20-year-old. Relative intensity may give a better indicator of the level of effort required for the individual and may be measured in energy expenditure (VO_2) relative to the person's peak VO_2, or HR relative to maximal HR, or as a percentage of HR reserve (220 − age − resting HR). Intensity may also be expressed as perceived exertion, often expressed on the Borg scale. The Borg scale was originally designed to be equivalent to the exertion perceived at a given HR in a 20-year-old person and ranges from 6 to 20. Moderate level exercise is usually defined as exercise leading to 11–14 on the Borg scale with some increase in HR and breathing and typically an energy expenditure of 3–6 METS, such as brisk walking. Vigorous exercise is defined as exercise in which the person exercising cannot lead a

TABLE 18.3 Absolute and Relative Exercise Intensities and Examples of Corresponding Activities

INTENSITY	METS	ABSOLUTE INTENSITY EXAMPLES	$\%VO_{2MAX}$	$\%HR_{MAX}$	RELATIVE INTENSITY RPE (BORG TEST SCORE)	TALK TEST
Low intensity, light effort	1.1–2.9	Walking < 4.7 km/h, light household work, light gardening	28–39	45–54	10–11	No changes in breathing rate or limitation in speaking
Moderate intensity, moderate effort	3–5.9	Walking briskly (4.8–6.5 km/h), slow cycling (15 km/h), painting/decorating, vacuuming, gardening (mowing lawn), golf (pulling clubs in trolley), tennis (doubles), ballroom dancing, water aerobics	40–59	55–69	12–13	Breathing is faster but compatible with speaking full sentences
High intensity, vigorous effort	6–7.9	Race-walking, jogging or running, bicycling > 15 km/h, heavy gardening (continuous digging or hovering), swimming laps, tennis (singles)	60–79	70–89	14–16	Breathing very hard, incompatible with carrying on a conversation comfortably
Very hard effort	8–9.9	Running fast	80–99	89–99	17–19	Talking not possible
Maximal effort	> 10	Maximum sprinting	100	100	20	Talking not possible

Note that for older persons a high relative intensity will be equivalent of a lower absolute intensity.
MET is estimated as the energy cost of a given activity divided by resting energy expenditure: 1 MET = 3.5 mL/kg per min oxygen consumption (VO_2).
$\%HR_{max}$, Percentage of measured or estimated maximum heart rate (220 – age); *METs*, metabolic equivalents; *RPE*, Borg rating of perceived exertion (6–20); $\%VO_{2max}$, percentage of measured VO_{2max}.
Modified from Norton K, Norton L, Sadgrove D. Position statement on physical activity and exercise intensity terminology. J Sci Med Sport. *2010;13(5):496–502; Howley ET. Type of activity: resistance, aerobic and leisure versus occupational physical activity.* Med Sci Sports Exerc. *2001;33(6 Suppl):S364–S369.*

conversation (the so-called "talk test"), has a significant increase in HR and breathing frequency, and the exercise is perceived as 14–16 on the Borg scale. High-intensity interval training includes intervals with rate of perceived exertion of 17–19 on the Borg scale. For individuals on β-blocker medication, it is important to consider the modification of HR response and preferably to guide training intensity on other relative intensity parameters. For older patients, deconditioned individuals, and patients with severe heart failure, a relative measure of intensity is more appropriate.

Aerobic Exercise and Cardiorespiratory Fitness

In healthy populations, physical activity has been shown to be strongly associated with longevity due to beneficial effects on a number of disease entities including coronary heart disease.

Cardiorespiratory fitness is strongly associated with cardiovascular and all-cause mortality outcomes.[67] A meta-analysis of 33 prospective studies and more than 100,000 healthy study participants in which a baseline exercise test was performed showed a beneficial effect of cardiorespiratory fitness on all-cause and coronary heart disease/CVD mortality.[60] The effect sizes were somewhat heterogeneous between studies, mainly due to study characteristics such as method of estimating cardiorespiratory fitness, method of adjustment, and duration of follow-up. The overall relative risk (RR) associated with each 1 MET increase in maximum aerobic capacity was 0.87 (0.84–0.90) for all-cause mortality and 0.85 (0.82–0.88) for coronary heart disease and CVD mortality.[60] The difference in expected maximum METs in a sedentary versus an active male aged 40 years is approximately 2 METs. Due to adjustment in several of the studies for factors that may be intermediary on the pathway from exercise to CVD, e.g., blood pressure, body weight, and diabetes, the beneficial effect of cardiorespiratory fitness is likely to be underestimated. The meta-analysis concluded that the minimum cardiorespiratory fitness level associated with significantly lower mortality and CVD risk in men and women, respectively, is 9 and 7 METs at age 40 years, 8 and 6 METs at age 50 years, and 7 and 5 METs at age 60 years.

Cardiorespiratory fitness is more strongly related to health outcomes than self-reported physical activity. A meta-analysis of studies from 1992 to 2007 summarized the association between physical activity and all-cause mortality and CVD mortality.[62] The analysis, which included over 800,000 individuals, found some heterogeneity and indication of publication bias, presumably partially due to considerable differences in methodology between the studies. The strongest associations with mortality outcomes were seen for studies based on objective assessment of exercise capacity. In these studies, the highest level of cardiorespiratory fitness was associated with an adjusted RR of 0.43 (0.33–0.57) for CVD mortality and of 0.59 (0.53–0.65) for all-cause mortality. Studies based on self-reported levels of physical activity, also comparing the highest with the lowest level, had a RR of 0.70 (0.66–0.74) for CVD mortality and 0.71 (0.66–0.76) for all-cause mortality. The beneficial effect was seen in both men and women. Greater effects of physical activity were seen in the statistical models only adjusted for age, consistent with the effect to be partially mediated through cardiovascular risk factors.

Whereas fitness measures are more objective and precise, measures of physical activity are normally summarized from questionnaire information and perhaps do not accurately capture the elements of the exercise expenditure. Although physical activity is a principal determinant of cardiorespiratory fitness, the correlation between physical activity and cardiorespiratory fitness is only modest.[68,69] Indeed, some physically active persons have relatively low cardiorespiratory fitness and, conversely, some relatively inactive persons have high cardiorespiratory fitness. Thus, there may be additional beneficial effects of cardiorespiratory fitness condition on constitutional, environmental, or genetic factors, although this remains to be proven.

Although cardiorespiratory fitness is a strong predictor of prognosis and provides information on the functional status of the patient with coronary heart disease, measurement of cardiorespiratory fitness is generally not a part of the cardiologist's assessment in chronic CVD, and it is rare to consider cardiorespiratory fitness when assessing individual patient risk. Cardiorespiratory fitness has been shown in primary prevention to be an independent predictor of risk, improving multiple metrics of risk prediction compared with a risk model of traditional risk factors.[70] In patients with coronary heart disease, cardiorespiratory fitness is also strongly associated with improved long-term outcome.[71]

Dosage: Intensity, Duration, and Frequency

The greatest health benefits of exercise are seen when progressing from sedentary to light physical activity. Beyond this, more daily exercise leads to a dose-dependent improvement in cardiorespiratory fitness,[72] and it has generally been assumed that more is better in terms of time spent exercising and intensity of the exercise. Recent epidemiologic evidence, however, suggests that moderate amounts of exercise are optimal to achieve longevity and protect against CVD. In a study pooling data from six prospective population studies comprising more than 600,000 participants and 116,000 deaths, the optimal level of physical activity for longevity was 22.5–40 MET-hours per week (equivalent of 4–8 hours of brisk walking) but the added benefit compared to light activity (1.5–3 hours of brisk walking) was modest: adjusted hazard ratios were 0.69 and 0.61, respectively, when comparing to the sedentary.[73] At the extreme end, among participants spending more than 75 MET-hours per week exercising, no additional benefit (but also no significant harm) was seen. Another population study (2015) also suggested a U-shaped relationship for jogging, with levelling off or even increased risk for strenuous joggers, although these findings were based on very few endpoints in the high activity group.[74]

Many studies do not distinguish between intensity of exercise and time spent exercising but summarize with measures such as total number of calories consumed or MET-hours, or use graded questionnaires that do not make a clear distinction. Studies attempting to distinguish between volume and intensity have generally shown that higher-intensity exercise yields more favorable effects on mortality and coronary heart disease risk factors than lower-intensity exercise, independent of the total time spent exercising or the total exercise volume.[63,75,76] A large 2015 study comprising more than 200,000 participants from Australia found greater mortality benefit from vigorous as compared with moderate intensity activities: for the same amount of weighted weekly time spent on exercise, doing vigorous activities 30% or more of the time was associated with a 13% mortality risk reduction when compared to being physically active but doing no vigorous activities.[77] Correspondingly, running also seems to be superior to walking not only at the same volume but also at lower volumes, being superior to walking by a factor of two to four in terms of mortality reduction at similar volumes of exercise.[78] In a study of more than 55,000 adults followed for 15 years, runners had 30% and 45% lower adjusted risks of all-cause and cardiovascular mortality, respectively. Surprisingly, however, there seemed to be no extra benefit from jogging more hours per week or MET-hours spent jogging. In contrast, the speed (intensity) of jogging seemed to be of importance.[79]

These findings, however, are not unequivocal. In one large study, whether the MET-hours were achieved by moderate or vigorous activity did not seem to impact the beneficial effect.[73] Also, results from the Harvard Alumni Health Study and Women's Health Initiative found little or no added benefit from increasing the percentage of exercise performed as vigorous exercise when keeping the total amount fixed with respect to all-cause or cardiovascular mortality.[80]

In summary, the evidence supports prevailing guideline recommendations of exercise for primary and secondary prevention in emphasizing that the most important step is to achieve some level of physical activity. Beyond this, optimal effect is achieved with increased activities of daily living and daily exercise of moderate or vigorous intensity.[11,19]

Interval Training

In recent years the trend of increasing intensity has also been implemented through high-intensity interval training. Independent of energy expenditure, vigorous physical activity is more efficient than moderate activity in inducing cardiorespiratory fitness and metabolic fitness.[75,81,82] High-intensity interval training has been very popular among athletes for decades because it leads to more rapid improvement in cardiorespiratory fitness. A 2015 meta-analysis of studies comparing interval training with moderate continuous training in patients with coronary heart disease confirmed that interval training was more efficient in achieving cardiorespiratory fitness.[83] Some studies have indicated the superiority of a high-intensity interval training to moderate aerobic training for a variety of outcomes such as glycemic control, metabolic syndrome, and heart failure.[84,85] Not all studies confirm this though[86] and more larger-scale, multicenter studies with extended follow-up are needed to determine whether high-intensity interval training is superior to moderate training in leading to sustainable effects on cardiorespiratory fitness and, ultimately, improved outcomes.

Although there is some evidence pointing toward a more beneficial effect of exercise of greater intensity, this should be weighed against the greater risk of muscular and other injuries and, in selected patients with coronary heart disease, the potential risk of adverse cardiac events. For some individuals, e.g., patients with reduced left ventricular ejection fraction or patients who have residual reversible ischemia, the risk/benefit ratio for vigorous or hard exercise may be reversed.

Walking

Walking is the most common type of physical activity in all populations worldwide. In a US adult population it has been estimated that walking constitutes almost 50% of overall physical activity, running and jogging constitute 14%, and other types of exercise—including bicycling, climbing stairs, working out (fitness), and organized sports—constitute the remainder.[87] Estimating the effect of walking, cycling, and other easily performed activities that are part of daily living is important for providing guidance on health-promoting physical activities for cardiac patients. Physical activity as a part of daily living and commuting is readily available to all and reduces the barriers to obtaining healthier lifestyles. Several meta-analyses have confirmed the effect of walking on mortality and coronary heart disease risk[63,88,89] with an estimated risk reduction of 30% for the highest versus lowest walking categories for both CVD and all-cause mortality.[88] However, a more moderate effect of 3% risk reduction with 1 hour of walking per week and 7% for 150 minutes per week was found in one meta-analysis.[63]

Both walking and cycling can be performed at low energy expenditure. The Women's Health Initiative, which included more than 75,000 participants, reported that MET-hours spent walking had additional benefits in terms of reducing cardiovascular risk.[90] A 2014 meta-analysis summarizing results from observational studies, comprising 14 studies and 280,000 participants for walking and seven studies with 187,000 participants for cycling, concluded that both cycling and walking were associated with reduced all-cause mortality risk: walking or cycling 11.25 MET-hours per week (the equivalent of 2–3 hours of brisk walking) was associated with a 10% reduced mortality risk with little further dose-response effect of higher MET-hours.[91] The meta-analysis only included studies that adjusted for other physical activity to ensure that the risk estimates were most likely attributable to the walking and cycling activity. Results were somewhat heterogeneous but the method of assessing walking intensity and quantity was also heterogeneous, as was adjustment for confounding factors.

When compared with jogging, walking has less benefit. This is consistent with more intense activity having more benefit on cardiovascular fitness and glucose metabolism. Studies comparing walking speed and quantity indicate that speed is superior in preventing development of the metabolic syndrome, preventing heart failure, and protecting against coronary heart disease.[92–94] Similarly, lower versus higher walking speed was associated with a threefold risk of CVD mortality but not an increased risk of cancer in a population sample aged above 65 years.[95] However, there are beneficial effects of walking at a lower speed. The Studies of a Targeted Risk Reduction Intervention through Defined Exercise intervention (STRRIDE) study indicated that even at low intensity, 30 minutes of walking each day can prevent weight gain in overweight subjects.[96]

Intervention studies of the effect of walking on cardiovascular risk factors have accumulated. Summarizing the results from 32 papers comparing walking intervention with no exercise, walking was concluded to improve aerobic capacity (3.0 mL/kg per min); reduce systolic (– 3.6 mm Hg) and diastolic (– 1.5 mm Hg) blood pressure; and reduce waist circumference (– 1.5 cm), weight (– 1.4 kg), percentage body fat (– 1.2%), and BMI (– 0.5 kg/m^2), but had no effect on blood lipids, including HDL-C.[97] Randomized controlled trials of walking intervention among patients with type 2 diabetes have shown improvement in glycemic control and BMI,[98] and speed of walking may be more important than time spent walking; in a cohort study with follow-up, healthy participants free of the metabolic syndrome at baseline had a 50% lower risk of developing the metabolic syndrome after 10 years if they had a fast walking speed, whereas walking more than 1 hour per day at low speed did not confer protection.[93]

Resistance Training

The majority of the evidence described pertains to aerobic exercise. With the ageing of the population with coronary heart disease, comorbidities and age-related functional decline play an increasing role. These enhance the importance of resistance training to maintain muscular strength in management of the patients and the overall treatment plan. The importance of including resistance training has been acknowledged in several recommendations,[65,99–101] and a combination of aerobic training with resistance training is thought to be more effective than aerobic training alone in improving body composition, strength, and some indicators of cardiovascular fitness.[102] Among patients with type 2 diabetes, a combination of aerobic and resistance training improved glycated hemoglobin (Hba1c) levels. This was not achieved by aerobic or resistance training alone.[103]

Resistance training can be performed in a cardiac rehabilitation setting and in fitness centers using weight machines but may also be performed at home with modes such as weight lifting exercises, elastic bands, or calisthenics. Resistance training with a heavy load may lead to a considerable increase in blood pressure. However, provided resting blood pressure is well controlled, patients without heart failure can safely perform resistance training. For patients with heart failure, training of smaller muscle groups separately, a smaller load, or a shorter duration may be recommended based on an individual evaluation.[100] Use of the Valsalva maneuver during resistance training increases blood pressure further and should be avoided in patients with heart failure. Documented beneficial effects of resistance training include improvements in blood pressure, glucose metabolism, and weight control. Resistance training also improves balance and coordination. In particular, for the increasing group of elderly patients with coronary heart disease, exercise including resistance training is important to maintain muscular strength and function and improved ability to perform activities of daily living through older age.

Sedentary Behavior

A distinction has been drawn between sedentary behavior and physical activity, with the former being defined not by level of physical activity but by time spent in a sedentary manner. The two are naturally interrelated, but whereas the traditional definition of exercise/physical activity refers to a separate activity recommended for 30 minutes of each day, sedentary behavior may refer to the remaining 23.5 hours of the day. More time spent being sedentary, in particular hours sitting or watching television, was associated with adverse cardiovascular risk factors, CVD outcomes, and all-cause mortality in several studies,[104–107] although some observational studies have not been able to confirm this.[108] Whether or not this is independent of time spent engaged in physical exercise remains to be studied further.[105,107] In particular, older adults spend many hours sitting. A 2015 review concluded that, based on self-report, almost 60% of older adults spent more than 4 hours per day sitting, and using objective validation the number of hours spent sitting was even higher.[109,110]

Nonexercise activities are activities of daily living not categorized as exercise, e.g., walking, moving around, standing, and fidgeting. Nonexercise activities, which can now be captured more accurately with accelerometers, increase energy expenditure and are associated with lower body weight, less abdominal obesity, better glycemic control, and lower metabolic score even after adjusting for moderate and vigorous exercise.[111] Bed-rest studies confirm these findings. In healthy young men with normal levels of activity, reducing the number of daily steps from an average of 10,501 to 1344 over 2 weeks resulted in marked increases in intra-abdominal fat, decreases in aerobic fitness, and impairments in several metabolic markers including insulin sensitivity.[112,113]

Although further studies are needed, these accumulated data show that among individuals who do not perform any exercise, the role of daily activities in reducing sedentary behavior and promoting cardiovascular health needs to be emphasized. The amount of time spent being sedentary can be minimized by active travelling (cycling, walking, or using public transportation), taking breaks from extended periods of sitting, and reducing screen time.

Mechanisms

The effects of exercise training are fundamentally the same in persons with and without CVD. Exercise leads to central and peripheral adaptations that improve the body's ability to consume oxygen for work. With regular exercise, peripheral adaptations are responsible for increased ability of the musculature to use oxygen to derive energy for the work performed without increasing cardiac output. Through central adaptations, maximal cardiac output can be improved mainly through adaptation of stroke volume, whereas the maximum HR is relatively fixed.

Aerobic exercise enhances the ability to deliver more energy peripherally at the same demand on the heart and vascular system by increasing energy efficiency. Aerobic exercise also results in improved endothelial function causing lower peripheral resistance and improved coronary microvascular function, thereby improving the oxygen supply for the heart during exercise. This means that the same level of work can be performed for a decreased myocardial oxygen demand (HR × systolic blood pressure). For patients with angina due to residual ischemia, these mechanisms are important because angina may occur at a higher threshold when the same load on the heart can sustain a greater level of body work. Exercise has further antithrombotic and fibrinolytic effects and also favors higher vagal balance with reduced risk of arrhythmia.[11] The preconditioning effect of exercise seen in animal studies, although not demonstrated in humans, may play a role in reducing the impact of coronary occlusion.[114]

Exercise exerts its effects in primary and secondary prevention of CVD through a number of beneficial effects on cardiovascular risk factors, including lowered systolic and diastolic blood pressure and lipids, and improved glycemic control by increasing insulin sensitivity and reducing abdominal adiposity. Exercise improves endothelial function, endogenous fibrinolysis, cardiac output, HR variability and autonomic control, and capillary and mitochondrial density. Exercise also decreases myocardial oxygen demand, platelet aggregation, and blood viscosity. Additionally, physically active individuals have a better quality of life, less depression and anxiety, and better sleep quality; report less stress; and are more prone to maintaining cognitive function at higher age.

Lipids

Exercise has consistently been shown in cross-sectional, prospective, and intervention studies to reduce levels of triglycerides and increase HDL-C but has little effect on total cholesterol or LDL-C levels. Although minor effects are seen on total LDL-C, exercise is associated with a shift in particle size toward larger, less atherogenic LDL-C particles. Similarly, exercise has a beneficial effect on HDL-C particle size, causing an increase mainly in the less atherogenic HDL-C2 particles.[115] Some effects of exercise on lipids are mediated via the weight-lowering effects, the decrease in fat mass, and the increase in lean body mass accompanying exercise training. The isolated effect of exercise is difficult to quantify. Effects of exercise and statin therapy are additive, as are other cardiovascular prevention strategies. Interestingly, patients with dyslipidemia who are fit but not on statin treatment have a lower mortality risk than patients with dyslipidemia on statins who are unfit.[116]

With statins and potential future general use of more potent LDL-C-reducing medication, the effects of exercise on HDL-C and triglycerides deserve attention to address residual risk. Mechanisms for affecting HDL-C and triglycerides are thought to be via increased activity of lipoprotein lipase, which in turn lowers very low-density lipoprotein cholesterol (VLDL-C) and triglyceride levels. The reduced availability of triglycerides causes an increase in HDL-C and increased size of LDL-C particles. Exercise also reduces hepatic lipase activity. Hepatic lipase activity leads to smaller HDL-C particles with higher turnover and thus less reverse cholesterol transport activity. Little is known of the effects of resistance training on lipids, although smaller, older studies indicate less effect on lipids than aerobic training.[117]

Inflammation, Body Weight, Blood Pressure, and Glycemic Control

Physical activity reduces blood pressure and prevents or delays development of hypertension, helps control body weight and reduces abdominal obesity, and improves insulin sensitivity, as well as glucose control in patients with diabetes. The clustering of cardiovascular risk factors in the metabolic syndrome is also beneficially affected by physical activity. In a Finnish trial of lifestyle counseling of individuals at high risk of developing diabetes, moderate and vigorous leisure time physical activity was associated with decreased likelihood of developing the metabolic syndrome and increased likelihood of its resolution.[118] Similarly, cardiorespiratory fitness is associated with reduced prevalence of metabolic syndrome and increased likelihood of resolve.[119] Persons with higher levels of physical activity generally have lower levels of inflammation, and intervention studies also indicate a small but significant decrease in inflammatory markers such as high-sensitivity C-reactive protein, tumor necrosis factor-alpha, and interleukins following exercise training. Some of the effects of physical activity on cardiovascular risk factors are partly mediated through weight control.

Intervention Studies

Exercise training is a cornerstone of cardiac rehabilitation and is discussed hereafter. In cardiac rehabilitation studies offering exercise training two to three times weekly over a period of 8 to 24 weeks, the effect size has been in the range of a 10% to 20% improvement in peak VO_2.

Exercise training is also beneficial in patients who are not fully revascularized. In a study of 101 males with angina and greater than 75% stenosis of one coronary artery randomized to PCI with stent or a 12-month exercise training program, after one year the exercise training group had a similar outcome to the PCI group regarding angina and improvement in myocardial perfusion at scintigraphy, and a better exercise capacity and event-free survival rate.[120] These effects occurred despite no changes in epicardial vessel stenosis at repeat angiography. Effects were presumably through improved microcirculation and development of collaterals. This was a relatively small, single-center trial and conclusions should be drawn with caution. However, the trial does indicate that in patients with epicardial stenosis not amenable to revascularization, exercise training may be a potential means of reducing ischemia, reducing symptoms, and improving prognosis.

BOX 18.2 Recommendation for Physical Activity for Adults

All adults should avoid inactivity:

- Some physical activity is better than none, and any amount of physical activity results in some health benefits.

For substantial health benefits:

- 150 min per week of moderate-intensity aerobic activity, or
- 75 min per week of vigorous-intensity aerobic physical activity, or
- an equivalent combination of moderate- and vigorous-intensity aerobic activity.
- Activity episodes should be at least 10 min in duration and spread throughout the week.

For more extensive health benefits:

- 300 min per week of moderate-intensity aerobic activity, or
- 150 min per week of vigorous-intensity aerobic physical activity, or
- an equivalent combination of moderate- and vigorous-intensity activity.

Combine with moderate- or high-intensity muscle-strengthening activities that involve all major muscle groups on 2 or more days per week.

Modified from Office of Disease Prevention and Health Practice, US Department of Health and Human Services: The 2008 Physical Activity Guidelines for Americans. <http://health.gov/paguidelines/guidelines/summary.aspx>

Recommendations Regarding Exercise

Exercise has profound health promoting effects. Consequently, assessment of a patient's habitual level of exercise and recommendation on how to achieve improved physical fitness should be a routine part of patient care in cardiovascular medicine. For all patients, the clinician should encourage 30 to 60 minutes of moderate-intensity aerobic activity daily. Such activity may include brisk walking supplemented by an increase in daily lifestyle activities (e.g., walking breaks at work, gardening, household work) to improve cardiorespiratory fitness and move patients out of the unfit, sedentary, high-risk cohort. For all cardiac patients, risk assessment with a physical activity history and/or an exercise test is recommended to guide prognosis and prescription. The clinician should also counsel patients to report and be evaluated for symptoms related to exercise.

Recommendations for exercise, whether for healthy adults, persons with increased cardiovascular risk such as patients with diabetes and hypertension, or patients who have already developed CVD, are summarized in Box 18.2. These recommendations also apply to older adults but may be modified to adapt to the individual's abilities.

Unfortunately, there is a large discrepancy between the recommendations for physical activity and what is actually practiced in the population. Among adults aged 60 years or more in the National Health and Nutrition Examination Survey (NHANES) study, 52% reported no leisure time physical activity.[121] A 2016 European multicenter data reported that approximately 60% of patients with coronary heart disease were sedentary or only had limited physical activity.[4] According to US data, less than 30% of individuals at high risk received counseling on physical activity by their physician.[122] For this reason the AHA has made regular exercise a focus for preventive medicine, adding a sedentary lifestyle to the modifiable CVD risk factors.[123]

Safety

Exercise in patients with coronary heart disease is generally safe, and the beneficial effects far outweigh the minor risks. However, during exercise training the risk of MI, cardiac arrhythmia, or sudden cardiac death is transiently increased. The risk has been estimated through summarizing data from a large number of cardiac rehabilitation trials with supervised training among patients with coronary heart disease.[124] The rate of cardiac arrest was 8.6 per million training hours, the rate of MI was 4.5 per million training hours, and the rate of cardiac death was 1.3 per million training hours.[125] This risk evaluation is based on cardiac patients who have had a symptom-limited exercise test performed before embarking on exercise. It is therefore recommended that patients with uncomplicated coronary heart disease, i.e., patients who are fully revascularized with no residual ischemia on a symptom-limited exercise test and who have a normal ejection fraction, undergo exercise training with no limitations following a cardiopulmonary exercise test that does not show ischemia or cardiac arrhythmias. Primarily to avoid musculoskeletal injury the exercise intensity and duration should be adapted to the individual's exercise capacity and usual level of exercise and gradually increased from there.

For subgroups such as patients with heart failure, including patients with device therapy, patients surviving cardiac arrest, patients with residual ischemia, and other groups, exercise training is also recommended but should initially be supervised and preceded by a symptom-limited maximal cardiopulmonary exercise test. The training program should be individually adapted. The exercise-based risk of adverse cardiac events during exercise is low, even in symptomatic patients with moderate to severe heart failure, as confirmed in the large Heart Failure: A Controlled Trial Investigating Outcomes of Exercise Training (HF-ACTION) trial.[126]

CARDIAC REHABILITATION

Cardiac rehabilitation is a multidisciplinary intervention offered to help heart patients increase cardiorespiratory fitness, reduce cardiac symptoms, improve health, and reduce the risk of future heart problems (Fig. 18.3). In addition to optimizing pharmacologic treatment and providing

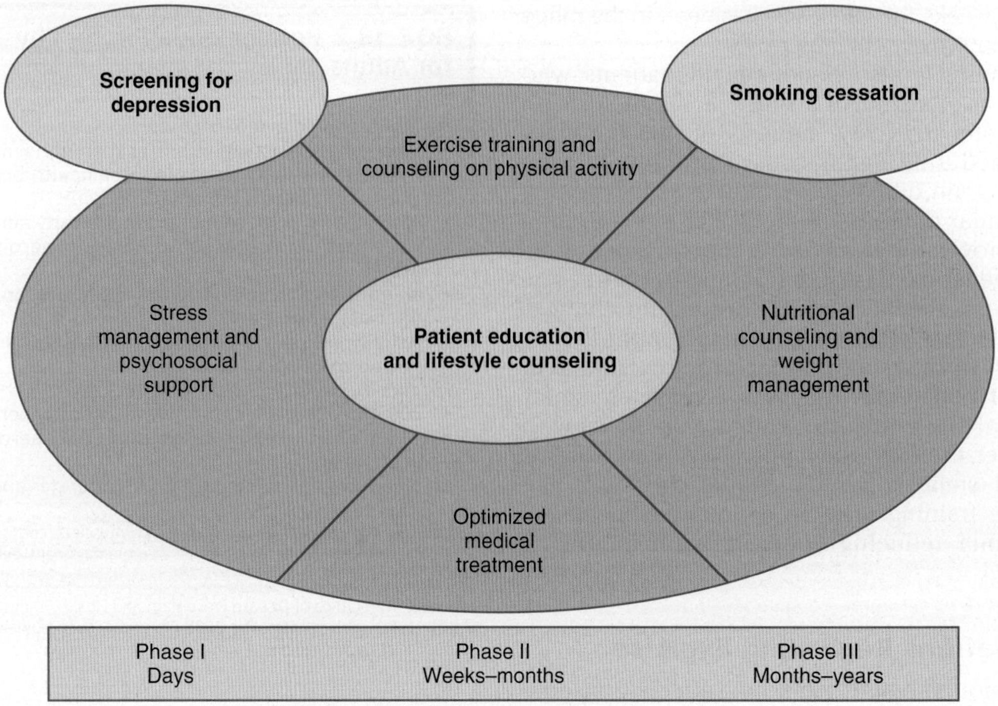

FIG. 18.3 Components of a cardiac rehabilitation program.

behavioral strategies to promote lifestyle change, cardiac rehabilitation includes education, counseling, psychosocial support, and commonly also a structured exercise program.

Other issues often raised by patients during cardiac rehabilitation include sexual and erectile dysfunction, alcohol consumption, and stress management. Depression and anxiety are commonly seen in patients with coronary heart disease, are associated with adverse cardiovascular prognosis, and represent barriers to lifestyle change and adherence to medication. Accordingly, it is recommended to screen all patients with coronary heart disease for depression and refer to adequate treatment.[127] Cardiac rehabilitation provides a good opportunity to perform the screening and necessary subsequent action, although it should be noted that randomized trials have so far failed to show survival benefit of treating depression in patients with coronary heart disease (see Chapter 26).

Cardiac rehabilitation is often divided into three phases. Phase 1 is initiated while the patient is still in the hospital and consists of early mobilization and brief counseling about the nature of the illness, the treatment, risk factors management, and the plan for follow-up. Phase 2 comprises the secondary prevention or cardiac rehabilitation program offered after hospital discharge, most commonly as a supervised ambulatory outpatient program of 3 to 6 months' duration. In some countries this may be a home-based, tele-monitored, or shorter residential program. Phase 3 reflects the lifetime maintenance of a healthy lifestyle and optimal risk factor control with the goal of halting or slowing the disease progression and maintaining an active and healthy life. In prevailing guidelines of cardiovascular societies worldwide, cardiac rehabilitation has received a class I recommendation and there is consensus that all eligible patients should be referred and encouraged to participate.

Definition and Core Components

Cardiac rehabilitation encompasses a multiteam effort with a core component being implementation of lifestyle changes. The importance of cardiac rehabilitation has increased, not least because of the limited time spent in hospital and the need for the patient to understand the disease and to understand that the lifelong implications depend on a structured ambulatory follow-up. Core components are education in understanding the disease; motivational counseling on nutrition, physical activity, and healthy lifestyle; exercise training; risk factor control (blood pressure, serum lipids, blood glucose, weight, and smoking); understanding of medication and lifelong lifestyle changes; and psychosocial support and stress alleviation. Because effective lifestyle changes depend critically on interaction and support of the patient's surroundings, cardiac rehabilitation should involve the family of the patient.[128] An exercise training program with the aim of improving cardiorespiratory fitness is regarded as beneficial for almost all patients after MI and revascularization.[129,130] Unfortunately, most studies indicate that sustainable changes are very difficult to achieve and require more than a brief cardiac rehabilitation.

Some components of secondary prevention and follow-up on coronary heart disease patients after acute events or revascularization may be provided in an individual ambulatory setting, but are best delivered as part of a team effort in integrated cardiac rehabilitation. Centralizing cardiac rehabilitation also ensures that the needs of specific patient groups, such as patients with devices implanted (cardiac resynchronization therapy [CRT], implantable cardioverter defibrillator [ICD], pacemaker), patients with heart failure, patients with peripheral arterial disease, and patients with comorbidities, are met. All patients with coronary heart disease can benefit from cardiac rehabilitation, and

TABLE 18.4 Physical Activity Counseling for Specific Patient Groups

CONDITION	ESTABLISHED/GENERALLY AGREED ISSUES
Post-ACS and post primary PCI	Assess: Risk must be assessed by physical activity history and exercise testing to guide prescription. Symptom-limited exercise testing after clinical stabilization; submaximal exercise stress testing in selected cases Recommend: After uncomplicated procedure, physical activity can start the next day. After a large and/or complicated myocardial damage, physical activity should start after clinical stabilization and be increased slowly, according to the symptoms. In the presence of preserved exercise capacity without symptoms, patient can resume routine physical activity for 30–60 min, such as brisk walking, supplemented by an increase in daily activities (such as walking breaks at work, gardening, or household work); otherwise, the patient should resume physical activity at 50% of maximal exercise capacity and gradually increase. Physical activity should be a combination of activities like walking, climbing stairs, cycling.
Stable CAD and post elective PCI	Assess: Exercise capacity and ischemia threshold by symptom limited exercise stress test, exercise or pharmacological imaging technique in symptomatic patients with un-interpretable ECG Recommend: See Table 18.3.
Post cardiac surgery, coronary artery and valve heart surgery	Assess: Exercise capacity to guide exercise prescription Submaximal exercise stress test as soon as possible A maximal exercise test after surgical wound stabilization Recommend: Physical activity counseling according to wound healing and exercise capacity; Table 18.3
Chronic heart failure	Assess: Peak exercise capacity by maximal symptom-limited cardiopulmonary exercise testing. For testing protocol, small increments 5–10 W per min on bicycle ergometer or modified Bruce or Naughton protocols on treadmill are indicated (in order to achieve max. exercise capacity in 8–12 min). Recommend: At least 30–60 min/day of moderate intensity exercise; Table 18.3
Cardiac transplantation	Assess: Peak exercise capacity by maximal symptom-limited cardiopulmonary exercise testing Recommend: Long-term dynamic and resistance exercise to prevent many side effects of immunosuppressive therapy Exercise intensity relies more on the perceived exertion (i.e., Borg scale) than on a specific HR due to impaired HR response in de-innervated heart. Individual adaptation of rate of increase in pace/intensity.

ACS, Acute coronary syndrome; *CAD*, coronary artery disease; *ECG*, electrocardiogram; *HR*, heart rate; *PCI*, percutaneous coronary intervention.
Modified from Corra U, Piepoli MF, Carre F, et al. Secondary prevention through cardiac rehabilitation: physical activity counselling and exercise training: key components of the position paper from the Cardiac Rehabilitation Section of the European Association of Cardiovascular Prevention and Rehabilitation. Eur Heart J. *2010;31(16):1967–1974.*

cardiac rehabilitation is recommended for patients following MI and revascularization, for patients with heart failure, and after valve replacement. Exercise-based cardiac rehabilitation has been expanded in some countries to patients with atrial fibrillation, patients with an assist device, and after heart transplantation. After CABG (and other conditions with sternum split), lower extremity exercise can be started early, and after 4 to 6 weeks, when the sternum has been stabilized, the patient can be engaged in exercise involving the upper extremities.

Cardiac rehabilitation has been offered as an in-patient service, as an out-patient service in a cardiology setting, as an out-patient service in communal settings, or as home-based training. The most studied type of cardiac rehabilitation is exercise-based cardiac rehabilitation in an out-patient, cardiology setting with a 12- to 24-week program two to three times weekly. The backbone of the training is continuous aerobic training of moderate to hard intensity. The effect on peak VO_2 is approximately 10% to 20% and is similar across age groups and gender.[86] Newer studies indicate a greater effect with interval training, as is well recognized from athletes. However, whether or not this translates into greater long-term benefits is not known. Studies also indicate that training should be supplemented with resistance training to achieve greater gain in exercise capacity and to counteract debility and frailty, particularly in older people and women with coronary heart disease, as previously discussed (Table 18.4).

Exercise-based cardiac rehabilitation is effective in reducing total and cardiovascular mortality and hospital admissions. From a previous systematic review and meta-analysis of exercise-based cardiac rehabilitation for coronary heart disease, which included 47 trials published up to 2009 and comprised more than 10,000 patients, cardiac rehabilitation was associated with longer-term reduced overall mortality (RR 0.87 [0.75–0.99]) and cardiovascular mortality (RR 0.74 [0.63–0.87]).[131] Exercise interventions differed in duration (1–30 months), frequency (1–7 times per week), time per session (20–90 min), and exercise intensity and type, the main component being moderate, continuous aerobic training. Participants were predominantly post-MI and CABG patients and results were relatively homogeneous across the studies. Of the ten studies that assessed effect on quality of life, seven found significant improvement following intervention. The patients included in the trials are, however, not representative of the current coronary heart disease population in need of cardiac rehabilitation as 88% were male and the mean age was 55 years. However, observational studies indicate similar effects of exercise training on exercise capacity in other patient groups, including women and the elderly. Community-based observational studies also confirm the beneficial effect of cardiac rehabilitation. Among patients receiving CABG, participants in cardiac rehabilitation had an adjusted mortality risk reduction of 44%, corresponding to a 10-year absolute risk reduction of 12.7% and a number needed to treat of eight. Similar results were seen for CABG combined with valve surgery.[132,133]

An updated meta-analysis including 63 trials and more than 14,000 participants with a median follow-up of 12 months confirmed a 36% reduction in cardiovascular mortality risk and an 18% reduction in risk of hospital admission for recurrent events but failed to find a significant effect on total mortality, MI, or revascularization. This study also confirmed an effect on quality of life measures.[134] There was a trend for later studies conducted in the era of contemporary medical therapy to have smaller mortality benefits.

Heart Failure

Particular care should be given to special groups with coronary heart disease. Exercise training in patients with heart failure has been shown to be beneficial, with an effect on exercise capacity, quality of life, and on adverse outcomes such as hospital admission and cardiac mortality. Meta-analyses of studies with more than 12 months of follow-up comparing exercise training with usual care among patients with systolic heart failure have concluded that exercise training leads to reduced total mortality (hazard ratio 0.88) and heart failure–specific admissions (hazard ratio 0.61). Exercise training also leads to improved quality of life.[135] This is consistent with (and dominated by) the findings from the large multicenter HF-ACTION trial. In this trial, symptomatic, stable congestive heart failure (CHF) patients with left ventricular ejection fraction 35% or below who were in the New York Heart Association (NYHA) group II–IV were randomized to a comprehensive, prolonged exercise intervention consisting of 36 supervised exercise sessions followed by home-based exercise versus usual care. Although the patients did not comply with the target of performing 90 minutes of exercise weekly, the intervention group had a reduced risk of the major outcome of mortality and hospital admission for heart failure. In prespecified adjusted analyses, hazard ratios were 0.89 ($p = 0.03$) for all-cause mortality or hospitalization, 0.91 ($p = 0.09$) for cardiovascular mortality or hospitalization, and 0.85 ($p = 0.03$) for cardiovascular mortality or heart failure hospitalization. A small but statistically significant effect was also seen on health status (Minnesota Living with Heart Failure Questionnaire).[126,136]

UPTAKE AND ADHERENCE TO LIFESTYLE CHANGES AND CARDIAC REHABILITATION

Lifestyle changes are complementary to medical treatment, they are inexpensive, have few if any side effects, and have numerous health benefits beyond cardiovascular disease. Yet they remain underutilized.

Adherence to lifestyle changes after acute coronary events has a rapid onset of effect. In the OASIS trial, more than 18,000 patients were followed after acute coronary events. The patients, who managed to give up smoking, and/or adhere to dietary recommendations and/or exercise one month after their event, had a significantly lower risk of repeat events within the subsequent 5 months. Diet and exercise adherence was associated with a 48% decreased risk of MI when compared with nonadherence, smoking cessation was associated with a 43% decreased risk, and never-smokers who adhered to diet and exercise recommendations had a 74% lower risk than the nonadherent to all three lifestyle factors. However, even though these patients were selected to be participants in a trial, only 29% were adherent to diet and exercise recommendations at 30 days. In comparison, more than 96% adhered to antiplatelet medication.[3]

Cardiac rehabilitation is an important component of recovery from coronary events but uptake and adherence to such programs are below recommended levels. In the EUROASPIRE IV study, a cross-sectional study of secondary prevention in 8000 patients with coronary artery disease undertaken more than 6 months after their event, only half of the patients (50.7%) had been offered cardiac rehabilitation and 81.3% of these had only attended half of the program. These figures were greater in comparison to less than one-third of eligible patients being offered cardiac rehabilitation in the EUROASPIRE III study[137,138] but are likely to give a very optimistic view of the status of secondary prevention because these were selected patients (participation rate 50%) in selected centers.[4] Indeed, other studies indicate lower participation rates. Surveys have found that less than 30% of eligible patients participate in cardiac rehabilitation and among those that do, many do not complete the program and only 50% continue exercise training 6 months after program completion.[139]

Unfortunately, most patients do not attend cardiac rehabilitation either because it is not offered or because they do not accept or adhere to the program. A 2014 Cochrane review of studies attempting to improve uptake of and/or adherence to cardiac rehabilitation identified 18 studies comprising 2505 participants. Interventions included structured nurse- or therapist-led contacts, early appointments after discharge, motivational letters, gender-specific programs, and intermediate-phase programs for older patients but were too heterogeneous for any meta-analysis to be performed. A number of the studies showed a positive effect on uptake and adherence but the overall conclusion was that the evidence was weak for efficient interventions to increase uptake and adherence and more quality studies targeting patient-identified barriers may increase the likelihood of success.[139]

Predictors of nonuptake are: (1) older age, (2) women, (3) comorbidities, (4) lower educational attainment, (5) socioeconomic deprivation, and (5) ethnicity, with blacks being less likely to participate than whites in the United States and patients of other ethnic origin being less likely to participate in Europe.[140] Patient-related factors associated with limited uptake and adherence are presented in Box 18.3. Addressing structural barriers is likely to increase uptake. It is universally accepted that automatic referral procedures for patients experiencing MI or revascularization would address some of these barriers. Strong endorsement from healthcare providers serves as a further catalyst,[141] as does minimizing the delay from discharge to the phase 2 rehabilitation[142] and implementing performance indicators.

BOX 18.3 Factors Associated with Referral and Enrollment in Cardiac Rehabilitation Programs

1. **Patient oriented factors**
   - female sex
   - older age
   - race/ethnic minority groups
   - lack of or limited health care insurance
   - low socioeconomic status
   - low educational attainment
   - low self efficacy
   - low health literacy
   - lack of perceived need for CR or secondary prevention
   - language
   - cultural beliefs and understanding of disease and treatment
   - work related factors (loss of salary, self-employment, etc.)
   - limited social support
   - home responsibilities
2. **Medical factors**
   - multiple comorbidities including depression and musculoskeletal problems
3. **Healthcare system factors**
   - lack of referral
   - lack of enrollment after referral
   - strength of endorsement by treating physician
   - patient provider relationship
   - program availability and characteristics
   - distance, public transportation, programs suitable for groups characterized by race, age and gender groups

CR, Cardiac rehabilitation.
From Balady GJ, Ades PA, Bittner VA, et al. Referral, enrollment, and delivery of cardiac rehabilitation/secondary prevention programs at clinical centers and beyond: a presidential advisory from the American Heart Association. *Circulation*. 2011;124(25):2951–2960.

References

1. Yusuf S, Hawken S, Ounpuu S, et al.: Effect of potentially modifiable risk factors associated with myocardial infarction in 52 countries (the INTERHEART study): case-control study, *Lancet* 364(9438):937–952, 2004.
2. Ford ES, Ajani UA, Croft JB, et al.: Explaining the decrease in U.S. deaths from coronary disease, 1980–2000, *N Engl J Med* 356(23):2388–2398, 2007.
3. Chow CK, Jolly S, Rao-Melacini P, et al.: Association of diet, exercise, and smoking modification with risk of early cardiovascular events after acute coronary syndromes, *Circulation* 121(6):750–758, 2010.
4. Kotseva K, Wood D, De BD, et al.: EUROASPIRE IV: a European Society of Cardiology survey on the lifestyle, risk factor and therapeutic management of coronary patients from 24 European countries, *Eur J Prev Cardiol* 23(6):636–648, 2016.
5. *Centers for Disease Control and Prevention*. http://www.cdc.gov/tobacco/data_statistics/fact_sheets/health_effects/tobacco_related_mortality/, 2016.
6. Centers for Disease Control and Prevention: *The Health Consequences of Smoking—50 Years of Progress: a Report of the Surgeon General*, Atlanta, GA, 2014, U.S. Department of Health and Human Services, Centers for Disease Control and Prevention, National Center for Chronic Disease Prevention and Health Promotion, Office on Smoking and Health.
7. Prescott E, Hippe M, Schnohr P, Hein HO, Vestbo J: Smoking and risk of myocardial infarction in women and men: longitudinal population study, *BMJ* 316(7137):1043–1047, 1998.
8. Law MR, Morris JK, Wald NJ: Environmental tobacco smoke exposure and ischaemic heart disease: an evaluation of the evidence, *BMJ* 315(7114):973–980, 1997.
9. He J, Vupputuri S, Allen K, et al.: Passive smoking and the risk of coronary heart disease—a meta-analysis of epidemiologic studies, *N Engl J Med* 340(12):920–926, 1999.
10. Lightwood JM, Glantz SA: Declines in acute myocardial infarction after smoke-free laws and individual risk attributable to secondhand smoke, *Circulation* 120(14):1373–1379, 2009.
11. Piepoli MF, Hoes AW, Agewall S, et al.: 2016 European guidelines on cardiovascular disease prevention in clinical practice, *Eur Heart J* 28:2375–2414, 2016.
12. Boffetta P, Straif K: Use of smokeless tobacco and risk of myocardial infarction and stroke: systematic review with meta-analysis, *BMJ* 339:b3060, 2009. http://dx.doi.org/10.1136/bmj.b3060.
13. Csordas A, Bernhard D: The biology behind the atherothrombotic effects of cigarette smoke, *Nat Rev Cardiol* 10(4):219–230, 2013.
14. Shields M, Wilkins K: *Smoking, smoking cessation and heart disease risk: a 16-year follow-up study*, 24(2):12–22, 2013.
15. National Cancer Institute U: *Changes in Cigarette-Related Disease Risks and Their Implication for Prevention and Control*. Smoking and Tobacco Control Monograph No. 8 [Bethesda, Md.]: U.S. Dept. of Health and Human Services, Public Health Service, National Institutes of Health, National Cancer Institute, 1991-; 1997.
16. Critchley J, Capewell S: Smoking cessation for the secondary prevention of coronary heart disease, *Cochrane Database Syst Rev* (1):CD003041, 2004.
17. Mohiuddin SM, Mooss AN, Hunter CB, et al.: Intensive smoking cessation intervention reduces mortality in high-risk smokers with cardiovascular disease, *Chest* 131(2):446–452, 2007.
18. Anthonisen NR, Skeans MA, Wise RA, et al.: The effects of a smoking cessation intervention on 14.5-year mortality: a randomized clinical trial, *Ann Intern Med* 142(4):233–239, 2005.
19. Eckel RH, Jakicic JM, Ard JD, et al.: 2013 AHA/ACC guideline on lifestyle management to reduce cardiovascular risk: a report of the American College of Cardiology/American Heart Association Task Force on Practice Guidelines, *Circulation* 129(25 Suppl 2):S76–S99, 2014.
20. Stead LF, Bergson G, Lancaster T: Physician advice for smoking cessation, *Cochrane Database Syst Rev* (2):CD000165, 2008. http://dx.doi.org/10.1002/14651858.CD000165.pub3.
21. Rice VH, Stead LF: Nursing interventions for smoking cessation, *Cochrane Database Syst Rev* (1):CD001188, 2008. http://dx.doi.org/10.1002/14651858.CD001188.pub3.
22. Heatherton TF, Kozlowski LT, Frecker RC, Fagerstrom KO: The Fagerstrom Test for Nicotine Dependence: a revision of the Fagerstrom Tolerance Questionnaire, *Br J Addict* 86(9):1119–1127, 1991.
23. Cahill K, Stevens S, Perera R, Lancaster T: Pharmacological interventions for smoking cessation: an overview and network meta-analysis, *Cochrane Database Syst Rev* 5:CD009329, 2013. http://dx.doi.org/10.1002/14651858.CD009329.pub2.
24. Stead LF, Perera R, Bullen C, et al.: Nicotine replacement therapy for smoking cessation, *Cochrane Database Syst Rev* 11:CD000146, 2012. http://dx.doi.org/10.1002/14651858.CD000146.pub4.
25. Rigotti NA, Clair C, Munafo MR, Stead LF: Interventions for smoking cessation in hospitalised patients, *Cochrane Database Syst Rev* 5:CD001837, 2012. http://dx.doi.org/10.1002/14651858.CD001837.pub3.
26. Chang PH, Chiang CH, Ho WC, et al.: Combination therapy of varenicline with nicotine replacement therapy is better than varenicline alone: a systematic review and meta-analysis of randomized controlled trials, *BMC Public Health* 15:689, 2015.
27. Leaviss J, Sullivan W, Ren S, et al.: What is the clinical effectiveness and cost-effectiveness of cytisine compared with varenicline for smoking cessation? A systematic review and economic evaluation, *Health Technol Assess* 18(33):1–120, 2014.
28. McRobbie H, Bullen C, Hartmann-Boyce J, Hajek P: Electronic cigarettes for smoking cessation and reduction, *Cochrane Database Syst Rev* 12:CD010216, 2014. http://dx.doi.org/10.1002/14651858.CD010216.pub2.
29. Wing RR, Bolin P, Brancati FL, et al.: Cardiovascular effects of intensive lifestyle intervention in type 2 diabetes, *N Engl J Med* 369(2):145–154, 2013.
30. Sjostrom L, Peltonen M, Jacobson P, et al.: Bariatric surgery and long-term cardiovascular events, *JAMA* 307(1):56–65, 2012.
31. Jensen MD, Ryan DH, Apovian CM, et al.: 2013 AHA/ACC/TOS guideline for the management of overweight and obesity in adults: a report of the American College of Cardiology/American Heart Association Task Force on Practice Guidelines and The Obesity Society, *Circulation* 129(25 Suppl 2):S102–S138, 2014.
32. Keys A: Coronary heart disease in seven countries, *Circulation* 41(Suppl 4):1–211, 1970.
33. Nordmann AJ, Suter-Zimmermann K, Bucher HC, et al.: Meta-analysis comparing Mediterranean to low-fat diets for modification of cardiovascular risk factors, *Am J Med* 124(9):841–851, 2011.
34. Sofi F, Abbate R, Gensini GF, Casini A: Accruing evidence on benefits of adherence to the Mediterranean diet on health: an updated systematic review and meta-analysis, *Am J Clin Nutr* 92(5):1189–1196, 2010.
35. Sofi F, Macchi C, Abbate R, Gensini GF, Casini A: Mediterranean diet and health status: an updated meta-analysis and a proposal for a literature-based adherence score, *Public Health Nutr* 17(12):2769–2782, 2014.
36. Hartley L, Igbinedion E, Holmes J, et al.: Increased consumption of fruit and vegetables for the primary prevention of cardiovascular diseases, *Cochrane Database Syst Rev* 6:CD009874, 2013. http://dx.doi.org/10.1002/14651858.CD009874.pub2.
37. Rees K, Hartley L, Flowers N, et al.: "Mediterranean" dietary pattern for the primary prevention of cardiovascular disease, *Cochrane Database Syst Rev* 8:CD009825, 2013. http://dx.doi.org/10.1002/14651858.CD009825.pub2.
38. Estruch R, Ros E, Salas-Salvado J, et al.: Primary prevention of cardiovascular disease with a Mediterranean diet, *N Engl J Med* 368(14):1279–1290, 2013.
39. Ornish D: Mediterranean diet for primary prevention of cardiovascular disease, *N Engl J Med* 369(7):675–676, 2013.
40. de Lorgeril M, Renaud S, Mamelle N, et al.: Mediterranean alpha-linolenic acid-rich diet in secondary prevention of coronary heart disease, *Lancet* 343(8911):1454–1459, 1994.
41. de Lorgeril M, Salen P, Martin JL, et al.: Mediterranean diet, traditional risk factors, and the rate of cardiovascular complications after myocardial infarction: final report of the Lyon Diet Heart Study, *Circulation* 99(6):779–785, 1999.
42. Mozaffarian D: Mediterranean diet for primary prevention of cardiovascular disease, *N Engl J Med* 369(7):673–674, 2013.
43. Kastorini CM, Milionis HJ, Esposito K, et al.: The effect of Mediterranean diet on metabolic syndrome and its components: a meta-analysis of 50 studies and 534,906 individuals, *J Am Coll Cardiol* 57(11):1299–1313, 2011.
44. Esposito K, Marfella R, Ciotola M, et al.: Effect of a Mediterranean-style diet on endothelial dysfunction and markers of vascular inflammation in the metabolic syndrome: a randomized trial, *JAMA* 292(12):1440–1446, 2004.
45. Esposito K, Maiorino MI, Ciotola M, et al.: Effects of a Mediterranean-style diet on the need for antihyperglycemic drug therapy in patients with newly diagnosed type 2 diabetes: a randomized trial, *Ann Intern Med* 151(5):306–314, 2009.
46. Esposito K, Maiorino MI, Di PC, Giugliano D: Adherence to a Mediterranean diet and glycaemic control in Type 2 diabetes mellitus, *Diabet Med* 26(9):900–907, 2009.
47. Esposito K, Maiorino MI, Bellastella G, et al.: A journey into a Mediterranean diet and type 2 diabetes: a systematic review with meta-analyses, *BMJ Open* 5(8):e008222, 2015. http://dx.doi.org/10.1136/bmjopen-2015-008222.
48. Kwok CS, Umar S, Myint PK, Mamas MA, Loke YK: Vegetarian diet, Seventh Day Adventists and risk of cardiovascular mortality: a systematic review and meta-analysis, *Int J Cardiol* 176(3):680–686, 2014.
49. Chowdhury R, Warnakula S, Kunutsor S, et al.: Association of dietary, circulating, and supplement fatty acids with coronary risk: a systematic review and meta-analysis, *Ann Intern Med* 160(6):398–406, 2014.
50. Rizos EC, Ntzani EE, Bika E, Kostapanos MS, Elisaf MS: Association between omega-3 fatty acid supplementation and risk of major cardiovascular disease events: a systematic review and meta-analysis, *JAMA* 308(10):1024–1033, 2012.
51. Chowdhury R, Kunutsor S, Vitezova A, et al.: Vitamin D and risk of cause specific death: systematic review and meta-analysis of observational cohort and randomised intervention studies, *BMJ* 348, 2014. g1903. http://dx.doi.org/10.1136/bmj.g1903.
52. Ford JA, MacLennan GS, Avenell A, et al.: Cardiovascular disease and vitamin D supplementation: trial analysis, systematic review, and meta-analysis, *Am J Clin Nutr* 100(3):746–755, 2014.
53. Manson JE, Bassuk SS: Vitamin D research and clinical practice: at a crossroads, *JAMA* 313(13):1311–1312, 2015.
54. Barton P, Andronis L, Briggs A, McPherson K, Capewell S: Effectiveness and cost effectiveness of cardiovascular disease prevention in whole populations: modelling study, *BMJ* 343, 2011. d4044. http://dx.doi.org/10.1136/bmj.d4044.
55. Holmes MV, Dale CE, Zuccolo L, et al.: Association between alcohol and cardiovascular disease: Mendelian randomisation analysis based on individual participant data, *BMJ* 349, 2014. http://dx.doi.org/10.1136/bmj.g4164. g4164.
56. Costanzo S, Di Castelnuovo A, Donati MB, Iacoviello L, de Gaetano G: Cardiovascular and overall mortality risk in relation to alcohol consumption in patients with cardiovascular disease, *Circulation* 121(17):1951–1959, 2010.
57. American Heart Association: *Alcohol and Heart Health*, 2016. http://www.heart.org/HEARTORG/HealthyLiving/HealthyEating/Nutrition/Alcohol-and-Heart-Health_UCM_305173_Article.jsp#.VsiOwvnhDIU Accessed sep 12 2016.

58. Berryman JW: Exercise is medicine: a historical perspective, *Curr Sports Med Rep* 9(4):195–201, 2010.
59. Morris JN, Heady JA, Raffle PA, Roberts CG, Parks JW: Coronary heart-disease and physical activity of work, *Lancet* 265(6795):1053–1057, 1953.
60. Kodama S, Saito K, Tanaka S, et al.: Cardiorespiratory fitness as a quantitative predictor of all-cause mortality and cardiovascular events in healthy men and women: a meta-analysis, *JAMA* 301(19):2024–2035, 2009.
61. Sofi F, Capalbo A, Cesari F, Abbate R, Gensini GF: Physical activity during leisure time and primary prevention of coronary heart disease: an updated meta-analysis of cohort studies, *Eur J Cardiovasc Prev Rehabil* 15(3):247–257, 2008.
62. Nocon M, Hiemann T, Muller-Riemenschneider F, et al.: Association of physical activity with all-cause and cardiovascular mortality: a systematic review and meta-analysis, *Eur J Cardiovasc Prev Rehabil* 15(3):239–246, 2008.
63. Samitz G, Egger M, Zwahlen M: Domains of physical activity and all-cause mortality: systematic review and dose-response meta-analysis of cohort studies, *Int J Epidemiol* 40(5):1382–1400, 2011.
64. Kohl III HW, Craig CL, Lambert EV, et al.: The pandemic of physical inactivity: global action for public health, *Lancet* 380(9838):294–305, 2012.
65. Smith Jr SC, Benjamin EJ, Bonow RO, et al.: AHA/ACCF Secondary Prevention and Risk Reduction Therapy for Patients with Coronary and Other Atherosclerotic Vascular Disease: 2011 update: a guideline from the American Heart Association and American College of Cardiology Foundation, *Circulation* 124(22):2458–2473, 2011.
66. Gulati M, Black HR, Shaw LJ, et al.: The prognostic value of a nomogram for exercise capacity in women, *N Engl J Med* 353(5):468–475, 2005.
67. Mora S, Redberg RF, Cui Y, et al.: Ability of exercise testing to predict cardiovascular and all-cause death in asymptomatic women: a 20-year follow-up of the lipid research clinics prevalence study, *JAMA* 290(12):1600–1607, 2003.
68. Schmidt MD, Cleland VJ, Thomson RJ, Dwyer T, Venn AJ: A comparison of subjective and objective measures of physical activity and fitness in identifying associations with cardiometabolic risk factors, *Ann Epidemiol* 18(5):378–386, 2008.
69. Dvorak RV, Tchernof A, Starling RD, et al.: Respiratory fitness, free living physical activity, and cardiovascular disease risk in older individuals: a doubly labeled water study, *J Clin Endocrinol Metab* 85(3):957–963, 2000.
70. Gupta S, Rohatgi A, Ayers CR, et al.: Cardiorespiratory fitness and classification of risk of cardiovascular disease mortality, *Circulation* 123(13):1377–1383, 2011.
71. Barons MJ, Turner S, Parsons N, et al.: Fitness predicts long-term survival after a cardiovascular event: a prospective cohort study, *BMJ Open* 5(10):e007772, 2015, http://dx.doi.org/10.1136/bmjopen-2015-007772.
72. Church TS, Earnest CP, Skinner JS, Blair SN: Effects of different doses of physical activity on cardiorespiratory fitness among sedentary, overweight or obese postmenopausal women with elevated blood pressure: a randomized controlled trial, *JAMA* 297(19):2081–2091, 2007.
73. Arem H, Moore SC, Patel A, et al.: Leisure time physical activity and mortality: a detailed pooled analysis of the dose-response relationship, *JAMA Intern Med* 175(6):959–967, 2015.
74. Schnohr P, O'Keefe JH, Marott JL, Lange P, Jensen GB: Dose of jogging and long-term mortality: the Copenhagen City Heart Study, *J Am Coll Cardiol* 65(5):411–419, 2015.
75. Swain D, Franklin BA: Comparison of cardioprotective benefits of vigorous versus moderate intensity aerobic exercise, *Am J Cardiol* 97(1):141–147, 2006.
76. Tanasescu M, Leitzmann MF, Rimm EB, et al.: Exercise type and intensity in relation to coronary heart disease in men, *JAMA* 288(16):1994–2000, 2002.
77. Gebel K, Ding D, Chey T, et al.: Effect of moderate to vigorous physical activity on all-cause mortality in middle-aged and older Australians, *JAMA Intern Med* 175(6):970–977, 2015.
78. Wen CP, Wai JP, Tsai MK, et al.: Minimum amount of physical activity for reduced mortality and extended life expectancy: a prospective cohort study, *Lancet* 378(9798):1244–1253, 2011.
79. Lee DC, Pate RR, Lavie CJ, et al.: Leisure-time running reduces all-cause and cardiovascular mortality risk, *J Am Coll Cardiol* 64(5):472–481, 2014.
80. Shiroma EJ, Sesso HD, Moorthy MV, Buring JE, Lee IM: Do moderate-intensity and vigorous-intensity physical activities reduce mortality rates to the same extent? *J Am Heart Assoc* 3(5):e000802, 2014, http://dx.doi.org/10.1161/JAHA.114.000802.
81. Janssen I, Ross R: Vigorous intensity physical activity is related to the metabolic syndrome independent of the physical activity dose, *Int J Epidemiol* 41(4):1132–1140, 2012.
82. Nokes N: Relationship between physical activity and aerobic fitness, *J Sports Med Phys Fitness* 49(2):136–141, 2009.
83. Elliott AD, Rajopadhyaya K, Bentley DJ, Beltrame JF, Aromataris EC: Interval training versus continuous exercise in patients with coronary artery disease: a meta-analysis, *Heart Lung Circ* 24(2):149–157, 2015.
84. Weston KS, Wisloff U, Coombes JS: High-intensity interval training in patients with lifestyle-induced cardiometabolic disease: a systematic review and meta-analysis, *Br J Sports Med* 48(16):1227–1234, 2014.
85. Wisloff U, Ellingsen O, Kemi OJ: High-intensity interval training to maximize cardiac benefits of exercise training? *Exerc Sport Sci Rev* 37(3):139–146, 2009.
86. Conraads VM, Pattyn N, De MC, et al.: Aerobic interval training and continuous training equally improve aerobic exercise capacity in patients with coronary artery disease: the SAINTEX-CAD study, *Int J Cardiol* 179:203–210, 2015.
87. Watson K, Frederick G, Harris C, Carlson S, Fulton J: U.S. adults' participation in specific activities: behavioral risk factor surveillance system—2011, *J Phys Act Health* 12(Suppl 1):S3–S10, 2015.
88. Hamer M, Chida Y: Walking and primary prevention: a meta-analysis of prospective cohort studies, *Br J Sports Med* 42(4):238–243, 2008.
89. Zheng H, Orsini N, Amin J, et al.: Quantifying the dose-response of walking in reducing coronary heart disease risk: meta-analysis, *Eur J Epidemiol* 24(4):181–192, 2009.
90. Manson JE, Greenland P, LaCroix AZ, et al.: Walking compared with vigorous exercise for the prevention of cardiovascular events in women, *N Engl J Med* 347(10):716–725, 2002.
91. Kelly P, Kahlmeier S, Gotschi T, et al.: Systematic review and meta-analysis of reduction in all-cause mortality from walking and cycling and shape of dose response relationship, *Int J Behav Nutr Phys Act* 11:132, 2014.
92. Saevereid HA, Schnohr P, Prescott E: Speed and duration of walking and other leisure time physical activity and the risk of heart failure: a prospective cohort study from the Copenhagen City Heart Study, *PLoS One* 9(3):e89909, 2014, http://dx.doi.org/10.1371/journal.pone.0089909.
93. Laursen AH, Kristiansen OP, Marott JL, Schnohr P, Prescott E: Intensity versus duration of physical activity: implications for the metabolic syndrome. A prospective cohort study, *BMJ Open* 2(5):e001711, 2012, http://dx.doi.org/10.1136/bmjopen-2012-001711.
94. Schnohr P, Scharling H, Jensen JS: Intensity versus duration of walking, impact on mortality: the Copenhagen City Heart Study, *Eur J Cardiovasc Prev Rehabil* 14(1):72–78, 2007.
95. Dumurgier J, Elbaz A, Ducimetiere P, et al.: Slow walking speed and cardiovascular death in well functioning older adults: prospective cohort study, *BMJ* 339, 2009. b4460 http://dx.doi.org/10.1136/bmj.b4460.
96. Slentz CA, Duscha BD, Johnson JL, et al.: Effects of the amount of exercise on body weight, body composition, and measures of central obesity: STRRIDE—a randomized controlled study, *Arch Intern Med* 164(1):31–39, 2004.
97. Murtagh EM, Nichols L, Mohammed MA, et al.: The effect of walking on risk factors for cardiovascular disease: an updated systematic review and meta-analysis of randomised control trials, *Prev Med* 72:34–43, 2015.
98. Qiu S, Cai X, Schumann U, et al.: Impact of walking on glycemic control and other cardiovascular risk factors in type 2 diabetes: a meta-analysis, *PLoS One* 9(10):e109767, 2014, http://dx.doi.org/10.1371/journal.pone.0109767.
99. Vanhees L, Geladas N, Hansen D, et al.: Importance of characteristics and modalities of physical activity and exercise in the management of cardiovascular health in individuals with cardiovascular risk factors: recommendations from the EACPR. Part II, *Eur J Prev Cardiol* 19(5):1005–1033, 2012.
100. Vanhees L, Rauch B, Piepoli M, et al.: Importance of characteristics and modalities of physical activity and exercise in the management of cardiovascular health in individuals with cardiovascular disease (Part III), *Eur J Prev Cardiol* 19(6):1333–1356, 2012.
101. Williams MA, Haskell WL, Ades PA, et al.: Resistance exercise in individuals with and without cardiovascular disease: 2007 update: a scientific statement from the American Heart Association Council on Clinical Cardiology and Council on Nutrition, Physical Activity, and Metabolism, *Circulation* 116(5):572–584, 2007.
102. Marzolini S, Oh PI, Brooks D: Effect of combined aerobic and resistance training versus aerobic training alone in individuals with coronary artery disease: a meta-analysis, *Eur J Prev Cardiol* 19(1):81–94, 2012.
103. Church TS, Blair SN, Cocreham S, et al.: Effects of aerobic and resistance training on hemoglobin A1c levels in patients with type 2 diabetes: a randomized controlled trial, *JAMA* 304(20):2253–2262, 2010.
104. Chomistek AK, Manson JE, Stefanick ML, et al.: Relationship of sedentary behavior and physical activity to incident cardiovascular disease: results from the Women's Health Initiative, *J Am Coll Cardiol* 61(23):2346–2354, 2013.
105. Katzmarzyk PT: Physical activity, sedentary behavior, and health: paradigm paralysis or paradigm shift? *Diabetes* 59(11):2717–2725, 2010.
106. Basterra-Gortari FJ, Bes-Rastrollo M, Gea A, et al.: Television viewing, computer use, time driving and all-cause mortality: the SUN cohort, *J Am Heart Assoc* 3(3):e000864, 2014, http://dx.doi.org/10.1161/JAHA.114.000864.
107. Warren TY, Barry V, Hooker SP, et al.: Sedentary behaviors increase risk of cardiovascular disease mortality in men, *Med Sci Sports Exerc* 42(5):879–885, 2010.
108. Pulsford RM, Stamatakis E, Britton AR, Brunner EJ, Hillsdon M: Associations of sitting behaviours with all-cause mortality over a 16-year follow-up: the Whitehall II study, *Int J Epidemiol* 44(6):1909–1916, 2015.
109. Harvey JA, Chastin SF, Skelton DA: How sedentary are older people? A systematic review of the amount of sedentary behavior, *J Aging Phys Act* 23(3):471–487, 2015.
110. Harvey JA, Chastin SF, Skelton DA: Prevalence of sedentary behavior in older adults: a systematic review, *Int J Environ Res Public Health* 10(12):6645–6661, 2013.
111. Healy GN, Matthews CE, Dunstan DW, Winkler EA, Owen N: Sedentary time and cardio-metabolic biomarkers in US adults: NHANES 2003–06, *Eur Heart J* 32(5):590–597, 2011.
112. Krogh-Madsen R, Thyfault JP, Broholm C, et al.: A 2-wk reduction of ambulatory activity attenuates peripheral insulin sensitivity, *J Appl Physiol (1985)* 108(5):1034–1040, 2010.
113. Olsen RH, Krogh-Madsen R, Thomsen C, Booth FW, Pedersen BK: Metabolic responses to reduced daily steps in healthy nonexercising men, *JAMA* 299(11):1261–1263, 2008.
114. Kavazis AN: Exercise preconditioning of the myocardium, *Sports Med* 39(11):923–935, 2009.
115. Irving BA, Nair KS, Srinivasan M: Effects of insulin sensitivity, body composition, and fitness on lipoprotein particle sizes and concentrations determined by nuclear magnetic resonance, *J Clin Endocrinol Metab* 96(4):E713–E718, 2011.
116. Kokkinos PF, Faselis C, Myers J, Panagiotakos D, Doumas M: Interactive effects of fitness and statin treatment on mortality risk in veterans with dyslipidaemia: a cohort study, *Lancet* 381(9864):394–399, 2013.
117. Durstine JL, Grandjean PW, Cox CA, Thompson PD: Lipids, lipoproteins, and exercise, *J Cardiopulm Rehabil* 22(6):385–398, 2002.
118. Ilanne-Parikka P, Laaksonen DE, Eriksson JG, et al.: Leisure-time physical activity and the metabolic syndrome in the Finnish diabetes prevention study, *Diabetes Care* 33(7):1610–1617, 2010.
119. Hassinen M, Lakka TA, Hakola L, et al.: Cardiorespiratory fitness and metabolic syndrome in older men and women: the dose responses to Exercise Training (DR's EXTRA) study, *Diabetes Care* 33(7):1655–1657, 2010.
120. Hambrecht R, Walther C, Mobius-Winkler S, et al.: Percutaneous coronary angioplasty compared with exercise training in patients with stable coronary artery disease: a randomized trial, *Circulation* 109(11):1371–1378, 2004.
121. Hughes JP, McDowell MA, Brody DJ: Leisure-time physical activity among US adults 60 or more years of age: results from NHANES 1999–2004, *J Phys Act Health* 5(3):347–358, 2008.
122. Ma J, Urizar Jr GG, Alehegn T, Stafford RS: Diet and physical activity counseling during ambulatory care visits in the United States, *Prev Med* 39(4):815–822, 2004.
123. Thompson PD, Buchner D, Pina IL, et al.: Exercise and physical activity in the prevention and treatment of atherosclerotic cardiovascular disease: a statement from the Council on Clinical Cardiology (Subcommittee on Exercise, Rehabilitation, and Prevention) and the Council on Nutrition, Physical Activity, and Metabolism (Subcommittee on Physical Activity), *Circulation* 107(24):3109–3116, 2003.
124. Thompson PD, Franklin BA, Balady GJ, et al.: Exercise and acute cardiovascular events placing the risks into perspective: a scientific statement from the American Heart Association Council on Nutrition, Physical Activity, and Metabolism and the Council on Clinical Cardiology, *Circulation* 115(17):2358–2368, 2007.
125. Lavie CJ, Thomas RJ, Squires RW, Allison TG, Milani RV: Exercise training and cardiac rehabilitation in primary and secondary prevention of coronary heart disease, *Mayo Clin Proc* 84(4):373–383, 2009.
126. O'Connor CM, Whellan DJ, Lee KL, et al.: Efficacy and safety of exercise training in patients with chronic heart failure: HF-ACTION randomized controlled trial, *JAMA* 301(14):1439–1450, 2009.
127. Lichtman JH, Bigger Jr JT, Blumenthal JA, et al.: Depression and coronary heart disease: recommendations for screening, referral, and treatment: a science advisory from the American Heart Association Prevention Committee of the Council on Cardiovascular Nursing, Council on Clinical Cardiology, Council on Epidemiology and Prevention, and Interdisciplinary Council on Quality of Care and Outcomes Research: endorsed by the American Psychiatric Association, *Circulation* 118(17):1768–1775, 2008.
128. Wood DA, Kotseva K, Connolly S, et al.: Nurse-coordinated multidisciplinary, family-based cardiovascular disease prevention programme (EUROACTION) for patients with coronary heart disease and asymptomatic individuals at high risk of cardiovascular disease: a paired, cluster-randomised controlled trial, *Lancet* 371(9629):1999–2012, 2008.
129. Piepoli MF, Corra U, Benzer W, et al.: Secondary prevention through cardiac rehabilitation: from knowledge to implementation. A position paper from the Cardiac Rehabilitation Section of the European Association of Cardiovascular Prevention and Rehabilitation, *Eur J Cardiovasc Prev Rehabil* 17(1):1–17, 2010.
130. Leon AS, Franklin BA, Costa F, et al.: Cardiac rehabilitation and secondary prevention of coronary heart disease: an American Heart Association scientific statement from the Council on Clinical Cardiology (Subcommittee on Exercise, Cardiac Rehabilitation, and Prevention) and the Council on Nutrition, Physical Activity, and Metabolism (Subcommittee on Physical Activity), in collaboration with the American Association of Cardiovascular and Pulmonary Rehabilitation, *Circulation* 111(3):369–376, 2005.

131. Heran BS, Chen JM, Ebrahim S, et al.: Exercise-based cardiac rehabilitation for coronary heart disease, *Cochrane Database Syst Rev* (7):CD001800, 2011. http://dx.doi.org/10.1002/14651858.CD001800.pub2.
132. Goel K, Pack QR, Lahr B, et al.: Cardiac rehabilitation is associated with reduced long-term mortality in patients undergoing combined heart valve and CABG surgery, *Eur J Prev Cardiol* 22(2):159–168, 2015.
133. Pack QR, Goel K, Lahr BD, et al.: Participation in cardiac rehabilitation and survival after coronary artery bypass graft surgery: a community-based study, *Circulation* 128(6):590–597, 2013.
134. Anderson L, Thompson DR, Oldridge N, et al.: Exercise-based cardiac rehabilitation for coronary heart disease, *Cochrane Database Syst Rev* 1:CD001800, 2016. http://dx.doi.org/10.1002/14651858.CD001800.pub3.
135. Taylor RS, Sagar VA, Davies EJ, et al.: Exercise-based rehabilitation for heart failure, *Cochrane Database Syst Rev* 4:CD003331, 2014. http://dx.doi.org/10.1002/14651858.CD003331.pub4.
136. Flynn KE, Pina IL, Whellan DJ, et al.: Effects of exercise training on health status in patients with chronic heart failure: HF-ACTION randomized controlled trial, *JAMA* 301(14):1451–1459, 2009.
137. Kotseva K, Wood D, De BG, et al.: EUROASPIRE III: a survey on the lifestyle, risk factors and use of cardioprotective drug therapies in coronary patients from 22 European countries, *Eur J Cardiovasc Prev Rehabil* 16(2):121–137, 2009.
138. Kotseva K, Wood D, De BG, et al.: Cardiovascular prevention guidelines in daily practice: a comparison of EUROASPIRE I, II, and III surveys in eight European countries, *Lancet* 373(9667):929–940, 2009.
139. Karmali KN, Davies P, Taylor F, et al.: Promoting patient uptake and adherence in cardiac rehabilitation, *Cochrane Database Syst Rev* 6:CD007131, 2014. http://dx.doi.org/10.1002/14651858.CD007131.pub3.
140. Gregory PC, LaVeist TA, Simpson C: Racial disparities in access to cardiac rehabilitation, *Am J Phys Med Rehabil* 85(9):705–710, 2006.
141. Lavie CJ, Arena R, Franklin BA: Cardiac rehabilitation and healthy life-style interventions. Editorial comment, *J Am Coll Cardiol* 67(1):13–15, 2016.
142. Balady GJ, Ades PA, Bittner VA, et al.: Referral, enrollment, and delivery of cardiac rehabilitation/secondary prevention programs at clinical centers and beyond: a presidential advisory from the American Heart Association, *Circulation* 124(25):2951–2960, 2011.

19 Obesity and the Obesity Paradox

Carl J. Lavie, Alban De Schutter, and Richard V. Milani

INTRODUCTION

After smoking, obesity is probably the second leading cause of preventable death in the United States and most of the westernized world.[1,2] The estimated prevalence of obesity is almost 80 million, with close to 130 million in the United States being overweight, and currently almost 10 million being severely obese.[1–4] In fact, during the past 50 years, the average life expectancy in the United States has been reduced by a full year due to the impact of obesity, partially offsetting gains made from reduced smoking and improvements in automobile safety (Fig. 19.1).[5,6] Therefore, attention directed at the prevention and treatment of obesity is especially needed.

Obesity appears to be a risk factor for cardiovascular (CV) disease (CVD) independently of age, lipid levels, blood pressure (BP), glucose levels, and left ventricular hypertrophy.[2–4] Certainly, obesity places a "heavy" toll on the CV system, negatively affecting many of the established CV and coronary heart disease (CHD) risk factors, including increasing BP and the prevalence of hypertension, worsening plasma lipid levels (in particular increasing triglyceride levels and reducing the cardioprotective high-density lipoprotein cholesterol [HDL-C] levels), increasing glucose levels and the risk of metabolic syndrome and type 2 diabetes mellitus (T2DM), and increasing levels of inflammation. Additionally, obesity has adverse effects on CV structure and function. Combined, these effects increase the risk of CVD, including CHD.

In this chapter, we review the effects of obesity on CHD risk factors and on the prevalence of CHD. We also review the impact of obesity on prognosis in patients with established CHD, including patients following revascularization procedures with percutaneous coronary intervention (PCI) and coronary artery bypass grafting (CABG). Finally, we will discuss the implications of weight loss in patients with CHD, especially in light of the so-called "obesity paradox."

MECHANISMS LINKING OBESITY WITH INCREASED CHD RISK

The adverse effects of obesity on CHD risk factors and CV structure and function are summarized in Box 19.1.[3,4] Excess body weight is one of the most powerful risk factors for increased BP and the development of hypertension, a major CHD risk factor. In a prospective examination of 35- to 75-year-old participants from the Framingham Heart Study, 34% of hypertension cases in men and 62% of hypertension cases in women were attributed to a body mass index (BMI) greater than or equal to 25 kg/m^2 based on the estimated population attributable risk.[7] In an analysis of patients with a self-reported BP higher than 140/90 mmHg in the Physicians' Health Study, which included over 13,500 healthy male physicians, an 8% increase in the risk of incident hypertension was noted for each one-unit increase in BMI during a median 14.5-year follow-up.[8] In this study, although incident hypertension was mostly associated with obesity at baseline, a weight gain of more than 5% in 8 years was also significantly associated with an increased hypertension risk in persons with normal baseline BMI.

Obesity is a leading cause of elevated blood glucose, metabolic syndrome, and T2DM. In an examination of data from the Behavioral Risk Factor Surveillance System from 1990 to 1998, the overall prevalence of T2DM increased by 33%, which was closely related to the increased prevalence of obesity.[9] In fact, a 9% increase in T2DM rate was noted for every 1 kg increase in weight. The association of obesity with insulin resistance and metabolic syndrome appears to significantly increase the risk of T2DM and CVD. Metabolic syndrome, which is defined by abdominal obesity, atherogenic dyslipidemia, hypertension, insulin resistance, and pro-inflammatory and prothrombotic states, is associated with a more than twofold increased risk of CHD, with an attributable risk of 37% in patients older than 50 years.[10,11] Alexander and colleagues[12] in 2003, in an analysis of the National Health and Nutrition Examination Survey, noted no increase in CHD prevalence in patients who had T2DM but no metabolic syndrome, whereas CHD risk was increased in patients with metabolic syndrome but without T2DM. The highest risk of CHD was noted in those with metabolic syndrome and T2DM. The higher risk is imposed by higher intra-abdominal fat, measured clinically as waist circumference (WC). WC was the strongest predictor of metabolic syndrome, was independently associated with each component of the metabolic syndrome, and was more strongly associated with metabolic syndrome than was BMI.[13,14]

Atherogenic dyslipidemia and metabolic syndrome in obesity is defined by elevated triglyceride levels, low levels of HDL-C, and increased proportions of small, dense

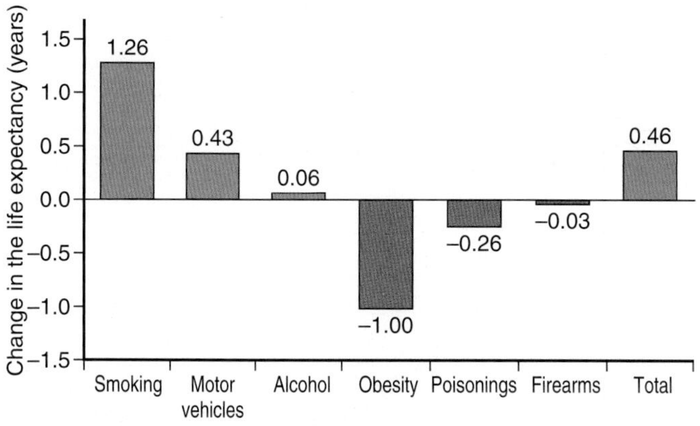

FIG. 19.1 The impact of behavioral changes on life expectancy between 1960 and 2010. *(Modified from Stewart ST, Cutler DM. The contribution of behavior change and public health to improved U.S. population health.* NBER Working Paper Series. *Working Paper 20631.* http://www.nber.org/papers/w20631. *October 2014; and from Stewart ST, Cutler DM. How behavioral changes have affected U.S. population health since 1960.* NBER Working Paper Series. *Working Paper 20631.* http://www.nber.org/aging health/2015no1/w20631. *March 2016.)*

BOX 19.1 Adverse Effects of Obesity

1. Insulin resistance
   - glucose intolerance
   - metabolic syndrome
   - type 2 diabetes mellitus
2. Dyslipidemia
   - elevated total cholesterol
   - elevated triglycerides
   - elevated LDL cholesterol
   - elevated non-HDL cholesterol
   - elevated apolipoprotein-B
   - elevated small, dense LDL particles
   - decreased HDL cholesterol
   - decreased apolipoprotein-A1
3. Hemodynamics
   - increased blood volume
   - increased stroke volume
   - increased arterial pressure
   - increased LV wall stress
   - pulmonary artery hypertension
4. Cardiac structure
   - LV concentric remodeling
   - LV hypertrophy (eccentric and concentric)
   - left atrial enlargement
   - RV hypertrophy
5. Cardiac function
   - LV diastolic dysfunction
   - LV systolic dysfunction
   - RV failure
6. Inflammation
   - increased C-reactive protein
   - overexpression of tumor necrosis factor
7. Neurohumoral
   - insulin resistance and hyperinsulinemia
   - leptin insensitivity and hyperleptinemia
   - reduced adiponectin
   - sympathetic nervous system activation
   - activation of renin–angiotensin–aldosterone system
   - overexpression of peroxisome proliferator-activator receptor
   - reduced levels of atrial and brain natriuretic peptide
8. Cellular
   - hypertrophy
   - apoptosis
   - fibrosis

HDL, High-density lipoprotein; *LDL,* low-density lipoprotein; *LV,* left ventricular; *RV,* right ventricular.

Reproduced with permission from Lavie CJ, De Schutter A, Parto P, et al. Obesity and prevalence of cardiovascular diseases and prognosis: the obesity paradox updated. *Prog Cardiovasc Dis* http://dx.doi.org/10.1016/j.pcad.2016.01.008 [Epub ahead of print].

low-density lipoprotein cholesterol (LDL-C), which is more atherogenic than the large, more buoyant LDL-C.[11] Increased circulating fatty acids are taken up by the liver, which results in increased production of triglyceride-rich particles, especially very-low-density lipoproteins. In the setting of high triglycerides, most of the LDL-C is produced in the small, dense form, which is more easily oxidized and more atherogenic.

Although the association of obesity with increased CVD has been established independently and in association with such major risk factors as hypertension, metabolic syndrome/T2DM, and atherogenic dyslipidemia, the exact mechanisms linking obesity, especially abdominal obesity, with insulin resistance and other factors influencing the risk of CVD have not been fully elucidated.[11] Fat-related hormones and cytokines, termed *adipokines*, are secreted by the adipocytes and macrophages in adipose tissue. Several clotting factors, including fibrinogen, von Willebrand factor, and factor VII and VIII, are increased in obesity and insulin resistance.[11] Plasminogen activator inhibitor type-I levels increase with BMI and WC, which may inhibit endogenous fibrinolysis.[11] Mechanisms involved with increasing BP include insulin-mediated vasoconstriction, increased insulin-mediated renal sodium reabsorption, insulin-related stimulation of the sympathetic nervous system, increased vasoconstriction related to elevated free fatty acids, and production of components of the renin-angiotensin-aldosterone system by adipose tissue.[11]

Leptin levels also increase in obesity, and chronically elevated leptin levels have been related to increased atherosclerosis, in-stent restenosis, and inflammation.[11,15] Interleukin-6, tumor necrosis factor, adiponectin, and C-reactive protein (CRP) may also be elevated and be involved in atherosclerosis and CHD events.[11]

ASSOCIATION OF OBESITY WITH CVD EVENTS

Considering the multiple pathogenic mechanisms associated with obesity described above, there is no surprise that obesity is related to increased risk of most CVD, including hypertension, heart failure (HF), atrial fibrillation (AF), as well as CHD and CHD events.[3,4,15] Many of these factors are associated with inflammation, prothrombotic states, and increased risk of atherosclerosis.[11] Many large prospective studies, including the Framingham Heart Study, the Nurses Health Study, and the Manitoba Study, have documented obesity as an independent predictor of CVD.[7,11,16,17] The potential relationship between BMI categories and incidence of non-ST-segment elevation myocardial infarction (NSTEMI) were assessed retrospectively in a cohort of over 110,000 patients with unstable angina and NSTEMI in which obesity was the strongest risk factor was associated with NSTEMI at younger age, ahead of tobacco abuse. In fact, compared with normal-weight individuals, the mean age incidence of NSTEMI was 3.5, 6.8, 9.4, and 12.0 years earlier in overweight (BMI 25–29.9 kg/m^2), Class I obesity (BMI 30–34.9 kg/m^2), Class II obesity (BMI 35–39.9 kg/m^2), and Class III obesity (BMI ≥ 40 kg/m^2), respectively.[18] Considering the increased prevalence of obesity and more severe obesity, there is concern for marked increases in the occurrence of acute CVD events in younger individuals in upcoming decades.

Several recent reports have also demonstrated that severe Class III obesity is a significant predictor of premature myocardial infarction (MI) at very young ages.[19–22] However, obesity, especially when only mild to moderate in severity, may have a different impact regarding infarct size and severity of coronary artery disease (CAD). In fact, recent data demonstrated that obese patients with MI had less severe CAD than thinner patients with MI.[23] Also, the size of MI in NSTEMI was different to that in ST-segment elevation MI (STEMI), with obese patients having greater infarct size in NSTEMI, but smaller infarct size in STEMI.[24]

IMPACT OF OBESITY ON PROGNOSIS IN CHD: THE OBESITY PARADOX

Given the well-known adverse effects of overweight and obesity on major CVD risk factors discussed above, not surprisingly almost all CVD, including CHD, is increased in the setting of higher weight. However, many studies of patients with established CVD, including hypertension, HF, AF, as well as CHD, have demonstrated surprisingly good prognosis in overweight and obese patients, which has been termed the *obesity paradox*.[3,4] In fact, despite challenges at the time of CV revascularization in obese patients, these patients have tended to have a better overall prognosis following revascularization with PCI and CABG, and following MI, compared with leaner patients, with similar findings seen in patients with stable CHD.[11,25]

Following Revascularization with PCI

Because of the higher prevalence of CAD, overweight and obese patients will frequently undergo coronary revascularization. In fact, population-based registries and databases have reported the prevalence of overweight and obesity to be as high as 70% among patients undergoing PCI or CABG.[26] Various risk stratification systems have described obesity as a risk factor for worse clinical outcomes after coronary revascularization due to increased wound infections, longer hospital stay, and higher postprocedure mortality among more obese patients, although this may apply more to CABG than to PCI, as CABG may be postponed or declined due to obesity.[11,25] However, there have been contradictory results in various studies describing the association between BMI and subsequent MI and CVD mortality, as well as other morbidity.

In PCI, establishing femoral access can be more difficult in obese patients, as is accomplishing hemostasis afterward; this may be less of an issue with more recent use of radial artery approach.[11] Thigh and pelvic hematoma recognition may be delayed, as are the other physical examination findings associated with acute blood loss in patients with obesity. Nevertheless, despite the potential for access complications in obese patients, several studies have suggested a protective effect associated with obesity with regards to bleeding and vascular complications of PCI, similar to the paradox observed with other outcomes. Several studies have suggested that underweight and normal-BMI patients have higher bleeding complications than obese patients. Although the highest risk of bleeding occurred in patients with the lowest BMIs, a bimodal relationship was observed with also a high complication rate in those with the highest BMIs (Fig. 19.2).[27] Patients were more likely to undergo radial artery access as BMI increased, and both obese and nonobese patients have less vascular complications with this approach. Nonradial access was the strongest independent predictor of vascular complications in obese patients with PCI. Potentially lower bleeding in obese patients could have been related to younger age, better renal function, and lower relative doses of antithrombotic agents that are not dosed according to body weight.

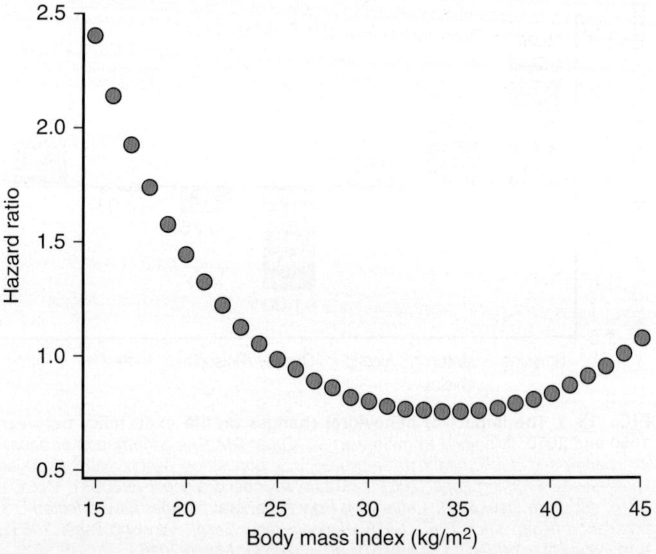

FIG. 19.2 Hazard ratio for mortality after percutaneous coronary intervention (median follow-up period, 2.1 years) according to body mass index. *(Reproduced with permission from Powell BD, Lennon RJ, Lerman A, et al. Association of body mass index with outcome after percutaneous coronary intervention.* Am J Cardiol. *2003;91:472–476.)*

TABLE 19.1 Mean Age of Patients Undergoing PCI and CABG in Various BMI Categories

	MEAN AGE (Y)	
BMI (kg/m²)	PCI	CABG
<20	69.3	67.9
20–24.9	65.0	64.6
25–29.9	62.3	64.0
30–34.9	60.1	61.9
≥35	58.3	60.5

BMI, Body mass index; *CABG,* coronary artery bypass graft; *PCI,* percutaneous coronary intervention.
Reproduced with permission from Sharma A, Vallakati A, Einstein AJ, et al. Relationship of body mass index with total mortality, cardiovascular mortality, and myocardial infarction after coronary revascularization: evidence from a meta-analysis. Mayo Clin Proc. *2014;89:1080-1100.*

We recently examined 26 studies of patients undergoing PCI, with data on age (Table 19.1) and major events (total mortality, CVD mortality, and MI; Table 19.2).[25] After a mean follow-up of approximately 1.7 years, compared with normal BMI subjects, the highest rate of mortality, CVD mortality, and MI occurred in underweight patients following PCI, being increased by 2.7-, 2.8-, and 1.9-fold, respectively. The overweight patients (BMI 25–29.9 kg/m^2) had the lowest risk, with significant reductions in total mortality and CVD mortality of 32% and 22%, respectively, with a trend for 6% lower risk of MI. The mildly obese had a significant 36% reduction in mortality and a trend for 6% lower CVD mortality, whereas those with BMI of 35 kg/m^2 or above had a trend for 19% lower mortality that was not statistically significant.

Following Revascularization with CABG

Paradoxical effects of obesity on outcomes after revascularization have been noted in the surgical literature as well.[11,25] In an earlier propensity-matched analysis of 6068 consecutive patients undergoing primary CABG from a single center during a 12-year period, two propensity models were derived

TABLE 19.2 Results Summary: Outcomes after Coronary Revascularization Procedures as per BMI

	LOW BMI	NORMAL BMI	OVERWEIGHT	OBESE	SEVERELY OBESE
Total mortality	2.59 (2.09–3.21)	1	0.72 (0.66–0.78)	0.73 (0.61–0.87)	0.78 (0.64–0.96)
PCI	2.65 (2.19–3.20)	1	0.68 (0.62–0.74)	0.64 (0.56–0.73)	0.81 (0.61–1.07)
CABG	2.66 (1.51–4.66)	1	0.83 (0.67–1.02)	0.92 (0.64–1.34)	0.76 (0.55–1.04)
Cardiac mortality	2.67 (1.63–4.39)	1	0.81 (0.68–0.95)	1.03 (0.69–1.55)	1.47 (0.74–2.89)
PCI	2.76 (1.67–4.56)	1	0.78 (0.66–0.93)	0.94 (0.62–1.44)	1.16 (0.66–2.03)
CABG	0.98 (0.06–16.97)	1	1.06 (0.52–2.13)	1.57 (0.49–5.1)	4.07 (1.4–11.85)
Myocardial infarction	1.79 (1.28–2.50)	1	0.92 (0.84–1.01)	0.99 (0.85–1.15)	0.93 (0.78–1.11)
PCI	1.85 (1.28–2.67)	1	0.94 (0.86–1.03)	1.04 (0.87–1.25)	0.96 (0.77–1.19)
CABG	1.47 (0.64–3.4)	1	0.85 (0.64–1.14)	0.84 (0.67–1.05)	0.89 (0.66–1.20)

BMI, Body mass index; *CABG*, coronary artery bypass graft; *PCI*, percutaneous coronary intervention.
Reproduced with permission from Sharma A, Vallakati A, Einstein AJ, et al. Relationship of body mass index with total mortality, cardiovascular mortality, and myocardial infarction after coronary revascularization: evidence from a meta-analysis. Mayo Clin Proc *2014;89:1080-1100.*

comparing all small patients with normal-size patients and all obese patients with normal-size patients, with an analysis made based on both body surface area (BSA) and BMI.[28] During follow-up, survival curves showed that mortality in very small patients with BSA less than 1.7 m^2 was higher than in normal-size patients despite less insulin dependence and greater use of all arterial grafts in the smaller patients. Mortality was also higher in slightly small patients (BSA 1.7–1.85 m^2) than in normal-size patients, as well as in very obese patients (BMI ≥ 36 kg/m^2), but worse survival was not noted in those with BMI 32–36 kg/m^2. Additionally, very small patients required significantly more transfusions and reoperations for bleeding, transfusion, and pulmonary edema, all of which may be secondary to greater on-pump hemodilution in smaller patients. Although not statistically significant, operative mortality was almost double in those with BSA less than 1.85 m^2. While operative mortality was not worse in very obese patients, the risk of postoperative complications was significantly higher (39% vs. 26%; $p < 0.001$), and very obese patients had a statistically higher rate of sternal wound infections, pulmonary edema, pneumonia, noncardiac reoperations, acute renal failure, AF, gastrointestinal problems, and longer postoperative hospital stays compared with normal-BMI patients undergoing CABG. Sternal wound complications also occurred more commonly in moderately obese patients. Wound infection and complications may be secondary to the increased incidence of T2DM that occurs with higher BMI, as well as decreased perfusion of adipose tissue.

In a retrospective analysis of 9862 patients who had CABG at a single institution over a 10-year period, obesity was not associated with increased mortality, MI, arrhythmias, stroke or infection.[29] However, morbidly obese patients (BMI ≥ 40 kg/m^2) with CABG had more re-exploration procedures. Additionally, obese patients with T2DM were noted to experience more atrial and ventricular dysrhythmias, increased ventricular tachycardia, renal insufficiency, respiratory failure, and leg wound infections compared with normal-BMI patients with T2DM.

Similar to our recent analysis of post-PCI patients, we also analyzed 12 CABG studies in over 60,000 patients.[25] The worst survival was noted in the underweight patients, with 2.7-fold higher mortality than normal BMI patients. Overweight, obese, and even severely obese patients had trends for lower total mortality and MI compared with normal-BMI patients, but there were slight trends of higher CV mortality in the overweight and obese patients and over fourfold higher CV mortality in the severely obese post-CABG (see Table 19.1).[25]

General CHD

In 2006, Romero-Corral and associates[30] reported a meta-analysis of 40 cohort studies of over 250,000 patients with CHD grouped according to BMI. The low-BMI patients had the highest mortality during a follow-up of nearly 4 years, while the obese had the lowest mortality risk. Overweight patients had the lowest risk on the adjusted analysis, while obese and even severely obese patients had no increased risk of mortality. Both underweight and severely obese patients (BMI ≥ 35 kg/m^2) had increased CV mortality, but even the severely obese did not have higher total mortality in this huge meta-analysis.

More recently, in a meta-analysis of 89 studies of over 1.3 million patients with CHD, by far the largest of such studies, Wang and colleagues[31] confirmed the general observations of earlier meta-analyses but also provided some very unique insights involving more long-term follow-up. Interestingly, the obesity paradox was evident during early follow-up, meaning better survival among the overweight and obese, which was even present in the severely obese patients. However, the better survival in obesity appears to disappear after 5 years, and those with Class II and III obesity (BMI ≥ 35 kg/m^2 and 40 kg/m^2, respectively) had a higher mortality during long-term follow-up. This higher mortality with severe obesity supports data from Flegal et al.[32] relating to a non-CHD population in primary prevention, which showed the best survival in the overweight patients, a trend toward better survival in mild, Class I obesity, but significantly higher mortality in those with more severe degrees of obesity.

On the one hand, some studies have recently demonstrated an increased risk for CHD patients with "normal weight obesity" or "normal weight central obesity," in which percent body fat (BF) or WC, respectively, is elevated, although BMI may be in the normal range.[33–35] On the other hand, we have demonstrated an obesity paradox even with increased WC when combined with low levels of cardiorespiratory fitness (discussed below), whereas there was excellent survival in all groups with preserved cardiorespiratory fitness.[36]

CHALLENGES WITH BMI AS A MEASURE OF ADIPOSITY

BMI represents total weight and is composed of weight from muscle, skeletal, and BF, which may be partly the reason for the sometimes paradoxical relationship between BMI and prognosis in CHD.[3,4] Clearly, there may be a discrepancy

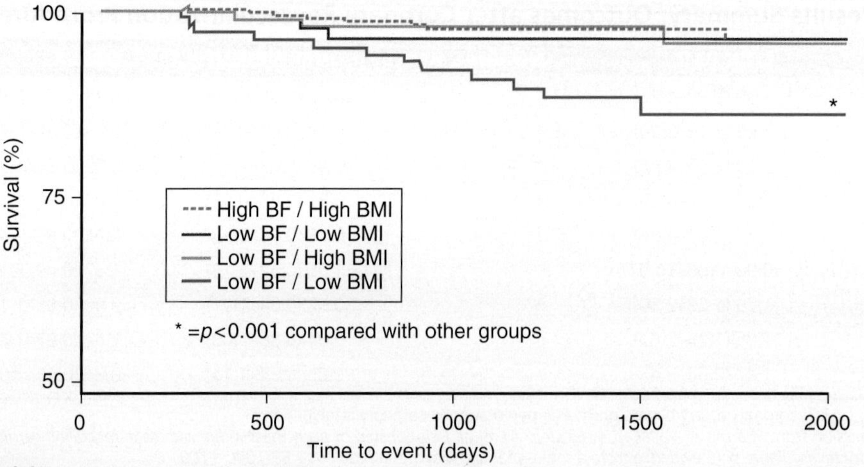

No. at risk:

High %BF High BMI	311	262	186	107	10
High %BF Low BMI	125	116	88	51	6
Low %BF High BMI	26	23	17	10	2
Low %BF Low BMI	119	110	81	46	12

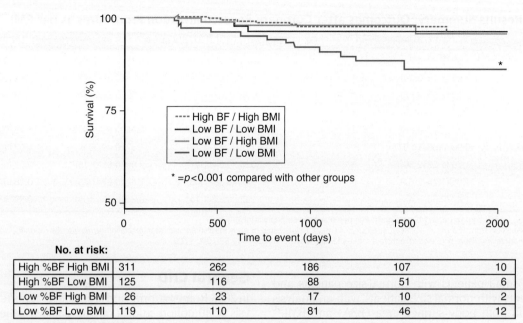

FIG. 19.3 Kaplan–Meier survival curves of 581 patients referred for cardiac rehabilitation by high and low body mass index (BMI) and body fat (BF) followed for 3 years for all-cause mortality. The outcome for the lean patients, i.e., the subgroup with both low BMI and BF was significantly worse than that for the other subpopulations. *(Reproduced with permission from Lavie CJ, De Schutter A, Patel D, et al. Body composition and coronary heart disease mortality: an obesity or a lean paradox?* Mayo Clin Proc. *2011;86:857–864.)*

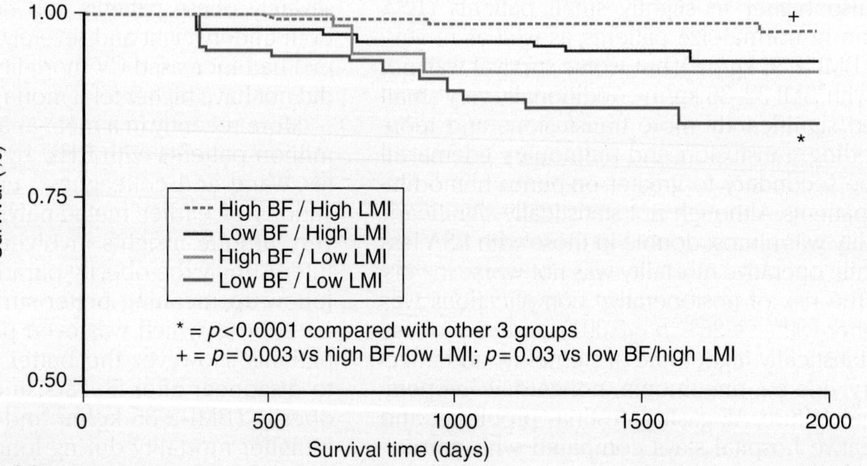

No. at risk:

High %BF High LMI	276	234	167	96	7
Low %BF High LMI	179	165	128	71	11
High %BF Low LMI	53	44	33	21	5
Low %BF Low LMI	62	58	40	25	7

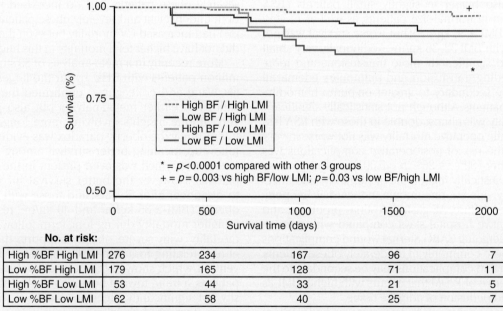

FIG. 19.4 Three-year survival based on body composition: low and high body fat (BF) and low and high lean mass index (LMI). Mortality was highest in the low BF/low LMI group (15%, or 9 of 62), followed by the high BF/low LMI group (5.7%, or 3 of 53), low BF/high LMI group (4.5%, or 8 of 179), and high BF/high LMI group (2.2%, or 6 of 270). *BF*, Body fat; *LMI*, lean mass index. *(Reproduced with permission from Lavie CJ, De Schutter A, Patel DA, et al. Body composition and survival in stable coronary heart disease: impact of lean mass index and body fat in the "obesity paradox."* J Am Coll Cardiol. *2012;60:1374–1380.)*

between that observed with BMI and other assessments of body adiposity, including BF, WC, and others. Nevertheless, we have demonstrated an obesity paradox in several studies using percent BF[37–40] and even with WC or central obesity, at least in the cohorts with central obesity and low cardiorespiratory fitness.[36]

Some studies, including our own, have raised the possibility that the association of less severe adiposity with worse clinical outcomes in CHD may represent a "lean paradox" more so than an overweight paradox or obesity paradox.[38,41,42] We have demonstrated this paradox in CHD cohorts with both low BMI as well as low BF, where both are independent predictors of higher mortality.[37–39] However, in a study of 581 CHD patients followed on average for over 3 years, we demonstrated that only those with both low BMI (<25 kg/m^2) and low BF (<25% in men and <35% in women) had higher mortality (Fig. 19.3).[38] In addition, we have demonstrated in 570 CHD patients that both low BF and low lean mass (or non-fat mass) was associated with worse survival (Fig. 19.4),[40] whereas the best survival was noted in CHD patients with both high lean mass and high BF, and those CHD patients with one of these two had an intermediate survival during 3-year follow-up. Many studies suggest that this represents more of an overweight paradox than a true obesity paradox,[38,41,42] as generally the overweight

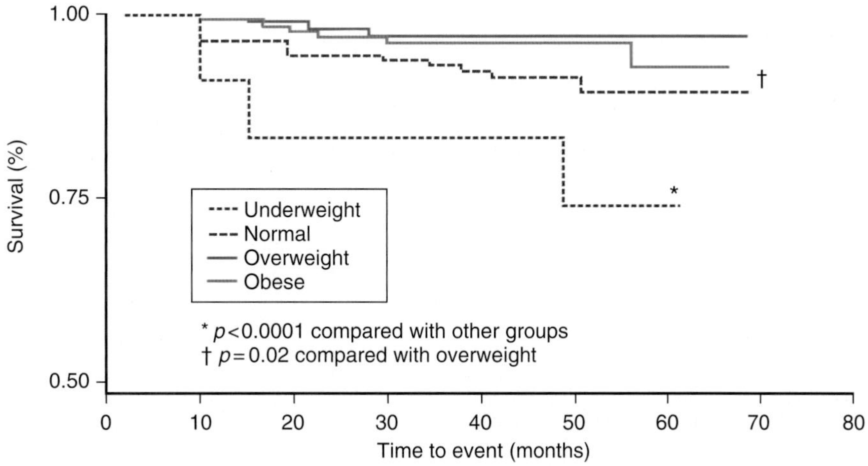

FIG. 19.5 Kaplan–Meier survival curves of 581 subjects by age and gender-adjusted body fat (BF) category. The underweight and normal BF categories had significantly worse prognosis than the overweight and obese categories. After adjustment for confounders, higher BF category was associated with lower mortality. *(Reproduced with permission from De Schutter A, Lavie CJ, Patel DA, et al. Relation of body fat categories by Gallagher classification and by continuous variables to mortality in patients with coronary heart disease.* Am J Cardiol. *2013;111:657–660.)*

groups by BMI or by BF classification often have the best survival (Fig. 19.5).[43]

Impact of Cardiorespiratory Fitness on the Obesity Paradox in CHD

Numerous studies have demonstrated the importance of fitness to predict CV and all-cause survival, including in cohorts with CHD.[3,4] In fact, levels of fitness may be one of the strongest predictors of prognosis in CHD patients. Additionally, cardiorespiratory fitness is an important predictor of prognosis in patients with obesity and markedly alters the relationship between adiposity and subsequent prognosis.[3,4,36,44]

Certainly, levels of fitness are typically lower in overweight and obese subjects compared with lean patients.[45] In a recent analysis of 5328 male nonsmokers referred for exercise stress testing (mean age 52 years), an inverse relationship between BMI and estimated cardiorespiratory fitness was observed.[46] Compared with 1370 normal-BMI subjects who had metabolic equivalent (MET) levels of 12.7 ± 3.0 METs, the 2333 overweight and 1625 obese subjects had lower levels of fitness (11.2 ± 2.5 and 9.7 ± 2.3 METs, respectively), indicating progressively lower estimated fitness with increase in BMI. Nevertheless, age- and gender-related cardiorespiratory fitness predicted survival equally well across BMI groups.

In a study of 9563 patients with CHD followed for almost 14 years for CVD and all-cause mortality, only those in the lowest tertile of age- and gender-related levels of cardiorespiratory fitness assessed on treadmill testing demonstrated an obesity paradox, which was present by all parameters of adiposity, including BMI, WC, and percent BF (Fig. 19.6).[36] However, CHD patients who were not in the bottom tertile of cardiorespiratory fitness had a good overall prognosis, and no obesity paradox was observed. In other words, patients who were not low-fit had a favorable prognosis regardless of their level of BMI, WC, and percent BF. This relationship between cardiorespiratory fitness, obesity status by BMI, and survival was also noted in a recent study of 18,000 veterans assessed by maximal treadmill testing.[47] These data all support the fact that fitness markedly alters the relationship between adiposity and subsequent prognosis in CHD patients.

POTENTIAL REASONS FOR AN OBESITY PARADOX IN CHD

There are several potential explanations for this puzzling obesity paradox in patients with CVD, which are summarized in Box 19.2. Initially when this paradox was recognized, it was thought that it must be due to unrecognized confounding factors, in addition to obvious ones, such as lower age, less smoking, and less chronic obstructive lung disease (COPD) in the heavier patients. In most studies, the age of the heavier patients is just 2–4 years lower, and this can easily be adjusted for in multivariate analyses. Also, many studies adjust for smokers, only assess nonsmokers, eliminate deaths during the first few years of follow-up, or even adjust for COPD.[38,40] Obese patients may present earlier at a less advanced disease stage, with more prevalent symptoms due to noncardiac reasons, including more deconditioning, more dyspnea due to restrictive lung issues, and edema due to more venous insufficiency, as well as having lower expression of natriuretic peptides, which may be particularly important in hypertension and HF, conditions that frequently coexist with CHD.[3,4,15] Obese patients also have lower levels of plasma renin activity at any given BP, and with higher levels of BP they can usually tolerate higher doses of many of the cardio-protective medications. None of the studies, however, are able to compensate adequately for nonpurposeful weight loss before study entry, a condition that would be expected to imply poor prognosis. Additionally, none of the studies can adjust for genetic risk that may be more relevant in lower-weight individuals. For example, the patient who has gained marked weight after their teens, which led to higher BP, dyslipidemia, glucose abnormalities, and inflammation, may not have developed CVD, including CHD, in the first place without the marked weight gain. However, the person who develops CVD at lower weight may do so from genetic predisposition. Although the thinner person may have a similar severity of CHD and lower risk factors, including lower BP and less hypertension, better lipid levels, lower blood sugar and prevalence of T2DM, along with lower CRP, their prognosis may be worse, possibly due to genetic predisposition. Finally, obese patients may have more metabolic reserve to fight chronic diseases, and although obese patients have higher BF, they often have a greater muscular strength than thinner people (discussed below).[3,4,15]

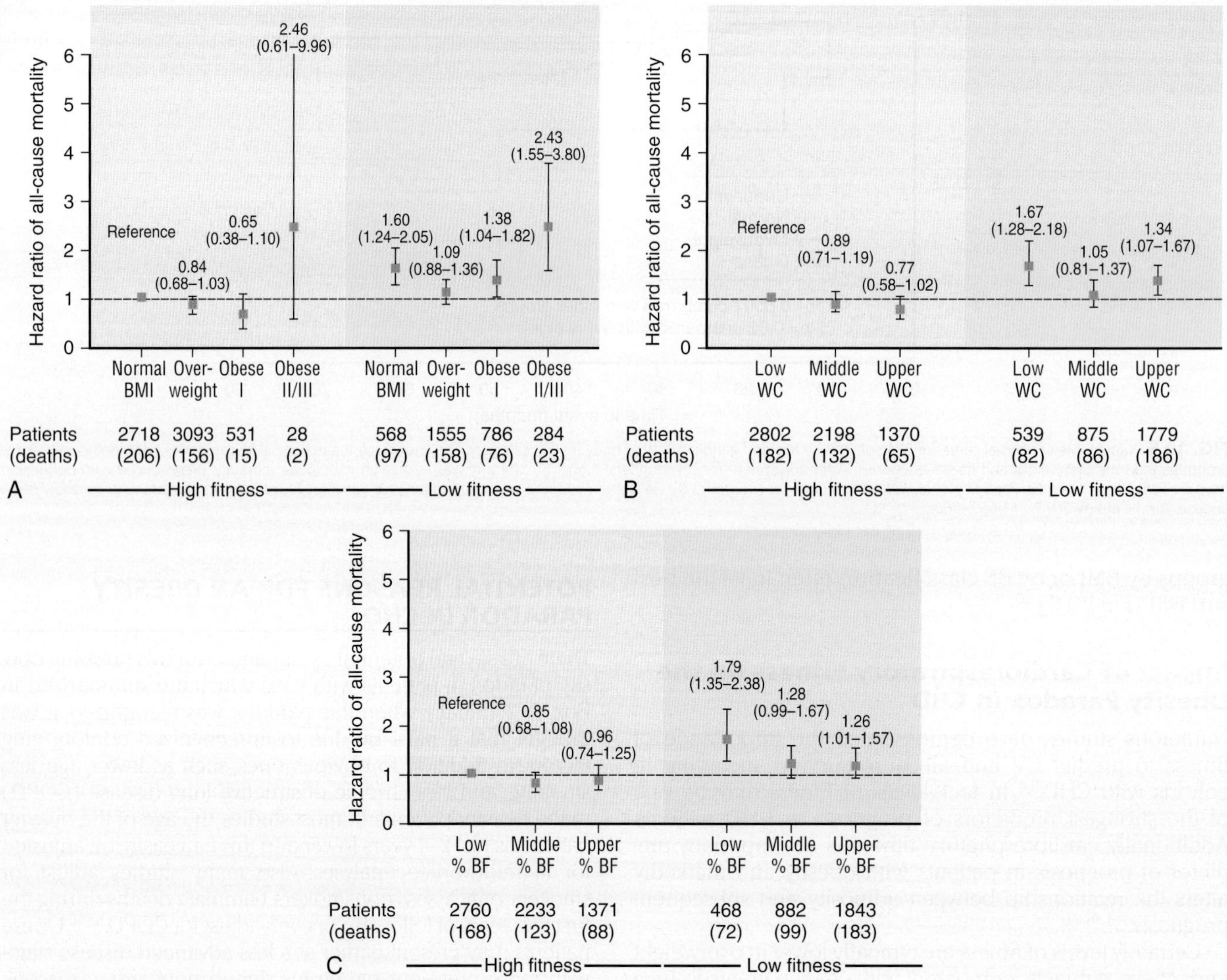

FIG. 19.6 A total of 9563 subjects stratified by **(A)** body mass index (BMI), **(B)** waist circumference (WC), and **(C)** body fat (BF) tertiles and followed for 13 years for all-cause mortality. Normal BMI, low WC, and low BF in the high-fitness group were used as reference groups. Boxplot represents hazard ratio and 95% confidence interval after adjustment for age, baseline examination year, physical activity, smoking, hyperlipidemia, diabetes, and family history of cardiovascular disease. *(Reproduced with permission from McAuley PA, Artero EG, Sui X, et al. The obesity paradox, cardiorespiratory fitness, and coronary heart disease.* Mayo Clin Proc. *2012;87:443–451.)*

BOX 19.2 Potential Reasons for the Obesity Paradox in CHD

1. Greater metabolic reserve including:
   - increased muscle mass and muscular strength
   - less cachectic
2. Earlier clinical presentation including:
   - earlier acute clinical presentation due to comorbidities, including restrictive lung disease, peripheral edema, etc.
   - younger age of presentation for medical care in general
   - increased medical screening due to obesity
   - higher usage of cardiac medications and higher doses due to medical screening
   - higher usage of cardiac medications due to higher rates of hypertension and hyperlipidemia
   - lower levels of plasma renin activity and atrial natriuretic peptides
   - less genetic predisposition to advanced CHD

CHD, Coronary heart disease.

IMPACT OF WEIGHT LOSS ON CHD

Despite the evidence indicating an obesity paradox in patients with CHD, there are still potential benefits of purposeful weight loss, especially when this occurs in the setting of increased physical activity, exercise training, and cardiac rehabilitation.[3,4,48–51] In a recent meta-analysis by Pack and colleagues[52] of 12 nonrandomized studies in 14 cohorts ($n > 35{,}000$), overall weight loss was actually associated with a significant 30% increase in major CVD events. On the one hand, observational weight loss (which is less likely to be intentional) appeared to be particularly deleterious, being associated with a marked 62% increase in major CVD events. On the other hand, presumed intentional weight loss, especially when combined with increased physical activity and exercise training, was associated with a significant 33% reduction in major CVD events. Although more studies of purposeful weight loss in CHD are clearly needed, purposeful weight loss in combination with increased exercise and formal cardiac rehabilitation presently seems beneficial. One of the potential disadvantages of weight loss, especially without increased exercise, is that BF is reduced but typically lean mass and muscle mass also decline, and this combination may be associated with a poor prognosis.[53,54] Since muscle mass, lean mass, and muscular strength are all important and are associated with benefits on CVD and CHD risk factors and survival, resistance training in combination with aerobic exercise to increase cardiorespiratory fitness seems to be particularly beneficial, since it combines improvements in cardiorespiratory fitness with preservation of lean mass, muscle mass, and muscular strength.[52–57] Cardiac rehabilitation programs are ideal settings to improve cardiorespiratory fitness and muscular strength with supervised exercise training following major CHD events, which may be particularly suited for obese CHD patients.[50,51,58,59]

PREVENTION OF OBESITY AND WEIGHT GAIN

During recent years, the origins of the obesity epidemic and progressive weight gain throughout life have been in considerable dispute.[4,60,61] However, regardless of this debate, it is generally widely accepted that increments in body weight and overall levels of adiposity are the result of chronic positive energy balance (i.e., energy expenditure < energy intake).[62,63] Many studies have suggested that energy or food intake, and especially sugar intake, is largely, if not completely, responsible for the obesity epidemic, blaming much of the obesity epidemic in the westernized world on poor dietary choices, fast foods, and excessive carbohydrate intake and sugar, especially sugary beverages.[64–68] One of the arguments to support this theory is that time spent in leisure-time physical activity has remained essentially unchanged in recent decades, supporting the conclusion that obesity is solely due to excessive energy or caloric intake.[62] However, this leisure-time physical activity represents a relatively small portion of total time per week, which is much more impacted by occupational-related activity or household management energy expenditure.[4]

Nevertheless, we have demonstrated very marked declines in occupational-related physical activity[62] and household management energy expenditure,[63] and dramatic declines in caloric expenditure in mothers, even more so in those with children under the age of 5 years.[69] In fact, the typical woman has a household management energy expenditure that is more than 1800 calories per week less than that of 5 decades ago,[63] and that of the average mother is 1500 calories per week less than 5 decades previously.[69] This suggests that females today would have to walk or jog 15–18 more miles per week to make up for the decline in energy expenditure elsewhere. Therefore, not only does the decline in energy expenditure lead to progressive weight gain, but since physical activity is the largest contributor to cardiorespiratory fitness, this decline in physical activity is impacting both obesity and overall fitness, as well as the weight of the next generation.[69–72]

In order to make up for the decrease in physical activity, reductions in caloric intake from all sources are needed, but particularly from carbohydrate and sugar for patients with low physical activity, high glucose and/or triglycerides, and those with metabolic syndrome and T2DM. However, increasing physical activity and exercise training are particularly needed to treat obesity and prevent weight regain after weight-loss programs.[48,49,57]

PHARMACOLOGIC TREATMENT OF OBESITY

A detailed review of currently approved pharmacologic approaches to obesity is beyond the scope of this chapter, particularly since none of the current agents have established efficacy and safety in patients with CHD.[73] Besides Orlistat, which is now available without a prescription, works as a lipase inhibitor to prevent fat absorption, and is not well-tolerated from a gastrointestinal standpoint, all the other agents have concerns about cardiac safety, including promoting valve disease or increasing BP and/or heart rate.[73,74] The available agents are listed in Table 19.3. Although none of these agents are specifically approved for patients with CHD, the pros and cons of the various medications versus severe obesity need to be considered, especially in patients who are not good candidates for bariatric surgery.

BARIATRIC SURGERY

Although a detailed review of bariatric surgery is beyond the scope of this chapter, considerable advances have been made in this area over recent decades.[73] In fact, even the 1991 National Institute of Health Consensus Development Conference panel on bariatric surgery recommended that for patients with a BMI of 40 kg/m^2 or above, or those with a BMI of 35 kg/m^2 or above who had associated high-risk comorbid conditions (such as cardiopulmonary disease or T2DM), this therapy is a reasonable consideration.[75] The U.S. Food and Drug Administration (FDA) has also approved the indication for laparoscopic adjustable gastric banding for a BMI of 30 kg/m^2 or above with a comorbidity.[73]

The three most common bariatric surgical procedures performed are laparoscopic adjustable gastric banding, laparoscopic sleeve gastrectomy, and Roux-en-Y gastric bypass with weight loss of 20–25%, 25–30%, and 30% at 5 years with

TABLE 19.3 Approved Obesity Medications

DRUG	MECHANISM	PROS	CONS
Orlistat	Lipase inhibitor. Blocks intestinal fat absorption.	Cardiac safety	Gastrointestinal side effects, weight loss relatively small, rare liver toxicity
Lorcaserin	Selective serotonin receptor agonist. Promotes satiety.	Relatively safe	Concern for valve disease, cannot take with many antidepressants
Phentermine & Topiramate	Stimulant. Reduces appetite.	Good weight loss	Teratogenic, potential to increase heart rate and blood pressure, suicidal thoughts
Bupropion & Naltrexone	Acts on hypothalamus to reduce hunger.	Good weight loss	Suicidal thoughts, concern about heart and CV system
Liraglutide	Glucagon-like peptide-1 agonist. Reduces appetite, increases satiety, and controls blood sugars.	Good weight loss and treats T2DM, clinical event reduction at lower dose in T2DM	Nausea and other gastrointestinal effects; pancreatitis, possible thyroid tumors, increases heart rate

CV, Cardiovascular; *T2DM*, type 2 diabetes mellitus.

these procedures, respectively.[73] Significant improvements in multiple obesity-related comorbidities have been reported, including T2DM, hypertension, dyslipidemia, obstructive sleep apnea, and quality of life, as well as long-term CVD events, especially in cohorts with T2DM.[73,76–78] Among the improved comorbidities, the prevention and treatment of T2DM has gained the most attention,[79] but a meta-analysis also suggested reductions in mortality by 30% to 45%.[73,80] Although large studies in patients with CVD, including CHD, have not been performed, small studies have suggested efficacy and safety in these patients.[4,73]

CONCLUSION

Obesity adversely impacts most CVD and CHD risk factors and may be an independent risk factor. Clearly, obese patients develop CVD at an accelerated rate, and this is certainly the case for CHD. Although obese patients may have increased rates of some complications early after revascularization procedures (especially with more severe obesity following CABG), risks of other complications (such as bleeding) are lower. Overall, the short- and medium-term prognosis regarding obesity is quite favorable and even better than in underweight and even normal-weight patients undergoing revascularization. However, long-term obese patients, particularly with moderate and severe degrees of obesity (BMI ≥ 35 kg/m^2), tend to have a less favorable prognosis. Weight loss is clearly needed in more severe obesity, and even in overweight and mildly obese patients seems to be advantageous when accomplished in the setting of increased cardiorespiratory fitness resulting from physical activity, exercise training, and especially cardiac rehabilitation.

References

1. Ogden CL, Carroll MD, Kit BK, Flegal KM: Prevalence of childhood and adult obesity in the United States, 2011–2012, *JAMA* 311:806–814, 2014.
2. Bastien M, Poirier P, Lemieux I, Després JP: Overview of epidemiology and contribution of obesity to cardiovascular disease, *Prog Cardiovasc Dis* 56:369–381, 2014.
3. Lavie CJ, De Schutter A, Parto P, et al. Obesity and prevalence of cardiovascular diseases and prognosis: the obesity paradox updated. *Prog Cardiovasc Dis*. doi: 10.1016/j.pcad.2016.01.008 [Epub ahead of print].
4. Lavie CJ, McAuley PA, Church TS, et al.: Obesity and cardiovascular diseases: implications regarding fitness, fatness, and severity in the obesity paradox, *J Am Coll Cardiol* 63:1345–1354, 2014.
5. Stewart ST, Cutler DM: The contribution of behavior change and public health to improved U.S. population health, *NBER Working Paper Series*, October 2014. Working Paper 20631. http://www.nber.org/papers/w20631.
6. Stewart ST, Cutler DM: How behavioral changes have affected U.S. population health since 1960, *NBER Working Paper Series*, March 2016. Working Paper 20631. http://www.nber.org/aging health/2015no1/w20631.
7. Wilson PWF, D'Agostino RB, Sullivan L, et al.: Overweight and obesity as determinants of cardiovascular risk: the Framingham Experience, *Arch Intern Med* 162:1867–1872, 2002.
8. Gelber RP, Gaziano JM, Manson JE, et al.: A prospective study of body mass index and the risk of developing hypertension in men, *Am J Hypertens* 20:370–377, 2007.
9. Mokdad AH, Ford ES, Bowman BA, et al.: Diabetes trends in the US: 1990–1998, *Diabetes Care* 23:1278–1283, 2000.
10. Lavie CJ, Milani RV, O'Keefe JH: Dyslipidemia intervention in metabolic syndrome: emphasis on improving lipids and clinical event reduction, *Am J Med Sci* 341:388–393, 2011.
11. Miller MT, Lavie CJ, White CJ: Impact of obesity on the pathogenesis and prognosis of coronary heart disease, *J Cardiometab Syndr* 3:162–167, 2008.
12. Alexander CM, Landsman PB, Teutsch SM, et al.: NCEP-defined metabolic syndrome, diabetes, and prevalence of coronary heart disease among NHANES III participants age 50 years and older, *Diabetes* 52:1210–1214, 2003.
13. Rader DJ: Effect of insulin resistance, dyslipidemia, and intra-abdominal adiposity on the development of cardiovascular disease and diabetes mellitus, *Am J Med* 120:S12–S18, 2007.
14. Carr DB, Utzschneider KM, Hull RL, et al.: Intra-abdominal fat is a major determinant of the National Cholesterol Education Program Adult Treatment Panel III criteria for the metabolic syndrome, *Diabetes* 53:2087–2094, 2004.
15. Lavie CJ, Milani RV, Ventura HO: Obesity and cardiovascular disease: risk factor, paradox, and impact of weight loss, *J Am Coll Cardiol* 53:1925–1932, 2009.
16. Hubert HB, Feinleib M, McNamara PM, et al.: Obesity as an independent risk factor for cardiovascular disease: a 26-year follow-up of participants in the Framingham Heart Study, *Circulation* 67:968–977, 1983.
17. Rabkin SW, Mathewson FA, Hsu PH: Relation of body weight to development of ischemic heart disease in a cohort of young North American men after a 26 year observation period: the Manitoba Study, *Am J Cardiol* 39:452–458, 1977.
18. Baker AR, Silva NF, Quinn DW, et al.: Human epicardial adipose tissue expresses a pathogenic profile of adipocytokines in patients with cardiovascular disease, *Cardiovasc Diabetol* 5:1, 2006.
19. Das SR, Alexander KP, Chen AY, et al.: Impact of body weight and extreme obesity on the presentation, treatment, and in-hospital outcomes of 50,149 patients with ST-segment elevation myocardial infarction: results from the NCDR (National Cardiovascular Data Registry), *J Am Coll Cardiol* 58:2642–2650, 2011.
20. Lavie CJ, Milani RV, Ventura HO: Impact of obesity on outcomes in myocardial infarction: combating the "obesity paradox", *J Am Coll Cardiol* 58:2651–2653, 2011.
21. Payvar S, Kim S, Rao SV, et al.: In-hospital outcomes of percutaneous coronary interventions in extremely obese and normal-weight patients: findings from the NCDR (National Cardiovascular Data Registry), *J Am Coll Cardiol* 62:692–696, 2013.
22. Buschur ME, Smith D, Share D, et al.: The burgeoning epidemic of morbid obesity in patients undergoing percutaneous coronary intervention: insight from the Blue Cross Blue Shield of Michigan Cardiovascular Consortium, *J Am Coll Cardiol* 62:685–691, 2013.
23. Cepeda-Valery B, Chaudhry K, Slipczuk L, et al.: Association between obesity and severity of coronary artery disease at the time of acute myocardial infarction: another piece of the puzzle in the "obesity paradox.", *Intl J Card* 176:247–249, 2014.
24. Cepeda-Valery B, Chaudhry K, Slipczuk L, et al.: Association between obesity and infarct size: insight into the obesity paradox, *Intl J Card* 167:604–606, 2013.
25. Sharma A, Vallakati A, Einstein AJ, et al.: Relationship of body mass index with total mortality, cardiovascular mortality, and myocardial infarction after coronary revascularization: evidence from a meta-analysis, *Mayo Clin Proc* 89:1080–1100, 2014.
26. Minutello RM, Chou ET, Hong MK, et al.: Impact of body mass index on in-hospital outcomes following percutaneous coronary intervention (report from the New York State Angioplasty Registry), *Am J Cardiol* 93:1229–1232, 2004.
27. Powell BD, Lennon RJ, Lerman A, et al.: Association of body mass index with outcome after percutaneous coronary intervention, *Am J Cardiol* 91:472–476, 2003.
28. Habib RH, Zacharias A, Schwann TA, et al.: Effects of obesity and small body size on operative and long-term outcomes of coronary artery bypass surgery: a propensity-matched analysis, *Ann Thorac Surg* 79:1976–1986, 2005.
29. Pan W, Hindler K, Lee V, et al.: Obesity in diabetic patients undergoing coronary artery bypass graft surgery is associated with increased postoperative morbidity, *Anesthesiology* 104:441–447, 2006.
30. Romero-Corral A, Montori VM, Somers VK, et al.: Association of bodyweight with total mortality and with cardiovascular events in coronary artery disease: a systematic review of cohort studies, *Lancet* 368:666–678, 2006.
31. Wang ZJ, Zhou YJ, Galper BZ, et al.: Association of body mass index with mortality and cardiovascular events for patients with coronary artery disease: a systematic review and meta-analysis, *Heart* 101:1631–1638, 2015.
32. Flegal KM, Kit BK, Orpana H, Graubard BL: Association of all-cause mortality with overweight and obesity using standard body mass index categories: a systematic review and meta-analysis, *JAMA* 309:71–82, 2013.
33. Coutinho T, Goel K, Corrêa de Sá D, et al.: Central obesity and survival in subjects with coronary artery disease: a systematic review of the literature and collaborative analysis with individual subject data, *J Am Coll Cardiol* 57:1877–1886, 2011.
34. Coutinho T, Goel K, Corrêa de Sá D, et al.: Combining body mass index with measures of central obesity in the assessment of mortality in subjects with coronary disease: role of "normal weight central obesity", *J Am Coll Cardiol* 61:553–560, 2013.
35. Goel K, Lopez-Jimenez F, De Schutter A, et al.: Obesity paradox in different populations: evidence and controversies, *Future Cardiol* 10:81–91, 2014.
36. McAuley PA, Artero EG, Sui X, et al.: The obesity paradox, cardiorespiratory fitness, and coronary heart disease, *Mayo Clin Proc* 87:443–451, 2012.
37. De Schutter A, Lavie CJ, Milani RV: The impact of obesity on risk factors and prevalence and prognosis of coronary heart disease: the obesity paradox, *Prog Cardiovasc Dis* 56:401–408, 2014.
38. Lavie CJ, De Schutter A, Patel D, et al.: Body composition and coronary heart disease mortality: an obesity or a lean paradox? *Mayo Clin Proc* 86:857–864, 2011.
39. Lavie CJ, Milani RV, Artham SM, et al.: The obesity paradox, weight loss, and coronary disease, *Am J Med* 122:1106–1114, 2009.
40. Lavie CJ, De Schutter A, Patel DA, et al.: Body composition and survival in stable coronary heart disease: impact of lean mass index and body fat in the "obesity paradox.", *J Am Coll Cardiol* 60:1374–1380, 2012.
41. Azimi A, Charlot MG, Torp-Pedersen C, et al.: Moderate overweight is beneficial and severe obesity detrimental for patients with documented atherosclerotic heart disease, *Heart* 99:655–660, 2013.
42. Lavie CJ, De Schutter A, Milani RV: Is there an obesity, overweight or lean paradox in coronary heart disease? Getting to the 'fat' of the matter, *Heart* 99:596–598, 2013.
43. De Schutter A, Lavie CJ, Patel DA, et al.: Relation of body fat categories by Gallagher classification and by continuous variables to mortality in patients with coronary heart disease, *Am J Cardiol* 111:657–660, 2013.
44. Barry VW, Baruth M, Beets MW, et al.: Fitness vs. fatness on all-cause mortality: a meta-analysis, *Prog Cardiovasc Dis* 56:382–390, 2014.
45. Alpert MA, Lavie CJ, Agrawal H, et al.: Cardiac effects of obesity: pathophysiologic, clinical and prognostic consequences—a review, *J Cardiopulm Rehabil Prev* 36:1–11, 2016.
46. Abudiab M, Aijaz B, Konecny T, et al.: Usefulness of function and aerobic capacity based on stress testing to predict outcomes in normal, overweight, and obese patients, *Mayo Clin Proc* 88:1427–1434, 2013.
47. Kokkinos P, Faselis C, Myers J, et al.: Cardiorespiratory fitness and the paradoxical BMI—mortality risk association in male veterans, *Mayo Clin Proc* 89:754–762, 2014.
48. Swift DL, Johannsen NM, Lavie CJ, et al.: The role of exercise and physical activity in weight loss and maintenance, *Prog Cardiovasc Dis* 56:441–447, 2014.
49. Ades PA, Savage PD: Potential benefits of weight loss in coronary heart disease, *Prog Cardiovasc Dis* 56:448–456, 2014.
50. Menezes AR, Lavie CJ, Milani RV, et al.: Cardiac rehabilitation in the United States, *Prog Cardiovasc Dis* 56:522–529, 2014.
51. Menezes AR, Lavie CJ, Forman DE, et al.: Cardiac rehabilitation in the elderly, *Prog Cardiovasc Dis* 57:152–159, 2014.
52. Pack QR, Rodriguez-Escudero JP, Thomas RJ, et al.: The prognostic importance of weight loss in coronary artery disease: a systematic review and meta-analysis, *Mayo Clin Proc* 89:1368–1377, 2014.
53. Artero EG, Lee DC, Lavie CJ, et al.: Effects of muscular strength on cardiovascular risk factors and prognosis, *J Cardiopulm Rehabil Prev* 32:351–358, 2012.
54. Lavie CJ, Forman DE, Arena R. Bulking up skeletal muscle to improve heart failure prognosis. *JACC Heart Fail*. doi: 10.1016/j.jchf.2015.12.005 [Epub ahead of print].
55. Jahangir E, De Schutter A, Lavie CJ: Low weight and overweightness in older adults: risk and clinical management, *Prog Cardiovasc Dis* 57:127–133, 2014.
56. Ortega FB, Lavie CJ, Blair SN: Obesity and cardiovascular disease, *Circ Res* 118:1752–1770, 2016.
57. Lavie CJ, Arena R, Swift DL, et al.: Exercise and the cardiovascular system: clinical science and cardiovascular outcomes, *Circ Res* 117:207–219, 2015.
58. Lavie CJ, Arena R, Franklin BA: Cardiac rehabilitation and healthy life-style interventions: rectifying program deficiencies to improve patient outcomes, *J Am Coll Cardiol* 67:13–15, 2016.
59. Grace SL, Bennett S, Ardern CI, et al.: Cardiac rehabilitation series: Canada, *Prog Cardiovasc Dis* 56:530–535, 2014.
60. McAllister EJ, Dhurandhar NV, Keith SW, et al.: Ten putative contributors to the obesity epidemic, *Crit Rev Food Sci Nutr* 49:868–913, 2009.
61. Hebert JR, Allison DB, Archer E, Lavie CJ, Blair SN: Scientific decision making, policy decisions, and the obesity pandemic, *Mayo Clin Proc* 88:593–604, 2013.

62. Church TS, Thomas DM, Tudor-Locke C, et al.: Trends over 5 decades in U.S. occupation-related physical activity and their associations with obesity, *PLoS One* 6:e19657, 2011.
63. Archer ER, Shook RP, Thomas DM, et al.: 45-Year trends in women's use of time and household management energy expenditure, *PLoS One* 8:e56620, 2013.
64. Swinburn B, Sacks G, Ravussin E: Increased food energy supply is more than sufficient to explain the US epidemic of obesity, *Am J Clin Nutr* 90:1453–1456, 2009.
65. Katan MB, Ludwig DS: Extra calories cause weight gain—but how much? *JAMA* 303:65–66, 2010.
66. Westerterp KR, Plasqui G: Physically active lifestyle does not decrease the risk of fattening, *PLoS One* 4:e4745, 2009.
67. DiNicolantonio JJ, O'Keefe JH, Lucan SC: Added fructose: a principal driver of type 2 diabetes mellitus and its consequences, *Mayo Clin Proc* 90:372–381, 2015.
68. DiNicolantonio JJ, Lucan SC, O'Keefe JH: The evidence for saturated fat and for sugar related to coronary heart disease, *Prog Cardiovasc Dis* 58:464–472, 2016.
69. Archer E, Lavie CJ, McDonald SM, et al.: Maternal inactivity: 45-year trends in mothers' use of time, *Mayo Clin Proc* 88:1368–1377, 2013.
70. Archer E: The childhood obesity epidemic as a result of nongenetic evolution: the maternal resources hypothesis, *Mayo Clin Proc* 90:77–92, 2015.
71. Archer E: In reply- Maternal, paternal, and societal efforts are needed to "cure" child obesity, *Mayo Clin Proc* 90:555–557, 2015.
72. Lavie CJ, Archer E, Jahangir E: Cardiovascular health and obesity in women: is cardiorespiratory fitness the answer? *J Womens Health* 25:657–658, 2016.
73. Kushner RF: Weight loss strategies for treatment of obesity, *Prog Cardiovasc Dis* 56:465–472, 2014.
74. Di Nicolantonio JJ, Chatterjee S, O'Keefe JH, Meier P: Lorcaserin for the treatment of obesity? A closer look at its side effects, *Open Heart* 1:e000173, 2014.
75. Gastrointestinal surgery for severe obesity: National Institutes of Health Consensus Development Conference Statement, *Am J Clin Nutr* 55:615S–619S, 1992.
76. Vest AR, Heneghan HM, Schauer PR, et al.: Surgical management of obesity and the relationship to cardiovascular disease, *Circulation* 127:945–959, 2013.
77. Buchwald H, Avidor Y, Braunwald E, et al.: Bariatric surgery: a systematic review and meta-analysis, *JAMA* 292:1724–1737, 2004.
78. Sjostrom L, Peltonen M, Jacobson P, et al.: Bariatric surgery and long-term cardiovascular events, *JAMA* 307:56–65, 2012.
79. Dixon JB, le Roux CW, Rubino F, et al.: Bariatric surgery for type 2 diabetes, *Lancet* 379:2300–2311, 2012.
80. Pontiroli AE, Morabito A: Long-term prevention of mortality in morbid obesity through bariatric surgery: a systematic review and meta-analysis of trials performed with gastric banding and gastric bypass, *Ann Surg* 253:484–487, 2011.

20 The Medical Treatment of Stable Angina

Lawrence Kwon and Clive Rosendorff

"... it is of all symptoms the most clamant, the most universal, and probably the most diagnostic, and one calling, above all others, on the resources of the doctor."

Sir James MacKenzie (1925)[1]

INTRODUCTION

The Context

Medical therapy of stable angina aims to address the key factor mediating myocardial ischemia: oxygen supply/demand imbalance. Pain is not the only symptom that a patient with myocardial ischemia may experience; there may also be severe fatigue, dyspnea, abdominal pain, nausea, sweating, and, occasionally, a sense of imminent death *(angor animi)*. Understanding cardiac pain requires knowledge of the interplay of ischemic, metabolic, and neurologic mechanisms. In this chapter, we will focus on ischemic and metabolic mechanisms and their therapy.

This chapter will not include a discussion of the clinical evaluation of a patient with stable angina, of lifestyle interventions, of antiplatelet, anticoagulant, and lipid-lowering drugs, and of revascularization strategies, all of which are dealt with in other chapters. Instead, we will focus on the narrower challenge of reducing the symptom of angina using pharmacologic agents, both traditional and novel.

Percutaneous Coronary Intervention Versus Optimal Medical Therapy for Symptomatic Ischemia

The Appropriate Use Criteria for Percutaneous Coronary Intervention (PCI) in Stable Ischemic Heart Disease recommend that patients take at least two classes of antianginal agents for symptomatic relief before PCI is considered.[2] Despite these recommendations, many patients undergo revascularization, partly stemming from psychological and emotional elements on the part of both patients and physicians.[3] Two groundbreaking studies, the Bypass Angioplasty Revascularization Investigation (BARI 2D) trial,[4] and Clinical Outcomes Utilizing Revascularization and Aggressive Drug Evaluation (COURAGE) trial,[5] compared optimal medical therapy plus revascularization versus optimal medical therapy alone to reduce mortality or major cardiovascular events.

BARI 2D compared PCI or coronary artery bypass grafting (both in addition to optimal medical therapy) versus optimal medical therapy alone in patients with type 2 diabetes mellitus. No difference was seen in 5-year mortality or in the endpoint of death between revascularization and optimal medical therapy without PCI.[4] Likewise, the COURAGE trial, with a mean follow-up of 4.6 years, revealed no significant difference in the survival rate between optimal medical therapy and PCI for the primary event rates, death, or percentage of subjects angina-free at 5 years,[5] nor was there any difference in survival after an extended 15-year follow-up.[6] On the other hand, a comprehensive network meta-analysis showed that coronary artery bypass grafting or PCI with one of the new generation drug-eluting stents resulted in reductions in death, death caused by myocardial infarction (MI), and repeat revascularization, compared to medical therapy.[7] There was no attempt to assess in these studies whether "medical treatment" was optimal medical therapy.

The ongoing ISCHEMIA (International Study of Comparative Health Effectiveness with Medical and Invasive Approaches) will also address this question.[8] In the meantime it is reasonable to recommend that PCI or coronary artery bypass grafting be reserved for patients whose angina limits daily activity despite optimal medical therapy, which includes at least two traditional antianginal medications in maximally tolerated dosage.

Decreasing Myocardial Oxygen Demand and Increasing Oxygen Supply

Pharmacologic prevention of symptoms of angina during periods of exertion has classically involved the use of agents that reduce myocardial oxygen demand and/or increase myocardial oxygen supply in response to exercise. Importantly, all available classes of traditional antianginal agents have similar effects on exercise duration. Thus, there is no clear indication that one drug is superior to the others based on this outcome.[9]

Management of patients with chronic stable angina has two main objectives: (1) symptomatic relief from ischemia; and (2) cardiovascular risk reduction and improvement of prognosis. These objectives are modulated by two different mechanisms: symptoms of ischemia are due to an insufficient oxygen supply/demand ratio, whereas acute coronary syndromes are due to vulnerable plaque erosion and rupture, resulting in thrombotic coronary occlusion.

Major determinants of myocardial oxygen demand are heart rate, contractility, and wall tension; minor determinants are basal metabolism and activation energy. Oxygen demand can be reduced by decreasing cardiac workload or by shifting myocardial metabolism to substrates that require less oxygen per unit of adenosine triphosphate (ATP) produced. Oxygen supply may be increased by coronary vasodilatation or by increasing the duration of myocardial perfusion during diastole by slowing the heart rate. Antianginal agents either reduce myocardial oxygen demand or increase myocardial oxygen supply to reduce symptoms of angina pectoris and signs of ischemia.

Traditional Anti-Ischemic Therapy

Traditional anti-ischemic therapy includes three antianginal agents: *nitrates*, *β-blockers*, and *calcium-channel blockers (CCBs)*. The traditional agents reduce anginal symptoms and prolong exercise duration and/or time to ST-segment depression on the electrocardiogram (ECG). Frequently, a combination of these drugs is necessary for symptom control, but hard data on the use of all three classes together are lacking. None of these drugs has been shown to be disease modifying: they do not change the risk of MI, sudden cardiac death, or all-cause mortality.[9] Although patients with stable coronary heart disease and preserved left ventricular function on optimal medical therapy may not have symptomatic relief with the addition of an angiotensin converting enzyme (ACE) inhibitor, there is evidence that ACE inhibitors reduce the rates of death from cardiovascular causes, MI, and coronary revascularization. Thus, we will be discussing ACE inhibitors as part of the traditional antianginal therapies.

Although efficacious, traditional anti-ischemic agents do not produce relief in all patients, and individual variation in responsiveness is well known. The combination of β-blockers with nitrates is favored because both agents lower myocardial oxygen demand and increase subendocardial blood flow through different mechanisms. The β-blockers prevent potential reflex tachycardia from nitrate-induced hypotension. In addition, by slowing the heart rate, β-blockers increase the duration of myocardial perfusion during diastole. Nitrates are vasodilators, thus they increase coronary perfusion and blunt any rise in left ventricular preload and end-diastolic pressure caused by the negative inotropic action of the β-blockers. β-Blockers combined with dihydropyridine CCBs improve exercise duration more than either alone and tolerance is usually acceptable, but the combination of β-blockers with non-dihydropyridine CCBs, such as verapamil and diltiazem, should be used with caution, and is contraindicated if there is left ventricular dysfunction or significant conduction system disease.

Novel Anti-Ischemic Therapy

Unfortunately, many patients with chronic angina remain symptomatic despite receiving the combination of two or more conventional drugs (β-blockers, nitrates, CCBs) at maximum tolerated dosages. Many patients with chronic angina also have concomitant comorbidities that make it difficult to up-titrate the dose or that contraindicate use of conventional antianginal drugs due to the fear of inducing dose-related adverse effects such as hypotension, bradycardia, or atrioventricular (AV) block. In addition, persistent angina occurs in approximately 10% to 25% of patients subjected to coronary bypass surgery and/or percutaneous interventions, and 60% to 80% require antianginal therapy 1 year after the procedure.

Novel antianginal medications include the following: (1) *ranolazine*, a drug that reduces myocardial ischemia by its action on the late sodium current; (2) *ivabradine*, a selective, heart rate slowing drug that inhibits the I_f current in pacemaker cells of the sinoatrial node; (3) *nicorandil*, a nicotinamide-nitrate ester that acts as an ATP-sensitive potassium channel opener, with nitric oxide donor capacity and antianginal properties that lead to direct coronary vasodilatation; (4) *trimetazidine*, a drug that inhibits β-oxidation of fatty acids, increases myocardial glucose utilization, and prevents reduction in ATP and phosphocreatine levels in response to hypoxia or ischemia; and (5) *molsidomine*, a drug that dilates venous capacitance vessels (reducing preload), dilates coronary arterial segments, exerts a platelet stabilizing effect by inhibiting thromboxane, and has a nitric oxide-donating effect.

These drugs have considerable potential as adjunctive therapy for angina, particularly in patients who are refractory to standard therapies, and they may be a primary therapeutic option in certain circumstances because they generally do not adversely affect blood pressure, pulse rate, or left ventricular systolic function. Thus, they offer an advantage in patients in whom conventional agents may induce symptomatic hypotension, inappropriate bradycardia, or worsening heart failure (HF). The clinical utility of each of these will be discussed later in this chapter.

Investigational Anti-Ischemic Therapy

Because of the inability of current antianginal drugs to optimally control chronic angina in all cases, such as in patients with severe coronary artery disease not amenable to revascularization, or with high risk of death and repeated hospital admissions, there is an unmet need for new drugs with different, but complementary, mechanisms of action devoid of the limitations of current treatments (with no or minimal hemodynamic effects) and that can be safely added to current therapy. In this chapter, in addition to addressing some of the newest prescribable antianginal drugs, we will briefly review drugs currently under development for the treatment of chronic angina.

Do Antianginal Drugs Prevent Coronary Events?

The choice of disease-modifying treatments that influence prognosis raises a few problems. The COURAGE study clearly demonstrated that all of these treatments should be used at the maximum tolerated doses, closest to those that have been proven to be effective in improving prognosis.[5] As the population ages patients with stable angina will have an increasing number of coexisting diseases, such as hypertension, diabetes, and dyslipidemia, which predispose to acute coronary syndromes. Different mechanisms of action for the anti-ischemic drugs allow treatment to be targeted to the individual patient, dependent on comorbidities and cardiac function. For example, in the absence of contraindications, β-blockers remain the reference treatment to prevent angina attacks and for the secondary prevention of MI. The most common coexisting cardiovascular risk factor is hypertension and, therefore, dihydropyridine CCBs have a role in combined treatment with β-blockers.

A combination of anti-ischemic drugs might improve the benefit of treatment with an additive or even synergistic effect. The findings of the Heart Outcomes Prevention Evaluation (HOPE)[10] and EURopean trial On reduction of cardiac events with Perindopril in stable coronary Artery disease (EUROPA),[11] discussed hereafter, support the use of an ACE inhibitor for the prevention of cardiovascular complications in all high-risk patients, including those with stable angina.

In all cases, the importance of risk profiling, management of comorbidities that increase the risk of cardiovascular events, such as hypertension, diabetes, and dyslipidemia, and aggressive lifestyle modification in all patients cannot be overstated.

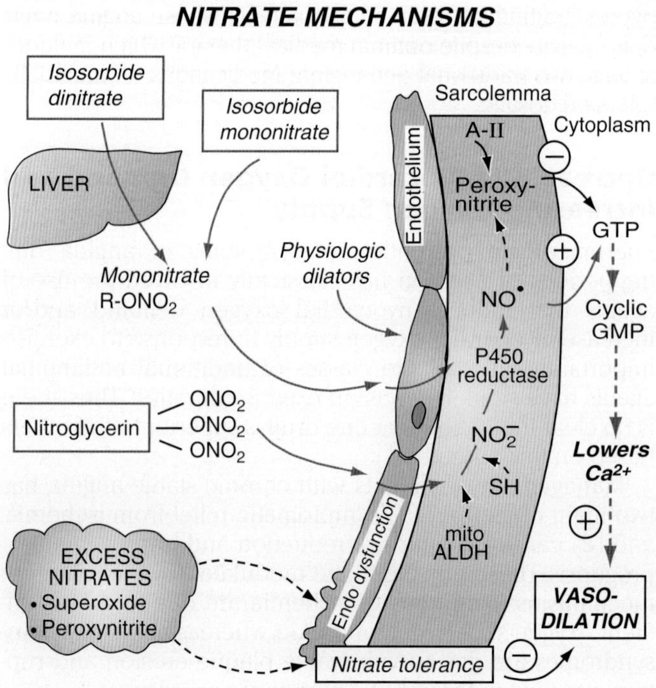

FIG. 20.1 Nitrate mechanisms. Exogenous nitrates are organic prodrugs that undergo enzymatic bioactivation to vasoactive nitric oxide (NO) in several steps. Nitroglycerin (GTN) produces NO via the action of mitochondrial aldehyde dehydrogenase-2 (mitoALDH). Isosorbide dinitrate (IDN) undergoes hepatic biotransformation to isosorbide mononitrate (IMN). IMN, bypassing the mitoALDH step, forms NO. NO relaxes vascular smooth muscle by activating guanylyl cyclase, leading to an increase in cyclic guanosine monophosphate (cGMP), which inhibits calcium entry into smooth muscle cells, causing vasorelaxation. Several mechanisms explain nitrate tolerance including the buildup of superoxide and peroxynitrite. Superoxide, likely the result of uncoupled endothelial nitric oxide synthase, and vascular NO form peroxynitrite, which inhibits soluble guanylyl cyclase and activates NO synthase uncoupling. *AII*, Angiotensin II; *GTP*, guanosine triphosphate. *(From Opie LH, Horowitz, JD, eds.* Drugs for the Heart. *8th ed. Philadelphia: WB Saunders; 2013:38–63 [Fig. 2.4].)*

TRADITIONAL ANTI-ISCHEMIC THERAPY

Nitrates

Mechanism of Action

Endogenous nitric oxide (NO) production is mediated by the enzyme nitric oxide synthase (NOS). In coronary artery disease, NO generation by NOS may be inhibited by ischemia, because NOS activity requires the availability of oxygen.[12] Nitrates are antianginal agents by virtue of their biotransformation to NO. Nitrates, by generating NO, are coronary vasodilators, reduce preload by venodilatation, and are arteriolar dilators. The arteriolar dilatation affects the arterial wave reflection from the periphery back to the aorta so that there is lowering of left ventricular afterload. Accordingly, aortic systolic pressure is reduced with little or no decrease in brachial systolic pressure. However, nitrates are better venous than arteriolar dilators probably because of reflex activation of the sympathetic nervous system, which limits arteriolar dilatation.

In experimental studies, NO also possesses antiatherogenic actions, reducing endothelial cell–leukocyte interaction, smooth muscle proliferation, and platelet adherence and aggregation (Fig. 20.1).[13,15-17] In one study, long-term supplementation with L-arginine, a precursor of NO, improved small-vessel coronary endothelial function in humans.[14]

The most commonly used nitrates are nitroglycerin (glyceryl trinitrate [GTN]), isosorbide dinitrate (IDN), and isosorbide-5-mononitrate (IMN). These may be available as sublingual, oral, sustained oral, buccal, oral spray, transdermal patch, and intravenous formulations. Exogenous nitrates are organic prodrugs that undergo enzymatic bioactivation to vasoactive NO in several steps. GTN produces NO via the action of mitochondrial aldehyde dehydrogenase-2 (mtALDH-2). IDN undergoes hepatic biotransformation to IMN. IMN, bypassing the miALDH-2 step, forms NO. NO relaxes vascular smooth muscle by activating guanylyl cyclase, leading to an increase in cyclic guanosine monophosphate (cGMP), which inhibits calcium entry into smooth muscle cells, causing vasorelaxation. NO also relaxes smooth muscle cells by inhibiting potassium channels and hyperpolarizing the membrane.

Endothelial dysfunction decreases production (or enhances inactivation) of NO. Organic nitrates, by their conversion to NO, have the ability to replenish deficient levels of NO in patients with coronary artery disease. In these patients, exogenous nitrate administration substitutes for the impaired activity of the endothelial L-arginine/NO pathway.[16,18]

Pharmacokinetics

Sublingual GTN is the nitrate of choice for acute angina attacks. GTN is rapidly absorbed from mucus membranes, skin, and the gastrointestinal tract and has a plasma half-life of only a few minutes. GTN is metabolized by a liver reductase enzyme to biologically active glyceryl dinitrate and biologically inactive glyceryl mononitrate. The elimination half-life of glyceryl dinitrate is 10-fold longer than the parent GTN, which may account for the antianginal effect lasting more than a few minutes.

Isosorbide mononitrate is bioavailable without any hepatic metabolism, whereas isosorbide dinitrate (IDN) needs to be converted in the liver to active mononitrates such as isosorbide mononitrate (IMN), with a half-life of 4 to 6 hours. IDN may also be given sublingually, but because IDN needs to undergo hepatic bioactivation, the onset of antianginal action is slower than for GTN. IDN and IMN are usually prescribed for daily oral administration for angina prophylaxis, but the development of tolerance is a significant problem.

Drug-Drug Interactions

The most important interaction is with the selective phosphodiesterase (PDE)-5 inhibitors, such as sildenafil, tadalafil, and vardenafil, which inhibit the degradation of cGMP and are used for the therapy of erectile dysfunction and sometimes for pulmonary arterial hypertension. The combination of nitrates and a PDE-5 inhibitor can cause serious hypotensive reactions and should not be taken on the same day. Alcohol and other vasodilators, including some antihypertensive drugs (eg, CCBs, α-blockers, hydralazine, minoxidil) may augment hypotension.

Side Effects

Common side effects include headaches, facial flushing, hypotension and syncope, and tachycardia. In hypertrophic cardiomyopathy, nitrates may exaggerate left ventricular outflow obstruction. Reduced venous return due to venous dilatation may compromise cardiac output in acute coronary syndromes, hypertrophic cardiomyopathy, constrictive pericarditis, and tight mitral or aortic stenosis.

Hemodynamics

Nitrates alleviate anginal symptoms by increasing myocardial oxygen supply and reducing oxygen demand. Increasing oxygen supply is achieved by (1) coronary vasodilatation; (2) venodilatation, thereby reducing cardiac filling pressure, lowering left ventricular diastolic pressure, and thus allowing for increased subendocardial myocardial perfusion; (3) preventing coronary artery vasospasm; and (4) replacing endogenous NO in vascular smooth muscle cells exhibiting endothelial dysfunction. Decreased myocardial oxygen demand occurs by (1) dilatation of venous capacitance vessels, reducing preload, and resulting in diminished systolic wall stress; and (2) reduction in systolic wall stress by reducing left ventricular afterload.[15,18]

Organic nitrates exert their maximal vasodilatory effect at the level of venous capacitance vessels. Large and medium-sized coronary arteries and their collateral vessels are affected, whereas arterioles with a diameter of less than 100 mm are relatively less affected.[16,17] The vasodilatory effect on epicardial coronary arteries with or without atherosclerotic coronary artery disease helps relieve coronary vasospasm.[12]

Antiaggregant Action of Nitrates

GTN exerts limited antithrombotic and antiplatelet effects in patients with stable angina, by an action on platelet cGMP. NO is a potent activator of platelet guanylyl cyclase, which increases platelet cGMP levels and leads to decreased fibrinogen binding to the glycoprotein IIb/IIIa receptor. Fibrinogen binding is essential for platelet aggregation, and its inhibition leads to impairment of platelet function.[18,19]

Ischemic Preconditioning

The term ischemic preconditioning describes a protective phenotype characterized by reduced sensitivity to ischemia and reperfusion injury following previous episodes of ischemia. Several lines of evidence from animal and human studies have demonstrated that the administration of GTN is associated with an increased ischemic threshold, as manifested by reduced infarct size, reduced ECG changes in the setting of percutaneous angioplasty, and reduced endothelial dysfunction after ischemia and reperfusion.[18]

Indications

Short-acting nitrates are often given to relieve acute anginal pain and can also be used prophylactically to improve exercise tolerance and prevent exercise-induced ischemia. The use of prophylactic GTN may be particularly appropriate for patients with predictable angina precipitated by exertion or specific activities. Short-acting nitrates may also be used to supplement long-acting nitrates when patients experience acute attacks. Long-acting nitrates, either as monotherapy or in combination with β-blockers or CCBs, are used to prevent or reduce the frequency of angina in patients with coronary artery disease.[18]

Some physicians recommend short-acting nitrates if angina occurs only a few times per week and long-acting nitrates if angina is more frequent. In patients who have angina with exertion, long-acting nitrates are sometimes preferred to prevent symptoms throughout the day. It is well known that continuous treatment with organic nitrates can lead to the development of tolerance, with loss of clinical efficacy. Tolerance can be reduced by nitrate-free intervals of 10–12 hours; therefore, it is not clinically feasible to provide continuous antianginal prophylaxis with any of the currently available long-acting nitrates.[18]

Dosage

Three different nitrates—GTN, IMN, IDN—are available in a variety of formulations including sublingual, buccal, oral, spray, ointment, and transdermal preparations. Short-acting nitrates are available as sublingual/buccal preparations, whereas long-acting preparations include oral-sustained forms and slow-release transdermal patches and ointments, which increase their duration of action (Table 20.1).

Among short-acting nitrates, sublingual GTN tablets are the standard initial therapy for effort-induced angina in the United States, whereas sublingual nitroglycerin spray is favored in most European countries as the preferred short-acting formulation. Sublingual GTN can be administered by metered dose spray that dispenses 0.4 mg of the drug. One to two sprays can be used at the start of an attack and up to three sprays can be used in a 15-minute period.

The onset of action of transdermal patches of nitroglycerin is 30 minutes, with duration of action of 8 to 14 hours. The transdermal patch comes in several sizes: each cm^2 of applied system delivers approximately 0.02 mg of nitroglycerin per hour. Thus, the 5-, 10-, 15-, 20-, 30-, and 40-cm^2 systems deliver approximately 0.1, 0.2, 0.3, 0.4, 0.6, and 0.8 mg

TABLE 20.1 Nitrates: Routes of Administration, Dosages, and Frequency of Dosing

NITRATES	ROUTES OF ADMINISTRATION	DOSAGES	FREQUENCY
Nitroglycerin (Glyceryl trinitrate)	Sublingual tablet	0.15–0.6 mg	As needed
	Sublingual spray	0.4 mg	As needed
• Nitrostat	Intravenous	5–400 μg/min	As needed
• Nitro-Bid	Sublingual tablet	0.3–0.6 mg	As needed
• Nitro-Dur	Ointment (topical) 2%	0.5–2 in (7.5–30 mg)	As needed
	Patch	1 Patch (2.5–15 mg)	2 × daily
Isosorbide mononitrate	Sublingual/oral tablet	10–40 mg	2 × daily
• Imdur	Sustained release	30–120 mg	1 × daily
• Monoket	Sustained release	5–20 mg	2 × daily
Isosorbide dinitrate	Sublingual/oral tablet	2.5–10 mg	Every 2–3 h
• Isordil	Sustained release tablet	5–40 mg	2–3 × daily
• Dilatrate-SR	Sustained release tablet	40–160 mg	2 × daily
Pentaerythrityl tetranitrate	Sublingual tablet	5–10 mg	As needed
	Oral tablet	10 mg	3 × daily
• Cardilate			

Prescribers are advised to check the approved dosages of the particular preparation of nitrates that they intend to prescribe. Usually the patient should be started on the lowest dose of any agent, with up-titration as necessary. Nitrate-free intervals of 10–12 hours will reduce tolerance.

of nitroglycerin per hour, respectively. The remainder of the nitroglycerin in each system serves as a reservoir and is not delivered in normal use. After 12 hours, for example, each system has delivered approximately only 6% of its original content of nitroglycerin.

Nitrate Resistance and Tolerance

Although acute treatment, including sublingual administration, is immediate and effective, the benefit of nitroglycerin has been limited because of *in vivo* tolerance that rapidly develops on continuous treatment. Nitroglycerin tolerance is manifested as a reduced vasodilatory response and the requirement of higher doses of the drug after continuous treatment. Tolerance is a major limiting factor in the use of nitrates. Traditionally, the pathogenesis of tolerance has been described as a result of metabolic or functional effects. The metabolic effect of organic nitrates declines during continuous use as a result of decreased biotransformation to NO or decreased activity of NO released by this process (end-organ tolerance). Functional effects consisting of counter-regulatory mechanisms to NO (called "pseudotolerance") may occur in response to nitrate therapy. For example, neurohormonal activation and plasma volume expansion may counterbalance or vitiate the therapeutic effects of nitrates.[19]

Several postulated mechanisms underlie nitrate tolerance[20–25]:

1. *Nitrate resistance* is sometimes associated with incremental impairment of endothelial function, largely due to generation of the superoxide anion (O_2^-) free radicals. Chronic continuous in vivo exposure to high doses of GTN sometimes induces incremental O_2^- generation with resulting evidence of redox stress. Prolonged nitrate therapy may result in the formation of peroxynitrite, which inhibits endothelial NOS, thus decreasing NO formation.
2. *True nitrate tolerance*
   (a) *Impaired nitrate bioactivation.* The activation of GTN is catalyzed by mitochondrial aldehyde dehydrogenase-2 (mtALDH-2) and, conversely, nitroglycerin can inactivate mtALDH-2. Nitrate tolerance may therefore reflect progressive inhibition of mtALDH-2 activity. Bioactivation of GTN also requires thiols or sulfhydryl-containing compounds. Interactions between GTN and sulfhydryl-containing receptors are necessary for vascular smooth muscle relaxation, and repeated administration of GTN results in sulfhydryl depletion and the development of tolerance.
   (b) *Formation of aldehydes.* Aldehydes are highly toxic compounds that generate reactive oxygen species (ROS), and are normally restricted by the action of ALDH. Because organic nitrates inactivate ALDH, including mtALDH-2, excessive production of ROS results, leading to endothelial dysfunction.
   (c) *Other enzymes* have been implicated in the vascular metabolism of GTN and other organic nitrates, including glutathione-S-transferase (GST), cytochrome P3A, other cytochrome P450 isoforms, and xanthine oxidoreductase (XOR).
   (d) *Reduced bioactivity of NOS.* Clear evidence now exists that GTN therapy has negative effects on the function of NOS, the enzyme responsible for the endothelial control of vascular tone.[23] GTN therapy appears to induce a dysfunctional state of NOS, in which the reductive activation of molecular oxygen to form O_2^- is not followed by oxidation of L-arginine and NO synthesis, resulting in the net generation of "NOS uncoupling." Uncoupling can be triggered by reduced bioavailability of tetrahydrobiopterin and/or L-arginine, cofactor and substrate, respectively, for NOS.
   (e) *Formation of peroxynitrite.* As an unstable structural isomer of nitrate, NO_3^-, peroxynitrite is a powerful oxidant that may influence nitrate resistance. Increased concentrations of peroxynitrite have been associated with prolonged nitrate therapy and may destabilize the metabolite isomer of nitroglycerin. This inhibits endothelial NOS, decreasing NO formation.

Strategies to Reduce Nitrate Tolerance

Various measures have been tried to prevent nitrate tolerance. The only effective approach to mitigate tolerance has been the use of "interval dosing" or "intermittent therapy," that is, dosing regimens or nitrate formulations that yield low or nitrate-free plasma concentrations for 10–12 hours per day.[26] One example is to prescribe 12-hour intervals of isosorbide mononitrate instead of the standard 7 hours, or

TABLE 20.2 Agents Postulated to Limit or Reverse Development of Nitrate Tolerance

AGENT	POTENTIAL MECHANISM(S) OF ACTION
ACE inhibitors	Prevention of NAD(P)H oxidase activation
Hydralazine	Inhibition of NAD(P)H oxidase
Ascorbic acid	Limitation of oxidative stress
Folic acid	Re-coupling of NO synthase
L-Arginine	Increased NO generation
N-Acetylcysteine	• Potentiation of nitrate bioconversion • Limitation of oxidative stress

ACE, Angiotensin-converting enzyme; *NAD(P)H,* reduced nicotinamide adenine dinucleotide (phosphate); *NO,* nitric oxide.
Modified from Table 1 in Horowitz J D: Amelioration of nitrate tolerance: matching strategies with mechanisms. J Am Coll Cardiol. *2003;41:2001.*

to recommend nitrate-free days. This approach, however, carries a risk for increased angina episodes during nitrate-free periods and precludes a continuous therapeutic effect.[18]

There have been some studies, either in animals or in small numbers of humans, which suggest other strategies for managing nitrate tolerance. Some human studies have suggested that vitamin E,[27] vitamin C,[28] and statins[29] are effective. In animal studies, pravastatin and atorvastatin prevented nitrate tolerance and vascular superoxide formation induced by subcutaneous GTN injections, an effect associated with increased basal cGMP levels that was abolished when rats received an inhibitor of eNOS concomitantly with GTN[25] (Table 20.2).

Folic acid can reverse endothelial dysfunction, possibly by restoring the bioavailability of tetrahydrobiopterin (a cofactor for NO synthase), arginine (its substrate), or both. This observation suggests a possible role of folic acid in preventing nitrate tolerance.[25]

Treatment for 5 to 10 days with L-arginine, the substrate for NO synthesis, can modify or prevent development of nitrate tolerance during continuous transdermal GTN use.[30]

Hydralazine may attenuate nitrate tolerance, perhaps by preventing superoxide generation. This relationship could contribute to the efficacy of combined nitrate-hydralazine therapy in patients with HF. Hydralazine is a vasodilator that also may overcome the effect of the formation of free radicals; indeed, the combination of nitrates and hydralazine has an established place in the treatment of HF.[31] In patients with angina pectoris, a β-blocker should be given in combination with hydralazine because of reflex sympathetic activation.

Clinical Utility of Nitrates

1. Short-acting nitrates for acute effort angina: *Sublingual GTN* 0.15 to 0.6 mg every 5 minutes until there is pain relief, up to a maximum of four to five tablets. Side effects are headaches and postural hypotension. *Sublingual IDN* 2.5 to 10 mg every 2 to 3 hours is recommended only if the patient is unresponsive to or intolerant of sublingual GTN. This is because dinitrate requires hepatic conversion to the active mononitrate, so the onset of antianginal action is slower (3–4 minutes) than with GTN, but the antianginal effects, however, last for up to 1 hour.
2. Long-acting nitrates for angina prophylaxis: *Oral sustained release IDN* is used at an initial dose 5–40 mg twice daily or three times daily, with a maintenance dose of 10–40 mg twice daily or three times daily. Tolerance is a major limiting factor, and several strategies have been proposed to limit tolerance, including interval dosing, and dosing-free days. *Oral sustained release IMN* carries similar dosage, indications, and effects as isosorbide dinitrate. Again, tolerance can be minimized by eccentric (twice daily or three times daily) dosing, or by the use of a slow-release preparation (Imdur), initial dose 30–60 mg daily, titrating up to 120 mg daily over 7 days. Rarely, 240 mg daily may be required.[32] *Transdermal nitroglycerin* patches permit the timed release of GTN over a 24-h period, but have not been shown to be superior to oral preparations.

Side Effects of Nitrates

Common side effects are hypotension, syncope, tachycardia, headache, and facial flushing. Less common is methemoglobinemia, treated with intravenous methylene blue. Contraindications include hypertrophic cardiomyopathy, where nitrates may increase outflow tract obstruction, constrictive pericarditis (because nitrates are potent venodilators and will reduce cardiac filling pressures), and concomitant administration on the same day with selective phosphodiesterase inhibitors (PDE-5) such as sildenafil, tadalafil, and vardenafil. A systolic blood pressure of less than 90 mm Hg is also a contraindication.

Conclusion

Organic nitrates, such as GTN, IMN, and IDN, when given acutely, have potent vasodilator effects, improving angina symptoms in patients with stable coronary artery disease. The mechanisms underlying vasodilation include intracellular bioactivation of the nitrates (IDN to IMN in the liver, GTN by vascular mitochondrial aldehyde dehydrogenase), the release of NO, and activation of the enzyme soluble guanylyl cyclase. Increasing cyclic guanosine-3′,5′-monophosphate (cGMP) leads to an activation of the cGMP-dependent kinase I, thereby causing the relaxation of the vascular smooth muscle by decreasing intracellular calcium concentration. The hemodynamic and anti-ischemic effects of organic nitrates are rapidly lost upon long-term (low-dose) administration due to the rapid development of tolerance and endothelial dysfunction, which in most cases is linked to impaired bioactivation by miALDH-2 and intracellular oxidative stress.

β-Blockers

Introduction

β-Adrenergic receptors are G-protein coupled transmembrane proteins. Their main antianginal action lies in the intracellular part of the β-receptor that is coupled to the G-protein complex: G_s (stimulatory) and G_i (inhibitory). Agonists bind to the ligand site and stimulate the β-adrenergic receptors (β_1, β_2, and β_3 subtypes). This binding triggers adenylyl cyclase, another transmembrane enzyme, to convert adenosine triphosphate to cyclic adenosine monophosphate, which acts as a second messenger, initiating a cascade of variable events that are organ dependent.[33,34] By interacting mainly with G_s, β_1-adrenoreceptor activation of adenylyl cyclase mediates the positive inotropic and chronotropic functions in cardiac myocytes. β_2-Adrenoreceptors interact with cardiomyocyte G_s and G_i; one of the G_i protein pathways may mediate the antiapoptotic effect of β_2-adrenoreceptors.[35] β_3-Adrenoreceptors couple with G_i only

TABLE 20.3 Classification and Physiologic Actions of β-Adrenergic Receptors and β-Blockers Used in Angina Pectoris

ACTIVATION		SELECTIVE BLOCKERS		NON-SELECTIVE BLOCKERS	
β_1	β_2	β_1	β_2	β_1, β_2	α_1, β_1, β_2 (VASODILATORS)
• SA node: Increased heart rate • Atria: Increased contractility and conduction velocity • AV node: increased automaticity and conduction velocity • His-Purkinje: increased automaticity and system conduction velocity • Ventricles: increased automaticity, contractility, and conduction velocity	• Peripheral, coronary and carotid arteries: dilation • Lungs: dilation of bronchi • Uterus: smooth muscle relaxation • Other: increased insulin release; increased liver and muscle glycogenolysis	• Atenolol • Bisoprolol • Metoprolol • Nebivolol	None	• Propranolol • Nadolol • Timolol • Celiprolol	• Carvedilol • Labetalol

Modified from Table 54.5 Physiologic Actions of β-Adrenergic Receptors in Douglas L. Mann MD, Douglas P. Zipes MD, et al. Braunwald's Heart Disease: A Textbook of Cardiovascular Medicine, *10th ed. Saunders, an imprint of Elsevier Inc., 2014.*

and activate NO, but not via the adenylyl cyclase pathway, to reduce vascular tone (Table 20.3).

Mechanism of Action and Pharmacology

β-Blockers exert several cardioprotective effects. Despite the action of β_1 inhibition in blocking adrenergically mediated coronary vasodilation, thus potentially reducing coronary blood flow, β_1 inhibition is most important for angina management. However, because nearly all of myocardial perfusion occurs in diastole, the slower heart rate with its longer diastolic filling time actually improves myocardial blood flow. In addition, by reducing cardiac output and by inhibiting renin release from juxtaglomerular cells, β-blockers lower blood pressure, thus reducing systolic wall stress.[34,35]

β_1-Selective blockers become less selective at higher doses and may begin to block β_2-adrenoreceptors in the tracheobronchial tree causing bronchospasm. Therefore, β-blockers, even β_1-selective blockers, are contraindicated in patients with bronchial asthma. However, at conventional doses, selective β_1-receptor blockers are not contraindicated in patients with chronic obstructive pulmonary disease (COPD) unless there is a significant bronchospastic component. Furthermore, β_1-selective blockers should be used with care in patients with peripheral arterial disease, as described hereafter.

The vasodilator activity of some of the newer-generation β-blockers is achieved through two pathways: either combined β- and α-adrenergic receptor blockade (eg, labetalol and carvedilol) or direct vasodilator activity through the activation of NOS and the release of NO (eg, nebivolol). Carvedilol may also ameliorate myocardial ischemic effects through inhibition of monocyte adhesion to the endothelium, by scavenging oxygen-free radicals, protection of endothelial function, direct vasodilation, and inhibition of oxidation of low-density lipoprotein, thus slowing the development of atherosclerotic plaques. Nebivolol exhibits greater selectivity for β_1-adrenergic receptors than other β-blockers. The NO potentiating, vasodilatory effect of nebivolol is unique among β-blockers and, at doses below 10 mg/d, does not inhibit the increase in heart rate normally seen with exercise.[36]

β-Blockers can also be classified according to their lipophilicity and hydrophilicity. Lipid-soluble β-blockers (eg, propranolol, timolol, metoprolol, oxprenolol) are absorbed completely by the small intestine, metabolized by the liver, and can penetrate the blood-brain barrier. Water-soluble β-blockers (eg, atenolol, sotalol, and nadolol) are absorbed incompletely through the gut and cleared by the kidneys. There are β-blockers (eg, betaxolol, bisoprolol, and pindolol) that are cleared partly by the liver and partly by the kidney. Some of the central nervous system side effects of β-blockers, such as depression and fatigue, have been linked to lipophilicity, but evidence for this is sparse.

Adverse Effects of β-Blockers

β-Blockers can increase insulin resistance and predispose patients to incident diabetes. In a network meta-analysis of 22 clinical trials with 143,153 participants who did not have diabetes at randomization, the risk of new-onset diabetes was most pronounced with diuretics and β-blockers (more so than with other classes of antihypertensive agents), implying a negative metabolic effect by the β-blockers.[37] β-Blockers may contribute to the development of diabetes by weight gain (as much as 1.2 kg in one study), attenuation of the β-receptor mediated release of insulin from pancreatic β-cells, and decreased blood flow through microcirculation in skeletal muscle tissue, which results in decreased insulin sensitivity.[38,39]

There may also be worsening by some, but not all, β-blockers of glycemic control in patients with established diabetes. In the GEMINI (Glycemic Effects in Diabetes Mellitus Carvedilol-Metoprolol Comparison in Hypertensives) trial,[39] diabetics newly treated with metoprolol had an increase in hemoglobin (Hgb) A1c, whereas treatment with carvedilol did not elevate Hgb A1c. This finding suggests not all β-blockers have an equally adverse effect on diabetes control. A caution in diabetic patients is that β-blockers may mask the tachycardia that signals hypoglycemia.[40]

Exercise endurance depends, in part, on a properly functioning sympathetic nervous system. β-Blockers may hamper exercise tolerance by antagonizing this effect. β-Blockers may also worsen depressive symptoms and induce sexual dysfunction. These drugs have been associated with Raynaud's phenomenon and aggravation of peripheral arterial disease. β_2-blockade inhibits the vasodilating effects of catecholamines in peripheral blood vessels and leaves the constrictor (α-adrenergic) receptors unopposed, thereby enhancing vasoconstriction. Severe peripheral arterial disease, with claudication or physical signs of poor peripheral perfusion, should be regarded as a contraindication to the use of β-blockers.[40–42]

Abrupt withdrawal of β-blockers after prolonged administration can result in increased total ischemic activity in patients with chronic stable angina. Chronic β-blocker therapy can be safely discontinued by slowly withdrawing the drug in a stepwise manner over the course of 2 to 3 weeks. If abrupt withdrawal of β-blockers is required, patients should be instructed to reduce exertion and manage angina episodes with sublingual nitroglycerin, substituting a calcium antagonist, or using both agents in combination.[42]

β-Blockers should not be prescribed for patients with bradycardia associated with third-degree heart block or sick-sinus syndrome or in untreated pheochromocytoma. They may mask the clinical signs of hyperthyroidism and precipitate thyroid storm with abrupt discontinuation.

The most common comorbid conditions cited for withholding β-blockers in elderly patients after myocardial ischemia are COPD and asthma.[43] The safety of β-blockers in COPD patients who do not have significant bronchospasm has been demonstrated, but their use in patients who have COPD and angina remains low. Patients diagnosed with COPD tend to be treated with inhalers despite lack of objective evidence of bronchospasm, including pulmonary function testing. Patients should not be denied the benefits of β-blockers if they do not have significant bronchospasm. It may be necessary to discontinue the drug in a few patients because of bronchoconstriction, but, from the published literature, the potential benefit appears large enough to warrant taking this small risk. Metoprolol, a cardioselective β-blocker with a short half-life, has been shown to be safe and effective in patients with COPD and may be the β-blocker of choice for initiating therapy.

β-Blockers and Cardioprotection

The use of β-blockers is recommended in patients with stable ischemic heart disease (SIHD) and reduced ejection fraction and/or history of myocardial ischemia or acute coronary syndrome within the last 3 years.

The role of β-blockers in the management of patients with HF with reduced ejection fraction is well established. The Metoprolol CR/XL Randomized Intervention Trial in Heart Failure (MERIT-HF), in patients with New York Heart Association (NYHA) class II to IV HF, showed a 34% reduction in mortality in patients treated with metoprolol succinate versus placebo.[44] The CarvedilOl ProspEctive RaNdomIzed CUmulative Survival (COPERNICUS) trial included patients with a left ventricular ejection fraction (LVEF) of less than 25%. Compared with placebo, carvedilol reduced mortality risk at 12 months by 38% and the risk of death or hospitalization for HF by 31%.[45]

Another longer-acting β-blocker, bisoprolol, showed similar long-term benefit on survival in patients with HF. The Cardiac Insufficiency Bisoprolol Study (CIBIS-II)[46] showed a 32% reduction in all-cause mortality in bisoprolol-treated patients with NYHA class III or IV HF caused by ischemic and nonischemic cardiomyopathy.

Although all three of these agents (metoprolol, carvedilol, and bisoprolol) are beneficial in patients with HF, the Carvedilol or Metoprolol European Trial (COMET)[47] demonstrated a 17% greater mortality reduction in favor of carvedilol compared with metoprolol XL, with mean daily doses of 85 and 42 mg/d, respectively. As a result of these studies, β-blockers, particularly metoprolol, carvedilol, and bisoprolol, are recommended for the long-term management of patients with angina and left ventricle (LV) systolic dysfunction.

On the other hand, there is insufficient evidence to support β-blockers to prevent coronary events in patients with normal ejection fraction and no history of symptomatic myocardial ischemia. Patients with ischemic heart disease from the Reduction of Atherothrombosis for Continued Health (REACH) registry ($n = 21{,}860$) were divided into three cohorts: prior MI, coronary artery disease (CAD) without MI, or those with CAD risk factors only. The study showed no significant difference in the primary composite outcome of cardiovascular death, nonfatal MI, and nonfatal stroke in patients on β-blockers versus those not on β-blockers for all three cohorts. Only in those with recent MI (≤1 year), was β-blocker use associated with a lower incidence of the secondary outcome, defined as the primary outcome plus hospitalization for atherothrombotic events or a revascularization procedure.[48]

β-Blockers and Atrial Fibrillation

In atrial fibrillation (AF) a rapid ventricular rate may be associated with angina. β-Blockers are well established as useful and effective agents for rate control in patients with AF. Whereas β-blockers have been shown to improve cardiovascular outcomes in HF with reduced ejection fraction, this action seems to be attenuated in the presence of AF. In a meta-analysis of four studies that enrolled patients with HF, 1677 of them with AF, half were treated with β-blocker, and half with placebo. In patients with sinus rhythm there was a significant reduction in mortality and HF hospitalizations, but not in those with AF.[49] In addition, whereas β-blockers predominantly slow AV conduction, they do not exhibit specific antifibrillation properties in the atria. Thus, there is no significant effect of acute administration of a β-blocker in eliciting the conversion of AF or flutter to sinus rhythm.[50]

Conclusion

The anti-ischemic and antiarrhythmic activities of β-blockers have made this class of agents, together with nitrates, the mainstay of angina therapy. Generally, β_1-selective blockers are preferred. Examples are metoprolol tartrate (short acting) or succinate (long acting), and bisoprolol. Carvedilol, a β-blocker with α-antagonist activity, and nebivolol, a β-blocker that also generates NO, add to the established benefits of this exceptional class of drugs in ameliorating angina. β-Blockers remain the standard of care after episodes of myocardial ischemia and in patients with HF with reduced ejection fraction. However, other than their antianginal and antihypertensive actions, there is a scarcity of evidence to support the use of β-blockers in patients with chronic ischemic heart disease who have a normal ejection fraction.[8] None of the relevant studies have demonstrated a prognostic advantage of β-blockers over other antianginal drugs for preventing adverse cardiovascular events. Future studies should assess the use of β-blockers combined with other therapies (ie, antiplatelets, statins, nitrates, additional classes of antihypertensive medications, and PCI) in these patients.

Calcium-Channel Blockers

Introduction

The actions of CCBs on coronary blood flow are complex. The change in blood flow that they induce depends on their actions at rest versus during exercise, effects on coronary perfusion pressure, variable changes in myocardial oxygen demand, autoregulation of coronary flow, and differential effects on diastolic perfusion time.[9]

Classification

Based on their chemical structure, CCBs fall into the following groups[15] (Table 20.4):

TABLE 20.4 Calcium Channel Blockers used for Ischemic Heart Disease

GENERIC NAME (TRADE NAME)	USUAL DAILY DOSAGE (MG)	PEAK RESPONSE (HR)	DURATION OF RESPONSE (HR)	COMMON SIDE EFFECTS
Dihydropyridines				
Amlodipine (Norvasc)	5–10 qd	6–12	24	Headache, flushing, edema
Felodipine (Plendil ER)	2.5 qd	2–5		
Nifedipine GITS (Procardia XL)	30–90 qd	4–6		
Nifedipine (Procardia, Adalat)	10–30 tid	0.1	4–6	Headache, hypotension, dizziness, flushing, edema
Nicardipine (Cardene)	20–40 tid	0.5–2	8	
Non-Dihydropyridines				
Diltiazem (Cardizem)	60–120 tid	2.5–4	8	Hypotension, bradycardia, dizziness, flushing, edema
Diltiazem CD (Cardizem CD)	240–280 qd	10	24	
Verapamil (Calan, Isoptin)	80–120 tid	6–8	8	
Verapamil SR (Calan SR, Isoptin SR)	120–240 bid	5	12–24	

bid, 2 times a day; *CD*, controlled diffusion; *CR*, controlled release; *ER and XL*, extended release; *GITS*, gastrointestinal therapeutic system; *qd*, once a day; *SR*, sustained release; *tid*, 3 times a day.
Modified from Weir MR, Hanes DS, Klassen DK, Wasser WG: Antihypertensive therapy. In Skoreci K, editor: Brenner and Rector's The Kidney, *ed10, Philadelphia, 2016, Elsevier. Table 50.15.*

1. Dihydropyridines (eg, amlodipine, nifedipine, nicardipine, felodipine). These act mainly on arterial vascular smooth muscle cells to dilate vessels, consequently lowering blood pressure.
2. Nondihydropyridines (divided into two subgroups):
   (a) Phenylalkylamines (eg, verapamil) act mainly on cardiac cells and have negative inotropic and negative chronotropic effects. They have less vasodilatory action than dihydropyridines and, hence, cause less reflex tachycardia.
   (b) Benzothiazepines (eg, diltiazem) combine the properties of dihydropyridines and phenylalkylamines. By exerting both cardiac depressant and vasodilatory actions, benzothiazepines are able to reduce arterial pressure without producing as much reflex cardiac stimulation as dihydropyridines.

Mechanism of Action

Transmembrane calcium influx occurs via a voltage-gated calcium channel consisting of four subunits: α_1, $\alpha_{2\delta}$, α_β, and α_γ. The α_1 subunit is the dominant component of calcium channels and constitutes the pore structure for ion conduction. Ten different α_1 subunits have been reported, each with a specific distribution and ion conductance of its channels. These distinct subunits characterize the channel properties of L-, N-, T-, P-, Q-, and R-type calcium channels. Of these channels, the L-type is the main target for CCBs. The L-type voltage-gated calcium channel is responsible for excitation-contraction coupling of skeletal, smooth, and cardiac muscle. L-type voltage-gated calcium channels are also involved in conduction of the pacemaker signal in the heart.[51] T-type calcium channels exhibit properties different from those of the L-type; they are involved in pacemaking and regulation of blood flow, but not in myocardial contraction.

All calcium antagonists cause dilatation of epicardial coronary vessels and arterial resistance vessels. Epicardial coronary vasodilatation is the primary mechanism responsible for the beneficial effect of calcium antagonists in relieving vasospastic angina.

CCBs in Angina

Nondihydropyridine CCBs reduce myocardial oxygen demand via their negative inotropic and chronotropic actions. Dihydropyridine CCBs are also postulated to improve the relative bioavailability of coronary artery nitric oxide and to improve endothelium-dependent vasodilator responses. These actions have led some to postulate that dihydropyridines favorably modify the natural history of atherosclerosis. Whether such an effect would be a direct pharmacologic effect of CCBs or secondary to their blood pressure-lowering effect is not clear.

All calcium-channel antagonists have similar antianginal efficacy. The choice of one agent or another is based primarily on pharmacodynamic characteristics, particularly whether or not a negative chronotropic effect is desired. The nondihydropyridines reduce heart rate, contractility, and blood pressure, thereby decreasing myocardial oxygen demand. The dihydropyridines are coronary vasodilators and also reduce myocardial oxygen demand by peripheral vasodilatation, thus lowering blood pressure and reducing myocardial wall tension.[9]

Other Actions

Dihydropyridine CCBs, but not phenylalkylamine CCBs, increase endogenous fibrinolytic activity.[52] Given the marked cellular changes associated with loss of normal calcium transport in atherosclerotic vessels, it has been proposed that CCBs slow the progression of CAD in addition to favorably effecting hemodynamics. Angiographic trials have shown significantly reduced formation of lesions in both patients with documented CAD and in animal models. In both in vitro and in vivo studies, amlodipine inhibited oxidative lipid damage.[53]

Smooth-muscle cell proliferation and migration are early hallmarks of atheroma. Amlodipine inhibits smooth muscle cell proliferation following cholesterol enrichment at concentrations several orders of magnitude lower than those needed to inhibit calcium. Thus, amlodipine may interfere with certain adverse effects induced by cholesterol, including atherogenic changes in vessels. In addition, tumor necrosis factor-α (TNF-α), a cytokine that is elevated in atherosclerosis, mediates inflammatory damage to vessel walls. Amlodipine has inhibited TNF-α-induced endothelial apoptosis in a dose-dependent manner.[53]

Clinical Evidence for the Efficacy of CCBs in Angina

Effective Treatment of Vasospastic Angina

CCBs are effective in the treatment of vasospastic angina. In one study, diltiazem (60 mg twice daily) reduced the mean frequency of vasospastic episodes during 72 hours from 43 to 5. In another randomized placebo-controlled study, patients were treated with either 10 mg of amlodipine once daily or placebo once daily for 4 weeks. The rate of vasospastic anginal episodes and the consumption of nitroglycerin tablets decreased significantly with amlodipine treatment.[54,55]

Cardioprotection

Trials, including ACTION (A Coronary disease Trial Investigating Outcome with Nifedipine)[55] and CAMELOT (Comparison of Amlodipine vs Enalapril to Limit Occurrences of Thrombosis),[56] have documented that CCBs are safe and beneficial for patients with CAD. ACTION did not support a beneficial effect of nifedipine on cardiovascular outcomes. A subset analysis of patients with concurrent angina and hypertension, however, found that an extended-release dosage formulation sustained blood concentrations of nifedipine over 24 hours (nifedipine gastrointestinal therapeutic system), significantly reducing the combined incidence of all-cause mortality, MI, refractory angina, HF, stroke, and peripheral revascularization by 13%.[57]

CAMELOT compared amlodipine or enalapril to placebo in normotensive patients with coronary artery disease (n = 1991). Although BP reduction was similar in the two active treatment groups, adverse cardiovascular events occurred less frequently in the amlodipine group than in the enalapril group. Compared with atenolol in patients with hypertension and coronary artery disease, verapamil caused less new-onset of diabetes mellitus, fewer angina attacks, and less depression.[56]

The Prospective Randomized Evaluation of the Vascular Effects of Norvasc Trial (PREVENT) was a 3-year multicenter, randomized, placebo-controlled trial that evaluated the effects of amlodipine on the development and progression of atherosclerotic lesions in coronary and carotid arteries among patients with CAD. Amlodipine therapy was associated with statistically significant slowing of carotid atherosclerosis progression, independent of blood pressure changes, and a reduced cardiovascular morbidity.[58]

The Coronary Angioplasty Amlodipine Restenosis Study (CAPARES) was performed in a similar patient population as that of the PREVENT trial. Amlodipine significantly reduced the incidence of repeat PCIs and clinical events after PCI, without reducing luminal loss.[59]

Pharmacokinetics

The pharmacokinetics of first-generation CCBs, including the nondihydropyridines verapamil and diltiazem, are similar. Even though the drugs are nearly completely absorbed after ingestion, their immediate bioavailability is offset by first-pass hepatic metabolism. Their onset of action is between 30 minutes and 2 hours, and their elimination half-lives range from 2 to 7 hours.

On the other hand, the second-generation CCBs, such as the dihydropyridine amlodipine, have a slower onset and longer duration of action, and a longer elimination half-life. These properties reduce the risk of reflex tachycardia and negative inotropy, thus making them relatively safe in patients with left ventricular dysfunction. The t_{max} of amlodipine is 6 to 12 hours, and the elimination half-life is 35 to 50 hours. A slower duration of action can be achieved by using medications with sustained release formulations or by a gastrointestinal therapeutic system, which is available for nifedipine.

Interactions of CCBs with Other Drug Classes

Nondihydropyridine CCBs interact with other negative chronotropic or inotropic agents, particularly β-blockers. They should generally not be coprescribed with β-blockers, particularly in patients with left ventricular dysfunction or failure.

CCBs inhibit the hepatic cytochrome CYPA4 enzyme and may raise blood levels of statins and numerous other drugs. Cimetidine and grapefruit juice may raise the effective level of CCBs. Because magnesium is a calcium antagonist, magnesium supplements may enhance the actions of CCBs, particularly nifedipine.

Adverse Effects of CCBs

One of the potential adverse effects of using CCBs with a short duration of action, such as short-acting nifedipine (20–40 minutes), is that of increased mortality risk in patients with CAD. Reasons for this effect include a precipitous fall in blood pressure, reflexively triggering increased sympathetic activity and tachyarrhythmias.

A dihydropyridine CCB can be added to optimal doses of β-blockers and nitrates, with an acceptable safety profile. Common side effects of CCBs are peripheral edema, headache, dizziness, and constipation. Ankle edema is not secondary to increased sodium retention but rather from arteriolar dilatation producing an increase in capillary hydrostatic pressure. With nondihydropyridine CCBs, bradycardia and heart block can occur in patients who have significant conduction disorders. For patients with severe systolic dysfunction, nondihydropyridine CCBs can worsen or precipitate congestive HF. CCBs can also suppress lower esophageal sphincter contraction and worsen gastroesophageal reflux disease.

Novel CCBs

CCBs with sustained activity and T/N-type calcium channel-blocking action could provide more beneficial effects than classic CCBs, and may expand the clinical utility of these agents. Among these novel CCBs are benidipine, cilnidipine, and efonidipine.

Benidipine

Benidipine may be more efficacious in vasospastic angina than other CCBs. A meta-analysis compared the actions of benidipine, amlodipine, nifedipine, and diltiazem alone or in combination on major adverse cardiovascular events (MACE) in vasospastic angina patients. The hazard ratio (HR) for the occurrence of MACE was significantly lower for benidipine than other CCBs, even after correcting for patient characteristics that could have affected the occurrence of MACE. Possible explanations for this result with benidipine are greater NO production; preservation of levels of tetrahydrobiopterin, an essential cofactor for NOS; and greater vasoselectivity.[54]

Cilnidipine

Cilnidipine is a dual blocker of L-type voltage-gated calcium channels in vascular smooth muscle and N-type calcium channels in sympathetic nerve terminals that supply blood vessels. Its reno-, neuro-, and cardioprotective effects have been demonstrated in clinical practice and in animal studies. In a study conducted in 2920 hypertensive patients, cilnidipine plus an angiotensin receptor blocker reduced heart rate significantly, particularly in patients with baseline heart rate greater than 75 beats per minute. In another study, cilnidipine relaxed arteries through calcium-channel antagonism and increased NO production by enhancing endothelial NOS in the human internal thoracic artery.[60]

Efonidipine

Efonidipine blocks both L- and T-type calcium channels. In isolated animal myocardial and vascular models, efonidipine exerted potent negative chronotropic and vasodilator effects but only a weak negative inotropic effect. In both animal models and patients, reduction of blood pressure was accompanied by no or minimum reflex tachycardia. The result was improved myocardial oxygen balance and maintenance of cardiac output. Thus, efonidipine, an L- and T-type dual CCB, appears to be promising as an antihypertensive and antianginal drug with organ-protective effects in the heart and kidney.[61]

Angiotensin Converting Enzyme Inhibitors, Angiotensin Receptor Blockers

Introduction

Whereas neither angiotensin converting enzyme (ACE) inhibitors nor angiotensin receptor blockers (ARBs) are usually regarded as antianginal drugs per se, they are included here because their antiarteriosclerotic, antiatherogenic, and vasodilator actions would clearly impact directly the severity and frequency of angina attacks.

ACE inhibitors are effective in reducing coronary events in high-risk patients and are recommended for consideration in patients with hypertension, diabetes, chronic kidney disease (CKD), and after myocardial ischemia. They have been proven to prevent and improve both ischemic HF and progression of CKD. When combined with thiazide diuretics, ACE inhibitors reduce the incidence of recurrent stroke.[62]

Pharmacology and Pharmacodynamics

Endothelial cells are major mediators of the multistage process of atherosclerosis, and local angiotensin II and bradykinin levels are crucial to the functioning of these cells. ACE converts the hormone angiotensin I to the active vasoconstrictor angiotensin II and also accelerates the metabolic degradation of bradykinin. Four angiotensin II receptors have been identified, AT_{1-4}. AT_1 receptors mediate vasoconstriction, aldosterone synthesis and secretion, cardiac hypertrophy, and vascular smooth muscle proliferation. The AT_2 receptor subtype is less well characterized, but there is evidence for its role in fetal tissue development, inhibition of cell differentiation, apoptosis, and possibly vasodilatation. AT_3 and AT_4 receptors are even less well characterized, but do not appear to affect vascular caliber, and in any case have as a ligand angiotensin IV, a metabolite of angiotensin II, and not angiotensin II itself.

Over 90% of ACE is found in tissue, only 10% in soluble form in plasma. Overexpression of tissue ACE in CAD disrupts the angiotensin II/bradykinin balance resulting in endothelial dysfunction. ACE inhibitors reduce the production of angiotensin II, which prevents vasoconstriction, reduces adhesion molecules and growth factors, decreases oxidative stress, and prevents apoptosis. A concomitant decrease in the degradation of bradykinin as a result of ACE inhibition contributes to vasodilation and an antiapoptotic action.

Classic Clinical Trials of ACE Inhibitors in Stable Coronary Artery Disease

ACE inhibitors are not considered to be primary therapy for angina; they do not immediately reduce the frequency or severity of angina attacks. However, several clinical studies have established ACE inhibitors, ARBs, and, in ischemic HF, aldosterone antagonists, as essential adjunctive therapy in many patients with coronary artery disease and angina. Their mode of action is to reduce the adverse impact of angiotensin II or aldosterone on the heart and vasculature, resulting in improved cardiovascular outcomes.

In the Heart Outcomes Prevention Evaluation (HOPE) study, which included 80% of subjects with a history of HF, and one-third with diabetes, treatment with ramipril versus placebo produced a 22% reduction in the composite endpoint of cardiovascular death, myocardial ischemia, and stroke in the ramipril-treated cohort. There was also a significant reduction in worsening angina (23.8% vs. 26.2%, risk ratio 0.89, 95% CI 0.82–0.96, $p < 0.004$).[10] In the EUROPA trial, 12,218 patients were randomized to the ACE inhibitor perindopril or placebo. Treatment with perindopril (target dose, 8 mg daily) was associated with a 20% relative risk reduction in the composite endpoint of cardiovascular death, myocardial ischemia, or cardiac arrest ($p < 0.003$).[11]

The QUinapril Ischemic Event Trial (QUIET) tested the hypothesis that quinapril 20 mg daily would reduce ischemic events (cardiac death, resuscitated cardiac arrest, nonfatal myocardial ischemia, coronary artery bypass grafting, coronary angioplasty, or hospitalization for angina pectoris) and angiographic progression of HF in patients without systolic left ventricular dysfunction. A similar (38%) incidence of ischemic events occurred in the quinapril and placebo groups.[63] Patients in the Prevention of Events with Angiotensin Converting Enzyme inhibition (PEACE) trial had stable CAD, angina (70% of the subjects), and normal or slightly reduced left ventricular function and were randomized to trandolapril or placebo. No difference between the groups was found in the incidence of the primary composite endpoint of cardiovascular death, myocardial ischemia, or coronary artery revascularization. The investigators concluded that ACE inhibitors might not be necessary as routine therapy in patients with low-risk ischemic heart disease with preserved left ventricular function, especially those who have received intensive treatment with revascularization and lipid-lowering agents.[64]

Thus, two large studies in high-cardiovascular-risk patients (HOPE and EUROPA) showed cardiovascular protective effects by ACE inhibitors, and two studies in lower-cardiovascular-risk patients (QUIET and PEACE) did not. In a 2009 meta-analysis of ACE inhibition versus angiotensin receptor blockade, Baker et al[65] reviewed nine trials and concluded that adding an ACE inhibitor to a standard regimen in patients with ischemic heart disease and preserved left ventricular function reduced total mortality and nonfatal myocardial ischemia at the expense of slightly increased syncope and cough. All but two ACE inhibitor trials found significantly fewer recurrent cardiac events using various agents. Most trials included few women (11–43%) and elderly patients (mean age 57 to 67 years). Whether the benefit associated with ACE inhibitors was a class effect was not clear. Despite these trial limitations, wider use of ACE inhibitors was supported in patients with ischemic heart disease and preserved left ventricular function.

One suggested mechanism for the beneficial action on cardiovascular outcomes of ACE inhibitors in patients with stable CAD and angina is blood pressure reduction. However, the reduction of blood pressure was quite modest in HOPE (3/2 mm Hg) and EUROPA (5/2 mm Hg). There is now some evidence from a EUROPA substudy for an alternative mode of action of ACE inhibitors. Serum from HF patients was found to significantly downregulate eNOS protein expression and activity significantly versus that of healthy controls ($p < 0.01$), most probably as a result of upregulation of tissue ACE. One year of treatment with perindopril upregulated eNOS protein expression and activity. In addition, von Willebrand factor, endothelial apoptosis, tissue angiotensin II, and tumor necrosis factor were all elevated in patients with HF and reversed by perindopril.[66] Thus, perindopril normalizes the angiotensin II/bradykinin balance, reduces inflammation, and prevents endothelial apoptosis. We do not know whether this activity is unique to perindopril or is a class effect of ACE inhibitors, and whether this is unique to patients with ischemic HF, or generalizable to all patients with CAD and stable angina.

Yet no study sought to assess whether or not an ACE inhibitor lessened the frequency and severity of angina as a primary outcome, until The Quinapril Anti-ischemia and Symptoms of Angina Reduction (QUASAR) trial,[67] a double-blind, randomized, placebo-controlled, parallel-group study. Subjects ($n = 336$), with stable angina but no left ventricular dysfunction or recent MI, were randomized to receive quinapril or placebo for a total of 16 weeks. Exercise-induced electrocardiographic changes, the Seattle Angina Questionnaire, and ambulatory ECG monitoring were the measured variables. There were no differences between the subjects treated with quinapril versus placebo in the time to induce a 1-mm ST-segment depression during an exercise treadmill test, in the mean value for the five scores of the Seattle Angina Questionnaire, or in the number of ischemic episodes seen on the ambulatory ECG.

Thus, ACE inhibitors should not be regarded as primary therapy for angina per se. However, there is abundant evidence to support their use to reduce adverse cardiovascular outcomes in patients with ischemic heart disease, particularly if the patients have hypertension, left ventricular dysfunction, or HF, have had a prior MI, or have diabetes or CKD.

Angiotensin Receptor Blockers in Stable Coronary Artery Disease

Several ARBs have been shown to reduce the incidence or severity of ischemic heart disease events, progression of renal disease in type 2 diabetes mellitus, and cerebrovascular events. ARBs are often considered to be an alternative therapy in individuals with cardiovascular disease who are intolerant of ACE inhibitors.

The Ongoing Telmisartan Alone and In Combination with Ramipril Global Endpoint Trial (ONTARGET) randomized 25,620 patients with vascular disease or high-risk diabetes (of whom 74% had a history of CAD) to the ACE inhibitor ramipril (10 mg/d), the ARB telmisartan (80 mg/d), or a combination of these two drugs. Although not the prespecified primary or secondary outcome, the authors recorded worsening or new angina. There was no difference between ramipril, telmisartan, and the combination in the incidence of this outcome measure.[68]

In the Telmisartan Randomised Assessment Study in ACE Intolerant Subjects with Cardiovascular Disease (TRANSCEND), patients with cardiovascular disease or diabetes with end-organ damage were randomized to telmisartan (80 mg daily) or placebo. HF patients were excluded from TRANSCEND. The composite of cardiovascular death, nonfatal myocardial ischemia, and stroke occurred in 13% of patients on telmisartan versus 14.8% of the placebo group ($p = 0.048$), and fewer patients in the telmisartan group had a cardiovascular hospitalization (30.3% vs 33%; $p = 0.025$). The investigators concluded that telmisartan exerted modest benefits on the composite endpoint of cardiovascular death, myocardial ischemia, and stroke.[69]

In the "Valsartan" in Acute Myocardial Infarction Trial (VALIANT), the ARB valsartan had effects similar to those of the ACE inhibitor captopril in reducing cardiovascular event endpoints. The combination of the ARB with the ACE inhibitor yielded an increase in adverse events with no incremental benefit for cardiovascular events.[70] Valsartan Antihypertensive Long-term Use Evaluation (VALUE) was a study of patients with hypertension and high cardiovascular risk. The rate of a composite outcome that included myocardial ischemia and HF in patients treated with valsartan was similar to that observed for the CCB amlodipine[71] However, there were important differences in blood pressure control in the early stages of the VALUE trial (a significant blood pressure difference in favor of amlodipine) that may have confounded outcomes for myocardial ischemia and especially stroke.[72]

There have also been some ARB trials with negative results. In one, the OPtimal Trial In Myocardial infarction with the Angiotensin II Antagonist Losartan (OPTIMAAL), beneficial cardiovascular outcomes were not shown.[73] The lack of benefit in patients with complicated MI may have been attributable to inadequate doses of losartan.

Though ARBs can be substituted in patients intolerant to ACE inhibitors, more studies of ARBs in patients with ischemic heart disease are needed.

Guideline Recommendations for ACE Inhibitors and ARBs

The most recent guidelines for the management of patients with chronic stable angina have the following recommendations for the role of ACE inhibitors and ARBs in patients with chronic stable angina:[73]

class I:

1. ACE inhibitors should be prescribed in all patients with stable ischemic heart disease who also have hypertension, diabetes mellitus, left ventricular ejection fraction 40% or less, or CKD, unless contraindicated. (Level of Evidence: A)
2. ARBs are recommended for patients with SIHD who have hypertension, diabetes mellitus, LV systolic dysfunction, or CKD and have indications for, but are intolerant of, ACE inhibitors. (Level of Evidence: A)

class IIa:

1. Treatment with an ACE inhibitor is reasonable in patients with both SIHD and other vascular disease. (Level of Evidence: B)
2. It is reasonable to use ARBs in other patients who are ACE inhibitor intolerant. (Level of Evidence: C)

NOVEL ANTI-ISCHEMIC THERAPY

Ranolazine

Mechanism of Action

Ranolazine is an effective antianginal and anti-ischemic drug that improves left ventricular diastolic function without altering global hemodynamics.[74] Early studies focused on the inhibitory properties of ranolazine with respect to fatty acid oxidation, which occurs under resting nonischemic conditions. By shifting adenosine triphosphate (ATP) production away from fatty acid oxidation ("partial fatty acid oxidation") toward carbohydrate oxidation, ranolazine reduces myocardial oxygen demand without impeding cardiac function.[75]

More recent studies question whether a clinical benefit of ranolazine is the ability to inhibit fatty acid oxidation, and offer alternative explanations for its efficacy.[76] Researchers report that cardiac function improves in the presence of less than or equal to 20 μM/L ranolazine, whereas inhibition of fatty acid oxidation requires higher drug concentrations (12% inhibition at 100 μM/L). It is now believed that the anti-ischemic action of ranolazine is mediated by the inhibition of the late inward sodium current (INa^+) across cardiac myocyte membranes, resulting in reduced intracellular Ca^{2+} overload.

Rapid activation of membrane sodium channels causes cardiac myocyte depolarization, leading to temporary intracellular accumulation of sodium (Fig. 20.2). Myocardial contraction follows the release of calcium ions (Ca^{2+}) from the sarcoplasmic reticulum, which induces binding of actin and myosin. Ranolazine acts on late INa^+ channels. In normal resting myocytes, where the contribution of late inward sodium current is minimal, ranolazine exerts little effect.[77,78] Late INa^+ channels are overexpressed in the presence of hypoxic conditions caused by ischemia. The drug improves regional left ventricular diastolic dysfunction and segmental ischemia by inhibiting intracellular Ca^{2+} overload. Pathological states such as myocardial ischemia, left ventricular hypertrophy, and HF can cause cellular injury due to excessive cytosolic Ca^{2+}. Ca^{2+} overload of myocardial cells increases arrhythmia risk and generates higher diastolic intramyocardial tension, consuming excessive oxygen. Higher diastolic forces compress blood vessels, reducing blood flow and oxygen delivery to the myocardium.[79]

The effects of ranolazine appear to occur regionally at ischemic myocardial segments rather than over the entire myocardium. Disrupting the "ischemic cascade," which begins with regional diastolic dysfunction, ranolazine reduces oxygen consumption in ischemic cells, exercise-induced ST-segment depression, and angina. Through this disruption of the ischemic cascade, ranolazine normalizes diastolic muscle relaxation and preserves myocardial oxygen balance and blood perfusion.

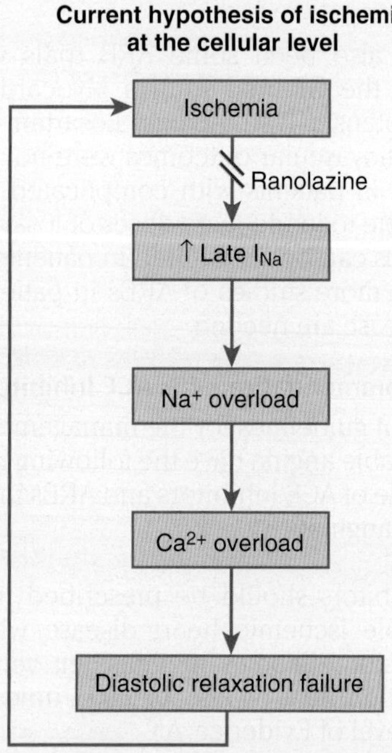

FIG. 20.2 Mechanism of action of ranolazine. Current hypothesis of some of the effects of myocardial ischemia. An enhanced late sodium current causes intracellular Na^+ overload, which increases intracellular calcium through the Na^+/Ca^{2+} exchanger. Cellular calcium overload causes an increase in the left ventricular diastolic tension. Myocardial contractile work, oxygen consumption, and compression of the vascular space during diastole may become abnormally elevated, exacerbating ischemia. Ranolazine inhibits the late INa^+ current. *(References: Ju YK, Saint DA, Gage PW. Hypoxia increases persistent sodium current in rat ventricular myocytes.* J Physiol. *1996;497(pt 2):337–347; Murphy E, Perlman M, London RE, Steenbergen C. Amiloride delays the ischemia-induced rise in cytosolic free calcium.* Circ Res. *1991;68:1250–1258.; Jansen MA, van Emous JG, Nederhoff MG, van Echteld CJ. Assessment of myocardial viability by intracellular 23Na magnetic resonance imaging.* Circulation. *2004;110:3457–3464.)*

Pharmacology

The pharmacokinetics of ranolazine are not affected by gender, diabetes mellitus, or congestive HF, and concentrations are not affected by food intake. Peak plasma levels occur 4 to 6 hours after an oral dose with 50% to 55% bioavailability. The drug is cleared by hepatic enzymes CYP3A4 (70–85%) and CYP2D6 (10–15%) and is also a substrate of P-glycoprotein, a widely expressed membrane transporter protein.

Because ranolazine prolongs the QT interval, it is contraindicated in patients with congenital or acquired long-QT syndrome or taking medications such as quinidine, sotalol, and antiarrhythmic agents that prolong the QT interval. An ECG should be obtained at baseline and follow-up to evaluate the drug's effect on QT interval. This appears not to be proarrhythmic; on the contrary, there are some data that ranolazine is antiarrhythmic.

Ranolazine clearance is reduced in renal insufficiency and diabetic patients with renal impairment should be closely monitored. Ranolazine is contraindicated in severe renal failure or moderate-to-severe hepatic impairment.

The most common adverse effects reported were nausea, headache, dizziness and constipation. At very high doses of up to 2000 mg/d, syncope and postural hypotension can occur due to α-adrenergic receptor blockade.

Clinical Drug-Drug Interactions of Importance

Ranolazine carries a risk of drug-drug interactions through cytochrome P450 enzymes. The drug is contraindicated in patients receiving potent CYP3A inhibitors (eg, itraconazole, ketoconazole, HIV protease inhibitors, clarithromycin) or CYP3A inducers (rifampin, rifabutin, rifapentin, phenobarbital, phenytoin, carbamazepine, diltiazem). Paroxetine may raise plasma ranolazine concentrations by a factor of 1.2 because of CYP2D6 inhibition. Ranolazine may nearly double levels of simvastatin because it is a mild inhibitor of CYP3A4 and CYP2D6. Verapamil may raise ranolazine levels up to threefold. Digoxin levels may rise 1.4- to 1.6-fold because of P-glycoprotein competition by ranolazine.

Evidence for Antianginal Efficacy

MARISA

The MARISA (Monotherapy Assessment of Ranolazine in Stable Angina) trial was a double-blind, crossover study of sustained-release ranolazine in three different doses: 500 mg, 1000 mg, or 1500 mg and placebo, each administered twice daily for 1 week in 191 high-risk patients with angina-limited exercise capacity. There was improvement in treadmill exercise duration, time to angina and time to 1 mm ST-segment depression at all doses with greater improvement at higher doses.[80]

CARISA

In the CARISA (Combination Assessment of Ranolazine in Stable Angina) study, 823 subjects were randomized into three groups: ranolazine; another antianginal therapy (atenolol, amlodipine, or diltiazem) in combination with ranolazine; and, placebo. After 12 weeks, the mean increase in exercise duration at trough was significantly greater for subjects treated with ranolazine than for subjects treated with placebo. Time to angina and ischemia (1 mm ST-depression) increased. A significant reduction in the frequency of anginal episodes and the use of sublingual nitrates was also observed.[81]

MERLIN

In a sub-study of patients with non-ST elevation acute coronary syndromes, and prior chronic angina, from the MERLIN-TIMI 36 (Metabolic Efficiency with Ranolazine for Less Ischemia in Non-ST-Elevation Acute Coronary Syndromes) trial, ranolazine was reported to reduce worsening angina (HR 0.77), the need for new antianginal therapy (HR 0.77), recurrent ischemia, and improvement in exercise duration during a standard exercise tolerance test, using the Bruce protocol. However, ranolazine was not effective in reducing the rate of the composite of cardiovascular death and MI. Thus, the MERLIN trial did not support the use of ranolazine in acute coronary syndrome, but added to previous safety data and provided additional support for ranolazine as antianginal therapy in chronic angina.[82]

ERICA

In ERICA (Efficacy of Ranolazine in Chronic Angina), a randomized, placebo-controlled trial, investigators enrolled 565 patients with stable CAD and recurring angina attacks (< three attacks in 1 week) being treated with amlodipine at a dose of 10 mg daily, with or without long-acting nitrates. Ranolazine was administered at a dose of 500 mg twice daily for 1 week, then titrated to 1000 mg twice daily for 6 weeks. For subjects in the ranolazine group, researchers reported a significant reduction in angina attacks, no meaningful changes in blood pressure or heart rate, and good tolerability, without syncope.[83]

TERISA

TERISA (Type 2 Diabetes Evaluation in Subjects with Chronic Stable Angina) assessed the efficacy of ranolazine on angina frequency and sublingual nitroglycerin use in 949 patients with type 2 diabetes, CAD, and chronic stable angina despite treatment. TERISA was an 8-week randomized, placebo-controlled trial. Over the final 6 weeks, the number of angina episodes in 1 week was significantly lower in patients on ranolazine than in patients receiving placebo, and there was no difference in the incidence of serious adverse effects between the ranolazine and placebo groups.[84]

RWISE

In contrast to the results of the trials mentioned previously, results from the Treatment With Ranolazine in Microvascular Coronary Dysfunction: Impact on Angina Myocardial Ischemia (RWISE) trial showed that ranolazine was not effective for angina associated with myocardial microvascular dysfunction. This was a study of oral ranolazine 500 to 1000 mg twice daily for 2 weeks versus placebo, and angina measured by the Seattle Angina Questionnaire (SAQ) and SAQ-7 (coprimaries), diary angina (secondary), stress myocardial perfusion reserve index, diastolic filling, and quality of life. Of 128 subjects (96% women), no treatment differences in outcomes were observed, except that ranolazine was associated with a decrease in stress heart rate.[85]

Conclusion

Clinical trial results show that ranolazine improves exercise stress test parameters (total duration, time to angina, and time to ST-segment depression) and reduces angina episodes and nitrate use among patients with chronic stable angina due to CAD. Ranolazine is effective as monotherapy and also when added to traditional antianginal pharmacotherapies as part of usual care for chronic stable angina. The drug appears to have a favorable safety profile, making it an attractive alternative for patients who cannot tolerate β-blockers or CCBs. Available data suggest that ranolazine should be considered for patients who experience persistent anginal symptoms despite use of traditional antianginal drugs.

Ivabradine

Introduction

Ivabradine, the first member of a group of specific heart rate lowering agents, was approved by the European Medicines Agency in 2005 for symptomatic stable angina and in 2012 for chronic HF in patients with an elevated heart rate.[85] Ivabradine was approved by the US Food and Drug Administration (FDA) in 2015 to reduce the risk of hospitalization for worsening HF in patients with stable, symptomatic, chronic HF. Ivabradine use is restricted to patients with LVEF of less than 35% who are in sinus rhythm with a resting heart rate of greater than 70 beats per minute and are either not receiving a β-blocker due to a contraindication or receiving maximally tolerated doses of a β-blocker.

Heart rate reduction is a recognized strategy for preventing myocardial ischemia and angina pectoris in patients with stable CAD. An elevated heart rate raises the mechanical load on the arterial wall and is associated with endothelial dysfunction and increased arterial stiffness. These consequences of an elevated heart rate may be atherogenic.[86] Lowering the heart rate confers numerous physiologic and pathophysiologic benefits. Among these are reduced myocardial oxygen demand through a reduction in cardiac workload and a rise in myocardial oxygen supply owing to diastolic prolongation[87,88] (Fig. 20.3).

Pharmacological Actions

Heart Rate Reduction

Ivabradine blocks trans-membrane f-channels and disrupts I_f ion current flow. This blockade and disruption prolong diastolic depolarization and slow sinoatrial node firing, which in turn lowers the heart rate in a dose-dependent manner. In patients with stable angina, ivabradine at doses of 2.5 mg,

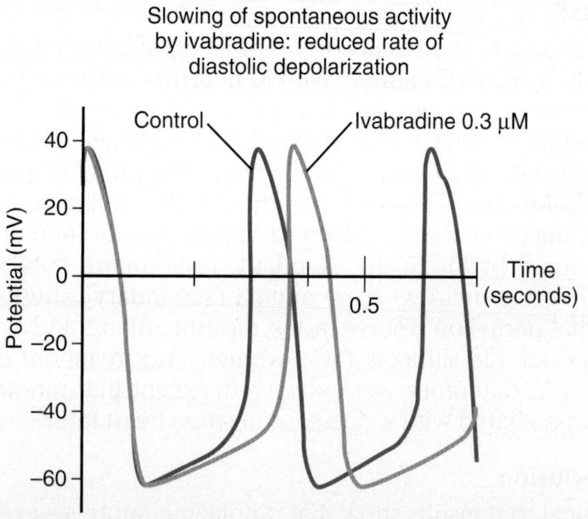

FIG. 20.3 Action of ivabradine on the sinoatrial node. Slowing of the spontaneous activity of the sinoatrial node by ivabradine. The I_f current is an inward Na^+/K^+ current that activates pacemaker cells of the sinoatrial node. Ivabradine selectively inhibits the hyperpolarization-activated, mixed Na^+/K^+ inward I_f current, which decreases rest and exercise heart rate and responsiveness. *(Modified from Nawarskas JJ, et al. Ivabradine: a unique and intriguing medication for treating cardiovascular disease.* Cardiol Rev. *2015;23:4:201–211.Fig. 3.)*

5 mg, and 10 mg twice daily reduced resting heart rate by approximately 7, 12, and 18 beats per minute, respectively. The specificity of ivabradine for the I_f current ensures that the drug exerts no direct effect on myocardial contractility, ventricular repolarization, or intracardiac conduction (Fig. 20.3).[87]

Improved Endothelial Function and Vascular Compliance

Ivabradine has been shown to reduce oxidative stress, protect and improve endothelial function, reduce atherosclerotic plaque formation, and preserve aortic compliance in mice. No functional interactions with calcium channels or intracellular mechanisms that regulate the reactivity of smooth muscle cells were observed. Hence, the beneficial effects on endothelial function occurred without altering muscle cell contractility. One clinical trial demonstrated significant improvement in left ventricular function and aortic elasticity in patients with reduced left ventricular ejection fraction.[88]

Efficacy of Ivabradine in the Therapy of Angina

The ASSOCIATE (evaluation of the antianginal efficacy and safety of the association of the I_f current inhibitor ivabradine with a β-blocker) study[89] verified the safety and efficacy of concomitantly administered β-blocker and ivabradine in patients with stable angina. Ivabradine significantly reduced resting and exercise HR, with improvement in exercise capacity (total exercise duration, time to limiting angina, angina onset, and 1 mm ST-segment depression, all with $p < 0.05$).

Similar results were reported in REDUCTION (reduction of heart rate in the treatment of stable angina with ivabradine); there were fewer angina episodes on ivabradine in patients older than 80 years.[86]

ADDITIONS (practical daily efficacy and safety of Procoralan in combination with β-blockers) was a 4-month evaluation of ivabradine studied in patients with stable angina on background β-blocker therapy. Patients in the ivabradine arm experienced more significant heart rate reductions with fewer anginal episodes per week and used nitrates less frequently. In a *post hoc* subgroup analysis, the benefits of ivabradine were consistent regardless of whether or not patients had received percutaneous intervention.[88]

Long-Term Outcomes

Long-term outcome results have been mixed. In SHIFT (Ivabradine and Outcomes in Chronic Heart Failure) there was a reduction in the risk of cardiovascular death and hospitalization due to worsening HF and improved quality of life in patients with chronic HF.[90]

BEAUTIFUL (morbidity-mortality evaluation of the I_f inhibitor ivabradine in patients with coronary disease and left ventricular dysfunction),[91] while documenting improved left ventricular end-systolic volume index after 12 months, found no improvement in cardiovascular outcomes in patients with left ventricular systolic dysfunction and stable CAD, nor in the primary composite outcome (cardiovascular death or admission for new-onset or worsening HF). In regard to adverse effects, the BEAUTIFUL Holter substudy showed that ivabradine did not have any significant adverse rhythm effects. In addition, in SIGNIFY (Study Assessing the Morbidity-Mortality Benefits of the I_f Inhibitor Ivabradine in Patients with Coronary Artery Disease),[92] ivabradine not only failed to significantly decrease the primary endpoint (composite of death from cardiovascular causes or nonfatal MI), but was associated with symptomatic and asymptomatic bradycardia and an increased incidence of AF.

Adverse Effects

Phosphenes, bradycardia, and AF are the primary adverse effects of ivabradine, phosphenes being the most common. A phosphene is a transient enhanced brightness in a limited area of the visual field. The brightness is triggered by a sudden change in light intensity. The onset usually occurs in the first 2 months of ivabradine treatment. Phosphenes are mild, transient, and do not affect the patient's ability to carry out normal activities. Other common adverse effects are headache, uncontrolled blood pressure, dizziness, ventricular extrasystoles, and first-degree AV block.[88]

Conclusion

Clinical trials have demonstrated the efficacy of ivabradine in angina, both alone and in combination with a β-blocker. Reduction in major adverse cardiovascular events has not been consistently demonstrated. There are also some significant side effects, particularly bradycardia, AF, and ocular phosphenes. Thus, ivabradine, although approved by the FDA to reduce the risk of hospitalization for worsening HF in patients with stable, symptomatic, chronic HF with reduced ejection fraction (< 35%), and in sinus rhythm, it has not been approved for the indication of angina.

The European Medicines Agency has approved ivabradine for chronic HF with systolic dysfunction, but also for the symptomatic treatment of chronic stable angina pectoris in CAD in adults with normal sinus rhythm and heart rate greater than or equal to 70 bpm, and who are unable to tolerate or with a contraindication to the use of β-blockers, or in combination with β-blockers in patients inadequately controlled with an optimal β-blocker dose.

The exact therapeutic niche of ivabradine is unclear. It remains to be determined which populations would most benefit from the drug and what the best combination with other antianginal agents would be.

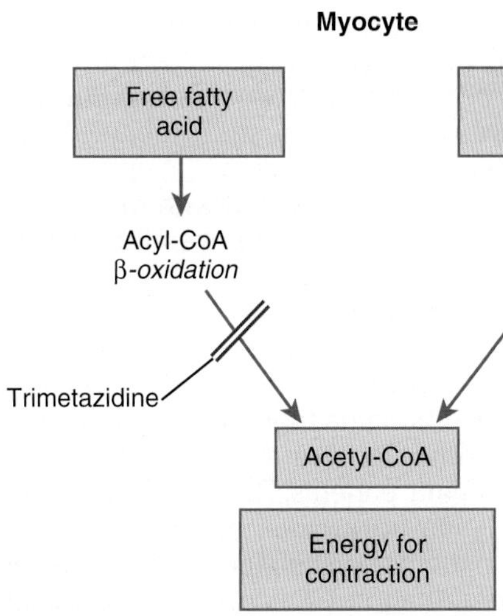

FIG. 20.4 Postulated mechanism of action of trimetazidine. Myocardial cells derive their energy via fatty acid and glucose metabolism. During ischemia the fatty acid pathway predominates. However, this pathway requires more oxygen than the glucose pathway. Theoretically, inhibition of fatty acid oxidation should promote a shift toward the more oxygen-efficient glucose pathway. A number of groups have reported experimental data showing that the antianginal trimetazidine is an inhibitor of partial fatty acid oxidation (pFOX). However, other investigators have not observed any inhibition with trimetazidine in other experimental models. Thus, inhibition of fatty acid oxidation as a major antianginal mechanism for trimetazidine remains to be definitively established. *(References: MacInnes A, Fairman DA, Binding P, et al. The antianginal agent trimetazidine does not exert its functional benefit via inhibition of mitochondrial long-chain 3-ketoacyl coenzyme A thiolase.* Circ Res. *2003;93:e26–e32; Lopaschuk GD, Barr R, Thomas PD, et al. Beneficial effects of trimetazidine in ex vivo working ischemic hearts are due to a stimulation of glucose oxidation secondary to inhibition of long-chain 3-ketoacyl coenzyme a thiolase.* Circ Res. *2003;93:e33–e37; Stanley WC. Myocardial energy metabolism during ischemia and the mechanisms of metabolic therapies.* J Cardiovasc Pharmacol Ther. *2004;9(suppl 1):S31–S45; Chaitman BR, Sano J. Novel therapeutic approaches to treating chronic angina in the setting of chronic ischemic heart disease.* Clin Cardiol. *2007;30(2 suppl 1):I25–I30.)*

Trimetazidine

Introduction

Trimetazidine (1-2,3,4-trimethoxybenzyl piperazine dihydrochloride), a member of the class of 3-ketoacyl coenzyme A thiolase (3-KAT) inhibitors, is a metabolic modulator that improves myocardial energetics at several levels. The drug inhibits β-oxidation of fatty acids; increases myocardial glucose utilization; prevents reduction in ATP and phosphocreatine levels in response to hypoxia or ischemia; preserves ionic pump function; minimizes free radical production; and protects against intracellular calcium overload and acidosis. Angina resulting from myocardial ischemia is associated with enhanced catecholamine release and increased lipolysis. This condition is also associated with an increase in circulating fatty acid levels, a relative increase in fatty acid oxidation (FAO), and therefore (through the "Randle cycle"), a reduced glucose oxidation (GO) rate (Fig. 20.4).[15]

Pharmacologic Actions

In patients with chronic angina, trimetazidine increases work capacity and delays the appearance of symptoms and electrocardiographic changes during exercise. Due to its absence of effect on heart rate and blood pressure, trimetazidine is a potentially useful agent for combination therapy with classic "hemodynamic" drugs for chronic treatment of angina pectoris. It can be added to standard antianginal therapy in patients who are refractory or intolerant to other drugs and are not suitable for revascularization. The addition of trimetazidine in patients receiving nifedipine or propranolol significantly improved the clinical status and reduced the number of ischemic episodes. These clinical effects were associated with prolongation of the exercise time and a delay in the appearance of ischemic symptoms and diagnostic ST-segment changes.[93]

Though trimetazidine has been approved for stable angina in many countries, the drug is not approved for use in the United States.

Efficacy of Trimetazidine for Angina

Several clinical trials have demonstrated potential benefits of trimetazidine in ischemic heart disease. In a multicenter, randomized, double-blind study of patients with chronic effort-induced angina and documented CAD, the combination of trimetazidine with propranolol was superior to the combination of nitrates with propranolol with regard to the number of ischemic attacks, exercise time, and time to onset of angina, and increased the maximum workload at peak exercise.[13]

Trimetazidine was compared to nifedipine in a double-blind study. Both drugs decreased the number of angina attacks and increased workload parameters without any significant difference between them. However, at a constant level of work, the rate-pressure product decreased with nifedipine but remained stable with trimetazidine.[15]

In other studies, results have been mixed. In several meta-analyses, trimetazidine was associated with a significant reduction in weekly angina episodes, and duration of exercise, and improved exercise time to 1 mm ST-segment depression compared with placebo.[15] However, in another meta-analysis of 23 randomized trials, trimetazidine was no more effective than other antianginal drugs in improving time to ST-segment depression or reducing weekly angina frequency, and no clear reduction in mortality or cardiovascular events was evident.[94]

Adverse Effects

Trimetazidine has a significant side effects profile, with the most common adverse reactions being nausea, vomiting, fatigue, dizziness, and myalgia. The drug can induce or increase parkinsonian symptoms: extrapyramidal rigidity, bradykinesia, and tremor. The mechanism responsible for these reactions is not known, but the presence of a piperazine nucleus in trimetazadine leads to the suggestion that a blockade of central D_2 dopamine receptors is involved.[95]

Conclusion

Trimetazidine may be beneficial in refractory angina, acute coronary syndrome, HF, and hypertrophic cardiomyopathy. However, trimetazidine lacks both widespread clinical experience and any guideline recommendation for the management of chronic stable angina. The European Medicines Agency limited the indication for trimetazadine to add-on therapy for patients inadequately controlled by first-line medications, and the drug has not been approved by the FDA for use in the United States.

Nicorandil

Introduction

Nicorandil (*N*-[2-(nitro-oxy) ethyl]-3-pyridine carboxamide) is a nicotinamide derivative coupled with a nitrate moiety. It functions as an NO donor and opens adenosine triphosphate-dependent potassium (KATP) channels.[96]

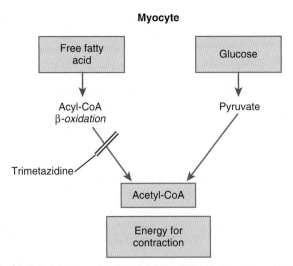

Mechanism of Action

Nitrate-Like Properties

Nicorandil prevents myocardial ischemia and angina symptoms through vasorelaxant effects on systemic and coronary vasculature. The nitrate component of the molecule reduces preload by acting on systemic venous vessels and dilates epicardial coronary arteries. Activation of soluble guanylyl cyclase increases cyclic guanosine monophosphate (cGMP) and activates protein kinase G, which lowers intracellular calcium and inhibits myosin light-chain kinase activity. These reactions result in vascular smooth muscle cell relaxation and vasodilatation. In patients with CAD, nicorandil dilates coronary arteries an average of 10% to 20%, primarily due to its nitrate component (Fig. 20.5).[96]

Nicotinamide Properties

Nicorandil, via its nicotinamide component, opens KATP channels and activates endothelial NOS, which improves endothelial function and provides cardioprotective effects.[97] Fibrinolysis is mediated by a balance between type I plasminogen activator (PAI-1) and tissue type plasminogen activator (tPA). Nicorandil may inhibit PAI-1, increasing endogenous fibrinolytic activity. Opening KATP channels in histiocytes increases intracellular Ca^{2+}, which upregulates PAI-1 synthesis. Nicorandil may also stabilize PAI-1 in platelet α-granules.[98]

Efficacy of Nicorandil in Stable Angina

Numerous clinical trials have evaluated nicorandil for symptomatic effort-induced angina. Nicorandil has been found to be similarly effective as conventional antianginal drugs. Nicorandil has equivalent side effects to other antiangina medications with no development of tolerance.

Two significant trials of nicorandil were the Study of Nicorandil in Angina Pectoris in the Elderly (SNAPE)[97] and the Symptomatic Stable Angina Pectoris (SWAN)[99] study. Both compared the anti-ischemic and antianginal effects of nicorandil and amlodipine in patients with stable angina. After 4 weeks of treatment, SNAPE reported similar results for nicorandil and amlodipine in increasing time to ischemia and time to angina and decreasing maximum ST-segment depression on a symptom-limited bicycle exercise test. In SWAN, the medications conferred similar time to symptom and total exercise duration.

The cardioprotective effects of nicorandil were evaluated in the Impact of Nicorandil in Angina (IONA)[100] and the Japanese Coronary Artery Disease (JCAD)[101] studies.

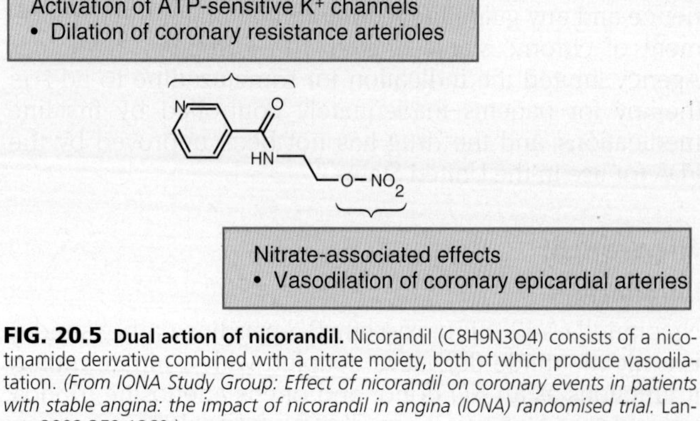

FIG. 20.5 Dual action of nicorandil. Nicorandil (C8H9N3O4) consists of a nicotinamide derivative combined with a nitrate moiety, both of which produce vasodilatation. *(From IONA Study Group: Effect of nicorandil on coronary events in patients with stable angina: the impact of nicorandil in angina (IONA) randomised trial.* Lancet. *2002;359:1269.)*

In IONA, patients with stable angina received nicorandil (20 mg daily) and had a significant reduction in cardiac events. The Japanese Coronary Artery Disease Study, a multicenter, prospective observational study, included patients with ischemic heart disease and significant epicardial coronary artery stenosis. They were treated with nicorandil over a 2.7-year period. A 35% reduction in overall mortality and 56% reduction in cardiac death were observed in nicorandil-treated patients versus controls.

In the Clinical European Studies in Angina and Revascularization (CESAR 2), nicorandil administered along with standard antiangina therapy showed a reduction in nonsustained ventricular and supraventricular arrhythmias in unstable angina patients. Rates of acute coronary syndromes and all cardiovascular events were lower in nicorandil-treated patients versus placebo controls. On the other hand, the combination of nicorandil and isosorbide dinitrate in patients with ischemic heart disease resulted in significantly worse flow-mediated dilatation (a marker of endothelial function) and carotid intima-medial thickness at 3 months.[102]

Nicorandil does not cause tachyphylaxis, impair endothelial function, or exacerbate angina. Its dual mode of action prevents the development of tolerance, and there is no rebound response to abrupt discontinuation of the drug.[96]

Nicorandil should be prescribed with caution in patients taking corticosteroids due to a small risk of gastrointestinal perforation, as this drug is primarily metabolized in the gastrointestinal tract. Sulfonylureas may antagonize the effects of nicorandil though closure of KATP channels.[96]

Conclusion

The European Society of Cardiology (ESC) guidelines[103] state "For second-line treatment it is recommended to add long-acting nitrates or ivabradine or nicorandil or ranolazine, according to heart rate, blood pressure and tolerance. (Class IIa, Level of Evidence B)" and may be considered in patients with microvascular angina with refractory symptoms (IIb/B). The National Institute for Health and Clinical Excellence (NICE) in the UK also recommends nicorandil for these purposes.[104] Nicorandil is EMA- but not FDA-approved.

Molsidomine

Introduction

Molsidomine has been available in Europe since 1977. It has not been approved by the FDA in the United States.

Pharmacological Actions

The mechanism of action of molsidomine is similar to nitrates. Molsidomine is metabolized in the liver to the active metabolite linsidomine, an unstable compound that releases endothelial NO upon decay. Molsidomine exerts a slight platelet antiaggregant effect but is indicated only to prevent angina attacks, not for the symptomatic relief of acute angina.[105,106]

Efficacy of Molsidomine in Angina Therapy

The largest study of molsidomine evaluated 533 patients. These patients received a placebo run-in phase followed by random assignment to two differing doses of molsidomine in a crossover design. Both doses of molsidomine resulted in significantly longer total exercise duration and fewer episodes of angina than placebo. Weekly angina episodes were reduced significantly in patients given either dose of molsidomine compared to angina frequency during the run-in phase.[107]

Though no head-to-head comparison of molsidomine versus nitrates has been performed, molsidomine has a similar hemodynamic profile to long-acting nitrates, with similar positive and negative effects, due to its nearly identical mechanism of action. In another study, molsidomine showed a 40% decline in efficacy after 14 days of use, suggesting the development of tolerance.[107]

Contraindications and Side Effects

As with nitrates, molsidomine should not be prescribed to patients taking type 5 phosphodiesterase inhibitors due to severe hypotension risk. The most common side effects are headache and hypotension. Hypotension risk increases as the dose increases.

INVESTIGATIONAL ANTI-ISCHEMIC THERAPY

Introduction

Newer, investigational, antianginal therapies range from pharmaceuticals to amino acids to hormone therapy. In addition, novel treatments such as chelation therapy, angiogenic growth factors, gene therapies, and cell-based therapies are discussed hereafter. Most have been tested in animal models, and very few in clinical trials, and those that have, have had small numbers included. Therefore, all of these postulated therapies should be regarded as speculative at best.

Allopurinol

Xanthine oxidase is a major source of O_2^- and is abundantly active in the vascular endothelium and plasma of patients with CAD. Its increased arterial activity reduces the availability of vascular NO and increases oxidative stress and endothelial dysfunction. Conversely, inhibition of xanthine oxidase reduces oxidative stress and improves endothelial function and cardiac contractility in patients with CAD. Allopurinol, by inhibiting xanthine oxidase, enhances calcium sensitivity in stunned trabeculae and exerts a positive inotropic effect. High-dose allopurinol was assessed in patients with angiographically documented stable CAD and LVEF less than 45%. The drug significantly prolonged the time to ST depression, total exercise time, and time to occurrence of chest pain. In addition, diastolic blood pressure during exercise dropped significantly, and the maximum tolerated rate-pressure product rose significantly.[108,109]

L-Arginine

L-Arginine, an amino acid, is a substrate of the enzyme eNOS and a key molecule in NO synthesis. L-Arginine theoretically improves coronary blood flow via NO-mediated, endothelium-dependent vasodilatation. Twenty-six patients with chest pain but without substantial CAD were randomly allocated to L-arginine or placebo. After 6 months, the coronary blood flow in response to acetylcholine in the subjects who were taking L-arginine increased compared with the placebo group, with similar improvement in patients' symptom scores in the L-arginine treatment group compared with the placebo group.[110]

However, a potentially lethal effect could occur in the presence of a high degree of eNOS uncoupling or tetrahydrobiopterin deficiency, as tetrahydrobiopterin is a required cofactor for the synthesis of NO by eNOS, the enzyme required for NO synthesis.[111]

L-Arginine has also been shown to modify or prevent the development of nitrate tolerance during continuous transdermal GTN therapy.[30]

Bosentan

Endothelin-1, in endothelial and vascular smooth muscle cells, is a potent vasoconstrictor shown to provoke coronary vasospasm. Bosentan is a competitive antagonist of endothelin-1 at the endothelin-A (ET-A) and endothelin-B (ET-B) receptors. One case report documented the efficacy of bosentan in treating refractory vasospastic angina.[112]

GLP-1 Mimetics and Analogs and DPP-4 Inhibitors

Glucagon-like peptide-1-amide (GLP-1), released from intestinal L cells in a glucose-dependent manner, increases glucose-stimulated pancreatic insulin secretion and myocardial glucose uptake by translocating glucose-transporting vesicles (GLUT-1 and GLUT-4) to the sarcolemma. The dipeptidyl peptidase-4 (DPP-4) enzyme inactivates GLP-1. The DPP-4 inhibitor sitagliptin has improved global and regional left ventricular performance and attenuated postischemic stunning during dobutamine stress ECG. GLP-1 mimetics and analogs and DPP-4 inhibitors represent a new approach for improving myocardial glucose uptake and regional and global left ventricular function.[113]

Mildronate

Mildronate reduces fatty acid oxidation to improve vascular tone. Long-term efficacy was assessed in 317 patients. At 12 months, mildronate improved time to ST-segment deviation, time to onset of angina, and total exercise duration by nearly 1 minute.[114]

Fasudil

Fasudil is used in Japan for treatment of cerebral vasospasm associated with subarachnoid hemorrhage. It inhibits the intracellular signaling enzyme Rho kinase, which is involved in vascular smooth muscle contraction (Fig. 20.6). Fasudil has been shown to dilate acetyl choline-induced coronary vasospasm in patients with vasospastic angina treated with nitroglycerin and to prevent myocardial ischemia in patients with microvascular angina.[115]

Estrogen/Progestogen

One study reported the effect of treatment with estradiol and norethisterone acetate on exercise tolerance and on the frequency and severity of ischemic attacks in postmenopausal women with stable angina pectoris. Estrogen/progestogen increased, and placebo decreased, time to 1 mm ST depression, and total exercise duration was significantly improved.[116]

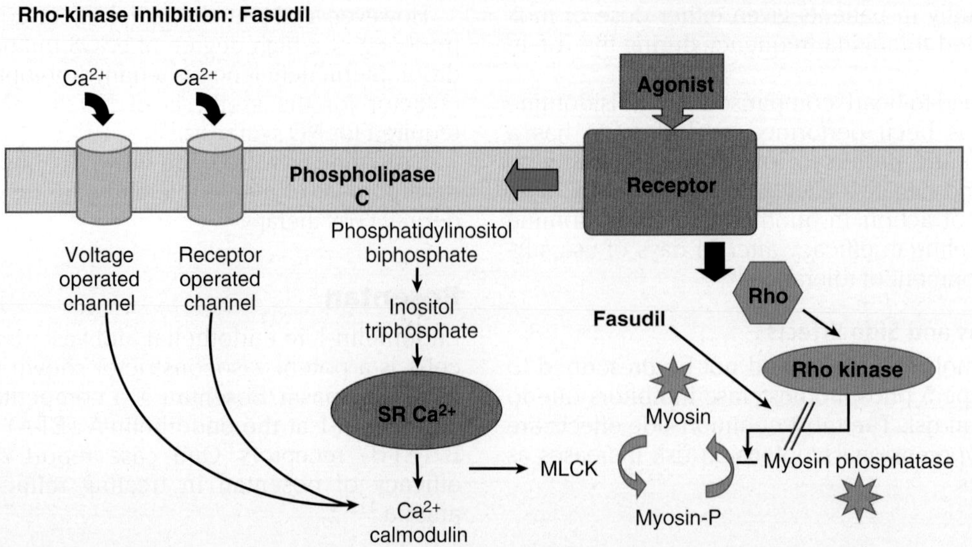

FIG. 20.6 Mechanism of action of fasudil. The role of calcium in activating myosin light chain kinase (MLCK) and phosphorylating myosin to cause contraction is well known. Dephosphorylation by myosin phosphatase causes subsequent dilation.[1] More recently, the involvement of Rho kinase has been identified. In the absence of increases in intracellular calcium, Rho (a member of the Ras superfamily of small G proteins) activates Rho kinase, which in turn deactivates myosin phosphatase. This causes accumulation of phosphorylated myosin. Fasudil inhibits this action, resulting in a decrease of vascular tone. *(From Seasholtz TM. The RHOad less traveled: the myosin phosphorylation-independent path from Rho kinase to cell contraction. Focus on Rho kinase mediates serum-induced contraction in fibroblast fibers independent of myosin LC20 phosphorylation.* Am J Physiol Cell Physiol. *2003;284:c596. Fig. 1.)*

Chelation Therapy

Chelation therapy is the intravenous infusion of disodium ethylene diamine tetraacetic acid (EDTA), with oral vitamins, minerals, electrolytes, and/or heparin. There has been no convincing evidence of improvement in exercise tolerance in patients with stable angina, but one study, the Trial to Assess Chelation Therapy (TACT) reported that, among stable patients with a history of MI, intravenous EDTA; compared with placebo, modestly reduced the risk of adverse cardiovascular outcomes, especially revascularization procedures. The authors concluded that "these results…are not sufficient to support the routine use of chelation therapy for treatment of patients who have had an MI."[117]

Angiogenic Growth Factors, Gene Therapies, and Cell-Based Therapies

Over the past decade, treatments have been sought that rebuild the vascular architecture or collaterals for treatment of refractory angina. These include angiogenic growth factors, gene therapies, and cell-based therapies.

Growth Factors/Gene Therapies

In several trials, vascular endothelial growth factor (VEGF) and fibroblast growth factor (FGF) have been administered either directly as proteins or via an adenovirus vector. None of the trials has been conclusive, though intracoronary administration of growth factors has been deemed safe.[118]

Vascular Endothelial Growth Factor

A high or low dose of recombinant human VEGF was injected into 178 patients with chronic angina, followed by either placebo or intravenous infusions on 3 subsequent days. Clinical angina improved significantly at 90 days.[106,118] After 120 days, patients given the high dose had experienced fewer angina attacks, but no effect on total exercise duration was noted.

Fibroblast Growth Factor 2

In the largest randomized controlled trial of fibroblast growth factor 2 (FGF-2) ($n = 337$), total exercise duration did not improve.[9]

Cell-Based Therapies

Administration of pluripotential stem cells can lead to therapeutic angiogenesis. In response to ischemia, bone marrow derived endothelial progenitor cells migrate and proliferate to form endothelial cells, resulting in neo-revascularization. In an early-phase trial of patients with refractory angina, injection of $CD34^+$ stem cells into the myocardium was associated with decreased frequency of angina attacks and increased total duration of exercise.[107]

COMPARATIVE EFFECTIVENESS OF DRUG CLASSES SINGLY AND IN COMBINATION IN THE TREATMENT OF STABLE ANGINA

Given that β-blockers have an established place in the therapy of stable angina, and given that other drugs (calcium channel blockers, ranolazine, ivabradine, and trimetazidine) also have proven efficacy, the question arises whether combinations of these agents may have greater efficacy than monotherapy in improving the symptoms of stable angina. This section reports the results of clinical trials comparing one agent with another and comparing combination therapy with monotherapy.

β-Blockers and Calcium-Channel Blockers

In a 1999 meta-analysis,[119] there were 31% fewer episodes of angina per week with β-blockers than with calcium antagonists. A more recent meta-analysis by Belsey et al.[120] examined 28 studies of a CCB added to a β-blocker and eight studies of a β-blocker added to a CCB. Results showed the addition of a CCB to a β-blocker produces a 21% reduction in the frequency of angina episodes, and the

21 Antiplatelet and Anticoagulant Drugs

Gregory Ducrocq and Philippe Gabriel Steg

INTRODUCTION

Chronic coronary artery disease (CAD) is a heterogeneous condition that encompasses patients with a history of acute coronary syndrome (ACS), patients with a history of coronary revascularization by percutaneous coronary intervention (PCI) or surgery, patients with stable angina symptoms, patients with silent myocardial ischemia, and asymptomatic patients without myocardial ischemia but with evidence of CAD by imaging. CAD is most often caused by obstructive atherosclerosis, although other mechanisms, such as vasospasm, may contribute. Across those various conditions, the role of anticoagulant and antiplatelet therapy is mainly to minimize the risk of a major adverse cardiac event, such as acute myocardial infarction (MI), stroke, or cardiovascular death, by preventing the occurrence or growth of an arterial thrombus as a consequence of plaque erosion or rupture. Because plaque erosion or rupture is ubiquitous in the coronary vasculature of patients with atherothrombosis,[1] antithrombotic therapies constitute a cornerstone of secondary prevention.

To prevent coronary thrombosis and acute coronary events in patients with chronic CAD, who represent a high-risk group,[2] a wide armamentarium of antithrombotic agents and strategies, ranging from single antiplatelet therapy to dual- or even triple-antithrombotic therapy and various anticoagulant agents, is available today.

With this growing number of options and combinations, the focus has shifted from using ever more potent agents to finding the optimal balance between thrombotic and bleeding risks on an individual level to select the optimal combination, intensity, and duration of treatment for each patient. Finally, CAD patients requiring oral anticoagulant (OAC) therapy for various conditions, such as atrial fibrillation, represent a growing proportion of patients with a specific benefit/risk balance regarding antithrombotic agents.

ANTIPLATELET AGENTS

Platelet-mediated thrombosis is a major pathophysiologic mechanism underlying coronary thrombosis.[3] Platelets adhere to ruptured or eroded plaques, are activated, aggregate, and release secondary messengers, which produce further thrombosis and vasoconstriction and serve as a surface for activation of the clotting cascade (Fig. 21.1). Therefore, inhibition of platelet activation or aggregation is a very effective method of preventing coronary thrombosis. The various existing antiplatelet agents can act at different points in the platelet to inhibit the cascade of platelet activation, amplification, and aggregation (see Fig. 21.1).

Aspirin

Aspirin (acetylsalicylic acid) has long been, and largely remains, the cornerstone of antithrombotic treatment for patients with chronic CAD.

Thromboxane receptors are expressed in platelets, inflammatory cells, the vascular wall, and atherosclerotic plaques.[4] Low doses of aspirin irreversibly block cyclooxygenase-1 (COX-1), the enzyme that promotes the synthesis of thromboxane A_2 from arachidonic acid, by acetylating a serine residue near the narrow catalytic site of the COX-1 channel.[5,6] When doses are increased, aspirin inhibits both COX-1 and COX-2, leading to antiinflammatory and analgesic effects, and it can also inhibit the formation of antiaggregatory prostacyclin. Therefore, low doses of aspirin are generally preferred.

Aspirin is rapidly absorbed in the stomach and upper small intestine. Plasma concentrations peak 30 to 40 minutes after the ingestion of uncoated aspirin. In contrast, after the administration of enteric-coated formulations, it can take up to 3 or 4 hours for plasma concentrations to reach their peak, and thromboxane inhibition can be less complete.[7] Aspirin has a half-life of 15 to 20 minutes in plasma. Despite the rapid clearance of aspirin from the circulation, its antiplatelet effect lasts for the life of a platelet. For its effect to be translated into prevention of thrombosis, inhibition of thromboxane generation needs to be greater than 95%.[8] It has been shown that daily administration of as low a dose as 30 mg of aspirin results in complete suppression of platelet thromboxane A_2 production after 1 week, through a cumulative process of fractional acetylation of unacetylated platelet COX-1 by successive daily doses of aspirin.[9] Therefore, regimens of 75 to 100 mg of aspirin daily usually exceed the minimal effective dose required for a full pharmacodynamic effect, accommodating some degree of interindividual variability in drug response. With a daily generation of approximately 10% of new platelets, near

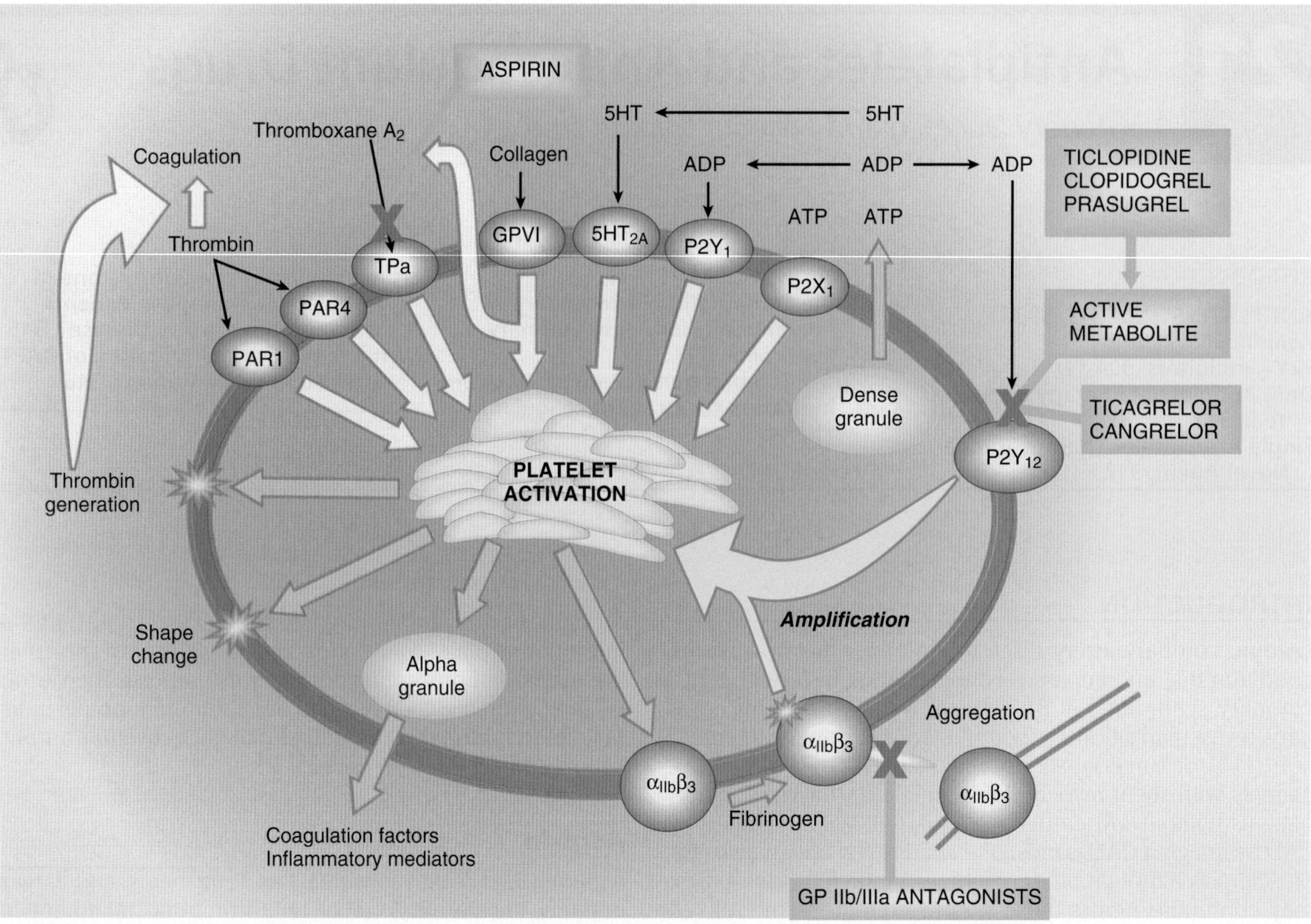

FIG. 21.1 Platelet activation and aggregation inhibitors. *ADP*, Adenosine diphosphate; *ATP*, adenosine triphosphate; *GP*, glycoprotein; *HT*, hydroxytryptamine; *PAR*, protease-activated receptor; *TP*, thromboxane A_2 receptor. *(From Storey RF. Biology and pharmacology of the platelet* $P2Y_{12}$ *receptor.* Curr Pharm Des. *2006;12:1255.)*

normal primary hemostasis can be recovered within 2 to 3 days after the last aspirin dose. A faster rate of platelet turnover has been reported in proinflammatory settings, such as diabetes[10]; this can reduce the aspirin-induced pharmacodynamic effect. In patients with diabetes, twice-daily administration of aspirin has been shown to result in greater platelet inhibition than once-daily administration.[11,12] However, the clinical implications of this observation remain to be demonstrated.

The benefit of aspirin in CAD patients has been documented extensively. A meta-analysis that included 287 studies evaluating antiplatelet agents (aspirin being the most represented), involving 135,000 patients, demonstrated that antiplatelet therapy reduced the combined outcomes of nonfatal MI, nonfatal stroke, and vascular death by one-third (Fig. 21.2A), and vascular mortality by one-sixth (with no apparent adverse effect on other deaths) across a broad group of patients with arterial diseases. In the same meta-analysis, doses of 75 to 150 mg appeared to be as effective as higher doses (Fig. 21.2B). Data from the CURRENT-OASIS 7 trial, which compared low doses (75–100 mg daily) and high doses (300–325 mg daily) of aspirin in ACS patients, found no reduction in efficacy with lower doses, but a reduction in the risk of major gastrointestinal bleeding (0.2% vs 0.4%; $p = 0.04$).[13]

$P2Y_{12}$ Inhibitors

$P2Y_{12}$ inhibitors act as antagonists of the platelet adenosine diphosphate (ADP) receptor $P2Y_{12}$, thereby inhibiting platelet aggregation. This pharmacologic class includes thienopyridines (ticlopidine, clopidogrel, and prasugrel) as well as ticagrelor (a cyclopentyl-triazolo-pyrimidine [CPTP] inhibitor) and cangrelor (a short-acting intravenous ADP inhibitor).

Ticlopidine

Ticlopidine was the first $P2Y_{12}$ inhibitor available. In a randomized trial of 650 patients with unstable angina, ticlopidine reduced MI by over 50% (5.1% vs 10.9%; $p = 0.006$) compared with "conventional therapy."[14] However, the clinical application of ticlopidine was hindered by its delayed onset of action and by the development of neutropenia (2.4%); for these reasons, ticlopidine use is currently largely abandoned.

Clopidogrel

Clopidogrel is a prodrug that needs to be transformed into an active metabolite. After absorption, 85% of clopidogrel is hydrolyzed by esterases into an inactive carboxylic acid; the remaining 15% undergoes a 2-step oxidation process via hepatic cytochrome P450 isoenzymes, mainly CYP2C19 (which is associated with both steps) and, to a lesser extent, CYP1A2, CYP2B6, CYP3A4, and CYP3A5.[15] The transient active thiol metabolite specifically and irreversibly binds to the platelet $P2Y_{12}$ receptor. Steady-state platelet function inhibition occurs after 5 to 7 days of clopidogrel maintenance dosing; for that reason, a loading dose is recommended to achieve more rapid inhibition.

Clopidogrel as Single Antiplatelet Therapy

The major randomized trial supporting the use of clopidogrel in chronic CAD patients was the Clopidogrel versus Aspirin in Patients at Risk of Ischaemic Events (CAPRIE)

Category of trial	No of trials with data	No (%) of vascular events: Allocated antiplatelet	No (%) of vascular events: Adjusted control	Observed-expected	Variance	% Odds reduction (SE)
Previous myocardial infarction	12	1345/9984 (13.5)	1708/10,022 (17.0)	−159.8	567.6	25 (4)
Acute myocardial infarction	15	1007/9658 (10.4)	1370/9644 (14.2)	181.5	519.2	30 (4)
Previous stroke/transient ischemic attack	21	2045/11,493 (17.8)	2464/11,527 (21.4)	−152.1	625.8	22 (4)
Acute stroke	7	1670/20,418 (8.2)	1858/20,403 (9.1)	−94.6	795.3	11 (3)
Other high risk	140	1638/20,359 (8.0)	2102/20,543 (10.2)	−222.3	737.0	26 (3)
Subtotal: all except acute stroke	188	6035/51,494 (11.7)	7644/51,736 (14.8)	−715.7	2449.6	25 (2)
All trials	**195**	**7705/71,912 (10.7)**	**9502/72,139 (13.2)**	**−810.3**	**3244.9**	**22 (2)**

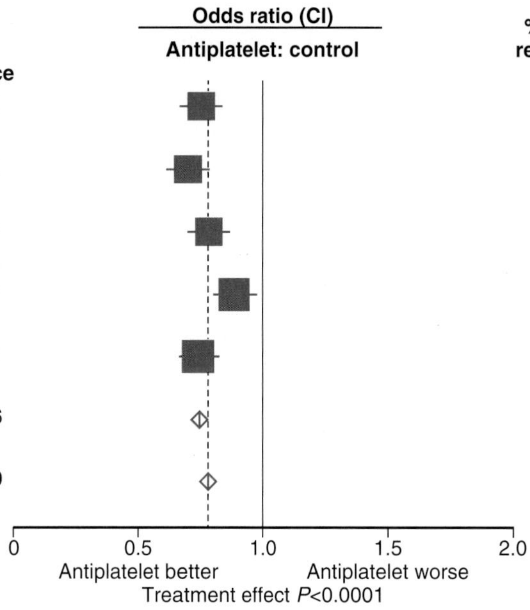

Heterogeneity of odds reductons between:
5 categories of trial: χ^2=21.4, df=4; P=0.0003
Acute stroke v other: χ^2=18.0, df=1; P=0.00002

A

Category of trial	No of trials with data	No (%) of vascular events: Regimen 1	No (%) of vascular events: Regimen 2	Observed-expected	Variance	% Odds reduction (SE)
Higher v lower aspirin doses:						
500–1500 mg *v* 75–325 mg*	7	227/1608 (14.1)	231/1589 (14.5)	−3.1	93.0	3 (10)
≥75 mg *v* < 75 mg†	3	254/1795 (14.2)	234/1775 (13.2)	8.5	104.3	−8 (10)
Subtotal	**10**	**481/3403 (14.1)**	**465/3364 (13.8)**	**5.4**	**197.3**	**−3 (7)**

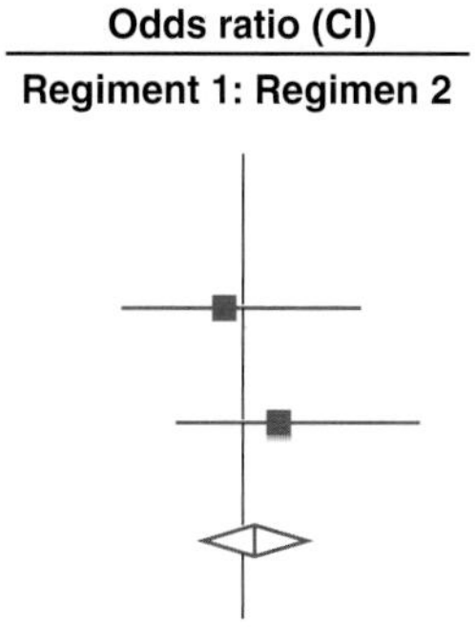

B

FIG. 21.2 **(A)** Benefit of aspirin in atherothrombotic patients according to clinical presentation. **(B)** Effect of different doses of aspirin on vascular events. *Includes one trial comparing 1400 mg/day *v* 350 mg/day, and another (excluding those with acute stroke) comparing 1000 mg/day *v* 300 mg/day among patients who were also given dipyridamole. †Includes two trials comparing 75-325 mg aspirin daily *v* <75 mg aspirin daily and one trial of 500-1500 mg aspirin daily *v* <75 mg aspirin daily. *CI*, Confidence interval; *SE*, standard error. *(From Antithrombotic Trialists Collaboration: Collaborative meta-analysis of randomised trials of antiplatelet therapy for prevention of death, myocardial infarction, and stroke in high risk patients.* BMJ. *2002;324:71.)*

trial,[16] which enrolled more than 19,000 stable patients with atherothrombosis (patients with previous ischemic stroke, previous MI, or peripheral arterial disease [PAD]). CAPRIE compared clopidogrel (75 mg daily) and aspirin (325 mg daily) in terms of reduction in risk of a composite outcome (ischemic stroke, MI, or vascular death). Patients assigned to clopidogrel had a significant but modest 8.7% relative reduction in the composite outcome compared with those assigned to aspirin (5.83% vs 5.32%, respectively; p = 0.043). There appeared to be some heterogeneity in benefit depending on subgroups (P for interaction = 0.042), with the largest relative benefit observed in patients with PAD (Fig. 21.3). Given the modest superiority, the cost of clopidogrel at the time, and the large evidence base for aspirin, aspirin has remained the first-line choice for antiplatelet therapy, but clopidogrel is an alternative for patients who are intolerant to aspirin.

Dual Antiplatelet Therapy with Aspirin and Clopidogrel

With the emergence of coronary stenting, it appeared that the combination of aspirin and an oral $P2Y_{12}$ receptor blocker was required to minimize the risk of stent thrombosis,[17–19] and dual antiplatelet therapy (DAPT) with aspirin and clopidogrel rapidly became the standard of care for patients undergoing

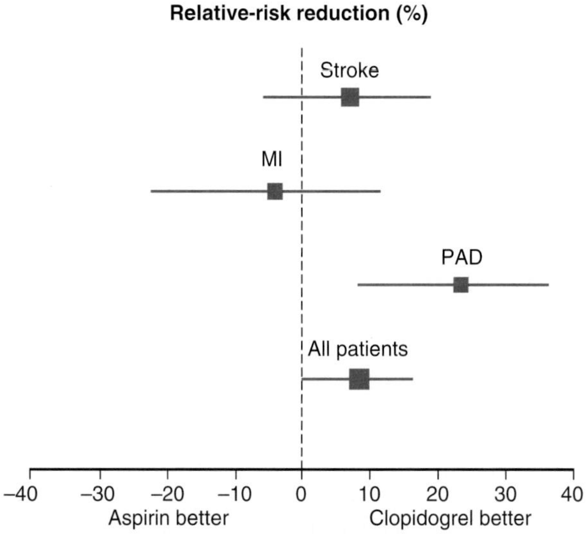

FIG. 21.3 Effect of clopidogrel compared with aspirin in the CAPRIE trial. *MI*, Myocardial infarction; *PAD*, peripheral arterial disease. *(From CAPRIE Steering Committee: A randomised, blinded trial of clopidogrel versus aspirin in patients at risk of is chaemic events (CAPRIE).* Lancet. *1996;348:1329.)*

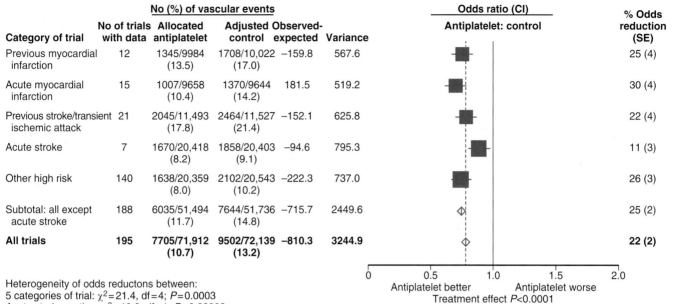

PCI. Subsequently, this combination was tested in ACS and its role was extended to secondary prevention.

Secondary Prevention after Acute Coronary Syndrome

In ACS patients, the benefit of DAPT with aspirin plus clopidogrel was established in the CURE randomized trial,[20] which enrolled more than 12,000 patients with non-ST-segment elevation (NSTE) ACS, who were assigned to clopidogrel or placebo on a background treatment of aspirin for up to 12 months. The primary outcome (composite of death from cardiovascular cause, nonfatal MI, or stroke) occurred in 9.3% of patients in the clopidogrel group and 11.4% in the placebo group ($p < 0.001$). Interestingly, the benefit of clopidogrel started early, but event curves continued to diverge for several months, suggesting continuous accrual of benefit from DAPT in secondary prevention (Fig. 21.4).

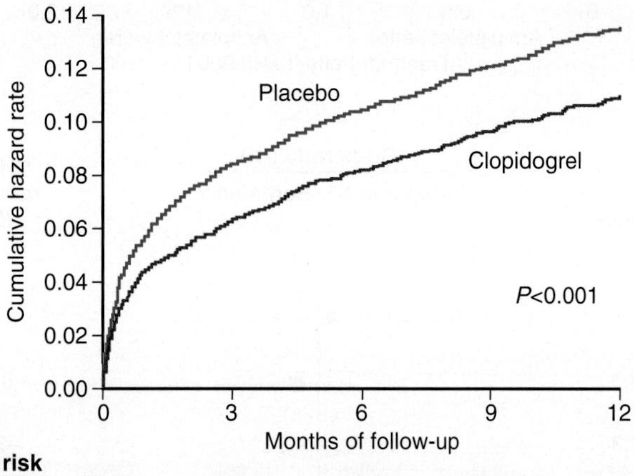

No. at risk

Placebo	6303	5780	4664	3600	2388
Clopidogrel	6529	5866	4779	3644	2418

FIG. 21.4 Cumulative hazard rates for the first primary outcome during the 12 months of the CURE trial. *(From Mehta SR, Yusuf S, Peters RJ, et al. Effects of pretreatment with clopidogrel and aspirin followed by long-term therapy in patients undergoing percutaneous coronary intervention: the PCI-CURE study.* Lancet. *2001;358:527.)*

The benefits of DAPT with aspirin plus clopidogrel were also demonstrated in ST-segment elevation MI (STEMI) in the CLARITY and COMMIT trials.[21,22] CLARITY[22] enrolled STEMI patients treated with thrombolysis who presented within 12 hours after symptom onset and were randomly assigned to receive clopidogrel (300-mg loading dose, followed by 75 mg once daily) or placebo. Clopidogrel reduced the primary outcome (a composite of either an occluded infarct-related artery, defined by a Thrombolysis In Myocardial Infarction [TIMI] flow grade of 0 or 1 on angiography, death, or recurrent MI before angiography) by 6.7% in absolute terms. COMMIT[21] randomized more than 45,000 Chinese patients within 24 hours of suspected acute MI to clopidogrel or placebo in addition to aspirin. Patients assigned to clopidogrel experienced a 9% relative reduction in the primary composite outcome of death, reinfarction, or stroke (2121 [9.2%] clopidogrel vs 2310 [10.1%] placebo; $p = 0.002$). There was also a 7% (95% confidence interval [CI] 1% to 13%) relative reduction in all-cause mortality (1726 [7.5%] vs 1845 [8.1%]; $p = 0.03$).

Although the follow-up periods in the CLARITY and COMMIT trials were 1 month, and despite the lack of solid data regarding the long-term benefit of clopidogrel compared with placebo after STEMI, international guidelines recommend 12 months of DAPT after STEMI, which is consistent with non-STEMI guidelines. After 12 months, treatment is generally scaled down to single antiplatelet therapy with low-dose aspirin.[23,24]

Stable Patients

The main trial testing DAPT with aspirin and clopidogrel in stable patients was the CHARISMA trial,[24a] which randomly assigned 15,603 stable patients to receive either clopidogrel or placebo, on top of aspirin. The population was somewhat heterogeneous: patients were eligible for enrollment if they had multiple atherothrombotic risk factors, or documented CAD, documented cardiovascular disease, or documented symptomatic PAD. Patients were not eligible if they had an established indication for clopidogrel therapy, such as recent ACS. After a median follow-up of 28 months, there

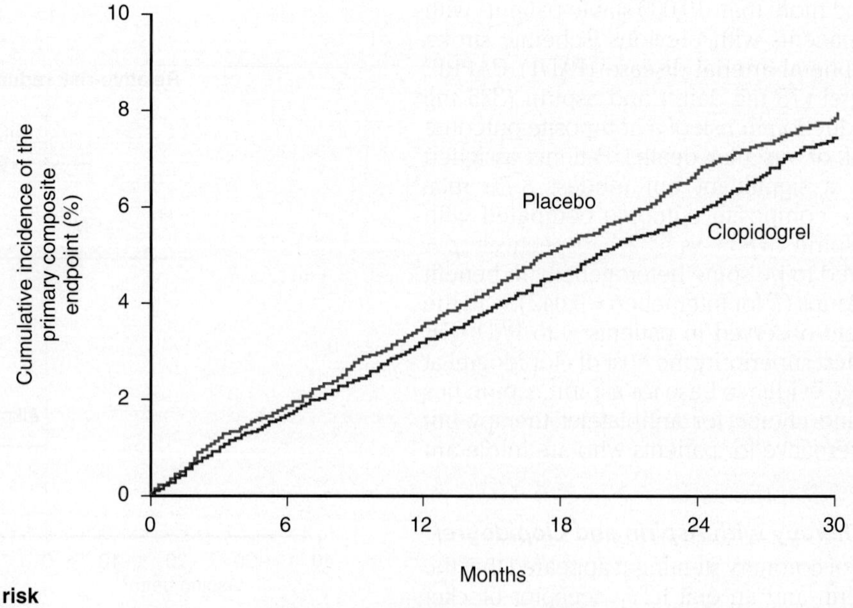

No. at risk

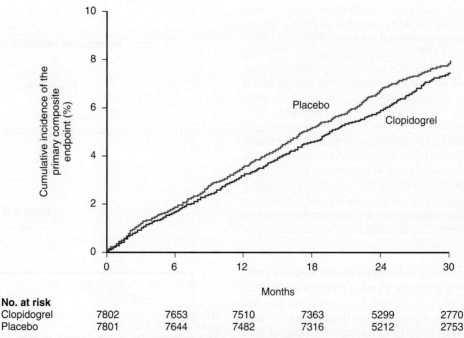

Clopidogrel	7802	7653	7510	7363	5299	2770
Placebo	7801	7644	7482	7316	5212	2753

FIG. 21.5 Kaplan-Meier curves for the primary composite endpoint (cardiovascular death, myocardial infarction, or stroke) in CHARISMA trial patients. *(From Bhatt, DL, Fox KAA, Hacke W, et al. Clopidogrel and aspirin versus aspirin alone for the prevention of atherothrombotic events.* N Engl J Med. *2006;354:1706.)*

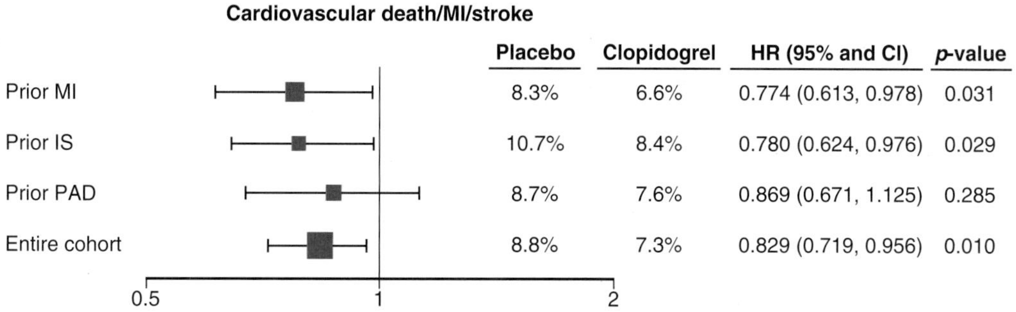

FIG. 21.6 Hazard ratios *(HRs)* for the primary endpoint in CHARISMA trial patients enrolled with prior myocardial infarction (MI), ischemic stroke (IS), or peripheral arterial disease (PAD). *CI,* Confidence interval. *(From Bhatt DL, Flather MD, Hacke W, et al. Patients with prior myocardial infarction, stroke, or symptomatic peripheral arterial disease in the CHARISMA trial.* J Am Coll Cardiol. *2007;49:19.)*

was no difference between the two treatment arms in terms of relative risk (0.93, 95% CI 0.83 to 1.05; $p = 0.22$) (Fig. 21.5).

There was an interaction between the treatment and the patient profile: patients with established atherothrombosis derived benefit from treatment with clopidogrel (hazard ratio [HR] 0.83, 95% CI 0.72 to 0.96; $p = 0.01$) (Fig. 21.6).[25] In contrast, patients with risk factors only derived no benefit (relative risk 1.20, 95% CI 0.91 to 1.59; $p = 0.20$).[24a] In a post hoc analysis,[25] including only patients with prior cardiovascular events (prior MI, ischemic stroke, or symptomatic PAD), the rate of cardiovascular death, MI, or stroke was lower in the clopidogrel plus aspirin arm than in the placebo plus aspirin arm: 7.3% versus 8.8% (HR 0.83, 95% CI 0.72 to 0.96; $p = 0.01$) (Fig. 21.7). Additionally, hospitalizations for ischemia were reduced (11.4% vs 13.2%; HR 0.86, 95% CI 0.76 to 0.96; $p = 0.008$).[25] There was no significant difference in the rate of severe bleeding (1.7% vs 1.5%; HR 1.12, 95% CI 0.81 to 1.53, $p = 0.50$). However, these subgroups and post hoc analyses of an overall negative trial were not deemed sufficient to change practice, and single antiplatelet therapy remained the recommendation for secondary prevention in patients with stable CAD.

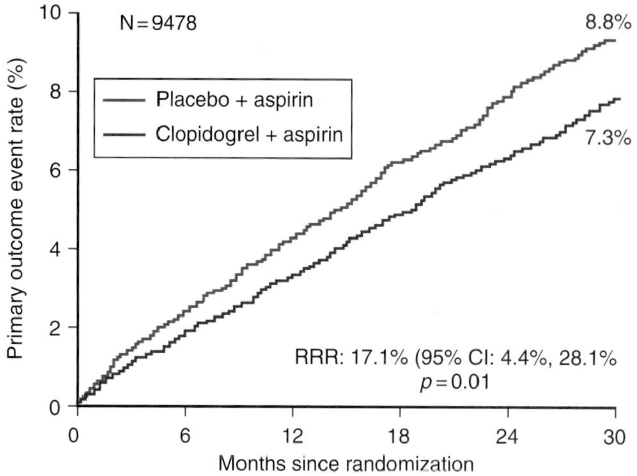

FIG. 21.7 Kaplan-Meier curves for the primary composite endpoint (cardiovascular death, myocardial infarction, or stroke) in the CHARISMA trial subanalysis of patients with documented atherothrombotic disease. *CI,* Confidence interval; *RRR,* relative risk reduction. *(From Bhatt DL, Flather MD, Hacke W, et al. Patients with prior myocardial infarction, stroke, or symptomatic peripheral arterial disease in the CHARISMA trial.* J Am Coll Cardiol. *2007;49:1982.)*

Limitations of Clopidogrel

Clopidogrel has substantial limitations, with a moderate antiplatelet effect and a delayed onset and offset of action. Moreover, the response to clopidogrel is highly variable. In a series of more than 500 patients, the response of subjects to clopidogrel was shown to follow a normal bell-shaped distribution (Fig. 21.8).[26]

Reduced effectiveness of clopidogrel has been shown in carriers of reduced-function alleles of particular enzymes, particularly the common variant CYP2C19*2. On clopidogrel, carriers of this variant have worse clinical outcomes than noncarriers.[27–29] The reduced response to clopidogrel among carriers of the reduced-function allele can, in part, be overcome with increased doses of clopidogrel.[28] However, trials have failed to show that altering the clopidogrel dose according to functional or genetic testing improves outcomes.[30–32]

Several trials have tried to adapt the clopidogrel dose according to platelet function testing or genotype. In the GRAVITAS trial, Price et al.[31] randomly assigned 2214 patients who had undergone PCI with at least one drug-eluting stent (DES) for the treatment of stable CAD. All patients were initially treated with aspirin plus clopidogrel. Platelet function was measured using the VerifyNow $P2Y_{12}$ test, 12 to 24 hours after PCI. Patients without high on-treatment reactivity (platelet reactivity units [PRUs] < 230) were kept on the standard clopidogrel dose (75 mg). Patients with high on-treatment reactivity (PRUs > 230) were randomized to receive a high clopidogrel dose (600 mg initial dose and 150 mg thereafter) or a standard clopidogrel dose (no additional loading dose, 75 mg daily). At 6 months, the primary endpoint (death from vascular cause, nonfatal MI, or stent thrombosis) occurred in 25 patients (2.3%) on high-dose clopidogrel compared with 25 patients (2.3%) on the standard clopidogrel dose (HR 1.01, 95% CI 0.58 to 1.76; $p = 0.97$). Severe or moderate bleeding was not increased with the high-dose regimen. Therefore, the use of the platelet function test to guide clopidogrel dosing failed to demonstrate superiority compared with a standard treatment strategy.

Other clinical trials have evaluated platelet treatment intensification, with a switch to more potent drugs rather than increasing the clopidogrel dose in patients with high on-treatment platelet reactivity; the results were also negative (see hereafter).

Prasugrel

Prasugrel is a second-generation thienopyridine that, like clopidogrel, requires conversion from an inactive form to an active metabolite by cytochrome p450 enzymes.[33] Compared with clopidogrel, prasugrel is metabolized more rapidly and completely to its active component. This difference in metabolism allows prasugrel to achieve a more rapid onset of action and a higher level of platelet inhibition (Fig. 21.9), as well as reduced interpatient variability.[33,34]

In the TRITON-TIMI 38 trial,[35] prasugrel was compared with clopidogrel in 13,608 ACS patients (both STEMI and

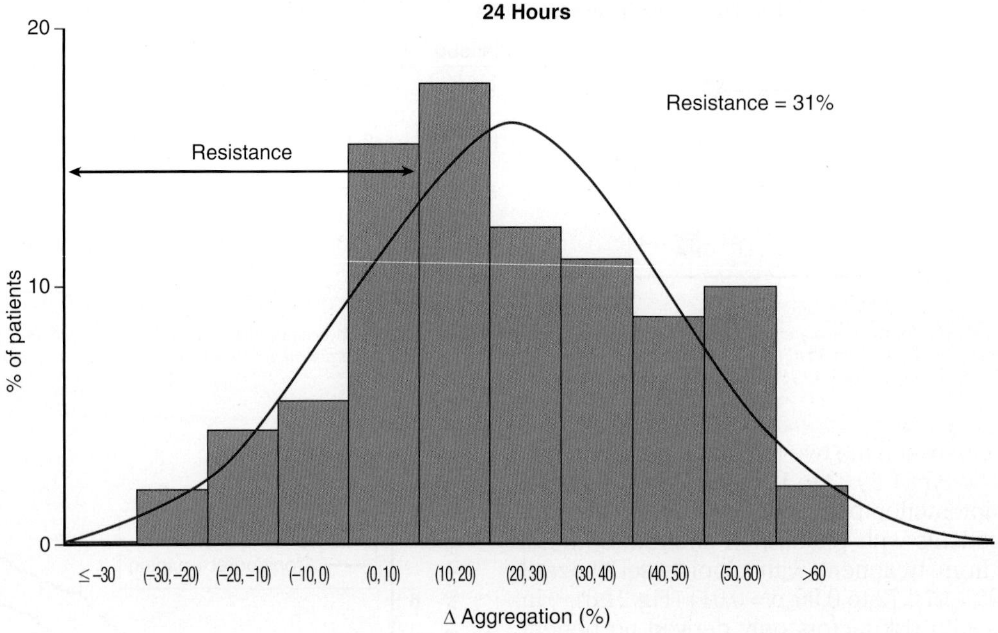

FIG. 21.8 Platelet aggregometry in response to adenosine diphosphate 24 hours after clopidogrel 300-mg loading dose. *(From Gurbel PA, Bliden KP, Hiatt BL, et al. Clopidogrel for coronary stenting: response variability, drug resistance, and the effect of pretreatment platelet reactivity.* Circulation. *2003;107:2908.)*

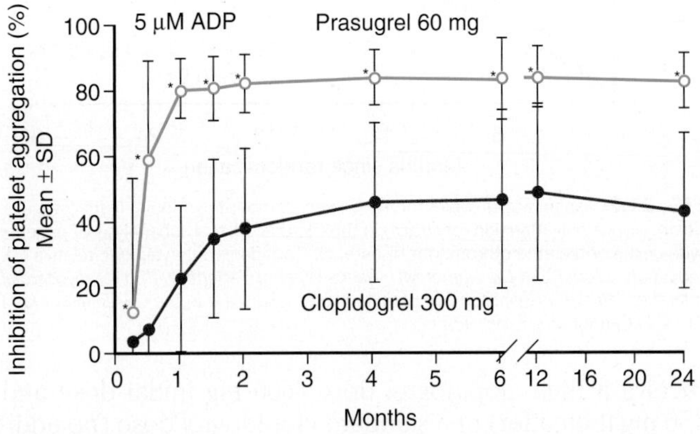

FIG. 21.9 Inhibition of platelet aggregation evaluated by aggregometry in response to 5 μM adenosine diphosphate (ADP) after a loading dose of prasugrel or clopidogrel in healthy subjects. *$p<0.01$. *SD*, Standard deviation. *(From Brandt JT, Payne CD, Wiviott SD, et al. A comparison of prasugrel and clopidogrel loading doses on platelet function: magnitude of platelet inhibition is related to active metabolite formation.* Am Heart J. *2007;153:66.e9.)*

NSTE ACS) scheduled for PCI, with a treatment duration ranging from 6 to 15 months. The primary efficacy composite endpoint of cardiovascular death, nonfatal MI, or nonfatal stroke was reduced by prasugrel (HR for prasugrel vs clopidogrel 0.81, 95% CI 0.73 to 0.90; $p < 0.001$). Conversely, major bleeding not related to coronary artery bypass graft (CABG) was increased by approximately a third (HR 1.32, 95% CI 1.03 to 1.68; $p = 0.03$) (Fig. 21.10). No differences in all-cause or cardiovascular mortality were observed between treatment arms.

A post hoc subgroup analysis of the TRITON-TIMI 38 trial showed that patients older than 75 years and with a body weight less than 60 kg derived no net clinical benefit from prasugrel and that in patients with previous stroke or transient ischemic attack (TIA), prasugrel was associated with net harm (Fig. 21.11). Therefore, prasugrel is contraindicated in patients with prior TIA or stroke, and there is a warning for patients aged over 75 years or with a body weight less than 60 kg.

In the TRITON-TIMI 38 trial, prasugrel was initiated in the acute phase and continued for up to 15 months. Secondary landmark analyses for efficacy, safety, and net clinical benefit were performed from randomization to day three, and from day three to the end of the trial. Significant reductions in ischemic events, including MI, stent thrombosis, and urgent target vessel revascularization, were observed with the use of prasugrel during the first three days and from day three to the end of the trial. TIMI major non-CABG bleeding rates were similar to clopidogrel during the first three days, but were higher with prasugrel from day three to the end of the study. Assessment of net clinical benefit favored prasugrel both early and late in the trial.[36] This trial therefore supports the use of prasugrel instead of clopidogrel in secondary prevention in ACS patients undergoing PCI, for approximately one year, after which treatment is scaled down to single antiplatelet therapy with aspirin.

However, the TRITON-TIMI 38 trial did not include medically managed patients. The TRILOGY trial[37] was therefore specifically designed to compare prasugrel with clopidogrel in patients presenting with NSTE ACS and managed without intervention. After a median follow-up of 17 months, the primary endpoint of death from cardiovascular causes, MI, or stroke among patients aged older than 75 years occurred in 13.9% of the prasugrel group and 16.0% of the clopidogrel group (HR in the prasugrel group 0.91, 95% CI 0.79 to 1.05; $p = 0.21$). This trial therefore does not support the use of prasugrel in NSTE ACS patients treated conservatively during the acute phase or in secondary prevention.

The use of prasugrel has not been evaluated in unselected stable patients. In the TRIGGER PCI trial,[32] patients with stable CAD who underwent PCI with at least one DES implantation had systematic evaluation of platelet reactivity on clopidogrel 75 mg with the VerifyNow $P2Y_{12}$ system. Patients with high platelet reactivity were randomly assigned to prasugrel 10 mg daily or clopidogrel 75 mg daily. The primary efficacy endpoint of cardiac death or MI at 6 months occurred in no patient on prasugrel versus one patient on clopidogrel. Given the low rate of ischemic events in this trial, the clinical utility of prasugrel based on platelet function evaluation in stable patients has not been established.

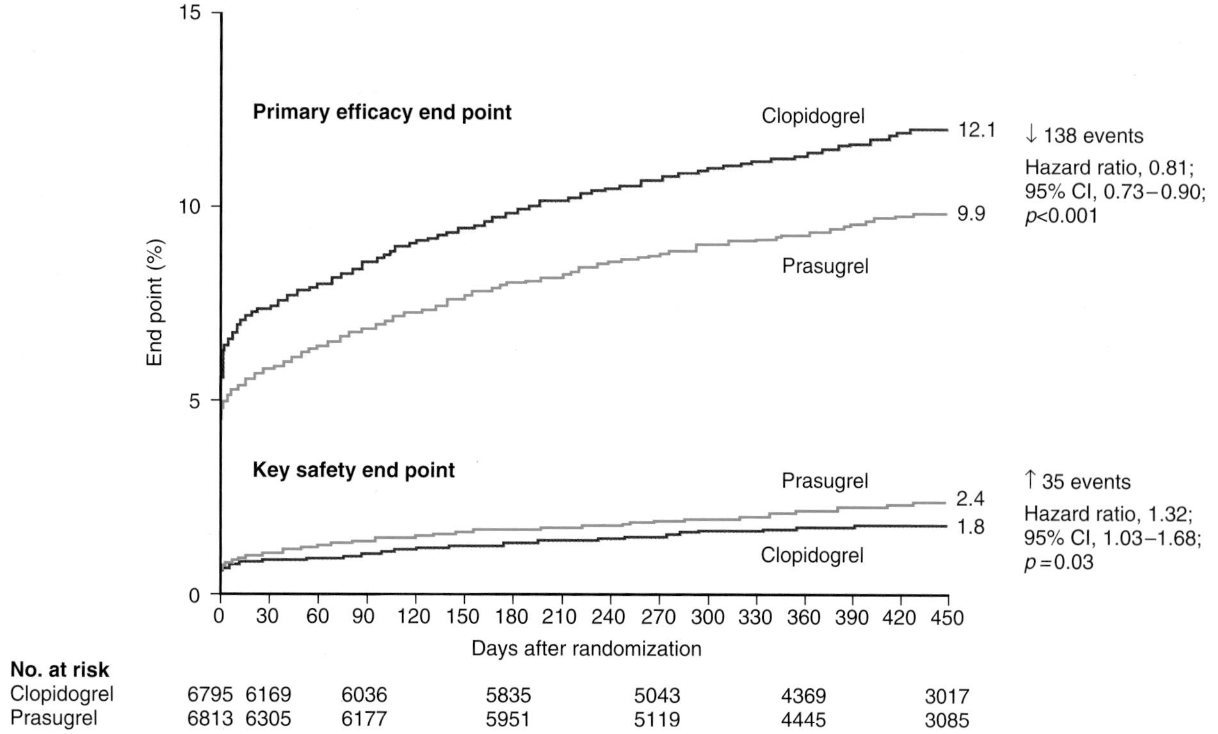

FIG. 21.10 Kaplan-Meier curves for the primary efficacy endpoint (cardiovascular death, nonfatal myocardial infarction, or nonfatal stroke) and the key safety endpoint (major bleeding) in patients on clopidogrel or prasugrel in the TRITON-TIMI 38 trial. *CI,* Confidence interval. *(From Wiviott SD, Braunwald E, McCabe CH, et al. Prasugrel versus clopidogrel in patients with acute coronary syndromes.* N Engl J Med. *2007;357:2001.)*

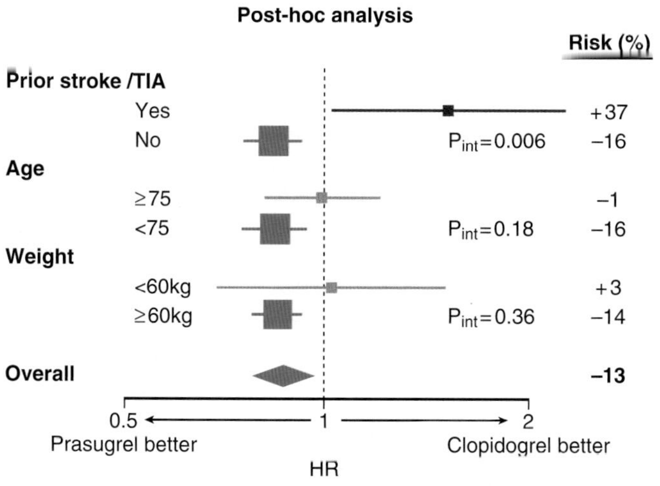

FIG. 21.11 Post hoc analysis of various subgroups deriving no benefit or harm from prasugrel versus clopidogrel in the TRITON-TIMI 38 trial. *HR,* Hazard ratio; P_{int}, *p* for interaction; *TIA,* transient ischemic attack. *(From Wiviott SD, Braunwald E, McCabe CH, et al. Prasugrel versus clopidogrel in patients with acute coronary syndromes.* N Engl J Med. *2007;357:2001.)*

Similarly, the ARCTIC trial[30] randomly assigned 2440 patients scheduled for coronary stenting (excluding STEMI patients) to a strategy of platelet function monitoring (assessed with VerifyNow and aspirin point-of-care assays), with drug adjustment (additional loading dose of clopidogrel or prasugrel followed by a daily maintenance dose of 150 mg of clopidogrel or 10 mg of prasugrel after the procedure) in patients with poor response to antiplatelet therapy, or to a conventional strategy without monitoring and drug adjustment. The primary endpoint occurred in 34.6% of the patients in the monitoring group versus 31.1% of those in the conventional-treatment group (HR 1.13, 95% CI 0.98 to 1.29; $p = 0.10$).

The results of the TRIGGER-PCI and ARCTIC trials do not support the use of prasugrel based on platelet function tests in stable patients. As a consequence, current guidelines do not support the routine use of a platelet function test to guide antiplatelet therapy.

Ticagrelor

Ticagrelor is a reversible and direct-acting oral antagonist of the ADP receptor $P2Y_{12}$. It has been demonstrated that ticagrelor provides faster onset and greater inhibition of platelet aggregation than does clopidogrel.[38,39] In the ONSET/OFFSET study, the onset and offset of platelet inhibition were compared between clopidogrel- and ticagrelor-treated patients. Ticagrelor achieved more rapid platelet inhibition than a loading dose of 600 mg of clopidogrel; this was sustained during the maintenance phase, and ticagrelor offset was faster after drug discontinuation (Fig. 21.12).[40]

Ticagrelor in Patients with Acute Coronary Syndrome

The clinical efficacy of ticagrelor in ACS patients was evaluated in the PLATO trial.[41] In this multicenter, double-blind, randomized trial, ticagrelor (180-mg loading dose and then 90 mg daily) was compared with clopidogrel (300- to 600-mg loading dose and then 75 mg daily) in 18,624 patients admitted to hospital with an ACS with or without ST-segment elevation. At 12 months, the primary endpoint (composite of death from cardiovascular causes, MI, or stroke) occurred in 9.8% of patients receiving ticagrelor compared with 11.7% of those receiving clopidogrel (HR 0.84, 95% CI 0.77 to 0.92; $p < 0.001$) (Fig. 21.13). Importantly, death from cardiovascular cause (a predefined secondary endpoint) was also reduced (4.0% vs 5.1%; HR 0.79, 95% CI 0.69 to 0.91; $p = 0.001$). No difference in the rates of major bleeding or transfusion was seen between the ticagrelor and clopidogrel groups (11.6% vs 11.2%; $p = 0.43$) when

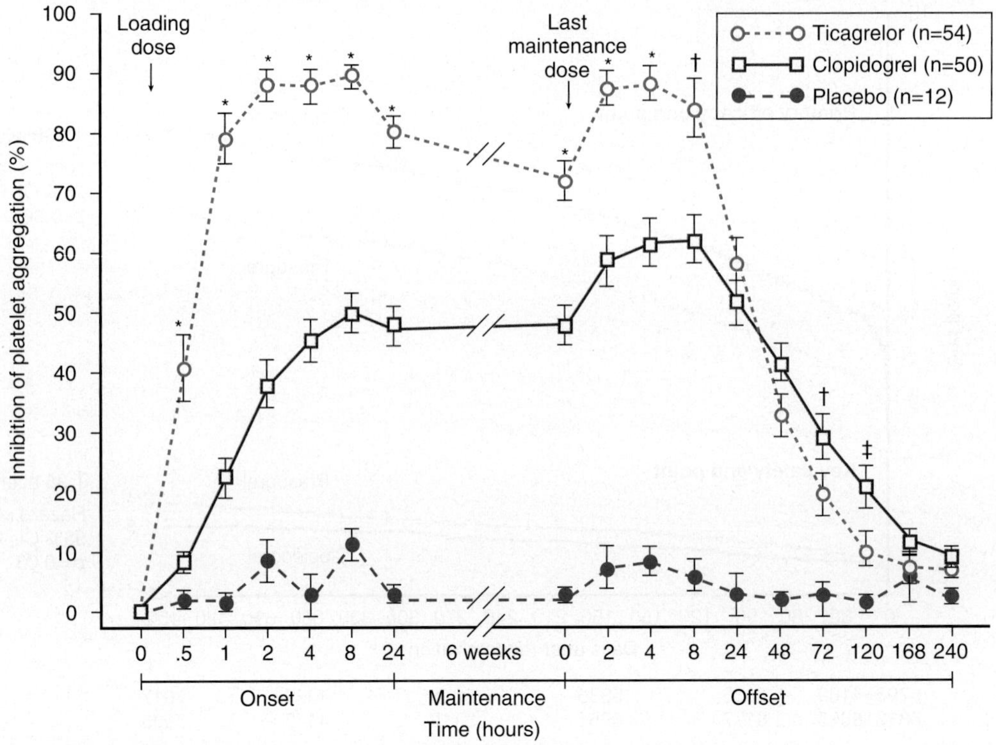

FIG. 21.12 Inhibition of platelet aggregation with ticagrelor versus clopidogrel. *$P<0.0001$, †$P<0.005$, ‡$P<0.05$, ticagrelor vs clopidogrel. *(From Gurbel PA, Bliden KP, Butler K, et al. Randomized double-blind assessment of the ONSET and OFFSET of the antiplatelet effects of ticagrelor versus clopidogrel in patients with stable coronary artery disease: the ONSET/OFFSET study.* Circulation. *2009;120:2577.)*

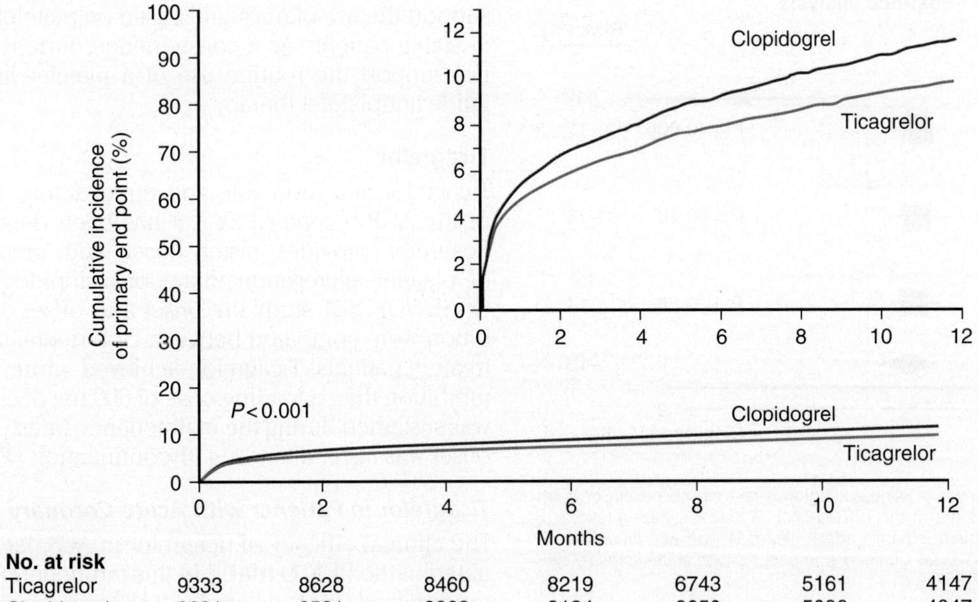

FIG. 21.13 Cumulative Kaplan-Meier estimate of the time of occurrence of the primary endpoint (composite of death from cardiovascular causes, myocardial infarction, or stroke) in the PLATO trial. *(From Wallentin L, Becker RC, Budaj A, et al. Ticagrelor versus clopidogrel in patients with acute coronary syndromes.* N Engl J Med. *2009;361:1045.)*

analyzed by intention to treat; however, this encompassed patients undergoing CABG surgery in whom bleeding rates were high. When non-CABG-related major bleeding was analyzed, ticagrelor increased bleeding (4.5% vs 3.8%; HR 1.19, 95% CI 1.02 to 1.38; $p = 0.03$).

Ticagrelor has specific side effects that are related to adenosine metabolism. Dyspnea was twice as frequent in patients given ticagrelor than in patients given clopidogrel, and led to treatment discontinuation in approximately 1% of patients.[41] The dyspnea was generally mild and transient (most episodes lasted < 1 week), occurred early after initiation, and was not associated with any abnormality on examination or on lung-function tests.[42] Holter monitoring detected more ventricular pauses during the first week in the ticagrelor group; however, these episodes were infrequent at 30 days and were rarely associated with symptoms.

Of note, an interaction ($p = 0.045$) was observed between treatment effect and enrollment region, with no benefit

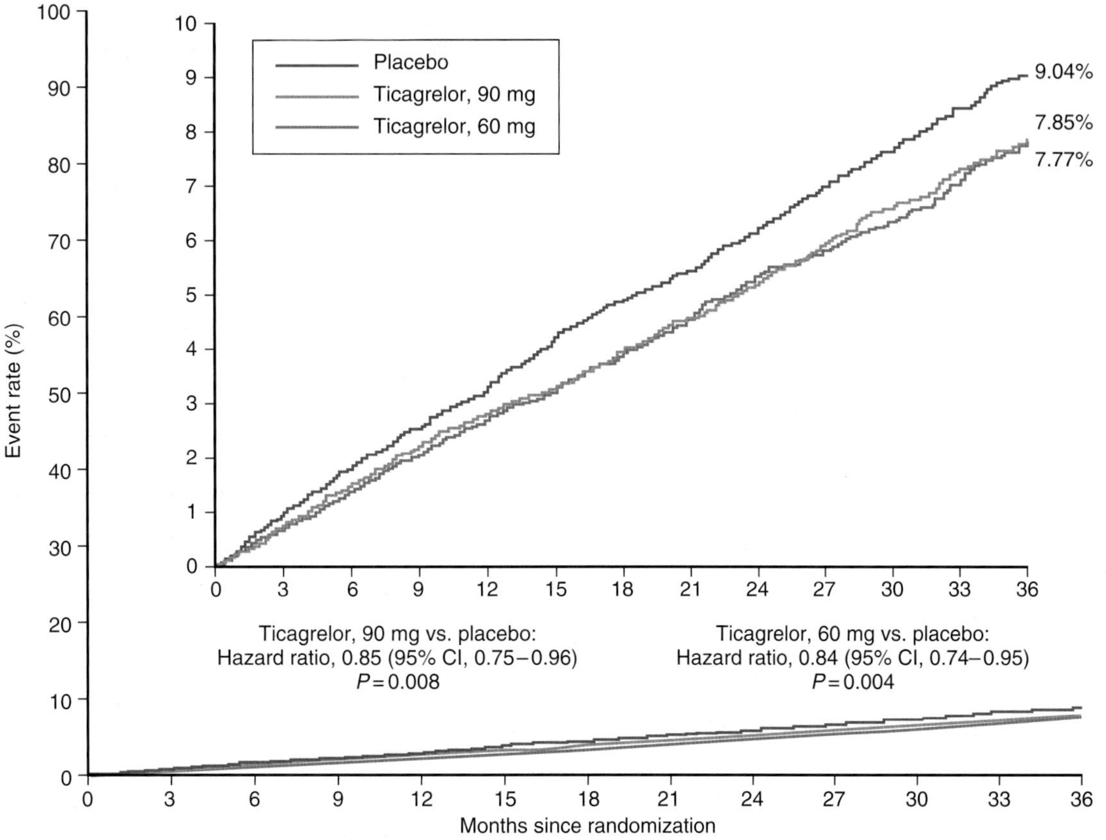

No. at risk													
Placebo	7067	6979	6892	6823	6761	6681	6508	6236	5876	5157	4343	3360	2028
Ticagrelor, 90 mg	7050	6973	6899	6827	6769	6719	6550	6272	5921	5243	4401	3368	2038
Ticagrelor, 60 mg	7045	6969	6905	6842	6784	6733	6557	6270	5904	5222	4424	3392	2055

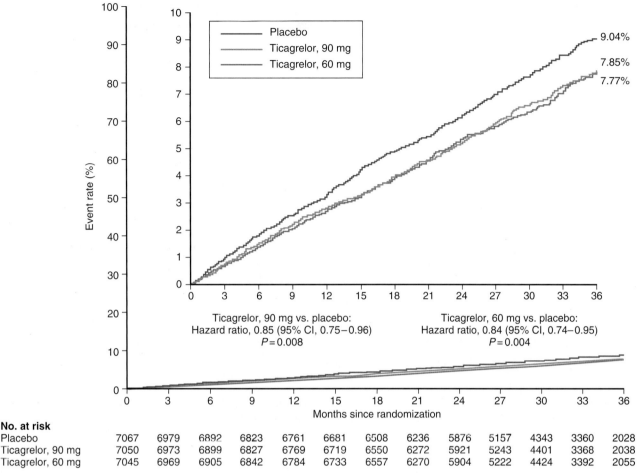

FIG. 21.14 Kaplan-Meier rates of cardiovascular death, myocardial infarction, and stroke over 3 years, according to study group, in the PEGASUS trial. *CI*, Confidence interval. *(From Bonaca MP, Bhatt DL, Cohen M, et al. Long-term use of ticagrelor in patients with prior myocardial infarction.* N Engl J Med. *2015;372:1791.)*

from ticagrelor in patients enrolled in North America. This interaction might result from a negative interaction between ticagrelor and the higher dose of aspirin usually used in the United States (> 150 mg) compared with other regions. This observation has led to a recommendation to use ticagrelor with low-dose aspirin (up to 150 mg).[43]

This trial therefore supports the use of ticagrelor instead of clopidogrel in secondary prevention in ACS patients undergoing PCI for up to 1 year, after which treatment is scaled down to single antiplatelet therapy with aspirin.

Ticagrelor in Stable Patients

In diabetic patients, the effectiveness of aspirin for the prevention of cardiovascular events is less firmly established than in the overall population,[44] possibly because of the accelerated turnover of platelets in these patients.[45,46] The THEMIS trial (NCT01991795, currently ongoing) aims to compare the effect of ticagrelor versus placebo on top of aspirin in patients with type 2 diabetes with either documented CAD or previous coronary revascularization. Patients with a history of MI or stroke are excluded, and therefore only stable patients are included.

Dual Antiplatelet Therapy Beyond 1 Year

The clopidogrel, prasugrel, and ticagrelor trials converge to show that DAPT combining aspirin and an oral $P2Y_{12}$ receptor blocker for up to one year is useful in secondary prevention. The potential benefit of DAPT beyond the first year after an ACS is less firmly established. Data come from several sources, including the PEGASUS trial[47] and many trials testing the optimal duration of DAPT after stenting (generally including both ACS and non-ACS patients).

PEGASUS[47] was a double-blind, international, randomized trial that included 21,162 patients who had had an MI 1 to 3 years previously and had one of several additional risk factors for atherothrombosis (age ≥ 65 years, diabetes mellitus requiring medication, a second prior spontaneous MI, multivessel CAD, or chronic renal dysfunction [defined as an estimated creatinine clearance of < 60 mL/min]). Patients were randomized to one of three arms: ticagrelor 90 mg twice daily; ticagrelor 60 mg twice daily; or placebo. All patients received low-dose aspirin. The median follow-up was 33 months. The primary endpoint (a composite of cardiovascular death, MI, or stroke) was reduced with the two ticagrelor doses, with Kaplan-Meier rates at 3 years of 7.85% in the group receiving 90 mg, 7.77% in the group receiving 60 mg, and 9.04% in the placebo group: HR for 90 mg of ticagrelor versus placebo 0.85, 95% CI 0.75 to 0.96 (p = 0.008); and HR for 60 mg of ticagrelor versus placebo 0.84, 95% CI 0.74 to 0.95 (p = 0.004) (Fig. 21.14). The primary safety endpoint (TIMI major bleeding rate) was higher with ticagrelor (2.60% with 90 mg and 2.30% with 60 mg) than with placebo (1.06%) ($p < 0.001$ for each dose versus placebo). All-cause death was not significantly different in the three groups. It appears, therefore, that the continuation of DAPT for more

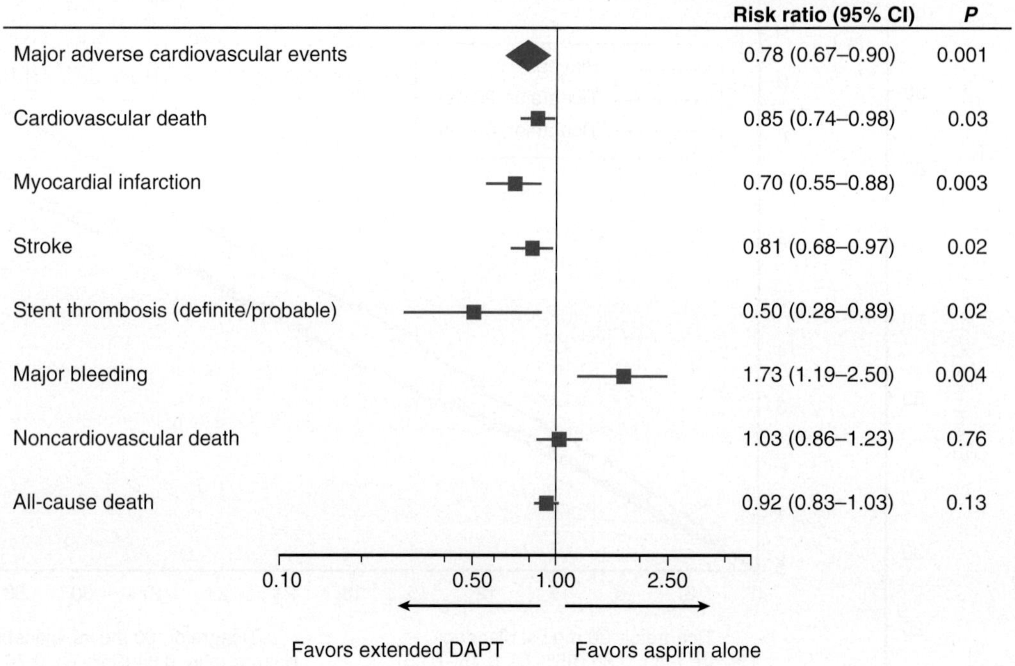

FIG. 21.15 Risk of individual cardiovascular and bleeding endpoints comparing extended dual antiplatelet therapy versus aspirin alone in patients with previous myocardial infarction. *CI*, Confidence interval. *(From Udell JA, Bonaca MP, Collet JP, et al. Long-term dual antiplatelet therapy for secondary prevention of cardiovascular events in the subgroup of patients with previous myocardial infarction: a collaborative meta-analysis of randomized trials.* Eur Heart J. *2016;37:390.)*

than one year after ACS may benefit some patients by reducing the rate of ischemic events. However, this reduction in ischemic events in a large population is counterbalanced by an increase in major bleeding, without clear benefit in terms of overall mortality reduction. Patients in whom DAPT is continued after one year have to be carefully selected; the tools allowing this selection remain to be created.

An additional analysis provides some insight into a subgroup of patients who may derive greater benefit from ticagrelor. Patients in the PEGASUS-TIMI 54 trial were categorized by time from last $P2Y_{12}$ inhibitor (≤ 30 days, > 30 to 360 days, > 360 days). The benefit of ticagrelor depended on the time from the last dose, with HRs (95% CIs) for ticagrelor (pooled doses) versus placebo of 0.73 (0.61 to 0.87), 0.86 (0.71 to 1.04), and 1.01 (0.80 to 1.27), respectively, by category (*p* trend for interaction = 0.001).[47a] The benefit of ticagrelor for long-term secondary prevention in patients with prior MI appears, therefore, to be more marked in patients continuing on or restarting after only a brief interruption of $P2Y_{12}$ inhibition. However, additional analyses are still needed to further clarify the profile of post-MI patients most likely to benefit from uninterrupted DAPT.

The DAPT study was a large trial (nearly 10,000 patients) that was powered to address the question of optimal DAPT duration after DES implantation.[48] In this trial, after 12 months of treatment with a thienopyridine (clopidogrel or prasugrel) and aspirin, patients who did not experience ischemic and bleeding events were randomized to receive thienopyridine continuation or placebo for another 18 months. In this trial, continued treatment with thienopyridine, versus placebo, reduced the rates of stent thrombosis (0.4% vs 1.4%; HR 0.29, 95% CI 0.17 to 0.48; $p < 0.001$) and major adverse cardiovascular and cerebrovascular events (4.3% vs 5.9%; HR 0.71, 95% CI 0.59 to 0.85; $p < 0.001$). The rate of moderate or severe bleeding was increased with continued thienopyridine treatment (2.5% vs 1.6%; $p = 0.001$). The rate of death from any cause was 2.0% in the group that continued thienopyridine therapy and 1.5% in the placebo group (HR 1.36, 95% CI 1.00 to 1.85; $p = 0.05$).

An additional analysis[49] examined the effect of continued thienopyridine on ischemic and bleeding events among patients initially presenting with versus without MI. In both groups, continued thienopyridine reduced MI (2.2% vs 5.2% [$p < 0.001$] for MI; 2.1% vs 3.5% [$p < 0.001$] for no MI; *p* for interaction = 0.15), but increased bleeding (1.9% vs 0.8% [$p = 0.005$] for MI; 2.6% vs 1.7% [$p = 0.007$] for no MI; *p* for interaction = 0.21). However, the reduction in major adverse cerebrovascular or cardiovascular events for continued thienopyridine was greater for patients with MI (3.9% vs 6.8%; $p < 0.001$) compared with those with no MI (4.4% vs 5.3%; $p = 0.08$) (*p* for interaction = 0.03).

In the PEGASUS and DAPT trials, prolonged DAPT reduced ischemic events, but increased bleeding, without a clear benefit in terms of mortality. Several smaller trials have evaluated the effect of long-term DAPT; these trials usually included a heterogeneous population. A meta-analysis[50] focusing on the subgroup of patients with previous MI included more than 33,000 patients. Extended DAPT decreased the risk of major adverse cardiovascular events compared with aspirin alone (6.4% vs 7.5%; risk ratio [RR] 0.78, 95% CI 0.67 to 0.90; $p = 0.001$) and reduced cardiovascular death (2.3% vs 2.6%; RR 0.85, 95% CI 0.74 to 0.98; $p = 0.03$), with no increase in noncardiovascular death (RR 1.03, 95% CI 0.86 to 1.23; $p = 0.76$) (Fig. 21.15).

It appears therefore that prolonged DAPT is of particular interest in patients with previous MI.

Single Antiplatelet Therapy with a Novel Agent

Several ongoing trials are evaluating the role of single antiplatelet therapy with ticagrelor after PCI. The GLOBAL LEADERS trial[51] and the TWILIGHT trial (NCT02270242) are evaluating ticagrelor monotherapy in an all-comer population of patients treated by PCI (including stable and ACS patients). The design of these trials is described in section titled Future Perspectives.

Vorapaxar

In addition to its role in the coagulation cascade, thrombin is a powerful inducer of platelet aggregation. Platelet responses to thrombin are mediated by surface G protein-coupled receptors, known as *protease-activated receptors* (PARs) or *thrombin receptors*. The PAR-1 subtype acts as the principal thrombin receptor on human platelets and is selectively blocked by vorapaxar. Importantly, PAR-1 blockade by vorapaxar spares other functions of thrombin, including coagulation, resulting in inhibition of thrombin-induced platelet activation, with a larger therapeutic index than that achieved by anticoagulant drugs.

Vorapaxar is a selective, orally active, potent, and competitive PAR-1 inhibitor, which is slowly eliminated (half-life of 159 to 311 hours). Vorapaxar has been evaluated in two large randomized trials: one in ACS, the TRACER trial,[52] and one in secondary prevention, the TRA 2P-TIMI 50 trial.[53]

TRACER[52] randomized nearly 13,000 patients with NSTE ACS to vorapaxar or placebo on top of DAPT (with aspirin plus clopidogrel). The trial was terminated early after a safety review. The primary endpoint of cardiovascular death, MI, stroke, recurrent ischemia with hospitalization, or urgent coronary revascularization was not reduced by vorapaxar (18.5% vs 19.9%; HR 0.92, 95% CI 0.85 to 1.01; $p = 0.07$), whereas there was an increase in the risk of bleeding. Rates of moderate and severe bleeding were 7.2% in the vorapaxar group and 5.2% in the placebo group (HR 1.35, 95% CI 1.16 to 1.58; $p < 0.001$). Intracranial hemorrhage rates were 1.1% and 0.2%, respectively (HR 3.39, 95% CI 1.78 to 6.45; $p < 0.001$).

In TRA 2P-TIMI 50,[53] more than 26,000 patients with a history of MI, stroke, or PAD were randomized to vorapaxar (2.5 mg daily) or placebo on top of standard therapy. At 3 years, the primary endpoint (a composite of cardiovascular death, MI, or stroke) had occurred in 1028 patients (9.3%) in the vorapaxar group and in 1176 patients (10.5%) in the placebo group (HR for the vorapaxar group 0.87, 95% CI 0.80 to 0.94; $p < 0.001$). Moderate or severe bleeding occurred in 4.2% of patients who received vorapaxar and 2.5% of those who received placebo (HR 1.66, 95% CI 1.43 to 1.93; $p < 0.001$). There was an increase in the rate of intracranial hemorrhage in the vorapaxar group (1.0% vs 0.5% in the placebo group; $p < 0.001$). Among patients with a history of stroke, the rate of intracranial hemorrhage in the vorapaxar group was 2.4% versus 0.9% in the placebo group ($p < 0.001$), with corresponding rates of fatal bleeding of 0.5% and 0.3% ($p = 0.46$). A prespecified subgroup analysis was performed to evaluate the safety and efficacy of vorapaxar in patients with previous MI.[54] Cardiovascular death, MI, or stroke occurred less frequently in the vorapaxar group (HR 0.80, 95% CI 0.72 to 0.89; $p < 0.0001$). Moderate or severe bleeding was more common with vorapaxar (HR 1.61, 95% CI 1.31 to 1.97; $p < 0.0001$). Intracranial hemorrhage occurred in 43 of 8880 patients (0.6%, 3-year Kaplan-Meier estimate) with vorapaxar versus 28 of 8849 (0.4%, 3-year Kaplan-Meier estimate) with placebo ($p = 0.076$).[54]

Another prespecified analysis focused on a group of patients with previous MI and no history of stroke or TIA, and with stratification on planned thienopyridine use.[55] In that analysis, vorapaxar reduced the composite of cardiovascular death, MI, and stroke compared with placebo, regardless of planned thienopyridine therapy: planned thienopyridine HR 0.80, 95% CI 0.70 to 0.91 ($p < 0.001$); no planned thienopyridine HR 0.75, 95% CI 0.60 to 0.94 ($p = 0.011$) (p for interaction = 0.67). Global Use of Strategies to Open Occluded Coronary Arteries (GUSTO) moderate or severe bleeding risk was increased with vorapaxar and was not significantly altered by planned thienopyridine use: planned HR 1.50, 95% CI 1.18 to 1.89 ($p < 0.001$); not planned HR 1.90, 95% CI 1.17 to 3.07 ($p = 0.009$) (p for interaction = 0.37).

These results have led to vorapaxar approval in secondary prevention in patients with previous MI or with PAD. However, given the risk of intracerebral hemorrhage in patients with previous stroke or TIA, it should not be used in this subset.

ANTICOAGULANTS

Triple Combination in Secondary Prevention after Acute Coronary Syndrome

Excess thrombin generation persists after ACS.[56] As a consequence, a combination of anticoagulant with antiplatelet agent is theoretically interesting. The combination of a vitamin K antagonist with aspirin has been shown, in the era antedating widespread use of PCI (and the attendant DAPT), to improve vascular outcomes after MI,[57] but at the expense of substantial increases in bleeding and inconvenience, because of the need for monitoring. In the era of DAPT, the benefit-risk ratio associated with the addition of anticoagulant therapy to DAPT is more uncertain. Several anticoagulants have been evaluated in this context.

Six of the new OACs have been tested in placebo-controlled phase II trials, which included patients with STEMI and NSTE ACS: ximelagatran (ESTEEM[58]), dabigatran etexilate (RE-DEEM[59]), rivaroxaban (ATLAS ACS-TIMI 46[60]), apixaban (APPRAISE[60a]), darexaban (RUBY-1[61]), and letaxaban (AXIOM-ACS[62]). These dose-finding studies were powered to evaluate safety, and the drugs were administered once or twice daily in multiple dosages for a maximum of 6 months. All of these trials showed a dose-dependent increase in bleeding. Only two agents have been evaluated in phase III trials: apixaban and rivaroxaban.

Apixaban

Apixaban is a direct factor Xa inhibitor. In the APPRAISE-2 trial,[63] 5 mg twice daily (the dose used to prevent thromboembolic complications in ACS patients) was compared with placebo, in addition to standard therapy, in patients with recent ACS. In this trial, which included more than 7000 patients, the addition of apixaban increased major bleeding. The primary safety outcome of TIMI major bleeding occurred in 46 of the 3673 patients (1.3%) who received at least one dose of apixaban (2.4 events/100 patient-years) and in 18 of the 3642 patients (0.5%) who received at least one dose of placebo (0.9 events/100 patient-years) (HR with apixaban 2.59, 95% CI 1.50 to 4.46; $p = 0.001$), without a significant reduction in ischemic events.

Rivaroxaban

Rivaroxaban is an OAC that directly and selectively inhibits factor Xa. The addition of very low doses of rivaroxaban to antiplatelet therapy was evaluated in the ATLAS ACS2-TIMI 51 trial[64]: more than 15,000 patients with a recent ASC were

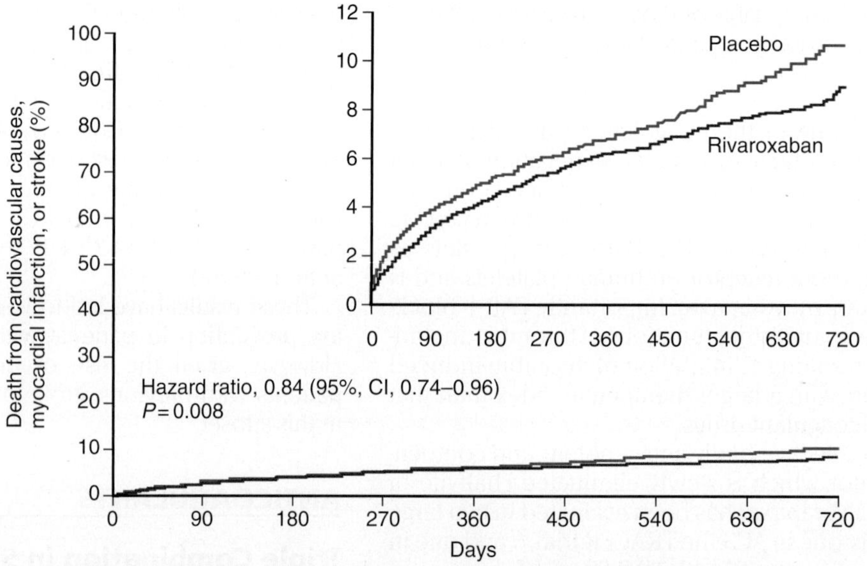

No. at risk

Rivaroxaban	10,229	8817	7797	6324	5137	3967	2830	1747	831
Placebo	5113	4437	3974	3253	2664	2059	1460	878	421

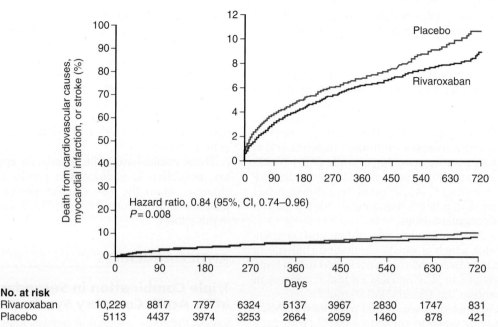

FIG. 21.16 Kaplan-Meier curves for the primary efficacy endpoint in the ATLAS ACS2-TIMI 51 trial. *CI,* Confidence interval. *(From Mega JL, Braunwald E, Wiviott SD, et al. Rivaroxaban in patients with a recent acute coronary syndrome.* N Engl J Med. *2012;366:9.)*

randomized to receive twice-daily doses of 2.5 mg or 5 mg of rivaroxaban or placebo. The primary outcome was a composite of cardiovascular death, MI, or stroke. It was reduced by rivaroxaban compared with placebo with both the twice-daily 2.5-mg dose (9.1% vs 10.7%; $p = 0.02$) and the twice-daily 5-mg dose (8.8% vs 10.7%; $p = 0.03$) (Fig. 21.16). Importantly, the twice-daily 2.5-mg dose of rivaroxaban reduced cardiovascular (2.7% vs 4.1%; $p = 0.002$) and all-cause mortality (2.9% vs 4.5%; $p = 0.002$). Rivaroxaban increased the rates of major bleeding not related to CABG (2.1% vs 0.6%; $p < 0.001$) and intracranial hemorrhage (0.6% vs 0.2%; $p = 0.009$), without a significant increase in fatal bleeding (0.3% vs 0.2%; $p = 0.66$) or other adverse events. The twice-daily 2.5-mg dose resulted in fewer fatal bleeding events than the twice-daily 5-mg dose (0.1% vs 0.4%; $p = 0.04$).

These results led the European Medicines Agency to approve rivaroxaban, coadministered with aspirin alone or with aspirin plus clopidogrel or ticlopidine for the prevention of atherothrombotic events in adult patients after an ACS with elevated cardiac biomarkers. Conversely, rivaroxaban was not approved by the US Food and Drug Administration for this indication, largely because of concerns regarding incomplete follow-up, as patients who discontinued the study drug were only followed for 30 days after stopping treatment.

Although encouraging, this trial only included patients receiving clopidogrel as a $P2Y_{12}$ inhibitor. The addition of low-dose rivaroxaban to new $P2Y_{12}$ inhibitors has not yet been evaluated. The ongoing GEMINI ACS1 trial (NCT02293395) is evaluating the risk of bleeding with rivaroxaban compared with aspirin, in addition to a $P2Y_{12}$ receptor antagonist (clopidogrel or ticagrelor), in patients with a recent ACS. Therefore, the exact role of rivaroxaban in the modern antithrombotic armamentarium remains to be clarified.

The role of low-dose rivaroxaban alone or combined with low-dose aspirin in stable patients with CAD or PAD is currently being evaluated versus aspirin alone in the COMPASS trial (NCT01776424). This very large trial (estimated 27,400 patients) includes patients with CAD or PAD. Patients requiring DAPT are excluded. Patients are randomized to one of three treatment arms: rivaroxaban 2.5 mg plus aspirin 100 mg once daily; rivaroxaban 5 mg twice daily; and aspirin 100 mg once daily. Patients who are not on proton-pump inhibitors will also be randomized to pantoprazole or placebo.

Triple Combination in Patients with an Indication for Oral Anticoagulant Therapy

Patients with an indication for OAC therapy (such as stroke prevention in atrial fibrillation or a mechanical valvular bioprosthesis) and with CAD present a real conundrum. The presence of atrial fibrillation is associated with an increased ischemic risk in CAD patients, but the combination of antiplatelet therapy with OAC therapy dramatically increases the bleeding risk.[65,66] Available data are scarce, but large ongoing trials should provide more information.

Currently Available Data

WOEST[67] was an open-label, multicenter, randomized, controlled trial that randomized 573 patients receiving OAC therapy and undergoing PCI (most of whom were stable) to either clopidogrel alone (double therapy) or clopidogrel plus aspirin (triple therapy). The primary endpoint was any bleeding at one year. Patients on double therapy experienced less bleeding at one year than patients on triple therapy (19.4% vs 44.4%; HR 0.36, 95% CI 0.26 to 0.50; $p < 0.0001$) (Fig. 21.17).

Surprisingly, there was actually an increase in ischemic events in patients receiving triple therapy (Fig. 21.18). This might be explained by the fact that patients who experience bleeding often require temporary or permanent withholding of antithrombotic agents. Although groundbreaking, this trial should be interpreted with caution. Firstly, this was a relatively modestly sized trial powered for bleeding. Secondly, the trial enrolled mostly stable patients, and it is uncertain whether the strategy outlined would be as safe in patients

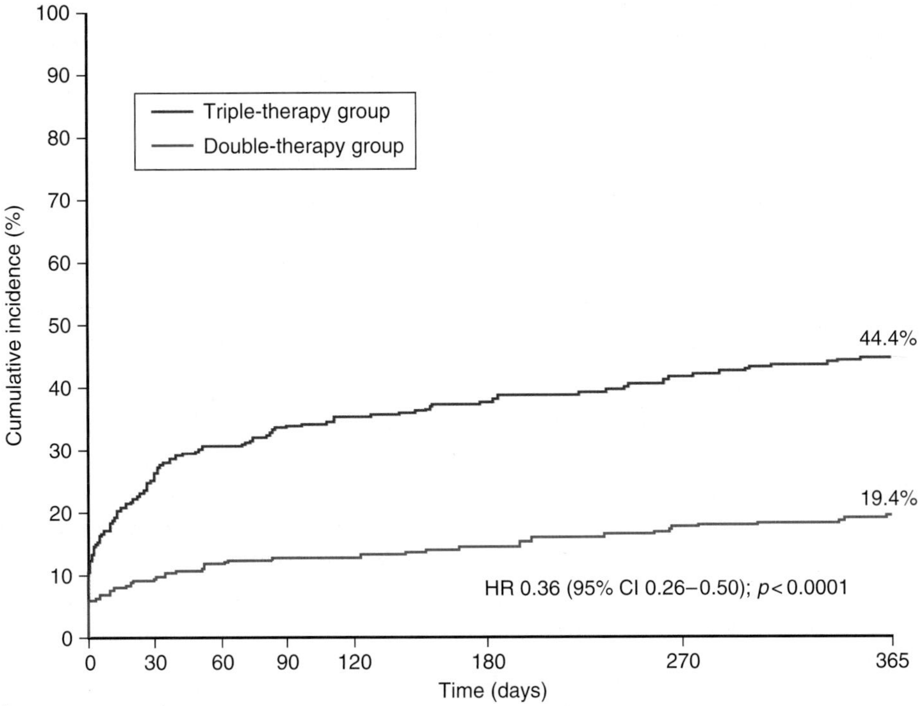

No. at risk

Triple therapy	284	210	194	186	181	173	159	140
Double therapy	279	253	244	241	241	236	226	208

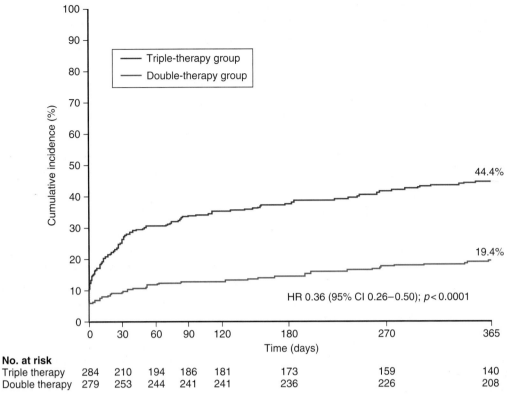

FIG. 21.17 Incidence of the primary endpoint (any bleeding) in the WOEST trial. *CI*, Confidence interval; *HR*, hazard ratio. *(From Dewilde WJ, Oirbans T, Verheugt FW, et al. Use of clopidogrel with or without aspirin in patients taking oral anticoagulant therapy and undergoing percutaneous coronary intervention: an open-label, randomised, controlled trial.* Lancet. *2013;381:1107.)*

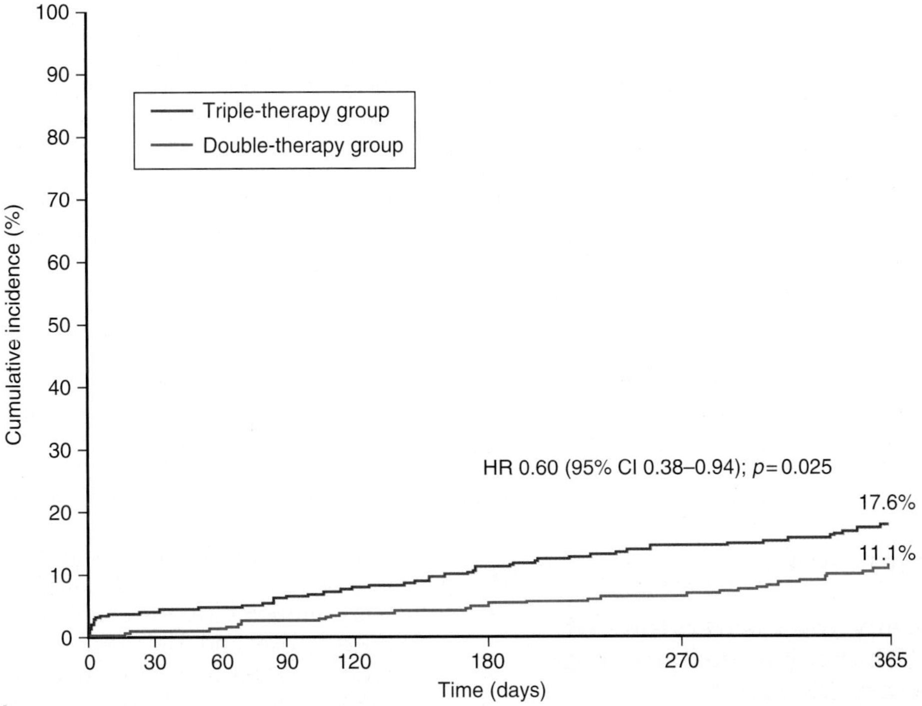

No. at risk

Triple therapy	284	272	270	266	261	252	242	223
Double therapy	279	276	273	270	266	263	258	234

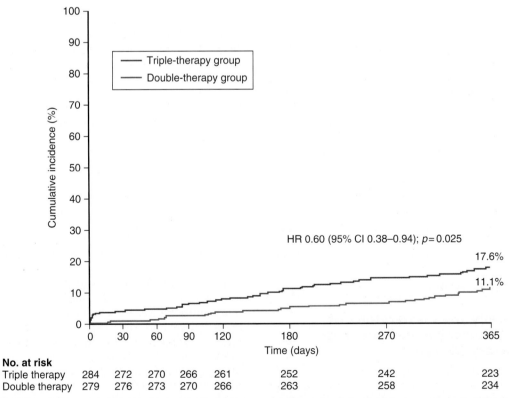

FIG. 21.18 Cumulative incidence of the secondary endpoint (death, myocardial infarction, stroke, target vessel revascularization, and stent thrombosis) in the WOEST trial. *CI*, Confidence interval; *HR*, hazard ratio. *(From Dewilde WJ, Oirbans T, Verheugt FW, et al. Use of clopidogrel with or without aspirin in patients taking oral anticoagulant therapy and undergoing percutaneous coronary intervention: an open-label, randomised, controlled trial.* Lancet. *2013;381:1107.)*

with ACS. Finally, the trial was done with vitamin K antagonists and does not provide an insight into the novel direct OACs, although the safety profile of the latter has generally been similar to, or better than, that of vitamin K antagonists.[68]

ISAR-TRIPLE[69] was a randomized, open-label trial that included 614 patients receiving OAC therapy who underwent DES implantation; they were assigned to either 6 weeks or 6 months of clopidogrel therapy. The primary endpoint was a composite of death, MI, definite stent thrombosis, stroke, or TIMI major bleeding at 9 months. The primary endpoint occurred in 30 patients (9.8%) in the 6-week group compared with 27 patients (8.8%) in the 6-month group (HR 1.14; 95% CI 0.68 to 1.91; $p = 0.63$), whereas the secondary endpoint of TIMI major bleeding occurred in 16 patients (5.3%) in the 6-week group compared with 12 patients (4.0%) in the 6-month group (HR 1.35, 95% CI 0.64 to 2.84; $p = 0.44$). The trial failed to demonstrate noninferiority of 6 weeks of therapy compared with 6 months of therapy, probably because of its modest size.

Upcoming Trials

Due to the evidence gap, several trials are currently being conducted.

MUSICA-2[70] is a multicenter, open-label, randomized trial including 300 patients that will test the hypothesis that DAPT compared with triple therapy in patients with nonvalvular atrial fibrillation at low-to-moderate risk of stroke ($CHADS_2$ score ≤ 2) after PCI and stenting reduces the risk of bleeding and is not inferior to triple therapy for preventing thromboembolic complications.

PIONEER AF-PCI[71] is an open-label, exploratory, multicenter trial that will randomize 2100 patients with atrial fibrillation undergoing PCI to one of three treatment arms: rivaroxaban 15 mg once daily plus clopidogrel 75 mg daily for 12 months (a WOEST trial-like strategy); or rivaroxaban 2.5 mg twice daily (with stratification to a prespecified duration of DAPT of 1, 6, or 12 months; an ATLAS trial-like strategy); or dose-adjusted vitamin K antagonist once daily (with stratification to a prespecified duration of DAPT of 1, 6, or 12 months; traditional triple therapy). The primary endpoint will be a composite of TIMI major bleeding, bleeding requiring medical attention, and minor bleeding.

RE-DUAL PCI is a multicenter, open-label trial that will include patients with nonvalvular atrial fibrillation presenting with an ACS and treated by PCI. Patients will be randomized to a dual antithrombotic therapy regimen of 110 mg dabigatran etexilate twice daily plus clopidogrel or ticagrelor, or 150 mg dabigatran etexilate twice daily plus clopidogrel or ticagrelor, or a triple antithrombotic therapy combination of warfarin plus clopidogrel or ticagrelor plus aspirin ≥ 100 mg once daily.

FUTURE PERSPECTIVES

Is Aspirin Really the Cornerstone of Antiplatelet Therapy in Patients with Coronary Artery Disease?

As previously described, the optimal duration of DAPT after PCI remains uncertain. However, as aspirin has been considered the cornerstone of antithrombotic therapy, new potent antiplatelet agents have not been evaluated as a single therapy. The GLOBAL LEADERS trial[51] randomized 16,000 all-comer patients, including ACS and stable patients, to ticagrelor 90 mg twice daily plus aspirin for 1 month followed by ticagrelor alone for 23 months versus conventional DAPT (ticagrelor or clopidogrel plus aspirin for 12 months followed by aspirin alone). Similarly, the TWILIGHT trial (NCT02270242) is randomizing 9000 patients and aims to determine the impact of antiplatelet monotherapy with ticagrelor alone versus DAPT with ticagrelor plus aspirin for 12 months in terms of reducing clinically relevant bleeding (efficacy) among high-risk patients undergoing PCI who have completed a 3-month course of aspirin plus ticagrelor. The secondary objective of this study is to determine the impact of antiplatelet monotherapy with ticagrelor alone versus DAPT with ticagrelor plus aspirin for 12 months in terms of reducing major ischemic adverse events (safety) among high-risk patients undergoing PCI who have completed a 3-month course of aspirin plus ticagrelor.

What Is the Optimal Duration of DAPT after Stent Implantation?

Stent implantation is associated with a risk of stent thrombosis, which is reduced, in part, by maintenance of DAPT. After bare-metal stent implantation, endothelialization occurs early, and DAPT is therefore recommended for up to one month.[72]

First generation DESs was associated with pathologic healing[73] and an increase in late and very late stent thrombosis.[74,75] For that reason, prolonged DAPT up to one year was initially recommended after DES implantation.[76] However, arterial healing has been considerably improved with second-generation DESs,[77] and this has resulted in improved safety and reduced stent thrombosis rates.[78,79] For this reason, shorter DAPT durations have been investigated with this new generation of DESs.

In the PRODIGY trial,[80] 2013 patients were randomized to 6 vs 24 months of DAPT after DES implantation. The risks of death, MI, cerebrovascular accident, and stent thrombosis did not differ between the study groups; however, there was a consistently greater risk of hemorrhage in the 24-month clopidogrel group.

In the ITALIC trial,[81] nearly 2000 patients were randomized to either 24 months or 6 months of DAPT after DES implantation. The primary endpoint was a composite of death, MI, urgent target vessel revascularization, stroke, and major bleeding at 12 months after stenting. There was no significant difference in the primary endpoint (24 months 1.5% vs 6 months 1.6%; $p = 0.85$) (Fig. 21.19). Noninferiority was demonstrated for 6-month versus 24-month DAPT, with an absolute risk difference of 0.11% (95% CI–1.04% to 1.26%; p for noninferiority = 0.0002). There were no significant differences in stent thrombosis or bleeding complications.

In the ISAR-SAFE trial,[82] 4000 patients were randomized to 6 or 12 months of DAPT after DES implantation. The primary endpoint was the composite of death, MI, stent thrombosis, stroke, and TIMI major bleeding at 9 months after randomization. In this trial, 6 months of DAPT was noninferior to 12 months (observed difference = –0.1%, upper limit of one-sided 95% CI = 0.5%, limit of noninferiority = 2%, p for noninferiority < 0.001).

These trials, in addition to others, suggest therefore that shorter DAPT durations are not inferior to longer DAPT durations (1 year or more) and are not, in particular, associated with increased stent thrombosis. However, the trials were relatively small and were probably underpowered to address the question of stent thrombosis, as the incidence of this complication is below 1%.

As mentioned previously, with nearly 10,000 patients, the DAPT trial[48] was powered to address the question of optimal DAPT duration after coronary stenting. After 12 months of treatment with a thienopyridine (clopidogrel or prasugrel) and aspirin, patients who did not experience ischemic or bleeding events were randomized to receive thienopyridine continuation or placebo for another 18 months. The coprimary efficacy endpoints were stent thrombosis and major adverse cardiovascular and cerebrovascular events (a composite of death, MI, or stroke) during the period from 12 to 30 months. The primary safety endpoint was moderate or severe bleeding. Continued treatment with thienopyridine, compared with placebo, reduced the rates of stent thrombosis (0.4% vs 1.4%; HR 0.29, 95% CI 0.17 to 0.48; $p < 0.001$) (Fig. 21.20) and major adverse cardiovascular and cerebrovascular events (4.3% vs 5.9%; HR 0.71, 95% CI 0.59 to 0.85; $p < 0.001$). The rate of MI was lower with thienopyridine treatment than with placebo (2.1% vs 4.1%; HR 0.47; $p < 0.001$). The rate of death from any cause was 2.0% in the group that continued thienopyridine therapy and 1.5% in the placebo group (HR 1.36, 95% CI 1.00 to 1.85; $p = 0.05$). The rate of moderate or severe bleeding was increased with continued thienopyridine treatment (2.5% vs 1.6%; $p = 0.001$). An elevated risk of stent thrombosis and MI was observed in both groups during the 3 months after discontinuation of thienopyridines.

This trial and the PEGASUS trial (see section on DAPT Beyond 1 Year) suggest that long-term DAPT might be beneficial for high-risk patients in whom ischemic risk exceeds bleeding risk, and deleterious in patients in whom bleeding risk exceeds ischemic risk. In particular, patients with previous MI seem to derive particular benefit from prolonged DAPT.

In a 2016 meta-analysis,[50] including more than 33,000 patients with previous MI, extended DAPT decreased the

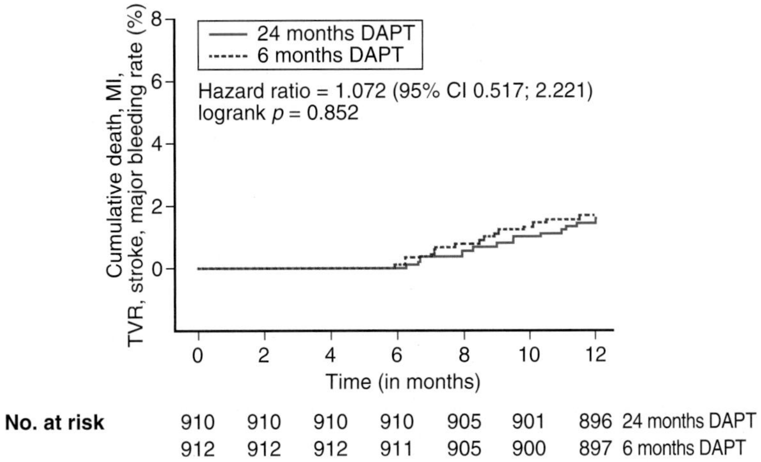

FIG. 21.19 Kaplan-Meier curves for the primary endpoint in the ITALIC trial. *DAPT,* Dual antiplatelet therapy; *MI,* myocardial infarction; *TVR,* target vessel revascularization. *(From Gilard M, Barragan P, Noryani AA, et al. 6- versus 24-month dual antiplatelet therapy after implantation of drug-eluting stents in patients nonresistant to aspirin: the randomized, multicenter ITALIC trial.* J Am Coll Cardiol. *2015;65:777.)*

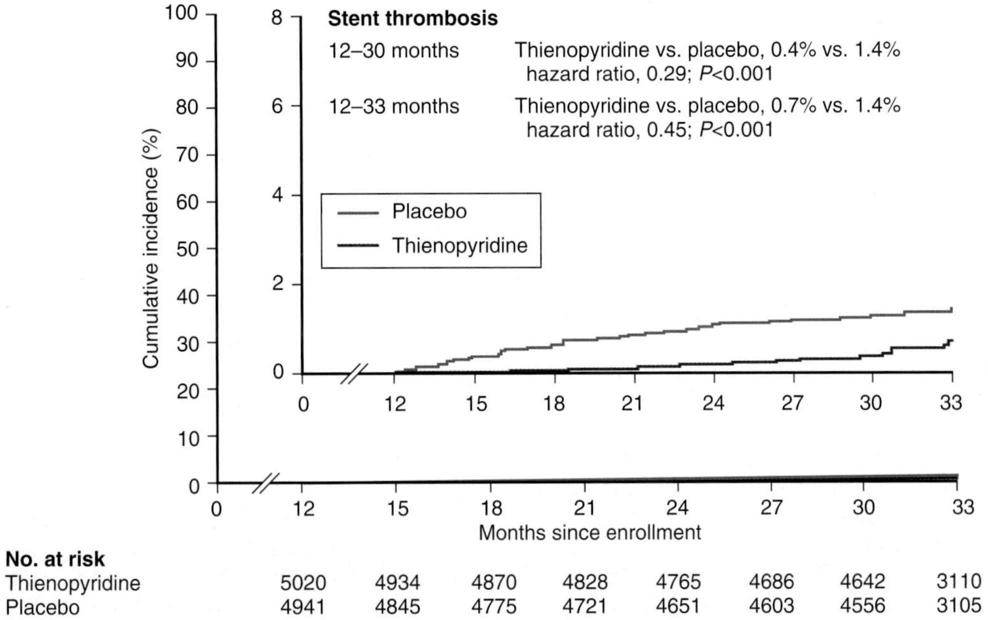

FIG. 21.20 Kaplan-Meier curves for stent thrombosis in the DAPT trial. *(From Mauri L, Kereiakes DJ, Yeh RW, et al. Twelve or 30 months of dual antiplatelet therapy after drug-eluting stents.* N Engl J Med. *2014;371:2155.)*

TABLE 21.1 The Dual Antiplatelet Therapy (DAPT) Score

VARIABLE	POINTS
Patient characteristics	
Age (years)	
≥ 75	−2
65 to < 75	−1
< 65	0
Diabetes mellitus	1
Current cigarette smoker	1
Prior PCI or prior MI	1
CHF or LVEF < 30%	2
Index procedure characteristics	
MI at presentation	1
Vein graft PCI	2
Stent diameter < 3 mm	1

CHF, Congestive heart failure; *LVEF*, left ventricular ejection fraction; *MI*, myocardial infarction; *PCI*, percutaneous coronary intervention.
(From Yeh RW, Secemsky EA, Kereiakes DJ, et al. Development and validation of a prediction rule for benefit and harm of dual antiplatelet therapy beyond 1 year after percutaneous coronary intervention. JAMA. *2016;315:1735.)*

TABLE 21.2 PARIS Risk Score for Major Bleeding

CHARACTERISTIC	POINTS
Age (years)	
< 50	0
50 to 59	+1
60 to 69	+2
70 to 79	+3
≥ 80	+4
BMI (kg/m²)	
< 25	+2
25 to 34.9	0
≥ 35	+2
Current smoking	
Yes	+2
No	0
Anemia	
Present	+3
Absent	0
CrCl < 60 mL/min	
Present	+2
Absent	0
Triple therapy on discharge	
Yes	+2
No	0

BMI, Body mass index; *CrCl*, creatinine clearance.
(From Baber U, Mehran R, Giustino G, et al. Coronary thrombosis and major bleeding After PCI with drug-eluting stents: risk scores from PARIS. J Am Coll Cardiol. *2016 May 17;67(19):2224-34.)*

risk of major adverse cardiovascular events compared with aspirin alone (6.4% vs 7.5%; RR 0.78, 95% CI 0.67 to 0.90; p = 0.001) and reduced cardiovascular death (2.3% vs 2.6%; RR 0.85, 95% CI 0.74 to 0.98; p = 0.03), with no increase in non-cardiovascular death (RR 1.03, 95% CI 0.86 to 1.23; p = 0.76). The resultant effect on all-cause mortality was an RR of 0.92 (95% CI 0.83 to 1.03; p = 0.13). Extended DAPT also reduced MI (RR 0.70, 95% CI 0.55 to 0.88; p = 0.003), stroke (RR 0.81, 95% CI 0.68 to 0.97; p = 0.02), and stent thrombosis (RR 0.50, 95% CI 0.28 to 0.89; p = 0.02). There was an increased risk of major bleeding (1.85% vs 1.09%; RR 1.73, 95% CI 1.19 to 2.50; p = 0.004), but not fatal bleeding (0.14% vs 0.17%; RR 0.91, 95% CI 0.53 to 1.58; p = 0.75).

It therefore appears that DAPT duration should currently be tailored according to the individual patient's risks. The DAPT score[83] is an attempt to address the problem of long-term treatment individualization according to ischemic and bleeding risks. Yeh et al.[83] have identified ischemic and bleeding risk determinants. Factors that were both ischemic and bleeding risk factors were eliminated from the model. The final score includes 10 items, with a negative ponderation for bleeding risk factors and a positive ponderation for ischemic risk factors (Table 21.1). According to the model, patients with a DAPT score less than 2 have an increased bleeding risk without ischemic reduction with prolonged DAPT, whereas patients with a DAPT score of 2 or greater have an ischemic risk reduction without an increased bleeding risk.

Similarly, risk scores for ischemic and major bleeding events after stent implantation have been derived from the PARIS trial[83a] and were validated in the ADAPT-DES registry.[84] The scores are presented in Tables 21.2 and 21.3.

Recent US guidelines[85] summarize the available evidence on DAPT duration as follows: in patients with stable CAD, clopidogrel should be given for at least 6 months. However, in patients who have tolerated DAPT without bleeding complication and who are not at high bleeding risk, continuation of DAPT may be reasonable. Conversely, in patients with stable CAD who develop a high risk of bleeding or significant overt

TABLE 21.3 PARIS Risk Score for Coronary Thrombotic Events

CHARACTERISTIC	POINTS
Diabetes mellitus	
None	0
Non–insulin-dependent	+1
Insulin-dependent	+3
Acute coronary syndrome	
No	0
Yes, Tn-negative	+1
Yes, Tn-positive	+2
Current smoking	
Yes	+1
No	0
CrCl < 60 mL/min	
Present	+2
Absent	0
Prior PCI	
Yes	+2
No	0
Prior CABG	
Yes	+2
No	0

CABG, Coronary artery bypass graft; *CrCl*, creatinine clearance; *PCI*, percutaneous coronary intervention; *Tn*, troponin.
(From Baber U, Mehran R, Giustino G, et al. Coronary thrombosis and major bleeding after PCI with drug-eluting stents: risk scores from PARIS. J Am Coll Cardiol. *2016 May 17;67(19):2224-34.)*

bleeding, discontinuation of a $P2Y_{12}$ inhibitor after 3 months may be reasonable. European guidelines are aligned with the US guidelines, as they recommend a DAPT duration of 6 months after DES implantation, but advise considering shorter durations in patients at high bleeding risk and longer durations in patients at high ischemic risk and low bleeding risk.

CONCLUSIONS

Long-term monotherapy with low-dose aspirin is still the cornerstone of antithrombotic therapy in patients with stable CAD. In patients who have experienced an MI or undergone stenting, a $P2Y_{12}$ inhibitor in addition to aspirin is clearly beneficial (with newer $P2Y_{12}$ oral inhibitors favored over clopidogrel in ACS patients), but there is lingering uncertainty about the optimal duration of such DAPT, which should probably be an individualized decision based on the patient's risk for ischemic events and bleeding, the procedure performed, and the patient's values and preferences. Risk scores, such as the DAPT or PARIS risk scores, may assist in clinical decision-making. Finally, in selected patients, the addition of low-dose rivaroxaban or vorapaxar to aspirin and clopidogrel may be considered in secondary prevention after MI.

References

1. Rioufol G, Finet G, Ginon I, et al.: Multiple atherosclerotic plaque rupture in acute coronary syndrome: a three-vessel intravascular ultrasound study, *Circulation* 106:804, 2002.
2. Steg PG, Bhatt DL, Wilson PW, et al.: One-year cardiovascular event rates in outpatients with atherothrombosis, *JAMA* 297:1197, 2007.
3. Falati S, Gross P, Merrill-Skoloff G, et al.: Real-time in vivo imaging of platelets, tissue factor and fibrin during arterial thrombus formation in the mouse, *Nat Med* 8:1175, 2002.
4. Feletou M, Vanhoutte PM, Verbeuren TJ: The thromboxane/endoperoxide receptor (TP): the common villain, *J Cardiovasc Pharmacol* 55:317, 2010.
5. Angiolillo DJ: The evolution of antiplatelet therapy in the treatment of acute coronary syndromes: from aspirin to the present day, *Drugs* 72:2087, 2012.
6. Patrono C: Aspirin as an antiplatelet drug, *N Engl J Med* 330:1287, 1994.
7. Patrono C, Garcia Rodriguez LA, Landolfi R, et al.: Low-dose aspirin for the prevention of atherothrombosis, *N Engl J Med* 353:2373, 2005.
8. Yu Y, Cheng Y, Fan J, et al.: Differential impact of prostaglandin H synthase 1 knockdown on platelets and parturition, *J Clin Invest* 115:986, 2005.
9. Patrono C, Ciabattoni G, Patrignani P, et al.: Clinical pharmacology of platelet cyclooxygenase inhibition, *Circulation* 72:1177, 1985.
10. Watala C, Golanski J, Pluta J, et al.: Reduced sensitivity of platelets from type 2 diabetic patients to acetylsalicylic acid (aspirin)—its relation to metabolic control, *Thromb Res* 113:101, 2004.
11. Capodanno D, Tamburino C, Sangiorgi GM, et al.: Impact of drug-eluting stents and diabetes mellitus in patients with coronary bifurcation lesions: a survey from the Italian Society of Invasive Cardiology, *Circ Cardiovasc Interv* 4:72, 2011.
12. Dillinger JG, Drissa A, Sideris G, et al.: Biological efficacy of twice daily aspirin in type 2 diabetic patients with coronary artery disease, *Am Heart J* 164:600, 2012.
13. Mehta SR, Bassand JP, Chrolavicius S, et al.: Dose comparisons of clopidogrel and aspirin in acute coronary syndromes, *N Engl J Med* 363:930, 2010.
14. Balsano F, Rizzon P, Violi F, et al.: Antiplatelet treatment with ticlopidine in unstable angina. A controlled multicenter clinical trial. The Studio della Ticlopidina nell'Angina Instabile Group, *Circulation* 82:17, 1990.
15. Kazui M, Nishiya Y, Ishizuka T, et al.: Identification of the human cytochrome P450 enzymes involved in the two oxidative steps in the bioactivation of clopidogrel to its pharmacologically active metabolite, *Drug Metab Dispos* 38:92, 2010.
16. CAPRIE Steering Committee: A randomised, blinded trial of clopidogrel versus aspirin in patients at risk of ischaemic events (CAPRIE), *Lancet* 348:1329, 1996.
17. Bertrand ME, Legrand V, Boland J, et al.: Randomized multicenter comparison of conventional anticoagulation versus antiplatelet therapy in unplanned and elective coronary stenting. The full anticoagulation versus aspirin and ticlopidine (FANTASTIC) study, *Circulation* 98:1597, 1998.
18. Schomig A, Neumann FJ, Kastrati A, et al.: A randomized comparison of antiplatelet and anticoagulant therapy after the placement of coronary-artery stents, *N Engl J Med* 334:1084, 1996.
19. Urban P, Macaya C, Rupprecht HJ, et al.: Randomized evaluation of anticoagulation versus antiplatelet therapy after coronary stent implantation in high-risk patients: the multicenter aspirin and ticlopidine trial after intracoronary stenting (MATTIS), *Circulation* 98:2126, 1998.
20. Fox KA, Mehta SR., Peters R, et al.: Benefits and risks of the combination of clopidogrel and aspirin in patients undergoing surgical revascularization for non-ST-elevation acute coronary syndrome: the Clopidogrel in Unstable angina to prevent Recurrent ischemic Events (CURE) Trial, *Circulation* 110:1202, 2004.
21. Chen ZM, Jiang LX, Chen YP, et al.: Addition of clopidogrel to aspirin in 45,852 patients with acute myocardial infarction: randomised placebo-controlled trial, *Lancet* 366:1607, 2005.
22. Sabatine MS, Cannon CP, Gibson CM, et al.: Addition of clopidogrel to aspirin and fibrinolytic therapy for myocardial infarction with ST-segment elevation, *N Engl J Med* 352:1179, 2005.
23. Levine GN, Bates ER, Bittl JA, et al.: 2016 ACC/AHA Guideline Focused Update on Duration of Dual Antiplatelet Therapy in Patients with Coronary Artery Disease: A Report of the American College of Cardiology/American Heart Association Task Force on Clinical Practice Guidelines: An Update of the 2011 ACCF/AHA/SCAI Guideline for Percutaneous Coronary Intervention, 2011 ACCF/AHA Guideline for Coronary Artery Bypass Graft Surgery, 2012 ACC/AHA/ACP/AATS/PCNA/SCAI/STS Guideline for the Diagnosis and Management of Patients with Stable Ischemic Heart Disease, 2013 ACCF/AHA Guideline for the Management of ST-Elevation Myocardial Infarction, 2014 AHA/ACC Guideline for the Management of Patients with Non-ST-Elevation Acute Coronary Syndromes, and 2014 ACC/AHA Guideline on Perioperative Cardiovascular Evaluation and Management of Patients Undergoing Noncardiac Surgery, *Circulation* 134:e123, 2016.
24. Roffi M, Patrono C, Collet JP, et al.: 2015 ESC Guidelines for the management of acute coronary syndromes in patients presenting without persistent ST-segment elevation: Task Force for the Management of Acute Coronary Syndromes in Patients Presenting Without Persistent ST-Segment Elevation of the European Society of Cardiology (ESC), *Eur Heart J* 37:267, 2016.

24a. Bhatt DL, Fox KA, Hacke W, et al.: Clopidogrel and aspirin versus aspirin alone for the prevention of atherothrombotic events, *N Engl J Med* 354:1706, 2006.

25. Bhatt DL, Flather MD, Hacke W, et al.: Patients with prior myocardial infarction, stroke, or symptomatic peripheral arterial disease in the CHARISMA trial, *J Am Coll Cardiol* 49:1982, 2007.
26. Gurbel PA, Bliden KP, Hiatt BL, et al.: Clopidogrel for coronary stenting: response variability, drug resistance, and the effect of pretreatment platelet reactivity, *Circulation* 107:2908, 2003.
27. Collet JP, Hulot JS, Pena A, et al.: Cytochrome P450 2C19 polymorphism in young patients treated with clopidogrel after myocardial infarction: a cohort study, *Lancet* 373:309, 2009.
28. Mega JL, Close SL, Wiviott SD, et al.: Cytochrome P-450 polymorphisms and response to clopidogrel, *N Engl J Med* 360:354, 2009.
29. Simon T, Verstuyft C, Mary-Krause M, et al.: Genetic determinants of response to clopidogrel and cardiovascular events, *N Engl J Med* 360:363, 2009.
30. Collet JP, Cuisset T, Range G, et al.: Bedside monitoring to adjust antiplatelet therapy for coronary stenting, *N Engl J Med* 367:2100, 2012.
31. Price MJ, Berger PB, Teirstein PS, et al.: Standard- vs high-dose clopidogrel based on platelet function testing after percutaneous coronary intervention: the GRAVITAS randomized trial, *JAMA* 305:1097, 2011.
32. Trenk D, Stone GW, Gawaz M, et al.: A randomized trial of prasugrel versus clopidogrel in patients with high platelet reactivity on clopidogrel after elective percutaneous coronary intervention with implantation of drug-eluting stents: results of the TRIGGER-PCI (Testing Platelet Reactivity in Patients Undergoing Elective Stent Placement on Clopidogrel to Guide Alternative Therapy with Prasugrel) study, *J Am Coll Cardiol* 59:2159, 2012.
33. Wiviott SD, Braunwald E, McCabe CH, et al.: Intensive oral antiplatelet therapy for reduction of ischaemic events including stent thrombosis in patients with acute coronary syndromes treated with percutaneous coronary intervention and stenting in the TRITON-TIMI 38 trial: a subanalysis of a randomised trial, *Lancet* 371:1353, 2008.
34. Brandt JT, Payne CD, Wiviott SD, et al.: A comparison of prasugrel and clopidogrel loading doses on platelet function: magnitude of platelet inhibition is related to active metabolite formation, *Am Heart J* 153:66.e9, 2007.
35. Wiviott SD, Braunwald E, McCabe CH, et al.: Prasugrel versus clopidogrel in patients with acute coronary syndromes, *N Engl J Med* 357:2001, 2007.
36. Antman EM, Wiviott SD, Murphy SA, et al.: Early and late benefits of prasugrel in patients with acute coronary syndromes undergoing percutaneous coronary intervention: a TRITON-TIMI 38 (TRial to Assess Improvement in Therapeutic Outcomes by Optimizing Platelet InhibitioN with Prasugrel-Thrombolysis In Myocardial Infarction) analysis, *J Am Coll Cardiol* 51:2028, 2008.
37. Roe MT, Armstrong PW, Fox KA, et al.: Prasugrel versus clopidogrel for acute coronary syndromes without revascularization, *N Engl J Med* 367:1297, 2012.
38. Husted S, Emanuelsson H, Heptinstall S, et al.: Pharmacodynamics, pharmacokinetics, and safety of the oral reversible P2Y12 antagonist AZD6140 with aspirin in patients with atherosclerosis: a double-blind comparison to clopidogrel with aspirin, *Eur Heart J* 27:1038, 2006.
39. Storey RF, Husted S, Harrington RA, et al.: Inhibition of platelet aggregation by AZD6140, a reversible oral P2Y12 receptor antagonist, compared with clopidogrel in patients with acute coronary syndromes, *J Am Coll Cardiol* 50:1852, 2007.
40. Gurbel PA, Bliden KP, Butler K, et al.: Randomized double-blind assessment of the ONSET and OFFSET of the antiplatelet effects of ticagrelor versus clopidogrel in patients with stable coronary artery disease: the ONSET/OFFSET study, *Circulation* 120:2577, 2009.
41. Wallentin L, Becker RC, Budaj A, et al.: Ticagrelor versus clopidogrel in patients with acute coronary syndromes, *N Engl J Med* 361:1045, 2009.
42. Storey RF, Becker RC, Harrington RA, et al.: Characterization of dyspnoea in PLATO study patients treated with ticagrelor or clopidogrel and its association with clinical outcomes, *Eur Heart J* 32:2945, 2011.
43. Mahaffey KW, Wojdyla DM, Carroll K, et al.: Ticagrelor compared with clopidogrel by geographic region in the Platelet Inhibition and Patient Outcomes (PLATO) trial, *Circulation* 124:544, 2011.
44. De Berardis G, Sacco M, Strippoli GF, et al.: Aspirin for primary prevention of cardiovascular events in people with diabetes: meta-analysis of randomised controlled trials, *BMJ* 339:b4531, 2009.
45. Capodanno D, Patel A, Dharmashankar K, et al.: Pharmacodynamic effects of different aspirin dosing regimens in type 2 diabetes mellitus patients with coronary artery disease, *Circ Cardiovasc Interv* 4:180, 2011.
46. Henry P, Vermillet A, Boval B, et al.: 24-hour time-dependent aspirin efficacy in patients with stable coronary artery disease, *Thromb Haemost* 105:336, 2011.
47. Bonaca MP, Bhatt DL, Cohen M, et al.: Long-term use of ticagrelor in patients with prior myocardial infarction, *N Engl J Med* 372:1791, 2015.

47a. Bonaca MP, Bhatt DL, Steg PG, et al.: Ischaemic risk and efficacy of ticagrelor in relation to time from P2Y12 inhibitor withdrawal in patients with prior myocardial infarction: insights from PEGASUS-TIMI 54, *Eur Heart J* 37:1133, 2016.

48. Mauri L, Kereiakes DJ, Yeh RW, et al.: Twelve or 30 months of dual antiplatelet therapy after drug-eluting stents, *N Engl J Med* 371:2155, 2014.
49. Yeh RW, Kereiakes DJ, Steg PG, et al.: Benefits and risks of extended duration dual antiplatelet therapy after PCI in patients with and without acute myocardial infarction, *J Am Coll Cardiol* 65:2211, 2015.
50. Udell JA, Bonaca MP, Collet JP, et al.: Long-term dual antiplatelet therapy for secondary prevention of cardiovascular events in the subgroup of patients with previous myocardial infarction: a collaborative meta-analysis of randomized trials, *Eur Heart J* 37:390, 2016.
51. Vranckx P, Valgimigli M, Windecker S, et al.: Long-term ticagrelor monotherapy versus standard dual antiplatelet therapy followed by aspirin monotherapy in patients undergoing biolimus-eluting stent implantation: rationale and design of the GLOBAL LEADERS trial, *EuroIntervention* 11, 2015. epub ahead of print.
52. Tricoci P, Huang Z, Held C, et al.: Thrombin-receptor antagonist vorapaxar in acute coronary syndromes, *N Engl J Med* 366:20, 2012.
53. Morrow DA, Braunwald E, Bonaca MP, et al.: Vorapaxar in the secondary prevention of atherothrombotic events, *N Engl J Med* 366:1404, 2012.
54. Scirica BM, Bonaca MP, Braunwald E, et al.: Vorapaxar for secondary prevention of thrombotic events for patients with previous myocardial infarction: a prespecified subgroup analysis of the TRA 2° P-TIMI 50 trial, *Lancet* 380:1317, 2012.
55. Bohula EA, Aylward PE, Bonaca MP, et al.: Efficacy and safety of vorapaxar with and without a thienopyridine for secondary prevention in patients with previous myocardial infarction and no history of stroke or transient ischemic attack: results from TRA 2° P-TIMI 50, *Circulation* 132:1871, 2015.
56. Merlini PA, Bauer KA, Oltrona L, et al.: Persistent activation of coagulation mechanism in unstable angina and myocardial infarction, *Circulation* 90:61, 1994.
57. Rothberg MB, Celestin C, Fiore LD, et al.: Warfarin plus aspirin after myocardial infarction or the acute coronary syndrome: meta-analysis with estimates of risk and benefit, *Ann Intern Med* 143:241, 2005.
58. Wallentin L, Wilcox RG, Weaver WD, et al.: Oral ximelagatran for secondary prophylaxis after myocardial infarction: the ESTEEM randomised controlled trial, *Lancet* 362:789, 2003.
59. Oldgren J, Budaj A, Granger CB, et al.: Dabigatran vs. placebo in patients with acute coronary syndromes on dual antiplatelet therapy: a randomized, double-blind, phase II trial, *Eur Heart J* 32:2781, 2011.
60. Mega JL, Braunwald E, Mohanavelu S, et al.: Rivaroxaban versus placebo in patients with acute coronary syndromes (ATLAS ACS-TIMI 46): a randomised, double-blind, phase II trial, *Lancet* 374:29, 2009.

60a. Alexander JH, Becker RC, Bhatt DL, et al.: Apixaban, an oral, direct, selective factor Xa inhibitor, in combination with antiplatelet therapy after acute coronary syndrome: results of the Apixaban for Prevention of Acute Ischemic and Safety Events (APPRAISE) trial, *Circulation* 119:2877, 2009.

61. Steg PG, Mehta SR, Jukema JW, et al.: RUBY-1: a randomized, double-blind, placebo-controlled trial of the safety and tolerability of the novel oral factor Xa inhibitor darexaban (YM150) following acute coronary syndrome, *Eur Heart J* 32:2541, 2011.
62. Goldstein S, Bates E, Bhatt D, et al.: Safety evaluation of the factor Xa inhibitor TAK-442 in subjects with acute coronary syndromes: phase 2 AXIOM-ACS trial results, *Eur Heart J* 32(abstract supplement):414, 2011. [abstract P2430].
63. Alexander JH, Lopes RD, James S, et al.: Apixaban with antiplatelet therapy after acute coronary syndrome, *N Engl J Med* 365:699, 2011.
64. Mega JL, Braunwald E, Wiviott SD, et al.: Rivaroxaban in patients with a recent acute coronary syndrome, *N Engl J Med* 366:9, 2012.
65. Lamberts M, Gislason GH, Olesen JB, et al.: Oral anticoagulation and antiplatelets in atrial fibrillation patients after myocardial infarction and coronary intervention, *J Am Coll Cardiol* 62:981, 2013.
66. Ruff CT, Bhatt DL, Steg PG, et al.: Long-term cardiovascular outcomes in patients with atrial fibrillation and atherothrombosis in the REACH Registry, *Int J Cardiol* 170:413, 2014.
67. Dewilde WJ, Oirbans T, Verheugt FW, et al.: Use of clopidogrel with or without aspirin in patients taking oral anticoagulant therapy and undergoing percutaneous coronary intervention: an open-label, randomised, controlled trial, *Lancet* 381:1107, 2013.
68. Ruff CT, Giugliano RP, Braunwald E, et al.: Comparison of the efficacy and safety of new oral anticoagulants with warfarin in patients with atrial fibrillation: a meta-analysis of randomised trials, *Lancet* 383:955, 2014.
69. Fiedler KA, Maeng M, Mehilli J, et al.: Duration of triple therapy in patients requiring oral anticoagulation after drug-eluting stent implantation: the ISAR-TRIPLE Trial, *J Am Coll Cardiol* 65:1619, 2015.
70. Sambola A, Montoro JB, Del Blanco BG, et al.: Dual antiplatelet therapy versus oral anticoagulation plus dual antiplatelet therapy in patients with atrial fibrillation and low-to-moderate thromboembolic risk undergoing coronary stenting: design of the MUSICA-2 randomized trial, *Am Heart J* 166:669, 2013.
71. Gibson CM, Mehran R, Bode C, et al.: An open-label, randomized, controlled, multicenter study exploring two treatment strategies of rivaroxaban and a dose-adjusted oral vitamin K antagonist treatment strategy in subjects with atrial fibrillation who undergo percutaneous coronary intervention (PIONEER AF-PCI), *Am Heart J* 169:472, 2015.
72. Windecker S, Kolh P, Alfonso F, et al.: 2014 ESC/EACTS Guidelines on myocardial revascularization: the Task Force on Myocardial Revascularization of the European Society of Cardiology (ESC) and the European Association for Cardio-Thoracic Surgery (EACTS) developed with the special contribution of the European Association of Percutaneous Cardiovascular Interventions (EAPCI), *Eur Heart J* 35:2541, 2014.
73. Nakazawa G, Finn AV, Vorpahl M, et al.: Coronary responses and differential mechanisms of late stent thrombosis attributed to first-generation sirolimus- and paclitaxel-eluting stents, *J Am Coll Cardiol* 57:390, 2011.
74. Camenzind E, Steg PG, Wijns W: Stent thrombosis late after implantation of first-generation drug-eluting stents: a cause for concern, *Circulation* 115:1440, 2007.
75. McFadden EP, Stabile E, Regar E, et al.: Late thrombosis in drug-eluting coronary stents after discontinuation of antiplatelet therapy, *Lancet* 364:1519, 2004.
76. Grines CL, Bonow RO, Casey Jr DE, et al.: Prevention of premature discontinuation of dual antiplatelet therapy in patients with coronary artery stents: a science advisory from the American Heart Association, American College of Cardiology, Society for Cardiovascular Angiography and Interventions, American College of Surgeons, and American Dental Association, with representation from the American College of Physicians, *J Am Coll Cardiol* 49:734, 2007.
77. Stefanini GG, Holmes Jr DR: Drug-eluting coronary-artery stents, *N Engl J Med* 368:254, 2013.
78. Serruys PW, Silber S, Garg S, et al.: Comparison of zotarolimus-eluting and everolimus-eluting coronary stents, *N Engl J Med* 363:136, 2010.
79. Stone GW, Rizvi A, Newman W, et al.: Everolimus-eluting versus paclitaxel-eluting stents in coronary artery disease, *N Engl J Med* 362:1663, 2010.
80. Valgimigli M, Campo G, Monti M, et al.: Short- versus long-term duration of dual-antiplatelet therapy after coronary stenting: a randomized multicenter trial, *Circulation* 125:2015, 2012.
81. Gilard M, Barragan P, Noryani AA, et al.: 6- versus 24-month dual antiplatelet therapy after implantation of drug-eluting stents in patients nonresistant to aspirin: the randomized, multicenter ITALIC trial, *J Am Coll Cardiol* 65:777, 2015.
82. Schulz-Schupke S, Byrne RA, Ten Berg JM, et al.: ISAR-SAFE: a randomized, double-blind, placebo-controlled trial of 6 vs. 12 months of clopidogrel therapy after drug-eluting stenting, *Eur Heart J* 36:1252, 2015.
83. Yeh RW, Secemsky EA, Kereiakes DJ, et al.: Development and validation of a prediction rule for benefit and harm of dual antiplatelet therapy beyond 1 year after percutaneous coronary intervention, *JAMA* 315:1735, 2016.
83a. Baber U, Mehran R, Giustino G, et al.: Coronary thrombosis and major bleeding after PCI with drug-eluting stents: risk scores from PARIS. *J Am Coll Cardiol.* 2016 May 17;67(19):2224-34.
84. Stone GW, Witzenbichler B, Weisz G, et al.: Platelet reactivity and clinical outcomes after coronary artery implantation of drug-eluting stents (ADAPT-DES): a prospective multicentre registry study, *Lancet* 382:614, 2013.
85. Levine GN, Bates ER, Bittl JA, et al.: 2016 ACC/AHA Guideline Focused Update on Duration of Dual Antiplatelet Therapy in Patients with Coronary Artery Disease: A Report of the American College of Cardiology/American Heart Association Task Force on Clinical Practice Guidelines, *J Am Coll Cardiol* 68:1082, 2016.

22 Prevention of Sudden Cardiac Death

Ayman A. Hussein and Mina K. Chung

INTRODUCTION

The relationship between coronary heart disease (CHD) and sudden cardiac death (SCD) has long been recognized, with an initial description by Leonardo Da Vinci in the 15th century of an SCD, which he witnessed and attributed at autopsy to a "parched and shrunk and withered . . . artery that feeds the heart."[1] Research over the past 50 years allowed improved characterization and understanding of CHD as a substrate for SCD. Many pathophysiologic processes underlying the vulnerability to SCD in CHD have been increasingly recognized, including the impact of CHD burden, vascular pathophysiology, the role of ischemia and scarring, the electrophysiologic abnormalities of the myocardial substrate, and the role of ischemic cardiomyopathy and left ventricular (LV) dysfunction. This has allowed significant advancements in medical and interventional therapies to prevent and treat SCD.

DEFINITION AND EPIDEMIOLOGY

SCD is defined as death from otherwise unexpected sudden circulatory collapse from a cardiovascular cause. Generally, this includes SCD events that are witnessed, occurring within 1 hour of change in clinical status, or nonwitnessed death, which has occurred within the preceding 24 hours.[2–4] As such, the estimates of SCD in the community have varied based on definitions and ascertainment of events.[5,6] In the United States, it is estimated that 300,000 to 350,000 SCD cases occur every year.[5]

The exact contribution of CHD to the population of SCD cases is not clearly defined and remains a subject of debate.[6] In fact, SCD estimates in the United States are largely based on the retrospective review of death certificates or extrapolation to the general population from smaller well-studied communities.[7–11] Nonetheless, it is generally accepted that approximately 80% of all SCD cases are related to CHD and that SCD accounts for approximately 50% of all deaths from CHD.[12] Improvements in primary and secondary prevention measures have led to significant declines in CHD-related mortality since the 1980s,[13,14] but the rates of sudden and unexpected deaths from CHD have declined to a lesser extent.[15,16] This reflects two challenging aspects in risk stratification: SCD is the initial clinical manifestation of CHD in a substantial proportion of SCD events, and accurate SCD risk prediction in patients with established CHD remains suboptimal.[12] As such, individual risk assessment in clinical practice remains difficult with the currently available tools and strategies.

Similarly, it remains difficult to ascertain age, gender, and racial differences in CHD-related SCD events. However, it is likely that similar trends would be observed due to the substantial contribution of CHD to the overall SCD burden. In general, the incidence of SCD increases with age regardless of gender or race.[17] However, by age groups, the proportion of overall deaths classified as SCDs appears to be more significant in the young.[18] Women, in general, have a lower incidence of SCD than do men[19,20] which may reflect the lower or delayed burden of CHD in women. There also appear to be some racial differences in SCD epidemiology. Black Americans are at higher risk compared to white Americans, and Hispanic Americans are at lower risk than are non-Hispanic Americans.[11,17,21,22] Whether these variations are related to genetic or socioeconomic differences is not clear.

PATHOPHYSIOLOGY

The pathophysiology of SCD is complex but is believed to reflect the interaction of the vascular substrate, the myocardial substrate, and systemic modulation.[23] SCD events typically require a substrate and a trigger, which lead to electrical instability and lethal ventricular arrhythmia, which result in hemodynamic collapse and death (Fig. 22.1). Both the substrate and the triggers are dynamic, contributing to the clinical challenges in risk stratification.

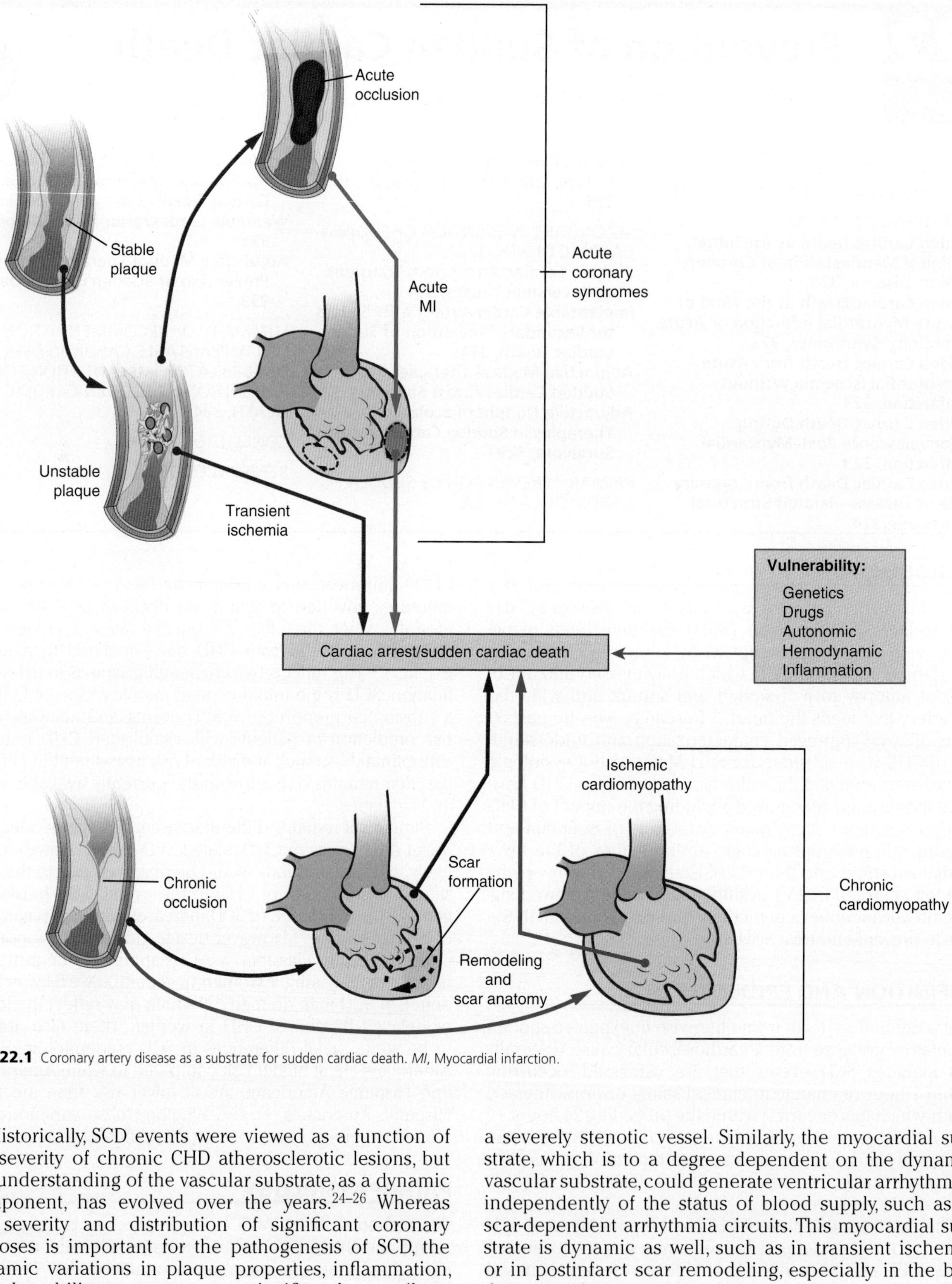

FIG. 22.1 Coronary artery disease as a substrate for sudden cardiac death. *MI*, Myocardial infarction.

Historically, SCD events were viewed as a function of the severity of chronic CHD atherosclerotic lesions, but the understanding of the vascular substrate, as a dynamic component, has evolved over the years.[24–26] Whereas the severity and distribution of significant coronary stenoses is important for the pathogenesis of SCD, the dynamic variations in plaque properties, inflammation, or vulnerability to rupture may significantly contribute to SCD. An unstable plaque, even in the absence of acute coronary syndrome (ACS) from significant lumen occlusion, may lead to spasm and could trigger arrhythmias. As such, the identification of a culprit vessel, especially postmortem, is not an easy task even in the presence of a severely stenotic vessel. Similarly, the myocardial substrate, which is to a degree dependent on the dynamic vascular substrate, could generate ventricular arrhythmias independently of the status of blood supply, such as in scar-dependent arrhythmia circuits. This myocardial substrate is dynamic as well, such as in transient ischemia or in postinfarct scar remodeling, especially in the border zones between scar and normal myocardium. The dynamic changes affecting the myocardium and its vulnerability to arrhythmias include mechanical stress and autonomic influences, which may result in transient ischemia or vulnerability of a static scar to electrical reentry and arrhythmogenesis.[23,27–29]

The contribution of CHD to SCD encompasses the spectrum of CHD and its effect on the myocardium as an arrhythmogenic substrate. Clinical settings include: (1) SCD as the initial clinical manifestation of CHD, (2) acute myocardial infarction (MI) or ACSs, (3) acute myocardial ischemia without infarction, (4) myocardial convalescence post-MI, and (5) CHD-related structural changes, such as scar formation or ventricular dilatation from prior infarction or chronic ischemia. In the latter, there is a particular role for the severity of LV dysfunction and heart failure in SCD pathogenesis.

It is estimated that approximately 25% of CHD-related SCD patients have evidence of myocardial necrosis on autopsy studies.[30,31] In sudden cardiac arrest survivors, biomarker evidence of MI is present in approximately 40% of patients,[32] which suggests that acute MI contributes to some but not all CHD-related SCD. In non-MI CHD-related SCD, the underlying mechanism is ventricular arrhythmia caused by ischemic or other arrhythmogenic triggers with an underlying diseased substrate.[16]

Sudden Cardiac Death as the Initial Clinical Manifestation of Coronary Heart Disease

This is perhaps the most challenging group for both clinicians and researchers. It is estimated that this first event category contributes approximately one-third of all SCD events, accounting for over 100,000 cases every year in the United States. Unfortunately, strategies are lacking for risk stratification and identification of subjects at risk in the general population. Risk assessment relies primarily on identifying high-risk pockets within low-risk groups. The presence of CHD risk factors carries a risk of future SCD even in the absence of clinically recognized CHD,[23,33] emphasizing the importance of risk factor control to prevent SCD in the general population.

Sudden Cardiac Death at the Time of Acute Myocardial Infarction or Acute Coronary Syndromes

This typically refers to the initial 24- to 48-hour period after the onset of an MI. Whereas it shares some features related to SCD from ischemia without infarction, elevated risk in this setting is characterized by a dynamic substrate, which is a manifestation of acute loss of blood supply; ischemia and cardiomyocyte death; abnormal local electrical activation patterns; reperfusion and dynamic heterogeneities in electrical properties in the infarct and peri-infarct zones; and systemic factors, such as inflammation, hemodynamic alterations, and neurohormonal alterations. The endpoint of these phenomena is predisposition to electrical reentry and vulnerability to ventricular arrhythmias.

The burden of arrhythmias in the acute phase of MI appears to have decreased with early interventions to restore blood flow that may reverse or at least stabilize the local arrhythmogenic process.[34]

Ventricular arrhythmias occurring in the early phase after an acute MI have been considered transient without prognostic implications for long-term risk of recurrence. This is likely related to the multitude and dynamic nature of factors that contribute to arrhythmogenesis in the acute phase of MI. However, it has been suggested in some studies that a cardiac arrest in the early phase of acute MI might indicate some long-term risk[35,36]; however, it remains unknown whether this is related to individual predisposition, recurrent ischemia, subsequent remodeling, or further deterioration in LV function. Nevertheless, ventricular arrhythmias in the first 48 hours after MI do not serve as an indication for defibrillator implantation for secondary prevention purposes.

Sudden Cardiac Death from Acute Myocardial Ischemia Without Infarction

SCD from acute myocardial ischemia without infarction is typically from a supply-demand mismatch that results in transient ischemia and increased arrhythmic risk. Scenarios include either plaque rupture with acute thrombosis limiting blood flow, or vasospasm resulting in the same, as well as high-grade stable lesions in the setting of a sudden increase in demand. The abnormalities in myocardial perfusion and associated regional variations in ischemia and reperfusion result in regional heterogeneities in electrical properties and cell membrane electrophysiology[37] with resultant vulnerability to triggered electrical activity, reentry, and SCD.

In transient ischemic states, both the ischemia and reperfusion phases are important in arrhythmogenesis, the former by creating electrical gradients across the myocardium and areas of inexcitability and the latter by affecting repolarization dispersion in affected areas.[37,38] Triggered activity from this phenomenon typically generates polymorphic ventricular tachycardia (VT) that can degenerate into ventricular fibrillation (VF) and SCD.

Sudden Cardiac Death During Convalescence Post–Myocardial Infarction

This phase typically starts beyond the first 48 hours after MI and extends for weeks, months, or even years with continuing vascular and myocardial remodeling. Ventricular arrhythmias that occur during this phase, in contrast to arrhythmic events in the early post-MI phase, are strongly associated with risk of clinical recurrence of ventricular arrhythmias and with SCD. This risk appears to be further increased by the degree of LV dysfunction and remains elevated despite modern therapies.[39,40]

Of note, not all SCD events in the early convalescence phase post-MI are arrhythmic in nature and many could be attributed to mechanical complications of the infarction, such as myocardial rupture.[41] Nonetheless, arrhythmic SCD risk in the early convalescence phase post-MI remains high and predicts later events.[40] However, defibrillator implants early after MI showed no significant benefit in terms of all-cause survival in two separate trials (Defibrillator in Acute Myocardial Infarction Trial [DINAMIT] and Immediate Risk Stratification Improves Survival Trial [IRIS]).[42,43] Although both trials showed a benefit of implantable cardioverter defibrillator (ICD) implantation in reduction of arrhythmic deaths, this was counterbalanced by a higher rate of nonarrhythmic death.

In the late convalescence period after MI, typically referring to months or years after the index event, there continues to be a risk of SCD likely related to ischemic cardiomyopathy, continued remodeling, and heart failure. This risk is lower than the early convalescence period but is primarily a function of the degree of LV dysfunction.[44]

Sudden Cardiac Death from Coronary Heart Disease–Related Structural Changes

Such changes include scar formation or ventricular dilatation from prior infarction or chronic ischemia. Whereas one-quarter of SCD cases occur in the first 3 months after an acute MI, half of all SCD cases occur beyond the year after the index event.[45,46] The incidence of SCD after acute MI appears to be similar in ST elevation and non-ST elevation MIs.[47] The risk is highest in the acute phase as previously noted but decreases gradually over time.[40,48]

A prior history of an MI increases the risk of SCD 4-fold in women and 10-fold in men.[49,50] The incidence rates of SCD after MI have declined over time with recent estimates of 1% per year in patients receiving optimal medical therapy and revascularization.[48,51,52] Despite improvements in overall mortality rates in MI survivors and the decline in SCD rates, there are still subsets of MI survivors who are considered to be at a particularly high risk.[40] The most powerful risk factors for SCD in chronic CHD are LV dysfunction and New York Heart Association (NYHA) functional class,[53] which thus form the basis for why these were used as entry criteria for clinical trials of ICDs and therefore are the primary factors affecting decisions for defibrillator implants for the primary prevention of SCD. The impact of these factors reflects their nature as clinical markers of CHD burden and the extent of damaged myocardium. However, whereas they identify high-risk subgroups in CHD, the absolute number of SCD cases from these subgroups account for only a minority of all CHD-related SCDs. Furthermore, many patients who receive defibrillators for primary prevention purposes never require therapy from their devices. These caveats emphasize the need for better strategies for risk stratification.

Risk stratification remains a topic of intense research. Multiple noninvasive markers have been evaluated for the purpose of improving individual risk prediction,[54] including clinical, imaging, electrophysiologic, genetic, and biologic markers. Although high-risk markers can be identified, clinical relevance is limited by an absence of evidence supporting use of these risk factors for selection of patients for risk-reducing therapies, such as ICD implantation. For example, in chronic ischemic heart disease and in post-MI patients, the presence of late potentials on signal-averaged electrocardiogram (ECG), reduced heart rate variability, and T-wave or repolarization alternans have been found to have significant associations with SCD, but available data have not supported incorporating these factors into the clinical criteria for ICD implantation (Table 22.1).[54]

Ischemic Cardiomyopathy, Heart Failure, and Sudden Cardiac Death

Ventricular arrhythmias are common in patients with heart failure and range from asymptomatic premature ventricular contractions to sustained VT, VF, or SCD. In patients with heart failure, progressive pump failure accounts for only one-third of all cardiovascular deaths, whereas SCD accounts for the other two-thirds and the latter is split equally between unexpected SCD or SCD during episodes of clinical worsening of heart failure.[55] The most common mechanism of SCD in this population is VT degenerating into VF.

The severity of heart failure correlates with higher overall mortality and absolute rates of SCD, but the proportion of total deaths classified as SCD decreases with worsening NYHA class. For example, in the Metoprolol CR/XL Randomized Intervention Trial in Congestive Heart Failure (MERIT-HF), NYHA class II, III, and IV were associated with 1-year mortality rates of 6.3%, 10.5%, and 18.6%, respectively, but the proportions of total deaths classified as SCDs were 64%, 59%, and 33%, respectively.[56] Also, not all sudden deaths in patients with heart failure are due to arrhythmia. In the Acute Infarction Ramipril Efficacy (AIRE) trial, only 39% of all SCD cases were thought to be due to arrhythmias.[57] Other observations in the literature suggest that arrhythmic SCD cases account for most but not all unwitnessed deaths and deaths occurring within 1 hour of onset of symptoms.[58]

SECONDARY PREVENTION OF SUDDEN CARDIAC DEATH

Secondary prevention aims to prevent SCD in patients who have survived a prior sudden cardiac arrest or sustained VT.[3]

Sudden Cardiac Arrest from Transient or Reversible Causes

Experts agree, based on available evidence,[3] that the primary goal of management in patients who survived a sudden cardiac arrest from a transient or reversible cause is to address the underlying condition or disease process. There are, however, caveats to this approach, and decision-making in clinical practice may not be straightforward. For example, it has been traditionally thought that ventricular arrhythmias in the setting of acute ischemia have low risk for future SCD and as such may not benefit from ICD implants. The reality is that these patients may have experienced a prior MI or have a significant burden of coronary disease and despite revascularization may still have a myocardial scar or large myocardial territory at risk that would be a substrate for recurrent ventricular arrhythmia. Studies have indeed demonstrated increased subsequent risks in patients with ventricular arrhythmias in the setting of acute ischemia.[35,59] Furthermore, in a subsequent analysis of the Antiarrhythmics Versus Implantable Defibrillators (AVID) trial, the mortality rate of patients who were included in the AVID registry but not randomized due to a transient or correctable cause for VT/VF was no different, or was perhaps even worse, than that of the population considered to have high-risk VT/VF in the randomized trial.[35]

As such, a careful approach to risk stratification and identification of both reversible and nonreversible causes on a case-by-case basis is valuable to optimize patient outcomes. In the specific setting of coronary disease, scar-dependent ventricular arrhythmias are mostly monomorphic tachycardia in nature, whereas arrhythmias related to acute ischemia are mostly polymorphic VT or VF. In general, patients with polymorphic VT or VF in the setting of acute ischemia should be treated with revascularization for the purpose of reducing the risk of SCD. Sustained monomorphic VTs in the setting of electrolyte abnormalities or antiarrhythmic drug use should be treated by identifying and correcting the underlying condition, but it is important not to assume that these were the only cause of sustained monomorphic VT.

Implantable Cardioverter Defibrillators for Secondary Prevention of Sudden Cardiac Death

The role of ICDs is well established for the purpose of secondary SCD prevention based on the results of randomized clinical trials (Table 22.2), which have demonstrated that implantation of ICDs in patients who have survived a sudden

TABLE 22.1 Summary of Noninvasive Risk-Stratification Techniques for Identifying Patients with Coronary Artery Disease Who Are at Risk for Sudden Cardiac Death

TECHNIQUE	CONCLUSION
Imaging	
LVEF	Low LVEF is a well-demonstrated risk factor for SCD. Although low LVEF has been effectively used to select high-risk patients for application of therapy to prevent sudden arrhythmic death, LVEF has limited sensitivity: the majority of SCDs occur in patients with more preserved LVEF.
ECG	
QRS duration	Most retrospective analyses show increased QRS duration is likely a risk factor for SCD. Clinical utility to guide selection of therapy has not been tested.
QT interval and QT dispersion	Data from some retrospective analyses show that abnormalities in cardiac repolarization are risk factors for SCD. Clinical utility to guide selection of therapy has not yet been tested.
SAECG	An abnormal SAECG is likely a risk factor for SCD, based predominantly on prospective analyses. Clinical utility to guide selection of therapy has been tested, but not yet demonstrated.
Short-term HRV	Limited data link impaired short-term HRV to increased risk for SCD. Clinical utility to guide selection of therapy has not yet been tested.
Long-Term Ambulatory ECG Recording (Holter)	
Ventricular ectopy and NSVT	The presence of ventricular arrhythmias (VPBs, NSVT) on Holter monitoring is a well-demonstrated risk factor for SCD. In some populations, the presence of NSVT has been effectively used to select high-risk patients for application of therapy to prevent sudden arrhythmic death. This may also have limited sensitivity.
Long-term HRV	Low HRV is a risk factor for mortality, but unlikely to be specific for SCD. Clinical utility to guide selection of therapy has been tested, but not demonstrated.
Heart rate turbulence	Emerging data show that abnormal heart rate turbulence is a likely risk factor for SCD. Clinical utility to guide selection of therapy has been tested, but not yet demonstrated.
Exercise Test/Functional Status	
Exercise capacity and NYHA class	Increasing severity of heart failure is a likely risk factor for SCD, although it may be more predictive of risk for progressive pump failure. Clinical utility to guide selection of therapy has not yet been tested.
Heart rate recovery and recovery ventricular ectopy	Limited data show that low heart rate recovery and ventricular ectopy during recovery are risk factors for SCD. Clinical utility to guide selection of therapy has not yet been tested.
T-wave alternans	A moderate amount of prospective data suggests that abnormal T-wave alternans is a risk factor for SCD. Clinical utility to guide selection of therapy has been evaluated, but the results to date are inconsistent.
BRS	A moderate amount of data suggests that low BRS is a risk factor for SCD. Clinical utility to guide selection of therapy has not yet been tested.

BRS, Baroreceptor sensitivity; *ECG*, electrocardiogram; *HRV*, heart rate variability; *LVEF*, left ventricular ejection fraction; *NSVT*, nonsustained ventricular tachycardia; *NYHA*, New York Heart Association; *SAECG*, signal-averaged ECG; *SCD*, sudden cardiac death; *VPB*, ventricular premature beats.
From Goldberger JJ, Cain ME, Hohnloser SH, et al. AHA/ACC/HRS scientific statement on noninvasive risk stratification techniques for identifying patients at risk for sudden cardiac death. J Am Coll Cardiol. *2008;52:1179–1199.*

TABLE 22.2 Randomized Clinical Trials of Implantable Cardioverter Defibrillators for Secondary Prevention of Sudden Cardiac Death and Which Included Patients with Chronic Coronary Disease

	N	% CHD	DESIGN	POPULATION	HR
AVID (1997)	1016	> 80%	ICD vs. class III AAD	Resuscitated VF, cardioverted VT, VT with syncope or VT with LVEF ≤ 40% and symptoms of hemodynamic compromise	0.62 ($p < 0.02$)
CASH (2000)	288	> 70%	ICD vs. amiodarone vs. metoprolol	Resuscitated cardiac arrest from documented sustained ventricular arrhythmias	0.77 ($p = 0.08$)
CIDS (2000)	659	> 80%	ICD vs. amiodarone	Resuscitated VF or VT or unmonitored syncope	0.80 ($p = 0.1$)

AAD, Antiarrhythmic drug; *CHD*, coronary heart disease; *HR*, hazard ratio of mortality with implantable cardioverter defibrillator implant; *ICD*, implantable cardioverter defibrillator; *LVEF*, left ventricular ejection fraction; *VF*, ventricular fibrillation; *VT*, ventricular tachycardia.

cardiac arrest or experienced sustained VT results in reductions in SCD and total mortality compared to antiarrhythmic medications.[3,60–67] An algorithm for ICD use for secondary prevention of SCD in patients with coronary artery disease (CAD) is presented in Fig. 22.2. The use of ICDs for secondary prevention of SCD within 40 days after MI or 90 days after coronary revascularization is shown in Figs. 22.3 and 22.4.

AVID: Antiarrhythmics Versus Implantable Defibrillators Trial

In the pivotal secondary prevention randomized trial, AVID,[60] 1016 patients with resuscitated VF, sustained VT with syncope or sustained VT with hemodynamic compromise or symptoms suggesting hemodynamic instability in the setting of LV dysfunction (left ventricular ejection fraction

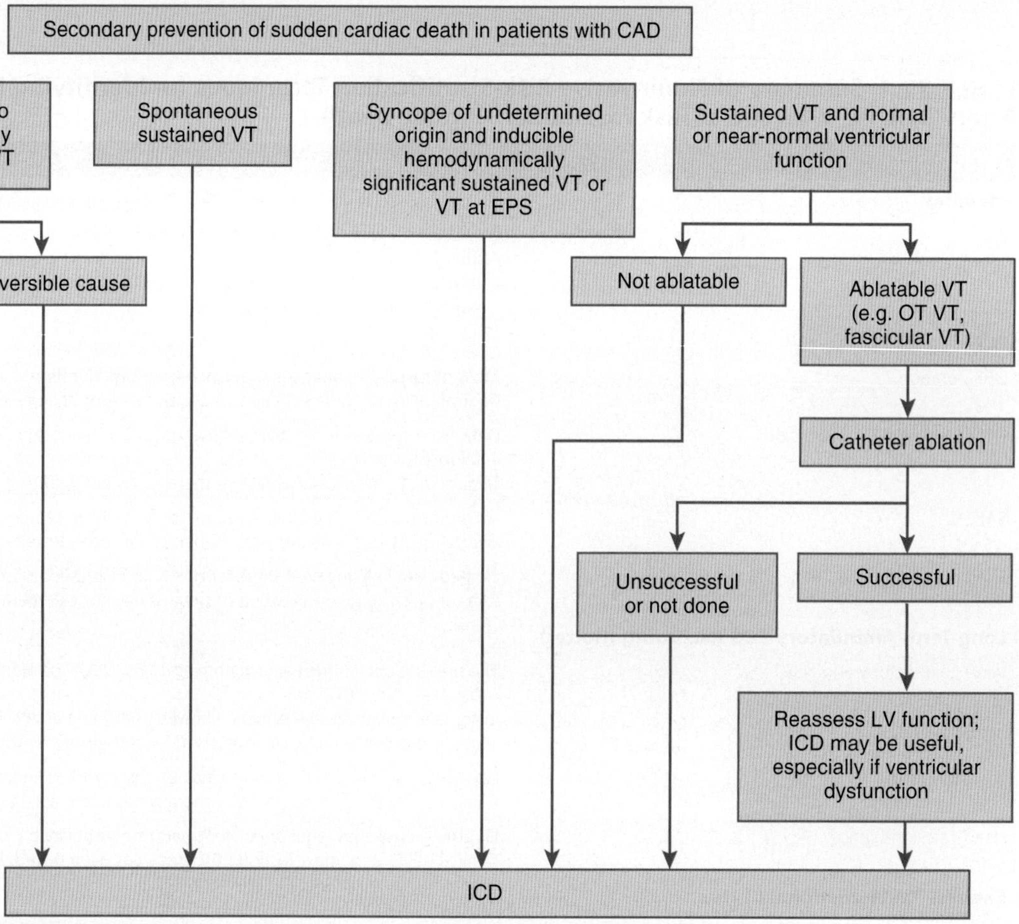

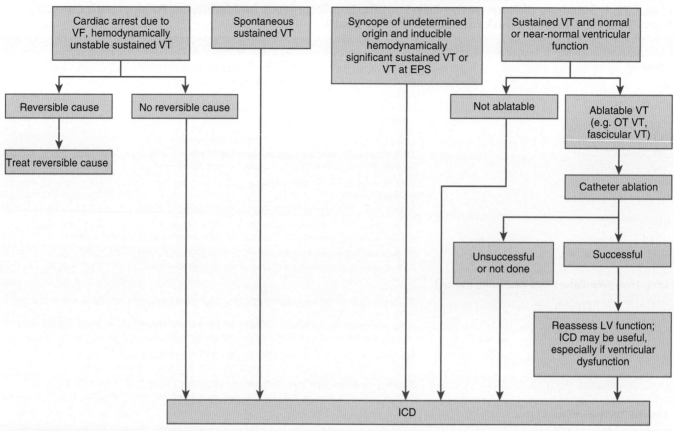

FIG. 22.2 Implantable cardioverter defibrillators for the secondary prevention of sudden cardiac death in patients with coronary artery disease. *CAD*, Coronary artery disease; *EPS*, electrophysiologic study; *ICD*, implantable cardioverter defibrillator; *LV*, left ventricular; *OT*, outflow tract; *VF*, ventricular fibrillation; *VT*, ventricular tachycardia. *(Modified from Olshansky B, Chung MK, Pogwizd S, Goldschlager N.* Arrhythmia Essentials. *Philadelphia: Elsevier; 2017.)*

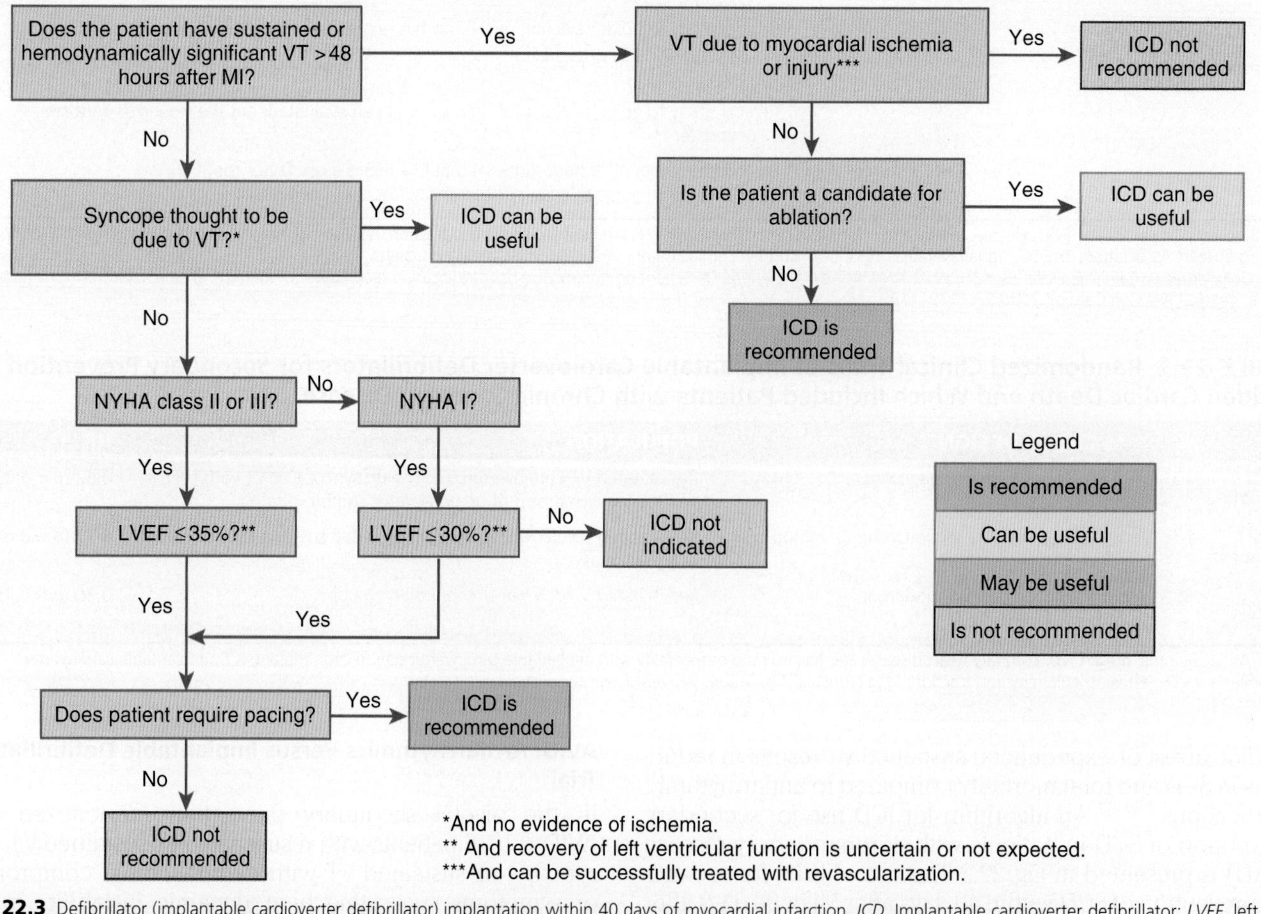

FIG. 22.3 Defibrillator (implantable cardioverter defibrillator) implantation within 40 days of myocardial infarction. *ICD*, Implantable cardioverter defibrillator; *LVEF*, left ventricular ejection fraction; *MI*, myocardial infarction; *NYHA*, New York Heart Association; *VT*, ventricular tachycardia. *(Modified with permission from Kusumoto FM, et al. HRS/ACC/AHA expert consensus statement on the use of implantable cardioverter-defibrillator therapy in patients who are not included or not well represented in clinical trials.* Heart Rhythm. *2014;11:1270–1313.)*

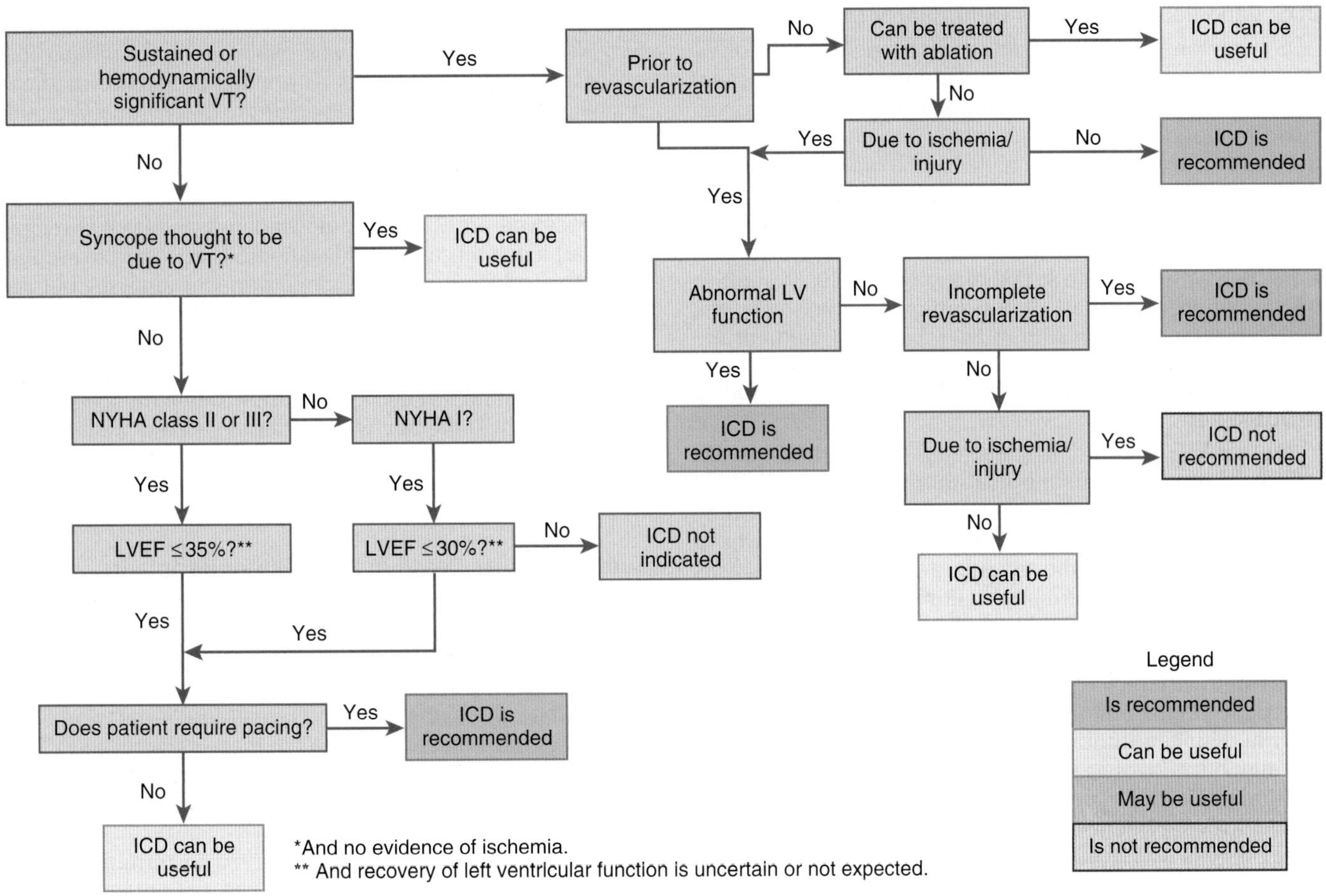

FIG. 22.4 Defibrillator (implantable cardioverter defibrillator) implantation within 90 days of revascularization. *ICD*, Implantable cardioverter defibrillator; *LVEF*, left ventricular ejection fraction; *NYHA*, New York Heart Association; *VT*, ventricular tachycardia. *(Modified with permission from Kusumoto FM, et al. HRS/ACC/AHA expert consensus statement on the use of implantable cardioverter-defibrillator therapy in patients who are not included or not well represented in clinical trials.* Heart Rhythm. *2014;11:1270–1313.)*

[LVEF] < 40%) were randomized to treatment with a defibrillator implant or antiarrhythmic medications sotalol or amiodarone. The primary endpoint of the trial was all-cause mortality. The majority of patients enrolled in this trial had coronary disease (81% in both arms), prior MI (67% in both arms), or significant LV dysfunction (median LVEF 31%).

The overall survival was greater with ICDs, with unadjusted estimates of 89.3% versus 82.3% in the antiarrhythmic drug group at 1 year, 81.6% versus 74.7% at 2 years, and 75.4% versus 64.1% at 3 years ($p < 0.02$). This corresponded to relative reductions in mortality of 39%, 24%, and 31% at 1, 2, and 3 years, respectively. In subset analyses, the benefit of defibrillator therapy was primarily in patients with CHD as the underlying cause of their arrhythmias. The trial was stopped prematurely due to the observed significant survival benefit with ICD implants. The primary effect of ICDs was prevention of arrhythmic death compared with antiarrhythmics, but the rates of nonarrhythmic death were equivalent in the treatment arms. To be noted also was that patients treated with antiarrhythmics appeared to be at greater risk of noncardiac death, such as deaths related to pulmonary or renal disease.[68]

A subsequent analysis of AVID[69] found that in patients with LVEF greater than 35%, there were no differences in outcomes between the treatment arms, whereas in patients with LVEF values between 20% and 35%, there was a clear and significant survival benefit of ICDs over medical therapy at 2 years (83% vs. 72%). The same extent of difference was observed in the small subset with LVEF less than 20% but the analysis did not have enough power to detect statistical difference.

CASH: Cardiac Arrest Survival in Hamburg Trial

CASH[65] was a prospective, multicenter, randomized trial for the comparison of implantable defibrillators versus antiarrhythmic drug therapy in survivors of cardiac arrest secondary to documented ventricular arrhythmias. The study randomized 349 survivors of cardiac arrest from documented VT or VF to treatment with an ICD, metoprolol, propafenone, or amiodarone. Assignment to propafenone was discontinued during the trial due to an observed 61% higher all-cause mortality rate in propafenone versus ICD patients upon follow-up of 11.3 months. The primary endpoint of the trial was all-cause mortality. Coronary disease was present in approximately 75% of the patients enrolled in the trial. Over a mean follow-up of 57 months, the all-cause death rates were 36.4% in the ICD arm and 44.4% in the amiodarone/metoprolol arm. The overall survival was higher in the ICD arm but did not reach statistical significance likely due to lack of power, as the mean LVEF was 46%, indicating a healthier population than in AVID, and accordingly the 19.6% 2-year mortality rate was under half that used to calculate trial sample size. Nevertheless, the secondary endpoint of SCD was significantly reduced with ICD implants compared to medical therapy (13% vs. 33%). The trial also noted that the benefit of ICD therapy appears to be primarily during the first 5 years after the index event.

CIDS: Canadian Implantable Defibrillator Study

CIDS[61] randomized 659 patients with resuscitated VF or VT or with unmonitored syncope to treatment with ICD implant or amiodarone. The primary outcome of the trial was all-cause mortality, and the secondary outcome was arrhythmic death. The proportion of patients with coronary disease exceeded 80% in both the ICD and medical therapy arms, with the majority having experienced a prior MI. Over 5 years of follow-up, the trial found a nonsignificant reduction in the risk of death with ICD therapy with a 19.7% relative risk reduction, as well as a nonsignificant reduction in the risk of arrhythmic death with 32.8% relative risk reduction.

Cumulative Data of Landmark Trials and Generalizability of Outcomes

Whereas AVID showed a statistically significant benefit with ICD implant versus medical therapy, CIDS and CASH showed a nonsignificant trend toward benefit, which may have reflected a beta error and lack of statistical power to detect significance in the magnitude of benefit that was observed, different patient populations, or longer follow-up time in CIDS. It is also possible that patients who were considered by their managing physicians to be better candidates for ICD therapy than antiarrhythmics may have been referred for defibrillator implant rather than enrollment in the trial with randomization. This would introduce a bias that may have favored the outcomes in the medical intervention arm.

Conclusive evidence regarding the benefit of ICDs in these patients was observed in a meta-analysis of the three major trials and a fourth trial with a smaller population (Fig. 22.5).[70] When combined in a meta-analysis, data showed that patients with ICDs had a survival advantage over those treated with medical therapy with a 25% reduction in relative risk. This was primarily related to a positive effect on SCD rates, with a 50% relative risk reduction from this mode in death with ICDs. An important observation is that of an absolute risk reduction of 7% in all-cause mortality, which translates into a number needed to treat of 15 that supersedes most clinical trials in modern cardiovascular medicine.

The findings were reproduced in a second meta-analysis of AVID, CIDS, and CASH with a 28% relative risk reduction in all-cause mortality and a 50% reduction in sudden arrhythmic death and a superior benefit in patients with LVEF below 35% compared to those with LVEF above 35%.[64] The generalizability of these benefits was explored by examining the effectiveness of defibrillators as applied in routine medical practice in a large cohort of patients from the National Veterans Administration database.[71] For 3 years the study followed 6996 patients with new-onset ventricular arrhythmia and preexisting ischemic heart disease and congestive heart failure, of which 1442 received an ICD. The main finding was that ICD recipients had lower all-cause (odds ratio 0.52) and cardiovascular mortality (odds ratio 0.56) in multivariable analyses but no difference in noncardiovascular mortality. These benefits were observed despite a significantly lower frequency of use of angiotensin-converting enzyme inhibitors (ACE-I), β-blockers, and statins. An important observation was that the magnitude of benefit of ICD therapy was similar to or even greater than that observed in the clinical trials, with a finding that one death was prevented in this population for every four to five patients receiving an ICD over three years of follow-up.

Sudden Cardiac Death in Defibrillator Recipients

SCD due to nonarrhythmic causes (such as pulseless electrical activity, pulmonary embolus, or aortic dissection) or SCD from terminal cardiac arrhythmias can still occur in ICD recipients. In the secondary prevention trials of SCD, up to one-third of all deaths in the ICD treatment arms were SCD. The most common cause of SCD in these patients was VT or VF, which is treated appropriately by a defibrillator shock but is followed by electromechanical dissociation and pulseless electrical activity.[72]

Refractory arrhythmias are observed in terminal stages of heart failure and may still occur in patients with ICDs despite the proper function of ICDs. In this population, further treatment options include advanced heart failure therapies and consideration for heart transplant. Other factors that could lead to SCD despite ICD implants include ventricular arrhythmias, which fall under the detection limit of the device, and very rarely failure of the ICD in detecting the arrhythmia or delivering appropriate therapy.

Adjunctive Medical Therapies in Sudden Cardiac Arrest Survivors

No medical therapy is considered to be an acceptable alternative to ICD implants in SCD survivors. That being said,

Study	Defibrillator n/N	Conventional n/N	RR (95% CI fixed)	Weight %	RR (95% CI fixed)
Wever 1995	4/29	11/31		3.7	0.39 (0.14, 1.08)
AVID 1997	80/507	122/509		42.3	0.66 (0.51, 0.85)
CASH 2000	36/99	84/189		20.1	0.82 (0.60, 1.11)
CIDS 2000	83/328	98/331		33.9	0.85 (0.67, 1.10)
Total (95% CI)	**203/963**	**315/1060**		**100.0**	**0.75 (0.64, 0.87)**

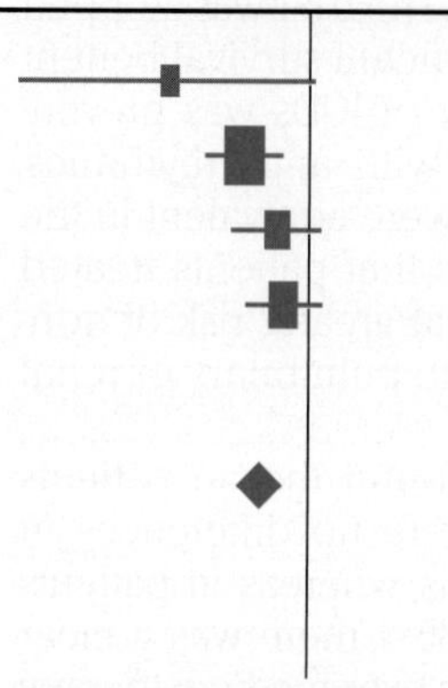

Test for heterogeneity chi-square = 3.97 df = 3 $p = 0.26$

Test for overall effect z = −3.75 $p = 0.26$

FIG. 22.5 All-cause mortality in pooled secondary prevention defibrillator trials. *CI*, Confidence interval; *df*, degree of freedom; *n/N*, sample/population size; *RR*, risk ratio. *(Reproduced with permission from Lee DS, Green LD, Liu PP, et al. Effectiveness of implantable defibrillators for preventing arrhythmic events and death: a meta-analysis.* J Am Coll Cardiol. *2003;41:1573–1582.)*

optimal medical therapy to address specific underlying conditions may contribute to further reductions in both cardiovascular mortality and SCD in this population.[3]

Antiarrhythmic Drugs

In patients who have survived a sudden cardiac arrest or experienced sustained ventricular arrhythmias but have declined ICD implants, antiarrhythmic drugs could be used as an alternative to ICDs to reduce arrhythmia burden. Among patients who receive ICDs for the secondary prevention of SCD, many experience recurrent ventricular arrhythmias that trigger appropriate defibrillator shocks. Antiarrhythmic medications may reduce the need for defibrillator shocks in these patients and therefore improve the quality of life. In this population with structural heart disease, antiarrhythmic medication options are limited to amiodarone, sotalol, or mexilitene,[3] with amiodarone being the preferred agent due to superior efficacy and lower proarrhythmic effects compared to sotalol. However, amiodarone's side effects profile with long-term use of this medication make sotalol and mexiletine acceptable alternatives in select scenarios, despite lower efficacy. Amiodarone can raise the defibrillation threshold, whereas sotalol may decrease it, and these effects may be important in patients with high defibrillation thresholds. Also, the potent β-blockade effects of sotalol can limit its use in patients with marginally or poorly compensated heart failure.

The need for adjunctive antiarrhythmic therapy in patients who have received an ICD for the secondary prevention of SCD is not uncommon and was reported to have been used in the ICD therapy arms in 22% of AVID patients at 2 years and 28% of CIDS patients at 5 years.[60,61]

The addition of antiarrhythmic medications aims primarily to improve quality of life and reduce shocks, but shock prevention has not been found to improve survival in a systematic review that included 6000 ICD recipients.[73]

In this population of patients, antiarrhythmic drugs might also be indicated for the treatment of supraventricular arrhythmias, which could lead to inappropriate defibrillator shocks, especially for atrial fibrillation. With modern programming, there have been reductions in the rates of inappropriate shocks, but control of supraventricular arrhythmias might improve quality of life for patients regardless of reduction of inappropriate shocks.

β-Blockers

Among patients with coronary disease, those with prior MI and LV dysfunction or heart failure may derive survival benefit from β-blocker therapy, which may also include improvement in SCD risk as a subset of modes of death. In patients with recurrent ventricular arrhythmias, β-blockers may suppress the adrenergic drive associated with these arrhythmias. Moreover, in many patients with heart failure, β-blocker therapy may prevent recurrent clinical heart failure episodes, which are known to be periods of increased risk of arrhythmia recurrence. Furthermore, β-blockers may reduce inappropriate shocks from atrial fibrillation or sinus tachycardia with rapid ventricular rates in these patients.

In patients who survived a sudden cardiac arrest but were not enrolled in AVID, β-blocker use was associated with a survival benefit.[74] The same study found that this protective effect was not prominent in patients already receiving amiodarone or a defibrillator.

Lipid-Lowering Medications

Patients with coronary disease should be treated with lipid-lowering agents in concordance with the corresponding clinical guidelines. The use of lipid-lowering agents for the purpose of reducing SCD remains controversial but available data suggest benefit.[75,76] In patients with CHD who have received an ICD in AVID, lipid-lowering therapy was found to be associated with a 60% relative reduction in the probability of VT/VF recurrence.[75] Another observational study showed that the use of lipid-lowering drugs was associated with a reduction of recurrences of ventricular arrhythmias in patients with coronary disease and ICD implants.[76]

To date, there are no clinical trial data to suggest an independent antiarrhythmic benefit from use of statins. Similarly, regarding antiarrhythmic benefits of fish oil, a meta-analysis showed no reduction in defibrillator discharges with use of fish oil or omega-3 fatty acids.[77]

Adjunctive Nonpharmacologic Therapies in Sudden Cardiac Arrest Survivors

Catheter Ablation

Catheter ablation is a treatment option for ventricular arrhythmias. In patients with CHD who had survived a sudden cardiac arrest, catheter ablation for ventricular arrhythmias could be performed as adjunctive therapy for frequent ventricular arrhythmias triggering ICD shocks, as an alternative for patients who decline ICD implantation, or in patients with cardiomyopathy and bundle branch reentrant VT, which is typically treated by ablation of the right bundle.

Catheter ablation has been associated with better outcomes for VTs from ischemic heart disease versus nonischemic substrate. In patients with prior MI, sustained monomorphic VTs typically originate from a scar substrate, primarily in the border zone areas of the scar where scar tissue is dispersed among surviving bundles of myocytes. This substrate is amenable to endocardial catheter ablation, which would ideally target the critical isthmus of reentry when addressing the clinical VT. Additional substrate modification is performed by many experts in the field.[78] A trial published in 2015[79] showed that an extensive substrate-based ablation approach is superior to ablation targeting only clinical and stable VTs in patients with ischemic cardiomyopathy presenting with tolerated VT. In our practice, every effort is made to map and target the clinical VT in addition to substrate modification.

Catheter ablation may also be effective for the treatment of VF that is triggered by premature ventricular depolarizations, especially if they appear to be uniform in morphology.[80] Such triggers could originate from the His-Purkinje system in patients with coronary disease, especially the posterior fascicle. Whereas ischemia in this territory could be the underlying cause of premature ventricular depolarizations leading to VF, there are instances with no identifiable revascularization target or persistence of the problem despite revascularization. Catheter ablation targeting the premature ventricular depolarization trigger may be successful in abolishing recurrent VF in these patients.

Catheter ablation has also been evaluated as a prophylactic adjunctive therapy in patients who had experienced sustained VT and received ICD therapy. A meta-analysis of these

TABLE 22.3 Randomized Clinical Trials of Defibrillators for Primary Prevention of Sudden Cardiac Death and Which Included Patients with Chronic Coronary Disease

	N	% CHD	DESIGN	POPULATION	TIMING	HR
MADIT (1996)	196	100%	ICD vs. conventional medical therapy	Prior MI; LVEF ≤ 35%; NSVT; inducible nonsuppressible sustained VT/VF at EPS	> 3 weeks post-MI > 2 months post-CABG > 3 months post-PTCA	0.46 (p = 0.009)
MUSTT (1999)	704	100%	EP-guided therapy with AADs or ICD or no AAD therapy	CAD; LVEF ≤ 40%; Asx NSVT; inducible sustained ventricular tachyarrhythmia	≥ 4 days post-MI or revascularization	0.40 (p < 0.001)
MADIT-II (2002)	1232	100%	ICD vs. conventional medical therapy	Prior MI LVEF ≤ 30%	> 1 month post-MI > 3 months post-revascularization	0.69 (p = 0.02)
SCDHeFT (2005)	2521	52%	ICD vs. amiodarone vs. placebo	NYHA FC II-III, LVEF ≤ 35%	> 3 months' heart failure	0.77 (p = 0.007)
CABGPatch (1997)	900	100%	Epicardial ICD vs. no ICD	CABG, LVEF ≤ 35%, abnormal SAECG	At time of CABG	1.07 (NS)
DINAMIT (2004)	674	100%	ICD vs. no ICD	Recent MI, LVEF ≤ 35% ↓HRV or average heart rate ≥ 80 bpm	6–40 days post-MI	1.08 (p = 0.7)
IRIS (2009)	898	100%	ICD vs. no ICD	Recent MI, LVEF ≤ 40% and heart rate > 90 bpm or NSVT > 150 bpm	3–31 days post-MI	1.04 (p = 0.8)

AAD, Antiarrhythmic drug; *Asx*, asymptomatic; *bpm*, beats per minute; *CABG*, coronary artery bypass graft surgery; *EP*, electrophysiologic; *EPS*, electrophysiology studies; *HR*, hazard ratio of mortality with implantable cardioverter defibrillator implant; *HRV*, heart rate variability; *ICD*, implantable cardioverter defibrillator; *LVEF*, left ventricular ejection fraction; *MI*, myocardial infarction; *NS*, nonsignificant; *NSVT*, nonsustained ventricular tachycardia; *NYHA FC*, New York Heart Association functional class; *PTCA*, percutaneous transluminal coronary angioplasty; *SAECG*, signal-averaged ECG; *VF*, ventricular fibrillation; *VT*, ventricular tachycardia.

studies[81] showed that prophylactic VT ablation decreased VT recurrence but had no effect on mortality.

Surgical Interventions

With advancements in defibrillator therapies and catheter intervention, surgery for ventricular arrhythmia is rarely performed nowadays and is typically reserved for patients with recurrent ventricular arrhythmias and defibrillator shocks who have failed adjunctive medical therapies and catheter ablation. Surgical approaches to ventricular arrhythmias in patients with prior MI include resection of the scar substrate or aneurysm surgery with or without concomitant mapping.

In refractory cases, cardiac transplantation may be indicated in select candidates. Conversely, in patients awaiting cardiac transplantation who experience a sudden cardiac arrest or sustained ventricular arrhythmias, ICD implantation may be used as a bridge to transplantation with resultant improvement in survival.[82–86]

PRIMARY PREVENTION OF SUDDEN CARDIAC DEATH

Primary prevention aims to prevent SCD in high-risk patients who have not experienced a prior sudden cardiac arrest or sustained VT.[3]

Implantable Cardioverter Defibrillators for Primary Prevention of Sudden Cardiac Death

In patients with CHD, the role of ICDs has been established by evidence from randomized trials in those with ischemic cardiomyopathy and heart failure (Table 22.3). This population has an increased risk of ventricular arrhythmia, and SCD may be the first manifestation of ventricular arrhythmia in this group.[3] Randomized trials support the use of ICDs in select high-risk patients for the purpose of primary prevention of SCD, whereas antiarrhythmic medication other than β-blockers does not appear to improve survival. An algorithm for use of ICDs in the primary prevention of SCD in patients with CAD is presented in Fig. 22.6. The use of ICDs for primary prevention of SCD within 40 days after MI or 90 days after coronary revascularization is included in Figs. 22.3 and 22.4.

MADIT: Multicenter Automatic Defibrillator Implantation Trial

MADIT[87] assessed whether prophylactic therapy with an implanted defibrillator, as compared with conventional medical therapy, would improve survival in certain high-risk patients. Eligibility criteria were NYHA functional class I, II, or III; prior MI; LVEF less than or equal to 35%; documented asymptomatic nonsustained VT; and inducible, nonsuppressible ventricular tachyarrhythmia upon electrophysiologic testing. The trial randomized 196 patients to receive an ICD or conventional medical therapy. Amiodarone was used in most patients in the medical intervention arm. During 27 months of follow-up, ICD implantation was associated with a 54% relative risk reduction in overall mortality, cardiac mortality, and arrhythmic deaths compared with medical therapy. Post hoc analyses of the MADIT trial suggested that this survival benefit is primarily in a select group with a higher risk profile, such as severely depressed LV function (LVEF < 26%), intraventricular conduction delay, and clinical heart failure requiring therapy.[88,89]

The trial was limited by the small size and low incidence of primary outcome events, as well as a potential referral bias with selection of patients who may not respond to antiarrhythmics, given that nonsupressibility in the electrophysiology laboratory with procainamide was an enrollment criterion. Moreover, the trial had concluded that there was no evidence to suggest that amiodarone, β-blockers, or any other antiarrhythmic therapy had a significant influence on the observed outcomes, but more patients in the defibrillator arm were taking β-blockers on both short- and long-term follow-up, and, as such, the possibility of residual confounding and possible survival benefit from β-blockers could not be ignored. Nonetheless, this remains a landmark trial that set grounds for larger trials with robust methodology and simpler risk stratification.

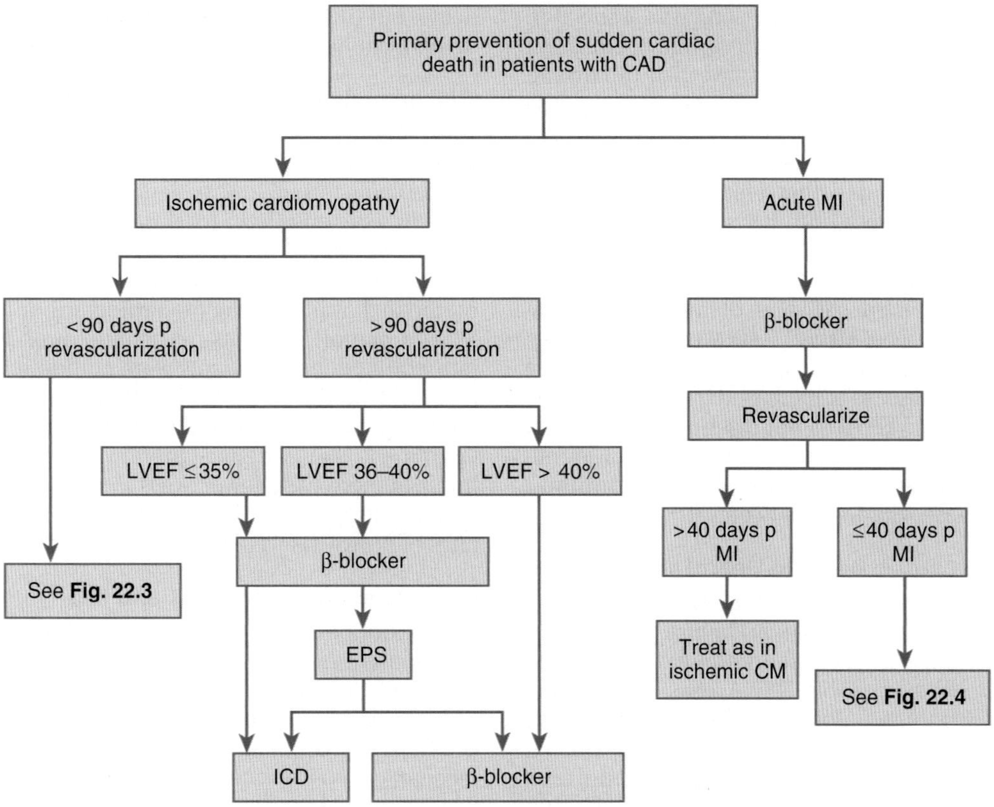

FIG. 22.6 Implantable cardioverter defibrillators for the primary prevention of sudden cardiac death in patients with coronary artery disease. *CAD*, Coronary artery disease; *CM*, cardiomyopathy; *EPS*, electrophysiology studies; *ICD*, implantable cardioverter defibrillator; *LVEF*, left ventricular ejection fraction; *MI*, myocardial infarction; *P*, post. *(Modified from Olshansky B, Chung MK, Pogwizd S, Goldschlager N.* Arrhythmia Essentials. *Philadelphia: Elsevier: 2018.)*

MADIT-II Trial

MADIT-II[90] was designed to evaluate the effect of ICDs in patients with reduced LV function and a prior MI. The trial randomized 1232 patients with a prior MI, which had occurred more than 30 days prior to enrollment (> 90 days if coronary bypass surgery was performed), and an LVEF of 30% or less to receive an ICD or conventional medical therapy. In contrast to the first MADIT trial, invasive electrophysiologic testing for risk stratification was not required in MADIT-II, and documentation of nonsustained VT was not an inclusion criterion. The primary endpoint of the trial was all-cause mortality. The trial was stopped early due to survival benefit in the ICD arm, observed after an average follow-up of 20 months. The all-cause mortality rates were 19.8% in the medical therapy arm and 14.2% in the ICD group with a relative risk reduction of 31%, which was statistically significant. In subgroup analyses, there seemed to be a benefit from ICD therapy regardless of age, sex, LVEF, NYHA class, and the QRS interval. The survival benefit with ICD implantation was primarily from reduction of SCD rates (3.8% vs. 10.0%).

Of note in the ICD group, more patients required hospitalization for clinical heart failure, which could have been related to improved survival and natural progression of myocardial dysfunction or the impact of unplanned right ventricular pacing with subsequent dyssynchrony.

CABG Patch: Coronary Artery Bypass Graft Patch Trial

CABG Patch[91] aimed to evaluate the effect on survival of prophylactic defibrillator implants at the time of coronary bypass graft surgery (CABG) in patients with coronary disease, LV dysfunction, and abnormalities on signal-averaged electrocardiograms. The study randomized 900 patients who were referred for elective bypass surgery and had LVEF of less than 36% and abnormal signal-averaged electrocardiograms to receive an epicardial ICD or no ICD at the time of surgery. During an average follow-up of 32 months, the study found no benefit in the ICD arm in terms of overall and cardiovascular mortality. It is possible that this could have been related to a survival benefit that bypass surgery provides regardless of ICD implantation, improvements in LV function after coronary bypass, or adverse effects from addition of an epicardial ICD system. In current clinical practice, ICDs are not recommended in the first 90 days after revascularization, and transvenous or subcutaneous ICDs have replaced the need for epicardial systems.

MUSTT: Multicenter Unsustained Tachycardia Trial

MUSTT[92] aimed to assess the utility of electrophysiologic testing to further guide therapy in certain patients at high risk for SCD. The trial was not primarily a defibrillator trial but provided significant insights about management of certain high-risk patients. MUSTT enrolled patients with a prior MI (which had occurred more than 4 days prior to enrollment), asymptomatic nonsustained VT at least 4 days post-MI or postrevascularization but within 6 months of enrollment, LVEF of 40% or less, and inducible sustained VT upon invasive electrophysiologic testing. Patients who met the enrollment criteria were randomized to receive either antiarrhythmic therapy, including drugs and implantable defibrillators, as indicated by the results of electrophysiologic testing, or no antiarrhythmic therapy. In this trial, ACE-I and β-blockers were administered if the patients could tolerate them. The primary endpoint was cardiac arrest or death from arrhythmia. After a median follow-up of 39 months, therapy guided by electrophysiologic testing was associated with a 27% relative risk reduction of the primary endpoint compared to standard therapy. The relative risk of cardiac arrest or death from arrhythmia was 76% lower among ICD recipients than among those patients discharged without an ICD, and this accounted for a large extent of the overall trial findings. The study concluded that electrophysiologically guided antiarrhythmic therapy with ICDs, but not with antiarrhythmic drugs, reduces the risk of sudden death in high-risk patients with coronary disease.

To further assess the prognostic value of inducible arrhythmia, a subsequent analysis of MUSTT[93] showed that both low ejection fraction and inducible tachyarrhythmias identified patients with coronary disease at increased mortality risk. The analysis suggested that LVEF does not discriminate between modes of death, whereas inducible tachyarrhythmia identifies patients in whom death is more likely to be arrhythmic, especially among those with LVEF between 30% and 40%.

SCD-HeFT: Sudden Cardiac Death in Heart Failure

SCD-HeFT[94] evaluated the impact of amiodarone versus defibrillator implants in patients with heart failure. The primary endpoint of SCD-HeFT was all-cause mortality. The trial randomly assigned 2521 patients with NYHA class II or III heart failure of at least 3 months' duration after treatment with ACE-I and β-blocker therapy (as tolerated) and LVEF of 35% or less to conventional medical therapy plus placebo, conventional therapy plus amiodarone, or conventional therapy plus a conservatively programmed, shock-only, single-lead ICD. The study included patients with either ischemic or nonischemic cardiomyopathy. Patients with coronary disease and ischemic cardiomyopathy comprised 52% of all enrolled patients. Over a median follow-up of 45.5 months, death rates were 29%, 28%, and 22% in the placebo, amiodarone, and ICD groups, respectively, which translated into similar mortality risks between amiodarone and placebo, but a survival benefit with ICDs compared to placebo with a relative risk reduction of 23%. The results did not vary based on whether patients had ischemic or nonischemic cardiomyopathy with an observed 21% relative risk reduction in the ischemic cardiomyopathy group. The survival benefit with ICD implant in this trial was primarily observed in NYHA class II but not class III patients in subgroup analyses.

DINAMIT: Defibrillator in Acute Myocardial Infarction Trial

The MADIT trials enrolled patients at least 3 weeks or 1 month after MI. DINAMIT[95] aimed to assess the benefit of early post-MI ICD implantation. The study enrolled 674 patients with recent MI (6 to 40 days), LVEF below 35%, and impaired cardiac autonomic function manifested by depressed heart-rate variability or an elevated average 24-hour heart rate (≥ 80 beats/minute) on Holter monitoring. The trial excluded any patients with sustained VT that occurred beyond 48 hours after MI, those with NYHA class IV heart failure, and those who had undergone CABG or three-vessel percutaneous coronary intervention post-MI. Enrolled patients were randomized to receive an ICD with conventional medical therapy or medical therapy alone. The primary endpoint of the trial was all-cause mortality, and a predefined secondary endpoint was the occurrence of arrhythmic death. During a mean follow-up of 30 months, the study found no difference in overall mortality between the treatment groups. ICD implantation was associated with a reduction in arrhythmic death, but this survival benefit was offset by an increase in death from nonarrhythmic causes in ICD recipients.

IRIS: Immediate Risk Stratification Improves Survival Trial

IRIS was the second trial[42] to assess the role of defibrillator implants in high-risk patients shortly after MI. In IRIS, 898 patients were enrolled 5 to 31 days after MI if they had at least one of two criteria: (1) LVEF less than or equal to 40% and a resting heart rate greater than or equal to 90 beats per minute on the first available electrocardiogram, or (2) nonsustained VT at a rate of 150 beats per minute or above during Holter monitoring. Eligible patients were randomly assigned to treatment with an ICD or to medical therapy alone. During a mean follow-up of 37 months, the overall mortality rates were similar in the ICD and medical therapy arms. Similar to DINAMIT findings, there were fewer SCDs in the ICD group than in the control group with a relative risk reduction of 69%, but the rates of non-SCDs were higher in the ICD arm.

Lack of Benefit in DINAMIT and IRIS

The lack of benefit in early post-MI ICD trials for the purpose of primary prevention of SCD compared to late post-MI trials could be attributed to a number of reasons including: (1) possible recovery of LV function, which could dilute the benefit of ICDs, (2) possibility of deaths from recurrent ischemia or mechanical complications,[96] both of which are not prevented by ICD implants, (3) the enrollment of patients with abnormal autonomic profiles, as reflected by reduced heart rate variability in DINAMIT and resting heart rate of 90 beats per minute or greater in IRIS, may have selected patients at risk of nonarrhythmic deaths, and possibly (4) additional risk from ICD implantation in the early post-MI period. Whereas these explanations are hypothetical in nature, the findings of DINAMIT and IRIS are the primary reason why, in current clinical practice guidelines, ICD implants are not routinely recommended for primary prevention purposes until at least 40 days after an MI.

Shock Avoidance in Implantable Cardioverter Defibrillator Therapy

There has been concern that inappropriate ICD shock therapies might affect survival. In a post hoc analysis of the Sudden Cardiac Death in Heart Failure Trial (SCDHeFT), appropriate and inappropriate shocks were associated with worse survival among subjects randomized to ICD therapy for primary prevention of SCD.[97] Several studies have shown that shocks can be reduced with appropriate programming,[98] and a landmark randomized study, Multicenter Automatic Defibrillator Implantation Trial Reduce Inappropriate Therapy (MADIT-RIT), showed that such programming can be associated with improved survival.[99] Recommendations for programming of ICD tachycardia detection and therapies are included in a 2015 expert consensus statement.[98]

Addition of Left Ventricular Lead to Defibrillators

The addition of an LV lead to defibrillators for the purpose of cardiac resynchronization therapy may be beneficial in select patients with ischemic heart disease with LVEF of 35% or less, heart failure, and a QRS duration of 120 milliseconds or greater.[100,101] The benefit appears to be greatest in patients with left bundle branch block with a QRS width of greater than 150 milliseconds.[102,103] Cardiac resynchronization therapy has been shown to improve survival[100,101,104–106] by primarily reducing mortality through a reduction in progression or worsening of heart failure and to a lesser extent from reduction of SCD. Limited data, however, suggest that a reduction in ventricular arrhythmia burden could result from reverse ventricular remodeling in cardiac resynchronization therapy (CRT) responders.[107]

Complications of Implantable Defibrillators

Complications related to defibrillator implants have decreased over the years, especially with the transition from abdominal device implants with epicardial leads placed via thoracotomy to prepectoral implants using the axillary, cephalic, or subclavian veins. The overall complication rates with device implantation procedures are in the range of 3% to 6% and half of them are considered to be major.[108–110] These complications include bleeding at the implant site, device pocket or systemic infections, pneumothorax, cardiac perforation, or lead dislodgement. Procedure-related death is rare and estimated to occur in 2 to 4 per 1000 implants.

Lead-related complications include endovascular infections, dislodgement, fracture, or insulation defects. Occlusion of the access vein may occur over time, which may preclude implantation of additional leads via the same route unless lead extraction is performed. Fibrosis at the lead tip has been described and may negatively interfere with pacing or defibrillation thresholds. Estimates of lead-related complications from the AVID trial were approximately 10%.[111]

Lead failure may result in failure to sense or pace, inappropriate shocks, inappropriate inhibition of pacing, or failure to defibrillate. Death from lead failure has been reported but is very rare.[112] Overall, lead failures are estimated to occur in 5% to 40% of cases at 10 years of follow-up,[113–115] and these have been typically related to lead diameter or design.

Tricuspid regurgitation remains a debated rare complication of leads and could be related to the lead itself passing through the valve or pacing-related dyssynchrony.

Pulse generator complications are uncommon, occur in less than 2% of implants, and include skin erosion, infection, migration, or premature battery depletion.[111] Pulse generator hardware or software issues are very rare. Pain at the implant site, decreased motility of the shoulder, or tendinitis have been observed but very rarely require device reintervention. Another rare complication is twiddler's syndrome, in which rotating the device in its pocket results in lead dislodgement or malfunction.[116]

Subcutaneous Defibrillators

Totally subcutaneous defibrillators (S-ICD) have been introduced to avoid inherent problems related to transvenous leads, including risks at the time of implant, risks of endovascular infections, and lead failures, as well as the full reliance of defibrillators on lead integrity and function. The S-ICD system consists of a pulse generator that is implanted in a left midaxillary position and connected to a totally subcutaneous lead, which has a shocking coil electrode that is usually positioned in a left parasternal position. The current device can deliver up to 80 joules, and successful defibrillation at 65 joules is typically needed to provide an adequate safety margin. Preimplant screening is necessary to ensure ability of the device to appropriately sense ventricular activation and to avoid inappropriate shocks. With proper screening, this device has been found to successfully detect ventricular arrhythmias during defibrillation threshold testing in 98% to 100% of cases and to successfully defibrillate in 95% to 100% of cases.[117–126]

This device was approved for use in the United States in September, 2012. It is best suited for patients at risk of endovascular infections and young patients who inherently require multiple system revisions or upgrades in their lifetime.

The caveat with S-ICD use is the inability to pace. Therefore, the S-ICD is not preferred in patients who have or who may develop indications for pacing, as well as those who need antitachycardia pacing. Similarly, patients with indications for CRT would benefit from a transvenous rather than a subcutaneous system.

Wearable Cardioverter Defibrillators

Wearable cardioverter defibrillators (WCDs) may be useful in patients who are at increased risk of SCD, but in whom implantation of an implantable defibrillator is deferred, such as in the early post-MI or postrevascularization period or in patients with active infection. In such patients, the WCD serves as a temporary alternative to ICDs for the purpose of SCD prevention and has demonstrated similar efficacy in terminating VT or VF.[127–132]

The caveat with wearable defibrillators is lack of pacing capabilities, and as such these cannot provide antitachycardia pacing or treat bradyarrhythmias. Nonetheless, they could be used as a bridge to the implantation of a permanent defibrillator or a bridge to a decision in cases where LV function is expected to improve. A randomized trial of early WCD use after MI in patients with LVEF of 35% or less is ongoing (https://clinicaltrials.gov/ct2/show/NCT01446965).

Adjunctive Medical Therapy in Primary Prevention of Sudden Cardiac Death

Optimal medical therapy to target underlying comorbidities is recommended in all patients who meet criteria for ICD implantation, ideally before the implant takes place.

β-Blockers

The use of β-blockers in patients with acute MI reduces both all-cause mortality and the risk of SCD.[133,134] Similarly, a substantial part of the benefit of β-blocker therapy in patients with ischemic cardiomyopathy and heart failure is related to a reduction in SCD rates.[56,135] This benefit is also observed in patients who have received ICD implants. In ICD recipients in MADIT-II, β-blocker therapy was associated with reduction in all-cause mortality and the risk of ventricular arrhythmia with a relative risk reduction of 52%.[136]

Angiotensin-Converting Enzyme Inhibitors and Angiotensin Receptor Blockers

There are conflicting data regarding the benefit of these agents for the purpose of prevention of arrhythmic death. Nonetheless, a meta-analysis that included 15,104 patients from 15 trials of acute MI showed modest benefit for reduction of SCD.[137] Angiotensin receptor blockers (ARBs) are generally used as alternative therapy in patients who cannot tolerate ACE-I, but available data suggest that they may not provide the same benefit in terms of reduction of SCD.[138]

Aldosterone Antagonists

Eplerenone has been studied in post-MI patients with LV dysfunction, heart failure, and/or diabetes mellitus and was shown to reduce all-cause mortality and SCD rates with a relative risk reduction of 21%.[139] Aldosterone antagonists

BOX 22.1 Current Guideline Recommendations for Defibrillator Implants in Patients with Coronary Disease

Class I: ICD implantation is indicated

- in patients who are survivors of cardiac arrest due to VF or hemodynamically unstable sustained VT after evaluation to define the cause of the event and to exclude any completely reversible causes,
- in patients with spontaneous sustained VT, whether hemodynamically stable or unstable,
- in patients with syncope of undetermined origin with clinically relevant, hemodynamically significant sustained VT or VF induced at electrophysiologic study,
- in patients with LVEF ≤ 35% due to prior MI who are at least 40 days post-MI and are in NYHA functional class II or III,
- in patients with LV dysfunction due to prior MI who are at least 40 days post-MI, have an LVEF ≤ 30%, and are in NYHA functional class I,
- in patients with nonsustained VT due to prior MI, LVEF ≤ 40%, and inducible VF or sustained VT at electrophysiologic study.

Class IIa: ICD implantation is reasonable

- for patients with sustained VT and normal or near-normal ventricular function,
- for nonhospitalized patients awaiting transplantation for advanced cardiomyopathy.

Class III: ICD implantation is not indicated

- for patients who do not have a reasonable expectation of survival with an acceptable functional status for at least 1 year, even if they meet ICD implantation criteria,
- for patients with incessant VT or VF,
- in patients with significant psychiatric illnesses that may be aggravated by device implantation or that may preclude systematic follow-up,
- for NYHA class IV patients with drug-refractory congestive heart failure who are not candidates for cardiac transplantation or CRT-D,
- for syncope of undetermined cause in a patient without inducible ventricular tachyarrhythmias,
- for patients with ventricular tachyarrhythmias due to a completely reversible disorder.

CRT-D, Cardiac resynchronization therapy defibrillator; *ICD*, implantable cardioverter defibrillator; *LV*, left ventricular; *LVEF*, left ventricular ejection fraction; *MI*, myocardial infarction; *NYHA*, New York Heart Association; *VF*, ventricular fibrillation; *VT*, ventricular tachycardia.

Modified from Epstein AE, DiMarco JP, Ellenbogen KA, et al. ACC/AHA/HRS 2008 guidelines for device-based therapy of cardiac rhythm abnormalities. *J Am Coll Cardiol.* 2008;51:e1–e62; and Epstein AE, DiMarco JP, Ellenbogen KA, et al. 2012 ACCF/AHA/HRS focused update incorporated into the ACC/AHA/HRS 2008 guidelines for device-based therapy of cardiac rhythm abnormalities. *J Am Coll Cardiol.* 2013;61:e6–e75.

have been suggested to exert an antiarrhythmic effect on the ventricles.[140] The antifibrotic effect of these drugs may account for at least some of their benefit.

Statins

The role of statins in the treatment of coronary disease, especially in post-MI patients, is well established, but their use for the purpose of primary prevention of arrhythmic death is not well established. Limited data suggest that part of the survival benefit from statins in these patients could be related to reduction in SCD.[75,141,142]

Antiarrhythmic Drugs

Clinical trials do not support the routine use of antiarrhythmics for the purpose of primary prevention of SCD[46,143–145] due to inefficacy and potential proarrhythmic effects.

SUMMARY OF RECOMMENDATIONS FOR IMPLANTABLE CARDIOVERTER DEFIBRILLATOR IMPLANTATION FOR PREVENTION OF SUDDEN CARDIAC DEATH

The current American College of Cardiology (ACC)/American Heart Association (AHA)/Heart Rhythm Society (HRS) guidelines for ICD implantation in patients with CHD are summarized in Box 22.1. A HRS/ACC/AHA expert consensus document[146] provides further guidance in terms of defibrillator implants for patients who were not well represented in clinical trials or guidelines (see Figs. 22.3 and 22.4).

CONCLUSIONS

CHD is associated with SCD risk. Medical therapies to address coronary disease and associated comorbid conditions are associated with a survival benefit that in part could be related to a reduction in the risk of SCD as a subset mode of death. Defibrillator implantation is the main therapy for primary prevention of SCD in select groups of patients with CHD as evidenced by multiple clinical trials and subsequently in clinical practice guidelines.[147]

References

1. MacCurdy E: *The Notebooks of Leonardo Da Vinci*, 1954. New York: Braziller.
2. Lopshire JC, Zipes DP: Sudden cardiac death: better understanding of risks, mechanisms, and treatment, *Circulation* 114:1134–1136, 2006.
3. European Heart Rhythm Association, Heart Rhythm Society, Zipes DP, et al.: ACC/AHA/ESC 2006 guidelines for management of patients with ventricular arrhythmias and the prevention of sudden cardiac death: a report of the American College of Cardiology/American Heart Association Task Force and the European Society of Cardiology Committee for Practice Guidelines (Writing Committee to Develop Guidelines for Management of Patients with Ventricular Arrhythmias and the Prevention of Sudden Cardiac Death), *J Am Coll Cardiol* 48:e247–e346, 2006.
4. Fishman GI, Chugh SS, Dimarco JP, et al.: Sudden cardiac death prediction and prevention: report from a National Heart, Lung, and Blood Institute and Heart Rhythm Society Workshop, *Circulation* 122:2335–2348, 2010.
5. Mozaffarian D, Benjamin EJ, Go AS, et al.: Heart disease and stroke statistics—2015 update: a report from the American Heart Association, *Circulation* 131:e29–e322, 2015.
6. Kong MH, Fonarow GC, Peterson ED, et al.: Systematic review of the incidence of sudden cardiac death in the United States, *J Am Coll Cardiol* 57:794–801, 2011.
7. Gillum RF: Sudden coronary death in the United States: 1980–1985, *Circulation* 79:756–765, 1989.
8. Escobedo LG, Zack MM: Comparison of sudden and nonsudden coronary deaths in the United States, *Circulation* 93:2033–2036, 1996.
9. Chugh SS, Jui J, Gunson K, et al.: Current burden of sudden cardiac death: multiple source surveillance versus retrospective death certificate-based review in a large U.S. community, *J Am Coll Cardiol* 44:1268–1275, 2004.
10. Cobb LA, Fahrenbruch CE, Olsufka M, Copass MK: Changing incidence of out-of-hospital ventricular fibrillation, 1980–2000, *JAMA* 288:3008–3013, 2002.
11. Zheng ZJ, Croft JB, Giles WH, Mensah GA: Sudden cardiac death in the United States, 1989 to 1998, *Circulation* 104:2158–2163, 2001.
12. Myerburg RJ: Sudden cardiac death: exploring the limits of our knowledge, *J Cardiovasc Electrophysiol* 12:369–381, 2001.
13. Ford ES, Ajani UA, Croft JB, et al.: Explaining the decrease in U.S. deaths from coronary disease, 1980–2000, *N Engl J Med* 356:2388–2398, 2007.
14. Rosamond WD, Chambless LE, Folsom AR, et al.: Trends in the incidence of myocardial infarction and in mortality due to coronary heart disease, 1987 to 1994, *N Engl J Med* 339:861–867, 1998.
15. Fox CS, Evans JC, Larson MG, Kannel WB, Levy D: Temporal trends in coronary heart disease mortality and sudden cardiac death from 1950 to 1999: the Framingham Heart Study, *Circulation* 110:522–527, 2004.
16. Huikuri HV, Castellanos A, Myerburg RJ: Sudden death due to cardiac arrhythmias, *N Engl J Med* 345:1473–1482, 2001.
17. Becker LB, Han BH, Meyer PM, et al.: Racial differences in the incidence of cardiac arrest and subsequent survival. The CPR Chicago Project, *N Engl J Med* 329:600–606, 1993.
18. Krahn AD, Connolly SJ, Roberts RS, Gent M: ATMA Investigators. Diminishing proportional risk of sudden death with advancing age: implications for prevention of sudden death, *Am Heart J* 147:837–840, 2004.
19. Kannel WB, Schatzkin A: Sudden death: lessons from subsets in population studies, *J Am Coll Cardiol* 5:141B–149B, 1985.
20. Cupples LA, Gagnon DR, Kannel WB: Long- and short-term risk of sudden coronary death, *Circulation* 85:11–18, 1992.
21. Cowie MR, Fahrenbruch CE, Cobb LA, Hallstrom AP: Out-of-hospital cardiac arrest: racial differences in outcome in Seattle, *Am J Public Health* 83:955–959, 1993.
22. Gillum RF: Sudden cardiac death in Hispanic Americans and African Americans, *Am J Public Health* 87:1461–1466, 1997.
23. Myerburg RJ, Junttila MJ: Sudden cardiac death caused by coronary heart disease, *Circulation* 125:1043–1052, 2012.
24. Fuster V, Badimon L, Badimon JJ, Chesebro JH: The pathogenesis of coronary artery disease and the acute coronary syndromes (2), *N Engl J Med* 326:310–318, 1992.
25. Furukawa T, Moroe K, Mayrovitz HN, et al.: Arrhythmogenic effects of graded coronary blood flow reductions superimposed on prior myocardial infarction in dogs, *Circulation* 84:368–377, 1991.
26. Mehta D, Curwin J, Gomes JA, Fuster V: Sudden death in coronary artery disease: acute ischemia versus myocardial substrate, *Circulation* 96:3215–3223, 1997.
27. Yan AT, Shayne AJ, Brown KA, et al.: Characterization of the peri-infarct zone by contrast-enhanced cardiac magnetic resonance imaging is a powerful predictor of post-myocardial infarction mortality, *Circulation* 114:32–39, 2006.

28. Schmidt A, Azevedo CF, Cheng A, et al.: Infarct tissue heterogeneity by magnetic resonance imaging identifies enhanced cardiac arrhythmia susceptibility in patients with left ventricular dysfunction, *Circulation* 115:2006–2014, 2007.
29. Tamaki S, Yamada T, Okuyama Y, et al.: Cardiac iodine-123 metaiodobenzylguanidine imaging predicts sudden cardiac death independently of left ventricular ejection fraction in patients with chronic heart failure and left ventricular systolic dysfunction: results from a comparative study with signal-averaged electrocardiogram, heart rate variability, and QT dispersion, *J Am Coll Cardiol* 53:426–435, 2009.
30. Adelson L, Hoffman W: Sudden death from coronary disease related to a lethal mechanism arising independently of vascular occlusion or myocardial damage, *JAMA* 176:129–135, 1961.
31. Farb A, Tang AL, Burke AP, et al.: Sudden coronary death. Frequency of active coronary lesions, inactive coronary lesions, and myocardial infarction, *Circulation* 92:1701–1709, 1995.
32. Greene HL: Sudden arrhythmic cardiac death—mechanisms, resuscitation and classification: the Seattle perspective, *Am J Cardiol* 65:4B–12B, 1990.
33. Deo R, Albert CM: Epidemiology and genetics of sudden cardiac death, *Circulation* 125:620–637, 2012.
34. Goldberg RJ, Yarzebski J, Spencer FA, et al.: Thirty-year trends (1975–2005) in the magnitude, patient characteristics, and hospital outcomes of patients with acute myocardial infarction complicated by ventricular fibrillation, *Am J Cardiol* 102:1595–1601, 2008.
35. Wyse DG, Friedman PL, Brodsky MA, et al.: Life-threatening ventricular arrhythmias due to transient or correctable causes: high risk for death in follow-up, *J Am Coll Cardiol* 38:1718–1724, 2001.
36. Askari AT, Shishehbor MH, Kaminski MA, et al.: The association between early ventricular arrhythmias, renin-angiotensin-aldosterone system antagonism, and mortality in patients with ST-segment-elevation myocardial infarction: insights from Global Use of Strategies to Open coronary arteries (GUSTO) V, *Am Heart J* 158:238–243, 2009.
37. Furukawa T, Bassett AL, Furukawa N, Kimura S, Myerburg RJ: The ionic mechanism of reperfusion-induced early afterdepolarizations in feline left ventricular hypertrophy, *J Clin Invest* 91:1521–1531, 1993.
38. Myerburg RJ, Kessler KM, Mallon SM, et al.: Life-threatening ventricular arrhythmias in patients with silent myocardial ischemia due to coronary-artery spasm, *N Engl J Med* 326:1451–1455, 1992.
39. Melgarejo-Moreno A, Galcera-Tomas J, Garcia-Alberola A, et al.: Incidence, clinical characteristics, and prognostic significance of right bundle-branch block in acute myocardial infarction: a study in the thrombolytic era, *Circulation* 96:1139–1144, 1997.
40. Solomon SD, Zelenkofske S, McMurray JJ, et al.: Sudden death in patients with myocardial infarction and left ventricular dysfunction, heart failure, or both, *N Engl J Med* 352:2581–2588, 2005.
41. Pouleur AC, Barkoudah E, Uno H, et al.: Pathogenesis of sudden unexpected death in a clinical trial of patients with myocardial infarction and left ventricular dysfunction, heart failure, or both, *Circulation* 122:597–602, 2010.
42. Steinbeck G, Andresen D, Seidl K, et al.: Defibrillator implantation early after myocardial infarction, *N Engl J Med* 361:1427–1436, 2009.
43. Hohnloser SH, Kuck KH, Dorian P, et al.: Prophylactic use of an implantable cardioverter-defibrillator after acute myocardial infarction, *N Engl J Med* 351:2481–2488, 2004.
44. Piccini JP, Al-Khatib SM, Hellkamp AS, et al.: Mortality benefits from implantable cardioverter-defibrillator therapy are not restricted to patients with remote myocardial infarction: an analysis from the Sudden Cardiac Death in Heart Failure Trial (SCD-HeFT), *Heart Rhythm* 8:393–400, 2011.
45. Marchioli R, Barzi F, Bomba E, et al.: Early protection against sudden death by n-3 polyunsaturated fatty acids after myocardial infarction: time-course analysis of the results of the Gruppo Italiano per lo Studio della Sopravvivenza nell'Infarto Miocardico (GISSI)-Prevenzione, *Circulation* 105:1897–1903, 2002.
46. Torp-Pedersen C, Moller M, Bloch-Thomsen PE, et al.: Dofetilide in patients with congestive heart failure and left ventricular dysfunction. Danish Investigations of Arrhythmia and Mortality on Dofetilide Study Group, *N Engl J Med* 341:857–865, 1999.
47. Berger CJ, Murabito JM, Evans JC, Anderson KM, Levy D: Prognosis after first myocardial infarction. Comparison of Q-wave and non-Q-wave myocardial infarction in the Framingham Heart Study, *JAMA* 268:1545–1551, 1992.
48. Adabag AS, Therneau TM, Gersh BJ, Weston SA, Roger VL: Sudden death after myocardial infarction, *JAMA* 300:2022–2029, 2008.
49. Albert CM, Chae CU, Grodstein F, et al.: Prospective study of sudden cardiac death among women in the United States, *Circulation* 107:2096–2101, 2003.
50. Kannel WB, Wilson PW, D'Agostino RB, Cobb J: Sudden coronary death in women, *Am Heart J* 136:205–212, 1998.
51. Huikuri HV, Tapanainen JM, Lindgren K, et al.: Prediction of sudden cardiac death after myocardial infarction in the beta-blocking era, *J Am Coll Cardiol* 42:652–658, 2003.
52. Makikallio TH, Barthel P, Schneider R, et al.: Frequency of sudden cardiac death among acute myocardial infarction survivors with optimized medical and revascularization therapy, *Am J Cardiol* 97:480–484, 2006.
53. Stevenson WG, Stevenson LW, Middlekauff HR, Saxon LA: Sudden death prevention in patients with advanced ventricular dysfunction, *Circulation* 88:2953–2961, 1993.
54. Goldberger JJ, Cain ME, Hohnloser SH, et al.: American Heart Association/American College of Cardiology Foundation/Heart Rhythm Society scientific statement on noninvasive risk stratification techniques for identifying patients at risk for sudden cardiac death. A scientific statement from the American Heart Association Council on Clinical Cardiology Committee on Electrocardiography and Arrhythmias and Council on Epidemiology and Prevention, *J Am Coll Cardiol* 52:1179–1199, 2008.
55. Narang R, Cleland JG, Erhardt L, et al.: Mode of death in chronic heart failure. A request and proposition for more accurate classification, *Eur Heart J* 17:1390–1403, 1996.
56. Effect of metoprolol CR/XL in chronic heart failure: Metoprolol CR/XL Randomised Intervention Trial in Congestive Heart Failure (MERIT-HF), *Lancet* 353:2001–2007, 1999.
57. Cleland JG, Erhardt L, Murray G, Hall AS, Ball SG: Effect of ramipril on morbidity and mode of death among survivors of acute myocardial infarction with clinical evidence of heart failure. A report from the AIRE Study Investigators, *Eur Heart J* 18:41–51, 1997.
58. Greenberg H, Case RB, Moss AJ, et al.: Analysis of mortality events in the Multicenter Automatic Defibrillator Implantation Trial (MADIT-II), *J Am Coll Cardiol* 43:1459–1465, 2004.
59. Viskin S, Halkin A, Olgin JE: Treatable causes of sudden death: not really "treatable" or not really the cause? *J Am Coll Cardiol* 38:1725–1727, 2001.
60. A comparison of antiarrhythmic-drug therapy with implantable defibrillators in patients resuscitated from near-fatal ventricular arrhythmias. The Antiarrhythmics versus Implantable Defibrillators (AVID) Investigators, *N Engl J Med* 337:1576–1583, 1997.
61. Connolly SJ, Gent M, Roberts RS, et al.: Canadian implantable defibrillator study (CIDS): a randomized trial of the implantable cardioverter defibrillator against amiodarone, *Circulation* 101:1297–1302, 2000.
62. Wever EF, Hauer RN, van Capelle FL, et al.: Randomized study of implantable defibrillator as first-choice therapy versus conventional strategy in postinfarct sudden death survivors, *Circulation* 91:2195–2203, 1995.
63. Siebels J, Kuck KH: Implantable cardioverter defibrillator compared with antiarrhythmic drug treatment in cardiac arrest survivors (the Cardiac Arrest Study Hamburg), *Am Heart J* 127:1139–1144, 1994.
64. Connolly SJ, Hallstrom AP, Cappato R, et al.: Meta-analysis of the implantable cardioverter defibrillator secondary prevention trials. AVID, CASH and CIDS studies. Antiarrhythmics vs Implantable Defibrillator study. Cardiac Arrest Study Hamburg. Canadian Implantable Defibrillator Study, *Eur Heart J* 21:2071–2078, 2000.
65. Kuck KH, Cappato R, Siebels J, Ruppel R: Randomized comparison of antiarrhythmic drug therapy with implantable defibrillators in patients resuscitated from cardiac arrest: the Cardiac Arrest Study Hamburg (CASH), *Circulation* 102:748–754, 2000.
66. Ezekowitz JA, Armstrong PW, McAlister FA: Implantable cardioverter defibrillators in primary and secondary prevention: a systematic review of randomized, controlled trials, *Ann Intern Med* 138:445–452, 2003.
67. Lee DS, Austin PC, Rouleau JL, et al.: Predicting mortality among patients hospitalized for heart failure: derivation and validation of a clinical model, *JAMA* 290:2581–2587, 2003.
68. Causes of death in the Antiarrhythmics Versus Implantable Defibrillators (AVID) Trial, *J Am Coll Cardiol* 34:1552–1559, 1999.
69. Domanski MJ, Sakseena S, Epstein AE, et al.: Relative effectiveness of the implantable cardioverter-defibrillator and antiarrhythmic drugs in patients with varying degrees of left ventricular dysfunction who have survived malignant ventricular arrhythmias. AVID Investigators. Antiarrhythmics Versus Implantable Defibrillators, *J Am Coll Cardiol* 34:1090–1095, 1999.
70. Lee DS, Green LD, Liu PP, et al.: Effectiveness of implantable defibrillators for preventing arrhythmic events and death: a meta-analysis, *J Am Coll Cardiol* 41:1573–1582, 2003.
71. Chan PS, Hayward RA: Mortality reduction by implantable cardioverter-defibrillators in high-risk patients with heart failure, ischemic heart disease, and new-onset ventricular arrhythmia: an effectiveness study, *J Am Coll Cardiol* 45:1474–1481, 2005.
72. Mitchell LB, Pineda EA, Titus JL, Bartosch PM, Benditt DG: Sudden death in patients with implantable cardioverter defibrillators: the importance of post-shock electromechanical dissociation, *J Am Coll Cardiol* 39:1323–1328, 2002.
73. Ha AH, Ham I, Nair GM, et al.: Implantable cardioverter-defibrillator shock prevention does not reduce mortality: a systemic review, *Heart Rhythm* 9:2068–2074, 2012.
74. Exner DV, Reiffel JA, Epstein AE, et al.: Beta-blocker use and survival in patients with ventricular fibrillation or symptomatic ventricular tachycardia: the Antiarrhythmics Versus Implantable Defibrillators (AVID) trial, *J Am Coll Cardiol* 34:325–333, 1999.
75. Mitchell LB, Powell JL, Gillis AM, et al.: Are lipid-lowering drugs also antiarrhythmic drugs? An analysis of the Antiarrhythmics versus Implantable Defibrillators (AVID) trial, *J Am Coll Cardiol* 42:81–87, 2003.
76. De Sutter J, Tavernier R, De Buyzere M, Jordaens L, De Backer G: Lipid lowering drugs and recurrences of life-threatening ventricular arrhythmias in high-risk patients, *J Am Coll Cardiol* 36:766–772, 2000.
77. Jenkins DJ, Josse AR, Beyene J, et al.: Fish-oil supplementation in patients with implantable cardioverter defibrillators: a meta-analysis, *CMAJ* 178:157–164, 2008.
78. Wissner E, Stevenson WG, Kuck KH: Catheter ablation of ventricular tachycardia in ischaemic and non-ischaemic cardiomyopathy: where are we today? A clinical review, *Eur Heart J* 33:1440–1450, 2012.
79. Di Biase L, Burkhardt JD, Lakkireddy D, et al.: Ablation of Stable VTs Versus Substrate Ablation in Ischemic Cardiomyopathy: the VISTA Randomized Multicenter Trial, *J Am Coll Cardiol* 66:2872–2882, 2015.
80. Knecht S, Sacher F, Wright M, et al.: Long-term follow-up of idiopathic ventricular fibrillation ablation: a multicenter study, *J Am Coll Cardiol* 54:522–528, 2009.
81. Mallidi J, Nadkarni GN, Berger RD, Calkins H, Nazarian S: Meta-analysis of catheter ablation as an adjunct to medical therapy for treatment of ventricular tachycardia in patients with structural heart disease, *Heart Rhythm* 8:503–510, 2011.
82. Jeevanandam V, Bielefeld MR, Auteri JS, et al.: The implantable defibrillator: an electronic bridge to cardiac transplantation, *Circulation* 86:276–279, 1992.
83. Grimm M, Wieselthaler G, Avanessian R, et al.: The impact of implantable cardioverter-defibrillators on mortality among patients on the waiting list for heart transplantation, *J Thorac Cardiovasc Surg* 110:532–539, 1995.
84. Bolling SF, Deeb GM, Morady F, et al.: Automatic internal cardioverter defibrillator: a bridge to heart transplantation, *J Heart Lung Transplant* 10:562–566, 1991.
85. Saba S, Atiga WL, Barrington W, et al.: Selected patients listed for cardiac transplantation may benefit from defibrillator implantation regardless of an established indication, *J Heart Lung Transplant* 22:411–418, 2003.
86. Lorga-Filho A, Geelen P, Vanderheyden M, et al.: Early benefit of implantable cardioverter defibrillator therapy in patients waiting for cardiac transplantation, *Pacing Clin Electrophysiol* 21:1747–1750, 1998.
87. Moss AJ, Hall WJ, Cannom DS, et al.: Improved survival with an implanted defibrillator in patients with coronary disease at high risk for ventricular arrhythmia. Multicenter Automatic Defibrillator Implantation Trial Investigators, *N Engl J Med* 335:1933–1940, 1996.
88. Mushlin AI, Hall WJ, Zwanziger J, et al.: The cost-effectiveness of automatic implantable cardiac defibrillators: results from MADIT. Multicenter Automatic Defibrillator Implantation Trial, *Circulation* 97:2129–2135, 1998.
89. Moss AJ, Fadl Y, Zareba W, et al.: Survival benefit with an implanted defibrillator in relation to mortality risk in chronic coronary heart disease, *Am J Cardiol* 88:516–520, 2001.
90. Moss AJ, Zareba W, Hall WJ, et al.: Prophylactic implantation of a defibrillator in patients with myocardial infarction and reduced ejection fraction, *N Engl J Med* 346:877–883, 2002.
91. Bigger Jr JT: Prophylactic use of implanted cardiac defibrillators in patients at high risk for ventricular arrhythmias after coronary-artery bypass graft surgery. Coronary Artery Bypass Graft (CABG) Patch Trial Investigators, *N Engl J Med* 337:1569–1575, 1997.
92. Buxton AE, Lee KL, Fisher JD, et al.: A randomized study of the prevention of sudden death in patients with coronary artery disease. Multicenter Unsustained Tachycardia Trial Investigators, *N Engl J Med* 341:1882–1890, 1999.
93. Buxton AE, Lee KL, Hafley GE, et al.: Relation of ejection fraction and inducible ventricular tachycardia to mode of death in patients with coronary artery disease: an analysis of patients enrolled in the multicenter unsustained tachycardia trial, *Circulation* 106:2466–2472, 2002.
94. Bardy GH, Lee KL, Mark DB, et al.: Amiodarone or an implantable cardioverter-defibrillator for congestive heart failure, *N Engl J Med* 352:225–237, 2005.
95. Hohnloser SH, Kuck KH, Dorian P, et al.: Prophylactic use of an implantable cardioverter-defibrillator after acute myocardial infarction, *N Engl J Med* 351:2481–2488, 2004.
96. Orn S, Cleland JG, Romo M, Kjekshus J, Dickstein K: Recurrent infarction causes the most deaths following myocardial infarction with left ventricular dysfunction, *Am J Med* 118:752–758, 2005.
97. Poole JE, Johnson GW, Hellkamp AS, et al.: Prognostic importance of defibrillator shocks in patients with heart failure, *N Engl J Med* 359:1009–1017, 2008.
98. Wilkoff BL, Fauchier L, Stiles MK, et al.: 2015 HRS/EHRA/APHRS/SOLAECE expert consensus statement on optimal implantable cardioverter-defibrillator programming and testing, *Heart Rhythm*, 13:e50-86, 2016.
99. Moss AJ, Schuger C, Beck CA, et al.: Reduction in inappropriate therapy and mortality through ICD programming, *N Engl J Med* 367:2275–2283, 2012.
100. Cleland JG, Daubert JC, Erdmann E, et al.: The effect of cardiac resynchronization on morbidity and mortality in heart failure, *N Engl J Med* 352:1539–1549, 2005.
101. Bristow MR, Saxon LA, Boehmer J, et al.: Cardiac-resynchronization therapy with or without an implantable defibrillator in advanced chronic heart failure, *N Engl J Med* 350:2140–2150, 2004.
102. Stavrakis S, Lazzara R, Thadani U: The benefit of cardiac resynchronization therapy and QRS duration: a meta-analysis, *J Cardiovasc Electrophysiol* 23:163–168, 2012.
103. Sipahi I, Carrigan TP, Rowland DY, Stambler BS, Fang JC: Impact of QRS duration on clinical event reduction with cardiac resynchronization therapy: meta-analysis of randomized controlled trials, *Arch Intern Med* 171:1454–1462, 2011.
104. Linde C, Abraham WT, Gold MR, et al.: Randomized trial of cardiac resynchronization in mildly symptomatic heart failure patients and in asymptomatic patients with left ventricular dysfunction and previous heart failure symptoms, *J Am Coll Cardiol* 52:1834–1843, 2008.

105. Moss AJ, Hall WJ, Cannom DS, et al.: Cardiac-resynchronization therapy for the prevention of heart-failure events, *N Engl J Med* 361:1329–1338, 2009.
106. Tang AS, Wells GA, Talajic M, et al.: Cardiac-resynchronization therapy for mild-to-moderate heart failure, *N Engl J Med* 363:2385–2395, 2010.
107. Barsheshet A, Wang PJ, Moss AJ, et al.: Reverse remodeling and the risk of ventricular tachyarrhythmias in the MADIT-CRT (Multicenter Automatic Defibrillator Implantation Trial-Cardiac Resynchronization Therapy), *J Am Coll Cardiol* 57:2416–2423, 2011.
108. Atwater BD, Daubert JP: Implantable cardioverter defibrillators: risks accompany the life-saving benefits, *Heart* 98:764–772, 2012.
109. Dodson JA, Lampert R, Wang Y, et al.: Temporal trends in quality of care among recipients of implantable cardioverter-defibrillators: insights from the National Cardiovascular Data Registry, *Circulation* 129:580–586, 2014.
110. Russo AM, Daugherty SL, Masoudi FA, et al.: Gender and outcomes after primary prevention implantable cardioverter-defibrillator implantation: findings from the National Cardiovascular Data Registry (NCDR), *Am Heart J* 170:330–338, 2015.
111. Kron J, Herre J, Renfroe EG, et al.: Lead- and device-related complications in the antiarrhythmics versus implantable defibrillators trial, *Am Heart J* 141:92–98, 2001.
112. Hauser RG, Abdelhadi R, McGriff D, Retel LK: Deaths caused by the failure of Riata and Riata ST implantable cardioverter-defibrillator leads, *Heart Rhythm* 9:1227–1235, 2012.
113. Eckstein J, Koller MT, Zabel M, et al.: Necessity for surgical revision of defibrillator leads implanted long-term: causes and management, *Circulation* 117:2727–2733, 2008.
114. van Rees JB, van Welsenes GH, Borleffs CJW, et al.: Update on small-diameter implantable cardioverter-defibrillator leads performance, *Pacing Clin Electrophysiol* 35:652–658, 2012.
115. Maisel WH, Kramer DB: Implantable cardioverter-defibrillator lead performance, *Circulation* 117:2721–2723, 2008.
116. Chaara J, Sunthorn H: Twiddler syndrome, *J Cardiovasc Electrophysiol* 25:659, 2014.
117. Bardy GH, Smith WM, Hood MA, et al.: An entirely subcutaneous implantable cardioverter-defibrillator, *N Engl J Med* 363:36–44, 2010.
118. Jarman JWE, Lascelles K, Wong T, et al.: Clinical experience of entirely subcutaneous implantable cardioverter-defibrillators in children and adults: cause for caution, *Eur Heart J* 33:1351–1359, 2012.
119. Jarman JWE, Todd DM: United Kingdom national experience of entirely subcutaneous implantable cardioverter-defibrillator technology: important lessons to learn, *Europace* 15:1158–1165, 2013.
120. Kobe J, Reinke F, Meyer C, et al.: Implantation and follow-up of totally subcutaneous versus conventional implantable cardioverter-defibrillators: a multicenter case-control study, *Heart Rhythm* 10:29–36, 2013.
121. Olde Nordkamp LRA, Dabiri Abkenari L, Boersma LVA, et al.: The entirely subcutaneous implantable cardioverter-defibrillator: initial clinical experience in a large Dutch cohort, *J Am Coll Cardiol* 60:1933–1939, 2012.
122. Lambiase PD, Barr C, Theuns DAMJ, et al.: Worldwide experience with a totally subcutaneous implantable defibrillator: early results from the EFFORTLESS S-ICD Registry, *Eur Heart J* 35:1657–1665, 2014.
123. Weiss R, Knight BP, Gold MR, et al.: Safety and efficacy of a totally subcutaneous implantable-cardioverter defibrillator, *Circulation* 128:944–953, 2013.
124. Aydin A, Hartel F, Schluter M, et al.: Shock efficacy of subcutaneous implantable cardioverter-defibrillator for prevention of sudden cardiac death: initial multicenter experience, *Circ Arrhythm Electrophysiol* 5:913–919, 2012.
125. Burke MC, Gold MR, Knight BP, et al.: Safety and efficacy of the totally subcutaneous implantable defibrillator: 2-year results from a pooled analysis of the IDE Study and EFFORTLESS Registry, *J Am Coll Cardiol* 65:1605–1615, 2015.
126. Dabiri Abkenari L, Theuns DAMJ, Valk SDA, et al.: Clinical experience with a novel subcutaneous implantable defibrillator system in a single center, *Clin Res Cardiol* 100:737–744, 2011.
127. Feldman AM, Klein H, Tchou P, et al.: Use of a wearable defibrillator in terminating tachyarrhythmias in patients at high risk for sudden death: results of the WEARIT/BIROAD, *Pacing Clin Electrophysiol* 27:4–9, 2004.
128. Reek S, Geller JC, Meltendorf U, et al.: Clinical efficacy of a wearable defibrillator in acutely terminating episodes of ventricular fibrillation using biphasic shocks, *Pacing Clin Electrophysiol* 26:2016–2022, 2003.
129. Chung MK, Szymkiewicz SJ, Shao M, et al.: Aggregate national experience with the wearable cardioverter-defibrillator: event rates, compliance, and survival, *J Am Coll Cardiol* 56:194–203, 2010.
130. Klein HU, Meltendorf U, Reek S, et al.: Bridging a temporary high risk of sudden arrhythmic death. Experience with the wearable cardioverter defibrillator (WCD), *Pacing Clin Electrophysiol* 33:353–367, 2010.
131. Epstein AE, Abraham WT, Bianco NR, et al.: Wearable cardioverter-defibrillator use in patients perceived to be at high risk early post-myocardial infarction, *J Am Coll Cardiol* 62:2000–2007, 2013.
132. Kutyifa V, Moss AJ, Klein H, et al.: Use of the wearable cardioverter defibrillator in high-risk cardiac patients: data from the Prospective Registry of Patients Using the Wearable Cardioverter Defibrillator (WEARIT-II Registry), *Circulation* 132:1613–1619, 2015.
133. Nuttall SL, Toescu V, Kendall MJ: Beta blockade after myocardial infarction. Beta blockers have key role in reducing morbidity and mortality after infarction, *BMJ* 320:581, 2000.
134. Friedman LM, Byington RP, Capone RJ, et al.: Effect of propranolol in patients with myocardial infarction and ventricular arrhythmia, *J Am Coll Cardiol* 7:1–8, 1986.
135. Packer M, Bristow MR, Cohn JN, et al.: The effect of carvedilol on morbidity and mortality in patients with chronic heart failure. U.S. Carvedilol Heart Failure Study Group, *N Engl J Med* 334:1349–1355, 1996.
136. Brodine WN, Tung RT, Lee JK, et al.: Effects of beta-blockers on implantable cardioverter defibrillator therapy and survival in the patients with ischemic cardiomyopathy (from the Multicenter Automatic Defibrillator Implantation Trial-II), *Am J Cardiol* 96:691–695, 2005.
137. Domanski MJ, Exner DV, Borkowf CB, et al.: Effect of angiotensin converting enzyme inhibition on sudden cardiac death in patients following acute myocardial infarction. A meta-analysis of randomized clinical trials, *J Am Coll Cardiol* 33:598–604, 1999.
138. Pitt B, Poole-Wilson PA, Segal R, et al.: Effect of losartan compared with captopril on mortality in patients with symptomatic heart failure: randomised trial—the Losartan Heart Failure Survival Study ELITE II, *Lancet* 355:1582–1587, 2000.
139. Pitt B, Remme W, Zannad F, et al.: Eplerenone, a selective aldosterone blocker, in patients with left ventricular dysfunction after myocardial infarction, *N Engl J Med* 348:1309–1321, 2003.
140. Ramires FJ, Mansur A, Coelho O, et al.: Effect of spironolactone on ventricular arrhythmias in congestive heart failure secondary to idiopathic dilated or to ischemic cardiomyopathy, *Am J Cardiol* 85:1207–1211, 2000.
141. Chiu JH, Abdelhadi RH, Chung MK, et al.: Effect of statin therapy on risk of ventricular arrhythmia among patients with coronary artery disease and an implantable cardioverter-defibrillator, *Am J Cardiol* 95:490–491, 2005.
142. Dickinson MG, Ip JH, Olshansky B, et al.: Statin use was associated with reduced mortality in both ischemic and nonischemic cardiomyopathy and in patients with implantable defibrillators: mortality data and mechanistic insights from the Sudden Cardiac Death in Heart Failure Trial (SCD-HeFT), *Am Heart J* 153:573–578, 2007.
143. Camm AJ, Pratt CM, Schwartz PJ, et al.: Mortality in patients after a recent myocardial infarction: a randomized, placebo-controlled trial of azimilide using heart rate variability for risk stratification, *Circulation* 109:990–996, 2004.
144. Singer I, Al-Khalidi H, Niazi I, et al.: Azimilide decreases recurrent ventricular tachyarrhythmias in patients with implantable cardioverter defibrillators, *J Am Coll Cardiol* 43:39–43, 2004.
145. Pratt CM, Eaton T, Francis M, et al.: The inverse relationship between baseline left ventricular ejection fraction and outcome of antiarrhythmic therapy: a dangerous imbalance in the risk-benefit ratio, *Am Heart J* 118:433–440, 1989.
146. Kusumoto FM, Calkins H, Boehmer J, et al.: HRS/ACC/AHA expert consensus statement on the use of implantable cardioverter-defibrillator therapy in patients who are not included or not well represented in clinical trials, *J Am Coll Cardiol* 64:1143–1177, 2014.
147. Epstein AE, DiMarco JP, Ellenbogen KA, et al.: ACC/AHA/HRS 2008 guidelines for device-based therapy of cardiac rhythm abnormalities: a report of the American College of Cardiology/American Heart Association Task Force on Practice Guidelines (Writing Committee to Revise the ACC/AHA/NASPE 2002 Guideline Update for Implantation of Cardiac Pacemakers and Antiarrhythmia Devices) developed in collaboration with the American Association for Thoracic Surgery and Society of Thoracic Surgeons, *J Am Coll Cardiol* 51:e1–e62, 2008.

23 Revascularization Approaches

Steven P. Marso

INTRODUCTION

The indications for coronary revascularization among patients with chronic coronary heart disease evolve as the scientific information accumulates and technology advances. The benefits associated with prompt coronary revascularization in reducing cardiovascular death and nonfatal myocardial infarction (MI) in patients presenting with acute coronary syndrome (ACS) are widely accepted.[1,2] However, there is little clinical evidence to demonstrate a reduction in hard clinical endpoints in patients with stable symptoms undergoing coronary revascularization.

Clinical data generally support and clinicians have traditionally accepted that coronary revascularization in patients with chronic stable ischemic heart disease (SIHD) is appropriate in patients at high risk for future cardiovascular events or with lifestyle-limiting symptoms.[3] Both the clinical guidelines[4] and the coronary revascularization appropriate use criteria[5] provide specific recommendations for clinicians considering a revascularization strategy among patients with SIHD.

Despite a nearly 70% decline in the age-standardized heart disease-related mortality over the last 40 years,[6] coronary vascular disease remains the leading cause of death since 1900 in the United States.[7] It has been estimated that approximately half of this reduced risk is directly attributable to improved medical treatment and coronary revascularization procedures.[8] The majority of this risk reduction is associated with improved medical therapy rather than coronary revascularization procedures. This improvement in estimated cardiovascular risk has been attenuated in recent years because of an increase in societal obesity and a concomitant increase in the prevalence of diabetes.

GOALS OF TREATMENT

The major goals when treating patients with chronic coronary artery disease (CAD) are to reduce symptoms, improve the quality of life (QoL), and reduce risk of death and MI. Risk factor modification and optimal medical therapy are foundational strategies. Despite the use of these evidence-based medical therapies, patients often have persistent symptoms and residual cardiovascular risk. Data from a large, multinational, longitudinal registry of outpatients estimate that 1 in 3 patients have active symptoms and 1 in 4 have objective evidence of ischemia,[9] and both are associated with future cardiovascular risk.

The decision to recommend coronary revascularization in patients with SIHD should be considered carefully. The discussion with the patient and family should include a transparent discussion of all treatment options, the anticipated benefits, and the risks of potential complications. In general, a discussion of an initial medical therapy approach should be discussed with the patient. In today's healthcare environment, it is widely accepted that patients with chronic stable angina should be initially offered evidence-based medical therapy that can be optimized over time. This would include pharmacologic antianginal therapy, lifestyle intervention, and therapies to mitigate future cardiovascular risk. When patients undergo cardiac catheterization and the anatomy is appropriate for percutaneous coronary intervention (PCI), the trend in the last decade has been to proceed with ad hoc PCI rather than deferring it. Ad hoc PCI occurs approximately 86% of the time in the United States.[10] For elective indications, deferring PCI allows one to consider alternative treatment strategies especially in the setting of high-risk multivessel CAD. Additionally, certain clinical scenarios are better suited for PCI whereas others are better suited for coronary artery bypass grafting (CABG). For example, patients who are medically noncompliant or who have recent gastrointestinal bleeding related to peptic ulcer disease may not be optimal candidates for long-term dual antiplatelet therapy and would be appropriate candidates to undergo CABG. On the other hand, patients with high clinical comorbidities or high frailty and three-vessel CAD coupled with impaired left ventricular (LV) dysfunction would be expected to have a survival benefit with CABG but may be too high risk and more appropriately referred for multivessel PCI. These and various other issues can often be better vetted with a *heart team approach*. This requires an interruption in the care process to enable a multidisciplinary team discussion and the willingness of busy practitioners to meet and discuss clinical cases. The heart team approach, especially in complex cases, is preferable.

Shared Decision-Making

Current guidelines recommend the use of a multidisciplinary heart team to facilitate decisions regarding coronary revascularization, percutaneous aortic valve replacement, and other high-risk cardiac procedures.[11] This decision-making process is best shared across a wide variety of individuals including the patient, the patient's family, the interventional cardiologist, the cardiac surgeon, the general cardiologist, and the primary care physician. It has been demonstrated that this clinical care paradigm is not only feasible but also appealing. Physicians who have known the patient over a prolonged period of time, often the general cardiologist and/or primary care physician, should play an important role in recommending therapies regarding coronary revascularization, whether it be CABG or PCI. Ideally the risk-benefit discussion during these heart team meetings would be provided by both the interventional cardiologist and the cardiac surgeon, who are best suited to provide an individualized risk-benefit assessment.

Coronary Revascularization: General Comments

Coronary revascularization procedures are common and costly, associated with an annual cost of $3.2 billion to Medicare.[12] The rates of coronary revascularization procedures in the United States are decreasing. Between 2001 and 2008 there was a 14% decrease in the annual rate of coronary revascularization procedures, which was principally driven by a 28%, reduction in CABG procedures and an unchanged PCI rate. After 2008, PCI rates in the United States

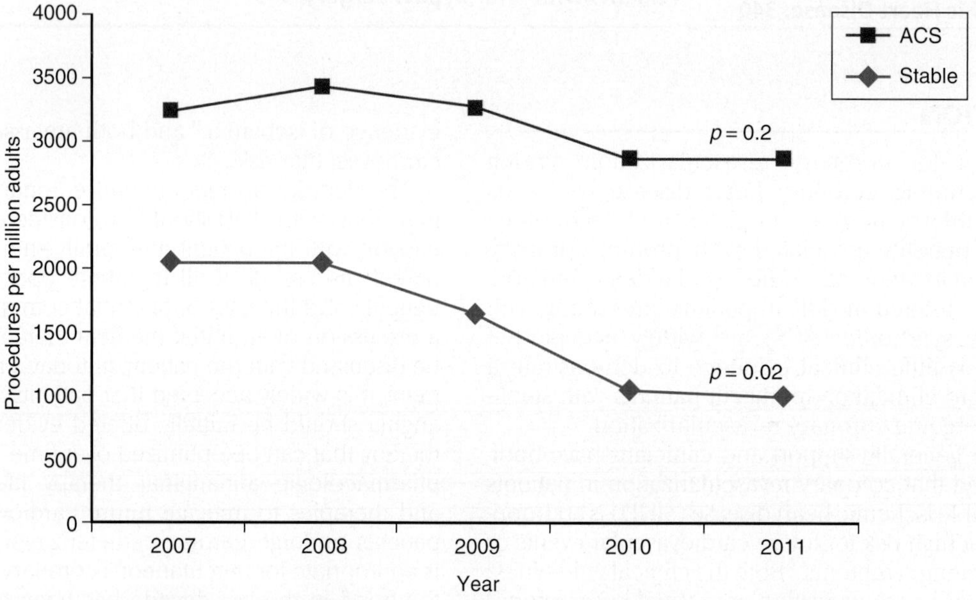

Annual % change*		2007	2008	2009	2010
	Stable	+0.6%	−19.3%	−36.6%	−5.7%
	ACS	+5.8%	−4.7%	−11.9%	−1.5%

A

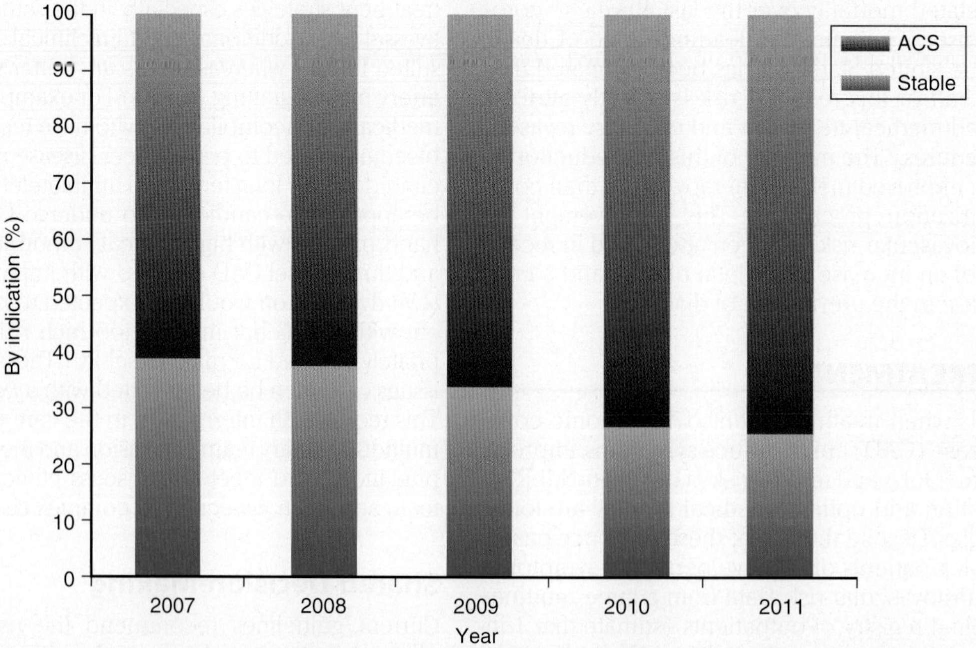

B

FIG. 23.1 Temporal changes in coronary revascularization procedures from 2007–2011 **(A)**. Frequency of PCI by indication: ACS or stable **(B)**. *ACS* = acute coronary syndrome. *(From Kim LK, Feldman DN, Swaminathan RV, et al. Rate of percutaneous coronary intervention for the management of acute coronary syndromes and stable coronary artery disease in the United States (2007 to 2011).* Am J Cardiol. *2014;114:1003–1010.)*

decreased by 28%, and much of this decline was in patients with SIHD[13] (Fig. 23.1).

Following publication of US national rates of "appropriate" coronary revascularization,[14] data from the Washington State Clinical Outcomes Assessment Program between 2010 and 2013 showed that the number of PCI procedures decreased substantially, which was driven by a 43% decline in the number of PCI procedures performed for elective indications. The majority of this decline occurred following the onset of state-wide measurement of PCI appropriateness.[15]

An estimated 500,000 PCI procedures are performed annually in the United States, and an equal number is performed in the rest of the world. The safety and efficiency of procedural techniques have evolved over the past 40 years. PCI is now considered a mature medical procedure. The physician-reported success rates are 99%, and the observed morbidity and mortality rates are approximately 1% to 2%. The complication rates for PCI procedures remain low despite an increasing complexity of lesions and higher-risk clinical demographics.

In 2010, 1488 facilities in the United States were enrolled in the American College of Cardiology National Cardiovascular Data Registry (ACC NCDR) CathPCI Registry, which captured approximately 85% of the PCI procedures performed. A 2012 analysis from this registry includes 1.1 million PCI patients and provides a cross-sectional description of the current state of coronary angiography and PCI in the United States.[10] Institutional and operator volumes for PCI procedures are often used as proxies for PCI quality. Both vary considerably across institutions, with approximately half of all ACC NCDR institutions performing fewer than 400 PCI procedures and 13% performing more than 1000 PCI procedures annually. Currently, 40% of patients are older than age 65 and 12% are older than 80, 80% of patients are overweight, 45% are obese, and 36% have a history of diabetes mellitus. Approximately half the patients underwent a preprocedural stress test, with myocardial perfusion imaging being most commonly performed. Fig. 23.2 shows the percent of patients by indications for diagnostic coronary angiography and PCI. Approximately 18% of patients underwent PCI for stable angina symptoms,

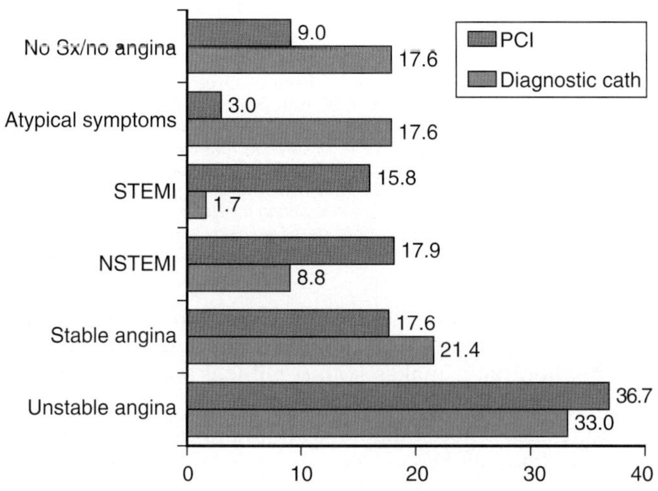

FIG. 23.2 Indications for diagnostic catheterization and percutaneous coronary intervention (PCI). *NSTEMI*, Non-ST elevation myocardial infarction; *STEMI*, ST elevation myocardial infarction; *Sx*, symptoms. *(From Dehmer GJ, Weaver D, Roe MT, et al. A contemporary view of diagnostic cardiac catheterization and percutaneous coronary intervention in the United States: a report from the CathPCI Registry of the National Cardiovascular Data Registry, 2010 through June 2011.* J Am Coll Cardiol. *2012;60(20):2017–2031.)*

while an additional 9% were asymptomatic. Radial artery access in the 2010 report was used in approximately 7% of PCI procedures. This percentage has steadily increased over the last 7 years, with transradial access rates now approaching 20% in the United States (but higher in many parts of the world). The observed in-hospital mortality rate was 0.72%, and in-hospital stroke rate was 0.17%. The most common noncardiac complication continues to be periprocedural bleeding. With the emergence of third- and fourth-generation drug-eluting stents (DESs), target vessel revascularization rates are low at 5% to 7%, and stent thrombosis rates are measurably lower with newer-generation DES platforms.[16]

Lesion progression is a well-recognized factor accounting for future cardiovascular risk following PCI. Approximately 20% of patients undergo repeat PCI within 3 years of the index PCI because of nonculprit lesion progression.[17] Similarly, the Providing Regional Observations to Study Predictors of Events in the Coronary Tree (PROSPECT) trial demonstrated that 50% of all major adverse cardiovascular events at 3 years occur solely as a function of nonculprit lesion progression.[18] Current PCI practices are designed to identify and effectively treat culprit lesions. Because of this, optimal medical therapy for secondary prevention is requisite among patients undergoing PCI.

Two major limitations of PCI remain: a higher than desirable frequency of incomplete revascularization related to complex disease and residual cardiovascular risk related to morbid and mortal events due to disease progression.

CABG is also very common and now performed approximately 400,000 times annually in the United States.[19] There has, however, been a steady decline in the frequency of CABG procedures performed in the United States. Until recently this decline has been associated with an increase in percutaneous coronary revascularization procedures. The most commonly used conduits are the left internal mammary artery (LIMA) and the greater saphenous veins. The use of the LIMA is now considered a quality indicator for CABG and has long been linked to higher long-term patency than saphenous venous grafts. Moreover clinical outcomes are improved with use of the LIMA.[20–22] Other arterial conduits such as the radial artery, the right internal mammary artery, and the gastroepiploic artery have been used and demonstrate improved patency rates compared with the saphenous venous grafts but are not routinely used in clinical practice.[23–25]

In general, a CABG procedure takes 3 to 4 hours, and the patient remains hospitalized for 5 to 7 days and recuperates for 6 to 12 weeks following discharge. The risk for perioperative morbidity and mortality has decreased over time. There is now nearly universal participation of CABG centers in the Society of Thoracic Surgeons National Adult Cardiac Surgery Database. Although the predicted risk of mortality has not changed over time, there has been a measurable reduction in the adjusted mortality rates in the last 10 years (Fig. 23.3).[20] This has been similarly true for perioperative stroke rates.

Stroke remains a serious complication following CABG. Risk factors include increasing age, concomitant peripheral or cerebrovascular disease, diabetes, and aortic atherosclerosis. Neurocognitive decline has also been described in the post-CABG population[26] and specifically linked to cardiopulmonary bypass. These studies have not been randomized controlled trials and the results are heterogeneous.[27,28] Thus the link between CABG and cognitive decline remains uncertain. The current belief is that neurocognitive dysfunction is related to a number of factors including the impact of major surgery coupled with long-term effects in patients

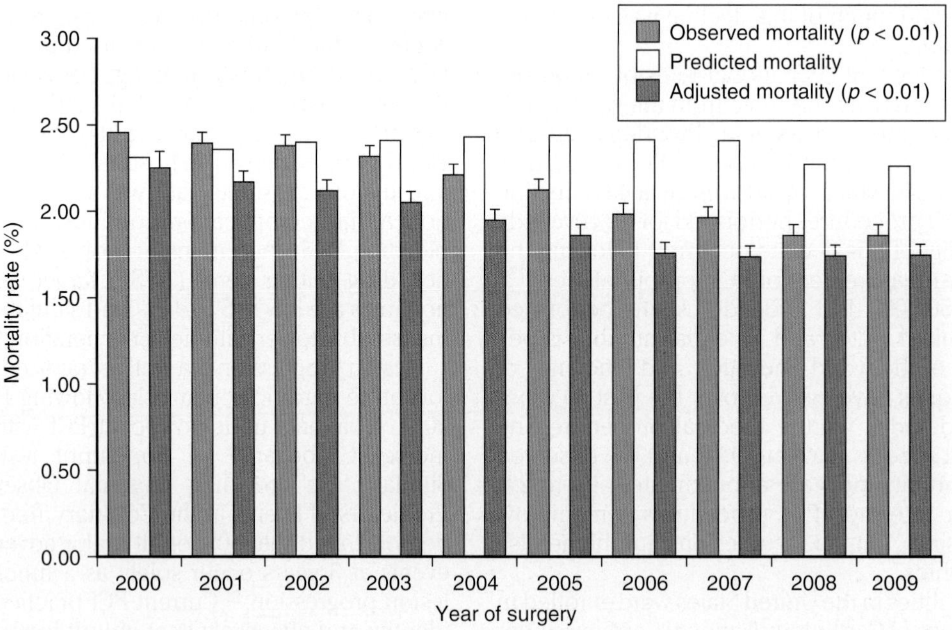

FIG. 23.3 Temporal decline in postoperative coronary artery bypass grafting mortality rates.

BOX 23.1 Medical Therapy for Secondary Prevention Following Coronary Artery Bypass Grafting (CABG)

Aspirin, 81 mg
P2Y12 receptor inhibitors if they were indicated prior to CABG (i.e. for acute coronary syndrome or prior percutaneous coronary intervention)
β-blocker use in patients with prior myocardial infarction, left ventricular systolic dysfunction
Lifelong high-intensity statin therapy
Angiotensin-converting enzyme inhibitors in patients with diabetes and/or left ventricular systolic dysfunction
Aldosterone antagonists in patients with left ventricular systolic dysfunction and heart failure symptoms or signs
Consideration for participating in short-term cardiac rehabilitation program

with cardiovascular risk factors and concomitant coronary artery and cerebrovascular disease.[19]

There remains a risk for native disease progression and bypass graft failure following CABG. Thus it is vitally important that clinicians ensure patients remain on appropriate medical therapy. A 2016 American Heart Association (AHA) scientific statement clarifies appropriate secondary prevention therapy following CABG (Box 23.1).[29] In addition to these recommendations, studies have suggested that P2Y12 receptor inhibition following CABG may be associated with improved graft patency.[30,31]

There has been significant interest in maintaining the benefits of CABG with the use of less-invasive approaches. These techniques require specialized training and are limited in that complete revascularization is achieved less often. The sustainability of these techniques remains uncertain. Off-pump surgery has also been studied; however, the results have been inconsistent with no clear advantage over on-pump surgery.[32–34] Hybrid surgical and percutaneous revascularization strategies have been explored in recent years. With this strategy patients undergo minimally invasive surgery with a LIMA usually to the left anterior descending artery and then subsequently undergo PCI to either the left circumflex or right coronary artery. Long-term data comparing this hybrid approach to conventional CABG are lacking, but this approach makes sound clinical sense in specific patient populations. Common appropriate use criteria for PCI and CABG for patients with multivessel disease are shown in Table 23.1.[35]

TABLE 23.1 Appropriate Use Criteria for Common Indications in Patients with Multivessel Coronary Disease

	CABG	PCI
Two-vessel CAD with proximal LAD stenosis	A	A
Three-vessel CAD with low CAD burden (i.e., 3 focal stenoses, low SYNTAX score)	A	A
Three-vessel CAD with intermediate to high CAD burden (i.e., multiple diffuse lesions, presence of CTO, or high SYNTAX score)	A	U
Isolated left main stenosis	A	U
Left main stenosis and additional CAD with low CAD burden (i.e., one to two vessel additional involvement, low SYNTAX score)	A	U
Left main stenosis and additional CAD with intermediate to high CAD burden (i.e., three vessel involvement, presence of CTO, or high SYNTAX score)	A	I

A, Appropriate, *I*, Inappropriate, *U*, Uncertain appropriateness.
CABG, Coronary artery bypass grafting; *CAD*, coronary artery disease; *CTO*, chronic total occlusion; *LAD*, left anterior descending artery; *PCI*, percutaneous coronary intervention; *SYNTAX*, Synergy Between PCI with TAXUS and Cardiac Surgery.
(From Patel MR, Dehmer GJ, Hirshfeld JW, et al. CCF/SCAI/STS/AATS/AHA/ASNC/HFSA/SCCT 2012 appropriate use criteria for coronary revascularization focused update: a report of the American College of Cardiology Foundation Appropriate Use Criteria Task Force, Society for Cardiovascular Angiography and Interventions, Society of Thoracic Surgeons, American Association for Thoracic Surgery, American Heart Association, American Society of Nuclear Cardiology, and the Society of Cardiovascular Computed Tomography. J Am Coll Cardiol. *2012;59:857–881.)*

Indications for Coronary Revascularization in Patients with Stable Ischemic Heart Disease

The goals of coronary revascularization, whether PCI or CABG, are to relieve symptoms, improve QoL, and mitigate

TABLE 23.2 Stress Test Findings

HIGH RISK (> 3% ANNUAL MORTALITY)	INTERMEDIATE RISK (1%–3% ANNUAL MORTALITY)	LOW RISK (< 1% ANNUAL MORTALITY)
Resting LVEF < 35%	Mild to moderate resting LVEF 35%–49%	Duke treadmill score ≥ 5
Duke treadmill score ≤ −11	Duke treadmill score 11–5	Normal or small myocardial perfusion defect
Exercise LVEF < 35%	Stress-induced moderate perfusion defect without LV dilation or increased lung uptake	Normal stress echocardiographic wall motion during stress testing
Stress-induced large perfusion defect	Limited exercise capacity. Echocardiographic ischemia or wall motion abnormality at higher doses of dobutamine	
Stress-induced multiple perfusion defects		
Large, fixed perfusion defect with LV dilation or increased lung uptake (thallium 201)		
Stress-induced moderate perfusion defect with LV dilation or increased lung uptake		
> 2 segments wall motion abnormality on dobutamine echocardiography		
Stress echocardiographic evidence of extensive ischemia		

LVEF, Left ventricular ejection fraction.

the risk of future complications related to atherosclerotic CAD such as cardiovascular mortality and nonfatal MI. These goals have not changed over the last several decades. However, the evidence base for coronary revascularization and medical therapy has greatly expanded over the past decade.[4,36] These newer data provide clinicians with additional insights when recommending therapy to patients with chronic stable heart disease.

Relief of Symptoms

Relief of symptoms and improvement in QoL are central benefits of coronary revascularization in the SIHD population.[37] Clinical data supporting sustained improved QoL following PCI in SIHD patients are varied. Study designs range from prospective nonrandomized data using pre-post analytic strategies with broad inclusion criteria to highly selected randomized controlled trials comparing PCI with medical and surgical therapies. Numerous noncomparative cohort studies demonstrate that PCI improves QoL and exercise capacity compared with pre-PCI assessment.[37] Many (but not all) of these studies suggest PCI reduces both angina and need for antianginal medications and improves both exercise capacity and health status. A meta-analysis including 7818 patients demonstrated that PCI was superior to medical therapy in reducing angina.[38] There was heterogeneity across these trials with shorter follow-up and earlier trials favoring PCI, whereas higher use of evidence-based therapies favored medical therapy. In general, factors associated with improved post-PCI QoL include increased frequency of baseline angina, greater extent of baseline myocardial ischemia, cardiac rehabilitation, and nonsmoking status. Lower socioeconomic status, unemployment, and numerous clinical comorbidities are associated with lower QoL after PCI.

In general, both CABG and PCI improve QoL. In the early weeks following coronary revascularization, PCI trends better than CABG, but this difference attenuates by 3 to 5 months.[37] In a collaborative meta-analysis of 10 randomized clinical trials comparing CABG with PCI,[39] CABG was superior to PCI in angina relief at 1 year in patients with multivessel disease. Most studies suggest CABG is superior to PCI in reducing angina and improving QoL, although the benefits of CABG diminish over many years of follow-up; this is likely related to vein graft failure and disease progression.

Coronary Revascularization to Reduce the Risk of Death and Nonfatal Myocardial Infarction

There are limited data to support the hypothesis that PCI reduces death and nonfatal MI in patients with low-risk SIHD. Selected trials have evaluated surgical revascularization for high-risk patients with three-vessel disease, left main disease, severe LV dysfunction, or severe ischemia.[38] Both clinicians and practice guidelines extrapolate these early clinical trial findings to justify coronary revascularization (both PCI and CABG) in high-risk SIHD patients. Risk is often estimated following a noninvasive stress test. Features of low-, intermediate-, and high-risk stress test findings are shown in Table 23.2.

Low-Risk Patients

Many clinical trials have compared medical therapy with coronary revascularization in low-risk patients with chronic stable angina. Without exception these trials were neutral with respect to hard cardiovascular endpoints.[40,41] Although these trials were largely conducted in the 1970s and 1980s and there have been major advances in medical, percutaneous, and surgical therapies since then, the overall findings are thought to be relevant today. In short, CABG was associated with improved symptoms but no measurable difference in survival or nonfatal MI.

Although many prior studies have failed to demonstrate a long-term benefit on death or MI following PCI or CABG in stable patients,[42–45] the Clinical Outcomes Utilizing Revascularization and Aggressive Drug Evaluation (COURAGE) trial is frequently cited as the landmark trial comparing medical therapy with PCI in SIHD patients. COURAGE evaluated the efficacy of PCI versus medical therapy in 2287 patients.[46] Patients with either a greater than 70% diameter stenosis of at least one coronary artery with objective evidence of ischemia or greater than 80% stenosis coupled with typical angina symptoms were eligible. Exclusions included Canadian Cardiovascular Society (CCS) class IV angina, markedly abnormal stress tests, significant congestive heart failure symptoms, LV ejection fraction less than 30%, or revascularization within the prior 6 months.

At 5 years, there was no difference in the primary endpoint of death or MI between PCI and the medical therapy group (odds ratio [OR] ratio 1.05, 95% confidence interval [CI] 0.87–1.27, $p = 0.62$). PCI patients had a lower rate of repeat revascularization and a lower need for antianginal medications than the medical therapy group during the first year.

There are a number of limitations to COURAGE that restrict generalizability to a broader SIHD population.[47] COURAGE enrolled a lower-risk population than had been expected, with an annual cardiovascular mortality rate of 0.4%. There was an exceptionally high screen failure rate: of the nearly 36,000 patients screened, only 2287 enrolled. Other limitations included a low burden of baseline angina and a 30% crossover rate from medical therapy to PCI. The 5-year medical adherence rate in COURAGE was exceptional; 94% for aspirin, 93% for statins, and 86% for β-blocker therapy. Moreover 70% of patients achieved the low-density lipoprotein (LDL) target and almost half of the patients with diabetes achieved the hemoglobin A_{1c} target of less than 7%. These rates exceed those seen in usual clinical practice.[48]

Substudy data from COURAGE support prior clinical studies and the evolving hypothesis that higher baseline myocardial ischemia is associated with higher future cardiovascular risk and that this risk may be attenuated with adequate coronary revascularization. In a single-center study preceding COURAGE of 5183 consecutive patients undergoing rest-stress single photon emission computed tomography (SPECT), the severity of stress perfusion abnormalities was associated with higher rates of MI and cardiovascular death.[49] A summed stress score of greater than 13 was associated with an annual MI risk of 4.2% and a mortality rate of 2.9% when compared with patients with low-risk scans, who had an annual event rate of less than 1%. This same group of investigators also demonstrated that early revascularization following stress testing was associated with a lower adjusted rate of cardiovascular mortality in selected high-risk patients (4.6% vs 1.3%, $p < 0.01$).[50] The benefits associated with early coronary revascularization appeared to be limited to those patients with the baseline ischemic burden of greater than 10%.

The COURAGE nuclear substudy ($n = 314$ of 2287) also explored the ischemic burden hypothesis.[51] Patients underwent sequential rest-stress myocardial perfusion imaging studies with SPECT at baseline and then 6 to 18 months following randomization. The baseline ischemic burden in these subjects was modest at 8%. Although both PCI and medical therapies reduced ischemia, the reduction was not robust, 2.7% and 0.5% in the PCI and medical therapy groups, respectively. Resolution of significant baseline ischemia, defined as greater than 5% reduction in ischemic burden and at least over 10% baseline ischemia, was associated with greater relief of angina and lower rates of death or nonfatal MI (13.4% vs 24.7%). Patients randomized to PCI were more likely to experience a 5% or greater reduction in ischemic myocardium (33% vs 19%, $p = 0.0004$). Lastly there was a graded relationship between the extent and severity of residual ischemia and the risk of future cardiovascular events. The rate of death or nonfatal MI ranged from 0% among those patients without residual ischemia to 39% for patients who after treatment had a 10% or greater residual ischemic burden. These data support the hypothesis that baseline ischemic burden is associated with risk and that this risk may be diminished with complete coronary revascularization if associated with a reduction in residual ischemic burden.

The ischemic burden hypothesis is being formally tested in the International Study of Comparative Health Effectiveness with Medical and Invasive Approaches (ISCHEMIA) (NCT01471522), which is designed to determine whether an invasive strategy is superior to a conservative strategy in reducing cardiovascular death or MI among patients with at least moderate ischemia on noninvasive imaging. ISCHEMIA is projected to enroll 8000 patients at 500 sites. In order to formally test the ischemia burden hypothesis, ISCHEMIA will need to have a very high frequency of complete revascularization and minimal residual ischemia in patients randomized to early angiography.

Cardiac troponin concentrations are used to risk stratify ACS patients for prompt revascularization but have not routinely been used to assess risk in patients with SIHD. High-sensitivity assays are now available to detect very low cardiac troponin levels in patients with stable heart disease. These low-level elevations are strongly associated with death, MI, and stroke in patients with SIHD.[52,53] In the Bypass Angioplasty Revascularization Investigation in Type 2 Diabetes Trial (BARI 2D), elevated troponin T concentrations (≥ 14 ng/L) at baseline were common (approximately 40% of people had an increased baseline value) and associated with increased 5-year risk of death, MI, and stroke (hazard ratio [HR], 1.85; 95% CI, 1.48–2.32; $p < 0.001$). However, increased levels did not associate with improved outcome following coronary revascularization. Presently, whereas elevated troponins are associated with risk in SIHD patients, the elevated risk does not appear to be modified by routine coronary revascularization.

Complex Patients and Lesions

CABG has been shown to be superior to medical therapy in patients with severe multivessel CAD. These clinical trials date back to the 1970s and 1980s. When the early trials including the Veterans Administration Cooperative Study,[54] the European Coronary Surgery Study,[40] and the Coronary Artery Surgery Study[55] are included in a large clinical database of over 2600 patients, CABG was associated with lower mortality at 5 years (10% vs 16%, $p < 0.001$), which extended to 10 years (26% vs 31%, $p = 0.003$) compared with medical therapy. The reduction in mortality was in general consistent across a variety of subgroups. However, the absolute benefit was greatest for patients at the highest risk including those with extensive CAD and those with moderate to severe LV systolic dysfunction. The clinical benefit of CABG is not realized in the first 1 to 2 years following surgery. Beyond this the benefit of CABG is apparent and divergent over time. Inclusion of these earlier trials is limited in that the background medical therapy is very different from current practices.

PCI is favored over medical therapy and CABG in patients presenting with an ACS, including non-ST segment elevation and ST segment elevation MI and in SIHD patients with physiologically important disease that is not extensive. The extent of disease has traditionally been quantified by number of diseased vessels. In patients with very complex coronary anatomy and acceptable clinical risk, CABG has been the preferred strategy. In this later group, the evidence base has expanded in recent years with publication of landmark trials, many of which have included patients with relatively complex coronary anatomy.

There are many strengths and limitations to both PCI and CABG. These treatment options are neither curative nor mutually exclusive when treating SIHD patients over the course of an individual's lifetime. CABG is considered the gold standard for treating complex multivessel CAD and is associated with a higher rate of complete revascularization and lower likelihood of repeat revascularization than is PCI.[45,56,57] The major advantage of CABG is a higher likelihood of complete revascularization and the ability to bypass a significant portion of the proximal epicardial coronary artery, mitigating the likelihood of future cardiovascular morbidity and mortality if the patient were to experience nonculprit proximal disease progression. The major limitation for CABG is the risk of vein graft degeneration over time and the perioperative complication rate, especially among those patients with multiple clinical comorbidities. The major advantages of PCI are its less invasive nature, the efficacy of PCI in the ACS population, and the ability to selectively treat the culprit lesion. The major limitations of PCI are a higher frequency of incomplete revascularization, the inability to prevent the clinical implications of nonculprit disease progression, a higher rate of repeat revascularization even in the DES era, and the technical challenges in very complex lesion subsets. In short, angiographic burden and lesion complexity limit the effectiveness of PCI, whereas clinical comorbidities limit the safety of CABG.

Comparisons of PCI and CABG in Patients with Multivessel Coronary Artery Disease

The Arterial Revascularization Therapies Study (ARTS),[58] Argentine Randomized Trial of Coronary Angioplasty with Stenting Versus Coronary Bypass Surgery in Patients with Multiple Vessel Disease (ERACI II), Medicine Angioplasty or Surgery Study for Multi-Vessel Coronary Artery Disease (MASS-II),[59] and Stent or Surgery (SoS)[60] compared CABG to bare metal stenting and were each included in a pooled patient level meta-analysis of 3051 patients.[61] At 5 years the incidence of death, MI, and stroke was similar (16.7% vs 16.9%; HR, 1.04, 95% CI, 0.86–1.27; $p = 0.69$), yet incomplete (89.4% vs 62.0%; $p < 0.001$) and repeat (29.0% vs 7.9%; $p < 0.001$) revascularizations were more frequent in the PCI population. There was a trend for improved mortality among diabetic patients randomized to CABG (12.4% vs 7.9%; $p = 0.09$). A larger meta-analysis spanning the percutaneous transluminal coronary angioplasty (PTCA) and stent era included 59,014 patients and demonstrated that risk-adjusted survival rates were improved in patients treated with CABG compared with those undergoing PCI.[62]

The very large and more contemporary Synergy Between Percutaneous Coronary Intervention with TAXUS and Cardiac Surgery (SYNTAX) trial compared PCI with DESs to CABG in 1800 patients with previously untreated complex three-vessel and/or left main CAD.[63] This trial incorporated a local heart team approach, which consisted of a cardiac surgeon and an interventional cardiologist. Each member reviewed the clinical case and coronary anatomy and each needed to agree that revascularization could be achieved with CABG or PCI. SYNTAX was powered as a noninferiority comparison of CABG and PCI with a primary endpoint of all-cause mortality, stroke, MI, or repeat revascularization. The 12-month primary endpoint occurred more commonly following PCI (17.8% vs 12.4%; $p = 0.002$), and thus noninferiority of PCI was not met. The difference was principally driven by higher repeat revascularization rates in the PCI-treated patients. The 12-month MI rates were similar; however, CABG was associated with a nearly fourfold increase in stroke (2.2% vs 0.6%; $p = 0.003$). At 5 years, PCI was associated with higher rates of death, stroke, MI, and repeat revascularization.[64] Nonrandomized studies from 2012 have suggested lower mortality rates for CABG patients with multivessel disease.[65]

A number of post hoc subgroup analyses from SYNTAX have been informative and have impacted both clinical practice and design of ongoing clinical trials.

Baseline SYNTAX Score

The SYNTAX score (Fig. 23.4) was designed to predict the postprocedural risk associated with PCI or surgical revascularization. It is a visual estimate of CAD burden and complexity. The SYNTAX score takes into account complex lesions including bifurcations, chronic total occlusions, thrombus, calcification, and small diffuse disease. The score ranges from 0 to greater than 60 in very complex coronary anatomy lesions. In the SYNTAX trial, higher SYNTAX scores differentiated outcomes between CABG and PCI.[63] There was no difference in endpoints for patients randomized to CABG across the entire range of SYNTAX scores. This was not the case for patients randomized to PCI where there was a significant interaction in the cumulative event rates between patients with low, intermediate, and higher SYNTAX scores. In patients with baseline SYNTAX scores of 0 to 22 the outcomes were comparable for CABG and PCI patients. CABG was associated with lower event rates with SYNTAX scores greater than 22. The SYNTAX calculator is online at www.syntaxscore.com.

Unprotected Left Main Disease

CABG has been the preferred strategy for treating patients with significant, unprotected left main disease. This treatment paradigm has evolved in recent years. PCI has moved from a class IIb to a class IIa indication for the treatment of left main disease among patients with lower SYNTAX scores.[66] In the SYNTAX trial, there were 705 patients with unprotected left main stenosis. This was a prespecified subgroup and the 5-year major adverse coronary and cerebrovascular events (MACCE) rate was 36.9% for PCI and 31.0% for CABG (HR, 1.23; 95% CI, 0.95–1.59; $p = 0.12$). The composite of death, stroke, and MI was similar for PCI (19.0%) and CABG (20.8%). The rates of graft occlusion (4.4%) and stent thrombosis (5.1%) were also similar. When the patients were dichotomized based on SYNTAX scores, the 5-year MACCE rates were similar for PCI and CABG in left main patients with SYNTAX scores 0 to 32. In this low SYNTAX score group, the major adverse cardiac events (MACE) rate was numerically lower (14.8% vs 19.8%) and the death rate significantly lower (17.9% vs 15.1%) in the PCI group. However, in patients with SYNTAX scores of 33 or higher, CABG was associated with significantly lower cardiovascular death (15.8% vs 5.9%) and revascularization (34.1% vs 11.6%) rates. Based largely on these data, it is commonly believed that the extent and complexity of disease downstream from the left main is more related to clinical outcomes than the extent and/or complexity of the left main disease itself.

The Evaluation of Everolimus Eluting Stent System Versus Coronary Artery Bypass Surgery for Effectiveness of Left Main Revascularization (EXCEL) clinical trial is projected to randomize 2600 patients with unprotected left main disease with low or intermediate SYNTAX scores to either PCI or CABG. The primary outcome will be the composite of death, MI, and stroke (EXCEL clinicaltrials.gov identifier NCT01205776. http//clinicaltrials.gov/ct2/show/study/NCT01205776).

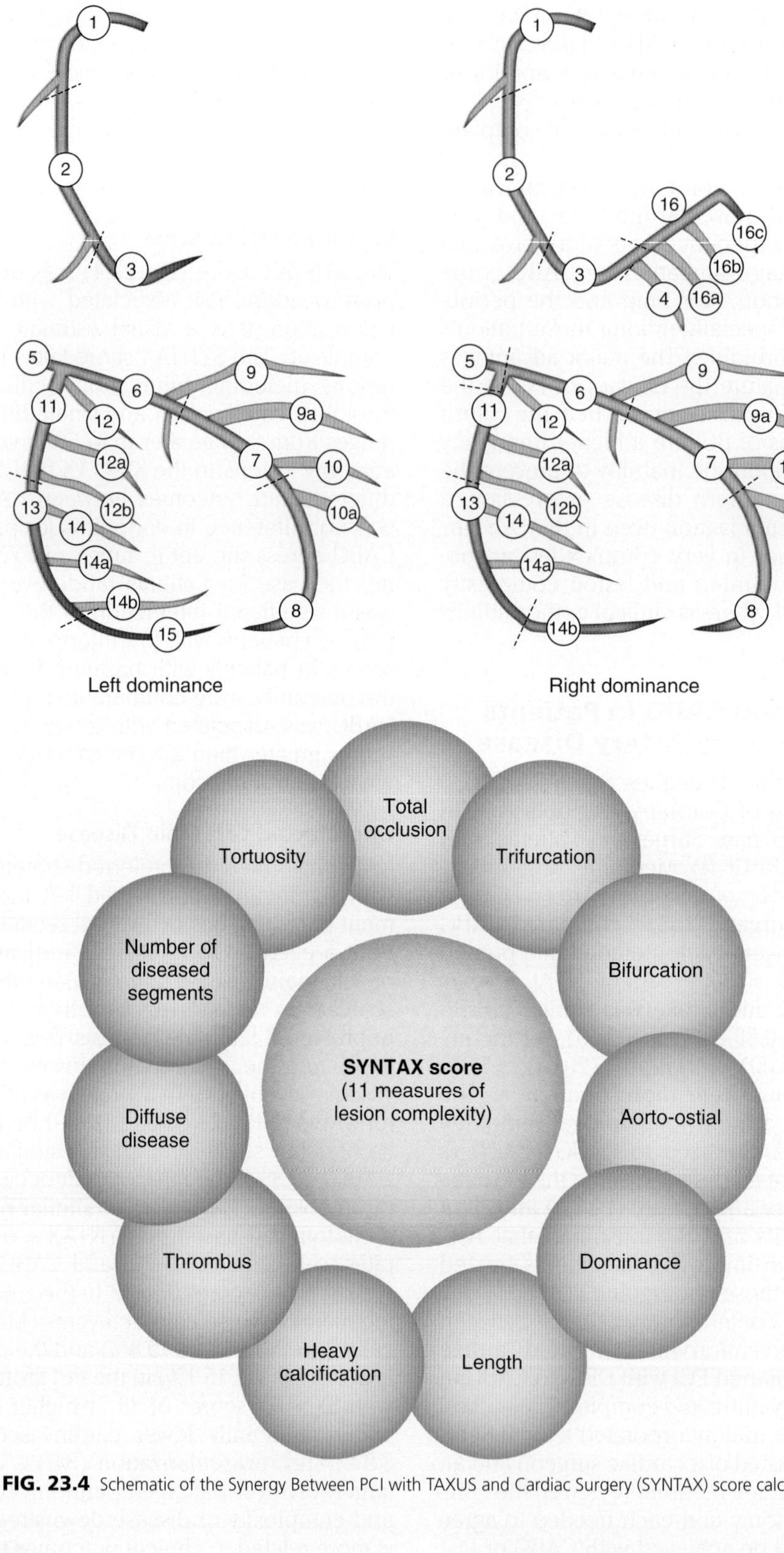

FIG. 23.4 Schematic of the Synergy Between PCI with TAXUS and Cardiac Surgery (SYNTAX) score calculation.

Diabetes Mellitus

Patients with diabetes (see Chapter 24) are often thought to have very complex coronary anatomy with a greater number of diseased vessels, lesion complexity, and smaller more diffusely diseased coronary arteries. Diabetes is very often a predictor of poor outcomes following both PCI and CABG. In general, clinical trial data suggest that CABG is superior to PCI in patients with type 2 diabetes mellitus with multivessel disease.[67] This recommendation dates back to the original BARI report.[68]

The BARI 2D trial compared coronary revascularization, either CABG or PCI, with medical therapy among patients with type 2 diabetes mellitus[69] and CCS class I or II angina. Whether patients underwent CABG or PCI was at the investigator's discretion. Patients with perceived need for immediate revascularization, left main disease, significant heart failure, or revascularization within 1 year of study entry were excluded. The 5-year all-cause mortality and MACE rates were similar between the medical therapy and coronary revascularization groups. Crossover approached 40%. CABG but not PCI was associated with a significant reduction in nonfatal MI.[70]

In the SYNTAX trial there were 296 patients with medically treated diabetes. In this substudy, the death, MI, stroke, and repeat revascularization rate was considerably higher in the PCI group (45.5% vs 23.6%; $p < 0.001$). This was driven by a twofold increase in all-cause mortality and a threefold increase in both repeat revascularization and MI rates. Stroke rates were comparable.[71]

The Future Revascularization Evaluation in Patients with Diabetes Mellitus: Optimal Management of Multivessel Disease (FREEDOM) trial was a dedicated large-scale randomized clinical trial comparing CABG with PCI in patients with diabetes mellitus. It randomized 1900 patients with diabetes and multivessel disease to undergo either PCI with DESs or CABG.[72] The 5-year rate of death, MI, or stroke occurred more frequently in the PCI-DES group (26.6% vs 18.7%; $p = 0.005$). CABG patients had significantly lower rates of nonfatal MI and all-cause mortality, whereas PCI patients had significantly fewer strokes. The 2- and 5-year results are shown in Fig 23.5.

FREEDOM and SYNTAX trials suggest greater treatment benefit of CABG in patients with increasing complexity of CAD. The treatment effect of CABG for patients with SYNTAX scores greater than 22 was numerically greater.[73] A similar numerical trend was seen in the 3-year results of the SYNTAX diabetes substudy. There is a consistent trend in the medical literature suggesting that, among patients with diabetes and complex multivessel CAD as assessed with the SYNTAX score, CABG lowers cardiovascular complications. On the basis of these clinical data the American College of Cardiology Foundation(ACCF)/AHA guidelines for the treatment of patients with SIHD give a class I recommendation favoring CABG over PCI for patients with multivessel CAD and concomitant diabetes mellitus.[74]

Ischemic Cardiomyopathy

Ischemic cardiomyopathy is a morbid condition with a 10-year mortality rate of 60%. These patients have a multitude of comorbidities including LV systolic dysfunction, impaired coronary hemodynamics, abnormal myocardial energetics, increased myocardial oxygen consumption, and altered myocardial lactate metabolism even in the absence of significant CAD. In such patients, the decision whether or not to perform coronary revascularization is difficult.

The Surgical Treatment for Ischemic Heart Failure (STICH) trial randomized 1212 patients with ischemic cardiomyopathy with an ejection fraction of less than 35% to either CABG or medical therapy. This was a complex patient population and included a high prevalence of patients with diabetes, previous MI, and New York Heart Association (NYHA) class II-III heart failure. At a median follow-up of 56 months, there was no significant difference in cardiovascular deaths between CABG and medical therapy.[75] The STITCH Extension Study was a 5-year extension that reported 10-year outcomes. The primary outcome of all-cause mortality occurred significantly less frequently in the CABG group (58.9% vs 66.1%; $p = 0.02$). This was driven by a significant reduction in both cardiovascular (40.5% vs 49.3%; $p = 0.006$) and noncardiovascular mortality (76.6% vs 87.0%; $p < 0.001$).[76] The median survival advantage was 1.44 years in the CABG group with a number needed to treat of 14 to prevent 1 death.

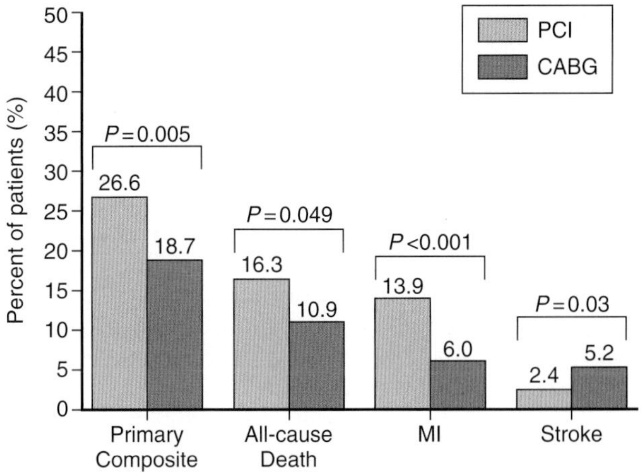

FIG. 23.5 Five-year outcomes from Synergy Between PCI with TAXUS and Cardiac Surgery (SYNTAX). *CABG*, Coronary artery bypass grafting; *PCI*, percutaneous coronary intervention. *(Data from Farkouh ME, Domanski M, Sleeper LA, et al. Strategies for multivessel revascularization in patients with diabetes.* N Engl J Med. *2012;367:2375–2384.)*

Patients with Chronic Kidney Disease

Patients with chronic kidney disease (CKD) are often excluded from clinical trials, yet this population has grown substantially in the past 10 years.[77] Although the risk of future cardiovascular events is substantial in the CKD population, there is a lower tendency to prescribe medical therapy and to perform stress tests, cardiac catheterizations, and revascularization procedures.[78] The 2014 European Society of Cardiology and the European Association for Cardio Thoracic Surgery guidelines on myocardial revascularization recommend CABG over PCI (class IIa) in patients with moderate-severe CKD and multivessel disease when surgical risk is acceptable.[79] These recommendations are based on nonrandomized large cohort studies. A large study from the New York State Registry (2015), however, suggests outcomes may be better following PCI.[80] Using propensity-score matching methodology involving 5920 patients with CKD, PCI was associated with a lower risk of death (HR, 0.55; 95% CI, 0.35–0.87) and stroke (HR, 0.2; 95% CI, 0.12–0.42) yet a higher risk of repeat revascularization (HR, 2.42; 95% CI, 2.05–2.85). In a small substudy of 243 patients on renal replacement therapy PCI was associated with higher rates of death (HR, 2.02; 95% CI, 1.40–2.93) and higher rates of repeat revascularization (HR, 2.44; 95% CI, 1.50–3.96) compared with CABG. These nonrandomized studies suggest PCI may be preferable in patients with CKD with the possible exception of patients on chronic renal replacement therapy.

Patients with Prior Bypass Surgery

Approximately 20% of PCI patients in the United States have a history of previous CABG.[81] There are a number of complex issues when intervening in patients with prior CABG ranging from the need to treat complex lesion subsets, including saphenous vein grafts, severe calcification, diffuse disease, bifurcation lesions, and chronic total occlusions. Patients with prior CABG are also high risk given advanced age, multivessel disease, and depressed LV systolic ejection fraction. Atheroembolization occurs more often following PCI of saphenous venous grafts because, in general, the atherosclerotic plaque in these grafts is more diffuse and friable, and patients have very thin fibrous caps and little or no calcification relative to native coronary atherosclerosis. This results in a higher frequency of atheroembolization, microvascular obstruction, no reflow, and postprocedural death or MI. No reflow can be treated with arterial vasodilators such as nitroprusside, verapamil, or adenosine. Embolic protection devices are generally considered effective in reducing the complications of atheroembolization in the setting of saphenous venous graft PCI. Many operators now preferentially treat obstructive coronary disease in the native coronary circulation rather than performing PCI on degenerated vein grafts, as it may be a safer, more effective, and more durable option than intervening on degenerated and/or occluded saphenous venous grafts.

Revascularization of Total Occlusions

Recent Occlusions Following ST Elevation Myocardial Infarction

Primary PCI for ST elevation myocardial infarction (STEMI) is the standard of care. However, approximately 1 in 3 patients does not receive prompt reperfusion therapy.[82] Observational studies have described an association between patent infarct-related artery after late presentation and improved outcomes, whereas others have not.[83–91]

The Occluded Artery Trial (OAT) enrolled 2166 patients with recent MI, ejection fraction less than 50%, and persistently occluded artery who were also beyond the traditional time period for myocardial salvage.[92] The primary endpoint was death, MI, or NYHA class IV heart failure. There was no difference between the PCI and medical therapy groups (17.2% vs 15.6%; HR, 1.16; 95% CI, 0.92–1.45; $p = 0.20$) respectively[92] with a mean follow-up of 3 years. The lack of benefit was consistent across subgroups. There was a numerical increase in the reinfarction rate in the PCI group that was greatest in the first 30 days but persisted through 5 years. Thus elective PCI does not reduce death or reinfarction in patients 3 to 28 days post MI with a persistently occluded infarct-related artery.

The Total Occlusion Study of Canada (TOSCA-2) was the angiographic substudy of OAT. The primary purpose was to establish the 1-year angiographic patency in OAT, which was approximately 82.7% in the PCI group compared with 25.2% in the medical group ($p < 0.0001$).[93] Patency of the infarct-related artery did not translate to an improvement in LV function or remodeling indices. The OAT nuclear substudy also showed no influence of baseline viability and the extent of LV remodeling as measured by end-systolic and diastolic volumes at 1 year. The ACC/AHA STEMI guidelines provide a class III recommendation for PCI of a totally occluded infarct artery greater than 24 hours after STEMI in patients who are asymptomatic and have one- or two-vessel disease if patients are stable and have no evidence of inducible cardiac ischemia.

Chronic Total Occlusions

OAT did not evaluate the efficacy of treating chronic total occlusions (CTOs). CTOs are occluded coronary arteries after thrombolysis with myocardial (TIMI) flow of 0 for 3 months or more. CTOs are found in 15% to 40% of diagnostic heart catheterizations.[94,95] There has been a significant increase in the number of CTO PCIs being performed worldwide. Expert operators are now achieving procedural success rates approaching 80% to 90% using what is now called the *hybrid approach*.[96] This approach utilizes both antegrade and retrograde approaches and subintimal techniques such as antegrade dissection reentry and reverse controlled antegrade and retrograde tracking to optimize successful crossing of the occlusion, while attempting to minimize procedural complications.

One of the major barriers to CTO PCI is the very high lesion complexity that is associated with prolonged, costly procedures that have a higher failure rate than standard PCI. The Japanese CTO score is commonly used to assess lesion complexity[97] (Table 23.3). A higher score is associated with higher technical failure rates and poor long-term outcomes.

The presence of developed collaterals is often cited as a major justification for not recommending coronary revascularization of a CTO segment. Studies demonstrate that myocardium subtended by collaterals to a CTO segment is nearly universally ischemic. Data from Werner et al. suggest that it is very uncommon to have normal blood flow downstream from collateralized CTO segments. In a registry of 59 patients without a prior Q-wave MI, fractional flow reserve (FFR) (see following discussion) values were less than 0.8, suggesting that collateralized myocardium is ischemic.[98]

CTOs are also associated with increased early and late cardiovascular risk following STEMI[99] and non-STEMI (NSTEMI).[100] There are a number of nonrandomized clinical studies including a 2015 meta-analysis[101,102] associating successful CTO PCI with improved survival, compared with a failed CTO PCI attempt. It should be noted that there are no data from adequately sized randomized controlled trials demonstrating that CTO PCI is associated with clinically meaningful and durable benefit.[102]

There is also an increasing body of literature establishing improved health status following successful CTO PCI in appropriately selected patients. CTO PCI is associated with at least as great an improvement in health status as is seen for PCI in non-CTO-PCI patients, despite a substantially lower success rate (85% vs 95%) in the CTO-PCI group.[103] Health status studies utilizing the Seattle Angina Questionnaire have shown an improvement in several domains including physical limitations, angina frequency, and treatment satisfaction.

CTO PCI is associated with higher procedural complications than is non-CTO PCI. In a recent large meta-analysis including over 18,000 CTO patients, CTO PCI was associated with a mortality rate of 0.2% and was associated with emergent coronary bypass grafting in 0.1%, stroke in 0.1%, MI in 2.5%, coronary perforation in 2.9%, tamponade in 0.3%, and contrast nephropathy in 3.8% of patients. Unsuccessful procedures were associated with higher mortality rates (1.5% vs 0.4% in successful procedures), and perforation leading to tamponade occurred in 1.7%. Unpublished data from the Outcomes, Patient Health Status, and Efficiency (OPEN) registry, which included a consecutive prospective study design with systematic collection of periprocedural complications and adjudication of important clinical outcomes and complications, demonstrated a

TABLE 23.3 The Japan Chronic Total Occlusion Score

	POINTS
Prior failed attempt	1
Angiographic evidence of heavy calcification	1
Bend within occluded segment	1
Blunt proximal cap	1
Length > 20 min	1

(From J Am Coll Cardiol Intv. 2011;4(2):213-221. doi:10.1016/j.jcin.2010.09.024.)

mortality rate approaching 1% and a major complication rate of 4% (JA Grantham, personal communication, 2016).

Complete Versus Incomplete Coronary Revascularization

The Coronary Artery Surgery Study (CASS) was one of the first to suggest that complete revascularization was associated with improved outcomes in patients with advanced CAD. Patients with severe angina and multivessel disease who received three or more grafts had improved survival when compared with those who received fewer grafts.[56] Clinical evidence since this early publication has not demonstrated a consistent benefit for complete revascularization, and current practice guidelines do not make firm recommendations on whether complete revascularization is essential. Whereas incomplete revascularization occurs significantly more frequently in PCI, it is not uncommon with CABG. In the New York State Registry, the frequency ranged from 45% to 89% in patients with multivessel CAD.[104] There are challenges when comparing outcomes of patients with complete versus incomplete revascularization. There are a number of higher-risk clinical comorbidities and technical issues that are associated with incomplete revascularization. Direct comparisons, even with sophisticated adjustment for residual confounding, are challenging.

However, incomplete revascularization is often associated with worse outcomes.[64] There was a high frequency of incomplete revascularization in both the CABG (43%) and PCI (48%) patients in the SYNTAX trial. There was a modest association between incomplete revascularization and increased adverse events in the SYNTAX trial that was primarily driven by the need for repeat revascularization. There was no clear association between harder cardiovascular endpoints such as death, MI, or stroke for those with incomplete revascularization following CABG, but a there was a modest association for patients randomized to PCI.[105]

A 2013 meta-analysis of both PCI and CABG studies identified 35 studies and 90,000 patients.[106] Complete revascularization occurred in approximately 50% of patients and was associated with a lower risk for mortality, MI, and need for repeat revascularization. The mortality benefit associated with complete revascularization was independent of whether patients underwent CABG or PCI. Following multivariable adjustment, complete revascularization remained a significant factor associated with lower mortality. Because of equipoise the concept of reasonable incomplete revascularization has been suggested as an alternative to an extreme approach of complete (or incomplete) revascularization.[107] This concept of reasonable incomplete revascularization hypothesizes that there is an acceptable magnitude of residual disease following a coronary revascularization procedure and that this residual disease burden would not be associated with future cardiovascular risk. Quantifying this residual disease burden is challenging and incompletely studied.

Standards for defining and quantifying complete revascularization are lacking. The residual SYNTAX score quantifies the amount of disease "left behind" following coronary revascularization. An Acute Catheterization and Urgent Intervention Triage Strategy (ACUITY) substudy using the residual SYNTAX score attempted to address this issue.[108] Only 40% of the patients had complete revascularization as defined by a residual SYNTAX score of 0. Incomplete revascularization was associated with older age, insulin-treated diabetes mellitus, hypertension, elevated cardiac biomarkers, and depressed LV ejection fraction. Higher residual SYNTAX score (indicating more incomplete revascularization) was associated with highly complex lesions, including severe calcification, chronic total occlusions, and bifurcation lesions.[108]

However, it should be noted that residual compared with baseline SYNTAX score was not a better discriminator of future cardiovascular risk. This study also showed that there was a very high likelihood of a residual SYNTAX score of greater than 8 in patients with higher baseline scores, suggesting that alternative strategies for coronary revascularization should be considered (e.g. CABG, hybrid procedures, or CTO PCI). Lastly, this study also suggests that complete revascularization is most important in patients with higher baseline SYNTAX scores. Whether there is an acceptable level of residual significant disease that is associated with lower risk is not known.

Revascularization of Intermediate Lesions

Angiographic assessment of the severity of coronary artery lesions is commonplace and the gold standard for quantifying the extent and complexity of CAD (see Chapter 14). Thus clinical practice and professional guidelines that influence revascularization approaches are predicated on anatomic criteria as assessed by coronary angiography. However, angiographic assessment of disease severity is limited. First, angiographic extent of disease does not always associate with future risk, and clinicians are often uncertain as to whether an angiographically defined lesion is significant or not. These borderline or intermediate lesions are often described as 50% to 70% diameter stenosis. Other imaging techniques such as intravascular ultrasound and optical coherence tomography are used to further define lesion severity; however, neither of these is associated with physiologic significance.

FFR is a practical diagnostic test used to assess the physiologic significance of a coronary artery stenosis. It is most commonly used in clinical practice to assess intermediate lesions. FFR-guided management in patients with SIHD is being used more often and is now a class I or class II guideline recommendation.[79,109]

Whereas invasive angiography remains the gold standard for the diagnosis and assessment of severity of CAD, the relationship between angiographic stenosis severity and coronary blood flow is complex. Assessing this significance with a, visual and/or quantification estimate of percent diameter stenosis is often discordant with the physiologic significance of that lesion whether assessed by noninvasive stress testing or FFR.[110]

There is a near linear relationship between perfusion pressure and blood flow when coronary resistance is minimized (with pharmacologic vasodilatation) within the physiologic blood pressure range.[111,112] Myocardial FFR is defined as the ratio of the maximum blood flow to the subtended myocardium in the presence of a given stenosis compared with maximal flow given the absence of this stenosis. Myocardial FFR is measured using a pressure-sensitive coronary wire with two hemodynamic pressure transducers. This wire is placed in such a fashion that the distal pressure transducer is distal to the lesion and the proximal hemodynamic pressure transducer is proximal to the lesion (in the aorta). FFR is calculated from the coronary pressure distal to the stenosis referred to as *Pd* and the aortic pressure referred to as *Pa* recorded simultaneously.

Induction of maximal vasodilation through pharmacologic hyperemia is critical when assessing FFR. The standard pharmacologic approach uses intravenous adenosine at a dose of 140 μg/kg per min. Adenosine is administered for 2 minutes, and the minimum FFR value typically occurs shortly after the onset of steady-state hyperemia. FFR is most often assessed using a 3-beat average that minimizes beat-to-beat variability.

FFR-Guided PCI in Patients with Stable Ischemic Heart Disease

Nonrandomized data suggested improved outcomes in patients undergoing FFR-guided PCI compared with angiography-guided decision-making.[113–117] Moreover, incorporating FFR versus using angiography alone appeared to be associated with reduced number of stents placed, lower MACE rate, and lower costs.[118] These clinical studies also suggested that deferring PCI based on an FFR of greater than 0.8 was safe.

The use of FFR has been tested in additional randomized controlled clinical trials. The Does Routine Pressure Wire Assessment Influence Management Strategy at Coronary Angiography for Diagnosis of Chest Pain? (RIPCORD) clinical trial was prospectively designed to assess whether FFR measurement during diagnostic coronary angiography would be associated with management decisions when compared with angiographic assessment.[119] In this trial 200 patients with chronic stable angina were randomized at 10 United Kingdom centers. RIPCORD demonstrated that the management plan, i.e. whether patients were referred to medical therapy, PCI, or CABG, changed in 26% of the population. Similar results were seen in a French registry.[120]

Coronary artery stenoses that are of intermediate angiographic severity are often not hemodynamically significant. The deferral of percutaneous coronary intervention (DEFER) study suggests that deferring intervention in lesions that are of intermediate severity and have FFR values greater than 0.75 is safe.[121] In this clinical trial, 325 patients were randomized to deferred or immediate PCI. In the immediate PCI arm, all patients underwent PCI independent of the FFR value. Those patients randomized to the deferral cohort only underwent PCI if the FFR value was less than 0.75. Deferral of PCI in patients with FFR greater than 0.75 was not associated with higher 5-year death and MI rates. The annual death or MI rate among patients with functionally nonsignificant lesions was less than 1% per year. DEFER suggests that intervention in a functionally nonsignificant lesion did not benefit the patient with respect to symptoms or outcomes. In addition, patients with increased risk of death or MI rate are those with a functionally significant abnormality as identified by an FFR of less than 0.75, which is consistent with prior observations with myocardial perfusion imaging (MPI) studies.[122–125]

The Fractional Flow Reserve versus Angiography for Guiding PCI in Patients with Multivessel Coronary Artery Disease (FAME-1 and FAME-2) clinical trials provided additional data supporting the routine use of FFR in selected patients undergoing coronary angiography.[126,127] Both trials demonstrated superiority of FFR- versus angiography-guided PCI with an approximate 30% reduction in the primary endpoint. FAME-1 randomized 1005 patients with multivessel disease in a 1:1 fashion to angiography- or FFR-guided PCI. The angiography-guided patients received more stents and more contrast agent, and the procedure was associated with higher costs of delivering care. In FAME-1, FFR-guidance had lower rates of the composite of death, nonfatal MI, and repeat revascularization versus usual care (13.2% vs 18.3%; $p = 0.02$). The difference in this composite was driven by numerical reduction in both repeat revascularization and nonfatal MI rates in the FFR group. The mortality rates were similar between the two study arms. There was no difference in freedom from angina in follow-up. Approximately 40% of the assessed lesions were not hemodynamically significant and thus PCI deferred. Data from FAME-1 suggest that one would need to treat 20 patients with FFR to prevent 1 adverse cardiovascular event in follow-up.

FAME-2 randomized patients with stable CAD in whom at least one stenosis was functionally significant (FFR ≤ 0.8). These patients were randomly assigned to FFR-guided PCI plus available medical therapy or best available medical therapy alone. The patients in whom all lesions assessed had an FFR value of greater than 0.8 were entered into a registry and also received guideline-based medical therapy. As in FAME-1, the primary composite endpoint was death, MI, or urgent revascularization. The data monitoring committee halted recruitment after enrolling 1220 patients because there were significant differences between groups in the percent of patients who had a primary endpoint. The composite primary endpoint occurred in 4.3% in the PCI group and 12.7% in the medical therapy group (HR, 0.32; 95% CI, 0.19–0.53; $p < 0.001$). This difference was driven by a lower rate of urgent revascularization in the PCI group (1.6% vs 11.1%; $p < 0.001$). A significant number of these repeat revascularizations were for urgent indications and were either prompted by MI or evidence of ischemia. The patients assigned to the registry had a similarly low frequency of the primary endpoint. Common indications for the use of FFR are summarized in Box 23.2.

The use of FFR in ACS remains controversial. This is partly driven by concerns regarding the diagnostic validity of FFR in ACS patients. Pharmacologic vasodilation is reduced in the culprit artery among ACS patients because of microvascular obstruction. This would likely lead to an unacceptably high false-negative rate and thus falsely reassuring FFR values in the culprit vessel.[128] However, trials are ongoing to evaluate the clinical utility of FFR in the nonculprit vessel. The Fractional flow reserve vs angiography in guiding management to optimize outcomes in non-ST-segment elevation myocardial infarction (FAMOUS-NSTEMI) clinical trial was a multicenter randomized trial utilizing routine FFR-guided management compared with standard management

BOX 23.2 Common Fractional Flow Reserve (FFR) Indications[109]

The adoption of FFR is a class I (level of evidence A) recommendation when prior evidence of ischemia is not available. FFR-guided PCI is a class IIa (level of evidence B) recommendation in patients with multivessel coronary artery disease (CAD).

When patients with a high pretest probability of CAD are referred for early invasive coronary angiography, the use of FFR has a class 1 recommendation (level of evidence C).

FFR should be considered for risk stratification among patients with inconclusive diagnosis on noninvasive testing or when there are conflicting results from different modalities (class IIa, level of evidence C).

Coronary revascularization of intermediate lesions in patients without ischemia and with an FFR > 0.8 is not recommended (class III recommendation, level of evidence B).

strategies in ACS patients.[129] The primary outcome compared the frequencies and differences in a proportion of patients allocated to medical management. The initial treatment decision was made after the coronary angiogram but before FFR measurement. Based on the FFR results, there was a higher proportion of patients treated medically in the FFR group compared with the angiography-guided group (22.7 vs 13.2%; $p = 0.02$). Although not adequately powered for clinical events, there was no difference in MACE rates between the two groups, and the costs were similar.[130]

Evolution in PCI Technology

There has been continuous and rapid innovation in device technology since the invention of coronary balloon angioplasty in the fall of 1977. These advances have led to improved safety, efficacy, and sustainability of PCI. The vessel response to high-pressure balloon inflation or stent deployment has been extensively studied and in general results in endothelial disruption, vascular inflammation, and medial stretch leading to vascular smooth muscle cell injury. This response to vessel injury coupled with clinical risk factors leads to significant clinical complications including stent thrombosis and restenosis. Innovation in stent design and improvements in the technical approach translate to an improved safety profile for PCI.

Plain old balloon angioplasty (POBA) revolutionized the approach to treating patients with obstructive CAD. However, these early procedures were limited. Balloon angioplasty was associated with both a very high acute vessel closure, driven by early elastic recoil and thrombosis, and restenosis in the first 6 months following the procedure. The rates of restenosis and late vessel closure were exceptionally high in the early balloon angioplasty era. Coronary stents were designed to overcome acute vessel recoil and to improve vessel patency. The stent scaffolding was designed to seal dissection flaps and provide improved vessel rigidity to prevent both early and late recoil. The WALLSTENT was a self-expanding stainless steel wire mesh structure and was the first coronary stent implanted in a human coronary artery in 1986.[131] This stent was very difficult to deliver and thus was limited for coronary intervention application. The next stent, and the first stent approved for use by the Food and Drug Administration (FDA), was the Palmaz-Shatz (Johnson & Johnson) stent in 1987. Unlike the WALLSTENT, this stent was on a balloon expandable stent delivery platform and was frequently used throughout the early 1990s. Since its inception, there has been a proliferation of new stent platforms. In general, coronary stents reduce early elastic recoil and restenosis compared with balloon angioplasty. Two large-scale randomized clinical trials established the superiority of bare metal stents (BMSs) over POBA.[132,133] The major limitations of these early stent platforms were the bulky nature of the platforms, the technical challenge associated with delivery, and the very high rates of acute and subacute stent thrombosis. Over the next several years the use of coronary stents increased substantially, such that by 2000 stents were used in over 85% of all PCI procedures.

In the early experience with BMSs, acute stent thrombosis occurred more commonly than anticipated. The use of dual antiplatelet therapy and adequately sizing stents and deploying stents under high pressure reduced the risk of acute stent thrombosis substantially by limiting the rate of malapposition and underexpansion. The major limiting factor for BMSs, even today, is that in-stent restenosis rates approach 20% to 30%.

Stent material and design have undergone substantial refinements in recent years[134] (Table 23.4). Early stents were composed of stainless steel because it is biologically inert. More recently cobalt-chromium alloys have replaced stainless steel, which allows for significantly thinner struts without compromising the radial strength. Cobalt-chromium stents in general are more trackable and deliverable than earlier prototypes. Recent iterations include platinum-chromium alloys, which allow for even thinner struts while retaining high radiopacity and radial strength.

DESs advanced the field substantively by reducing the rate of in-stent restenosis. However, initial approaches to coating stents with compounds such as gold, diamond, phosphorylcholine, and heparin to limit inflammation, platelet activation, thrombosis, and vascular smooth muscle cell proliferation were unsuccessful. It was not until BMSs were coated with specific antiproliferative agents such as sirolimus or paclitaxel that a clinical benefit was realized in limiting in-stent restenosis.[135–138]

Sirolimus is an immunosuppressive compound that acts by receptor inhibition of the mammalian target of rapamycin (mTOR), which results in cessation of the cell cycle progression in the late G1 to S phase and thus inhibits vascular smooth muscle cell proliferation.[135] Paclitaxel inhibits cell proliferation and migration by disrupting cellular microtubules delivery.[139]

In general, these antiproliferative agents are embedded within the polymer and coated on the surface of intracoronary stents. The elution kinetics allow the antiproliferative agent to slowly elute over days to several weeks following deployment. Initial randomized controlled trial data demonstrated a significant reduction in neointima formation and improved vessel patency over 1-year follow-up. Similar to early BMS outcomes, there were signals that DES placement was associated with increased risk of stent thrombosis. These early reports[140] were confirmed by larger registries.[141] The mechanism for in-stent thrombosis is related to delayed endothelialization due to either the presence of the anti-restenotic agents and/or a hypersensitivity reaction to the polymer. With improved stent design, polymers, and compliance with longer-term dual antiplatelet therapy, the risk for stent thrombosis including very late stent thrombosis has diminished substantially over time.

The newer DES platforms include modified antiproliferative agents including everolimus (PROMUS Element, Boston Scientific; Xience V, Abbot Vascular) and zotarolimus (Endeavor and Resolute, Medtronic). Everolimus is a derivative of sirolimus and similarly inhibits mTOR. Overall, everolimus-eluting stent platforms are superior in safety and efficacy when compared with first-generation DESs.[142–144] A meta-analysis of 11 randomized controlled trials comparing everolimus- with serolimus-eluting stents demonstrated a reduction in both definite stent thrombosis and need for repeat revascularization favoring the everolimus-eluting stent platforms. There was no difference in the risk of MI or cardiovascular mortality.[145]

Future applications for innovative drug or stent delivery platforms include directional drug delivery, biodegradable polymers, and biodegradable stent platforms. Directional drug delivery stent platforms have been developed such that the antiproliferative agent is coated only on the abluminal surface of the stent, thereby leaving the luminal surface as

TABLE 23.4 Available Stents

	CYPHER	TAXUS EXPRESS	ENDEAVOR	RESOLUTE	XIENCE V	PROMUS ELEMENT	BIOMATRIX
Manufacturer	Cordis	Boston Scientific	Medtronic	Medtronic	Abbott Vascular	Boston Scientific	Biosensors
Platform	Bx-Velocity	Express	Driver	Driver	Vision	Omega	Gazelle
Design	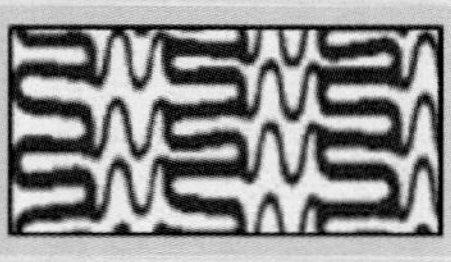	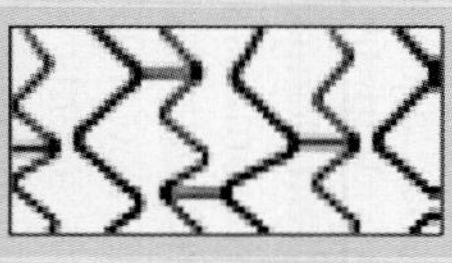	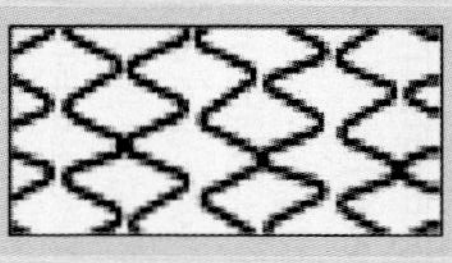	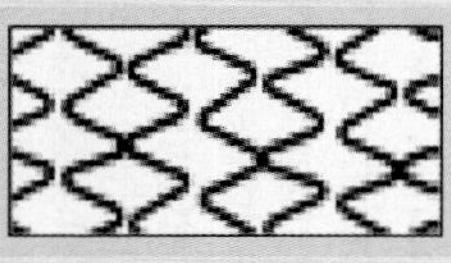	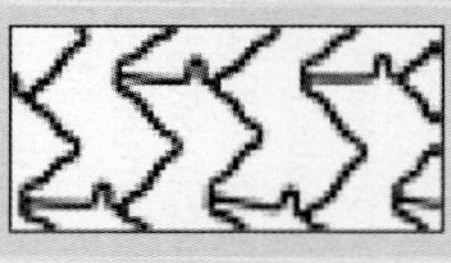	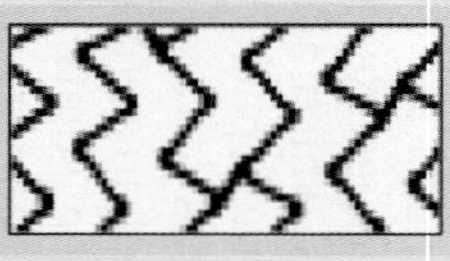	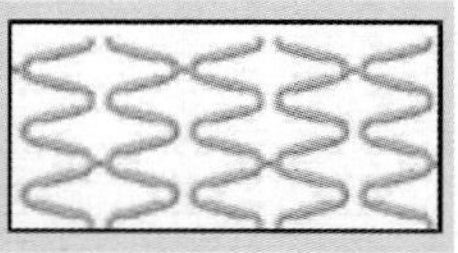
Material	SS	SS	MP35N CoCr	MP35N CoCr	L605 CoCr	PtCr	SS
Thickness of struts (μm)	140	132	91	91	81	81	112
Polymers	PEVA, PMBA	SIBS	PC	BioLinx	PBMA, PVDF-HFP	PBMA, PVDF-HFP	PLA
Polymer thickness (μm)	12.6	16	4.1	4.1	7.6	6	10
Drug	Sirolimus	Paclitaxel	Zotarolimus	Zotarolimus	Everolimus	Everolimus	Biolimus
Drug concentration (μg/cm^2)	140	100	100	100	100	100	156
Drug release in 4 weeks (%)	80	< 10	100	70	80	80	45
Late lumen loss (mm)*	0.17[137]	0.39[138]	0.61[148]	0.27[149]	0.16[142]	0.15[150]	0.13[151]

*Late lumen loss varies depending on trial population, timing of angiography, and study era. The values are indicative only, based on pivotal trials (referenced) of these stents.
CoCr, Cobalt-chromium; *HFP*, hexafluropropylene; *PC*, phosphorylcholine; *PEVA*, polyethylene-co-vinyl acetate; *PLA*, polylactic acid; *PMBA*, poly (n-butyl methacrylate); *PtCr*, platinum-chromium; *PVDF*, poly-vinylidene fluoride; *SIBS*, poly (styrene-b-isobutylene-b-styrene); *SS*, stainless steel.
(From Iqbal J, Gunn J, Serruys PW. Coronary stents: historical development, current status and future directions. Br Med Bull. *2013;106:193–211.)*

bare metal or for an alternative coating strategy to enhance endothelialization or prevent platelet adhesion. There are very few stent platforms utilizing this strategy. Biodegradable polymers offer many potential benefits compared with conventional DES platforms. In general, the release of the drug occurs during the degradation of the polymer. Once the drug is fully eluted and the polymer fully degraded, only a BMS platform remains. There are several stent platforms using biodegradable polymers. The biodegradable polymer stent currently available for use in the United States is the Synergy stent (Boston Scientific).

There has been extensive research and development dedicated to bioresorbable stent scaffolds.[146] Metallic drug-eluting stents, although very effective, are associated with incomplete endothelialization, polymer hypersensitivity, neoatherosclerosis, and stent fractures. Moreover, the target vessel failure rate ranges between 2% and 4% annually. Fully bioresorbable scaffolds were designed to provide mechanical support and drug delivery followed by complete scaffold bioresorption and complete return to vascular structure and function. These design features were an attempt to improve on the current metallic DES platforms. The goal therefore was to provide similar 1-year outcomes compared with contemporary metallic DESs coupled with improved long-term outcomes. The perceived benefits and limitations of bioresorbable stent platforms are shown in Box 23.3. The prototype bioresorbable stent platform is the Absorb Bioresorbable Vascular Scaffold (BVS) (Abbott Vascular) stent. Complete bioresorption is necessary to fully recover vascular structure and function. Although the rate of resorption varies as a function of the stent platform, drug elution typically occurs over approximately 3 months and bioresorption occurs over 12 to 36 months. BVS is associated with an increase in both the internal and external elastic lamina areas and vessel lumen area over 12 to 18 months. The polymeric struts are ultimately replaced by collagen and vascular smooth muscle cells, which retract over time. In general, there is expansive remodeling associated with bioresorbable stent placement. The registry and randomized controlled trial data with Absorb demonstrate that return of vasomotion, increased lumen, and expansive adaptive remodeling are seen by year 1 with complete scaffold resorption by year 3.[146] Randomized controlled trial data of Absorb BVS compared with Xience DES demonstrate that Absorb was noninferior for the primary endpoint of target lesion failure at 1 year. In the early registries there was a signal for a greater rate of scaffold thrombosis with Absorb compared with historic rates using contemporary DES platforms.[147] The greatest risk appeared in the first 30 days following implantation and in small vessels (< 2.5 mm, visual estimate). Next-generation fully bioabsorable stents are under development with the goal of substantially decreasing strut diameter to improve the scaffold profile and lower stent thrombosis risk.

BOX 23.3 Mechanisms That May Reduce Very Late Events with Vascular Bioresorbable Scaffolds (BRSs)

- Restoration of cyclic pulsality and normal vasomotion
  - Normalization of shear stress and cyclic strain
  - Restoration of normal vessel curvature
  - Reduced risk of very late polymer reactions
  - Avoidance/resolution of stent malapposition
  - Avoidance/resolution of late strut fractures
  - Reduced neoatherosclerosis
  - Unjailing of side branches
  - Formation of a (neomedia) cap over lipid-rich plaque
  - Plaque regression
- Advantages of vascular BRSs
  - Unjails covered side branches, restoring access
  - Avoids full metal jacket, restoring late bypass surgery options
  - Allows treatment of in-stent restenosis without necessitating a permanent additional metal layer
  - Facilitates noninvasive imaging follow-up without artifacts
  - Addresses physician's and patient's desires to avoid a permanent implant
- Disadvantages of first-generation vascular BRSs
  - Some devices require cold storage and specific deployment techniques
  - Thicker/wider struts with larger crossing profile (more difficult to deliver)
  - Greater attention to procedural technique required
  - Greater risks of acute strut fracture compared with metallic drug-eluting stents
  - Intraluminal scaffold dismantling
  - Higher early rates of scaffold thrombosis and target vessel-related myocardial infarction, particularly in small vessels

From Kereiakes DJ, Onuma Y, Serruys PW, et al. Bioresorbable vascular scaffolds for coronary revascularization. *Circulation.* 2016;134(2):168–182.

CONCLUSIONS

Despite major advances in medical therapies, patients continue to have residual symptoms and cardiovascular risk, and thus coronary revascularization remains an essential component of management for many. The use of a multidisciplinary heart team to facilitate decision-making regarding the method of coronary revascularization is preferable, especially in the setting of either high clinical risk or advanced/complex CAD. Relief of symptoms remains a central benefit of coronary revascularization in patients with SIHD. There are robust data suggesting that PCI improves the QoL in appropriately selected patients. CABG is also very effective in improving QoL, although when compared with PCI, QoL improves earlier following PCI than CABG. However, this benefit attenuates and CABG is superior to PCI in reducing angina and improving QoL at 1 year in patients with complex multivessel CAD. There are fewer data demonstrating that coronary revascularization reduces death and nonfatal MI in low-risk patients. It is generally accepted that coronary revascularization in patients at higher clinical risk is appropriate and reduces future risk. The ischemic burden hypothesis postulates that coronary revascularization will improve event-free survival rates among patients with high baseline ischemia. This is currently being tested in the ISCHEMIA clinical trial. CABG is generally preferred in patients with advanced CAD as assessed by the baseline SYNTAX score, in unprotected left main disease with a SYNTAX score of greater than 32, in patients with diabetes mellitus and multivessel CAD, and among patients with ischemic cardiomyopathy. PCI is generally preferred in patients following an ACS with one- or two-vessel CAD, in patients with advanced clinical risk or frailty, which is associated with a very high postoperative risk, and in patients who have had prior bypass surgery. FFR-guided management in patients with SIHD is being used with increased frequency and is recommended by practice guidelines. When there is uncertainty regarding lesion severity or when patients have not undergone preprocedural stress testing, FFR is very often informative and appropriate. The major advances in the near term for patients with chronic SIHD will be the continued advancement of complex coronary artery procedures including CTO PCI, as well as the introduction of bioresorbable stent platforms.

References

1. Keeley EC, Boura JA, Grines CL: Primary angioplasty versus intravenous thrombolytic therapy for acute myocardial infarction: a quantitative review of 23 randomised trials, *Lancet* 361:13–20, 2003.
2. Amsterdam EA, Wenger NK, Brindis RG, et al.: 2014 AHA/ACC Guideline for the Management of Patients With Non–ST-Elevation Acute Coronary Syndromes: a report of the American College of Cardiology/American Heart Association Task Force on Practice Guidelines, *Circulation* 130:e344–e426, 2014.
3. Members C, Gibbons RJ, Abrams J, et al.: ACC/AHA 2002 Guideline Update for the Management of Patients With Chronic Stable Angina—summary article: a report of the American College of Cardiology/American Heart Association Task Force on Practice Guidelines (Committee on the Management of Patients with Chronic Stable Angina), *Circulation* 107:149–158, 2003.
4. Fihn SD, Gardin JM, Abrams J, et al.: 2012 ACCF/AHA/ACP/AATS/PCNA/SCAI/STS Guideline for the Diagnosis and Management of Patients With Stable Ischemic Heart Disease: a report of the American College of Cardiology Foundation/American Heart Association Task Force on Practice Guidelines, and the American College of Physicians, American Association for Thoracic Surgery, Preventive Cardiovascular Nurses Association, Society for Cardiovascular Angiography and Interventions, and Society of Thoracic Surgeons, *Circulation* 126:e354–e471, 2012.
5. GROUP CRW, Patel MR, Dehmer GJ, et al.: ACCF/SCAI/STS/AATS/AHA/ASNC 2009 Appropriateness Criteria for Coronary Revascularization: a report of the American College of Cardiology Foundation Appropriateness Criteria Task Force, Society for Cardiovascular Angiography and Interventions, Society of Thoracic Surgeons, American Association for Thoracic Surgery, American Heart Association, and the American Society of Nuclear Cardiology: Endorsed by the American Society of Echocardiography, the Heart Failure Society of America, and the Society of Cardiovascular Computed Tomography, *Circulation* 119:1330–1352, 2009.
6. Ma J, Ward EM, Siegel RL, et al.: Temporal trends in mortality in the United States, 1969–2013, *JAMA* 314:1731–1739, 2015.
7. Mozaffarian D, Benjamin EJ, Go AS, et al.: Heart disease and stroke statistics–2015 update: a report from the American Heart Association, *Circulation* 131:e29–e322, 2015.
8. Ford ES, Ajani UA, Croft JB, et al.: Explaining the decrease in U.S. deaths from coronary disease, 1980–2000, *N Engl J Med* 356:2388–2398, 2007.
9. Steg PG, Greenlaw N, Tendera M, et al.: Prevalence of anginal symptoms and myocardial ischemia and their effect on clinical outcomes in outpatients with stable coronary artery disease: data from the International Observational CLARIFY Registry. *JAMA Intern Med* 174:1651–1659, 2014.
10. Dehmer GJ, Weaver D, Roe MT, et al.: A contemporary view of diagnostic cardiac catheterization and percutaneous coronary intervention in the United States: a report from the CathPCI Registry of the National Cardiovascular Data Registry, 2010 through June 2011, *J Am Coll Cardiol* 60:2017–2031, 2012.
11. Fihn SD, Blankenship JC, Alexander KP, et al.: 2014 ACC/AHA/AATS/PCNA/SCAI/STS focused update of the guideline for the diagnosis and management of patients with stable ischemic heart disease: a report of the American College of Cardiology/American Heart Association Task Force on Practice Guidelines, and the American Association for Thoracic Surgery, Preventive Cardiovascular Nurses Association, Society for Cardiovascular Angiography and Interventions, and Society of Thoracic Surgeons, *J Am Coll Cardiol* 64:1929–1949, 2014.
12. Epstein AJ, Polsky D, Yang F, et al.: Coronary revascularization trends in the United States, 2001–2008, *JAMA* 305:1769–1776, 2011.
13. Kim LK, Feldman DN, Swaminathan RV, et al.: Rate of percutaneous coronary intervention for the management of acute coronary syndromes and stable coronary artery disease in the United States (2007 to 2011), *Am J Cardiol* 114:1003–1010, 2014.
14. Chan PS, Patel MR, Klein LW, et al.: Appropriateness of percutaneous coronary intervention, *JAMA* 306:53–61, 2011.
15. Bradley SM, Bohn CM, Malenka DJ, et al.: Temporal trends in percutaneous coronary intervention appropriateness: insights from the Clinical Outcomes Assessment Program, *Circulation* 132:20–26, 2015.
16. Palmerini T, Biondi-Zoccai G, Della Riva D, et al.: Stent thrombosis with drug-eluting stents: is the paradigm shifting? *J Am Coll Cardiol* 62:1915–1921, 2013.
17. Park MW, Seung KB, Kim PJ, et al.: Long-term percutaneous coronary intervention rates and associated independent predictors for progression of nonintervened nonculprit coronary lesions, *Am J Cardiol* 104:648–652, 2009.
18. Stone GW, Maehara A, Lansky AJ, et al.: A prospective natural-history study of coronary atherosclerosis, *N Engl J Med* 364:226–235, 2011.
19. Alexander JH, Smith PK: Coronary-artery bypass grafting, *N Engl J Med* 374:1954–1964, 2016.
20. ElBardissi AW, Aranki SF, Sheng S, et al.: Trends in isolated coronary artery bypass grafting: an analysis of the Society of Thoracic Surgeons adult cardiac surgery database, *J Thorac Cardiovasc Surg* 143:273–281, 2012.
21. Hlatky MA, Boothroyd DB, Reitz BA, et al.: Adoption and effectiveness of internal mammary artery grafting in coronary artery bypass surgery among Medicare beneficiaries, *J Am Coll Cardiol* 63:33–39, 2014.
22. Tabata M, Grab JD, Khalpey Z, et al.: Prevalence and variability of internal mammary artery graft use in contemporary multivessel coronary artery bypass graft surgery: analysis of the Society of Thoracic Surgeons National Cardiac Database, *Circulation* 120:935–940, 2009.
23. Kelly R, Buth KJ, Legare JF: Bilateral internal thoracic artery grafting is superior to other forms of multiple arterial grafting in providing survival benefit after coronary bypass surgery, *J Thorac Cardiovasc Surg* 144:1408–1415, 2012.
24. Suma H, Tanabe H, Takahashi A, et al.: Twenty years experience with the gastroepiploic artery graft for CABG, *Circulation* 116:I188–I191, 2007.
25. Acar C, Ramsheyi A, Pagny JY, et al.: The radial artery for coronary artery bypass grafting: clinical and angiographic results at five years, *J Thorac Cardiovasc Surg* 116:981–989, 1998.
26. Newman MF, Kirchner JL, Phillips-Bute B, et al.: Longitudinal assessment of neurocognitive function after coronary-artery bypass surgery, *N Engl J Med* 344:395–402, 2001.
27. Shroyer AL, Grover FL, Hattler B, et al.: On-pump versus off-pump coronary-artery bypass surgery, *N Engl J Med* 361:1827–1837, 2009.
28. Hlatky MA, Bacon C, Boothroyd D, et al.: Cognitive function 5 years after randomization to coronary angioplasty or coronary artery bypass graft surgery, *Circulation* 96:II-11–14, 1997. discussion II-5.
29. Kulik A, Ruel M, Jneid H, et al.: Secondary prevention after coronary artery bypass graft surgery: a scientific statement from the American Heart Association, *Circulation* 131:927–964, 2015.
30. Gao G, Zheng Z, Pi Y, et al.: Aspirin plus clopidogrel therapy increases early venous graft patency after coronary artery bypass surgery: a single-center, randomized, controlled trial, *J Am Coll Cardiol* 56:1639–1643, 2010.
31. Deo SV, Dunlay SM, Shah IK, et al.: Dual anti-platelet therapy after coronary artery bypass grafting: is there any benefit? A systematic review and meta-analysis, *J Card Surg* 28:109–116, 2013.
32. Lamy A, Devereaux PJ, Prabhakaran D, et al.: Off-pump or on-pump coronary-artery bypass grafting at 30 days, *N Engl J Med* 366:1489–1497, 2012.
33. Lamy A, Devereaux PJ, Prabhakaran D, et al.: Effects of off-pump and on-pump coronary-artery bypass grafting at 1 year, *N Engl J Med* 368:1179–1188, 2013.
34. Diegeler A, Borgermann J, Kappert U, et al.: Off-pump versus on-pump coronary-artery bypass grafting in elderly patients, *N Engl J Med* 368:1189–1198, 2013.
35. Patel MR, Dehmer GJ, Hirshfeld JW, et al.: ACCF/SCAI/STS/AATS/AHA/ASNC/HFSA/SCCT 2012 appropriate use criteria for coronary revascularization focused update: a report of the American College of Cardiology Foundation Appropriate Use Criteria Task Force, Society for Cardiovascular Angiography and Interventions, Society of Thoracic Surgeons, American Association for Thoracic Surgery, American Heart Association, American Society of Nuclear Cardiology, and the Society of Cardiovascular Computed Tomography, *J Am Coll Cardiol* 59:857–881, 2012.
36. Fraker Jr TD, Fihn SD, Gibbons RJ, et al.: 2007 chronic angina focused update of the ACC/AHA 2002 guidelines for the management of patients with chronic stable angina: a report of the American College of Cardiology/American Heart Association Task Force on Practice Guidelines Writing Group to develop the focused update of the 2002 guidelines for the management of patients with chronic stable angina, *Circulation* 116:2762–2772, 2007.
37. Blankenship J, Naidu SS, Rao SV, et al.: Clinical expert consensus statement on best practices in the cardiac catheterization laboratory: Society for Cardiovascular Angiography and Interventions, *Catheter Cardiovasc Interv* 80:456–464, 2012.
38. Wijeysundera HC, Nallamothu BK, Krumholz HM, et al.: Meta-analysis: effects of percutaneous coronary intervention versus medical therapy on angina relief, *Ann Intern Med* 152:370–379, 2010.
39. Hlatky MA, Boothroyd DB, Bravata DM, et al.: Coronary artery bypass surgery compared with percutaneous coronary interventions for multivessel disease: a collaborative analysis of individual patient data from ten randomised trials, *Lancet* 373:1190–1197, 2009.
40. Varnauskas E: Twelve-year follow-up of survival in the randomized European Coronary Surgery Study, *N Engl J Med* 319:332–337, 1988.
41. Varnauskas E, Lorimer AR, Karlsson T: The role of early surgery following myocardial infarction. European Coronary Surgery Bypass Group, *Br J Clin Pract* 46:238–242, 1992.
42. Bavry AA, Kumbhani DJ, Rassi AN, et al.: Benefit of early invasive therapy in acute coronary syndromes: a meta-analysis of contemporary randomized clinical trials, *J Am Coll Cardiol* 48:1319–1325, 2006.
43. Henderson RA, Pocock SJ, Clayton TC, et al.: Seven-year outcome in the RITA-2 trial: coronary angioplasty versus medical therapy, *J Am Coll Cardiol* 42:1161–1170, 2003.
44. Parisi AF, Folland ED, Hartigan P: A comparison of angioplasty with medical therapy in the treatment of single-vessel coronary artery disease. Veterans Affairs ACME Investigators, *N Engl J Med* 326:10–16, 1992.
45. Hoffman SN, TenBrook JA, Wolf MP, et al.: A meta-analysis of randomized controlled trials comparing coronary artery bypass graft with percutaneous transluminal coronary angioplasty: one- to eight-year outcomes, *J Am Coll Cardiol* 41:1293–1304, 2003.
46. Boden WE, O'Rourke RA, Teo KK, et al.: Optimal medical therapy with or without PCI for stable coronary disease, *N Engl J Med* 356:1503–1516, 2007.
47. Kereiakes DJ, Teirstein PS, Sarembock IJ, et al.: The truth and consequences of the COURAGE trial, *J Am Coll Cardiol* 50:1598–1603, 2007.
48. Steinberg BA, Steg PG, Bhatt DL, et al.: Comparisons of guideline-recommended therapies in patients with documented coronary artery disease having percutaneous coronary intervention versus coronary artery bypass grafting versus medical therapy only (from the REACH International Registry), *Am J Cardiol* 99:1212–1215, 2007.
49. Hachamovitch R, Berman DS, Shaw LJ, et al.: Incremental prognostic value of myocardial perfusion single photon emission computed tomography for the prediction of cardiac death: differential stratification for risk of cardiac death and myocardial infarction, *Circulation* 97:535–543, 1998.
50. Hachamovitch R, Hayes SW, Friedman JD, et al.: Comparison of the short-term survival benefit associated with revascularization compared with medical therapy in patients with no prior coronary artery disease undergoing stress myocardial perfusion single photon emission computed tomography, *Circulation* 107:2900–2907, 2003.
51. Shaw LJ, Berman DS, Maron DJ, et al.: Optimal medical therapy with or without percutaneous coronary intervention to reduce ischemic burden: results from the Clinical Outcomes Utilizing Revascularization and Aggressive Drug Evaluation (COURAGE) trial nuclear substudy, *Circulation* 117:1283–1291, 2008.
52. Omland T, de Lemos JA, Sabatine MS, et al.: A sensitive cardiac troponin T assay in stable coronary artery disease, *N Engl J Med* 361:2538–2547, 2009.
53. de Lemos JA, Drazner MH, Omland T, et al.: Association of troponin T detected with a highly sensitive assay and cardiac structure and mortality risk in the general population, *JAMA* 304: 2503–2512, 2010.
54. Eleven-year survival in the Veterans Administration randomized trial of coronary bypass surgery for stable angina: The Veterans Administration Coronary Artery Bypass Surgery Cooperative Study Group, *N Engl J Med* 311:1333–1339, 1984.
55. Coronary Artery Surgery Study (CASS): A randomized trial of coronary artery bypass surgery. Survival data, *Circulation* 68:939–950, 1983.
56. Bell MR, Gersh BJ, Schaff HV, et al.: Effect of completeness of revascularization on long-term outcome of patients with three-vessel disease undergoing coronary artery bypass surgery. A report from the Coronary Artery Surgery Study (CASS) Registry, *Circulation* 86:446–457, 1992.
57. van den Brand MJ, Rensing BJ, Morel MA, et al.: The effect of completeness of revascularization on event-free survival at one year in the ARTS trial, *J Am Coll Cardiol* 39:559–564, 2002.
58. Serruys PW, Ong AT, van Herwerden LA, et al.: Five-year outcomes after coronary stenting versus bypass surgery for the treatment of multivessel disease: the final analysis of the Arterial Revascularization Therapies Study (ARTS) randomized trial, *J Am Coll Cardiol* 46:575–581, 2005.
59. Hueb W, Lopes NH, Gersh BJ, et al.: Five-year follow-up of the Medicine, Angioplasty, or Surgery Study (MASS II): a randomized controlled clinical trial of 3 therapeutic strategies for multivessel coronary artery disease, *Circulation* 115:1082–1089, 2007.
60. Booth J, Clayton T, Pepper J, et al.: Randomized, controlled trial of coronary artery bypass surgery versus percutaneous coronary intervention in patients with multivessel coronary artery disease: six-year follow-up from the Stent or Surgery Trial (SoS), *Circulation* 118:381–388, 2008.
61. Daemen J, Boersma E, Flather M, et al.: Long-term safety and efficacy of percutaneous coronary intervention with stenting and coronary artery bypass surgery for multivessel coronary artery disease: a meta-analysis with 5-year patient-level data from the ARTS, ERACI-II, MASS-II, and SoS trials, *Circulation* 118:1146–1154, 2008.
62. Hannan EL, Racz MJ, Walford G, et al.: Long-term outcomes of coronary-artery bypass grafting versus stent implantation, *N Engl J Med* 352:2174–2183, 2005.
63. Serruys PW, Morice MC, Kappetein AP, et al.: Percutaneous coronary intervention versus coronary-artery bypass grafting for severe coronary artery disease, *N Engl J Med* 360:961–972, 2009.
64. Head SJ, Davierwala PM, Serruys PW, et al.: Coronary artery bypass grafting vs. percutaneous coronary intervention for patients with three-vessel disease: final five-year follow-up of the SYNTAX trial, *Eur Heart J* 35:2821–2830, 2014.

65. Weintraub WS, Grau-Sepulveda MV, Weiss JM, et al.: Comparative effectiveness of revascularization strategies, *N Engl J Med* 366:1467–1476, 2012.
66. Levine GN, Bates ER, Blankenship JC, et al.: 2011 ACCF/AHA/SCAI Guideline for Percutaneous Coronary Intervention: a report of the American College of Cardiology Foundation/American Heart Association Task Force on Practice Guidelines and the Society for Cardiovascular Angiography and Interventions, *Circulation* 124:e574–e651, 2011.
67. Deb S, Wijeysundera HC, Ko DT, et al.: Coronary artery bypass graft surgery vs percutaneous interventions in coronary revascularization: a systematic review, *JAMA* 310:2086–2095, 2013.
68. Comparison of coronary bypass surgery with angioplasty in patients with multivessel disease: The Bypass Angioplasty Revascularization Investigation (BARI) Investigators, *N Engl J Med* 335:217–225, 1996.
69. Group BDS, Frye RL, August P, et al.: A randomized trial of therapies for type 2 diabetes and coronary artery disease, *N Engl J Med* 360:2503–2515, 2009.
70. Chaitman BR, Hardison RM, Adler D, et al.: The Bypass Angioplasty Revascularization Investigation 2 Diabetes randomized trial of different treatment strategies in type 2 diabetes mellitus with stable ischemic heart disease: impact of treatment strategy on cardiac mortality and myocardial infarction, *Circulation* 120:2529–2540, 2009.
71. Mohr FW, Morice MC, Kappetein AP, et al.: Coronary artery bypass graft surgery versus percutaneous coronary intervention in patients with three-vessel disease and left main coronary disease: 5-year follow-up of the randomised, clinical SYNTAX trial, *Lancet* 381:629–638, 2013.
72. Farkouh ME, Domanski M, Sleeper LA, et al.: Strategies for multivessel revascularization in patients with diabetes, *N Engl J Med* 367:2375–2384, 2012.
73. Dangas GD, Farkouh ME, Sleeper LA, et al.: Long-term outcome of PCI versus CABG in insulin and non-insulin-treated diabetic patients: results from the FREEDOM trial, *J Am Coll Cardiol* 64:1189–1197, 2014.
74. Hillis LD, Smith PK, Anderson JL, et al.: 2011 ACCF/AHA Guideline for Coronary Artery Bypass Graft Surgery. A report of the American College of Cardiology Foundation/American Heart Association Task Force on Practice Guidelines. Developed in collaboration with the American Association for Thoracic Surgery, Society of Cardiovascular Anesthesiologists, and Society of Thoracic Surgeons, *J Am Coll Cardiol* 58:e123–e210, 2011.
75. Velazquez EJ, Lee KL, Deja MA, et al.: Coronary-artery bypass surgery in patients with left ventricular dysfunction, *N Engl J Med* 364:1607–1616, 2011.
76. Velazquez EJ, Lee KL, Jones RH, et al.: Coronary-artery bypass surgery in patients with ischemic cardiomyopathy, *N Engl J Med* 374(16):1511–1520, 2016.
77. Collins AJ, Li S, Gilbertson DT, et al.: Chronic kidney disease and cardiovascular disease in the Medicare population, *Kidney Int Suppl* S24–S31, 2003.
78. Reddan DN, Szczech LA, Tuttle RH, et al.: Chronic kidney disease, mortality, and treatment strategies among patients with clinically significant coronary artery disease, *J Am Soc Nephrol* 14:2373–2380, 2003.
79. Authors/Task Force Members, Windecker S, Kolh P, et al.: 2014 ESC/EACTS guidelines on myocardial revascularization: The Task Force on Myocardial Revascularization of the European Society of Cardiology (ESC) and the European Association for Cardio-Thoracic Surgery (EACTS) developed with the special contribution of the European Association of Percutaneous Cardiovascular Interventions (EAPCI), *Eur Heart J* 35:2541–2619, 2014.
80. Bangalore S, Guo Y, Samadashvili Z, et al.: Revascularization in patients with multivessel coronary artery disease and chronic kidney disease: everolimus-eluting stents versus coronary artery bypass graft surgery, *J Am Coll Cardiol* 66:1209–1220, 2015.
81. Vora AN, Dai D, Gurm H, et al.: Temporal trends in the risk profile of patients undergoing outpatient percutaneous coronary intervention: a report from the National Cardiovascular Data Registry's CathPCI Registry, *Circ Cardiovasc Interv* 9:e003070, 2016.
82. Eagle KA, Goodman SG, Avezum A, et al.: Practice variation and missed opportunities for reperfusion in ST-segment-elevation myocardial infarction: findings from the Global Registry of Acute Coronary Events (GRACE), *Lancet* 359:373–377, 2002.
83. Topol EJ, Califf RM, Vandormael M, et al.: A randomized trial of late reperfusion therapy for acute myocardial infarction. Thrombolysis and Angioplasty in Myocardial Infarction-6 Study Group, *Circulation* 85:2090–2099, 1992.
84. Dzavik V, Beanlands DS, Davies RF, et al.: Effects of late percutaneous transluminal coronary angioplasty of an occluded infarct-related coronary artery on left ventricular function in patients with a recent (< 6 weeks) Q-wave acute myocardial infarction (Total Occlusion Post-Myocardial Infarction Intervention Study [TOMIIS]–a pilot study), *Am J Cardiol* 73:856–861, 1994.
85. Horie H, Takahashi M, Minai K, et al.: Long-term beneficial effect of late reperfusion for acute anterior myocardial infarction with percutaneous transluminal coronary angioplasty, *Circulation* 98:2377–2382, 1998.
86. Yousef ZR, Redwood SR, Bucknall CA, et al.: Late intervention after anterior myocardial infarction: effects on left ventricular size, function, quality of life, and exercise tolerance: results of the Open Artery Trial (TOAT Study), *J Am Coll Cardiol* 40:869–876, 2002.
87. Steg PG, Thuaire C, Himbert D, et al.: DECOPI (DEsobstruction COronaire en Post-Infarctus): a randomized multi-centre trial of occluded artery angioplasty after acute myocardial infarction, *Eur Heart J* 25:2187–2194, 2004.
88. Cigarroa RG, Lange RA, Hillis LD: Prognosis after acute myocardial infarction in patients with and without residual anterograde coronary blood flow, *Am J Cardiol* 64:155–160, 1989.
89. Galvani M, Ottani F, Ferrini D, et al.: Patency of the infarct-related artery and left ventricular function as the major determinants of survival after Q-wave acute myocardial infarction, *Am J Cardiol* 71:1–7, 1993.
90. Lamas GA, Flaker GC, Mitchell G, et al.: Effect of infarct artery patency on prognosis after acute myocardial infarction. The Survival and Ventricular Enlargement Investigators, *Circulation* 92:1101–1109, 1995.
91. Puma JA, Sketch Jr MH, Thompson TD, et al.: Support for the open-artery hypothesis in survivors of acute myocardial infarction: analysis of 11,228 patients treated with thrombolytic therapy, *Am J Cardiol* 83:482–487, 1999.
92. Hochman JS, Lamas GA, Buller CE, et al.: Coronary intervention for persistent occlusion after myocardial infarction, *N Engl J Med* 355:2395–2407, 2006.
93. Dzavik V, Buller CE, Lamas GA, et al.: Randomized trial of percutaneous coronary intervention for subacute infarct-related coronary artery occlusion to achieve long-term patency and improve ventricular function: the Total Occlusion Study of Canada (TOSCA)-2 trial, *Circulation* 114:2449–2457, 2006.
94. Fefer P, Knudtson ML, Cheema AN, et al.: Current perspectives on coronary chronic total occlusions: the Canadian Multicenter Chronic Total Occlusions Registry, *J Am Coll Cardiol* 59:991–997, 2012.
95. Jeroudi OM, Alomar ME, Michael TT, et al.: Prevalence and management of coronary chronic total occlusions in a tertiary Veterans Affairs hospital, *Catheter Cardiovasc Interv* 84:637–643, 2014.
96. Brilakis ES, Grantham JA, Rinfret S, et al.: A percutaneous treatment algorithm for crossing coronary chronic total occlusions, *JACC Cardiovasc Interv* 5:367–379, 2012.
97. Morino Y, Abe M, Morimoto T, et al.: Predicting successful guidewire crossing through chronic total occlusion of native coronary lesions within 30 minutes: the J-CTO (Multicenter CTO Registry in Japan) score as a difficulty grading and time assessment tool, *JACC Cardiovasc Interv* 4:213–221, 2011.
98. Werner GS, Surber R, Ferrari M, et al.: The functional reserve of collaterals supplying long-term chronic total coronary occlusions in patients without prior myocardial infarction, *Eur Heart J* 27:2406–2412, 2006.
99. Claessen BE, Dangas GD, Weisz G, et al.: Prognostic impact of a chronic total occlusion in a non-infarct-related artery in patients with ST-segment elevation myocardial infarction: 3-year results from the HORIZONS-AMI trial, *Eur Heart J* 33:768–775, 2012.
100. Gierlotka M, Tajstra M, Gasior M, et al.: Impact of chronic total occlusion artery on 12-month mortality in patients with non-ST-segment elevation myocardial infarction treated by percutaneous coronary intervention (from the PL-ACS Registry), *Int J Cardiol* 168:250–254, 2013.
101. Hoebers LP, Claessen BE, Elias J, et al.: Meta-analysis on the impact of percutaneous coronary intervention of chronic total occlusions on left ventricular function and clinical outcome, *Int J Cardiol* 187:90–96, 2015.
102. Galassi AR, Brilakis ES, Boukhris M, et al.: Appropriateness of percutaneous revascularization of coronary chronic total occlusions: an overview, *Eur Heart J*, 37:2692–2700, 2016.
103. Safley DM, Grantham JA, Hatch J, et al.: Quality of life benefits of percutaneous coronary intervention for chronic occlusions, *Catheter Cardiovasc Interv* 84:629–634, 2014.
104. Hannan EL, Wu C, Walford G, et al.: Incomplete revascularization in the era of drug-eluting stents: impact on adverse outcomes, *JACC Cardiovasc Interv* 2:17–25, 2009.
105. Head SJ, Mack MJ, Holmes Jr DR, et al.: Incidence, predictors and outcomes of incomplete revascularization after percutaneous coronary intervention and coronary artery bypass grafting: a subgroup analysis of 3-year SYNTAX data, *Eur J Cardiothorac Surg* 41:535–541, 2012.
106. Garcia S, Sandoval Y, Roukoz H, et al.: Outcomes after complete versus incomplete revascularization of patients with multivessel coronary artery disease: a meta-analysis of 89,883 patients enrolled in randomized clinical trials and observational studies, *J Am Coll Cardiol* 62:1421–1431, 2013.
107. Dauerman HL: Reasonable incomplete revascularization, *Circulation* 123:2337–2340, 2011.
108. Genereux P, Palmerini T, Caixeta A, et al.: Quantification and impact of untreated coronary artery disease after percutaneous coronary intervention: the residual SYNTAX (Synergy Between PCI with TAXUS and Cardiac Surgery) score, *J Am Coll Cardiol* 59:2165–2174, 2012.
109. Montalescot G, Sechtem U, Achenbach S, et al.: 2013 ESC guidelines on the management of stable coronary artery disease, *Eur Heart J* 34:2949, 2013.
110. De Bruyne B, Fearon WF, Pijls NH, et al.: Fractional flow reserve-guided PCI for stable coronary artery disease, *N Engl J Med* 371:1208–1217, 2014.
111. Koolen JJ, Pijls NH: Coronary pressure never lies, *Cathet Cardiovasc Interv* 72:248–256, 2008.
112. Spaan JA, Piek JJ, Hoffman JI, et al.: Physiological basis of clinically used coronary hemodynamic indices, *Circulation* 113:446–455, 2006.
113. Park SJ, Ahn JM, Park GM, et al.: Trends in the outcomes of percutaneous coronary intervention with the routine incorporation of fractional flow reserve in real practice, *Eur Heart J* 34:3353–3361, 2013.
114. Frohlich GM, Redwood S, Rakhit R, et al.: Long-term survival in patients undergoing percutaneous interventions with or without intracoronary pressure wire guidance or intracoronary ultrasonographic imaging: a large cohort study, *JAMA Int Med* 174:1360–1366, 2014.
115. Li J, Elrashidi MY, Flammer AJ, et al.: Long-term outcomes of fractional flow reserve-guided vs. angiography-guided percutaneous coronary intervention in contemporary practice, *Eur Heart J* 34:1375–1383, 2013.
116. Depta JP, Patel JS, Novak E, et al.: Outcomes of coronary stenoses deferred revascularization for borderline versus nonborderline fractional flow reserve values, *Am J Cardiol* 113:1788–1793, 2014.
117. Depta JP, Patel JS, Novak E, et al.: Risk model for estimating the 1-year risk of deferred lesion intervention following deferred revascularization after fractional flow reserve assessment, *Eur Heart J* 36:509–515, 2015.
118. Di Serafino L, De Bruyne B, Mangiacapra F, et al.: Long-term clinical outcome after fractional flow reserve- versus angio-guided percutaneous coronary intervention in patients with intermediate stenosis of coronary artery bypass grafts, *Am Heart J* 166:110–118, 2013.
119. Curzen N, Rana O, Nicholas Z, et al.: Does routine pressure wire assessment influence management strategy at coronary angiography for diagnosis of chest pain? The RIPCORD study, *Circ Cardiovasc Interv* 7:248–255, 2014.
120. Van Belle E, Rioufol G, Pouillot C, et al.: Outcome impact of coronary revascularization strategy reclassification with fractional flow reserve at time of diagnostic angiography: insights from a large French multicenter fractional flow reserve registry, *Circulation* 129:173–185, 2014.
121. Pijls NH, van Schaardenburgh P, Manoharan G, et al.: Percutaneous coronary intervention of functionally nonsignificant stenosis: 5-year follow-up of the DEFER Study, *J Am Coll Cardiol* 49:2105–2111, 2007.
122. Beller GA, Zaret BL: Contributions of nuclear cardiology to diagnosis and prognosis of patients with coronary artery disease, *Circulation* 101:1465–1478, 2000.
123. Pavin D, Delonca J, Siegenthaler M, et al.: Long-term (10 years) prognostic value of a normal thallium-201 myocardial exercise scintigraphy in patients with coronary artery disease documented by angiography, *Eur Heart J* 18:69–77, 1997.
124. Lee KL, Pryor DB, Pieper KS, et al.: Prognostic value of radionuclide angiography in medically treated patients with coronary artery disease. A comparison with clinical and catheterization variables, *Circulation* 82:1705–1717, 1990.
125. Shaw LJ, Iskandrian AE: Prognostic value of gated myocardial perfusion SPECT, *J Nucl Cardiol* 11:171–185, 2004.
126. Tonino PA, De Bruyne B, Pijls NH, et al.: Fractional flow reserve versus angiography for guiding percutaneous coronary intervention, *N Engl J Med* 360:213–224, 2009.
127. De Bruyne B, Pijls NH, Kalesan B, et al.: Fractional flow reserve-guided PCI versus medical therapy in stable coronary disease, *N Engl J Med* 367:991–1001, 2012.
128. Cuculi F, De Maria GL, Meier P, et al.: Impact of microvascular obstruction on the assessment of coronary flow reserve, index of microcirculatory resistance, and fractional flow reserve after ST-segment elevation myocardial infarction, *J Am Coll Cardiol* 64:1894–1904, 2014.
129. Layland J, Oldroyd KG, Curzen N, et al.: Fractional flow reserve vs. angiography in guiding management to optimize outcomes in non-ST-segment elevation myocardial infarction: the British Heart Foundation FAMOUS-NSTEMI randomized trial, *Eur Heart J* 36:100–111, 2015.
130. Layland J, Rauhalammi S, Watkins S, et al.: Assessment of fractional flow reserve in patients with recent non-ST-segment-elevation myocardial infarction comparative study with 3-T stress perfusion cardiac magnetic resonance imaging, *Circ Cardiovasc Interv* 8:e002207, 2015.
131. Sigwart U, Puel J, Mirkovitch V, et al.: Intravascular stents to prevent occlusion and restenosis after transluminal angioplasty, *N Engl J Med* 316:701–706, 1987.
132. Serruys PW, de Jaegere P, Kiemeneij F, et al.: A comparison of balloon-expandable-stent implantation with balloon angioplasty in patients with coronary artery disease. Benestent Study Group, *N Engl J Med* 331:489–495, 1994.
133. Fischman DL, Leon MB, Baim DS, et al.: A randomized comparison of coronary-stent placement and balloon angioplasty in the treatment of coronary artery disease. Stent Restenosis Study Investigators, *N Engl J Med* 331:496–501, 1994.
134. Morton AC, Crossman D, Gunn J: The influence of physical stent parameters upon restenosis, *Pathol Biol (Paris)* 52:196–205, 2004.
135. Poon M, Marx SO, Gallo R, et al.: Rapamycin inhibits vascular smooth muscle cell migration, *J Clin Invest* 98:2277–2283, 1996.
136. Morice MC, Serruys PW, Sousa JE, et al.: A randomized comparison of a sirolimus-eluting stent with a standard stent for coronary revascularization, *N Engl J Med* 346:1773–1780, 2002.
137. Moses JW, Leon MB, Popma JJ, et al.: Sirolimus-eluting stents versus standard stents in patients with stenosis in a native coronary artery, *N Engl J Med* 349:1315–1323, 2003.

138. Stone GW, Ellis SG, Cox DA, et al.: A polymer-based, paclitaxel-eluting stent in patients with coronary artery disease, *N Engl J Med* 350:221–231, 2004.
139. Axel DI, Kunert W, Goggelmann C, et al.: Paclitaxel inhibits arterial smooth muscle cell proliferation and migration in vitro and in vivo using local drug delivery, *Circulation* 96:636–645, 1997.
140. Laskey WK, Yancy CW, Maisel WH: Thrombosis in coronary drug-eluting stents: report from the meeting of the Circulatory System Medical Devices Advisory Panel of the Food and Drug Administration Center for Devices and Radiologic Health, December 7-8, 2006, *Circulation* 115:2352–2357, 2007.
141. Luscher TF, Steffel J, Eberli FR, et al.: Drug-eluting stent and coronary thrombosis: biological mechanisms and clinical implications, *Circulation* 115:1051–1058, 2007.
142. Stone GW, Midei M, Newman W, et al.: Comparison of an everolimus-eluting stent and a paclitaxel-eluting stent in patients with coronary artery disease: a randomized trial, *JAMA* 299:1903–1913, 2008.
143. Palmerini T, Biondi-Zoccai G, Della Riva D, et al.: Stent thrombosis with drug-eluting and bare-metal stents: evidence from a comprehensive network meta-analysis, *Lancet* 379:1393–1402, 2012.
144. Stone GW, Rizvi A, Newman W, et al.: Everolimus-eluting versus paclitaxel-eluting stents in coronary artery disease, *N Engl J Med* 362:1663–1674, 2010.
145. Park KW, Kang SH, Velders MA, et al.: Safety and efficacy of everolimus- versus sirolimus-eluting stents: a systematic review and meta-analysis of 11 randomized trials, *Am Heart J* 165, 2013. 241–50.e4.
146. Kereiakes DJ, Onuma Y, Serruys PW, et al.: Bioresorbable vascular scaffolds for coronary revascularization, *Circulation* 134:168–182, 2016.
147. Raber L, Brugaletta S, Yamaji K, et al.: Very late scaffold thrombosis: intracoronary imaging and histopathological and spectroscopic findings, *J Am Coll Cardiol* 66:1901–1914, 2015.
148. Fajadet J, Wijns W, Laarman GJ, et al.: Randomized, double-blind, multicenter study of the Endeavor zotarolimus-eluting phosphorylcholine-encapsulated stent for treatment of native coronary artery lesions: clinical and angiographic results of the ENDEAVOR-II trial, *Circulation* 114:798–806, 2006.
149. Serruys PW, Silber S, Garg S, et al.: Comparison of zotarolimus-eluting and everolimus-eluting coronary stents, *N Engl J Med* 363:136–146, 2010.
150. Meredith IT, Verheye S, Dubois CL, et al.: Primary endpoint results of the EVOLVE trial: a randomized evaluation of a novel bioabsorbable polymer-coated, everolimus-eluting coronary stent, *J Am Coll Cardiol* 59:1362–1370, 2012.
151. Windecker S, Serruys PW, Wandel S, et al.: Biolimus-eluting stent with biodegradable polymer versus sirolimus-eluting stent with durable polymer for coronary revascularisation (LEADERS): a randomised non-inferiority trial, *Lancet* 372:1163–1173, 2008.

24 Managing Chronic Coronary Artery Disease in Patients with Diabetes

Nikolaus Marx and Sebastian Reith

INTRODUCTION

Patients with diabetes mellitus—both type 1 and type 2—exhibit an increased risk of developing cardiovascular disease (CVD) with its sequelae of myocardial infarction, stroke, and heart failure. Compared to patients without diabetes, the management of coronary artery disease (CAD) in patients with diabetes includes different strategies in CV risk reduction, as well as various interventional options. In addition, because type 2 diabetes is much more common and a growing epidemic worldwide, a wealth of data exists for patients with type 2 diabetes, with only little evidence available regarding the relationship between type 1 diabetes and CAD. Accordingly, this chapter will mainly focus on type 2 diabetes.

CARDIOVASCULAR RISK IN TYPE 1 DIABETES

CV risk in patients with type 1 diabetes is characterized by more frequent and earlier occurrence of CV events than in populations without diabetes. CVD prevalence rates in type 1 diabetes vary between 3% and 12.4%.[1–4] The Pittsburgh Epidemiology of Diabetes Complications (EDC) study demonstrated that the incidence of major CVD events in young adults (age 28 to 38 years) with type 1 diabetes was 0.98% per year and surpassed 3% per year after age 55 years, making it the leading cause of death in this population.[3–5] In addition, data from the UK General Practice Research Database (GPRD), including 7400 patients with type 1 diabetes with a mean age 33 years and a mean duration of diabetes 15 years, suggest that type 1 diabetes is associated with markedly increased adjusted hazard ratios (HRs) for major coronary heart disease (CHD) events during 4.7 years of follow-up in men (adjusted HR 3.6; 95% confidence interval [CI] 2.8–4.6) and women (adjusted HR 9.6; 95% CI 6.4–14.5). These rates are similar to the relative risks (RRs) associated with type 2 diabetes.[1]

CARDIOVASCULAR RISK IN TYPE 2 DIABETES MELLITUS

In the late 1990s Haffner et al published epidemiologic data showing that patients with diabetes and no history of myocardial infarction (MI) have a similar risk of developing an MI over the next 7 years as do nondiabetic subjects after their first MI.[6] These data raised the hypothesis that diabetes may be seen as a CHD equivalent. This study was carried out when current cardiovascular therapies, such as statins and renin-angiotensin-aldosterone system (RAAS) blockers, were not yet implemented. Since then large CV outcome trials examining lipid-lowering strategies, antihypertensive therapies, and RAAS inhibition have led to an overall reduction of CV morbidity and mortality in patients with diabetes.[7] However, recent data published from the Emerging Risk Factor Collaboration showed that, despite extensive CV risk management with state-of-the-art therapy, the presence of diabetes still doubles the risk for CV death. Furthermore, the presence of diabetes together with a history of MI leads to a 4-fold risk increase versus subjects without diabetes or MI. This translates into a 6-year reduced life expectancy for a 60-year old man with diabetes and a loss of 12 years in a person with diabetes and a prior MI.[8] These data underscore the necessity for additional strategies to reduce CV risk in patients with diabetes.

RISK FACTOR MANAGEMENT

The reduction of CV risk in patients with diabetes is in general not different from patients without diabetes. However, given the increased absolute risk a very thorough approach is mandatory.

Lifestyle Intervention

The basis for risk reduction in patients with diabetes, as in nondiabetic subjects, is lifestyle intervention. Lifestyle intervention has been shown to prevent the development of CVD in primary prevention, but the benefit of lifestyle intervention including diet, physical activity, and weight loss is less well established in patients with existing chronic CAD. However, general aspects are covered by various guidelines such as the American Heart Association (AHA), American Diabetes Association, and European Society of Cardiology (ESC)/European Association for the Study of Diabetes (EASD)[9,10]: these include recommendations for smoking cessation, ideally guided by structured advice or a specially developed program, as well as a Mediterranean diet with fruit, vegetables, and olive oil. To what extent weight loss reduces CV risk in patients with existing CAD has not been established. Due to the lack of evidence, current guidelines do not recommend supplementation with vitamins or micronutrients to reduce CV risk in this population. With respect to physical activity, moderate to vigorous physical activity, at least 150 min/week, is recommended to prevent vascular disease in patients that can exercise.

Glucose Control

In patients with type 2 diabetes mellitus intensive glucose control can reduce microvascular complications such as retinopathy or nephropathy.[11–13] The effect on macrovascular events in patients with diabetes and chronic CAD is less well established. The United Kingdom Prospective Diabetes Study (UKPDS) was the first large study examining the effect of an intensive glucose control regimen on macrovascular events; the study compared conventional versus intensive therapy in 3867 patients with newly diagnosed type 2 diabetes and no history of CVD. Intensive therapy significantly reduced microvascular events such as nephropathy and retinopathy, but after a follow-up of 10 years only a nonsignificant reduction in macrovascular events such as MI was found.[12] Only after an additional 10 years of follow-up did the initial intensive therapy translate into a significant decrease in macrovascular events.[14] These results, albeit difficult to interpret because of the nature of this nonprespecified follow-up analysis, suggested that early intervention with a stringent glucose control strategy may eventually reduce macrovascular events in patients with diabetes without a history of CV disease.

Over the last decade various CV outcome trials in high-risk patients with diabetes have assessed the effect of a tight glucose control strategy compared with standard therapy on the incidence of CV events.[11,15,16] The Action to Control Cardiovascular Risk in Diabetes (ACCORD) Trial examined whether an intensive glucose control with the HbA_{1c} target of less than 6.5% (46 mmol/mol) compared with standard therapy with an HbA_{1c} target of less than 7.5% (58 mmol/mol) reduced CV events in 10,251 patients with type 2 diabetes. A very aggressive glucose-lowering approach with various combination therapies including insulin and up to 5 oral antidiabetic drugs was chosen to bring the HbA_{1c} value to target. After 3.5 years the study was stopped prematurely due to a higher mortality in the intensive treatment arm. The primary endpoint of MI, stroke, and CV death was not significantly different between groups, despite a significant difference in HbA_{1c} of 7.5% in the standard therapy and 6.4% in the intensive glucose-lowering group. Increased mortality associated with intensive therapy was mainly observed in subjects with multiple CV risk factors, as well as in those subjects in whom HbA_{1c} lowering was very difficult.

The Action in Diabetes and Vascular Disease: PreterAx and Diamicron Modified Release Controlled Evaluation (ADVANCE) trial included 11,140 patients and tested whether intensive glucose-lowering therapy with an HbA_{1c} target below 6.5% compared with standard therapy with an HbA_{1c} target according to local guidelines might reduce the primary combined endpoint of macrovascular (MI, stroke, or CV death) and microvascular (nephropathy or retinopathy) events.[17] The therapeutic algorithm in this trial to reduce HbA_{1c} levels was less aggressive than in ACCORD, and after a follow-up of 4.3 years the two groups significantly differed with an HbA_{1c} of 7.3% versus 6.5%. This HbA_{1c} difference translated into significant 10% RR reduction for microvascular events (p =0.013) but did not have a significant effect on the combined macrovascular endpoint. In contrast to ACCORD, there was no increase in mortality in this study.

The third trial, the Veterans Affairs Diabetes Trial (VADT), was a smaller trial randomizing 1791 patients with type 2 diabetes to intensive or standard glucose therapy with an HbA_{1c} target of 6.0% in the intensive group and 9.0% in the standard group.[16] Despite a highly significant difference in glucose control with an HbA_{1c} of 8.5% in the standard group and 7.0% in the intensive group, no reduction of the combined primary endpoint of MI, stroke, CV death, CHD intervention, or amputation was achieved. Patients in these three studies had a long duration of diabetes and a large proportion had preexisting CVD and a high number of associated risk factors such as hypertension or dyslipidemia. A meta-analysis of ACCORD, ADVANCE, and VADT suggested that an HbA_{1c} reduction of 1% may lead to a 15% RR reduction in nonfatal MI but no benefit on stroke and all-cause mortality.[18] Further analyses suggested that patients with a short duration of diabetes, no history of CVD, and low HbA_{1c} at baseline may still benefit from an intensive glucose-lowering therapy.[19,20] However, lower HbA_{1c} targets should only be achieved without increasing the risk for hypoglycemia; in addition, weight gain and uncontrolled combination therapy of oral antidiabetic medication and/or insulin should be avoided.

Hemoglobin A_{1c} Targets

Current guidelines from various diabetes and heart professional associations favor an individualized strategy for HbA_{1c} target based on age, history, duration of diabetes, and presence of CVD as well as other comorbidities and the risk of hypoglycemia. In general, a near-normal HbA_{1c} level below 7% (53 mmol/L) should be achieved to decrease microvascular complications. A tighter blood glucose control with an HbA_{1c} target less than 6.5 might be appropriate in selected subjects with a short duration of diabetes and a low risk of hypoglycemia. For older patients with diabetes as well as those with preexisting CV disease, less stringent HbA_{1c} lowering to a target less than or equal to 8% is recommended.[9,10]

Glucose-Lowering Agents

Most guidelines[9,10] recommend metformin as the first-line therapy for glucose-lowering because of its weight-loss effect and low risk of hypoglycemia.[21] In addition, data from the UKDPS suggested a beneficial effect on CV outcome: in the subgroup of 753 overweight patients metformin significantly reduced the risk of MI versus conventional therapy by 39%.[13] Such data were confirmed in two meta-analyses suggesting reduced CVD in patients treated with metformin.[22,23] The majority of patients with type 2 diabetes require combination therapy to achieve glycemic targets. Metformin can be combined with any other antidiabetic drug including sulfonylureas (SUs), α-glucosidase inhibitors, pioglitazone, glucagon-like peptide 1 (GLP1)-receptor agonists, dipeptidyl peptidase 4 (DPP4)-inhibitors, sodium-glucose cotransporter-2 (SGLT2)-inhibitors, and insulin. Of note, any of these agents can be used as monotherapy in subjects in whom metformin is contraindicated or not tolerated.

The PROspective pioglitAzone Clinical Trial In macroVascular Events (PROACTIVE) analyzed whether addition of pioglitazone or placebo to baseline antihyperglycemic therapy has an effect on CV events. It showed no benefit on the combined primary endpoint of all-cause mortality, nonfatal MI, acute coronary syndrome (ACS), coronary artery bypass graft (CABG), percutaneous coronary intervention (PCI), stroke, major leg amputation, or major leg revascularization. However, because this endpoint included non-CV composites such as reduction of leg amputation or revascularization—events that are unlikely to be reduced by medical therapy alone—a principal secondary endpoint was predefined. Pioglitazone significantly reduced this secondary outcome of MI, stroke, and CV mortality (HR 0.84; 95% CI, 0.72–0.98; $p = 0.027$) versus placebo.[24] For another thiazolidinedione, rosiglitazone, no such effects have been observed.[25,26] However, PROACTIVE showed an increase in heart failure, a class effect of these insulin-sensitizing agents.[27] The Study to Prevent Non-Insulin Dependent Diabetes Mellitus (STOP-NIDDM) showed a 49% RR reduction of CV events by acarbose versus placebo in patients with impaired glucose tolerance.[28,29] Still, this was not the primary endpoint of this study and the study population did not have manifest diabetes. Therefore, the effect of acarbose on CV events is currently being tested in a large CV outcome trial in China, the Acarbose Cardiovascular Evaluation (ACE), enrolling patients with established type 2 diabetes.

Conflicting data exist with respect to the effects of SUs on CV events. The University Group Diabetes Program (UGDP) was the first study conducted in the 1960s that raised concerns about the safety of the first-generation SU tolbutamide. It showed a significant increase of overall and CV mortality in subjects receiving tolbutamide versus placebo.[30,31] Still, this study was not designed or powered to test CV safety, and it has been criticized because the results were not corrected for higher preexisting CV risk in the tolbutamide group versus the placebo group.[32] In addition, it is unclear to what extent the findings of this study can be applied to current clinical practice, given the fact that modern diabetes management including a multifactorial approach was not applied. It is also unclear whether these findings apply to modern SUs. In contrast to the findings in UGDP, UKPDS demonstrated that tolbutamide, glyburide, and glimepiride were not associated with adverse CV events.[12] Other trials of longer-term duration also indicated that SUs are not associated with an increased CV risk when compared head-to-head with other agents, such as thiazolidinediones, DPP4-inhibitors, metformin, or GLP1-analogs.[33–39] In addition, a large meta-analysis of 40 randomized controlled trials of glucose-lowering drugs found no increased risk of macrovascular events and all-cause mortality in second-generation SUs versus other oral agents or placebo.[40] However, most of the trials included in this meta-analysis were not designed or powered to examine CV events. Moreover, the inconsistent reporting of adverse events and the short-term duration of these studies make it difficult to make final conclusions on the effect of SUs on CV events. Interestingly several observational studies have shown higher rates of all-cause and CV mortality associated with SU monotherapy or in combination with metformin compared with metformin monotherapy, but this was not confirmed in other studies.[41–44] Overall, there is an absence of conclusive outcome data on the impact of SUs on CV events. The ongoing Cardiovascular Outcome Trial of Linagliptin Versus Glimepiride in Type 2 Diabetes (CAROLINA) trial may shed more light on this issue.[45–47]

Newer Treatment Options

Over the last years, multiple novel antidiabetic therapies have come to the market and the Food and Drug Administration (FDA) and Europe, the Middle East, and Africa (EMEA) requirements have made it mandatory for the industry to perform CV outcome trials to show safety. The FDA required a demonstration of noninferiority of these agents versus placebo with regard to CV events, utilizing a noninferiority margin of 1.3. This has led to carrying out and publishing results of large CV outcome trials in patients with type 2 diabetes and high CV risk. So far, three large CV outcome trials with DPP4-inhibitors, three large trials with GLP1-receptor agonist, and the first outcome trial for an SGLT-2-inhibitor have been published. The three DPP4-inhibitor trials, SAVOUR (saxagliptin),[48] EXAMINE (alogliptin),[49] and TECOS (sitagliptin),[50] examined in a high-risk population of patients with a long duration of diabetes, prior CVD, and/or various risk factors whether the addition of the given drug increases CV risk versus placebo (Table 24.1).

These trials were designed as noninferiority trials and did not show an increased CV risk of any of these DPP4-inhibitors. Of note, they were designed to achieve glycemic equipoise between groups, not to examine whether a difference in HbA_{1c} levels in the two treatment arms translates into a reduction of CV events. Interestingly, SAVOUR-TIMI showed a significant increase in hospitalization for heart failure in patients treated with saxagliptin versus placebo,[48,51] whereas such a significant signal was not found in the two other trials of DPP4-inhibitors. Three similar trials were performed with GLP-1 receptor agonists. The ELIXA trial confirmed CV safety of lixisenatide versus placebo without showing a portenial benefit with respect to CV events.[52,53]

In contrast, the LEADER cardiovascular outcome trial testing the effect of the long acting GLP1 receptor agonist Liraglutide showed a significant reduction of the primary endpoint of cardiovascular death, myocardial infarction and stroke and the results were mainly driven by a significant reduction of cardiovascular death. In addition Liraglutide reduced overall mortality in a population of 9340 patients with diabetes and high cardiocardiovascular risk.[53a]

Most recently SUSTAIN 6 was reported. This study examined once weekly Semaglutide in 3297 patients with type 2 diabetes and high cardiovascular risk. Compared to placebo Semaglutide significantly reduced the combined cardiovascular endpoint of cardiovascular death, non-fatal myocardial infarction and non-fatal stroke. Interestingly this result was mainly driven by a significant 39% reduction of non-fatal stroke. The trend for myocardial infarction was statistically not significant NEJM 2016 inline). A similar trial with the GLP-1

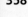

TABLE 24.1 Baseline Characteristics of Published Dipeptidyl Peptidase 4 Inhibitor Outcome Trials

	SAVOR (SAXAGLIPTIN)	EXAMINE (ALOGLIPTIN)	TECOS (SITAGLIPTIN)
Participants (*N*)	16,500	5400	14,724
Age (years)	65	61	66
Diabetes duration (years)	12	7.2	9.4
BMI (kg/m^2)	31	29	29
A_{1C} (%)	8.0	8.0	7.3
Prior CVD (%)	78	~100	100
Hypertension (%)	81	83	86
Prior insulin use (%)	41	30	23
Comparator	Placebo	Placebo	Placebo

BMI, Body mass index; *CVD,* cardiovascular disease.

TABLE 24.2 Cardiovascular (CV) Outcome Trials with SGLT2-Inhibitors

TRIAL	EMPA-REG OUTCOME	CANVAS	DECLARE-TIMI 58	VERTIS
Clinicaltrials.gov	NCT01131676	NCT01032629	NCT01730534	NCT01986881
Intervention	Empagliflozin vs placebo (2:1)	Canagliflozin vs placebo (2:1)	Dapagliflozin vs placebo (1:1)	Ertugliflozin vs placebo (2:1)
Primary outcome measure	CV death, nonfatal MI, nonfatal stroke	CV death, nonfatal MI, nonfatal stroke	CV death, nonfatal MI, nonfatal ischemic stroke	CV death, nonfatal MI, nonfatal stroke
Participants (*N*)	7020	4417	17,276	3900
Patients	T2D; established CV disease	T2D; high CV risk	T2D; high CV risk	T2D; established CV disease
Follow-up (years)	3	6–7 years	4–5 years	5–7 years
Results reporting (estimated)	2015	2017 (estimated)	2019 (estimated)	2020 (estimated)

CANVAS, Canagliflozin Cardiovascular Assessment Study; *DECLARE-TIMI 58,* Dapagliflozin Effect on Cardiovascular Events—TIMI 58; *EMPA-REG OUTCOME,* Empagliflozin Cardiovascular Outcome Event Trial in Type 2 Diabetes Mellitus Patients; *T2D,* type 2 diabetes mellitus; *VERTIS,* Randomized, Double-Blind, Placebo-Controlled, Parallel Group Study to Assess Cardiovascular Outcomes Following Treatment with Ertugliflozin in Subjects with Type 2 Diabetes Mellitus and Established Vascular Disease.

receptor agonist lixisenatide versus placebo confirmed this drug's safety, without showing a potential benefit with respect to CV events.[52,53]

Empagliflozin

SGLT-2-inhibitors are a new class of antidiabetic drugs that block the SGLT-2-receptor in the proximal tubule of the kidney, thus leading to increased urinary excretion of glucose along with sodium. The first published CV outcome trial to assess the effect of an SGLT-2-inhibitor was EMPA-REG, testing whether empagliflozin versus placebo influences the incidence of CV events. In a high-risk population of patients with type 2 diabetes and prior CVD, the study first tested in a hierarchical fashion the requirements of regulatory agencies for noninferiority with regard to major adverse CV events (MACEs), (ie, CV death, MI, and stroke), and then subsequently the drug's superiority versus placebo. A total of 7020 patients with a long duration of diabetes (> 10 years in 57%) and CVD were followed for a mean of 3.1 years;[54] 75% of the patients had CAD and approximately 50% of them had multivessel disease; 46% had prior MI; and approximately 10% had a history of cardiac failure. The patient population in EMPA-REG was very well treated: more than 75% were on a statin, more than 95% received antihypertensive therapy, and approximately 90% were on anticoagulant/antiplatelet drugs. This translated into good risk factor management with a mean blood pressure of 135/77 mm Hg and mean low-density lipoprotein cholesterol (LDL-C) of 2.2 mmol/L. Taken together, this study tested the effect of an SGLT-2-inhibitor in a very-high-risk population of patients with type 2 diabetes on top of standard of care and well-controlled risk factors. Unexpectedly, it showed a significant 14% reduction of the primary endpoint of CV death, MI, and stroke, a significant 38% reduction of CV mortality, and a significant 32% reduction of overall mortality, translating into a number-needed-to-treat of 39 over 3.1 years to prevent 1 CV death. In addition, empagliflozin significantly reduced hospitalizations for heart failure with separation of the curves after only a few weeks. These findings were consistent in all subgroups.[55]

For the first time this study showed in a prospective randomized controlled trial (RCT) in a population of patients with diabetes and CVD that an antidiabetic drug reduces CV events as well as CV and overall mortality. The mechanisms of these unexpected findings are unclear but given only minor differences in HbA_{1c} between groups the glucose-lowering properties of empagliflozin are unlikely to be responsible. Other mechanisms such as weight loss, reduction of blood pressure, sodium depletion, reduced oxidative stress and arterial stiffness, and reduction in sympathetic nerve activation are currently being discussed as potential mechanisms.[55a] So far, only data for the effects of empagliflozin on CV risk are available. Because many of these mechanistic effects have also been described for other SGLT2-inhibitors, it will be interesting to see the results of the ongoing CV outcome trials with dapagliflozin, canagliflozin, and ertugliflozin to find out whether the beneficial CV outcome effects reported from the EMPA-REG trial are a class effect or unique to empagliflozin (Table 24.2).

Cardiovascular Risks Associated with Hypoglycemia

Both insulin and SUs can lead to hypoglycemia in patients with diabetes. Severe hypoglycemia is defined as an event

TABLE 24.3 Pharmacologic Treatment Options for Type 2 Diabetes Mellitus

DRUG	EFFECT	WEIGHT CHANGE	HYPOGLYCEMIA (MONOTHERAPY)	COMMENTS
Metformin	Insulin sensitizer	Neutral/loss	No	Gastrointestinal side effects, lactic acidosis, vitamin B_{12} deficiency Contraindications: low eGFR, hypoxia, dehydration
Sulphonylurea	Insulin provider	Increase	Yes	Allergy, risk for hypoglycemia and weight gain
Meglitinides	Insulin provider	Increase	Yes	Frequent dosing, risk for hypoglycemia
α-Glucosidase inhibitor	Glucose absorption inhibitor	Neutral	No	Gastrointestinal side effects, frequent dosing
Pioglitazone	Insulin sensitizer	Increase	No	Heart failure, edema, fractures, urinary bladder cancer
GLP-1 agonist	Insulin provider	Decrease	No	Gastrointestinal side effects, pancreatitis Injectable
DPP4-inhibitor	Insulin provider	Neutral	No	Pancreatitis
Insulin	Insulin provider	Increase	Yes	Risk for hypoglycemia and weight gain Injectable
SGLT2-inhibitors	Blocks renal glucose absorption in the proximal tubuli	Decrease	No	Urinary tract infections

eGFR, Estimated glomerular filtration rate; *GLP-1*, glucagon-like peptide-1; *SGLT2*, sodium glucose cotransporter 2.
(From Ryden L, Grant PJ, Anker SD, et al. ESC Guidelines on diabetes, pre-diabetes, and cardiovascular diseases developed in collaboration with the EASD: the task force on diabetes, pre-diabetes, and cardiovascular diseases of the European Society of Cardiology (ESC) and developed in collaboration with the European Association for the Study of Diabetes (EASD). Eur Heart J. *2013;34(39):3035–3087.)*

requiring external assistance for recovery, whereas milder episodes may be treated by the patient alone. Clinical trials in patients with type 2 diabetes raised concerns about an increased risk for CV events after hypoglycemic events. In the previously mentioned trials, ACCORD, ADVANCE, and VADT, the rates of severe hypoglycemia were substantially higher in patients with intensive versus standard therapy. In ACCORD severe hypoglycemic events occurred in 16.2% versus 5.1%, in ADVANCE 2.7% versus 1.5%, and in VADT 21.2% versus 9.7% in the intensive glucose target groups versus control groups.[9] After publication of these data, intensive discussions have taken place to what extent severe hypoglycemic events contribute to CV events and excess mortality. To date it is recognized that hypoglycemia is a serious and common complication of diabetes treatment and is associated with CV events and mortality. Several mechanisms such as cardiac arrhythmias due to abnormal cardiac repolarization in high-risk patients, for example, those with CAD or cardiac autonomic neuropathy, increased thrombotic tendency/decreased thrombolysis, CV changes induced by catecholamines, and silent myocardial ischemia, have been discussed to link hypoglycemia with CV events. Although clear causality is as yet unproven, the avoidance of hypoglycemia is one of the key goals in diabetes therapy. Because a direct causal link with death or CV events has not been shown so far, hypoglycemia may serve as a marker of a patient's overall vulnerability to adverse clinical outcomes. Therefore, patients treated with SUs or insulin should be carefully monitored with respect to hypoglycemic events and, whenever possible, other agents that do not cause hypoglycemia should be used.[9,10] Table 24.3 summarizes therapeutic pharmacologic options to treat type 2 diabetes.

Lipid Lowering

Dyslipidemia in Patients with Diabetes

Patients with diabetes exhibit a characteristic dyslipidemia with usually moderately elevated LDL-C, high triglycerides, and low high-density lipoprotein (HDL)-C levels.[56] In patients with diabetes, total LDL concentrations may be misleading with respect to atherogenicity because patients with diabetes usually exhibit a higher proportion of small dense LDL particles that are more susceptible to oxidation and glycation, thus directly promoting atherogenesis.[57] However, to date there are no data suggesting that therapeutic strategies that lead to changes in LDL particle size reduce CV events.

Both clinical and epidemiologic studies suggest that elevated triglycerides and low HDL-C levels are associated with an increased CV risk, especially in patients with diabetes.[58,59] Despite this, therapeutic strategies to reduce triglyceride levels or to raise HDL-C levels in patients with diabetes seem less effective for risk reduction than lowering LDL-C. For decades, the class of lipid-lowering fibric acid derivatives such as fenofibrate or gemfibrozil was seen as the ideal therapy to address the characteristic dyslipidemia in patients with diabetes because these drugs reduce triglycerides and increase HDL-C. However, large clinical outcome trials did not support this assumption: in the FIELD study fenofibrate had no significant effect on the primary endpoint of CV death and nonfatal MI versus placebo, but it reduced total CV events with an RR reduction of 10% (HR 0.9; 95% CI 0.80–0.99; p =0.035).[60–62] The ACCORD trial examined whether the addition of fenofibrate to simvastatin versus placebo would lead to reduced CV events in 5519 patients with diabetes. Overall, fenofibrate did not show a significant effect on CV outcome. In a prespecified subgroup of patients with a characteristic diabetic dyslipidemia (triglycerides > 2.3 mmol/L [> 204 mg/dL] and HDL-C < 0.9 mmol [< 34 mg/dL)] fenofibrate significantly reduced CV events by 27%.[63] In both studies fenofibrate markedly reduced triglycerides but had only a minor effect on HDL-C. Subsequent meta-analyses of different fibrate trials showed a benefit on major CV events but no effect on CV mortality.[64,65] Therefore, current guidelines conclude that the combination therapy of statin plus fibrate provides no additional CV benefit beyond a statin therapy alone and should as such not be recommended.[9,10]

Low-Density Lipoprotein Cholesterol Lowering

Studies over the last three decades have revealed that LDL-C lowering is among the most potent strategies to reduce CV events in patients with diabetes. However, to date there is controversy about the strategy: the American guidelines are in favor of a "fire-and-forget" approach,[66] whereas the European guidelines propose a "treat-to-target" concept.[67] In patients with diabetes, the American guidelines distinguish two groups: those between 40 and 75 years of age and a high CV risk (10-year risk assessed by new pooled cohort equations > 7.5%) and a moderate-risk group with a 10-year risk less than 7.5%. In patients with diabetes in the high-risk group a high-intensity LDL-C reduction of at least 50% with a potent statin such as high-dose atorvastatin (80 mg[40]) or rosuvastatin (20 to 40 mg) is recommended, whereas subjects in the moderate-risk group should receive a less-intensive statin therapy to achieve an LDL-C reduction between 30% and 50%. This less-intensive daily therapy includes atorvastatin 10 to 20 mg, rosuvastatin 5 to 10 mg, simvastatin 20 to 40 mg, pravastatin 40 to 80 mg, pitavastatin 2 to 4 mg, or lovastatin 40 mg. In the US guidelines no target LDL-C levels are recommended. The American guidelines are based on statin RCTs only, whereas the European guidelines included RCTs, population epidemiology, and genetic epidemiology as a basis for their recommendations. Therefore the European guidelines recommend that patients are categorized based on their CV risk, and, depending on their individual risk, LDL-C target values are recommended. All patients with diabetes belong to the very-high-risk group, and ESC guidelines recommend an LDL-C target below 70 mg/dL (< 1.8 mmol/L) in these subjects.

Since publication of these guidelines, another large lipid-lowering CV outcome trial, Improved Reduction of Outcomes: Vytorin Efficacy International Trial (IMPROVE-IT), has presented results.[68,69] IMPROVE-IT examined whether ezetimibe, an inhibitor of the cholesterol transporter NPC1L1, which reduces intestinal cholesterol absorption, added to simvastatin versus simvastatin alone may affect CV event incidence in a population of 18,144 post-ACS patients with LDL-C levels above target. After a mean follow-up of 5.7 years, the addition of ezetimibe to simvastatin led to a reduction of LDL-C to 53.7 mg/dL (1.4 mmol/L) versus 69.5 mg/dL (1.8 mmol/L) in the simvastatin-alone group. This LDL-C reduction translated into a significant 6.7% RR reduction for the primary combined endpoint of CV death, MI, stroke, hospitalization for unstable angina, or revascularization with a number-needed-to-treat of 52 to prevent 1 event. Further subgroup analyses of IMPROVE-IT showed that the significant benefit in the overall population is mainly driven by a highly significant effect in patients with diabetes (European Society of Cardiology 2015 Congress. Presented August 30, 2015). Abstract 1947). These data challenge current lipid-lowering guidelines: first of all, IMPROVE-IT shows that a nonstatin lipid-lowering strategy can reduce CV events in high-risk patients. In addition, it demonstrates that further lowering of LDL-C to levels below the currently recommended targets translates into a further reduction of CV events, raising the hypothesis that "the lower, the better" strategy may apply for LDL-C reduction. In summary, lowering LDL-C is a very potent strategy to reduce CV risk in patients with diabetes and CAD independent of a fire-and-forget or treat-to-target strategy. The ESC/EASD guidelines recommend LDL-C target values less than 70 mg/dL in patients with diabetes mellitus and CAD.[10]

Novel strategies, such as inhibition of PCSK9[70] with antibodies such as alirocumab or evolocumab (both approved in Europe and the United States), have shown promising results in various patient populations including those with diabetes. In subjects with familial hypercholesterolemia, as well as in high-CV-risk patients with LDL-C levels not at target with currently available lipid-lowering drugs, these antibodies have been shown to exhibit a very potent LDL-C-lowering effect.[71,72] In patients with diabetes, subgroup analyses of phase III trials showed that PCSK9 inhibition is as effective as in nondiabetic subjects. Two large outcome trials, ODYSSEY Outcome and FOURIER, are examining whether the reduction of LDL-C by PCSK9 inhibition with alirocumab or evolocumab translates into a reduction of CV events. Both trials enrolled a large proportion of patients with diabetes, and the results will provide further insights into the effect of intensive LDL-C lowering in the high-risk population of patients with diabetes and CVD.

Various clinical trials have shown that statin use may increase the risk of incident diabetes in patients without diabetes. A large meta-analysis suggested that statin therapy is associated with a slightly increased RR (9%) of development of diabetes[73]; still the risk is low in absolute terms and does not outweigh the benefit with respect to the reduction in coronary events.

Therapies to Increase High-Density Lipoprotein Cholesterol in Patients with Type 2 Diabetes

Current guidelines do not recommend HDL-C-raising strategies in the lipid management of patients with diabetes. Over the last few years various approaches have been developed to increase HDL-C but no trial showed a significant reduction in CV events. The Atherothrombosis Intervention in Metabolic Syndrome with Low HDL/High Triglycerides: Impact on Global Health Outcomes (AIM-HIGH) trial compared niacin versus placebo in statin-treated patients with known CV disease. It had a large subgroup of patients with diabetes (34%). After 2 years niacin raised HDL-C from 35 mg/dL to 42 mg/dL, lowered triglycerides from 164 mg/dL to 122 mg/dL, and decreased LDL-C from 74 mg/dL to 62 mg/dL. However, AIM-HIGH was terminated after a mean follow-up of 3 years because of futility.[74] The primary endpoint of CV events or hospitalization for unstable angina did not differ among groups. In the subgroup of patients with diabetes the data were similar with no significant effect on CV outcome in niacin-treated patients. In addition, the Treatment of HDL to Reduce the Incidence of Vascular Events (HPS2-THRIVE) trial confirmed these data by showing that the addition of extended-release niacin/laropiprant to simvastatin (or ezetimibe/simvastatin) did not reduce the risk of CV events.[75]

Inhibition of cholesteryl ester transfer protein (CETP) was another strategy to increase HDL levels. Two large outcome trials (with the CETP inhibitors torcetrapib and dalcetrapib) did not show a reduction of CV events despite a 30% to 40% increase in HDL-C.[76,77] Clinical and experimental data suggest that this may be due to abnormal functional characteristics of HDL particles in patients with diabetes and/or CVD, suggesting that HDL function may be more important than the overall number of measured HDL particles.[78–80] Thus, current recommendations suggest that only lifestyle modification is indicated to address low HDL in patients with diabetes.

Blood Pressure Lowering

Hypertension is one of the CV risk factors associated with diabetes, and in patients with type 2 diabetes more than 60% have arterial hypertension.[81,82] Various pathophysiologic mechanisms such as increased renal sodium reabsorption due to hyperinsulinemia, increased sympathetic activity, and RAAS activation are thought to contribute to arterial hypertension in these patients.[83] Both hypertension and diabetes are additive risk factors for CVD,[84] and various data suggest that the presence of hypertension in subjects with diabetes leads to a 4-fold increase in CV risk.[6] Over the last decades blood pressure targets in patients with diabetes have changed and are still a matter of debate. The first trial to suggest stringent blood pressure lowering in patients with diabetes was the High-Potential Optimal Treatment (HOT) Trial. It showed that diastolic targets below 80 mm Hg significantly decreased CV risk versus a less stringent strategy with diastolic targets less than 100 or less than 90 mm Hg. Still, the mean diastolic blood pressure in the first group was still above 80 mm Hg and the mean systolic blood pressure was 144 mm Hg.[85]

Data from UKPDS published in 1998 showed that reduction of mean blood pressure from 154/87 mm Hg to 144/82 mm Hg led to a 24% reduction in CV events.[86] In addition, post-hoc UKPDS data suggest that a blood pressure drop of 10 mm Hg decreases diabetes-related mortality by 15%. The lowest systolic blood pressure achieved in this context was approximately 120 mm Hg.[87] The results from these studies suggested that there may be no threshold for the beneficial effect of BP lowering. These data were in contrast to those from the ACCORD trial in which 2700 patients with type 2 diabetes were randomized to intensive (mean systolic blood pressure at study end: 119 mm Hg) versus standard therapy (mean systolic blood pressure at study end: 134 mm Hg) over a mean follow-up of 4.7 years. There was no significant effect of the intensive therapy on the primary composite endpoint of nonfatal MI, nonfatal stroke, or CV death. Still, the incidence of fatal or nonfatal strokes was significantly reduced in the intensive therapy group, translating into a number-needed-to-treat for over 5 years of 98 to prevent 1 stroke event.[88] However, the intensive blood pressure-lowering approach significantly increased serious adverse events from 8.3% versus 3.3% with a significant increase in hypotension, syncope, arrhythmia, and hyperkalemia, as well as renal failure and a decrease of glomerular filtration rate below 30 mL/min per 1.73 m^2. These data from ACCORD showing an increase in serious adverse events do not support a reduction of systolic blood pressure below 130 mm Hg.

A 2011 meta-analysis including 13 RCTs and 37,736 patients with diabetes, impaired fasting glucose, or impaired glucose tolerance suggests that intensive blood pressure control (with a systolic blood pressure ≤135 mm Hg in this group) compared with a standard group (systolic blood pressure ≤140 mm Hg) leads to a 10% relative reduction in overall mortality and a 17% reduction of stroke incidence. However, this meta-analysis confirmed the ACCORD observation that more intensive blood pressure control leads to an up to 20% increase in serious adverse events.[89] These trials and analyses set the basis for the ESC guideline recommendation that patients with diabetes should achieve a blood pressure target of less than 140/85 mm Hg. In certain subgroups, including those with nephropathy and overt proteinuria, further reduction of systolic blood pressure to targets below 130 mm Hg may be considered, but the evidence to support this recommendation is scarce. In addition, the risk/benefit balance of intensive blood pressure management needs to be carefully considered individually with special attention in elderly patients and those with a long duration of diabetes.[10]

The management of blood pressure in patients with diabetes, as in nondiabetic subjects, includes lifestyle intervention with salt restriction and weight loss, as well as pharmacologic treatment. Lifestyle intervention is recommended for all patients with hypertension but it is often insufficient to adequately control blood pressure, making pharmacologic intervention necessary.

Pharmacologic Intervention to Lower Blood Pressure in Patients with Diabetes

In principle, all blood pressure–lowering agents can be used to treat patients with diabetes to a blood pressure target of less than 140/85 mm Hg. However, several RCTs enrolled large subgroups of patients with diabetes and demonstrated that blockade of the RAAS by angiotensin-converting enzyme (ACE) inhibitors or angiotensin receptor blockers provides the largest benefit in the reduction of CV events in these high-risk patients—in particular in patients with overt proteinuria.[90–93] Good evidence exists that for initial therapy, ACE inhibitors rather than calcium-channel blockers should be used to prevent or retard the occurrence of microalbuminuria in these patients.[94] A combination of ACE inhibitors and angiotensin receptor blockers did not show any CV benefit versus ACE inhibition alone in the ONTARGET trials and was even associated with more adverse events, suggesting that this combination therapy should not be used for blood pressure lowering.[95] The Aliskiren Trial in Type-2 Diabetes Using Cardio-renal Endpoints (ALTITUDE), examining the addition of the renin inhibitor aliskiren to RAAS blockade in patients with diabetes at high CV and renal events risk, did not show a reduction in CV events but an increase in adverse events, suggesting that this combination therapy should also be avoided.[96,97]

Other important points taken into consideration in antihypertensive therapy in patients with diabetes are the metabolic effects of various blood pressure–lowering agents. As such, thiazides and β-blockers are associated with an increased risk for the development of type 2 diabetes compared with RAAS inhibitors or calcium-channel blockers.[98] However, it is not known whether β-blockers and/or thiazides have similar effects in patients with prevalent type 2 diabetes, and the clinical importance of these adverse metabolic effects remains undetermined. Based on the unfavorable metabolic effects of diuretics and β-blockers, these agents should be avoided as first-line therapy in subjects with metabolic syndromes or high risk for diabetes.[10] Despite this, in patients with established diabetes the beneficial effect of blood pressure lowering seems to outweigh the potential negative metabolic effects by far and therefore diuretics and β-blockers should be used as combination therapy once RAAS inhibition is established. The Avoiding Cardiovascular Events through Complication Therapy in Patients Living with Systolic Hypertension (ACCOMPLISH) trial compared addition of the calcium-channel blocker amlodipine versus hydrochlorothiazide on top of an ACE inhibitor. The study had 11,506 patients, including 6946 patients with diabetes. In the diabetic subgroup, there was a significant reduction of the primary endpoint of CV death and CV events in the amlodipine arm. These data suggest that once RAAS inhibition has been established, the second-line drug should be a calcium-channel blocker given the neutral metabolic effects and favorable results seen in ACCOMPLISH.[99] Overall, current blood pressure targets are only achieved in a subset of patients with diabetes, underscoring the necessity to improve blood pressure lowering therapies in them.

Antiplatelet Therapy in Patients with Diabetes

In patients with diabetes platelet function is disturbed leading to a more frequent response to subthreshold stimuli, increased platelet turnover, and accelerated thrombopoiesis of hyperreactive platelets.[100] Various factors such as hyperglycemia itself with glycation of platelet membrane proteins, oxidative stress with increased reactive oxygen species production, formation of advance glycation end products, and endothelial dysfunction with the release of mediators that affect platelet activity may be crucial in this context. Conflicting data exist for the benefit of aspirin therapy in primary prevention in patients with diabetes: various CV outcome trials[101,102] as well as large meta-analyses[103,104] suggest a limited net benefit of aspirin in primary prevention when assessing reduced CV events compared with increased bleeding risk. Therefore, current guidelines do not uniformly recommend low-dose aspirin in primary prevention. The most recent ACC/AHA guideline in 2015 states that low-dose aspirin (75 to 162 mg/day) is reasonable among those with a 10-year CV risk of at least 10% without an increase of bleeding (class II b, level of evidence B) and that low-dose aspirin is reasonable in adults with diabetes mellitus at intermediate risk (10-year CV risk 5% to 10% [ACC/AHA class II b level of evidence C]).[9] In contrast, the ESC and EASD guidelines in 2013 state that antiplatelet therapy with aspirin in patients with diabetes and low risk is not recommended (class III) and antiplatelet therapy for primary prevention may be considered in high-risk patients with diabetes on an individual basis with a class II b level C recommendation.[10]

In secondary prevention it is recommended that patients with diabetes receive low-dose aspirin similar to what is recommended in patients without diabetes. The evidence for this statement stems from the Anti-platelet Trialists' Collaboration (ACT) showing that aspirin leads to a clear CV benefit in patients with preexisting systemic CVD, both in the presence or absence of diabetes. This analysis included more than 4000 patients with diabetes in RCTs and showed that aspirin clearly reduced CV events (nonfatal MI, nonfatal stroke, and CV death) in them.[105] In case of aspirin intolerance clopidogrel is recommended as an alternative antiplatelet therapy. In the setting of stable CAD current data do not support the use of novel antiplatelet agents such as prasugrel or ticagrelor.

In the ACT trial of 1000 patients with diabetes, aspirin reduced 42 vascular events in secondary prevention. In addition, interesting analyses of the ACT trial suggest that low-dose aspirin (75 to 150 mg/day) seems to be as effective as higher doses (150 mg/day). Moreover, low-dose aspirin was associated with a lower risk of bleeding complications than the higher dose.[106] These data were supported by an observational analysis from the Clopidogrel for High Atherothrombotic Risk and Ischemic Stabilisation, Management Avoidance (CHARISMA) trial demonstrating that aspirin doses above 100 mg/day are not associated with increased efficacy compared with a lower dose. In addition, CHARISMA suggests an increased, albeit not significant, risk of CV death, MI, and stroke (adjusted HR 1.16, 95% CI 0.93–1.14) as well as an increased risk of severe or life-threatening bleeding (adjusted HR 1.3, 95% CI 0.83–2.04) when aspirin doses above 100 mg/day were combined with clopidogrel.[107] These data were supported by a 2010 trial examining the optimal aspirin dose also showing that a higher aspirin dose is not effective in reducing CV events but may increase the risk of bleeding.[108] Table 24.4 summarizes the current recommendation of the ESC/EASD on risk factor management in diabetes.

TABLE 24.4 Summary of Treatment Targets for Managing Patients with Diabetes Mellitus or Impaired Glucose Tolerance (IGT) and Coronary Artery Disease

Blood pressure (mm Hg) In nephropathy	< 140/85 Systolic < 130
Glycemic control HbA_{1c} (%)*	Generally < 7.0 (53 mmol/mol) On an individual basis < 6.5–6.9% (48-52 mmol/mol)
Lipid profile LDL-C	Very-high-risk patients < 1.8 mmol/L (< 70 mg/dL) or reduced by at least 50% High-risk patients < 2.5 mmol/L (< 100 mg/dL)
Platelet stabilization	Patients with CVD and DM: aspirin 75 to 160 mg/day
Smoking Passive smoking	Cessation obligatory None
Physical activity	Moderate to vigorous ≥ 150 min/week
Weight	Aim for weight stabilization in overweight or obese patients based on calorie balance and weight reduction in subjects with IGT to prevent development of T2DM
Dietary habits Fat intake (% of dietary energy) Total Saturated Monounsaturated fatty acids Dietary fiber intake	< 35% < 10% > 10% > 40 g/day (or 20 g/1000 kcal per day)

CVD, Cardiovascular disease; *DM,* diabetes mellitus; *HbA_{1c},* glycated hemoglobin A_{1c}; *LDL-C,* low-density lipoprotein cholesterol; *T2DM,* type 2 diabetes mellitus.
*Diabetes Control and Complication Trial standard.

CORONARY REVASCULARIZATION IN PATIENTS WITH CAD AND DIABETES

In diabetes, long-standing impaired glucose metabolism, as well as associated risk factors, affect the CV system at the level of epicardial vessels (macrovascular disease) and the small capillaries in the peripheral segments of target vessels (microvascular disease).[109] The macrovascular involvement results in the development of advanced atherosclerosis with a subsequently enhanced risk of CAD, cerebrovascular disease, and peripheral arterial disease. Consequently, CAD is the leading cause of death in patients with diabetes.[6,109] The predominant therapeutic option in symptomatic patients with diabetes with stable CAD remains coronary revascularization, either by PCI or CABG. However, clinical outcomes in patients with diabetes and CAD are reported to be worse than in patients without diabetes. Moreover, as previously outlined, several investigations have demonstrated that patients with diabetes without a history of CV events have the same chance of MI as patients who do not have diabetes but who have previous coronary events.[6] In addition, patients with diabetes are at a significantly higher risk of recurrent CV events after PCI, in particular, in-stent restenosis, target vessel revascularization, MI, acute and subacute stent thrombosis, and death, and they have a poorer prognosis following ACS.[6,110–112] After CABG, patients with diabetes are particularly prone to sternal wound infections, acute kidney injury, heart failure, or death.[113,114]

The main aim of coronary revascularization in patients with diabetes with stable CAD is improvement of symptoms and prognosis.[115] According to current guidelines the first-line treatment is medical treatment including anti-ischemic drugs. However, the optimal revascularization strategy particularly in the high-risk population of diabetes patients remains controversial. Thus, careful evaluation of the general treatment indication and consecutively of the optimal therapeutic strategy is of particular importance in this specific patient cohort.

OPTIMAL MEDICAL TREATMENT VERSUS CORONARY REVASCULARIZATION

Despite the growing prevalence of diabetes in Western countries, the widespread and consequent use of CV drugs for primary and secondary prevention has led to a reduction of mortality of approximately 50% during the last decades.[116] There have been dramatic improvements and evolutions in fundamental medical management and adjunctive therapy of CAD, and moreover vast advances in revascularization techniques and materials have been made. Optimal medical treatment (OMT) aims to target the different components involved in the development of atherosclerosis and atherothrombosis with a specific focus on a strict control of lifestyle risk factors.[117,118] These include weight control, cessation of smoking, diet programs, implementation of balanced life rhythms, and pharmacologic control of arterial hypertension, hyperlipidemia, and, in the presence of diabetes, adequate glucose control as previously outlined.

However, studies examining OMT versus a revascularization strategy in patients with diabetes with stable CAD are scarce. In the Medicine, Angioplasty, or Surgery Study (MASS II), 611 patients with stable CAD, including 190 patients with diabetes, were randomized into three treatment arms (pharmacologic treatment, PCI, and CABG) with a follow-up of 5 years. Whereas mortality rates during the follow-up period were not different in the nondiabetic cohort, a revascularization approach using PCI or CABG led to a significantly lower mortality rate among patients with diabetes (p =0.039).[119]

In the Bypass Angioplasty Revascularization Investigation 2 Diabetes (BARI-2D) trial, 2368 patients with diabetes and relevant CAD were randomized to either immediate revascularization (CABG, n = 347 or PCI, n = 765) in addition to OMT or to OMT alone. Relevant CAD was defined as more than 50% stenosis with positive stress test or more than 70% stenosis with typical chest pain. In the overall study cohort, no significant survival difference in terms of freedom from major adverse cardiac and cerebrovascular events (MACCEs) or death was seen between revascularization and OMT groups (88.3% vs 87.8%, p =0.97) at 5-year follow-up. However, in the CABG stratum, which had more advanced CAD, a significantly higher rate of freedom from MACCEs and death was observed with surgical revascularization versus OMT alone (77.5% vs 69.6%, p =0.01). In contrast, in the PCI stratum there was no difference in freedom from MACCEs (77% vs 78.9%, p =0.15) between PCI and OMT.[120] Thus, BARI-2D demonstrated that OMT is a reasonable therapeutic option in patients with diabetes and less advanced CAD independent of the presence of ischemia. Moreover, regarding the indirect comparison between CABG and PCI in this trial, overall mortality was significantly lower with CABG than with PCI at 5-year follow-up (19.4% vs 34.5%, p =0.003) and after 10 years of follow-up (42.1% vs 54.5%, p =0.025), respectively.[120] This suggests that in patients with more extensive CAD and proven ischemia, CABG may be the preferred treatment modality, whereas in low-risk patients with diabetes (less advanced CAD on angiogram, stable clinical situation, normal left ventricular function) and reliable compliance to medical therapy, a conservative pharmacologic approach may be rational.[120] Thus both MASS II and BARI-2D outline superiority of CABG versus OMT alone.[119,120] In consecutive trials the need for consequent adherence to OMT as an important prerequisite to successful PCI and CABG has been stressed.[121]

In contemporary clinical practice a large number of patients with diabetes fail to achieve the prespecified OMT aims, despite the dramatic recent developments and the proven advantages of OMT. A pooled analysis of current trials with a total of 5034 patients with diabetes,[122] including the diabetic subgroups of the Clinical Outcomes Utilizing Revascularization and Aggressive Drug Evaluation (COURAGE),[123] the BARI-2D,[120] and the Future Revascularization Evaluation in Patients with Diabetes Mellitus: Optimal Management of Multi-Vessel Disease (FREEDOM) trial,[124] investigated the achievement of the four main targets of OMT with disillusioning results: only 18% of patients in COURAGE, 23% of patients in BARI-2D, and 8% of patients in FREEDOM reached all four prespecified treatment targets at 1-year follow-up. The role and modes of antithrombotic therapy in patients with diabetes undergoing PCI for stable CAD are not different from those for persons without diabetes.[125] Dual antiplatelet therapy, aspirin and a P2Y12 inhibitor, is an established therapy after stent implantation.[126,127] However, patients with diabetes frequently have an insufficient platelet response to clopidogrel.[128] Hence, the new, potent P2Y12 inhibitors prasugrel and ticagrelor may offer an advantage especially in patients with diabetes. The beneficial effect of prasugrel has been shown in the Trial To Assess Improvement in Therapeutic Outcomes By Optimizing Platelet Inhibition by Prasugrel (TRITON-TIMI 38) in patients with ACS. TRITON-TIMI 38 demonstrated a significant reduction of MACEs, a finding that was pronounced in the subgroup of patients with diabetes.[129] In the Platelet Inhibition and Patient Outcomes (PLATO) study, ticagrelor similarly indicated a benefit in terms of MACE reduction when compared with clopidogrel; however, the treatment benefit was not statistically significant in the diabetic cohort.[130] Both TRITON-TIMI 38 and PLATO were conducted in patients with ACS. Due to the lack of comparable data in populations with stable CAD, elective PCI, and/or diabetes, clopidogrel currently remains the recommended antiplatelet substance in these clinical constellations.

Coronary Revascularization in Patients with Diabetes

The concurrent presence of diabetes in patients with multivessel CAD bears an enhanced risk of in-stent restenosis after PCI and subsequently may result in a worse prognosis following CABG in contrast to patients without diabetes.[131] This refers largely to the aggressive nature of the disease with smaller coronary arteries affected in a diffuse manner, and consequently CABG has been the preferred treatment strategy in patients with diabetes requiring coronary revascularization. Numerous trials have demonstrated an efficacy benefit (less repeat revascularization) and moreover a safety benefit (lower mortality) with CABG than with PCI in patients with diabetes.[132–134] The advantages of CABG in patients with diabetes reflect reductions in CV events caused by both nonculprit and culprit lesions. Treatment with PCI usually focuses mainly on the coronary culprit lesion, whereas angiographically and/or functionally nonsignificant nonculprit lesions are generally not treated. However, data from the PROGRESS trial have indicated that particularly those lesions that appear rather mild angiographically have a tendency to rupture in the future due to enhanced plaque vulnerability and plaque burden.[135] In contrast, CABG offers complete treatment of culprit and nonculprit lesions throughout the bypassed segments. Thus, CABG provides an effective protection against secondary CV events due to rupture of initially nonflow-limiting but unstable plaques and thereby avoids the occurrence of concomitant CV events such as MI and sudden cardiac death.

Percutaneous Coronary Intervention with Balloon Angioplasty Versus Coronary Artery Bypass Grafting in Patients with Diabetes

In a subgroup analysis of the Early Bypass Angioplasty Revascularization Investigation (BARI) including 353 patients with diabetes mellitus, the revascularization strategies of CABG versus PCI with plain old balloon angioplasty (POBA) were compared. There was a survival benefit for CABG over PCI (80.6% vs 65.5%, p =0.003).[136] A more recent meta-analysis comprising 68 RCTs and a total of 24,015 patients with diabetes compared CABG with different modes of PCI (POBA, bare metal stent [BMS], first- and second-generation drug-eluting stents [DESs]). In the overall study cohort CABG was associated with numerically lower rates of both death (RR 0.8, 95% CI 0.55–1.23) and MI (RR 0.86, 95% CI 0.28–2.86); however, the difference was not statistically significant.[137]

Percutaneous Coronary Intervention Using Bare Metal Stent or First-Generation Drug-Eluting Stent Versus Coronary Artery Bypass Graft in Patients with Diabetes

In 2005 the Arterial Revascularizaton Therapies Study (ARTS) compared PCI using BMS with CABG. However, it did not primarily focus on patients with diabetes, and only a small diabetic subcohort of 208 patients was available for evaluation. In this subcohort PCI using BMS compared with CABG was found to have numerically, but not statistically significant, higher rates of overall mortality (13.4% vs 8.3%, p =0.27) and MI (10.7% vs 7.3%, p =0.47) at 5-year follow-up. However, rates for repeat revascularization (42.9% vs 10.4%, p <0.001) and MACCE (54.5% vs 25%, p < 0.001) were significantly higher in the PCI group than in the CABG group.[138]

As previously mentioned the BARI-2D trial addressed the question of revascularization in a diabetic patient cohort comparing OMT alone versus OMT plus revascularization therapy (either CABG or PCI). Within the PCI group the stent types were 56% BMS and 35% DES. Despite indicating a treatment benefit in favor of CABG over PCI, this study had a major limitation in that it did not directly compare CABG and PCI. This has subsequently led to several further RCTs comparing CABG with PCI with the use of first-generation DES.[132,133,139] In the Coronary Artery Revascularization in Diabetes (CARDia) trial, 510 patients with diabetes were enrolled and randomized to either PCI or CABG. The results did not show any differences regarding the primary composite endpoint of death, MI between the two strategies (PCI 13.0% vs CABG 10.5%, p =0.39).[133] However, when adding repeat revascularization to the composite endpoint, there was a relevant benefit favoring CABG (11.3% vs 19.3% with PCI, p =0.016) at 1-year follow-up.[137] A relevant limitation of the CARDia trial was the mixed use of BMS (31%) and first-generation sirolimus-eluting stent (SES) within the PCI arm.[133]

In the Veterans Affairs Coronary Artery Revascularization in Diabetes Study (VA CARDS), a small study enrolling 198 patients, most patients received a first-generation DES (60% SES or paclitaxel-eluting stent [PES]) while approximately 20% received a second-generation cobalt-chromium everolimus-eluting stent (CoCr-EES). Thus, VA CARDS was considered as a trial mainly comparing CABG with first-generation DES. It showed a significant reduction of overall mortality from 21% with PCI to 5% with CABG at 2 years of follow-up.[139]

A subcohort of the Synergy Between Percutaneous Coronary Intervention with Taxus and Cardiac Surgery (SYNTAX) trial, consisting of 452 patients with diabetes with left main or 3-vessel disease, similarly demonstrated higher rates of MACCEs with PCI using PES compared with CABG at 1 year (26% vs 14.2%, p =0.003) and after 5 years of follow-up (46.5% vs 29.6%, p <0.001). These findings were predominantly related to a higher rate of repeat revascularization within the PCI group at 1 year (PCI 20.3% vs CABG 6.4%, p < 0.001) and 5 years (PCI 35.3% vs CABG 14.6%, p <0.001).[140,141] Regarding the anatomic severity according to the SYNTAX score, a treatment benefit with CABG was only seen in those patients with diabetes and complex disease (SYNTAX score ≥33); whereas in intermediate and less complex CAD no differences in terms of the composite endpoint were demonstrated.[132] However, as SYNTAX and ARTS were not performed specifically in a diabetic population, the limited number of patients in these subgroups limits conclusions that can be drawn. The ARTS trial only used a historic control group,[134] the CARDia trial was stopped early due to low enrollment and was conclusively underpowered for true evaluation,[133] and the diabetic subgroup analysis of the SYNTAX trial was initially not designed to test differences in mortality.[132] Hence, these studies did not provide sufficient evidence to clearly endorse one of the two revascularization strategies.[116] Moreover, apart from current clinical practice CARDia, VA CARDS, and the diabetic subcohort of SYNTAX did not use newer-generation DES. Instead, predominantly BMS or first-generation DES were implanted and compared with CABG.[132,133,139]

As a consequence of these limitations, the FREEDOM study was designed.[124] This prospective multicenter study has emerged as a true landmark trial and the only RCT that was adequately powered to compare PCI and CABG in an exclusive cohort limited to patients with diabetes and multivessel disease. However, as in previous trials, first-generation DES (SES: 51% and PES: 43%) and not second-generation stents were implanted, which is different than the current standard of care in interventional cardiology. In FREEDOM, which enrolled 1900 patients with diabetes, the primary composite endpoint (all-cause mortality, nonfatal MI, or nonfatal stroke) was lower in patients treated by CABG compared with PCI at 1-year (CABG 18.7% vs PCI 26.6%, p =0.005)[124] and 5-year follow-up (CABG 11.8% vs PCI 16.8%, p =0.004).[142] Of note, this was related to significant differences in overall mortality (CABG 10.9% vs PCI 16.3%, p =0.049) and rate of MI (CABG 6.0% vs PCI 13.9%, p <0.001) at 5 years. Moreover, the incidences of repeat revascularization at 1 year after initial revascularization were significantly higher in the PCI than the CABG group (12.6% vs 4.8%, p <0.01). However, the rate of strokes was conversely higher in the CABG group (5.2 vs 2.4%, p =0.03) and no difference concerning cardiac-specific mortality was found (DES 10.9% vs CABG 6.8%, p =0.12). FREEDOM was still limited by the relatively low inclusion rate of women (28.6%), patients with an ejection fraction below 40% (2.5%), and patients with less advanced CAD (35.5%), defined as a SYNTAX score less than 22.[124,142]

Still, prior to SYNTAX and FREEDOM, lesion anatomy was hardly characterized and scores for lesion severity were not used at all.[121] Thus, stratification of patient cohorts according to the predescribed SYNTAX score tertiles of coronary lesion severity strengthens the impact of both the SYNTAX diabetic substudy analysis as well as the FREEDOM trial.[124,132,140] Unlike previous trials, the baseline characteristics in the FREEDOM cohort targeted a high-risk diabetic population with rather advanced and complex CAD, as characterized by an 83.3% rate of multivessel disease, an average number of lesions of 5.7 ± 2.2, an average lesion length of 77.6 mm ± 33.8 mm, and an average SYNTAX score of 26.2 ± 8.6. Unlike SYNTAX, FREEDOM documented good adherence to concomitant medication in both groups: specifically, in the PCI group approximately 90% of patients received dual antiplatelet therapy for at least 12 months. Furthermore, FREEDOM showed superiority of CABG over PCI in all categories of the SYNTAX score with no significant subgroup interaction (p =0.58).[124] Table 24.5 lists a survey of randomized trials on revascularization in patients with diabetes.

Consequently, the results of the FREEDOM trial had an important impact on clinical practice and current guideline recommendations. For patients with diabetes with stable CAD, the 2014 ACC/AHA guideline renewed its previous recommendation in favor of CABG over PCI from class II A to class I, in particular if a left inferior mammary artery graft can be anastomosed to the left anterior ascending artery, provided the patient is a good candidate for surgery.[143] Similarly the 2014 ESC/EACTS guideline on myocardial revascularization updated its previous recommendation of CABG over PCI in patients with diabetes and multivessel disease with an acceptable surgical risk to a class 1 recommendation with a level of evidence A.[141] Table 24.6 summarizes the specific recommendations for revascularization in patients with diabetes.[141]

However, these guideline recommendations have to be considered differentially and carefully. Overall evidence still remains rare and derives mostly, with the exception of the FREEDOM trial,[124] from observational studies and registry data or from diabetic subgroups of larger study cohorts with few RCTs. Also, despite the latest improvements in stent technologies, including the second-generation DES and most recently bioresorbable vascular scaffolds (BVSs), these new devices have not been incorporated in any trials comparing DES and CABG to date.[144] According to current data it is unquestionable that the regular use of newest generation DES may result in a substantial reduction of both angiographic restenosis and need for repeat revascularization[145] compared with BMSs. Moreover, a hierarchical pattern regarding the restenosis potential of an individual comparator can be observed in a large network meta-analysis with focus on the specific PCI modality.[137] A gradual decline of the rate of repeat revascularization with the applied PCI technique from POBA (341% increase toward CABG), to BMS (218% increase), to first-generation PES (81% increase) and first-generation SES (47% increase) was observed.[137] In contrast, second-generation CoCr-EES as a comparator for CABG was not associated with statistically significant excess repeat revascularization.[137] Despite the indirect comparison with other stent types, the CoCr-EES was the only stent that was not associated with statistically significant excess repeat revascularization in comparison with CABG.[137] Thus, presumably the more efficacious a certain stent is in terms of risk reduction, the less pronounced the resulting net benefit with CABG[146] may be. However, these meta-analyses may not fully account for between-trial differences due to the nature of study designs, and thus data have to be interpreted with caution.[137] Nevertheless, this indirect comparison is at least hypothesis-generating and thus indicates that the efficacy gap between CABG and PCI in patients with diabetes is probably lessened with the use of newer-generation DESs. This reflects the necessity for large RCTs comparing state-of-the-art PCI and new-generation DES with current CABG technology.

The 2015 Bypass Surgery Versus Everolimus-Eluting Stent Implantation for Multi-Vessel Coronary Artery Disease (BEST) trial is the only randomized study that explores CABG with the newer-generation DES as comparator.[147] This prospective, open-label RCT was designed to prove noninferiority of second-generation DES (EES) compared with CABG. However, the trial was stopped prematurely after slow enrollment of only 880 of the initially planned 1776 patients. Thus, the statistical power of the predescribed primary endpoint, defined as death, MI, and repeat revascularization, is inadequate. Second, the primary endpoint did not prove noninferiority for PCI compared with CABG (PCI 11% vs CABG 7.9%, p =0.32 for noninferiority). Consequently, all of the further analysis regarding the data of the BEST trial would only be hypothesis-generating.[147,148] In a subgroup analysis of the BEST trial including patients with diabetes (n = 363), there was a significantly higher rate of primary endpoints among those assigned to PCI compared with CABG (19.2% vs 9.1%, p =0.007).[147]

The latest observational registry study of 18,446 propensity-matched patients with multivessel disease, compared PCI using new-generation CoCr-EES (n = 9223) with CABG (n = 9223). It revealed no difference in the primary endpoint of all-cause mortality between PCI and CABG (PCI 3.1% vs CABG 2.9%, p =0.50). In accordance with previous studies, the investigators found a higher need for repeat revascularization (PCI 7.2% vs CABG 3.1%, p <0.001) and a

TABLE 24.5 Randomized Trials on Revascularization in Patients with Diabetes

		BASIC CHARACTERISTICS					PRIMARY ENDPOINT			MAXIMUM CLINICAL FOLLOW-UP					
YEAR OF PUBLICATION	STUDY(REF. NUMBER)	*N*	MEAN AGE (YEARS)	WOMEN (%)	MVD (%)	MEAN EF (%)	DEFINITION	YEARS	RESULTS	YEARS	DEATH	CV DEATH	M	REVASC	STROKE
Revascularization vs MT															
2009	BARI-2D[120]	2368	62	30	31	57	Death	5	11.7% vs 12.2%	5	11.7% vs 12.2%	5.9% vs 5.7%	11.5% vs 14.3%	—	2.6% vs 2.8%
CABG vs MT															
2009	BARI-2D[120]	763	63	24	52	57	Death	5	13.6% vs 16.4%	5	13.6% vs 16.4%	8.0% vs 9.0%	10.0% vs 17.6%	—	1.9% vs 2.6%
PCI vs MT															
2009	BARI-2D[120]	1605	62	33	20	57	Death	5	10.8% vs 10.2%	5	10.8% vs 10.2%	5.0% vs 4.2%	12.3% vs 12.6%	—	2.9% vs 2.9%
PCI vs CABG															
2013	SYNTAX[d,140]	462	65	29	100	—	Death, MI, stroke, or repeat revascularization	1	26.0% vs 14.2%[a] Sx score 0–22: 20.3% vs 18.3%; Sx-score 23–32: 26.0% vs 12.9%; Sx score ≥ 33: 32.4% vs 12.2%[a]	5	19.5% vs 12.9%	12.7% vs 6.5%[a]	9.0% vs 5.4%	35.3% vs 14.6%[a]	3.0% vs 4.7%
2010	CARDia,[133] (DES/BMS vs CABG)	510	64	26	93	—	Death, MI, or stroke	1	13.0% vs 10.5%	1	3.2% vs 3.2%	—	9.8% vs 6.0%[a]	11.8% vs 2.0%[a]	0.4% vs 2.8%
2012	FREEDOM[124] (DES vs CABG)	1900	63	29	100	66	Death, MI, or stroke	3.8	26.6% vs 18.7%[a] Sx score 0–22: 23% vs 17%; Sx score 23–32: 27% vs 18%;[a] Sx score ≥ 33: 31% vs 23%	3.8	16.3% vs 10.9%[a]	10.9% vs 6.8%	13.9% vs 6.0%[a]	12.6% vs 4.8%[a] (at 1y)	2.4% vs 5.2%
2013	VA-CARDS[139] (DES vs CABG)	207	62	1	—	—	Death or MI	2	18.4% vs 25.3%	2	21% vs 5.0%[a]	10.8% vs 5.0%	6.2% vs 15.0%	18.9% vs 19.5%	1.0% vs. 1.2%

[a]$p < 0.05$; [b]Randomization stratified by revascularization modality; [c]3-vessel disease; [d]subgroup analysis.

BMS, Bare-metal stent; *CABG,* coronary artery bypass grafting; *CV,* cardiovascular; *DES,* drug-eluting stent; *EF,* ejection fraction; *MI,* myocardial infarction; *MT,* medical therapy; *MVD,* multivessel disease; *PCI,* percutaneous coronary intervention; *PES,* paclitaxel-eluting stent; *Revasc,* revascularization; *SES,* stirolimus-eluting stent; *Sx score,* SYNTAX score.

(Adapted from Windecker S, Kolh P, Alfonso F, et al. 2014 ESC/EACTS guidelines on myocardial revascularization: the task force on myocardial revascularization of the European Society of Cardiology (ESC) and the European Association of Cardio-Thoracic Surgery (EACTS): developed with the special contribution of the European Association of Percutaneous Interventions (EAPCI). Eur Heart J. *2014; 35(37):2541–2619.)*

TABLE 24.6 Specific Recommendations for Revascularization in Patients with Diabetes

RECOMMENDATION(REF. NUMBER)	CLASS[a]	LEVEL[b]
In stable patients with multivessel CAD and/or ischemia, revascularization is indicated to reduce cardiac adverse events.[16]	I	B
In patients with stable multivessel CAD and an acceptable surgical risk, CABG is recommended over PCI.[20]	I	A
In patients with stable multivessel CAD and SYNTAX score, PCI should be considered as an alternative to CABG.[38]	IIa	B
New-generation DES are recommended over bare-metal stents.[70]	I	A
Bilateral mammary artery grafting should be considered.[61]	IIa	B
In patients on metformin, renal function should be carefully monitored for 2 or 3 days after coronary angiography/PCI.[141]	I	C

CABG, Coronary artery bypass grafting; *CAD*, coronary artery disease; *DESs*, drug-eluting stents; *PCI*, percutaneous coronary intervention.
[a]Class of recommendation.
[b]Level of evidence.
(Adapted from Windecker S, Kolh P, Alfonso F, et al. 2014 ESC/EACTS guidelines on myocardial revascularization: the task force on myocardial revascularization of the European Society of Cardiology (ESC) and the European Association of Cardio-Thoracic Surgery (EACTS): developed with the special contribution of the European Association of Percutaneous Interventions (EAPCI). Eur Heart J. *2014; 35(37):2541–2619.)*

higher rate of MI (PCI 1.9%/year vs CABG 1.1%/year, p <0.001) with PCI. Conversely, a higher rate of stroke (PCI 0.7% vs CABG 1.0%, p <0.001) with CABG was documented.[149] However, the higher rate of MI within the PCI group turned out to be statistically insignificant in the subgroup of patients with complete revascularization. This confirms previous findings showing that incomplete revascularization is associated with a significant increase of rates of MI and death.[149–151] In a subgroup analysis, 8096 patients with diabetes (39.3% of the entire study cohort) with propensity-matched scores were included. In the short term (within 30 days) EES compared with CABG was associated with a lower risk of both death (HR = 0.58, p =0.04) and stroke (HR = 0.14, p < 0.0001), but a higher risk of MI (HR = 2.44, p = 0.02). In the long term, EES compared with CABG was associated with no differences in the risk of death (HR = 1.12, p = 0.16), a lower risk of stroke (HR = 0.76, p = 0.04), a higher risk of MI (HR = 1.64, p < 0.0001), and a higher rate of repeat revascularization (HR = 2.42, p < 0.0001). However, concordant with the findings in the general population, the higher risk of MI was only seen in patients undergoing incomplete coronary revascularization with PCI.[152]

The currently ongoing Evaluation of the Xience Everolimus-Eluting Stent versus Coronary Artery Bypass Surgery for Effectiveness of Left Main Revascularization (EXCEL) trial compares CABG with PCI using CoCr-EES in patients with unprotected left main stenosis and may provide new insights into the role of revascularization strategies in patients with left main disease (ClinicalTrials.gov Identifier: NCT01205776). Although this study does not focus exclusively on a cohort of patients with diabetes, it may further contribute to the debate regarding the best therapeutic revascularization modality in patients with stable CAD.[146]

Advances in recent CABG technology include minimally invasive direct coronary artery bypass, regular use of arterial grafts with patency rates of more than 80% after 10 years,[153] and contemporary perioperative care. Particularly, diabetes does not seem to have a negative effect on the patency of either internal mammary artery or venous grafts.[154] However, graft selection in patients with diabetes remains controversial. Whereas nonrandomized analyses indicate an advantage of bilateral internal thoracic artery in patients with diabetes,[155] other studies pronounce the enhanced risk of sternal wound infections and mediastinitis, especially in diabetic patients on insulin therapy.[156,157] The use of radial artery conduits in patients with diabetes versus patients without diabetes offers a greater risk for vascular spasm and may be associated with impaired endothelial function.[158] In an RCT comparing radial grafts and venous saphenous grafts for CABG, the investigators found a significantly lower patency rate of radial arterial grafts compared with venous saphenous grafts in patients with diabetes. In contrast, in patients without diabetes the results were opposite.[159] Moreover, approximately 50% of patients with moderate to poor glucose control after CABG had no diabetes diagnosis in the preoperative assessment. This may inevitably result in inadequate perioperative glucose control, which is an established predictor of more in-hospital morbidity and mortality.[160] Despite the current evidence in favor of CABG in patients with diabetes and CAD, in daily clinical practice, in contrast to clinical trials, other parameters may substantially influence a reasonable and patient-orientated decision. These factors include the individual stroke risk, frailty, renal and pulmonary function, patient preference, and both operator and center experience with the respective revascularization modality.[116]

Bare Metal Stents Versus First- and Second-Generation Drug-Eluting Stents in Patients with Diabetes

Several RCTs, registries, and pooled meta-analyses have compared PCI with BMS versus first-generation DES in chronic CAD in patients with diabetes and have thereby focused on both efficacy (as assessed by a reduced repeat revascularization rate) and safety (as assessed by the rate of death, MI, or stent thrombosis). The Diabetes and Sirolimus-Eluting Stent (DIABETES)[161] and the Sirolimus-Eluting Stent in the Treatment of Diabetic Patients with De Novo Native Coronary Artery Lesions (SCORPIUS)[162] trials have demonstrated a significant benefit by use of first-generation SES compared with BMS. In DIABETES at 270-day follow-up comparing SES to BMS a reduction of repeat revascularization (SES 6.3% vs BMS 31.3%, p <0.001) and MACCE (SES 10.0% vs BMS 36.3%, p <0.001) was seen.[161] Similarly, 5-year follow-up data from the SCORPIUS trial demonstrated a reduction in repeat revascularization (SES 12.0% vs BMS 28.0%, p = 0.005) and MACCE (SES 34% vs BMS 49%, p =0.02).[162] However, the MACCE reduction was mainly attributed to a decreased rate of repeat revascularization in both trials, whereas no significant differences in strong endpoint parameters such as mortality, cardiac death, MI, or stent thrombosis were reported.[161,162] Thus, in summary SES performed better than BMS in patients with CAD and diabetes. However, a survival benefit from use of SES has not been shown. Similar results were also seen when comparing the other first-generation PES with BMS. The TAXUS-IV trial demonstrated superiority of PES in terms of significantly lower rates of in-stent restenosis and repeat revascularization versus BMS (PES 7.4% vs BMS 20.9%).[163] However, the implementation of second-generation DESs into the current treatment standard of chronic CAD with an optimized safety and efficacy profile has dramatically changed the therapeutic approach, especially in patients with diabetes and multivessel disease.

In a large meta-analysis of 126 RCTs including 258,544 patient-years of follow-up, the new-generation DES, the zotarolimus-eluting stent Resolute (ZES-R), the platinum-chromium (PtCr EES), and the CoCr-EES have emerged as the most efficacious stents for reducing the risk of repeat target vessel revascularization (TVR) in comparison to PCI with BMS.[164] Another large pooled analysis confirmed these findings in an exclusive population of patients with diabetes, encompassing 42 trials with 22,844 patient-years of follow-up: Bangalore et al demonstrated beneficial efficacy and safety of various first- and second-generation DES compared with BMS in patients with diabetes.[165] There was no increased risk of stent thrombosis, including very late stent thrombosis with any type of DES. The investigators found a significant reduction in TVR independent of the type of DES used; however, the extent of this effect varied with the different DES. Regarding efficacy outcomes, the different DES exhibited a progressive increase in TVR reduction (reduction of TVR vs BMS: ZES 37%, PES 53%, SES 62%, and EES 69%) with the EES appearing to be the most efficacious DES. None of the DES revealed an increased risk of any safety parameters versus BMS.[165]

Accordingly, this largest meta-analysis in patients with diabetes[165] confirms a previous meta-analysis comparing first-generation DES with BMS in 3852 patients with diabetes,[166] which had similarly demonstrated improved efficacy with comparable mortality rates for the first-generation DES (PES and SES) versus BMS. Hence, the data derived from Banaglore et al[165] transfer these former findings in patients with diabetes into the era of new-generation DES. A pooled analysis of the Clinical Evaluation of the Xience V Everolimus Eluting Coronary Stent System (SPIRIT) trial also demonstrated a significant reduction in death and the combination of death and MI for CoCr-EES in comparison with first-generation PES in a general population.[167] Similarly, the SYNTAX trial and a pooled analysis of four trials demonstrated lower incidences of CV events with EES versus PES in a general population.[137,168] On the contrary, among patients with diabetes there were no significant differences between the two stent types according to any safety and efficacy parameters.[168] Although multiple RCTs and meta-analyses have demonstrated superiority of newer-generation DES compared with first-generation DES, these findings still have to be interpreted carefully as data comparison between the different stent types and generations in these trials was indirect and therefore inherent to and limited by this type of analysis.[145,165] Based on these findings, current opinion is that PES are inferior to the so-called *limus*-eluting stents in a general patient population. However, regarding patients with diabetes, the controversy is still ongoing. In this specific patient cohort, data from large RCTs, medium-sized trials, pooled analyses, and registries demonstrated efficacy and safety values for PES that are apparently similar to those of the limus-eluting stents, including SES, ZES, and EES.[169,170]

Because of the lack of large RCTs with direct comparison of the different stent types in patients with diabetes, a debate has arisen as to whether diabetes may actually be the Achilles heel of limus-eluting stents.[171] This refers to the pathophysiologic background of limus-eluting stents, because in patients with diabetes an attenuation of the mammalian target of the rapamycin (mTOR) signaling pathway has been observed. This suggests that stents eluting the drug rapamycin (known as *sirolimus*) or its analogs (everolimus and zotarolimus)—generally termed limus-eluting stents—may be potentially less effective in diabetics. Theoretically, it may eventually make the PES an attractive option in this cohort.[172] This hypothesis is underpinned by the observation of an increasing gradient of event rates among different patient cohorts treated with EES: with the lowest event rate in patients without diabetes, an intermediate event rate in non–insulin-dependent diabetes mellitus (NIDDM) patients, and the highest event rate in insulin-dependent diabetes mellitus (IDDM) patients.[168] In contrast, after PES implantation a similar gradient of event rates was not apparent.

However, more recent data support the superiority of EES over PES in patients with diabetes. Kaul et al demonstrated that PCI with PES is inferior to EES in a cohort of 1830 patients with diabetes.[173] In comparison to PES, EES was associated with significantly lower rates of the primary endpoint target vessel failure (EES 2.9% vs PES 5.6%, p = 0.005) as well as the secondary endpoints of MI (EES 1.2% vs PES 3.2%, p =0.004), stent thrombosis (EES 0.4% vs PES 2.1%, p =0.002), and TVR (EES 1.2% vs PES 3.4%, p =0.002) at 1-year follow-up. These results offer for the first time evidence concerning the efficacy and safety of EES in direct comparison with first-generation PES in a specific patient population with diabetes.[173] This is of particular importance as the existing landmark revascularization trials in patients with diabetes, namely FREEDOM[124] and BARI-2D,[120] were conducted predominantly with first-generation DES, namely PES and SES. Thus, the results of this most current investigation may raise the question of whether the results of the FREEDOM and BARI-2D trials could have yielded different results if they had been performed using new-generation EESs.[149,174]

Moreover, recently the question about the most effective second-generation DES has arisen. To date solely two RCT head-to-head comparisons between the new-generation EES and ZES are available, and they are in a general patient population. In the Randomized Comparison of a Zotarolimus-Eluting Stent with an Everolimus-Eluting Stent (RESOLUTE All Comers) trial[175] and the Prospective Randomized Trial of Zotarolimus-Eluting Stents and Everolimus-Eluting Stents in Patients With Coronary Artery Disease (TWENTE) trial, no significant differences in efficacy and safety between ZES and EES after 2 years were seen.[176] However, with a relatively small number of patients with diabetes in RESOLUTE All Comers (23.4%) and TWENTE (21.6%), both studies were markedly underpowered to compare clinical outcomes in this subgroup. Park et al presented the first head-to-head comparison between EES and the Resolute ZES (R-ZES) in 1855 patients with diabetes.[177] After unrestricted implantation of the two second-generation DES, both EES and ZES showed comparable and low incidences of target lesion failure (EES 3.7% vs ZES 3.5%, p =0.899) and stent thrombosis (EES 0.8% vs ZES 0.1%, p =0.1) at 1-year. Moreover, composite endpoints, defined as all-cause mortality, any MI, and any revascularization, were similar (EES 9.1% vs ZES 10.2%, p = 0.416). This suggests an excellent efficacy and safety profile of both new-generation DES in patients with diabetes.[177] Current European guidelines on myocardial revascularization have recommended the use of DES as the preferred device in patients with diabetes (class 1, level of recommendation A),[141] whereas current American guidelines on the management of stable CAD do not specifically mention a favored stent subtype for revascularization in patients with diabetes.[143]

Second-Generation Drug-Eluting Stents and Bioresorbable Vascular Scaffolds in Patients with Diabetes

Bioresorbable vascular scaffolds (BVSs) represent a new and promising approach to the treatment of CAD as they offer temporary vessel support and drug delivery to the vessel wall.[178] In the ABSORB cohort B trial using the everolimus-eluting BVS system, a promising incidence rate of MACE (10%) without any occurrence of scaffold thrombosis at the 3-year follow-up was described in a general patient population.[179] However, to date there is still a paucity of data regarding the use of BVSs in patients with diabetes. Similarly, there is a lack of sufficient data on head-to-head comparisons of the various second-generation DES, EES, ZES, and everolimus-eluting BVSs in patients with diabetes. The first direct comparison between EES and BVS in diabetic patients was recently presented by Muramatsu et al, who performed a pooled analysis of the ABSORB and SPIRIT trials.[180]

First, there were no differences in terms of the primary endpoint, defined as a composite of death, target vessel MI, and TVR at 1-year between patients with (n = 136) and without diabetes (n = 415) (3.7% vs 5.1%, p = 0.64) treated with the BVS. This finding deserves specific consideration, because virtually every previous PCI study has demonstrated higher event rates in patients with diabetes than in patients without diabetes.[168,181] Secondly, there were no differences in the predescribed primary endpoint within the diabetic cohort between those treated with a BVS and those treated with a new-generation EES (n = 882) (3.9% vs 6.4%, p = 0.38).[180] Although these findings still need to be interpreted with caution due to the small sample size, they suggest that BVS in patients with diabetes is feasible, safe, and effective in the treatment of noncomplex coronary lesions.

SPECIFIC CHARACTERISTICS OF REVASCULARIZATION THERAPY IN PATIENTS WITH INSULIN-DEPENDENT AND PATIENTS WITH NON–INSULIN-DEPENDENT DIABETES

Currently, there is insufficient evidence whether the superiority of CABG for patients with diabetes is independent of glucose-lowering therapy and glucose control quality. Approximately one-quarter of patients with diabetes in the United States are treated with insulin (IDDM), and they exhibit a higher risk for complications after any type of coronary revascularization versus patients without diabetes and patients with NIDDM. Chronic hyperglycemia is considered the common denominator in both patients with IDDM and NIDDM.[116] The pathophysiologic impact of hyperglycemia involves systemic inflammation, endothelial dysfunction, hemostatic abnormalities, and increased cellular oxidative stress, all resulting in changes at the macro- and microvascular level.[116,182] Previous data have demonstrated that patients with IDDM undergoing CABG bear an enhanced risk of in-hospital mortality and wound infections.[183,184] Post-PCI IDDM patients are at particularly high risk of PCI and stent thrombosis in combination with reduced 1-year survival versus patients with NIDDM.[142] Subgroup analyses of patients with diabetes from two large-scale trials have explored the treatment benefit of CABG according to insulin requirement by comparing outcomes stratified by insulin treatment and using the SYNTAX score as a surrogate for coronary disease complexity. These studies yielded discordant findings.[140,142] Whereas the subgroup analysis of the SYNTAX trial, comprising 452 patients with diabetes, suggested a greater benefit for CABG over PCI in the IDDM group (n = 182) than the NIDDM group (n = 270),[140] a subanalysis of patients with diabetes in the FREEDOM trial showed a numerically decreased effect size of CABG over PCI in the IDDM group.[142] The latter trial explored outcomes of 1850 patients with diabetes categorized into an IDDM group (n = 602, 32.5%) and an NIDDM group.[142] Irrespective of the assigned treatment strategy, CABG (n = 277) or PCI with a DES (n = 325), IDDM patients had a worse clinical prognosis than NIDDM patients. Within the subgroup of IDDM, a significantly higher rate of MACE (death, MI, or stroke) occurred versus NIDDM patients (IDDM 28.7% vs NIDDM 19.5%, p < 0.001) at 5-year follow-up. These findings held true even after adjustments for clinical demographics, angiographic complexity as assessed by the SYNTAX score, and mode of revascularization therapy (adjusted HR 1.35; 95% CI 1.06–1.73). The risk of stroke increased similarly in both groups.[116,142] These findings indicate that CABG remains superior to PCI after adjustment for diabetes status, need for insulin therapy, and SYNTAX score.[116,142] However, both subanalyses were underpowered to reliably evaluate the hypothesis of treatment effects of CABG versus PCI by insulin status.[185] Thus, owing to the current lack of strong data, in patients with diabetes the use of insulin should not influence the choice of revascularization strategy (CABG vs PCI) as they presumably will derive treatment benefits that are comparable to those expected in the overall trial population of the FREEDOM and SYNTAX studies.[185]

The influence of insulin treatment in patients with diabetes regarding different DES is an additional point of interest. Stone et al[168] reported an increasing gradient of 2-year event rates among patients treated with a new-generation EES, with the lowest event rate in subjects without diabetes, an intermediate event rate in patients with NIDDM, and an elevated event rate in patients with IDDM. In contrast, among patients treated with a first-generation PES, the 2-year rates of adverse events were independent of diabetes status or insulin treatment. Furthermore, ischemia-driven target lesion revascularization (TVR) was reduced in patients with NIDDM assigned to EES versus PES (EES 3.7% vs PES 6.3%, p = 0.04), whereas in patients with IDDM a trend for a higher TVR rate was shown (EES 10.8% vs PES 5.5%, p = 0.08). Thus, this investigation suggests a significant interaction in patients with diabetes between insulin requirement and stent type for the occurrence of ischemia-driven TVR at 2 years (p = 0.01).[168]

CLINICAL DECISION-MAKING IN PATIENTS WITH MULTIVESSEL DISEASE WITH DIABETES

Various key variables have been established that might influence decision-making to select the most effective therapeutic approach in patients with diabetes and multivessel disease.[145] These parameters comprise the extent, anatomy, and lesion characteristics of CAD as assessed by the SYNTAX score, the surgical risk as assessed by the logistic EuroSCORE,[186] the EuroSCORE II,[187] or the Society of Thoracic Surgeons (STS) score,[188] the patient's age, preexisting comorbidities, and preference, and the operator's experience. The level of care can be optimized by the routine implementation of multidisciplinary teams.[189] The current European and American guidelines strengthen the need for a local multidisciplinary "heart team," consisting of a noninvasive cardiologist, an interventional cardiologist, and a cardiac surgeon with a class 1 recommendation (level of evidence C) for patients in whom therapeutic decision-making appears to be difficult.[141,143]

With particular regard to patients with diabetes, decision-making becomes even more complex and challenging. Diabetes is a systemic disease with rather diffuse atherosclerotic effects on the coronary vessels, characterized by smaller vessel diameters and longer lesions. As mechanical revascularization strategies usually address specific local lesions, they all have limited longevity.[160] Therefore, special attention has to be directed to optimized glycemic control. Moreover, a reasonable risk stratification is necessary, differentiating between low- and moderate-risk CAD and high-risk CAD. Thus, asymptomatic or mildly symptomatic patients with less severe CAD (single-vessel or 2-vessel not involving the proximal left anterior descending artery) are candidates for a conservative pharmacologic approach.[120]

However, if despite an optimal antidiabetic and anti-ischemic first-line pharmacologic therapy, clinical symptoms persist, and/or complex or 3-vessel CAD is present, revascularization strategies have to be considered.[143] At that point a pretreatment multidisciplinary team should discuss the individual case and consider the available treatment options and associated risks.[189] A collaboration of invasive cardiologists, noninvasive cardiologists, and cardiac surgeons is considered optimal to interpret all available information and provide a well-balanced discussion regarding the most effective and patient-oriented decision on myocardial revascularization.[189] Therefore the heart team uses a number of risk stratification tools such as the STS score and the logistic EuroSCORE or the EuroSCORE II. Both surgical and anatomic scores (SYNTAX score) should be used for final decision-making before any myocardial revascularization procedure.[189] One of the major aspects with respect to lesion severity and complexity is the capability to achieve complete revascularization. Complete revascularization in multivessel CAD is clearly associated with a better outcome than incomplete revascularization. Thus, a large meta-analysis in a general population of 37,116 patients with multivessel disease who had either complete (n = 11,596) or incomplete revascularization (n = 25,520) demonstrated a lower risk of mortality (RR) 0.82, $p = 0.05$) and nonfatal MI (RR 0.67, $p < 0.01$) for complete revascularization.[190] Another meta-analysis with 89,883 patients demonstrated that incomplete revascularization is more often found with PCI than with CABG (56% vs 25%, $p < 0.001$).[191] In addition, complete revascularization was associated with a lower long-term mortality (RR 0.71, $p < 0.001$), a lower rate of MI (RR 0.78, $p = 0.001$), and a lower rate of repeat coronary revascularization (RR 0.74, $p < 0.001$) compared with incomplete revascularization.[191] However, once complete revascularization is achieved, the rate of MACCEs during follow-up may not be different between CABG and PCI.[192] Moreover, currently there is a lack of data regarding different effects of complete and incomplete revascularization in an exclusively diabetic cohort.

Recently the so-called functional SYNTAX score, which recalculates the anatomic SYNTAX score by only incorporating ischemia-producing lesions as determined by fractional flow reserve, may challenge clinical decision-making by better discriminating the risk for adverse events in patients with complex CAD and particularly CV-high-risk patients with diabetes.[193] Another development has been the introduction of the redefined and validated SYNTAX II score. The absence of an individualized approach and of clinical parameters to help decision-making had been considered major limitations of the standard SYNTAX score. Hence, on the basis of the anatomically defined SYNTAX score, the SYNTAX II score has recently been defined and validated.[194] This score uses two anatomic and six clinical variables to predict 4-year mortality after CABG or PCI. The clinical variables include patient age, creatinine clearance, left ventricular ejection fraction, peripheral vascular disease, female gender, and chronic obstructive pulmonary disease.[194] The integration of clinical covariables into an established anatomic assessment of CAD severity may offer a more reliable instrument of risk stratification for patients with complex and multivessel disease. This applies particularly for the CV-high-risk population with diabetes.

References

1. Soedamah-Muthu SS, Fuller JH, Mulnier HE, et al.: High risk of cardiovascular disease in patients with type 1 diabetes in the U.K.: a cohort study using the general practice research database, *Diabetes Care* 29(4):798–804, 2006.
2. Soedamah-Muthu SS, Fuller JH, Mulnier HE, et al.: All-cause mortality rates in patients with type 1 diabetes mellitus compared with a non-diabetic population from the UK general practice research database, 1992-1999, *Diabetologia* 49(4):660–666, 2006.
3. Schram MT, Chaturvedi N, Fuller JH, et al.: Pulse pressure is associated with age and cardiovascular disease in type 1 diabetes: the Eurodiab Prospective Complications Study, *J Hypertens* 21(11):2035–2044, 2003.
4. Pambianco G, Costacou T, Ellis D, et al.: The 30-year natural history of type 1 diabetes complications: the Pittsburgh Epidemiology of Diabetes Complications Study experience, *Diabetes* 55(5):1463–1469, 2006.
5. Waden J, Forsblom C, Thorn LM, et al.: A1C variability predicts incident cardiovascular events, microalbuminuria, and overt diabetic nephropathy in patients with type 1 diabetes, *Diabetes* 58(11):2649–2655, 2009.
6. Haffner SM, Lehto S, Rönnemaa T, et al.: Mortality from coronary heart disease in subjects with type 2 diabetes and in nondiabetic subjects with and without prior myocardial infarction, *N Engl J Med* 339:229–234, 1998.
7. Gregg EW, Williams DE, Geiss L: Changes in diabetes-related complications in the United States, *N Engl J Med* 371(3):286–287, 2014.
8. Emerging Risk Factors Collaboration, Di Angelantonio E, Kaptoge S, et al.: Association of cardiometabolic multimorbidity with mortality, *JAMA* 314(1):52–60, 2015.
9. Fox CS, Golden SH, Anderson C, et al.: Update on prevention of cardiovascular disease in adults with type 2 diabetes mellitus in light of recent evidence: a scientific statement from the American Heart Association and the American Diabetes Association, *Circulation* 132(8):691–718, 2015.
10. Ryden L, Grant PJ, Anker SD, et al.: ESC Guidelines on diabetes, pre-diabetes, and cardiovascular diseases developed in collaboration with the EASD: the task force on diabetes, pre-diabetes, and cardiovascular diseases of the European Society of Cardiology (ESC) and developed in collaboration with the European Association for the Study of Diabetes (EASD), *Eur Heart J* 34(39):3035–3087, 2013.
11. ADVANCE Collaborative Group, Patel A, MacMahon S, et al.: Intensive blood glucose control and vascular outcomes in patients with type 2 diabetes, *N Engl J Med* 358:2560–2572, 2008.
12. Intensive blood-glucose control with sulphonylureas or insulin compared with conventional treatment and risk of complications in patients with type 2 diabetes (UKPDS 33). UK Prospective Diabetes Study (UKPDS) Group, *Lancet* 352:837–853, 1998.
13. Effect of intensive blood-glucose control with metformin on complications in overweight patients with type 2 diabetes (UKPDS 34). UK Prospective Diabetes Study (UKPDS) Group, *Lancet* 352:854–865, 1998.
14. Holman RR, Paul SK, Bethel MA, et al.: 10-year follow-up of intensive glucose control in type 2 diabetes, *N Engl J Med* 359(15):1577–1589, 2008.
15. Group AS, Buse JB, Bigger JT, et al.: Action to Control Cardiovascular Risk in Diabetes (ACCORD) trial: design and methods, *Am J Cardiol* 99(12A):21i–33i, 2007.
16. Duckworth W, Abraira C, Moritz T, et al.: Glucose control and vascular complications in veterans with type 2 diabetes, *N Engl J Med* 360(2):129–139, 2009.
17. Patel A, MacMahon S, Chalmers J, et al.: ADVANCE Collaborative Group. Intensive blood glucose control and vascular outcomes in patients with type 2 diabetes, *N Engl J Med* 358:2560–2572, 2008.
18. Control G, Turnbull FM, Abraira C, et al.: Intensive glucose control and macrovascular outcomes in type 2 diabetes, *Diabetologia* 52(11):2288–2298, 2009.
19. Kelly TN, Bazzano LA, Fonseca VA, et al.: Systematic review: glucose control and cardiovascular disease in type 2 diabetes, *Ann Intern Med* 151(6):394–403, 2009.
20. Ray KK, Seshasai SR, Wijesuriya S, et al.: Effect of intensive control of glucose on cardiovascular outcomes and death in patients with diabetes mellitus: a meta-analysis of randomised controlled trials, *Lancet* 373(9677):1765–1772, 2009.
21. Inzucchi SE, Bergenstal RM, Buse JB, et al.: Management of hyperglycemia in type 2 diabetes: a patient-centered approach: position statement of the American Diabetes Association (ADA) and the European Association for the Study of Diabetes (EASD), *Diabetes Care* 35(6):1364–1379, 2012.
22. Bennett WL, Maruthur NM, Singh S, et al.: Comparative effectiveness and safety of medications for type 2 diabetes: an update including new drugs and 2-drug combinations, *Ann Intern Med* 154(9):602–613, 2011.

23. Lamanna C, Monami M, Marchionni N, et al.: Effect of metformin on cardiovascular events and mortality: a meta-analysis of randomized clinical trials, *Diabetes Obes Metab* 13(3):221–228, 2011.
24. Dormandy JA, Charbonnel B, Eckland DJA, et al.: Secondary prevention of macrovascular events in patients with type 2 diabetes in the PROactive Study (PROspective pioglitAzone Clinical Trial In macroVascular Events): a randomised controlled trial, *Lancet* 366:1279–1289, 2005.
25. Home PD, Pocock SJ, Beck-Nielsen H, et al.: Rosiglitazone evaluated for cardiovascular outcomes in oral agent combination therapy for type 2 diabetes (RECORD): a multicentre, randomised, open-label trial, *Lancet* 373:2125–2135, 2009.
26. Home PD, Pocock SJ, Beck-Nielsen H, et al.: Rosiglitazone evaluated for cardiovascular outcomes—an interim analysis, *N Engl J Med* 357(1):28–38, 2007.
27. Erdmann E, Charbonnel B, Wilcox RG, et al.: Pioglitazone use and heart failure in patients with type 2 diabetes and preexisting cardiovascular disease: data from the PROactive study (PROactive 08), *Diabetes Care* 30(11):2773–2778, 2007.
28. Chiasson JL, Josse RG, Gomis R, et al.: Acarbose for prevention of type 2 diabetes mellitus: the STOP-NIDDM randomised trial, *Lancet* 359(9323):2072–2077, 2002.
29. Chiasson JL, Josse RG, Gomis R, et al.: Acarbose treatment and the risk of cardiovascular disease and hypertension in patients with impaired glucose tolerance: the STOP-NIDDM trial, *JAMA* 290(4):486–494, 2003.
30. Meinert CL, Knatterud GL, Prout TE, et al.: A study of the effects of hypoglycemic agents on vascular complications in patients with adult-onset diabetes. II. Mortality results, *Diabetes* 19(Suppl):789–830, 1970.
31. A study of the effects of hypoglycemia agents on vascular complications in patients with adult-onset diabetes. VI. Supplementary report on nonfatal events in patients treated with tolbutamide, *Diabetes* 25(12):1129–1153, 1976.
32. Seltzer HS: A summary of criticisms of the findings and conclusions of the University Group Diabetes Program (UGDP), *Diabetes* 21(9):976–979, 1972.
33. Kahn SE, Haffner SM, Heise MA, et al.: Glycemic durability of rosiglitazone, metformin, or glyburide monotherapy, *N Engl J Med* 355(23):2427–2443, 2006.
34. Garber A, Henry RR, Ratner R, et al.: Liraglutide, a once-daily human glucagon-like peptide 1 analogue, provides sustained improvements in glycaemic control and weight for 2 years as monotherapy compared with glimepiride in patients with type 2 diabetes, *Diabetes Obes Metab* 13(4):348–356, 2011.
35. Seck T, Nauck M, Sheng D, et al.: Safety and efficacy of treatment with sitagliptin or glipizide in patients with type 2 diabetes inadequately controlled on metformin: a 2-year study, *Int J Clin Pract* 64(5):562–576, 2010.
36. Mazzone T, Meyer PM, Feinstein SB, et al.: Effect of pioglitazone compared with glimepiride on carotid intima-media thickness in type 2 diabetes: a randomized trial, *JAMA* 296(21):2572–2581, 2006.
37. Nissen SE, Nicholls SJ, Wolski K, et al.: Comparison of pioglitazone vs glimepiride on progression of coronary atherosclerosis in patients with type 2 diabetes: the PERISCOPE randomized controlled trial, *JAMA* 299(13):1561–1573, 2008.
38. Gerstein HC, Miller ME, Byington RP, et al.: Action to control cardiovascular risk in diabetes study group. Effects of intensive glucose lowering in type 2 diabetes, *N Engl J Med* 358:2545–2559, 2008.
39. Gallwitz B, Rosenstock J, Rauch T, et al.: 2-year efficacy and safety of linagliptin compared with glimepiride in patients with type 2 diabetes inadequately controlled on metformin: a randomised, double-blind, non-inferiority trial, *Lancet* 380(9840):475–483, 2012.
40. Selvin E, Bolen S, Yeh HC, et al.: Cardiovascular outcomes in trials of oral diabetes medications: a systematic review, *Arch Intern Med* 168(19):2070–2080, 2008.
41. Johnson JA, Majumdar SR, Simpson SH, et al.: Decreased mortality associated with the use of metformin compared with sulfonylurea monotherapy in type 2 diabetes, *Diabetes Care* 25(12):2244–2248, 2002.
42. Morgan CL, Poole CD, Evans M, et al.: What next after metformin? A retrospective evaluation of the outcome of second-line, glucose-lowering therapies in people with type 2 diabetes, *J Clin Endocrinol Metab* 97(12):4605–4612, 2012.
43. Simpson SH, Majumdar SR, Tsuyuki RT, et al.: Dose-response relation between sulfonylurea drugs and mortality in type 2 diabetes mellitus: a population-based cohort study, *CMAJ* 174(2):169–174, 2006.
44. Tzoulaki I, Molokhia M, Curcin V, et al.: Risk of cardiovascular disease and all cause mortality among patients with type 2 diabetes prescribed oral antidiabetes drugs: retrospective cohort study using UK general practice research database, *BMJ* 339, 2009. b4731.
45. Marx N, Rosenstock J, Kahn SE, et al.: Design and baseline characteristics of the CARdiovascular Outcome Trial of LINAgliptin Versus Glimepiride in Type 2 Diabetes (CAROLINA(R)), *Diab Vasc Dis Res* 12(3):164–174, 2015.
46. Rosenstock J, Marx N, Johansen OE, et al.: Cardiovascular effects of diabetes drugs: making the dark ages brighter with Carolina, *Ann Intern Med* 158(6):499, 2013.
47. Rosenstock J, Marx N, Kahn SE, et al.: Cardiovascular outcome trials in type 2 diabetes and the sulphonylurea controversy: rationale for the active-comparator CAROLINA trial, *Diab Vasc Dis Res* 10(4):289–301, 2013.
48. Scirica BM, Bhatt DL, Braunwald E, et al.: Saxagliptin and cardiovascular outcomes in patients with type 2 diabetes mellitus, *N Engl J Med* 369(14):1317–1326, 2013.
49. White WB, Cannon CP, Heller SR, et al.: Alogliptin after acute coronary syndrome in patients with type 2 diabetes, *N Engl J Med* 369(14):1327–1335, 2013.
50. Green JB, Bethel MA, Armstrong PW, et al.: Effect of sitagliptin on cardiovascular outcomes in type 2 diabetes, *N Engl J Med* 373(3):232–242, 2015.
51. Scirica BM, Braunwald E, Raz I, et al.: Heart failure, saxagliptin, and diabetes mellitus: observations from the SAVOR-TIMI 53 randomized trial, *Circulation* 130(18):1579–1588, 2014.
52. Bentley-Lewis R, Aguilar D, Riddle MC, et al.: Rationale, design, and baseline characteristics in evaluation of lixisenatide in acute coronary syndrome, a long-term cardiovascular end point trial of lixisenatide versus placebo, *Am Heart J* 169(5), 2015. 631–8e7.
53. Pfeffer MA, Claggett B, Diaz R, et al.: Lixisenatide in patients with type 2 diabetes and acute coronary syndrome, *N Engl J Med* 373(23):2247–2257, 2015.
53a. Marso SP, Daniels GH, Brown-Frandsen K, et al: Liraglutide and cardiovascular outcomes in type 2 diabetes, *N Engl J Med* 28(4):311–322, 2016.
54. Zinman B, Inzucchi SE, Lachin JM, et al.: Rationale, design, and baseline characteristics of a Randomized, Placebo-Controlled Cardiovascular Outcome Trial of Empagliflozin (EMPA-REG OUTCOME), *Cardiovasc Diabetol* 13:102, 2014.
55. Zinman B, Wanner C, Lachin JM, et al.: Empagliflozin, cardiovascular outcomes, and mortality in type 2 diabetes, *N Engl J Med* 373(22):1092–1094, 2015.
55a. McGuire DK, Marx N, Sodium-glucose cotransporter-2 inhibition for the reduction of cardiovascular events in high-risk patients with diabetes mellitus, *Eur Heart J*, 2016 May 5. pii: ehw110. [Epub ahead of print].
56. Cannon CP: Mixed dyslipidemia, metabolic syndrome, diabetes mellitus, and cardiovascular disease: clinical implications, *Am J Cardiol* 102:5L–9L, 2008.
57. Soran H, Durrington PN: Susceptibility of LDL and its subfractions to glycation, *Curr Opin Lipidol* 22(4):254–261, 2011.
58. Chapman MJ, Ginsberg HN, Amarenco P, et al.: Triglyceride-rich lipoproteins and high-density lipoprotein cholesterol in patients at high risk of cardiovascular disease: evidence and guidance for management, *Eur Heart J* 32(11):1345–1361, 2011.
59. Miller M, Stone NJ, Ballantyne C, et al.: Triglycerides and cardiovascular disease: a scientific statement from the American Heart Association, *Circulation* 123(20):2292–2333, 2011.
60. Keech A, Simes RJ, Barter P, et al.: Effects of long-term fenofibrate therapy on cardiovascular events in 9795 people with type 2 diabetes mellitus (the FIELD study): randomised controlled trial, *Lancet* 366(9500).1849–1861, 2005.
61. Keech AC, Mitchell P, Summanen PA, et al.: Effect of fenofibrate on the need for laser treatment for diabetic retinopathy (FIELD study): a randomised controlled trial, *Lancet* 370(9600):1687–1697, 2007.
62. Scott R, O'Brien R, Fulcher G, et al.: Effects of fenofibrate treatment on cardiovascular disease risk in 9,795 individuals with type 2 diabetes and various components of the metabolic syndrome: the Fenofibrate Intervention and Event Lowering in Diabetes (FIELD) study, *Diabetes Care* 32(3):493–498, 2009.
63. Group AS, Ginsberg HN, Elam MB, et al.: Effects of combination lipid therapy in type 2 diabetes mellitus, *N Engl J Med* 362(17):1563–1574, 2010.
64. Bruckert E, Labreuche J, Deplanque D, et al.: Fibrates effect on cardiovascular risk is greater in patients with high triglyceride levels or atherogenic dyslipidemia profile: a systematic review and meta-analysis, *J Cardiovasc Pharmacol* 57(2):267–272, 2011.
65. Jun M, Foote C, Lv J, et al.: Effects of fibrates on cardiovascular outcomes: a systematic review and meta-analysis, *Lancet* 375(9729):1875–1884, 2010.
66. Stone NJ, Robinson JG, Lichtenstein AH, et al.: 2013 ACC/AHA guideline on the treatment of blood cholesterol to reduce atherosclerotic cardiovascular risk in adults: a report of the American College of Cardiology/American Heart Association task force on practice guidelines, *Circulation* 129(25 Suppl 2):S1–S45, 2014.
67. Reiner Z, Catapano AL, De Backer G, et al.: ESC/EAS Guidelines for the management of dyslipidaemias, *Rev Esp Cardiol* 64(12):1168e1–e60, 2011.
68. Cannon CP, Blazing MA, Giugliano RP, et al.: Ezetimibe added to statin therapy after acute coronary syndromes, *N Engl J Med* 372(25):2387–2397, 2015.
69. Cannon CP, Giugliano RP, Blazing MA, et al.: Rationale and design of IMPROVE-IT (IMProved Reduction of Outcomes: vytorin Efficacy International Trial): comparison of ezetimbe/simvastatin versus simvastatin monotherapy on cardiovascular outcomes in patients with acute coronary syndromes, *Am Heart J* 156(5):826–832, 2008.
70. Lambert G, Charlton F, Rye KA, et al.: Molecular basis of PCSK9 function, *Atherosclerosis* 203(1):1–7, 2009.
71. Robinson JG, Farnier M, Krempf M, et al.: Efficacy and safety of alirocumab in reducing lipids and cardiovascular events, *N Engl J Med* 372(16):1489–1499, 2015.
72. Sabatine MS, Giugliano RP, Wiviott SD, et al.: Efficacy and safety of evolocumab in reducing lipids and cardiovascular events, *N Engl J Med* 372(16):1500–1509, 2015.
73. Sattar N, Preiss D, Murray HM, et al.: Statins and risk of incident diabetes: a collaborative meta-analysis of randomised statin trials, *Lancet* 375(9716):735–742, 2010.
74. Investigators A-H, Boden WE, Probstfield JL, et al.: Niacin in patients with low HDL cholesterol levels receiving intensive statin therapy, *N Engl J Med* 365(24):2255–2267, 2011.
75. Group HTC, Landray MJ, Haynes R, et al.: Effects of extended-release niacin with laropiprant in high-risk patients, *N Engl J Med* 371(3):203–212, 2014.
76. Barter PJ, Caulfield M, Eriksson M, et al.: Effects of torcetrapib in patients at high risk for coronary events, *N Engl J Med* 357(21):2109–2122, 2007.
77. Schwartz GG, Olsson AG, Abt M, et al.: Effects of dalcetrapib in patients with a recent acute coronary syndrome, *N Engl J Med* 367(22):2089–2099, 2012.
78. Landmesser U: Coronary artery disease: HDL and coronary heart disease–novel insights, *Nat Rev Cardiol* 11(10):559–560, 2014.
79. Luscher TF, Landmesser U, von Eckardstein A, et al.: High-density lipoprotein: vascular protective effects, dysfunction, and potential as therapeutic target, *Circ Res* 114(1):171–182, 2014.
80. Riwanto M, Rohrer L, von Eckardstein A, et al.: Dysfunctional HDL: from structure-function-relationships to biomarkers, *Handb Exp Pharmacol* 224:337–366, 2015.
81. Nilsson PM, Cederholm J: Diabetes, hypertension, and outcome studies: overview 2010, *Diabetes Care* 34(Suppl 2):S109–S113, 2011.
82. Nilsson PM, Cederholm J, Zethelius BR, et al.: Trends in blood pressure control in patients with type 2 diabetes: data from the Swedish National Diabetes Register (NDR), *Blood Press* 20(6):348–354, 2011.
83. Redon J, Cifkova R, Laurent S, et al.: Mechanisms of hypertension in the cardiometabolic syndrome, *J Hypertens* 27(3):441–451, 2009.
84. Hypertension in Diabetes Study (HDS): II. Increased risk of cardiovascular complications in hypertensive type 2 diabetic patients, *J Hypertens* 11:319–325, 1993.
85. Hansson L, Zanchetti A, Carruthers SG, et al.: Effects of intensive blood-pressure lowering and low-dose aspirin in patients with hypertension: principal results of the Hypertension Optimal Treatment (HOT) randomised trial. HOT Study Group, *Lancet* 351(9118):1755–1762, 1998.
86. Tight blood pressure control and risk of macrovascular and microvascular complications in type 2 diabetes: UKPDS 38. UK Prospective Diabetes Study Group, *BMJ* 317(7160):703–713, 1998.
87. Adler AI, Stratton IM, Neil HA, et al.: Association of systolic blood pressure with macrovascular and microvascular complications of type 2 diabetes (UKPDS 36): prospective observational study, *BMJ* 321(7258):412–419, 2000.
88. Group AS, Cushman WC, Evans GW, et al.: Effects of intensive blood-pressure control in type 2 diabetes mellitus, *N Engl J Med* 362(17):1575–1585, 2010.
89. Bangalore S, Kumar S, Lobach I, et al.: Blood pressure targets in subjects with type 2 diabetes mellitus/impaired fasting glucose: observations from traditional and Bayesian random-effects meta-analyses of randomized trials, *Circulation* 123(24):2799–2810, 2011.
90. Lindholm LH, Hansson L, Ekbom T, et al.: Comparison of antihypertensive treatments in preventing cardiovascular events in elderly diabetic patients: results from the Swedish Trial in Old Patients with Hypertension-2. STOP Hypertension-2 Study Group, *J Hypertens* 18(11):1671–1675, 2000.
91. Niskanen L, Hedner T, Hansson L, et al.: Reduced cardiovascular morbidity and mortality in hypertensive diabetic patients on first-line therapy with an ACE inhibitor compared with a diuretic/beta-blocker-based treatment regimen: a subanalysis of the Captopril Prevention Project, *Diabetes Care* 24(12):2091–2096, 2001.
92. Ostergren J, Poulter NR, Sever PS, et al.: The Anglo-Scandinavian Cardiac Outcomes Trial: blood pressure-lowering limb: effects in patients with type II diabetes, *J Hypertens* 26(11):2103–2111, 2008.
93. Weber MA, Bakris GL, Jamerson K, et al.: Cardiovascular events during differing hypertension therapies in patients with diabetes, *J Am Coll Cardiol* 56(1):77–85, 2010.
94. Ruggenenti P, Fassi A, Ilieva AP, et al.: Preventing microalbuminuria in type 2 diabetes, *N Engl J Med* 351(19):1941–1951, 2004.
95. ONTARGET Investigators, Yusuf S, Teo KK, et al.: Telmisartan, ramipril, or both in patients at high risk for vascular events, *N Engl J Med* 358(15):1547–1559, 2008.
96. Parving HH, Brenner BM, McMurray JJ, et al.: Cardiorenal end points in a trial of aliskiren for type 2 diabetes, *N Engl J Med* 367(23):2204–2213, 2012.
97. Parving HH, Brenner BM, McMurray JJ, et al.: Baseline characteristics in the Aliskiren Trial in Type 2 Diabetes Using Cardio-Renal Endpoints (ALTITUDE), *J Renin Angiotensin Aldosterone Syst* 13(3):387–393, 2012.
98. Allcock DM, Sowers JR: Best strategies for hypertension management in type 2 diabetes and obesity, *Curr Diab Rep* 10(2):139–144, 2010.
99. Jamerson K, Weber MA, Bakris GL, et al.: Benazepril plus amlodipine or hydrochlorothiazide for hypertension in high-risk patients, *N Engl J Med* 359(23):2417–2428, 2008.

100. Ferroni P, Basili S, Falco A, et al.: Platelet activation in type 2 diabetes mellitus, *J Thromb Haemost* 2(8):1282–1291, 2004.
101. Belch J, MacCuish A, Campbell I, et al.: The prevention of progression of arterial disease and diabetes (POPADAD) trial: factorial randomised placebo controlled trial of aspirin and antioxidants in patients with diabetes and asymptomatic peripheral arterial disease, *BMJ* 337, 2008. a1840.
102. Ogawa H, Nakayama M, Morimoto T, et al.: Low-dose aspirin for primary prevention of atherosclerotic events in patients with type 2 diabetes: a randomized controlled trial, *JAMA* 300(18):2134–2141, 2008.
103. De Berardis G, Lucisano G, D'Ettorre A, et al.: Association of aspirin use with major bleeding in patients with and without diabetes, *JAMA* 307(21):2286–2294, 2012.
104. De Berardis G, Sacco M, Strippoli GF, et al.: Aspirin for primary prevention of cardiovascular events in people with diabetes: meta-analysis of randomised controlled trials, *BMJ* 339, 2009. b4531.
105. Collaborative overview of randomised trials of antiplatelet therapy–I: prevention of death, myocardial infarction, and stroke by prolonged antiplatelet therapy in various categories of patients. Antiplatelet Trialists' Collaboration, *BMJ* 308(6921):81–106, 1994.
106. Antithrombotic Trialists C: Collaborative meta-analysis of randomised trials of antiplatelet therapy for prevention of death, myocardial infarction, and stroke in high risk patients, *BMJ* 324(7329):71–86, 2002.
107. Steinhubl SR, Bhatt DL, Brennan DM, et al.: Aspirin to prevent cardiovascular disease: the association of aspirin dose and clopidogrel with thrombosis and bleeding, *Ann Intern Med* 150(6):379–386, 2009.
108. CURRENT-OASIS 7 Investigators, Mehta SR, Bassand JP, et al.: Dose comparisons of clopidogrel and aspirin in acute coronary syndromes, *N Engl J Med* 363(10):930–942, 2010.
109. Libby P, Theroux P: Pathophysiology of coronary artery disease, *Circulation* 111:3481–3488, 2005.
110. Norhammar A, Malmberg K, Diderholm E, et al.: Impact of diabetes on long-term-prognosis in patients with unstable angina and non-Q-wave myocardial infarction: results of the OASIS (Organization to Assess Strategies for Ischemic Syndromes) Registry, *Circulation* 102:1014–1019, 2000.
111. Harskamp RE, Park DW: Percutaneous coronary intervention in patients with diabetes: should choice of stents be influenced? *Expert Rev Cardiovasc Ther* 11:541–553, 2013.
112. Mehran R, Dangas GD, Kobayashi Y, et al.: Short- and long-term results after multivessel stenting in patients with diabetes, *J Am Coll Cardiol* 43:1348–1354, 2004.
113. McAlister FA, Man J, Bistritz L, et al.: Diabetes and coronary artery bypass surgery: an examination of perioperative glycemic control and outcomes, *Diab Care* 26:1518–1524, 2003.
114. Lawrie GM, Morris Jr GC, Glaeser DH, et al.: Influence of diabetes mellitus on the results of coronary bypass surgery. Follow-up of 212 diabetic patients ten to 15 years after surgery, *JAMA* 256:2967–2971, 1986.
115. Piccolo R, Giustino G, Mehran R, et al.: Stable coronary artery disease: revascularization and invasive strategy, *Lancet* 386:702–713, 2015.
116. Giustino G, Dangas GD: Surgical revascularization versus percutaneous coronary intervention and optimal medical therapy in patients with diabetes with multi-vessel coronary artery disease, *Prog Cardiovasc Dis* 306–315, 2015.
117. Brown TM, Voeks JH, Bittner V, et al.: Achievement of optimal medical therapy goals for U.S. adults with coronary artery disease: results from the REGARDS study, *J Am Coll Cardiol* 63:1626–1633, 2014.
118. Maron DJ, Boden WE, O'Routke RA, et al.: Intensive multifactorial intervention for stable coronary artery disease: optimal medical therapy in the COURAGE trial, *J Am Coll Cardiol* 55:1348–1358, 2010.
119. Soares PR, Hueb WA, Lemos PA, et al.: Coronary revascularization (surgical or percutaneous) decreases mortality after the first year in diabetic subjects but not in non-diabetic subjects with multivessel disease: an analysis from the Medicine, Angioplasty or Surgery Study (MASS II), *Circulation* 114(Suppl):1420–1424, 2006.
120. BARI 2D Study Group, Frye RL, August P, et al.: A randomized trial of therapies for type 2 diabetes and coronary artery disease, *N Engl J Med* 360(24):2503–2515, 2009.
121. Luthra S, Leiva-Juarez MM, Taggart DP: Systematic review for stable coronary artery disease in patients with diabetes, *Ann Thorac Surg* 100:2383–2397, 2015.
122. Farkouh ME, Boden WE, Bittner V, et al.: Risk factor control for coronary artery disease secondary prevention in large randomized trials, *J Am Coll Cardiol* 61(15):1607–1615, 2013.
123. Shaw LJ, Berman DS, Maron DJ, et al.: Optimal medical therapy with or without percutaneous coronary intervention to reduce ischemic burden: results from the Clinical Outcomes Utilizing Revascularization and Aggressive Drug Evaluation (COURAGE) trial, *Circulation* 117(110):1283–1291, 2008.
124. Farkouh ME, Dangas GD, Leon MB, et al.: Design of the Future Revascularization Evaluation in patients with Diabetes mellitus: optimal management of Multivessel disease (FREEDOM) trial, *Am Heart J* 155:215–223, 2008.
125. Ryden L, Grant PJ, Anker SD, et al.: ESC guidelines on diabetes, pre-diabetes and cardiovascular diseases developed in collaboration with the EASD, *Eur Heart J* 34:3035–3087, 2013.
126. Mauri L, Kereiakes DJ, Yeh RW, et al.: Twelve or 30 months of dual antiplatelet therapy after drug-eluting stents, *N Engl J Med* 371:2155–2166, 2014.
127. Giustino G, Baber U, Sartori S, et al.: Duration of dual antiplatelet therapy after drug-eluting stent implantation: a systematic review and meta-analysis of randomized controlled trials, *J Am Coll Cardiol* 65:1298–1310, 2015.
128. Wu ZK, Wang JJ, Wang T, et al.: Clopidogrel resistance in patients with coronary artery disease and metabolic syndrome: the role of hyperglycemia and obesity, *J Geriatr Cardiol* 12(4):378–382, 2015.
129. Wiviott SD, Braunwald E, Angiolillo DJ, et al.: Greater clinical benefit of more intensive oral antiplatelet therapy with prasugrel in patients with diabetes mellitus in the Trial to Assess Improvement in Therapeutic Outcomes by Optimizing Platelet Inhibition with Prasugrel-Thrombolysis in Myocardial Infarction 38, *Circulation* 118(16):1626–1636, 2008.
130. James S, Angiolillo DJ, Cornel JH, et al.: Ticagrelor versus clopidogrel in patients with acute coronary syndromes and diabetes: a substudy from the PLATelet inhibition and Outcomes (PLATO) trial, *Eur Heart J* 31(24):3006–3016, 2010.
131. Niles NW, McGrath PD, Malenka D, et al.: Survival of patients with diabetes and multivessel coronary artery disease after surgical or percutaneous coronary revascularization: results of a large regional prospective study. Northern New England Cardiovascular Disease Study Group, *J Am Coll Cardiol* 37(4):1008–1015, 2001.
132. Banning A, Westaby S, Morice MC, et al.: Diabetic and nondiabetic patients with left main and/or 3-vessel coronary artery disease: comparison of outcomes with cardiac surgery and paclitaxel-eluting stents, *J Am Coll Cardiol* 55(11):1067–1075, 2010.
133. Kapur A, Hall RJ, Malik IS, et al.: Randomized comparison of percutaneous coronary intervention with coronary artery bypass grafting in patients with diabetes. 1-year results of the CARDIa (Coronary Artery Revascularization in Diabetes) trial, *J Am Coll Cardiol* 55(5):432–440, 2010.
134. Onuma Y, Wykrzykowska JJ, Garg S, et al.: 5-year follow-up of coronary revascularization in patients with diabetes with multivessel coronary artery disease: insights from ARTS (Arterial Revascularization Therapy Study)-II and ARTS-I trials, *JACC Cardiovasc Interv* 4(3):317–323, 2011.
135. Stone GW, Maehara A, Lansky AJ, et al.: A prospective natural-history study of coronary atherosclerosis, *N Engl J Med* 364(3):226–235, 2011.
136. The Bypass Angioplasty Revascularization Investigation (BARI) Investigators: Comparison of coronary bypass surgery with angioplasty in patients with multivessel disease, *N Engl J Med* 335(4):217–225, 1996.
137. Bangalore S, Toklu B, Feit F, et al.: Outcomes with coronary artery bypass graft surgery versus percutaneous coronary intervention for patients with diabetes mellitus: can newer generation drug-eluting stents bridge the gap? *Circulation Cardiovasc Interv* 7(4):518–525, 2014.
138. Serruys PW, Ong AT, van Herwerden LA, et al.: Five-year outcomes after coronary stenting versus bypass surgery for the treatment of multivessel disease: the final analysis of the Arterial Revascularization Therapies Study (ARTS) randomized trial, *J Am Coll Cardiol* 46(4):575–581, 2005.
139. Kamalesh M, Sharp TG, Tang XC, et al.: Percutaneous coronary intervention versus coronary bypass surgery in United States veterans with diabetes, *J Am Coll Cardiol* 61(8):808–816, 2013.
140. Kappetein AP, Head SJ, Morice MC, et al.: Treatment of complex coronary artery disease in patients with diabetes: 5-year results comparing outcomes of bypass suregery and percutaneous coronary intervention in the SYNTAX trial, *Eur Cardiothorac Surg* 43(5):1006–1013, 2013.
141. Windecker S, Kolh P, Alfonso F, et al.: 2014 ESC/EACTS guidelines on myocardial revascularization: the task force on myocardial revascularization of the European Society of Cardiology (ESC) and the European Association of Cardio-Thoracic Surgery (EACTS): developed with the special contribution of the European Association of Percutaneous Interventions (EAPCI), *Eur Heart J* 35(37):2541–2619, 2014.
142. Dangas GD, Farkouh ME, Sleeper LA, et al.: Long-term outcome of PCI versus CABG in insulin and non-insulin-treated diabetic patients: results from the FREEDOM trial, *J Am Coll Cardiol* 64(12):1189–1197, 2014.
143. Fihn SD, Blankenship JC, Alexander KP, et al.: 2014 ACC/AHA/AATS/PCNA/SCAI/STS focused update of the guideline for the diagnosis and management of patients with stable ischemic heart disease: a report of the American College of Cardiology/American Heart Association task force on practice guidelines, and the American Association for Thoracic Surgery, Preventive Cardiovascular Nurses Association, Society for Cardiovascular Angiography and Interventions, and Society of Thoracic Surgeons, *Circulation* 130(19):1749–1767, 2014.
144. Toklu B, Bangalore S: Comparison of coronary artery graft surgery and percutaneous coronary intervention in patients with diabetes, *Curr Treat Options Cardiovasc Med* 17:21, 2015.
145. Bangalore S, Kumar S, Fusaro M, et al.: Short- and long-term outcomes with drug-eluting and bare metal coronary stents: a mixed-treatment comparison analysis of 117.762 patient-years of follow-up from randomized trials, *Circulation* 125:2873–2891, 2012.
146. Herbison P, Wong CK: Has the difference in mortality between percutaneous coronary intervention and coronary bypass grafting in people with heart disease and diabetes changed over the years? A systematic review and meta-regression, *BMJ Open* 5(12):e010055, 2015.
147. Park SJ, Ahn JM, Kim YH, et al.: Trial of everolimus-eluting stents or bypass surgery for coronary disease, *N Engl J Med* 372(13):1204–1212, 2015.
148. Buchanan GL, Chieffo A, Colombo A: Is there still a survival advantage to bypass surgery over percutaneous intervention in the modern era? *Prog Cardiovasc Dis* 58(3):335–341, 2015.
149. Bangalore, Guo Y, Samadashvili, et al.: Everolimus-eluting stents or bypass surgery for multivessel coronary disease, *N Engl J Med* 372:1213–1222, 2015.
150. Hannan EL, Wu C, Watford G, et al.: Incomplete revascularization in the era of drug-eluting stents: impact on adverse outcomes, *JACC Cardiovasc Interv* 2:17–25, 2009.
151. Genereux P, Palmerini T, Caixeta A, et al.: Quantification and impact of untreated coronary artery disease after percutaneous coronary intervention: the residual SYNTAX score, *J Am Coll Cardiol* 59:2165–2174, 2012.
152. Bangalore S, Guo Y, Samadashvili Z, et al.: Everolimus eluting stents versus coronary artery bypass graft surgery for patients with diabetes mellitus and multivessel disease, *Circ Cardiovasc Interv* 8(7):e002626, 2015.
153. Tector AJ, Schmahl TM, Janson B, et al.: The internal mammary artery graft. Its longevity after coronary bypass, *JAMA* 246:2181–2183, 1981.
154. Schwartz L, Kip KE, Frye RL, et al.: Coronary bypass graft patency in patients with diabetes in the Bypass Angioplasty Revascularization Investigation (BARI), *Circulation* 106:2652–2658, 2002.
155. Kinoshita T, Asai T, Nishimura O, et al.: Off-pump bilateral versus single skeletonized internal thoracic artery grafting in patients with diabetes, *Ann Thorac Surg* 90:1173–1179, 2010.
156. Dorman MJ, Kurlansky PA, Traad EA, et al.: Bilateral internal mammary artery grafting enhances survival in diabetic patients: a 30-year follow-up of propensity score-matched cohorts, *Circulation* 126:2935–2942, 2012.
157. Nakano J, Okabayashi H, Hanyu M, et al.: Risk factors for wound infection after off-pump coronary artery bypass grafting: should bilateral internal thoracic arteries be harvested in patients with diabetes? *J Thorac Cardiovasc Surg* 135:540–545, 2008.
158. Choudhary BP, Antoniades C, Brading AF, et al.: Diabetes mellitus as a predictor for radial artery vasoreactivity in patients undergoing coronary artery bypass grafting, *J Am Coll Cardiol* 50:1047–1053, 2007.
159. Goldman S, Sethi GK, Holman W, et al.: Radial artery grafts versus saphenous vein grafts in coronary artery bypass surgery: a randomized trial, *JAMA* 305:167–174, 2011.
160. Aronnson D, Edelmann ER: Coronary artery disease and diabetes mellitus, *Heart Failure Clin* 12:117–133, 2016.
161. Sabate M, Jimenez-Quevedo P, Angiolillo DJ, et al.: Randomized comparison of sirolimus-eluting stent versus standard stent for percutaneous revascularization in diabetic patients: the Diabetes and Sirolimus-Eluting Stent (DIABETES) trial, *Circulation* 112:2175–2183, 2005.
162. Sinning JM, Baumbart D, Werner N, et al.: Five-year results of the multicenter randomized controlled open-label study of the CYPHER Sirolimus-Eluting Stent in the Treatment of Diabetic Patients with DeNovo Native Coronary Artery Lesions (SCORPIUS) study: a German multicenter investigation on the effectiveness of sirolimus-eluting stents in diabetic patients, *Am Heart J* 163:446–453, 2012.
163. Hermiller JB, Raizner A, Cannon L, et al.: Outcomes with the polymer-based paclitaxel-eluting TAXUS stent in patients with diabetes mellitus: the TAXUS trial, *J Am Coll Cardiol* 45(8):1172–1179, 2005.
164. Bangalore S, Toklu B, Fusaro M, et al.: Bare metal stents, durable polymer drug eluting stents, and biodegradable polymer drug eluting stents for coronary artery disease: mixed treatment comparison meta-analysis, *BMJ* 347, f6625: 2013.
165. Bangalore S, Kumar S, Fusaro M, et al.: Outcomes with various drug eluting or bare metal stents in patients with diabetes mellitus: mixed treatment comparison analysis of 22,844 patient years of follow-up from randomized trials, *BMJ* 345:e5170, 2012.
166. Stettler C, Allemann S, Wandel S, et al.: Drug eluting and bare metal stents in people with and without diabetes: a collaborative network meta-analysis, *BMJ* 337, 2008. a1331.
167. Dangas GD, Serruys PW, Kereiakes DJ, et al.: Meta-analysis of everolimus-eluting versus paclitaxel-eluting stents bin coronary artery disease: final 3-year results of the SPIRIT clinical trials program (Clinical Evaluation of the Xience V Everolimus Eluting Coronary Stent System in the Treatment of Patients With De Novo Native Coronary Artery Lesions), *JACC Cardiovasc Interv* 6:914–922, 2013.
168. Stone GW, Kedhi E, Kereiakes DJ, et al.: Differential clinical responses to everolimus-eluting and paclitaxel-eluting coronary stents in patients with and without diabetes, *Circulation* 124(8): 893–900, 2011.
169. Daemen J, Garcia-Garcia HM, Kukreja N, et al.: The long-term value of sirolimus- and paclitaxel-eluting stents over bare metal stents in patients with diabetes mellitus, *Eur Heart J* 28:26–32, 2007.
170. Stankovic G, Cosgrave J, Chieffo A, et al.: Impact of sirolimus-eluting and paclitaxel-eluting stents on outcome in patients with diabetes mellitus and stenting in more than one coronary artery, *Am J Cardiol* 98:362–366, 2006.

171. Kastrati A, Massberg S, Ndrepepa G, et al.: Is diabetes the Achilles' heel of limus-eluting stents? *Circulation* 124:869–872, 2011.
172. Ost A, Svensson K, Ruishalme I, et al.: Attenuated mTOR signaling and enhanced autophagy in adipocytes from obese patients with type 2 diabetes, *Mol Med* 16:235–246, 2010.
173. Kaul U, Bangalore S, Ashok Seth MHA, et al.: Paclitaxel-eluting versus everolimus-eluting coronary stents in diabetes, *N Engl J Med* 373:1709–1719, 2015.
174. Bangalore S, Guo Y, Samadashvili Z, et al.: Everolimus-eluting stents versus coronary artery bypass graft surgery for patients with diabetes mellitus and multivessel disease, *Circ Cardiovasc Interv* 8(7):e002626, 2015.
175. Silber S, Windecker S, Vranckx P, et al.: Unrestricted randomized use of two new generation drug-eluting coronary stents: 2-year patient-related versus stent-related outcomes from the RESOLUTE All Comers trial, *Lancet* 377:1241–1247, 2011.
176. Tandjung K, Sen H, Lam MK, et al.: Clinical outcome following stringent discontinuation of dual antiplatelet therapy after 12 months in real-world patients treated with second-generation zotarolimus-eluting Resolute and everolimus-eluting Xience V stents: 2-year follow-up of the randomized TWENTE trial, *J Am Coll Cardiol* 61:2406–2416, 2013.
177. Park KW, Lee JM, Kang SH, et al.: Everolimus-eluting XIENCE V/PROMUS versus zotarolimus-eluting RESOLUTE stents in patients with diabetes, *JACC Cardiovasc Interv* 7:471–481, 2014.
178. Onuma Y, Serruys PW: Bioresorbable scaffold: the advent of a new era in percutaneous coronary and peripheral revascularization? *Circulation* 123:779–797, 2011.
179. Serruys PW, Onuma Y, Garcia-Garcia HM, et al.: Dynamics of the vessel wall changes following the implantation of the Absorb everolimus-eluting bioresorbable vascular scaffold: a multi-imaging modality study at 6, 12, 24 and 36 months, *EuroIntervention* 9(11):1271–1284, 2014.
180. Muramatsu T, Onuma Y, van Geuns RJ, et al.: One-year clinical outcomes of diabetic patients treated with everolimus-eluting bioresorbable vascular scaffolds: a pooled analysis of the ABSORB and the SPIRIT trials, *JACC Cardiovasc Interv* 7:482–493, 2014.
181. Schoos MM, Clemmensen P, Dangas GD: Second generation drug-eluting stents and bioresorbable vascular scaffolds in patients with diabetes, *JACC Cardiovasc Interv* 7(5):494–496, 2014.
182. Fang ZY, Prins JB, Marwick TH: Diabetic cardiomyopathy: evidence, mechanisms, and therapeutic implications, *Endocr Rev* 25:543–567, 2004.
183. Lazar HL, Fitzgerald C, Gross S, et al.: Determinants of length of stay after coronary artery bypass graft surgery, *Circulation* 92:II20–II24, 1995.
184. Carson JL, Scholz PM, Chen AY, et al.: Diabetes mellitus increases short-term-mortality and morbidity in patients undergoing coronary artery bypass graft surgery, *J Am Coll Cardiol* 40:418–423, 2002.
185. Marso SP, McGuire DK: Coronary revascularization strategies in patients with diabetes and multivessel coronary artery disease: has the final chapter been written? *J Am Coll Cardiol* 64(12):1198–1201, 2014.
186. Roques F, Michel P, Goldstone AR, et al.: The logistic EuroSCORE, *Eur Heart J* 24:881–882, 2003.
187. Nashef SA, Roques F, Sharples LD, et al.: EuroSCORE II, *Eur Cardiothorac Surg* 41:734–744, 2012.
188. Shahian DM, O'Brien SM, Filardo G, et al.: The Society of Thoracic Surgeons 2008 cardiac surgery risk models: part 1 coronary artery bypass grafting, *Ann Thorac Surg* 88:S2–S22, 2009.
189. Head SJ, Kaul S, Mack MJ, et al.: The rationale for heart team decision-making for patients with stable, complex coronary artery disease, *Eur Heart J* 34:2510–2518, 2013.
190. Aggarwal V, Rajpathak S, Singh M, et al.: Clinical outcomes based on completeness of revascularization in patients undergoing percutaneous coronary intervention: a meta-analysis of multivessel coronary artery disease studies, *EuroIntervention* 7(9):1095–1102, 2012.
191. Garcia S, Sandoval Y, Roukoz H, et al.: Outcomes after complete versus incomplete revascularization of patients with multivessel coronary artery disease: a metaanalysis of 89883 patients enrolled in randomized clinical trials and observational studies, *J Am Coll Cardiol* 62(16):1421–1431, 2013.
192. Sarno G, Garg S, Onuma Y, et al.: Impact of completeness of revascularization on the five-year outcome in percutaneous coronary intervention and coronary artery bypass graft patients (from the ARTS-II study), *Am J Cardiol* 106:1369–1375, 2010.
193. Nam CW, Mangiacapra F, Entjes R, et al.: Functional SYNTAX score for risk assessment in multivessel coronary artery disease, *J Am Coll Cardiol* 58(12):1211–1218, 2011.
194. Farooq V, van Klaveren D, Steyerberg EW, et al.: Anatomical and clinical characteristics to guide decision making between coronary artery bypass surgery and percutaneous coronary intervention for individual patients: development and validation of SYNTAX score II, *Lancet* 381:639–650, 2013.

25 Angina in Patients with Evidence of Myocardial Ischemia and No Obstructive Coronary Artery Disease

Puja K. Mehta, Janet Wei, and C. Noel Bairey Merz

INTRODUCTION

Treatment of angina and evidence of myocardial ischemia on stress testing with no obstructive coronary artery disease (CAD) by angiography is a challenge. Previously referred to as *cardiac syndrome X*, this syndrome was believed to have a benign cardiovascular prognosis; however data from the NHLBI-Women's Ischemia Syndrome Evaluation (WISE) and other studies demonstrate that up to 50% of these patients have coronary microvascular dysfunction (CMD), which carries an adverse cardiovascular prognosis.[1,2] Patients with CMD are more likely to be mid-life women, who have a high frequency of atherosclerosis on intravascular coronary ultrasound (IVUS), and face a 2.5% annual adverse cardiac event rate,[3] which includes myocardial infarction (MI), stroke, congestive heart failure, and sudden cardiac death. This rate of adverse events is notably higher compared with asymptomatic community controls. In addition to WISE, other studies in Europe and Canada have also reported on the elevated risk of adverse outcomes among those with ischemia and no obstructive CAD.[4,5] Whereas coronary endothelial dysfunction and impaired microvascular vasodilatory reserve are of particular importance in the pathophysiology of ischemic heart disease in women, a recent study demonstrated that CMD may be highly prevalent in both men and women, although this remains to be confirmed by larger prospective studies.[6] In addition to microvascular dysfunction, diagnoses to consider in patients with persistent angina and no obstructive CAD include coronary vasospasm (Prinzmetal angina) with and without myocardial bridging,[7] abnormal cardiac nociception, as well as noncardiac etiologies. It is important for the clinician to keep in mind the wide differential diagnosis of patients who present with chest pain and are found to have no obstructive CAD (Fig. 25.1).

Whereas CMD can be detected noninvasively by positron emission tomography (PET),[8] stress cardiac magnetic resonance (CMR) imaging,[9,10] and stress echo Doppler coronary flow reserve (CFR), depending on individual center expertise, the gold standard for its diagnosis is invasive coronary reactivity testing. Therapeutic success typically anchors on diagnostic certainty; coronary reactivity testing using intracoronary infusions of adenosine, acetylcholine, and nitroglycerin to assess microvascular and macrovascular (epicardial) endothelial and nonendothelial function (Table 25.1) should be considered in patients with signs and symptoms of ischemia if no obstructive CAD is found. Coronary reactivity testing can be safely performed in catheterization laboratories with experienced operators.[11–13] Both the endothelial-[12] and nonendothelial-dependent[11] abnormalities stratify patients at risk for future cardiovascular events, as well as characterizing mechanistic pathways to direct therapy.[1]

Two of the issues in diagnosis and, ultimately, treatment in symptomatic patients with ischemia but no obstructive CAD are the confusion in terminology in the literature to describe this group of patients, and the lack of standardized diagnostic criteria. To address these, the Coronary Vasomotion Disorders International Study Group (COVADIS) investigators have proposed international standards for the diagnostic criteria of coronary vasomotor disorders with the aim to facilitate research in this field and improve care in this patient population.[14] Large, randomized, placebo-controlled therapeutic outcome trials are lacking, and current US guidelines do not specifically address diagnosis and treatment of CMD.[15,16]

Therapeutic lifestyle change, low-dose aspirin, and lipid-lowering therapy are recommended due to the high prevalence of coronary atherosclerosis and risk of adverse cardiac events. Evidence collected in predominantly general cardiac syndrome X patients has investigated the use of β-blockers, angiotensin-converting enzyme inhibitors (ACE-I), L-arginine, nitrates, calcium-channel blockers, ranolazine, xanthine derivatives, α-blockers, enhanced external counterpulsation, cognitive behavioral therapy, tricyclic medication, and neurostimulation to improve symptoms, stress test parameters, and endothelial function with variable results. Treatment of patients should focus on two main goals: (1) antiatherosclerotic and anti-ischemic therapy to reduce adverse cardiac event risk, and (2) relief of angina to improve quality of life.

This chapter provides an overview of CMD and discusses currently available diagnostic methods of its detection, as

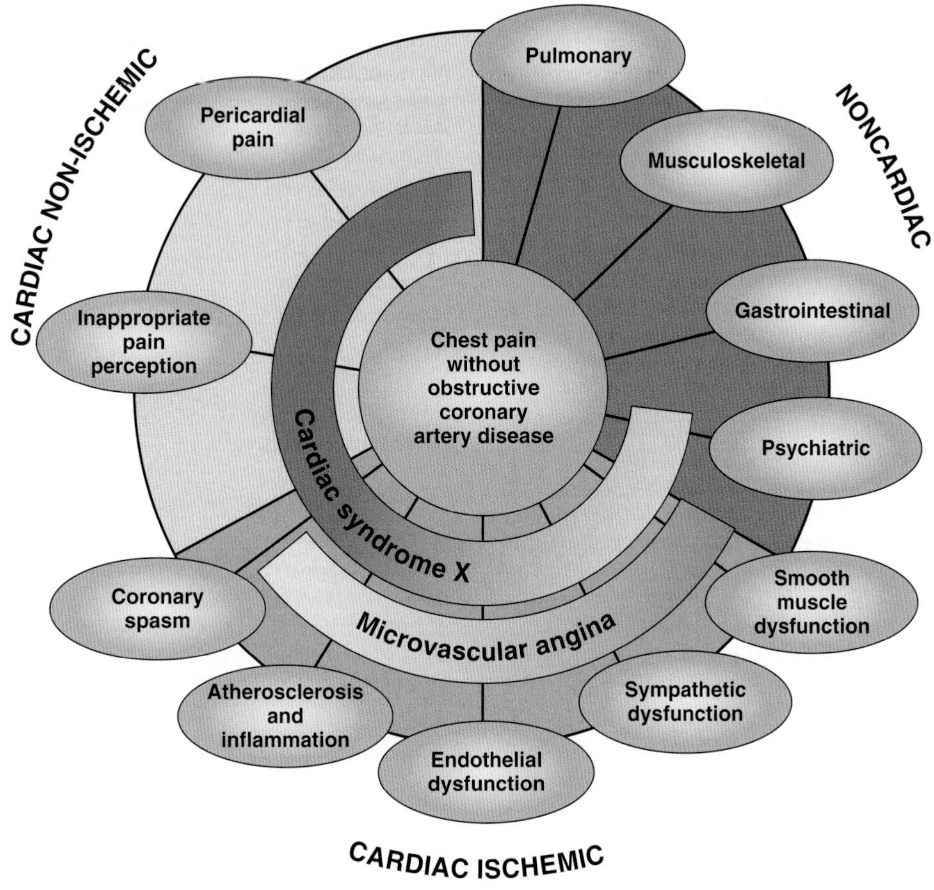

FIG. 25.1 Differential diagnosis of chest pain without obstructive coronary artery disease. Clinician should keep in mind the wide differential diagnosis for patients who present with chest pain and no obstructive coronary artery disease (CAD) and note that features can overlap. *(From Marinescu MA, Löffler AI, Ouellette M, et al. Coronary microvascular dysfunction, microvascular angina, and treatment strategies.* JACC Cardiovasc Imaging. *2015;8:210–220.)*

TABLE 25.1 Components of Coronary Reactivity Testing

	MICROVASCULAR DYSFUNCTION	MACROVASCULAR DYSFUNCTION
Nonendothelial dependent	Reduced CFR to adenosine (CFR ≤ 2.5)	Abnormal vasoreactivity to nitroglycerin (% diameter change < 20%)
Endothelial dependent	Reduced CBF to acetylcholine (% change in CBF ≤ 50%)	Abnormal vasoreactivity to acetylcholine (% diameter change < 5%)

CBF, Coronary blood flow; *CFR*; coronary flow reserve.

well as pharmacologic and nonpharmacologic interventions that can be utilized for these patients, with the understanding that the best approach is to develop a regimen based on individual patient needs and characteristics. Given the unfolding knowledge, we propose that existing unstable angina/non–ST elevation MI guidelines for the treatment of cardiac syndrome X[15] and chronic stable angina guidelines[16] from the American Heart Association (AHA)/American College of Cardiology (ACC) be modified to include the therapeutic strategies reviewed here (Box 25.1).

TERMINOLOGY

Cardiac syndrome X is an outdated term that described the triad of typical anginal chest pain, evidence of ischemia by

BOX 25.1 Treatment of Patients with Angina, Evidence of Myocardial Ischemia, and No Obstructive Coronary Artery Disease*

1. Coronary Microvascular Dysfunction
   - Abnormal Endothelial Function
     - ACE-I
     - HMG CoA reductase inhibitors (statins)
     - L-arginine supplementation
     - aerobic exercise
     - EECP for refractory angina
   - Abnormal Nonendothelial Function
     - β-blockers/medications with α- and β-blocking properties
     - nitrates
   - Antianginal
     - ranolazine
     - ivabradine
     - xanthine derivatives
     - nicorandil
2. Abnormal Smooth Muscle Function (Prinzmetal Angina)
   - calcium-channel blockers
   - nitrates
3. Abnormal Cardiac Nociception
   - low-dose tricyclic medication
   - spinal cord stimulation
   - stellate ganglion blockade
   - cognitive behavioral therapy

ACE-I, Angiotensin-converting enzyme inhibitors; *EECP*, enhanced external counterpulsation.
*Proposed modification of existing American College of Cardiology /American Heart Association unstable angina and stable angina guidelines.[15,16]

a positive exercise stress testing with ≥ 0.1 mV ST-segment depression, and normal-appearing coronary arteries on angiography. In 1973, Harvey Kemp first coined "cardiac syndrome X" in his editorial[17] on a study by Arbogast and Bourassa. In their study, Arbogast and Bourassa compared two groups of patients who developed angina with atrial pacing: those with angiographically normal–appearing coronary arteries (group X) versus those with obstructive coronary atherosclerosis.[18] A stricter definition consists of the following criteria: (1) exercise-induced, angina-like chest discomfort; (2) evidence of ischemia by ST-segment depression on electrocardiography during the anginal episode; (3) normal appearing coronary arteries on angiography; (4) no evidence of spontaneous or inducible epicardial coronary vasospasm; and (5) absence of cardiac structural pathology or systemic diseases, such as left ventricular hypertrophy, valvular heart disease, cardiomyopathy, or diabetes.

Historically, cardiac syndrome X patients formed an ill-defined subgroup of angina patients who were believed to have a benign syndrome with a good cardiovascular prognosis and were often dismissed from ongoing cardiac care. Despite decades of work in Europe and the United States, cardiac syndrome X remains a challenge to the practicing clinician, with no large randomized treatment or major adverse cardiac events (MACE) outcome trials. This is partly due to a lack of standardized diagnostic criteria and partly due to the diversity of mechanistic pathways that play a role in the pathophysiology of this heterogeneous disorder. Since the mid-2000s, with advances in diagnostic imaging modalities and invasive techniques to assess coronary physiology/flow and myocardial perfusion, it has become clear that at least 50% of cardiac syndrome X patients have CMD. The use of the term cardiac syndrome X is now considered *outdated* when referring to patients who have objective evidence of myocardial ischemia and no obstructive atherosclerosis.

Since 2013, the term *MINOCA* has been used to describe "myocardial infarction and no obstructive coronary artery disease" when the cause is not clear.[19] Criteria for MINOCA include the universal definition of MI by troponin rise and ischemic symptoms or electrocardiogram (ECG) changes, and no significant coronary stenosis (> 50% or more in epicardial coronary arteries).[20] The prevalence of MINOCA is estimated to be anywhere from 2% to 10%[19] and is more likely to occur in women and those younger in age compared to those who present with obstructive CAD.[21–23] A diagnosis of MINOCA should prompt the clinician to consider other causes of MI such as myocarditis, cardiomyopathy, coronary vasospasm, CMD, or a thrombotic disorder, as outlined by Pasupathy et al.[20] in Table 25.2. Most recently, the term *ANOCA* has been proposed to refer to those patients with "angina and no obstructive coronary artery disease."

TABLE 25.2 Diagnostic Considerations in the Evaluation of Myocardial Infarction with Nonobstructive Coronary Arteries (MINOCA)

CLINICAL DISORDER	DIAGNOSTIC INVESTIGATION
Noncardiac Disorders	
Renal impairment	Serum creatinine
Pulmonary embolism	CTPA or ventilation/perfusion imaging
Cardiac Disorders	
Myocardial Disorders	
Cardiomyopathy (takotsubo, dilated, hypertrophic)	Left ventriculography, Echo, CMR
Myocarditis	CRP, CMR, EMB
Myocardial trauma or injury	History (trauma, chemotherapy), CMR
Tachyarrhythmia-induced infarct	Arrhythmia monitoring
Coronary Disorders	
Concealed coronary dissection (aortic dissection involving valve, spontaneous coronary dissection)	Echo, CT angiogram
Sympathomimetic-induced spasm	Drug screen (eg, cocaine)
Epicardial coronary spasm	ACh provocation testing
Microvascular spasm	ACh provocation testing
Microvascular dysfunction	CFR
Coronary slow flow phenomenon	TIMI frame count
Plaque disruption/coronary thrombus	Intravascular ultrasound
Coronary emboli	Echo (left ventricular or valvular thrombus)
Thrombotic Disorders	
Factor V Leiden	Thrombophilia disorder screen
Protein C & S deficiency	

Ach, Acetylcholine; *CMR*, cardiac magnetic resonance imaging; *CRP*, C-reactive protein; *CT*, computed tomography; *CTPA*, computed tomography pulmonary angiogram; *EMB*, endomyocardial biopsy; *TIMI*, Thrombolysis In Myocardial Infarction.

(From Pasupathy S, Tavella R, Beltrame JF. The what, when, who, why, how and where of Myocardial Infarction with Non-Obstructive Coronary Arteries (MINOCA). Circ J. *2015;80:11–16.)*

EPIDEMIOLOGY

The finding of no obstructive CAD in the setting of acute coronary syndrome (ACS), unstable angina, and stable ischemic heart disease is more prevalent in women compared with men (Table 25.3).[1,24,25] In the Coronary Artery Surgery Study (CASS) of 25,000 men and women with signs or symptoms of myocardial ischemia who underwent coronary angiography, 39% of women and 11% of men demonstrated no obstructive CAD.[26] In a 2008 retrospective Canadian cohort of 32,856 patients suspected of ischemic heart disease who underwent coronary angiography, 23.3% of women versus 7.1% of men ($p < 0.001$) had angiographically normal coronary arteries; women with no obstructive CAD were over four times more likely than men to be readmitted to the hospital for symptoms/ACS within 6 months.[24] In the US National Cardiovascular Data Registry (NCDR) of patients undergoing coronary angiography for stable angina ($n = 375{,}886$), 51.2% of women had no obstructive CAD compared with 33.3% of men,[27] and based on these NCDR data, it has been estimated that approximately 3 million American women have CMD. Among the 168,322 women in the NCDR, black women had the lowest rate of significant obstructive CAD compared with Hispanic, Native American, Asian, and white, non-Hispanic women (41.7% vs 45.3%, 55%, 53%, and 50%, respectively). Numerous factors have been proposed to explain this sex difference in the presentation of ischemic heart disease.[28] Due to a diffuse pattern of plaque deposition throughout the artery, and outward positive remodeling of the arterial wall, without having one specific clear area of stenosis in the artery, these lesions are not amenable to percutaneous interventions, and thus the patient gets falsely labeled as "no significant CAD." In the WISE study of women with signs and symptoms of ischemia and no obstructive CAD on angiography, intravascular ultrasound demonstrated atherosclerotic plaque in up to 80% of the women.[29]

TABLE 25.3 Prevalence of No Obstructive Coronary Artery Disease in Women Compared to Men

	NO./TOTAL (%)		
	Women	Men	*p* Value
Acute Coronary Syndrome			
GUSTO	343/1768 (19.4)	394/4638 (8.4)	< 0.001
TIMI 18	95/555 (17)	99/1091 (9)	< 0.001
Unstable angina	252/826 (30.5)	220/1580 (13.9)	< 0.001
TIMI IIIa	30/113 (26.5)	27/278 (8.3)	< 0.001
MI without ST-segment elevation	41/450 (9.1)	55/1299 (4.2)	0.001
MI with ST-segment elevation	50/492 (10.2)	119/1759 (6.8)	0.02

GUSTO, Global Utilization of Streptokinase and t-PA for Occluded Coronary Arteries; *MI*, myocardial infarction; *TIMI*, Thrombosis In Myocardial Infarction.
From Bugiardini R, Bairey Merz CN. Angina with "normal" coronary arteries: a changing philosophy. JAMA. *2005;293:477–484.*

Symptoms

Stable angina is the most frequent initial manifestation of ischemic heart disease in women whereas acute MI and sudden death are more common initial presentations in men.[30,31] Women report more angina than men,[31a] in part due to higher somatic awareness in women.[31b] Whereas both men and women experience typical and atypical anginal symptoms, approximately half of men have typical symptoms versus one-third of women.[31c] In a recent large multi-center study of symptomatic men and women with suspected CAD, chest pain was the primary symptom in approximately three-fourths of both men and women, although more women characterized the pain as crushing, pressure, squeezing, or tightness.[31d] Patients with CMD may have both typical and atypical symptoms of angina. In addition to exercise-induced or exertional symptoms, they may report symptoms at rest and prolonged symptoms. Dyspnea with exertion is common, and should be considered an angina equivalent. Because routine cardiac stress testing is designed to detect obstructive CAD, CMD can be missed.[31e] Given the atypical symptoms and nondiagnostic testing results, these patients may be misdiagnosed as having a psychiatric or gastrointestinal cause of their symptoms. Endothelial dysfunction, smooth muscle dysfunction, impaired microvascular vasodilatory capacity, elevated resting vasomotor tone, and abnormal cardiac nociceptive abnormality contribute to various degrees in an individual patient.[31f] Given the high burden of cardiovascular risk factors and associated morbidity, it is reasonable to empirically treat for CMD if diagnostic testing for its detection is not available.[31e]

Persistent chest pain at 1 year after angiography in women with no obstructive CAD predicts cardiovascular events, with twice the rate of composite events [nonfatal MI, stroke, heart failure, and cardiovascular (CV) death] compared to those without persistent chest pain.[32] It is estimated that approximately 50% of women who present for chest pain evaluation continue to have symptoms at 5 years.[33] These patients present repeatedly to clinicians and emergency rooms seeking answers for their persistent symptoms and have considerable associated anxiety due to the absence of a clear diagnosis; they undergo repeated cardiac testing, contributing to high healthcare costs. In the WISE study of 883 women, those with no obstructive CAD had an average lifetime cost estimate of $767,288 (95% confidence interval [CI] $708,480–$826,097), with expenses increasing as the number of vessels with CAD increased (Fig. 25.2).[33]

Medical conditions such as depression and anxiety can also contribute to angina and need to be appropriately addressed and managed, as patients with persistent chest pain but no coronary obstruction have a higher prevalence of depression and anxiety and are more likely to need psychiatric medication.[28] Along with esophageal dysmotility disorders, a panic disorder should also be considered in those with recurrent chest pain that is out of proportion to objective evidence of ischemia found on testing. In one study of symptomatic patients with angiographically normal coronary arteries, 34% were found to meet Diagnostic and Statistical Manual of Mental Disorders criteria for having a panic disorder.[34] In a pilot study from Amsterdam of 20 patients with chest pain and no obstructive CAD on angiography who were screened with State Scale and Trait Scale of the State-Trait Anxiety Inventory, those with high anxiety had more ischemia on myocardial perfusion imaging compared to those with low anxiety.[35] In 2014, Vaccarino et al. reported a sex difference in mental stress–related myocardial ischemia in patients with a history of MI. Mental stress–induced ischemia was more common in younger women (age ≤ 50 years) compared to age-matched men, and this sex difference was not evident in those older than age 50 years.[36] Mental stress has been associated with coronary endothelial dysfunction,[37–39] and younger women may be particularly susceptible to adverse cardiac effects of mental stress.

PATHOPHYSIOLOGY

Symptomatic ischemic heart disease in those with no obstructive CAD represents a heterogeneous group of disorders with varying pathophysiologic mechanisms that often overlap (Fig. 25.3). The normal endothelium is a protective barrier, antithrombotic and antiinflammatory, and also mediates vascular smooth muscle cell vasodilatation. The majority of coronary vascular resistance is determined by the coronary microvasculature; under normal physiologic conditions, only 10% of resistance is determined by epicardial coronary arteries.[40,41] Whereas various autonomic, neurohormonal, and metabolic mechanisms influence myocardial blood flow, coronary endothelial dysfunction plays an important role in coronary vasodilator reserve.[42] A diagnosis of coronary endothelial dysfunction can help direct the clinician to currently available treatments that target the endothelium, although large randomized controlled trials specifically in well-phenotyped patients with CMD are lacking. In symptomatic women with no obstructive CAD who underwent coronary reactivity testing, those who had a history of MI were found to have more coronary endothelial dysfunction compared to those with no history of MI.[43] In addition to functional vascular abnormalities related to endothelial and microvascular dysfunction,

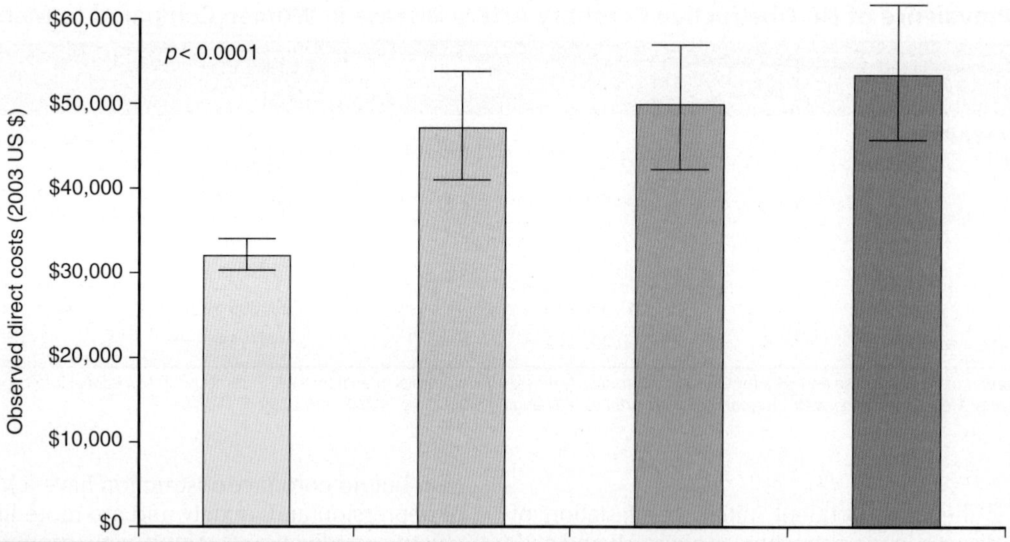

Cost components	Nonobstructive CAD	1 vessel CAD	2 vessel CAD	3 vessel CAD
Outpatient	6.7%	5.8%	14.3%	14.8%
Drug	32.6%	29.5%	27.0%	25.5%
Hospitalization	60.7%	64.7%	58.7%	59.7%

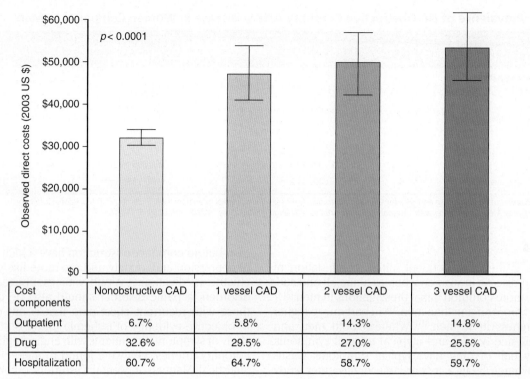

FIG. 25.2 No obstructive coronary artery disease is associated with high healthcare costs. As the severity of coronary artery disease (CAD) increases, healthcare costs increase; however, no obstructive CAD has a high healthcare cost that is comparable to obstructive CAD. *CAD,* Coronary artery disease. *(Shaw LJ, Merz CN, Pepine CJ, et al. The economic burden of angina in women with suspected ischemic heart disease: results from the National Institutes of Health–National Heart, Lung, and Blood Institute–sponsored Women's Ischemia Syndrome Evaluation.* Circulation. *2006;114:894–904.)*

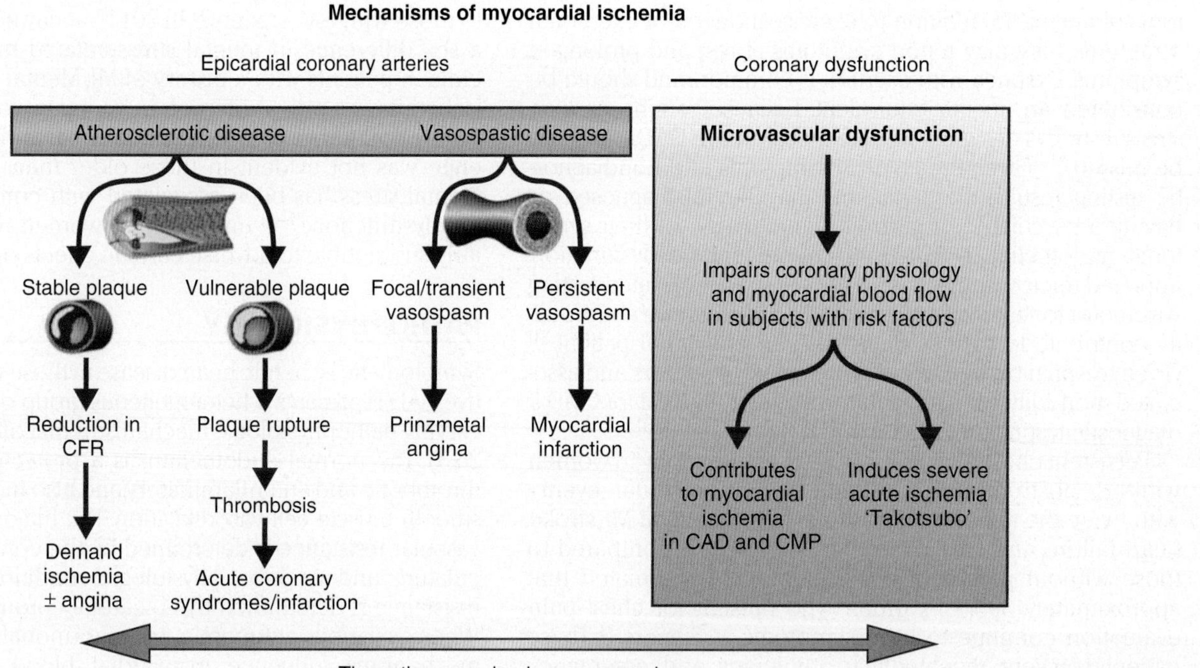

FIG. 25.3 Mechanisms of myocardial ischemia. Various structural and functional abnormalities that lead to ischemia can overlap. *CAD,* Coronary artery disease; *CFR,* coronary flow reserve; *CMP,* cardiomyopathy. *(From Crea F, Camici PG, Bairey Merz CN. Coronary microvascular dysfunction: an update.* Eur Heart J. *2014;35:1101–1111.)*

plaque erosion and microembolization may play a greater role in ischemic heart disease in women.[28,44,45]

Endothelial function is affected by aging, oxidative stress, changes in hormonal status, and conditions such as hypertension and diabetes. Bone marrow–derived endothelial progenitor cells have been shown to be important in vascular repair, and reduced numbers or regenerative capacity of these cells may play a role in microvascular dysfunction.[46] Patients with microvascular dysfunction are more likely to have hypertension, insulin resistance, and hyperlipidemia compared to the general population; in the WISE study, traditional cardiac risk factors appeared to be modestly related

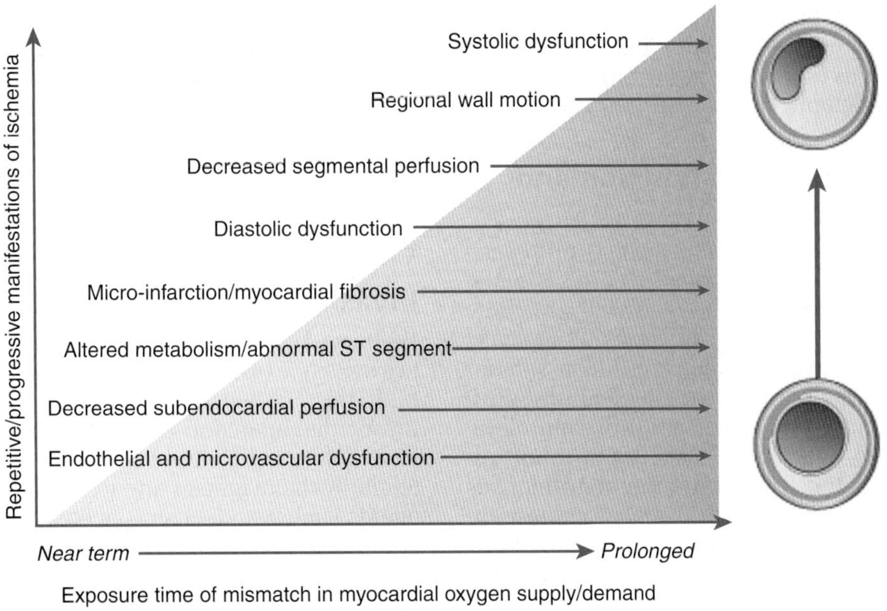

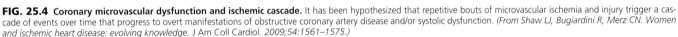

FIG. 25.4 Coronary microvascular dysfunction and ischemic cascade. It has been hypothesized that repetitive bouts of microvascular ischemia and injury trigger a cascade of events over time that progress to overt manifestations of obstructive coronary artery disease and/or systolic dysfunction. *(From Shaw LJ, Bugiardini R, Merz CN. Women and ischemic heart disease: evolving knowledge.* J Am Coll Cardiol. *2009;54:1561–1575.)*

to CMD when diagnosed by invasive coronary reactivity testing or when diagnosed by abnormal myocardial perfusion reserve index (MPRI) on CMR imaging. In 100 women suspected of ischemic heart disease (mean age 54 ± 10 years) with no obstructive CAD and with intravascular ultrasound–measured atherosclerosis, waist circumference and systolic blood pressure were independently associated with plaque presence and severity, after adjustment for multiple factors including age, diabetes, family history of CAD, hyperlipidemia, hormone replacement, and tobacco smoking.[47]

Impaired sympathovagal balance determined by heart rate variability, and altered baroreflex sensitivity, has also been implicated in patients with cardiac syndrome X.[48,49] Abnormal cardiac adrenergic nerve function measured by ^{123}I-*meta*-iodobenzylguanidine (*m*IBG) nuclear planar imaging in patients with cardiac syndrome X compared to normal patients has been reported previously.[50]

It has been hypothesized that CMD can lead to decreased subendocardial perfusion and that repetitive bouts of microvascular ischemia may lead to microinfarctions, fibrosis, and diastolic dysfunction, with progressive myocardial injury and systolic dysfunction (Fig. 25.4). In 2014, acetylcholine-induced coronary microvascular spasm was associated with diastolic dysfunction determined by echocardiography in patients with no obstructive CAD.[51] We have demonstrated that in a cohort of women who underwent invasive coronary reactivity testing for the diagnosis of CMD, over one-third had elevated left ventricular end diastolic pressures > 15 mmHg.[51a] Given the current epidemic of heart failure with preserved ejection fraction, which also has a female predominance, a mechanistic link between CMD and heart failure with preserved ejection fraction (HFpEF) has been proposed and is under investigation.[52]

Coronary Microvascular Dysfunction with Significant Coronary Artery Disease

CMD may occur concomitantly with significant obstructive coronary atherosclerosis. This may become evident when patients remain symptomatic despite percutaneous coronary intervention; in such cases, coronary vasospasm related to stent placement and/or CMD should be suspected. The phenomenon of no-reflow after intervention is associated with worse prognosis, and no-reflow is believed to occur due to abnormal microvascular function. CMD cannot be excluded as a cause of angina in those with obstructive CAD, because in the same patient, angina can occur due to dynamic epicardial stenosis and/or microvascular dysfunction and/or coronary spasm. This point is emphasized in the 2013 European Society of Cardiology (ECS) guidelines on the management of stable coronary artery disease. For the diagnosis of microvascular angina, the ECS guidelines provide a class IIa recommendation for dobutamine stress echocardiography and IIb for invasive coronary reactivity testing.[53] In contrast, the current US ACC/AHA guidelines on stable ischemic heart disease do not address specifics of diagnostic testing for CMD.[54]

Coronary Microvascular Dysfunction with Structural and Infiltrative Myocardial Disease

Studies on patients with cardiac syndrome X often excluded patients with structural heart disease such as hypertrophic cardiomyopathy (HCM) or dilated cardiomyopathy. The WISE study also excluded those with structural heart disease and/or cardiomyopathy. CMD has been demonstrated in those with hypertrophic and infiltrative cardiomyopathies such as amyloidosis. Whereas a diagnosis of microvascular dysfunction is typically made in those patients where structural heart disease such as HCM is excluded, one should note that patients with HCM have been shown to have a low CFR compared to healthy individuals. HCM patients with a low CFR had higher 3-year event rates compared to those with normal flow reserve (79% vs 17%, $p < 0.0001$).[55] Furthermore, those HCM patients who were asymptomatic but had an abnormal CFR had a 10-fold increased risk of events (including death, unstable angina, nonfatal MI, hospitalizations for heart failure, syncope, atrial fibrillation, and implantable cardioverter defibrillator implantations). A majority of HCM patients have been shown to have abnormal CFR by echocardiography.[55]

Coronary Microvascular Dysfunction and Takotsubo Cardiomyopathy

Also known as *stress-induced cardiomyopathy* or *broken heart syndrome*, Takotsubo cardiomyopathy (TTC) is much more common in women compared to men, with a majority of cases occurring in postmenopausal women.[56] Typically associated with a catecholamine surge due to a stressor (which can be emotional distress or physical stress), it resembles acute coronary syndrome, with troponin elevation and ECG changes. Obstructive CAD is not found on angiography and characteristic wall motion abnormalities are noted, with basal hyperkinesis and apical akinesis or hypokinesis. Reverse forms of TTC with apical hyperkinesis and basal akinesis, as well as biventricular forms, have also been described.[57] Previously thought to have a good prognosis because it is a reversible cardiomyopathy, recent data indicate that it may not be as benign.[58] Whereas various mechanisms are under investigation in TTC, including cardiac adrenergic dysfunction and multivessel spasm, impaired coronary endothelial function and vascular reactivity has been demonstrated in those patients with a history of TTC.[59] Vascular disorders such as Raynaud's and migraine, which tend to be more common in women, are also associated with TTC, implicating a more generalized vascular endothelial dysfunction.[60]

Coronary Slow Flow Phenomenon

When contrast is injected into the coronary ostia, if there is a delay in the opacification of the coronary artery, this microvascular dysfunction-related phenomenon[61] is described as coronary slow flow phenomenon, which occurs in 1–3% of coronary angiograms. It is generally defined as Thrombolytic In Myocardial Infarction (TIMI) grade 2 flow in the absence of obstructive CAD, with a transit time of three or more heart beats for contrast to travel to distal vessels. The TIMI frame count[62] has also been used to define coronary slow flow,[63] and this phenomenon of slower opacification is more often observed in men when coronary angiography is performed in the setting of acute coronary syndrome. It can present with rest or exertional pain, and abnormal microvascular resistance has been implicated. On endomyocardial biopsy of symptomatic patients with coronary slow flow, small vessel medial hypertrophy, myointimal proliferation, and endothelial abnormalities have been reported.[64] Similar to microvascular angina, patients may present with recurrent chest pain and undergo repeat hospitalizations. In the WISE study of women with no obstructive CAD, a longer TIMI frame count independently predicted hospitalization for angina.[65] Nitrates are not particularly helpful in slow flow because they are epicardial vasodilators, with little impact on microvascular tone.[66] Dipyridamole is a vasodilator that has been studied in coronary slow flow,[67] and the newer generation β-blocker nebivolol has been shown to improve CFR in patients with coronary slow flow. Nebivolol is a unique β-blocker as it potentiates nitric oxide effects leading to vasodilation and is also an antioxidant. The T-type calcium-channel blocker (CCB) mibrefradil (not available in the United States) has been shown to improve TIMI frame count and angina frequency by 56% compared to placebo in patients with coronary slow flow, which implicates smooth muscle dysfunction in coronary slow flow phenomenon.[68]

DIAGNOSTIC TESTING

Invasive Coronary Reactivity Testing

Patients who continue to have angina and have some objective evidence of myocardial ischemia or injury (such as abnormal stress testing or history of non–ST-segment elevation myocardial infarction [NSTEMI]), and who are suspected to have CMD, can be offered invasive coronary reactivity testing to clarify the diagnosis and to help guide therapy. Vasoactive agents such as adenosine, acetylcholine, and nitroglycerin can be used to test endothelial and nonendothelial macro- and microvascular function. In response to acetylcholine and nitroglycerin, coronary artery diameter changes can be assessed by quantitative coronary angiography. At time of printing, there are no guideline-recommended or standardized protocols for assessing coronary microvascular function, and centers that perform coronary reactivity testing have their own individual protocols.

Coronary reactivity testing can be helpful to clarify the etiology of symptoms in patients with objective evidence of ischemia who do not have obstructive CAD. Briefly, a Doppler flow wire is placed in the epicardial coronary vessel, and the hyperemic response to a potent vasodilator (typically adenosine) is noted by change in coronary flow velocity (Fig. 25.5). The intracoronary dose of adenosine used in the WISE study to assess myocardial flow reserve (18–36 μg) tests the nonendothelial-dependent microvascular response. In the WISE study of 159 symptomatic women (mean age 52.9 years) who underwent coronary reactivity testing for suspected CMD, 47% had a CFR ≤2.5 after intracoronary adenosine.[69] We have reported that low- and high-dose intracoronary adenosine (18 μg vs 36 μg) produced

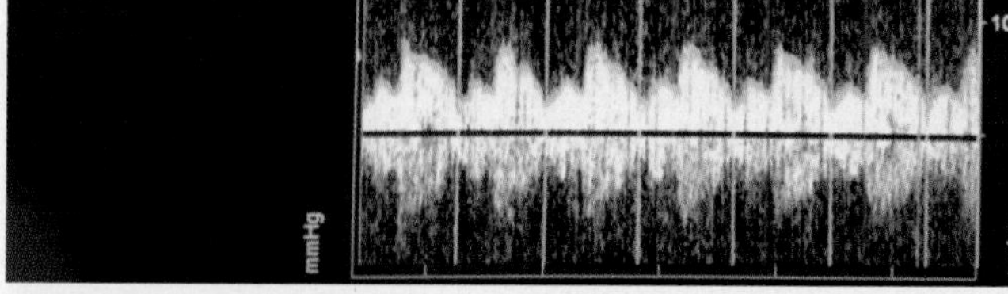

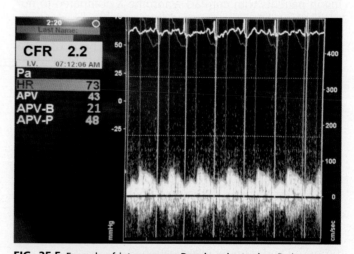

FIG. 25.5 Example of intracoronary Doppler wire tracing. During coronary physiology studies, a Doppler wire is placed in the coronary artery and coronary flow velocity is obtained, along with coronary flow reserve (CFR) in response to adenosine. Figure depicts average coronary flow peak velocity of 48 cm/s and an abnormal CFR of 2.2 in response to adenosine.[13] *APV*, Doppler average peak velocity; *CFR*, coronary flow reserve; *HR*, heart rate; *Pa*, mean aortic pressure. *(From Wei J, Mehta PK, Johnson BD, et al. Safety of coronary reactivity testing in women with no obstructive coronary artery disease: results from the NHLBI-sponsored WISE (Women's Ischemia Syndrome Evaluation) study.* JACC Cardiovasc Interv. *2012;5:646–653.)*

similar augmentation in coronary flow velocity,[70] and 47% of women demonstrate abnormal adenosine response with CFR ≤2.5.[13]

To test the coronary endothelial-dependent response, intracoronary acetylcholine in increasing concentrations is typically used, and coronary diameter change is noted visually and by quantitative coronary angiography. Acetylcholine stimulates the healthy endothelium to release nitric oxide, which in turn mediates vascular smooth muscle cell relaxation via cyclic guanosine monophosphate (cGMP). It must be noted that the entire epicardial vessel should be assessed in response to intracoronary acetylcholine because distal vasoconstriction can often be missed if one is focused only on the proximal segments of the epicardial vessel. Failure to dilate in response to acetylcholine indicates impaired endothelial function (Fig. 25.6). In the WISE study of women with no obstructive CAD who underwent coronary reactivity testing, 58% of patients had epicardial coronary endothelial dysfunction.[13] Coronary blood flow can be calculated by the following equation that incorporates the diameter change as well as flow velocity change to acetylcholine: Coronary blood flow = Pi x [vessel diameter/2]^2 x (average peak velocity/2).[2] Whereas designations of endothelial- versus nonendothelial-dependent responses are helpful conceptually, one must recognize that there is significant overlap in these mechanistic pathways. Piek et al.[71] have shown that coronary flow capacity, which combines CFR and maximal hyperemic average peak flow velocity, improves prediction of major adverse cardiovascular outcomes, compared with CFR alone.[71]

In the Coronary Artery Spasm as a Frequent Cause for Acute Coronary Syndrome (CASPAR) study, approximately 50% of patients with acute coronary syndrome with no obstructive CAD were found to have coronary vasospasm on intracoronary acetylcholine provocation testing.[72] Ong et al.[73] have also reported a high percentage of patients with microvascular spasm, defined in their study as electrocardiographic changes indicative of ischemia, and reproduction of patient symptoms in response to acetylcholine, without overt epicardial spasm seen on angiography.

In a study by Hasdai et al. in 203 patients (158 women, 45 men; mean age 51 years) without evidence of obstructive CAD, over 50% had an abnormal coronary reactivity testing result (11.3% had an abnormal adenosine response, 29.2% had an abnormal acetylcholine response, and 18% had abnormalities in response to both adenosine and acetylcholine).[2]

Currently, coronary reactivity testing is performed selectively at specialized centers. The approach used in our center is shown in Fig. 25.7. We have reported on the safety of coronary reactivity testing[13] using intracoronary adenosine (18 μg and 36 μg), acetylcholine (graded infusions of 0.364 μg and 36.4 μg over 3 min), and nitroglycerin (200 μg) in the left coronary artery. When performed by experienced operators in 293 women in the WISE study, there were no reactivity testing–related deaths, and two serious adverse events (0.7%; one dissection and one MI from spasm); MACE rate at 5.4 years of follow-up in this study was 8.2%.[13] In a European study of 921 patients (362 men) with no obstructive CAD who underwent intracoronary acetylcholine provocation testing (with graded doses of 2, 20, 100, and 200 μg infused over 3 min in the left coronary artery), no fatal or serious adverse complications were reported.[73] In this study, 1% of the patients (n = 9) had minor complications, including nonsustained ventricular tachycardia, paroxysmal atrial fibrillation, symptomatic bradycardia, and catheter-induced proximal right coronary artery spasm.[73]

Noninvasive Imaging Modalities

Exercise Treadmill Testing

In a 2014 consensus statement from the AHA on evaluation of women with suspected ischemic heart disease, exercise treadmill testing (ETT) remains as first-line, since it is widely available, relatively inexpensive, and provides excellent prognostic information based on metabolic equivalents of task (METS) achieved and functional capacity[74] (Fig. 25.8). Reproduction of symptoms during an ETT is important to consider when interpreting the ETT. ST-segment depression on exercise ECG testing or during an anginal episode can indicate ischemia related to obstructive CAD or microvascular dysfunction. A positive ETT with no obstructive CAD on angiography can lead to a conclusion of "false-positive" ETT; however, CMD should be considered as an etiology in such patients.

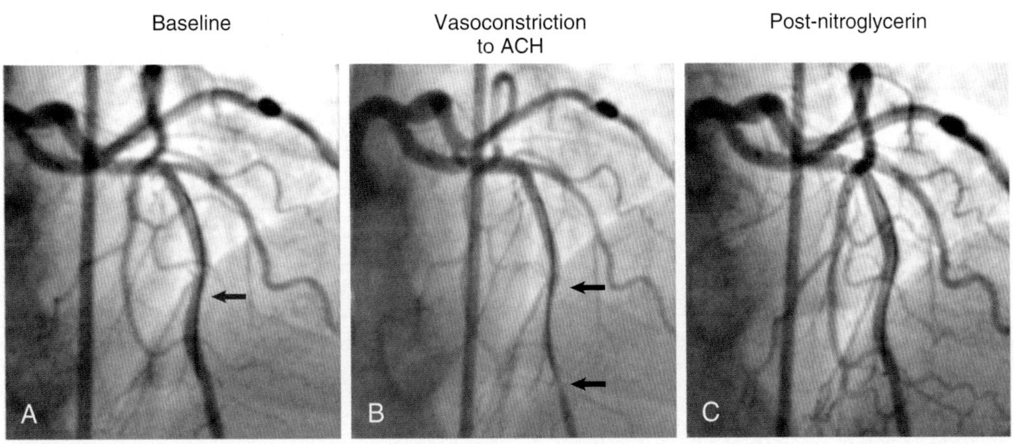

FIG. 25.6 Intracoronary provocation testing. Panel A in the Figure demonstrates a Doppler flow wire in the left anterior descending artery (*red arrow*). In response to intracoronary acetylcholine infusion, there is abnormal vasoconstriction (panel B, *black arrows*), which is resolved by intracoronary nitroglycerin (panel C). *ACH*, Acetylcholine. (*From Wei J, Mehta PK, Johnson BD, et al. Safety of coronary reactivity testing in women with no obstructive coronary artery disease: results from the NHLBI-sponsored WISE (Women's Ischemia Syndrome Evaluation) study.* JACC Cardiovasc Interv. *2012;5:646–653.*)

Stress Echocardiography

CFR can be measured via Doppler echocardiography, although this method is typically not utilized in routine clinical practice in the United States. Those with low CFR on dobutamine stress echo have less favorable prognosis compared to those with normal flow reserve on stress echo.[75] In a study of 1660 men and women with normal stress echocardiograms, CFR was measured in the left anterior descending artery in response to dipyridamole. Those with a low CFR ($\leq$ 2.0) had a high annualized event rate compared to those with CFR $\geq$ 2.0 (Fig. 25.9).[76]

Myocardial contrast echocardiography is an additional tool for detection of myocardial perfusion abnormalities and quantification of coronary blood flow, although its clinical use has been limited.[77,78] Myocardial contrast echocardiography uses intravenous microbubbles to generate time versus acoustic intensity curves, allowing calculation of myocardial blood flow velocity.[79] Myocardial contrast echocardiography can help evaluate microvascular volume, velocity, and coronary microvascular flow reserves in patients with CMD.[80]

Cardiac Positron Emission Tomography Imaging

In addition to detection of ischemia, rest/stress cardiac PET imaging can provide quantification of absolute myocardial blood flow and measurement of CFR for detection of CMD. Pharmacologic stress agents include dipyridamole, adenosine, regadenoson, or dobutamine, and nuclear tracers include rubidium-82 or N-13 ammonia. Since PET imaging is combined with computed tomography (CT), a coronary calcium score can be calculated, which can aid in additional CV risk stratification. PET-CT is not widely available in the United States, and when it is available, is often not covered by insurance. However, because PET is less likely to have attenuation artifacts than single-photon emission computed tomography (SPECT) in patients who are obese [body mass index (BMI) > 40 kg/m^2], have large breasts or breast implants, or chest wall deformity, cardiac PET imaging may be preferred in these populations and has been shown to provide incremental prognostic value in all patients irrespective of BMI.[81]

PET CFR is calculated as the ratio of absolute myocardial blood flow at peak hyperemia to resting myocardial blood

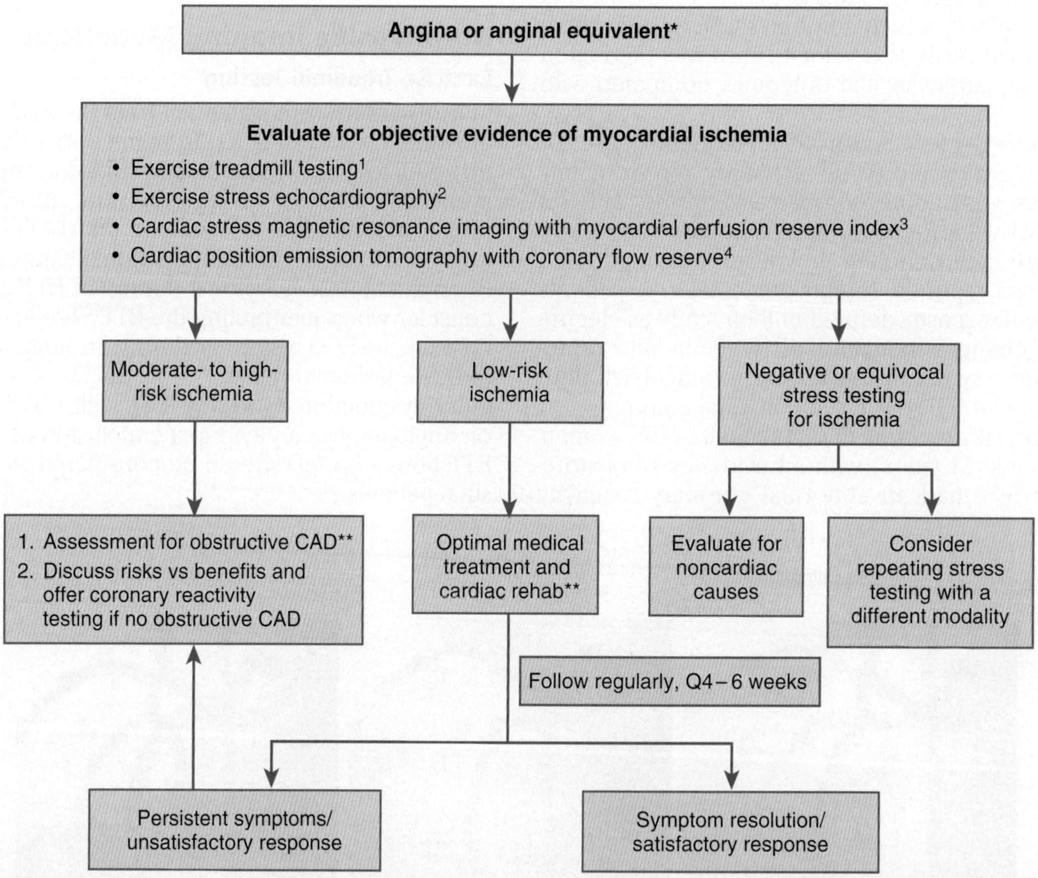

FIG. 25.7 Approach to diagnose coronary microvascular dysfunction in patients with suspected ischemia, preserved ejection fraction, and no structural heart disease.^ This is one example of an approach that is used to help guide the clinician regarding whether or not coronary reactivity testing would be helpful in a symptomatic patient at our center. US guidelines that specifically address coronary microvascular dysfunction and coronary reactivity testing are not available at this time.
[1] If patient is able to exercise and no contradictions
[2] If patient is able to exercise and has good windows for ultrasonography
[3] Consider if exercise treadmill testing (ETT) and stress echo are not an option or equivocal; benefit of no radiation and expertise is available at our center
[4] Consider if ETT and stress echo are not an option or equivocal; expertise available at our center, is a low radiation testing protocol, and can provide coronary calcium score
* Includes atypical symptoms
**Follow American College of Cardiology / American Heart Association stable ischemic heart disease guidelines
^ Does not apply in the acute setting or acute coronary syndrome within 4–6 weeks. Only applies to stable ischemic heart disease patients.
CAD, Coronary artery disease.

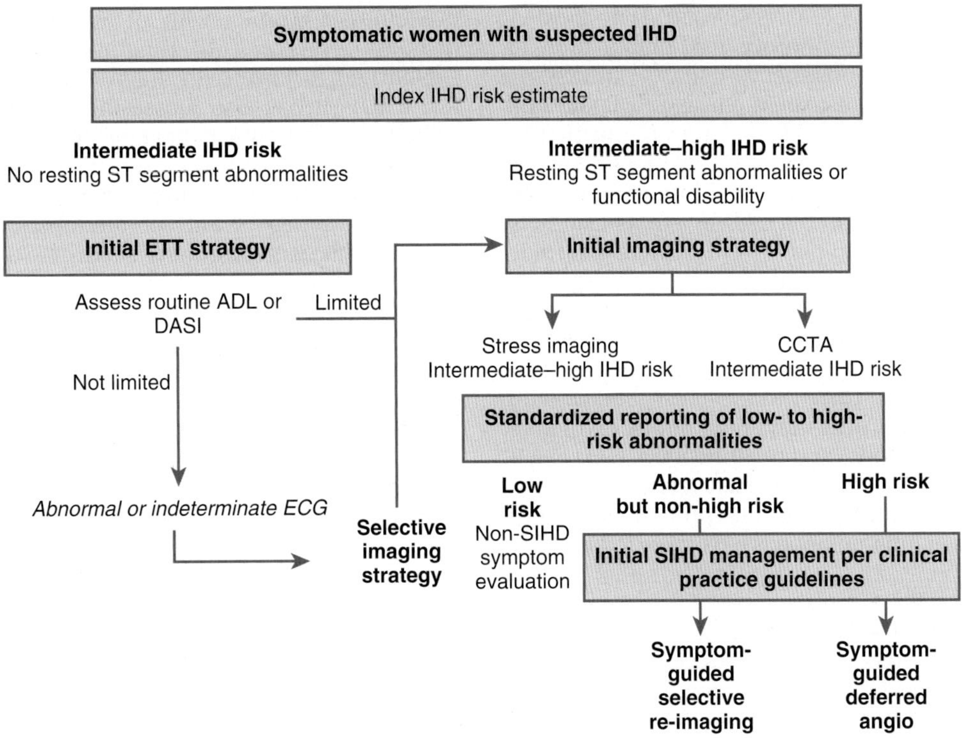

FIG. 25.8 Evaluation algorithm for intermediate- and intermediate- to high-risk women suspected of ischemic heart disease. For an intermediate-risk woman who can exercise, exercise treadmill testing remains the first-line recommended test for evaluation of ischemic heart disease in the recently proposed American Heart Association consensus statement. *ADL*, Activities of daily living; *CCTA*, cardiac computed tomography angiography; *DASI*, Duke activity score index; *ECG*, electrocardiogram; *ETT*, exercise treadmill testing; *IHD*, ischemic heart disease; *SIHD*, stable ischemic heart disease. *(Reproduced with permission from Mieres JH, Gulati M, Bairey Merz N, et al. Role of noninvasive testing in the clinical evaluation of women with suspected ischemic heart disease: a consensus statement from the American Heart Association.* Circulation. *2014;130:350–379. 2014, American Heart Association, Inc.)*

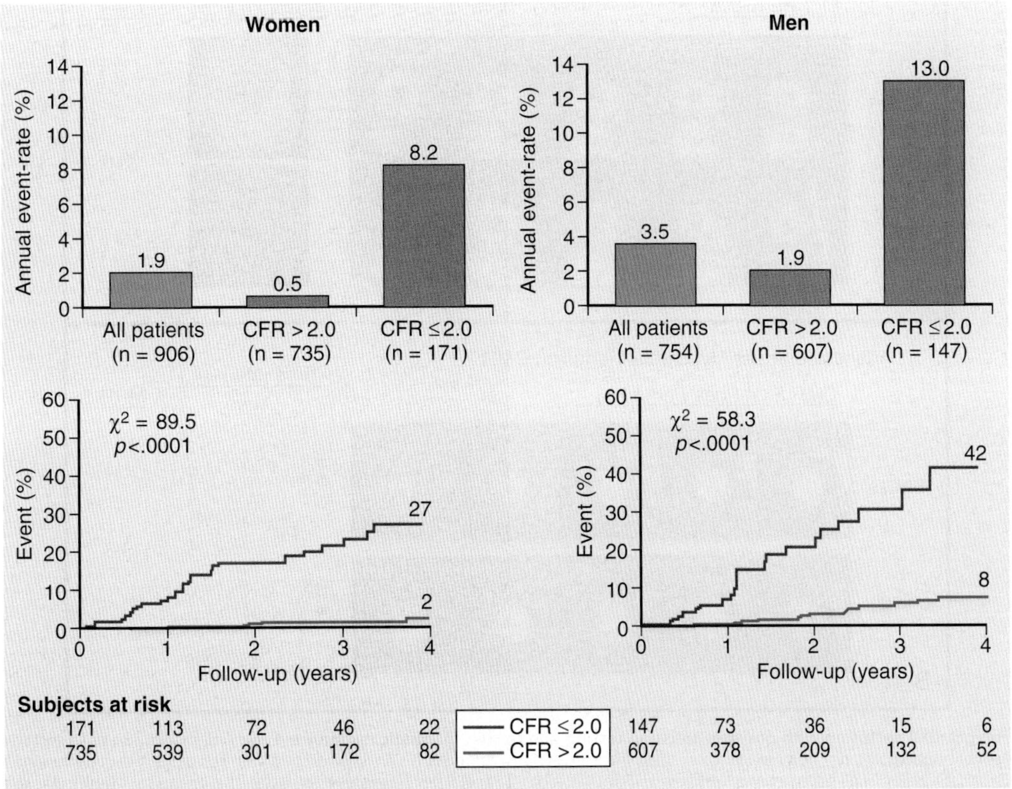

FIG. 25.9 A low coronary flow reserve is associated with higher event rate in women and men. Similar to invasively determined abnormal coronary flow reserve (CFR) and associated adverse prognosis, cardiac positron emission testing–determined low CFR is also associated with adverse events in men and women compared to those with normal CFR. *CFR*, Coronary flow reserve. *(From Cortigiani, L, Rigo F, Gherardi S, et al. Prognostic effect of coronary flow reserve in women versus men with chest pain syndrome and normal dipyridamole stress echocardiography.* Am J Cardiol. *2010;106:1703–1708.)*

flow, using automated image analysis tools[82] (Fig. 25.10A). PET CFR has been used to improve risk stratification in patients with and without obstructive CAD.[83,84] In a study of 73 patients undergoing rest/stress cardiac PET and coronary CT angiography, 38% of vessels with nonobstructive CAD had abnormal regional CFR of < 2.0.[85] PET CFR has also been shown to provide prognostic information in both men and women with and without CAD. In a recent study of 405 men and 813 women who underwent rest/stress cardiac PET for evaluation of ischemia, microvascular dysfunction (defined as CFR < 2.0) was highly prevalent in both men (51%) and women (53%); those with low CFR had worse CV outcomes than those with normal CFR.[6] PET-determined flow reserve has also been used to evaluate patients with chronic inflammatory disorders (systemic lupus erythematosus or rheumatoid arthritis) and no obstructive CAD or CV risk factors; CFR was found to be inversely related to disease duration and high-sensitivity C-reactive protein, consistent with the concept that inflammation is a risk factor for microvascular dysfunction.[86]

Cardiac Magnetic Resonance Imaging

CMR imaging can provide a comprehensive assessment of ischemic heart disease, including function, perfusion, and viability, and is an emerging modality for the evaluation of angina in the setting of no obstructive CAD. Prior work with phosphorus-31 nuclear CMR spectroscopy has demonstrated that an abnormal phosphocreatine/adenosine triphosphate ratio, indicative of ischemia, predicted cardiovascular outcomes in women without obstructive CAD.[87] Whereas first-pass perfusion CMR using pharmacologic stress is well established to have high diagnostic accuracy for obstructive CAD,[88] it has also increasingly been shown to detect ischemia in patients without obstructive CAD.[9,10,89,90] CMR subendocardial perfusion defects are frequently present in patients with abnormal stress testing and normal epicardial coronary arteries[89,91] and are the most common finding in women with acute coronary syndrome and normal epicardial coronary arteries.[92] Although visual subendocardial defects can be challenging to interpret in the setting of the "dark rim" image artifact, high resolution CMR sequences have now been able to optimize this detection.[93] The severity of ischemia can be assessed in a semiquantitative method, as time–intensity curves for ischemic myocardium demonstrate a reduced upslope and peak intensity compared to curves for normal myocardium[94,95] (Fig. 25.10B). In the WISE study, CMR MPRI was predictive of having an abnormal invasive coronary reactivity testing; an MPRI threshold of 1.84 predicted an abnormal coronary reactivity testing result with moderate sensitivity (73%) and specificity (74%).[9] A recent randomized, placebo-controlled trial of ranolazine in CMD patients demonstrated that improvement in angina correlated with improvement in MPRI.[96] Although MPRI is a validated semiquantitative myocardial perfusion assessment, it is not a direct measure of CFR, and absolute myocardial blood flow quantification methods are still being developed.[97] Further studies are needed to demonstrate the prognostic and therapeutic values of CMR.

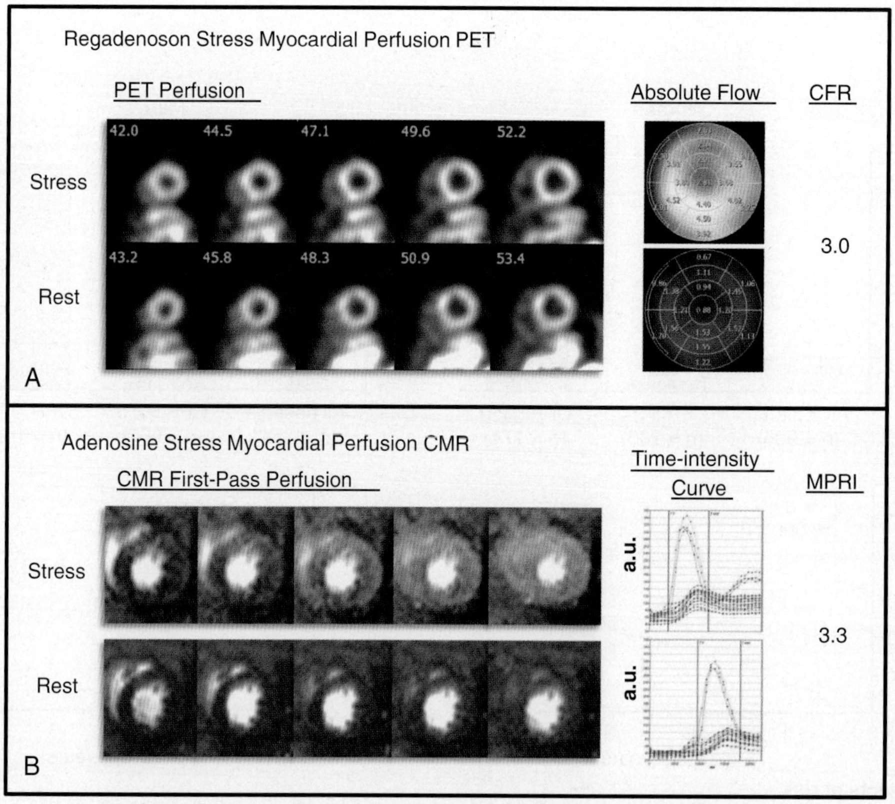

FIG. 25.10 Normal myocardial perfusion with positron emission testing and cardiac magnetic resonance. Panel A demonstrates serial short axis left ventricular slices from apex to base in a patient undergoing rest and regadenoson-stress myocardial perfusion positron emission testing with rubidium. Visual perfusion is normal, and coronary flow reserve of 3.0 is normal (stress flow 3.45 mL/g per min, rest flow 1.18 mL/g per min). Panel B demonstrates first-pass perfusion in a mid-ventricular slice in a patient undergoing adenosine-stress and rest myocardial perfusion cardiac magnetic resonance with gadolinium. Visual perfusion is normal, and myocardial perfusion reserve index 3.3 is normal (derived from the maximum upslope of the time-intensity curves of the myocardium and left ventricular cavity at stress and rest). *CFR*, Coronary flow reserve; *MPRI*, myocardial perfusion reserve index; *PET*, positron emission tomography.

THERAPEUTIC STRATEGIES

Antiatherosclerotic Therapy

Therapeutic Lifestyle Change

Due to a high burden of cardiac risk factors and coronary atherosclerosis in patients with angina,[1] evidence of ischemia, and no obstructive CAD, lifestyle changes to aggressively modify risk factors are important. Advisement for increased physical activity, smoking cessation, and incorporating a heart healthy diet is the cornerstone of a complete strategy. Physician counseling with the help of ancillary staff, including a nutritionist, and cardiac rehabilitation is ideal; angina is an approved diagnosis for cardiac rehabilitation for most healthcare insurers. Because patients often limit their physical activity to minimize their symptoms, they should be encouraged to work with a cardiac rehabilitation program to battle their fear of precipitating angina and improve their exercise tolerance. Physical conditioning has been demonstrated to be effective for increased exercise capacity and symptom relief in these patients.[98] Exercise improves endothelial function in those with CAD[99] and improves myocardial perfusion reserve in those with history of MI.[100] A 2015 trial in 70 nondiabetic patients with CMD (defined as impaired CFR in response to IV dipyridamole or adenosine by echocardiography) randomized to aerobic interval training or low calorie diet (800–1000 kcal/day) demonstrated that both interventions resulted in improvement in CFR.[101]

Antiplatelet Agents

A majority of patients with CMD have endothelial dysfunction and, whereas angiography shows no significant plaque burden, IVUS has demonstrated coronary atherosclerosis in most patients.[1] Therefore, ACC/AHA chronic stable angina guidelines[16] can be extrapolated to include use of antiplatelet agents such as aspirin in patients with evidence of ischemia and no obstructive CAD.

Lipid-Lowering Therapy

Therapy with statins can be used in patients who qualify by the presence of risk factors, evidence of atherosclerosis, or endothelial dysfunction. Statins have been shown to improve endothelial dysfunction, exercise-induced ischemia, and exercise tolerance, and in combination with ACE-I have been shown to improve angina.[102,103] Due to the high prevalence of subclinical coronary atherosclerosis in patients with CMD,[28] application of the current ACC/AHA[104] recommendations for low-density lipoprotein (LDL) cholesterol lowering are appropriate; in patients with ACSs, history of MI, stable angina, or coronary revascularization, a moderate or high-intensity statin is recommended. Additionally, in patients with ACS, further reduction of LDL cholesterol levels with ezetimibe has been shown to reduce cardiovascular events,[105] suggesting that other interventions to reduce LDL cholesterol may be beneficial in this population. The PCSK9 inhibitors alirocumab[106] and evolocumab[107] have been shown to achieve lower LDL cholesterol levels than statins (and augment LDL cholesterol lowering in patients on maximal intensity statin therapy), and can be used in higher-risk patients in whom statin therapy did not achieve sufficient LDL cholesterol lowering or who have statin intolerance. These novel agents are promising to reduce cardiovascular events, and longer-term follow-up is ongoing to evaluate safety and event reduction.

Antianginal Therapy

β-Blockers

β-blockers reduce the number and severity of anginal episodes and improve exercise tolerance in patients with CMD.[108,109] For angina precipitated by heightened sympathetic activity including mental stress, propranolol has been shown to reduce the number of ischemic episodes per day by a reduction in ST-segment depression.[108] Newer generation β-blockers (carvedilol and nebivolol) stimulate the release of nitric oxide from the endothelial cells and, because of their antioxidant properties,[110] lead to vasodilation and decrease peripheral vascular resistance,[111] and show promise in treatment of microvascular dysfunction. Carvedilol has been shown to improve CFR in those with dilated cardiomyopathy, and nebivolol has been shown to improve CFR in those with CAD.[112–114] Erdamar et al. showed that in patients with cardiac syndrome X, nebivolol significantly lowered serum myeloperoxidase activity, lowered malondialdehyde, and increased superoxide dismutase activity when compared to metoprolol.[111] Interestingly, both endothelial function and exercise stress test parameters improved more with nebivolol than metoprolol.

In contrast, in a 2016 reported randomized trial of nebivolol versus atenolol in men and women ($n = 24$) with angina and nonobstructive CAD, nebivolol did not significantly improve microvascular or endothelial function despite its known antioxidant properties. Surprisingly, those on nebivolol demonstrated plaque progression and constrictive remodeling by intravascular ultrasound at 1 year, which was attributed to a higher number of low shear stress segments in the nebivolol arm determined by computational fluid dynamics.[115]

Angiotensin-Converting Enzyme Inhibitors

ACE-I improve CFR and exercise duration in patients with cardiac syndrome X.[116] In a randomized trial of quinapril versus placebo in women with microvascular dysfunction in the WISE study, CFR improved in those women with lower baseline flow reserve values who were randomized to quinapril, and resulted in improved angina measured by Seattle Angina Questionnaire.[117] For those who are not tolerant of ACE-I, the addition of angiotensin receptor blockers as a therapeutic benefit in patients with microvascular dysfunction is speculative. Aldosterone antagonists such as spironolactone and eplerenone may be helpful in those with microvascular dysfunction who are found to have high left ventricular end diastolic pressures, although addition of eplerenone to ACE-I did not result in improvement in coronary microvascular function in a WISE substudy.[118]

L-Arginine

L-arginine is a precursor of nitric oxide, and its use over 6 months led to improved endothelial function and symptoms in patients with no obstructive CAD.[119] In another study in patients with Prinzmetal angina, L-arginine supplementation was associated with improvement in angina.[120] Randomized trials of L-arginine in CMD are needed before it can be recommended routinely for clinical care.

Nitrates

Nitrates can have a mixed vasodilatory effect on the microcirculation. There are no large randomized controlled trials exploring the role of nitrates specifically in patients with CMD. An observational study in 99 patients with cardiac syndrome X[121] showed that nitrates were effective antianginal therapy in 40–50% of the patients; there are no clear data showing that one nitrate preparation is better than another. Even though the effects of nitrates on angina duration and frequency are not always predictable in patients with CMD, it is clear that for many patients they provide relief. Many patients, but not all, develop nitrate tolerance after sustained use of the drug, and it is important to advise the patient regarding a nitrate-free interval of at least 12 hours per day.

Calcium-Channel Blockers

CCBs are first-line therapy for Prinzmetal angina and are effective at reducing coronary vasomotor tone as well as myocardial oxygen demand.[122] Several randomized and nonrandomized CCB studies have shown that diltiazem, verapamil, and nifedipine reduce episodes of Prinzmetal angina.[123–125] Whereas CCBs have also been shown to improve angina and exercise tolerance in patients with CMD,[126,127] in one study, diltiazem failed to improve CFR.[128] Several randomized clinical trials comparing β-blockers, nitrates, and CCBs[1] demonstrate β-blockers are most effective overall in this patient group. Specifically, in patients with cardiac syndrome X, atenolol was found to improve angina compared to amlodipine or isosorbide-5-mononitrate, and propranolol was found to be more effective than verapamil in reducing the number of angina episodes.[108,109] β-blockers can worsen symptoms in the minority of patients with epicardial coronary spasm.[15]

Ranolazine

Ranolazine is an antianginal, anti-ischemic agent that alters the late sodium current and reduces calcium overload in the myocyte.[129] In patients with chronic stable angina refractory to other antianginal therapy, the addition of ranolazine reduces angina and increases exercise time and time to ST-segment depression.[130,131] Ranolazine has also been specifically tested in patients with CMD and no obstructive CAD. In a small trial ranolazine demonstrated angina improvement measured by the Seattle Angina Questionnaire compared to placebo.[132] However, a larger subsequent mechanistic trial (RWISE) showed that ranolazine did not have a significant impact on angina in the overall cohort; nevertheless, patients with more severe CMD improved.[96] Angina and CMR myocardial perfusion reserve index were related in this trial, which indicated that continued investigation of other strategies to improve coronary microvascular function should be performed. One potential contributor to the null findings in RWISE is that patients were optimally treated with secondary prevention and antianginal medications, which is typically not the community standard of care, where this population of patients is often undiagnosed and undertreated.

Given the lack of significant hemodynamic effect, ranolazine can be considered in patients who have lower blood pressures and thus cannot tolerate the usual dosages of β-blockers or calcium-channel blockers.

Ivabradine

Ivabradine is a novel antianginal that selectively inhibits the funny channels [$I_{(f)}$] in the sinoatrial node, thereby reducing heart rates.[133–135] Approved in the United States for treatment of chronic stable angina in patients with normal sinus rhythm, it may be used in those who require heart rate reduction and are unable to tolerate β-blockers. It has been shown to be as effective as atenolol in a randomized double-blind trial in patients with stable angina.[136] Ivabradine was reported to be well tolerated, with the most common side effect of brightness in areas of the visual field (phosphenes).

α-Blockers

α_1-Blockers, such as doxazosin, block α-mediated vascular smooth muscle cell vasoconstriction. In a study of doxazosin versus placebo, there was no improvement in myocardial blood flow in response to dipyridamole in 28 patients with cardiac syndrome X.[137] Doxazosin also failed to result in an improvement in angina or exercise duration, or to show an improvement in ischemia by ECG.[138]

Xanthine Derivatives

Commonly used to treat bronchial asthma due to its phosphodiesterase inhibitory actions, aminophylline is also a nonselective adenosine receptor antagonist, which may be of benefit in patients with angina and ischemia as adenosine mediates cardiac pain. Emdin et al.[139] showed that acute administration of aminophylline leads to an improvement in effort angina and ischemia by ECG in eight cardiac syndrome X patients, and additional studies are needed.

Other Agents

Various other agents have been studied in symptomatic patients with no obstructive CAD, and some have shown more promise than others. In 20 symptomatic patients with no obstructive CAD who received the centrally acting α-agonist clonidine (0.1 mg BID for 3 weeks) versus placebo, there was no significant reduction in episodes of chest pain.[140] Nicorandil, an adenosine triphosphate–sensitive nitrate-potassium channel agonist, is an antianginal that has been shown to improve peak exercise capacity in patients with cardiac syndrome X, but failed to significantly improve exercise-induced ST changes.[141,142] The Rho kinase inhibitor, fasudil, has been studied in patients with chronic stable angina due to its ability to inhibit smooth muscle vasoconstriction and has been shown to increase ischemic threshold and exercise duration in these patients;[143,144] its use is currently limited to Japan and China. Phosphodiesterase inhibitors, which inhibit cGMP degradation by blocking phosphodiesterase, also have a potential role in the treatment of refractory angina, however there are no current clinical trials in microvascular patients. Phosphodiesterase inhibitors are contraindicated with nitrates and nicorandil due to hypotension. Perhexiline inhibits carnitine palmitoyltransferase and promotes greater myocardial carbohydrate utilization; it is also a vasodilatory agent with antianginal properties but is associated with neurotoxicity and hepatotoxicity at high plasma doses. Within the therapeutic range, it is an effective antianginal that also improves exercise tolerance,[145,146] but it is primarily used in Australia and New Zealand.[147,148] Trimetazidine is an agent that inhibits cardiomyocyte free fatty acid beta-oxidation and promotes glucose oxidation; this shift in metabolism reduces acidosis and also allows the ischemic cell to preserve energy.[149] Whereas it is an anti-ischemic, antianginal agent and has shown benefit in chronic stable angina,[150] results in cardiac syndrome X patients have been mixed.[151–153]

Enhanced External Counterpulsation

Enhanced external counterpulsation (EECP) is a noninvasive, Food and Drug Administration (FDA) approved treatment for management of refractory angina and consists of several sessions per week for optimal benefit. In several studies conducted in patients with CAD, EECP has been shown to improve functional capacity, anginal class, and time to ST-segment depression during exercise stress testing,[154–156] with sustained benefit reported.[157] In a report by Kronhaus et al.[158] in 30 patients with cardiac syndrome X and persistent angina, EECP therapy was effective in reducing angina as demonstrated by a reduction in Canadian Cardiovascular Society (CCS) angina and improved regional ischemia. This improvement was sustained in 87% of patients at almost 12 months. Diastolic augmentation of myocardial perfusion via inflation of pneumatic cuffs on lower extremities during EECP has been shown to improve collateral blood flow, as well as endothelial function, and a neurohormonal mechanism has been proposed.[159–161]

Stem Cell Therapy

Stem cell therapy remains experimental and has focused on patients with obstructive CAD and refractory angina[162,163] or postinfarction left ventricular dysfunction.[164] Stem cell studies have not targeted patients with angina and no obstructive CAD. However, preclinical stem cell therapy studies often consider an important treatment goal to be the restoration of impaired coronary microvascular function.[165] Microvascular rarefaction, which is defined as a reduced number of arterioles and capillaries,[166] may play a role in coronary microvascular angina[167] and may be reversed with intracoronary cardiosphere-derived cells as shown in an animal study.[168]

Cognitive Behavioral Therapy and Group Support

Cognitive behavioral therapy may be used as an adjunctive modality to treat refractory angina or for those patients who ask for nontraditional, nonpharmacologic ways to manage their angina.[15] A 2009 study showed that an 8 week program of the cognitive behavioral approach of autogenic training improved symptom frequency and severity in women with ischemia and nonobstructive coronary arteries.[169] In a study of 49 women with cardiac syndrome X, who were randomized to usual care or 12 monthly group-support meetings, group support helped reduce healthcare demands and maintained social support for these individuals.[170]

Abnormal Cardiac Nociception

In some patients with persistent chest pain, abnormal cardiac nociceptive abnormality can be the dominant cause of pain, with enhanced pain perception to stimuli. Cannon et al.[171] demonstrated that catheter manipulation in the right heart, atrial pacing, and intracoronary contrast injection reproduced chest pain in 29 out of 36 patients (81%) with no obstructive CAD. In this group, there was no relationship observed between cutaneous pain threshold testing and cardiac sensitivity. Others have also demonstrated enhanced visceral pain perception in patients with chest pain and no obstructive CAD.[172,173] It is unclear whether the enhanced pain sensitivity is due to abnormal cardiac nerve function or a problem with central pain processing.

Low-Dose Tricyclic Antidepressant Medication

Low-dose tricyclic antidepressant medication (imipramine, amitriptyline) can be used successfully in some patients with continued chest pain despite the above-mentioned therapies.[140] The mechanism of action for tricyclic medication is not yet completely understood, but it improves symptoms in patients with abnormal cardiac pain perception (nociception) and may have an effect via its modulation of norepinephrine uptake; it also has anticholinergic and α-antagonist effects, which may contribute to its analgesic effect.

Neural Modulation and Left Stellate Ganglion Blockade

Neurostimulation is an alternative treatment strategy for those with refractory angina due to abnormal cardiac nociception. The mechanism of this form of therapy is not entirely clear, but it has been found to increase resting blood flow in patients with normal coronary arteries.[174] Spinal cord stimulation is effective in reducing duration and frequency of angina; its anti-ischemic effect is likely due to reduced myocardial oxygen consumption.[175–177] Whereas it has not specifically been studied in a microvascular population with no obstructive CAD, left stellate ganglion blockade has been shown to be effective in patients with refractory angina despite multiple coronary interventions.[178,179]

Postmenopausal Hormone Therapy

The incidence of ischemic heart disease (IHD) increases after menopause, along with increased prevalence of cardiovascular risk factors such as diabetes, hypertension, and hyperlipidemia. In addition to declining estrogen levels, an altered ratio of testosterone/estrogen may contribute to increased risk. The majority of patients with CMD with no obstructive CAD are women who are of peri- or postmenopausal age, and estrogen has been implicated in the pathogenesis of microvascular dysfunction. Estrogen has beneficial effects on the vasculature as demonstrated in basic science studies,[180,181] and observational studies have suggested that hormone therapy may be of benefit in IHD.[182] Transdermal estrogen has been shown to improve coronary vascular reactivity in women with angina and no obstructive CAD,[183] and 17-β–estradiol attenuated acetylcholine-induced coronary vasoconstriction in the nonstenotic segments in women with CAD.[184]

However, in the Heart and Estrogen/Progestin Replacement Study (HERS) in 2763 postmenopausal women with coronary heart disease randomized to combination estrogen/progesterone versus placebo, there was no benefit of hormone therapy on MI or heart disease mortality, and there was an increased risk of deep venous thrombosis and pulmonary embolism. In the subsequent randomized Women's Health Initiative (WHI) trial,[185] which tested estrogen combined with progestin versus placebo, hormone therapy was associated with adverse cardiovascular outcomes. In 646 postmenopausal women suspected of ischemia who underwent coronary angiography in the WISE study, there was no independent relationship between estrogen exposure time and angiographic CAD or major outcomes.[186] In the Kronos Early Estrogen Prevention Study (KEEPS),[187] hormone therapy reduced vasomotor symptoms, but there was no difference in carotid intima-media thickness or coronary artery calcifications in women at 4 years. The route of delivery of hormone therapy may also be important, since oral estrogen is metabolized in the liver, whereas transdermal estrogens bypass first-pass metabolism. Current recommendations by the North American Menopause Society and several other organizations recommend that if hormone therapy is needed, it should be used for the shortest duration of time and for treatment of vasomotor symptoms only and not for primary CVD prevention.

CONCLUSIONS

Management of patients who have persistent angina, evidence of myocardial ischemia, and no obstructive CAD can be a treatment challenge for physicians. Cardiac syndrome X is an outdated term that is no longer used, as it is now evident that CMD plays a role in at least half of these patients. CMD is associated with adverse cardiovascular outcomes, and while it can be detected with modern invasive and imaging modalities, it remains underdiagnosed for many reasons. Invasive coronary reactivity testing can be performed in patients with recurrent symptoms to test endothelial- and nonendothelial-dependent vasomotor function, to help clarify the diagnosis of CMD, and to guide therapy. Therapeutic lifestyle change, low-dose aspirin, and lipid-lowering therapy are recommended due to the high prevalence of coronary atherosclerosis and elevated risk of adverse cardiac events. Limited evidence collected in predominantly general cardiac syndrome X patients supports the use of traditional pharmacologic antianginal, anti-ischemic medications, as well as strategies such as enhanced external counterpulsation, cognitive behavioral therapy, tricyclic medication, and neurostimulation to improve symptoms. Whereas some intermediate outcome trials in patients with ischemia and no obstructive CAD exist, large clinical outcome trials and specific guidelines are needed for patients with CMD.

References

1. Bugiardini R, Bairey Merz CN: Angina with "normal" coronary arteries: a changing philosophy, *JAMA* 293:477–484, 2005.
2. Hasdai D, Holmes Jr DR, Higano ST, Burnett Jr JC, Lerman A: Prevalence of coronary blood flow reserve abnormalities among patients with nonobstructive coronary artery disease and chest pain, *Mayo Clin Proc* 73:1133–1140, 1998.
3. Gulati M, Cooper-DeHoff RM, McClure C, et al.: Adverse cardiovascular outcomes in women with nonobstructive coronary artery disease: a report from the Women's Ischemia Syndrome Evaluation Study and the St James Women Take Heart Project, *Arch Intern Med* 169:843–850, 2009.
4. Jespersen L, Hvelplund A, Abildstrøm SZ, et al.: Stable angina pectoris with no obstructive coronary artery disease is associated with increased risks of major adverse cardiovascular events, *Eur Heart J* 33:734–744, 2012.
5. Sedlak TL, Lee M, Izadnegahdar M, et al.: Sex differences in clinical outcomes in patients with stable angina and no obstructive coronary artery disease, *Am Heart J* 166:38–44, 2013.
6. Murthy VL, Naya M, Taqueti VR, et al.: Effects of sex on coronary microvascular dysfunction and cardiac outcomes, *Circulation* 129:2518–2527, 2014.
7. Corban MT, Hung OY, Eshtehardi P, et al.: Myocardial bridging: contemporary understanding of pathophysiology with implications for diagnostic and therapeutic strategies, *J Am Coll Cardiol* 63:2346–2355, 2014.
8. Gould KL, Johnson NP, Bateman TM, et al.: Anatomic versus physiologic assessment of coronary artery disease. Role of coronary flow reserve, fractional flow reserve, and positron emission tomography imaging in revascularization decision-making, *J Am Coll Cardiol* 62:1639–1653, 2013.
9. Thomson LE, Wei J, Agarwal M, et al.: Cardiac magnetic resonance myocardial perfusion reserve index is reduced in women with coronary microvascular dysfunction. A National Heart, Lung, and Blood Institute-sponsored study from the Women's Ischemia Syndrome Evaluation, *Circ Cardiovasc Imaging* 8, 2015.
10. Shufelt CL, Thomson LEJ, Goykhman P, et al.: Cardiac magnetic resonance imaging myocardial perfusion reserve index assessment in women with microvascular coronary dysfunction and reference controls, *Cardiovasc Diagn Ther* 3:153–160, 2013.
11. Pepine CJ, Anderson RD, Sharaf BL, et al.: Coronary microvascular reactivity to adenosine predicts adverse outcome in women evaluated for suspected ischemia results from the National Heart, Lung and Blood Institute WISE (Women's Ischemia Syndrome Evaluation) study, *J Am Coll Cardiol* 55:2825–2832, 2010.
12. von Mering GO, Arant CB, Wessel TR, et al.: Abnormal coronary vasomotion as a prognostic indicator of cardiovascular events in women: results from the National Heart, Lung, and Blood Institute-Sponsored Women's Ischemia Syndrome Evaluation (WISE), *Circulation* 109:722–725, 2004.
13. Wei J, Mehta PK, Johnson BD, et al.: Safety of coronary reactivity testing in women with no obstructive coronary artery disease: results from the NHLBI-sponsored WISE (Women's Ischemia Syndrome Evaluation) study, *JACC Cardiovasc Interv* 5:646–653, 2012.
14. Beltrame JF, Crea F, Kaski JC, et al.: International standardization of diagnostic criteria for vasospastic angina, *Eur Heart J*, 2015.
15. Anderson JL, Adams CD, Antman EM, et al.: ACC/AHA 2007 guidelines for the management of patients with unstable angina/non ST-elevation myocardial infarction: a report of the American College of Cardiology/American Heart Association Task Force on Practice Guidelines (Writing Committee to Revise the 2002 Guidelines for the Management of Patients With Unstable Angina/Non ST-Elevation Myocardial Infarction): developed in collaboration with the American College of Emergency Physicians, the Society for Cardiovascular Angiography and Interventions, and the Society of Thoracic Surgeons: endorsed by the American Association of Cardiovascular and Pulmonary Rehabilitation and the Society for Academic Emergency Medicine, *Circulation* 116:e148–e304, 2007.
16. Fraker Jr TD, Fihn SD: 2002 Chronic Stable Angina Writing Committee. 2007 chronic angina focused update of the ACC/AHA 2002 Guidelines for the management of patients with chronic stable angina: a report of the American College of Cardiology/American Heart Association Task Force on Practice Guidelines Writing Group to develop the focused update of the 2002 Guidelines for the management of patients with chronic stable angina, *Circulation* 116:2762–2772, 2007.
17. Kemp Jr HG: Left ventricular function in patients with the anginal syndrome and normal coronary arteriograms, *Am J Cardiol* 32:375–376, 1973.
18. Arbogast R, Bourassa MG: Myocardial function during atrial pacing in patients with angina pectoris and normal coronary arteriograms. Comparison with patients having significant coronary artery disease, *Am J Cardiol* 32:257–263, 1973.
19. Beltrame JF: Assessing patients with myocardial infarction and nonobstructed coronary arteries (MINOCA), *J Intern Med* 273:182–185, 2013.
20. Pasupathy S, Tavella R, Beltrame JF: The what, when, who, why, how and where of Myocardial Infarction with Non-Obstructive Coronary Arteries (MINOCA), *Circ J* 80:11–16, 2015.
21. Patel MR, Chen AY, Peterson ED, et al.: Prevalence, predictors, and outcomes of patients with non-ST-segment elevation myocardial infarction and insignificant coronary artery disease: results from the Can Rapid risk stratification of Unstable angina patients Suppress ADverse outcomes with Early implementation of the ACC/AHA Guidelines (CRUSADE) initiative, *Am Heart J* 152:641–647, 2006.
22. Larsen AI, Galbraith PD, Ghali WA, et al.: Characteristics and outcomes of patients with acute myocardial infarction and angiographically normal coronary arteries, *Am J Cardiol* 95:261–263, 2005.
23. Bugiardini R, Manfrini O, De Ferrari GM: Unanswered questions for management of acute coronary syndrome: risk stratification of patients with minimal disease or normal findings on coronary angiography, *Arch Intern Med* 166:1391–1395, 2006.
24. Humphries KH, Pu A, Gao M, Carere RG, Pilote L: Angina with "normal" coronary arteries: sex differences in outcomes, *Am Heart J* 155:375–381, 2008.
25. Anderson RD, Pepine CJ: Gender differences in the treatment for acute myocardial infarction: bias or biology? *Circulation* 115:823–826, 2007.
26. Kemp HG, Kronmal RA, Vlietstra RE, Frye RL: Seven year survival of patients with normal or near normal coronary arteriograms: a CASS registry study, *J Am Coll Cardiol* 7:479–483, 1986.
27. Shaw LJ, Shaw RE, Merz CN, et al.: Impact of ethnicity and gender differences on angiographic coronary artery disease prevalence and in-hospital mortality in the American College of Cardiology-National Cardiovascular Data Registry, *Circulation* 117:1787–1801, 2008.
28. Shaw LJ, Bugiardini R, Merz CN: Women and ischemic heart disease: evolving knowledge, *J Am Coll Cardiol* 54:1561–1575, 2009.
29. Khuddus MA, Pepine CJ, Handberg EM, et al.: An intravascular ultrasound analysis in women experiencing chest pain in the absence of obstructive coronary artery disease: a substudy from the National Heart, Lung and Blood Institute–Sponsored Women's Ischemia Syndrome Evaluation (WISE), *J Interv Cardiol* 23:511–519, 2010.
30. Sullivan AK, Holdright DR, Wright CA, et al.: Chest pain in women: clinical, investigative, and prognostic features, *BMJ* 308:883–886, 1994.
31. Fihn SD, Gardin JM, Abrams J, et al.: 2012 ACCF/AHA/ACP/AATS/PCNA/SCAI/STS guideline for the diagnosis and management of patients with stable ischemic heart disease: a report of the American College of Cardiology Foundation/American Heart Association Task Force on Practice Guidelines, and the American College of Physicians, American Association for Thoracic Surgery, Preventive Cardiovascular Nurses Association, Society for Cardiovascular Angiography and Interventions, and Society of Thoracic Surgeons, *Circulation* 126:e354–e471, 2012.

31a. Davis KB, Chaitman B, Ryan T, et al.: Comparison of 15-year survival for men and women after initial medical or surgical treatment for coronary artery disease: a CASS registry study. Coronary Artery Surgery Study, *J Am Coll Cardiol* 25(5):1000–1009, 1995 Apr.

31b. Barsky AJ, Peekna HM, Borus JF: Somatic Symptom Reporting in Women and Men, *Journal of General Internal Medicine* 16(4):266–275, 2001.

31c. Alexander KP, Shaw LJ, Shaw LK, Delong ER, Mark DB, Peterson ED: Value of exercise treadmill testing in women, *J Am Coll Cardiol* 32(6):1657–1664, 1998 Nov 15. Erratum in: *J Am Coll Cardiol* 33(1):289; 1999 Jan.

31d. Hemal K, Pagidipati NJ, Coles A, et al. Sex Differences in Demographics, Risk Factors, Presentation, and Noninvasive Testing in Stable Outpatients With Suspected Coronary Artery Disease: Insights From the PROMISE Trial. *JACC Cardiovasc*

31e. Crea F, Camici PG: Bairey Merz CN. Coronary microvascular dysfunction: an update, *Eur Heart J* 35:1101–1111, 2014.

31f. Phan A, Shufelt C, Merz CN: Persistent chest pain and no obstructive coronary artery disease, *JAMA* 301(14):1468-1474; 2009 Apr 8.

32. Johnson BD, Shaw LJ, Pepine CJ, et al.: Persistent chest pain predicts cardiovascular events in women without obstructive coronary artery disease: results from the NIH-NHLBI-sponsored Women's Ischaemia Syndrome Evaluation (WISE) study, *Eur Heart J* 27:1408–1415, 2006.
33. Shaw LJ, Merz CN, Pepine CJ, et al.: The economic burden of angina in women with suspected ischemic heart disease: results from the National Institutes of Health–National Heart, Lung, and Blood Institute–sponsored Women's Ischemia Syndrome Evaluation, *Circulation* 114:894–904, 2006.
34. Beitman BD, Mukerji V, Lamberti JW, et al.: Panic disorder in patients with chest pain and angiographically normal coronary arteries, *Am J Cardiol* 63:1399–1403, 1989.
35. Vermeltfoort IA, Raijmakers PG, Odekerken DAM, et al.: Association between anxiety disorder and the extent of ischemia observed in cardiac syndrome X, *J Nucl Cardiol* 16:405–410, 2009.
36. Vaccarino V, Shah AJ, Rooks C, et al.: Sex differences in mental stress-induced myocardial ischemia in young survivors of an acute myocardial infarction, *Psychosom Med* 76:171–180, 2014.
37. Dakak N, Quyyumi AA, Eisenhofer G, Goldstein DS, Cannon 3rd RO: Sympathetically mediated effects of mental stress on the cardiac microcirculation of patients with coronary artery disease, *Am J Cardiol* 76:125–130, 1995.
38. Ramadan R, Sheps D, Esteves F, et al.: Myocardial ischemia during mental stress: role of coronary artery disease burden and vasomotion, *J Am Heart Assoc* 2:e000321, 2013. http://dx.doi.org/10.1161/JAHA.113.000321.
39. Wei J, Rooks C, Ramadan R, et al.: Meta-analysis of mental stress-induced myocardial ischemia and subsequent cardiac events in patients with coronary artery disease, *Am J Cardiol* 114:187–192, 2014.
40. Beltrame JF, Crea F, Camici P: Advances in coronary microvascular dysfunction, *Heart Lung Circ* 18:19–27, 2009.
41. Gould KL, Lipscomb K, Hamilton GW: Physiologic basis for assessing critical coronary stenosis. Instantaneous flow response and regional distribution during coronary hyperemia as measures of coronary flow reserve, *Am J Cardiol* 33:87–94, 1974.
42. Quyyumi AA, Cannon 3rd RO, Panza JA, Diodati JG, Epstein SE: Endothelial dysfunction in patients with chest pain and normal coronary arteries, *Circulation* 86:1864–1871, 1992.
43. Mian Z, Wei J, Bharadwaj M, et al.: Prior myocardial infarction is associated with coronary endothelial dysfunction in women with signs and symptoms of ischemia and no obstructive coronary artery disease, *Int J Cardiol* 207:137–139, 2016.
44. Yahagi K, Davis HR, Arbustini E, Virmani R: Sex differences in coronary artery disease: pathological observations, *Atherosclerosis* 239:260–267, 2015.
45. Falk E, Nakano M, Bentzon JF, Finn AV, Virmani R: Update on acute coronary syndromes: the pathologists' view, *Eur Heart J* 34:719–728, 2013.
46. Mohandas R, Sautina L, Li S, et al.: Number and function of bone-marrow derived angiogenic cells and coronary flow reserve in women without obstructive coronary artery disease: a substudy of the NHLBI-sponsored Women's Ischemia Syndrome Evaluation (WISE), *PLoS One* 8:e81595, 2013. http://dx.doi.org/10.1371/journal.pone.0081595.

47. Khaliq A, Johnson BD, Anderson RD, et al.: Relationships between components of metabolic syndrome and coronary intravascular ultrasound atherosclerosis measures in women without obstructive coronary artery disease: the NHLBI-Sponsored Women's Ischemia Syndrome Evaluation Study, *Cardiovasc Endocrinol* 4:45–52, 2015.
48. Adamopoulos S, Rosano GMC, Ponikowski P, et al.: Impaired baroreflex sensitivity and sympathovagal balance in syndrome X, *Am J Cardiol* 82:862–868, 1998.
49. Gulli G, Cemin R, Pancera P, et al.: Evidence of parasympathetic impairment in some patients with cardiac syndrome X, *Cardiovasc Res* 52:208–216, 2001.
50. Lanza GA, Giordano A, Pristipino C, et al.: Abnormal cardiac adrenergic nerve function in patients with syndrome X detected by [123I]metaiodobenzylguanidine myocardial scintigraphy, *Circulation* 96:821–826, 1997.
51. Arrebola-Moreno AL, Arrebola JP, Moral-Ruiz A, et al.: Coronary microvascular spasm triggers transient ischemic left ventricular diastolic abnormalities in patients with chest pain and angiographically normal coronary arteries, *Atherosclerosis* 236:207–214, 2014.
51a. Wei J, Mehta PK, Shufelt C, et al.: Diastolic dysfunction measured by cardiac magnetic resonance imaging in women with signs and symptoms of ischemia but no obstructive coronary artery disease, *Int J Cardiol* 220:775–780, 2016 Oct 1.
52. Wei J, Nelson MD, Szczepaniak EW, et al.: Myocardial steatosis as a possible mechanistic link between diastolic dysfunction and coronary microvascular dysfunction in women, *Am J Physiol Heart Circ Physiol* 310:H14–H19, 2016.
53. Montalescot G, Sechtem U, Achenbach S, et al.: 2013 ESC guidelines on the management of stable coronary artery disease: the Task Force on the management of stable coronary artery disease of the European Society of Cardiology, *Eur Heart J* 34:2949–3003, 2013.
54. Fihn SD, Blankenship JC, Alexander KP, et al.: 2014 ACC/AHA/AATS/PCNA/SCAI/STS focused update of the guideline for the diagnosis and management of patients with stable ischemic heart disease: a report of the American College of Cardiology/American Heart Association Task Force on Practice Guidelines, and the American Association for Thoracic Surgery, Preventive Cardiovascular Nurses Association, Society for Cardiovascular Angiography and Interventions, and Society of Thoracic Surgeons, *Circulation* 130:1749–1767, 2014.
55. Cortigiani L, Rigo F, Gherardi S, et al.: Prognostic implications of coronary flow reserve on left anterior descending coronary artery in hypertrophic cardiomyopathy, *Am J Cardiol* 102:1718–1723, 2008.
56. Sharkey SW, Maron BJ: Epidemiology and clinical profile of Takotsubo cardiomyopathy, *Circ J* 78:2119–2128, 2014.
57. Eitel I, von Knobelsdorff-Brenkenhoff F, Bernhardt P, et al.: Clinical characteristics and cardiovascular magnetic resonance findings in stress (takotsubo) cardiomyopathy, *JAMA* 306:277–286, 2011.
58. Pelliccia F, Parodi G, Greco C, et al.: Comorbidities frequency in Takotsubo syndrome: an international collaborative systematic review including 1109 patients, *Am J Med* 128(654):e11–e19, 2015.
59. Patel SM, Lerman A, Lennon RJ, Prasad A: Impaired coronary microvascular reactivity in women with apical ballooning syndrome (Takotsubo/stress cardiomyopathy), *Eur Heart J Acute Cardiovasc Care* 2:147–152, 2013.
60. Scantlebury DC, Prasad A, Rabinstein AA, Best PJ: Prevalence of migraine and Raynaud phenomenon in women with apical ballooning syndrome (Takotsubo or stress cardiomyopathy), *Am J Cardiol* 111:1284–1288, 2013.
61. Beltrame JF, Limaye SD, Horowitz JD: The coronary slow flow phenomenon—a new coronary microvascular disorder, *Cardiology* 97:197–202, 2002.
62. Gibson CM, Cannon CP, Daley WL, et al.: TIMI frame count: a quantitative method of assessing coronary artery flow, *Circulation* 93:879–888, 1996.
63. Yaymaci B, Dagdelen S, Bozbuga N, et al.: The response of the myocardial metabolism to atrial pacing in patients with coronary slow flow, *Int J Cardiol* 78:151–156, 2001.
64. Mosseri M, Yarom R, Gotsman MS, Hasin Y: Histologic evidence for small-vessel coronary artery disease in patients with angina pectoris and patent large coronary arteries, *Circulation* 74:964–972, 1986.
65. Petersen JW, Johnson BD, Kip KE, et al.: TIMI frame count and adverse events in women with no obstructive coronary disease: a pilot study from the NHLBI-sponsored Women's Ischemia Syndrome Evaluation (WISE), *PLoS One* 9:e96630, 2014. http://dx.doi.org/10.1371/journal.pone.0096630.
66. Mangieri E, Macchiarelli G, Ciavolella M, et al.: Slow coronary flow: clinical and histopathological features in patients with otherwise normal epicardial coronary arteries, *Cathet Cardiovasc Diagn* 37:375–381, 1996.
67. Kurtoglu N, Akcay A, Dindar I: Usefulness of oral dipyridamole therapy for angiographic slow coronary artery flow, *Am J Cardiol* 87:777–779, 2001. A8.
68. Beltrame JF, Turner SP, Leslie SL, et al.: The angiographic and clinical benefits of mibefradil in the coronary slow flow phenomenon, *J Am Coll Cardiol* 44:57–62, 2004.
69. Reis SE, Holubkov R, Conrad Smith AJ, et al.: Coronary microvascular dysfunction is highly prevalent in women with chest pain in the absence of coronary artery disease: results from the NHLBI WISE study, *Am Heart J* 141:735–741, 2001.
70. Petersen JW, Mehta PK, Kenkre TS, et al.: Comparison of low and high dose intracoronary adenosine and acetylcholine in women undergoing coronary reactivity testing: results from the NHLBI-sponsored Women's Ischemia Syndrome Evaluation (WISE), *Int J Cardiol* 172:e114–e115, 2014.
71. van de Hoef TP, Echavarría-Pinto M, van Lavieren MA, et al.: Diagnostic and prognostic implications of coronary flow capacity: a comprehensive cross-modality physiological concept in ischemic heart disease, *JACC Cardiovasc Interv* 8:1670–1680, 2015.
72. Ong P, Athanasiadis A, Borgulya G, Voehringer M, Sechtem U: 3-year follow-up of patients with coronary artery spasm as cause of acute coronary syndrome: the CASPAR (coronary artery spasm in patients with acute coronary syndrome) study follow-up, *J Am Coll Cardiol* 57:147–152, 2011.
73. Ong P, Athanasiadis A, Borgulya G, et al.: Clinical usefulness, angiographic characteristics, and safety evaluation of intracoronary acetylcholine provocation testing among 921 consecutive white patients with unobstructed coronary arteries, *Circulation* 129:1723–1730, 2014.
74. Mieres JH, Gulati M, Bairey Merz N, et al.: Role of noninvasive testing in the clinical evaluation of women with suspected ischemic heart disease: a consensus statement from the American Heart Association, *Circulation* 130:350–379, 2014.
75. Ahmari SA, Bunch TJ, Modesto K, et al.: Impact of individual and cumulative coronary risk factors on coronary flow reserve assessed by dobutamine stress echocardiography, *Am J Cardiol* 101:1694–1699, 2008.
76. Cortigiani L, Rigo F, Gherardi S, et al.: Prognostic effect of coronary flow reserve in women versus men with chest pain syndrome and normal dipyridamole stress echocardiography, *Am J Cardiol* 106:1703–1708, 2010.
77. Kaul S: Myocardial contrast echocardiography: a 25-year retrospective, *Circulation* 118:291–308, 2008.
78. Thomas JD: Myocardial contrast echocardiography perfusion imaging: still waiting after all these years, *J Am Coll Cardiol* 62:1362–1364, 2013.
79. Vogel R, Indermühle A, Reinhardt J, et al.: The quantification of absolute myocardial perfusion in humans by contrast echocardiography: algorithm and validation, *J Am Coll Cardiol* 45:754–762, 2005.
80. Galiuto L, Sestito A, Barchetta S, et al.: Noninvasive evaluation of flow reserve in the left anterior descending coronary artery in patients with cardiac syndrome X, *Am J Cardiol* 99:1378–1383, 2007.
81. Chow BJ, Dorbala S, Di Carli MF, et al.: Prognostic value of PET myocardial perfusion imaging in obese patients, *JACC Cardiovasc Imaging* 7:278–287, 2014.
82. Nakazato R, Heo R, Leipsic J, Min JK: CFR and FFR assessment with PET and CTA: strengths and limitations, *Curr Cardiol Rep* 16:484, 2014.
83. Beller GA: Enhanced risk stratification with noninvasive measurement of coronary flow reserve using positron emission tomography, *Circulation* 126:1808–1811, 2012.
84. Murthy VL, Naya M, Foster CR, et al.: Improved cardiac risk assessment with noninvasive measures of coronary flow reserve, *Circulation* 124:2215–2224, 2011.
85. Naya M, Murthy VL, Blankstein R, et al.: Quantitative relationship between the extent and morphology of coronary atherosclerotic plaque and downstream myocardial perfusion, *J Am Coll Cardiol* 58:1807–1816, 2011.
86. Recio-Mayoral A, Mason JC, Kaski JC, et al.: Chronic inflammation and coronary microvascular dysfunction in patients without risk factors for coronary artery disease, *Eur Heart J* 30:1837–1843, 2009.
87. Johnson BD, Shaw LJ, Buchthal SD, et al.: Prognosis in women with myocardial ischemia in the absence of obstructive coronary disease: results from the National Institutes of Health-National Heart, Lung, and Blood Institute-Sponsored Women's Ischemia Syndrome Evaluation (WISE), *Circulation* 109:2993–2999, 2004.
88. Greenwood JP, Maredia N, Younger JF, et al.: Cardiovascular magnetic resonance and single-photon emission computed tomography for diagnosis of coronary heart disease (CE-MARC): a prospective trial, *Lancet* 379:453–460, 2012.
89. Panting JR, Gatehouse PD, Yang G-Z, et al.: Abnormal subendocardial perfusion in cardiac syndrome X detected by cardiovascular magnetic resonance imaging, *N Engl J Med* 346:1948–1953, 2002.
90. Lanza GA, Buffon A, Sestito A, et al.: Relation between stress-induced myocardial perfusion defects on cardiovascular magnetic resonance and coronary microvascular dysfunction in patients with cardiac syndrome X, *J Am Coll Cardiol* 51:466–472, 2008.
91. Pilz G, Klos M, Ali E, et al.: Angiographic correlations of patients with small vessel disease diagnosed by adenosine-stress cardiac magnetic resonance imaging, *J Cardiovasc Magn Reson* 10(8), 2008.
92. Reynolds HR, Srichai MB, Iqbal SN, et al.: Mechanisms of myocardial infarction in women without angiographically obstructive coronary artery disease, *Circulation* 124:1414–1425, 2011.
93. Motwani M, Jogiya R, Kozerke S, Greenwood JP, Plein S: Advanced cardiovascular magnetic resonance myocardial perfusion imaging: high-spatial resolution versus 3-dimensional whole-heart coverage, *Circ Cardiovasc Imaging* 6:339–348, 2013.
94. Goykhman P, Mehta PK, Agarwal M, et al.: Reproducibility of myocardial perfusion reserve - variations in measurements from post processing using commercially available software, *Cardiovasc Diagn Ther* 2:268–277, 2012.
95. Hsu LY, Groves DW, Aletras AH, Kellman P, Arai AE: A quantitative pixel-wise measurement of myocardial blood flow by contrast-enhanced first-pass CMR perfusion imaging: microsphere validation in dogs and feasibility study in humans, *JACC Cardiovasc Imaging* 5:154–166, 2012.
96. Bairey Merz CN, Handberg EM, Shufelt CL, et al.: A randomized, placebo-controlled trial of late Na current inhibition (ranolazine) in coronary microvascular dysfunction (CMD): impact on angina and myocardial perfusion reserve, *Eur Heart J* 37:1504–1513, 2015.
97. Motwani M, Kidambi A, Uddin A, et al.: Quantification of myocardial blood flow with cardiovascular magnetic resonance throughout the cardiac cycle, *J Cardiovasc Magn Reson* 17(4), 2015.
98. Eriksson BE, Tyni-Lennè R, Svedenhag J, et al.: Physical training in Syndrome X: physical training counteracts deconditioning and pain in Syndrome X, *J Am Coll Cardiol* 36:1619 1625, 2000.
99. Hambrecht R, Wolf A, Gielen S, et al.: Effect of exercise on coronary endothelial function in patients with coronary artery disease, *N Engl J Med* 342:454–460, 2000.
100. Lee BC, Chen SY, Hsu HC, et al.: Effect of cardiac rehabilitation on myocardial perfusion reserve in postinfarction patients, *Am J Cardiol* 101:1395–1402, 2008.
101. Olsen RH, Pedersen LR, Jürs A, et al.: A randomised trial comparing the effect of exercise training and weight loss on microvascular function in coronary artery disease, *Int J Cardiol* 185:229–235, 2015.
102. Pizzi C, Manfrini O, Fontana F, Bugiardini R: Angiotensin-converting enzyme inhibitors and 3-hydroxy-3-methylglutaryl coenzyme A reductase in cardiac syndrome X: role of superoxide dismutase activity, *Circulation* 109:53–58, 2004.
103. Fabian E, Varga A, Picano E, et al.: Effect of simvastatin on endothelial function in cardiac syndrome X patients, *Am J Cardiol* 94:652–655, 2004.
104. Stone NJ, Robinson JG, Lichtenstein AH, et al.: 2013 ACC/AHA guideline on the treatment of blood cholesterol to reduce atherosclerotic cardiovascular risk in adults: a report of the American College of Cardiology/American Heart Association Task Force on Practice Guidelines, *J Am Coll Cardiol* 63:2889–2934, 2014.
105. Cannon CP, Blazing MA, Giugliano RP, et al.: Ezetimibe added to statin therapy after acute coronary syndromes, *N Engl J Med* 372:2387–2397, 2015.
106. Robinson JG, Farnier M, Krempf M, et al.: Efficacy and safety of alirocumab in reducing lipids and cardiovascular events, *N Engl J Med* 372:1489–1499, 2015.
107. Sabatine MS, Giugliano RP, Wiviott SD, et al.: Efficacy and safety of evolocumab in reducing lipids and cardiovascular events, *N Engl J Med* 372:1500–1509, 2015.
108. Bugiardini R, Borghi A, Biagetti L, Puddu P: Comparison of verapamil versus propranolol therapy in syndrome X, *Am J Cardiol* 63:286–290, 1989.
109. Lanza GA, Colonna G, Pasceri V, Maseri A: Atenolol versus amlodipine versus isosorbide-5-mononitrate on anginal symptoms in syndrome X, *Am J Cardiol* 84:854–856, 1999. A8.
110. Kalinowski L, Dobrucki LW, Szczepanska-Konkel M, et al.: Third-generation beta-blockers stimulate nitric oxide release from endothelial cells through ATP efflux: a novel mechanism for antihypertensive action, *Circulation* 107:2747–2752, 2003.
111. Erdamar H, Sen N, Tavil Y, et al.: The effect of nebivolol treatment on oxidative stress and antioxidant status in patients with cardiac syndrome-X, *Coron Artery Dis* 20:238–244, 2009.
112. Sugioka K, Hozumi T, Takemoto Y, et al.: Early recovery of impaired coronary flow reserve by carvedilol therapy in patients with idiopathic dilated cardiomyopathy: a serial transthoracic Doppler echocardiographic study, *J Am Coll Cardiol* 45:318–319, 2005.
113. Xiaozhen H, Yun Z, Mei Z, Yu S: Effect of carvedilol on coronary flow reserve in patients with hypertensive left-ventricular hypertrophy, *Blood Press* 19:40–47, 2010.
114. Togni M, Vigorito F, Windecker S, et al.: Does the beta-blocker nebivolol increase coronary flow reserve? *Cardiovasc Drugs Ther* 21:99–108, 2007.
115. Hung OY, Molony D, Corban MT, et al.: Comprehensive assessment of coronary plaque progression with advanced intravascular imaging, physiological measures, and wall shear stress: a pilot double-blinded randomized controlled clinical trial of nebivolol versus atenolol in nonobstructive coronary artery disease, *J Am Heart Assoc* 5:e002764, 2016. http://dx.doi.org/10.1161/JAHA.115.002764.
116. Chen JW, Hsu NW, Wu TC, Lin SJ, Chang MS: Long-term angiotensin-converting enzyme inhibition reduces plasma asymmetric dimethylarginine and improves endothelial nitric oxide bioavailability and coronary microvascular function in patients with syndrome X, *Am J Cardiol* 90:974–982, 2002.
117. Pauly DF, Johnson BD, Anderson RD, et al.: In women with symptoms of cardiac ischemia, nonobstructive coronary arteries, and microvascular dysfunction, angiotensin-converting enzyme inhibition is associated with improved microvascular function: a double-blind randomized study from the National Heart, Lung and Blood Institute Women's Ischemia Syndrome Evaluation (WISE), *Am Heart J* 162:678–684, 2011.
118. Bavry AA, Handberg EM, Huo T, et al.: Aldosterone inhibition and coronary endothelial function in women without obstructive coronary artery disease: an ancillary study of the National Heart, Lung, and Blood Institute-sponsored Women's Ischemia Syndrome Evaluation, *Am Heart J* 167:826–832, 2014.

119. Lerman A, Burnett Jr JC, Higano ST, McKinley LJ, Holmes Jr DR: Long-term L-arginine supplementation improves small-vessel coronary endothelial function in humans, *Circulation* 97:2123–2128, 1998.
120. Glueck CJ, Valdes A, Bowe D, Munsif S, Wang P: The endothelial nitric oxide synthase T-786c mutation, a treatable etiology of Prinzmetal's angina, *Transl Res* 162:64–66, 2013.
121. Kaski JC, Rosano GM, Collins P, et al.: Cardiac syndrome X: clinical characteristics and left ventricular function. Long-term follow-up study, *J Am Coll Cardiol* 25:807–814, 1995.
122. Stone PH: Calcium antagonists for Prinzmetal's variant angina, unstable angina and silent myocardial ischemia: therapeutic tool and probe for identification of pathophysiologic mechanisms, *Am J Cardiol* 59:101B–115B, 1987.
123. Parodi O, Simonetti I, Michelassi C, et al.: Comparison of verapamil and propranolol therapy for angina pectoris at rest: a randomized, multiple-crossover, controlled trial in the coronary care unit, *Am J Cardiol* 57:899–906, 1986.
124. Pepine CJ, Feldman RL, Whittle J, Curry RC, Conti CR: Effect of diltiazem in patients with variant angina: a randomized double-blind trial, *Am Heart J* 101:719–725, 1981.
125. Yasue H, Omote S, Takizawa A, et al.: Exertional angina pectoris caused by coronary arterial spasm: effects of various drugs, *Am J Cardiol* 43:647–652, 1979.
126. Cannon 3rd RO, Watson RM, Rosing DR, Epstein SE: Efficacy of calcium channel blocker therapy for angina pectoris resulting from small-vessel coronary artery disease and abnormal vasodilator reserve, *Am J Cardiol* 56:242–246, 1985.
127. Ozcelik F, Altun A, Ozbay G: Antianginal and anti-ischemic effects of nisoldipine and ramipril in patients with syndrome X, *Clin Cardiol* 22:361–365, 1999.
128. Sutsch G, Oechslin E, Mayer I, Hess OM: Effect of diltiazem on coronary flow reserve in patients with microvascular angina, *Int J Cardiol* 52:135–143, 1995.
129. Chaitman BR: Ranolazine for the treatment of chronic angina and potential use in other cardiovascular conditions, *Circulation* 113:2462–2472, 2006.
130. Chaitman BR, Pepine CJ, Parker JO, et al.: Effects of ranolazine with atenolol, amlodipine, or diltiazem on exercise tolerance and angina frequency in patients with severe chronic angina: a randomized controlled trial, *JAMA* 291:309–316, 2004.
131. Stone PH, Gratsiansky NA, Blokhin A, et al.: Antianginal efficacy of ranolazine when added to treatment with amlodipine: the ERICA (Efficacy of Ranolazine in Chronic Angina) trial, *J Am Coll Cardiol* 48:566–575, 2006.
132. Mehta PK, Goykhman P, Thomson LE, et al.: Ranolazine improves angina in women with evidence of myocardial ischemia but no obstructive coronary artery disease, *JACC Cardiovasc Imaging* 4:514–522, 2011.
133. Sulfi S, Timmis AD: Ivabradine–the first selective sinus node I(f) channel inhibitor in the treatment of stable angina, *Int J Clin Pract* 60:222–228, 2006.
134. Fox K, Ford I, Steg PG, et al.: Ivabradine for patients with stable coronary artery disease and left-ventricular systolic dysfunction (BEAUTIFUL): a randomised, double-blind, placebo-controlled trial, *Lancet* 372:807–816, 2008.
135. Swedberg K, Komajda M, Böhm M, et al.: Ivabradine and outcomes in chronic heart failure (SHIFT): a randomised placebo-controlled study, *Lancet* 376:875–885, 2010.
136. Tardif JC, Ford I, Tendera M, et al.: Efficacy of ivabradine, a new selective I(f) inhibitor, compared with atenolol in patients with chronic stable angina, *Eur Heart J* 26:2529–2536, 2005.
137. Rosen SD, Lorenzoni R, Kaski JC, Foale RA, Camici PG: Effect of alpha1-adrenoceptor blockade on coronary vasodilator reserve in cardiac syndrome X, *J Cardiovasc Pharmacol* 34:554–560, 1999.
138. Botker HE, Sonne HS, Schmitz O, Nielsen TT: Effects of doxazosin on exercise-induced angina pectoris, ST-segment depression, and insulin sensitivity in patients with syndrome X, *Am J Cardiol* 82:1352–1356, 1998.
139. Emdin M, Picano E, Lattanzi F, L'Abbate A: Improved exercise capacity with acute aminophylline administration in patients with syndrome X, *J Am Coll Cardiol* 14:1450–1453, 1989.
140. Cannon 3rd RO, Quyyumi AA, Mincemoyer R, et al.: Imipramine in patients with chest pain despite normal coronary angiograms, *N Engl J Med* 330:1411–1417, 1994.
141. Hongo M, Takenaka H, Uchikawa S, et al.: Coronary microvascular response to intracoronary administration of nicorandil, *Am J Cardiol* 75:246–250, 1995.
142. Chen JW, Lee WL, Hsu NW, et al.: Effects of short-term treatment of nicorandil on exercise-induced myocardial ischemia and abnormal cardiac autonomic activity in microvascular angina, *Am J Cardiol* 80:32–38, 1997.
143. Vicari RM, Chaitman B, Keefe D, et al.: Efficacy and safety of fasudil in patients with stable angina: a double-blind, placebo-controlled, phase 2 trial, *J Am Coll Cardiol* 46:1803–1811, 2005.
144. Fukumoto Y, Mohri M, Inokuchi K, et al.: Anti-ischemic effects of fasudil, a specific Rho-kinase inhibitor, in patients with stable effort angina, *J Cardiovasc Pharmacol* 49:117–121, 2007.
145. White HD, Lowe JB: Antianginal efficacy of perhexiline maleate in patients refractory to beta-adrenoreceptor blockade, *Int J Cardiol* 3:145–155, 1983.
146. Cole PL, Beamer AD, McGowan N, et al.: Efficacy and safety of perhexiline maleate in refractory angina. A double-blind placebo-controlled clinical trial of a novel antianginal agent, *Circulation* 81:1260–1270, 1990.
147. Lee L, Horowitz J, Frenneaux M: Metabolic manipulation in ischaemic heart disease, a novel approach to treatment, *Eur Heart J* 25:634–641, 2004.
148. Ashrafian H, Horowitz JD, Frenneaux MP: Perhexiline, *Cardiovasc Drug Rev* 25:76–97, 2007.
149. Kantor PF, Lucien A, Kozak R, Lopaschuk GD: The antianginal drug trimetazidine shifts cardiac energy metabolism from fatty acid oxidation to glucose oxidation by inhibiting mitochondrial long-chain 3-ketoacyl coenzyme A thiolase, *Circ Res* 86:580–588, 2000.
150. Peng S, Zhao M, Wan J, et al.: The efficacy of trimetazidine on stable angina pectoris: a meta-analysis of randomized clinical trials, *Int J Cardiol* 177:780–785, 2014.
151. Rogacka D, Guzik P, Wykretowicz A, et al.: Effects of trimetazidine on clinical symptoms and tolerance of exercise of patients with syndrome X: a preliminary study, *Coron Artery Dis* 11:171–177, 2000.
152. Nalbantgil S, Altintig A, Yilmaz H, et al.: The effect of trimetazidine in the treatment of microvascular angina, *Int J Angiol* 8:40–43, 1999.
153. Leonardo F, Fragasso G, Rossetti E, et al.: Comparison of trimetazidine with atenolol in patients with syndrome X: effects on diastolic function and exercise tolerance, *Cardiologia* 44:1065–1069, 1999.
154. Stys TP, Lawson WE, Hui JCK, et al.: Effects of enhanced external counterpulsation on stress radionuclide coronary perfusion and exercise capacity in chronic stable angina pectoris, *Am J Cardiol* 89:822–824, 2002.
155. Arora RR, Chou TM, Jain D, et al.: The multicenter study of enhanced external counterpulsation (MUST-EECP): effect of EECP on exercise-induced myocardial ischemia and anginal episodes, *J Am Coll Cardiol* 33:1833–1840, 1999.
156. Urano H, Ikeda H, Ueno T, et al.: Enhanced external counterpulsation improves exercise tolerance, reduces exercise-induced myocardial ischemia and improves left ventricular diastolic filling in patients with coronary artery disease, *J Am Coll Cardiol* 37:93–99, 2001.
157. Lawson WE, Hui JCK, Zheng ZS, et al.: Three-year sustained benefit from enhanced external counterpulsation in chronic angina pectoris, *Am J Cardiol* 75:840–841, 1995.
158. Kronhaus KD, Lawson WE: Enhanced external counterpulsation is an effective treatment for syndrome X, *Int J Cardiol* 135:256–257, 2009.
159. Beck DT, Martin JS, Casey DP, et al.: Enhanced external counterpulsation improves endothelial function and exercise capacity in patients with ischaemic left ventricular dysfunction, *Clin Exp Pharmacol Physiol* 41:628–636, 2014.
160. Loh PH, Cleland JG, Louis AA, et al.: Enhanced external counterpulsation in the treatment of chronic refractory angina: a long-term follow-up outcome from the International Enhanced External Counterpulsation Patient Registry, *Clin Cardiol* 31:159–164, 2008.
161. Lawson WE, Barsness G, Michaels AD, et al.: Effectiveness of repeat enhanced external counterpulsation for refractory angina in patients failing to complete an initial course of therapy, *Cardiology* 108:170–175, 2007.
162. Losordo DW, Schatz RA, White CJ, et al.: Intramyocardial transplantation of autologous CD34+ stem cells for intractable angina: a phase I/IIa double-blind, randomized controlled trial, *Circulation* 115:3165–3172, 2007.
163. van Ramshorst J, Bax JJ, Beeres SL, et al.: Intramyocardial bone marrow cell injection for chronic myocardial ischemia: a randomized controlled trial, *JAMA* 301:1997–2004, 2009.
164. Malliaras K, Makkar RR, Smith RR, et al.: Intracoronary cardiosphere-derived cells after myocardial infarction: evidence of therapeutic regeneration in the final 1-year results of the CADUCEUS trial (CArdiosphere-Derived aUtologous stem CElls to reverse ventricUlar dySfunction), *J Am Coll Cardiol* 63:110–122, 2014.
165. Kanazawa H, Tseliou E, Malliaras K, et al.: Cellular postconditioning: allogeneic cardiosphere-derived cells reduce infarct size and attenuate microvascular obstruction when administered after reperfusion in pigs with acute myocardial infarction, *Circ Heart Fail* 8:322–332, 2015.
166. Antonios TF, Singer DR, Markandu ND, Mortimer PS, MacGregor GA: Structural skin capillary rarefaction in essential hypertension, *Hypertension* 33:998–1001, 1999.
167. Pries AR, Badimon L, Bugiardini R, et al.: Coronary vascular regulation, remodelling, and collateralization: mechanisms and clinical implications on behalf of the working group on coronary pathophysiology and microcirculation, *Eur Heart J* 36:3134–3146, 2015.
168. Gallet R, de Couto G, Simsolo E, et al.: Cardiosphere-derived cells reverse heart failure with preserved ejection fraction (HFpEF) in rats by decreasing fibrosis and inflammation, *J Am Coll Cardiol: basic to Translational Science* 1:14–28, 2016.
169. Asbury EA, Kanji N, Ernst E, Barbir M, Collins P: Autogenic training to manage symptomology in women with chest pain and normal coronary arteries, *Menopause* 16:60–65, 2009.
170. Asbury EA, Webb CM, Collins P: Group support to improve psychosocial well-being and primary-care demands among women with cardiac syndrome X, *Climacteric* 14:100–104, 2011.
171. Cannon 3rd RO, Quyyumi AA, Schenke WH, et al.: Abnormal cardiac sensitivity in patients with chest pain and normal coronary arteries, *J Am Coll Cardiol* 16:1359–1366, 1990.
172. Chauhan A, Mullins PA, Thuraisingham SI, et al.: Abnormal cardiac pain perception in syndrome X, *J Am Coll Cardiol* 24:329–335, 1994.
173. Pasceri V, Lanza GA, Buffon A, et al.: Role of abnormal pain sensitivity and behavioral factors in determining chest pain in syndrome X, *J Am Coll Cardiol* 31:62–66, 1998.
174. Chauhan A, Mullins PA, Thuraisingham SI, et al.: Effect of transcutaneous electrical nerve stimulation on coronary blood flow, *Circulation* 89:694–702, 1994.
175. Lanza GA, Sestito A, Sgueglia GA, et al.: Effect of spinal cord stimulation on spontaneous and stress-induced angina and "ischemia-like" ST-segment depression in patients with cardiac syndrome X, *Eur Heart J* 26:983–989, 2005.
176. Borjesson M, Andrell P, Mannheimer C: Spinal cord stimulation for long-term treatment of severe angina pectoris: what does the evidence say? *Future Cardiol* 7:825–833, 2011.
177. Odenstedt J, Linderoth B, Bergfeldt L, et al.: Spinal cord stimulation effects on myocardial ischemia, infarct size, ventricular arrhythmia, and noninvasive electrophysiology in a porcine ischemia-reperfusion model, *Heart Rhythm* 8:892–898, 2011.
178. Chester M, Hammond C, Leach A: Long-term benefits of stellate ganglion block in severe chronic refractory angina, *Pain* 87:103–105, 2000.
179. Wiener L, Cox JW: Influence of stellate ganglion block on angina pectoris and the post-exercise electrocardiogram, *Am J Med Sci* 252:289–295, 1966.
180. Sudhir K, Jennings GL, Funder JW, Komesaroff PA: Estrogen enhances basal nitric oxide release in the forearm vasculature in perimenopausal women, *Hypertension* 28:330–334, 1996.
181. Haynes MP, Russell KS, Bender JR: Molecular mechanisms of estrogen actions on the vasculature, *J Nucl Cardiol* 7:500–508, 2000.
182. Grodstein F, Stampfer M: The epidemiology of coronary heart disease and estrogen replacement in postmenopausal women, *Prog Cardiovasc Dis* 38:199–210, 1995.
183. Roqué M, Heras M, Roig E, et al.: Short-term effects of transdermal estrogen replacement therapy on coronary vascular reactivity in postmenopausal women with angina pectoris and normal results on coronary angiograms, *J Am Coll Cardiol* 31:139–143, 1998.
184. Collins P, Rosano GM, Sarrel PM, et al.: 17 beta-Estradiol attenuates acetylcholine-induced coronary arterial constriction in women but not men with coronary heart disease, *Circulation* 92:24–30, 1995.
185. Manson JE, Hsia J, Johnson KC, et al.: Estrogen plus progestin and the risk of coronary heart disease, *N Engl J Med* 349:523–534, 2003.
186. Merz CN, Johnson BD, Berga SL, et al.: Total estrogen time and obstructive coronary disease in women: insights from the NHLBI-sponsored Women's Ischemia Syndrome Evaluation (WISE), *J Womens Health (Larchmt)* 18:1315–1322, 2009.
187. Wolff EF, He Y, Black DM, et al.: Self-reported menopausal symptoms, coronary artery calcification, and carotid intima-media thickness in recently menopausal women screened for the Kronos early estrogen prevention study (KEEPS), *Fertil Steril* 99:1385–1391, 2013.

26 Depression, Anxiety, and Stress

Lauren Wasson, Obi Emeruwa, and Karina W. Davidson

INTRODUCTION

Many patients with chronic coronary heart disease (CHD) have clinically significant depression: a costly, disease-accelerating comorbidity that is associated with compromised health-related quality of life and reduced quality-adjusted life years (QALYs). Depression is also associated with an increased risk of recurrent acute coronary syndrome (ACS) events, doubled all-cause mortality, and larger healthcare costs. Many of these patients also have clinically significant anxiety and stress. Given these observational data, many advisory and professional societies have suggested screening patients with CHD for negative emotions and providing comprehensive treatment if clinical levels of distress are detected.

The overarching goal of this chapter is to provide cardiologists with the state-of-the-art evidence for the aforementioned assertions and provide practical advice on screening, counseling, and treating depression, anxiety, and stress in patients with CHD. We begin by providing an overview of the professional guidelines and advisories on this topic. We then discuss the evidence on the epidemiology, screening, and treatment of these negative emotions in CHD patients. We end by providing some context for the current debates among scientists, practitioners, and professional organizations on the usefulness of managing negative emotions in CHD patients.[1]

Few cardiologists and other healthcare providers have implemented the recommendations to screen all patients with CHD for depression, anxiety, and stress, and treat these conditions if they are found.[2,3] The top barriers in the implementation of these recommendations include lack of time to assess and manage depression, insufficient depression education networks, and lack of evidence from randomized controlled trials (RCTs) to support these recommendations.[4,5] Yet, mandatory universal screening of depression in patients with CHD (or any patient) is recommended. As of 2014, the National Quality Forum introduced universal depression screening as a quality metric for all patients with a health encounter[6]; successful depression management at 6 and 12 months are quality metrics that will take effect in the near future. Thus, in the United States, patients with CHD will soon require screening for depression, and, if they are found to have clinically impairing depression, they will need to be followed up. With these changes looming in the United States and many other parts of the world, we provide an overview of the science, tools, and controversies on this topic.

PROFESSIONAL SOCIETY GUIDELINES/ ADVISORIES/STATEMENTS

Depression

The strength of observational findings linking depression to CHD outcomes has led many professional societies to advise routine depression screening for CHD patients and referral for treatment if indicated. However, it is important to note that there are no RCTs on this subject to inform these recommendations. Furthermore, although RCTs have shown that treatment can improve depression in some instances, it has not been clearly shown to lead to improved CHD outcomes.[7]

American Heart Association

In 2008, the American Heart Association (AHA) issued a science advisory endorsed by the American Psychiatric Association (APA) that recommended administering a depression screening questionnaire to ACS patients and referring those who screen positive to a professional qualified to diagnose and manage depression according to the algorithm in Fig. 26.1.[8] Boxes 26.1 and 26.2 detail the recommended screening questionnaires.[8,9] The United States Preventative Services Task Force (USPSTF) and AHA/APA guidelines recommend the Patient Health Questionnaire-2 (PHQ-2) yes/no version as the initial screen, as it has been validated as more sensitive and easier to administer than the PHQ-2 multiple choice screening questionnaire.[9] This advisory effectively expanded the scope of the previous year's release of evidence-based guidelines for cardiovascular disease prevention in women, which suggested that screening women at risk of CHD for depression

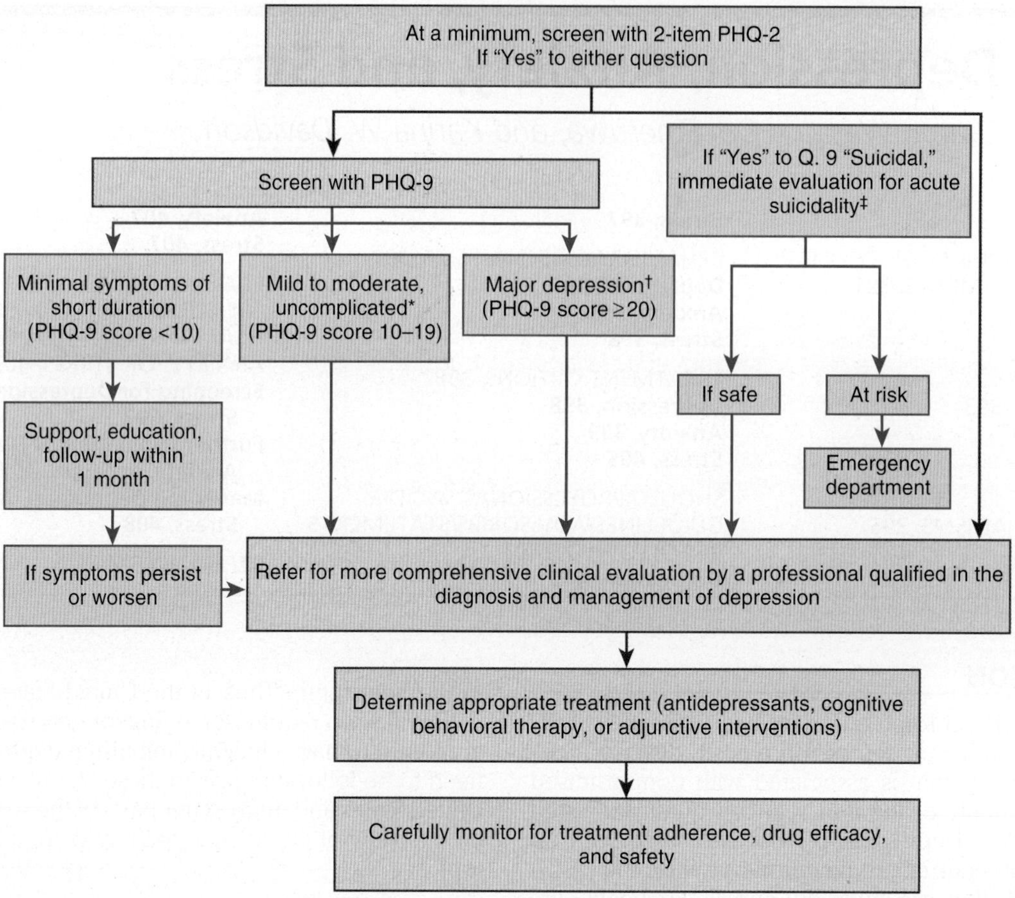

FIG. 26.1 American Heart Association's advisory for depression detection and treatment. *Meets diagnostic criteria for major depression, has a PHQ-9 score of 10–19, has had no more than 1 or 2 prior episodes of depression, and screens negative for bipolar disorder, suicidality, significant substance abuse, or other major psychiatric problems. †Meets the diagnostic criteria for major depression and 1) has a PHQ-9 score >20; or 2) has had 3 or more prior depressive episodes; or 3) screens positive for bipolar disorder, suicidality, significant substance abuse, or other major psychiatric problem. ‡If "Yes" to Q.9 "suicidal," immediately evaluate for acute suicidality. If safe, refer for more comprehensive clinical evaluation; if at risk for suicide, escort the patient to the emergency department. *PHQ*, Patient Health Quesionaire. *(From Lichtman JH, Bigger JT Jr, Blumenthal JA, et al. Depression and coronary heart disease: recommendations for screening, referral, and treatment: a science advisory from the American Heart Association Prevention Committee of the Council on Cardiovascular Nursing, Council on Clinical Cardiology, Council on Epidemiology and Prevention, and Interdisciplinary Council on Quality of Care and Outcomes Research. Circ 118, 1768–1775, 2008.)*

BOX 26.1 American Heart Association's Advisory for Depression Detection and Treatment: Patient Health Questionnaire-9 (PHQ-9) Depression Screening Scales

Over the past 2 weeks, how often have you been bothered by any of the following problems?

1. Little interest or pleasure in doing things.
2. Feeling down, depressed, or hopeless.
3. Trouble falling asleep, staying asleep, or sleeping too much.
4. Feeling tired or having little energy.
5. Poor appetite or overeating.
6. Feeling bad about yourself, feeling that you are a failure, or feeling that you have let yourself or your family down.
7. Trouble concentrating on things such as reading the newspaper or watching television.
8. Moving or speaking so slowly that other people could have noticed. Or being so fidgety or restless that you have been moving around a lot more than usual.
9. Thinking that you would be better off dead or that you want to hurt yourself in some way.

Courtesy of MacArthur Foundation Initiative on Depression and Primary Care. PRIME-MD Patient Health Questionnaire - 1999 Pfizer Inc. MacArthur Toolkit 2006 3CM, LLC. Used with permission. Available at http://www.depression-primarycare.org/.

and referring/treating when indicated was a class IIa (weight of evidence/opinion is in favor of usefulness/efficacy), level B (limited evidence from single randomized trial or other

BOX 26.2 PHQ-2 Yes/No Version

During the past month, have you often been bothered by:

1. Feeling down, depressed, or hopeless? (yes/no)
2. Little interest or pleasure in doing things? (yes/no)

From Whooley MA, Avins AL, Miranda J, et al. Case-finding instruments for depression. Two questions are as good as many. *J Gen Intern Med.* 1997;12(7):439–445.

randomized studies) recommendation.[10,11] The 2008 AHA advisory did specifically note that, at the time of its issuance, there was no direct evidence linking the treatment of depression with improved cardiac outcomes.[8]

The AHA/American College of Cardiology (ACC) released secondary prevention guidelines for CHD patients in 2011 that provide a class IIa, level B recommendation that patients with recent myocardial infarction (MI) or coronary artery bypass graft (CABG) be screened for depression.[12] These guidelines acknowledged that treating depression has not been shown to improve CHD outcomes but issued a class IIb, level C recommendation for treating depression with the logic that it may have clinical benefits other than improved CHD outcomes.[12]

In 2014, the AHA issued a scientific statement formally recognizing depression as a risk factor for poor post-ACS outcomes, including all-cause mortality, cardiac mortality, and composite endpoints (cardiac or all-cause mortality and nonfatal cardiac events).[13] This conclusion was based on a systematic review that identified prospective studies showing a strong and consistent observational association between depression and CHD outcomes, a lack of other explanations for this association, and the existence of a plausible biologic mechanism to account for this association.[13]

American Academy of Family Practitioners

In 2009, the American Academy of Family Practitioners (AAFP) published guidelines for the detection and management of post-MI depression.[14] It issued four specific guidelines based on review of published evidence. First, it recommended using any standardized symptom checklist to screen post-MI patients for depression during the index hospitalization and at regular intervals thereafter. Second, it recommended treating post-MI depression in order to improve symptoms. These recommendations were issued as level A with the specific note that they were based on RCTs showing improvement in depression outcomes but not cardiac outcomes, "though the evidence does not yet exclude the possibility of a small benefit."[14] The third and fourth recommendations suggested selective serotonin reuptake inhibitors (SSRIs) (level A) and/or psychotherapy (level B) for treating depression.

European Societies

The European Guidelines on Cardiovascular Disease Prevention in Clinical Practice are issued by a task force of the European Society of Cardiology and other societies. In 2012, the guidelines stated that depression contributes to both incident CHD and poor CHD outcomes. The guidelines made class IIa, level B recommendations that depression be assessed by a clinical interview or standardized questionnaire, and that tailored clinical management for depression be considered with the goal of improving CHD outcomes and enhancing quality of life.[15]

The British healthcare system,[16] via the National Institute of Health and Care Excellence (NICE), endorses depression screening in CHD patients and referral for treatment if depression is detected.

Anxiety

European Societies

The 2012 European prevention guidelines also state that anxiety contributes to both incident CHD and poor CHD outcomes. The guidelines included anxiety in the class IIa, level B recommendations, suggesting that anxiety be screened for via clinical interview or standardized questionnaire and tailored clinical management should be given, with the goal of improving CHD outcomes and enhancing quality of life.[15]

Stress

European Societies

The 2012 guidelines also state that stress at work and in family life increases the risk of both incident CHD and poor CHD outcomes. The guidelines provide a class IIa, level B recommendation to screen and provide tailored clinical management for stress, with the goal of improving CHD outcomes and enhancing quality of life.[15]

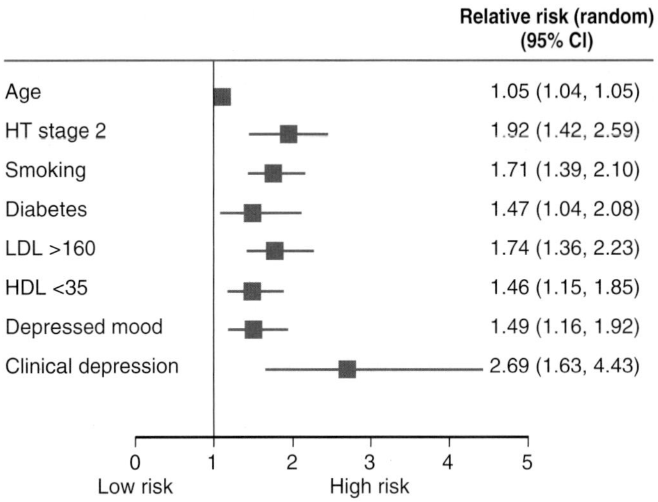

FIG. 26.2 Risk ratios of depressive symptoms and clinical depression (for death due to cardiac disease and myocardial infarction [MI]) and traditional cardiovascular-risk factors (for death due to cardiac disease, MI, coronary artery insufficiency, and development of angina). *CI*, Confidence interval; *HDL*, high-density lipoprotein; *HT*, hypertension; *LDL*, low-density lipoprotein. *(From Rozanski A, Blumenthal JA, Davidson KW, et al. The epidemiology, pathophysiology, and management of psychosocial risk factors in cardiac practice: the emerging field of behavioral cardiology.* J Am Coll Cardiol. *2005;45(5):637–651.)*

Both stress and anxiety have not been the focus of guidelines or consensus statements; however, interest in this topic seems to be increasing.[17,18]

EPIDEMIOLOGY

Depression

Depression is the leading cause of "years of life lived with disability" worldwide and significantly compromises quality of life and life expectancy when it coexists with a chronic medical disorder.[19] This is particularly true for CHD, as depression has been associated with an increased risk of developing CHD and worse outcomes among CHD patients.[19–21] Large epidemiologic studies have convincingly demonstrated that depression is a predictor for occurrence and recurrence of CHD. Depressive symptoms alone also predict CHD risk, but stronger effect sizes have been observed for major depressive disorder (MDD) compared with depressive mood, suggesting a dose-response relationship.[8,19]

Depression and Incident Coronary Heart Disease

In many studies with varied cohorts, depressive symptoms were associated with an increased risk of developing CHD. Depressive symptoms confer a relative risk of CHD ranging from 0.98 to 3.5 in different studies and a combined overall risk ranging from 1.6 to 5.4 compared with nondepressed patients in systematic reviews.[7,21] MDD is associated with an even greater risk of incident MI with an odds ratio of approximately 4.5.[21] The risk associated with depressive symptoms or clinical depression is perhaps even greater than that associated with traditional cardiovascular risk factors, as seen in Fig. 26.2.[22,23]

Depression among Patients with Coronary Heart Disease

Depression is one of the more frequently encountered chronic diseases among general medical patients, with a prevalence ranging from approximately 5% to 15%.[13,19] Depression is even more prevalent among CHD patients (Fig.

26.3).[24] As many as 20% of CHD patients meet the diagnostic criteria for MDD by The Diagnostic and Statistical Manual of Mental Disorders (DSM) criteria and 30% to 50% have significant patient-reported depressive symptoms.[14,19,20,25] The increased prevalence of depression extends past the immediate post-MI period.[14] Importantly, both clinically diagnosed depression and depressive symptoms predict increased cardiac risk. Approximately 7 million Americans living with CHD also have clinically significant depression, and half a million new such cases are added to this public health burden annually.[19]

Prognosis Associated with Depression in Patients with Coronary Heart Disease

Compared with nondepressed post-MI patients, depressed post-MI patients have more medical comorbidities and cardiac complications and higher mortality rates.[7,8,19,21] Observational studies show that ACS patients with depressive symptoms are at a two-fold higher risk of MI recurrence.[8,13,19,20] As seen in Fig. 26.4, depressive symptoms in CHD patients are at par with conventional CHD prognostic factors for predicting death and CHD recurrence.[19]

The AHA formally recognizes depression as a risk factor for poor outcomes among ACS patients based on its systematic literature review showing depression is a risk factor for all-cause mortality, cardiac mortality, and composite endpoints (cardiac or all-cause mortality and nonfatal cardiac events) after ACS.[13] Others have argued, however, that depression may be a risk marker rather than a risk factor because there is no trial evidence that treating depression alters the prognosis, making it more analogous to high-density lipoprotein or C-reactive protein (CRP).[26]

Impact of Depression on Health-Related Quality of Life

Depression is more strongly associated with health-related quality of life and health status than a single health condition such as angina, arthritis, asthma, or diabetes.[27] Depression clearly predicts impoverished health-related quality of life independent of traditional predictors of quality of life, specifically among patients with stable CHD and those with a recent ACS. In several studies of multiple predictors of quality of life in CHD patients, depression was the most important even when other predictors such as demographic and social variables, severity of disease, ejection fraction, and ischemia were assessed.[19,20] Recent ACS patients with a history of depression have twice the rate of angina, triple the physical limitations, and almost triple the risk of diminished health-related quality of life.[19] There have been calls to improve quality of

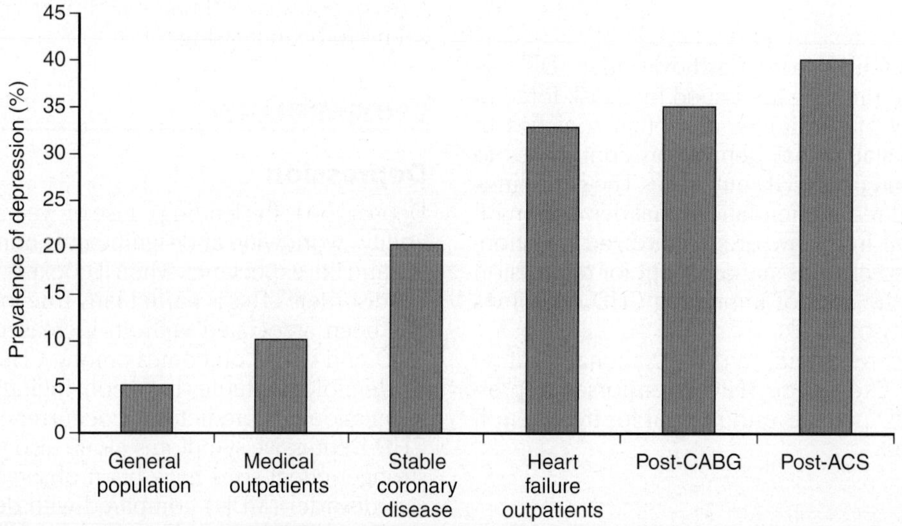

FIG. 26.3 The prevalence of depression across the patient spectrum. *ACS*, Acute coronary syndrome; *CABG*, coronary artery bypass graft. *(Data from Whooley MA. Depression and cardiovascular disease: healing the broken-hearted.* JAMA. *2006;295(24):2874–2881.)*

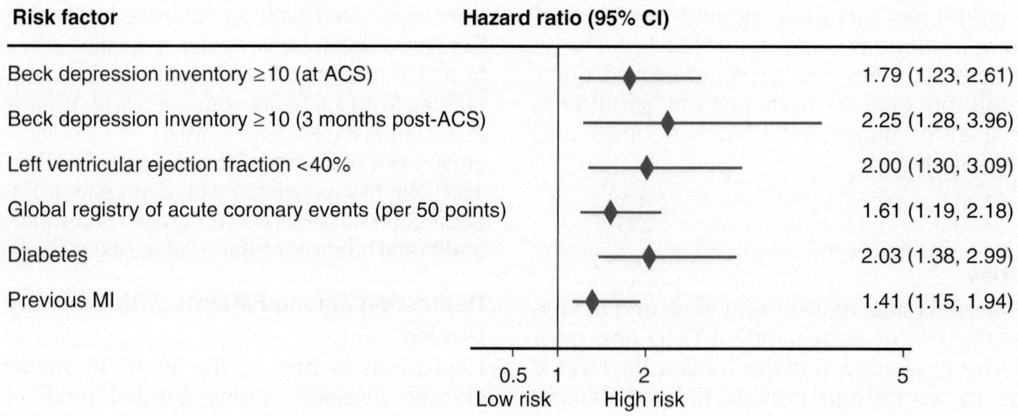

FIG. 26.4 Hazard ratios of depressive symptoms and traditional cardiovascular risk factors. *ACS*, Acute coronary syndrome; *CI*, confidence interval; *MI*, myocardial infarction. *(From Davidson KW. Depression and coronary heart disease.* ISRN Cardiol. *2012;2012:743813.)*

life in post-ACS patients, rather than continuing to focus on extending life of diminished quality. Some suggest that treating depression could answer this call.

Costs Associated with Depression

Depression has long been associated with high costs of medical utilization, many lost days of productivity, and reduced work performance. Patients who have a chronic medical condition, such as CHD, with depression have significantly more ambulatory visits, emergency room visits, days in bed due to illness, and functional disability. Annual healthcare costs were almost 41% higher and 5-year healthcare costs were almost 53% higher in depressed post-MI patients compared with nondepressed post-MI patients.[19,20]

Anxiety

Anxiety disorders are highly prevalent, with nearly 20% of Americans suffering from any anxiety disorder — a rate that is likely mirrored in CHD patients.[28] Some prospective studies have shown an increased risk of cardiovascular events among patients with anxiety symptoms and suggest that the increased risk exists even with simple phobias and nonclinical anxiety levels with a graded-response relationship.[28]

Stress

The literature relating stress and CHD is equivocal, perhaps due to differing definitions and conceptualizations of what constitutes "stress," as well as which CHD outcomes have been examined.[29] However, recent studies have indicated that stress is associated with incident CHD. Self-reported individual stressors are associated with incident CHD with risk ratios in excess of 1.6.[29] A meta-analysis of six prospective observational cohort studies showed that patient self-reported stress was associated with incident CHD at 6 months, with an aggregate relative risk of 1.27 (95% confidence interval [CI] 1.12–1.45).[30]

Specific stressors such as social isolation, stress at work, and marital problems have also been individually associated with incident CHD with risk ratios of approximately 1.5 in individual studies. Meta-analyses have shown that job strain and loneliness/isolation also increase the risk of incident CHD.[31] Not only is perceived stress a risk factor for CHD, but the perception that stress is affecting one's health is also a risk factor.[32]

Stress may also be associated with, poor prognosis in established CHD patients, although the evidence is limited.[31] Financial and job strains are examples of stressors that are related to recurrent CHD-related events.[33,34]

BIOLOGIC MECHANISMS

Depression

Many biologic mechanisms have been proposed to explain the association between depression and incident and recurrent CHD (Fig. 26.5 and Fig. 26.6). Dysregulations of several physiologic systems in depression are implicated in the depression–CHD link, including platelet reactivity,

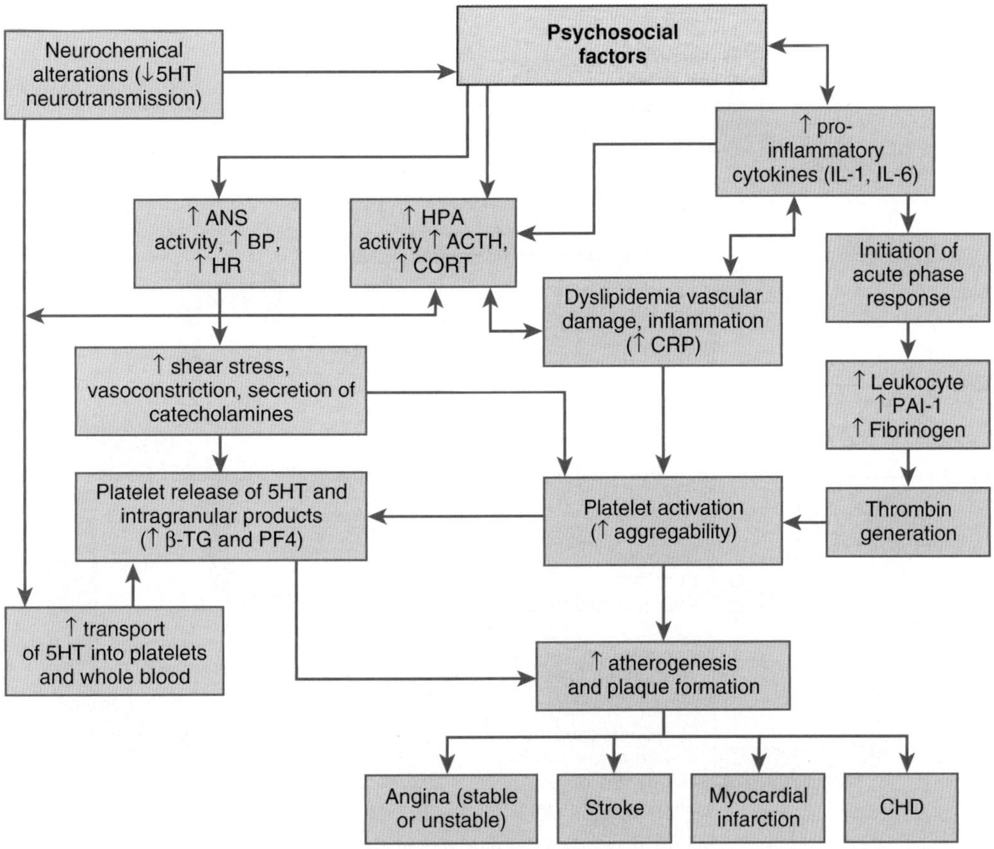

FIG. 26.5 Proposed physiologic mechanisms and pathways linking psychosocial factors and atherogenesis and related outcomes. *5HT,* Serotonin; *ACTH,* adrenocorticotropin; *ANS,* autonomic nervous system; *BP,* blood pressure; *CHD,* coronary heart disease; *CORT,* cortisol; *CRP,* C-reactive protein; *HPA,* hypothalamic-pituitary-adrenal; *HR,* heart rate; *IL,* interleukin; *PAI-1,* plasminogen activator inhibitor 1; *PF4,* platelet factor 4; *TG,* thromboglobulin; *WBC,* white blood cell. *(From Everson-Rose SA, Lewis TT. Psychosocial factors and cardiovascular diseases.* Annu Rev Public Health. *2005;26:469–500.)*

inflammation, autonomic imbalance, sleep architecture disruption, circadian rhythm disruption, anabolic/catabolic hormonal imbalance, and others. However, the evidence remains equivocal regarding the specific biologic dysregulations responsible for the link between depression and CHD. Although many promising mechanisms are briefly reviewed hereafter, there is little direct human evidence that any of these are causally involved in the pathogenesis of CHD in depression. A recent review of animal studies[35] suggests that most of these mechanisms are plausible, but human experiments and trials are required to conclusively implicate a biologic mechanism in the depression–ACS recurrence association.[19]

Platelet Reactivity

Several case-controlled studies have demonstrated platelet hyperreactivity in CHD patients, and CHD patients with MDD have exhibited higher levels of platelet factor 4 and β-thromboglobulin (β-TG)—markers of platelet aggregation—and platelet/endothelial cell adhesion molecule-1 when compared with CHD patients without MDD.[8,19]

Inflammation

Elevated levels of inflammatory biomarkers, including CRP, soluble intercellular adhesion molecule 1 (sICAM1), soluble vascular cell adhesion molecule-1, and tumor necrosis factor-α, are associated with an increased risk of cardiovascular events in patients with known CHD. Several cross-sectional studies have linked depression to chronic inflammation—as measured by CRP or sICAM1 levels—both in otherwise healthy participants and in post-ACS patients shortly after the index event.[8,19] Proinflammatory cytokines may contribute to coronary atherosclerosis.[7]

Autonomic Dysregulation

Autonomic dysregulation is characterized by increased activation of the sympathetic nervous system (SNS), which usually acts in concert with a reduced activation of the parasympathetic nervous system (PNS). Excess SNS activity produces many effects that contribute to CHD: high blood pressure, increased myocardial oxygen demand, platelet activation, increased myocyte apoptosis, and arrhythmias. Both elevated SNS activity and reduced PNS activity have been implicated in depression and CHD recurrence. Furthermore, CHD patients with depressive symptoms have been shown to have greater SNS activity as measured by higher norepinephrine excretion levels compared with CHD patients without depressive symptoms.[19]

Sleep Architecture Disruption

Depression and sleep architecture disruption are closely linked, although the specific dysregulated polysomnographic

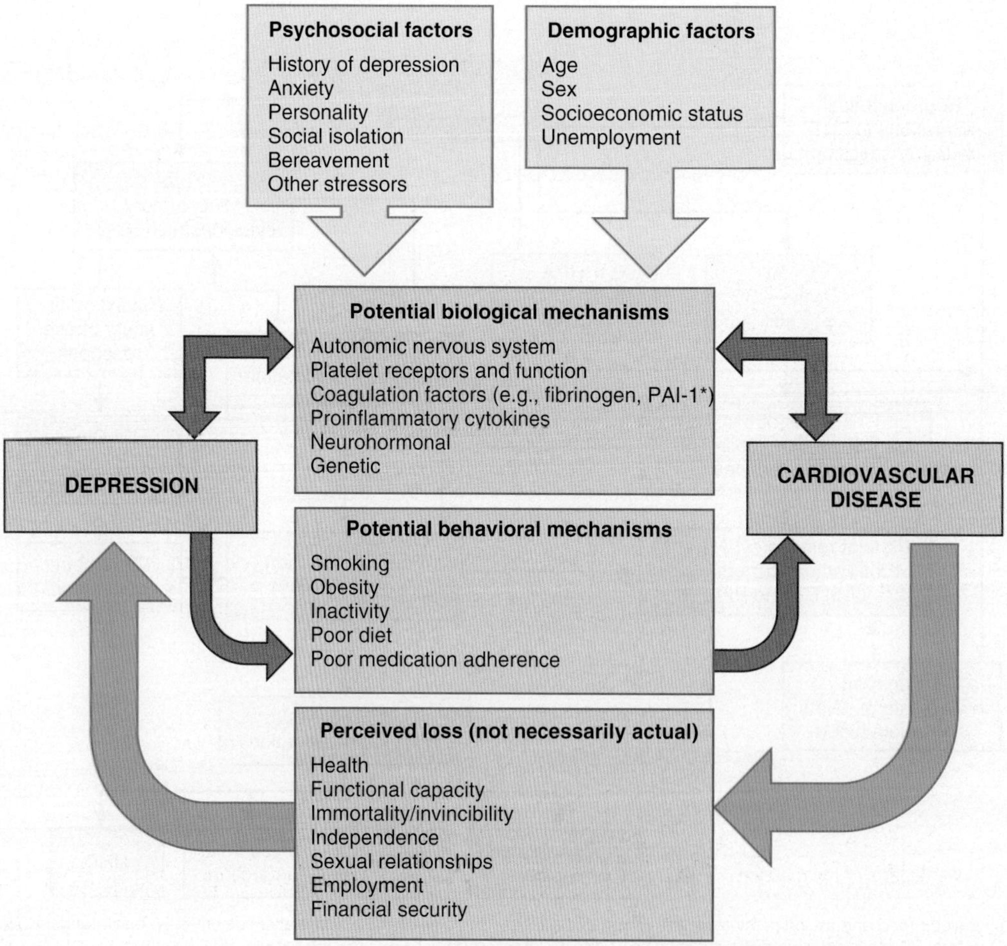

FIG. 26.6 Potential factors that could explain the relationship between cardiovascular disease and depression. **PAI-1*, Plasminogen activator inhibitor 1. *(From Hare DL, Toukhsati SR, Johansson P, et al. Depression and cardiovascular disease: a clinical review.* Eur Heart J. *2014;35(21):1365–1372.)*

parameters are unclear. Studies have shown that reduced rapid eye movement (REM) latency—the time from sleep onset to the first occurrence of REM—is the most frequently reported sleep dysregulation that distinguishes MDD patients from individuals without MDD. REM sleep is characterized by pronounced surges of SNS, which may be of sufficient magnitude to stimulate thrombotic processes, to increase hemodynamic stress on vessel walls conducive to plaque rupture, and to alter cardiac electrophysiologic properties. These autonomic surges may be responsible for cardiac events witnessed during REM sleep in humans. Importantly, this REM-induced cardiac sympathetic dominance is enhanced in individuals with a recent MI. Additionally, the total sleep time is consistently decreased in depressed patients and those prone to depressive episodes. Although there is a lack of prospective epidemiologic studies on the dimensions of sleep architecture and CHD recurrence, there is epidemiologic evidence that short sleep duration is predictive of ACS.[19]

Circadian Rhythm Disruption

Endogenous circadian rhythms regulate daily variations in most of the hormonal, physiologic, and psychologic variables implicated in depression and ACS. The systems with the most prominent variations are thermoregulation and melatonin secretion. There is evidence that the majority of cardiovascular events, including MIs, show a marked circadian rhythmicity with a peak incidence between 6:00 AM and 2:00 PM. However, in depressed patients, who often have circadian dysregulation, most MIs occur between 10:00 PM and 6:00 AM. Thus, circadian rhythm disruption in depressed patients may help elucidate some of the pathways by which these patients are at an increased risk of recurrent cardiovascular events.[19]

Hypothalamic-Pituitary-Adrenal Axis

The hypothalamic-pituitary-adrenal (HPA) axis, the major stress axis through which cortisol is released by the adrenal gland when stimulated by adrenocorticotropin (ACTH), has been studied extensively in depressed patients. Depressed patients exhibit elevated circulating plasma levels of ACTH and cortisol, elevated urinary cortisol concentration, and altered circadian rhythm of cortisol. Prospective studies among acute MI patients have shown that very high levels of cortisol (> 2000 nmol/L) predict mortality.[19]

Anxiety

The neurobiology underlying anxiety has not been examined or elucidated as extensively as that of depression, but some biologic alterations have been identified, such as markers of platelet reactivity, inflammation, autonomic dysregulation, and HPA system hyperactivity.

Platelet Reactivity

Panic disorder patients, like depressed patients, have been observed to have elevated plasma platelet factor 4 and β-TG concentrations.[28]

Inflammation

Inflammatory markers, including CRP and fibrinogen, are elevated among patients with anxiety with a dose-response relationship such that increased levels of inflammatory markers are associated with higher levels of anxiety.[28]

Autonomic Dysregulation

Increased anxiety has been associated with an increased risk of hypertension in prospective cohort studies, which suggests SNS hyperactivity. However, further research is needed to clarify this association.[28]

Hypothalamic-Pituitary-Adrenal Axis

Similar to depressed patients, patients with post-traumatic stress disorder (PTSD), a specific anxiety disorder, exhibit HPA system hyperactivity. Corticotropin-releasing factor concentrations are increased in the cerebrospinal fluid of patients with anxiety and/or PTSD.[28] Panic disorder patients do not seem to have consistent HPA system alterations, and there are insufficient data on HPA axis function in patients with other specific anxiety disorders.[28]

Stress

Similar to depression and anxiety, the mechanism linking stress with CHD outcomes is likely multifactorial and includes platelet reactivity, inflammation, autonomic dysregulation, and increased HPA axis activity.[30,31] Because an acute response to stress is transient hypertension, it has been hypothesized that a response to chronic stress is persistent hypertension.[31]

Additionally, acute cardiac events may be triggered by acute emotional stress. A meta-analysis showed that ACS that is preceded by anger, stress, or depressed mood in the past 24 hours has a pooled relative risk of nearly 2.5.[31] The risk may increase further with high-intensity emotional stressors such as death of a significant person or a diagnosis of cancer.[31] Similarly, Takotsubo (or stress) cardiomyopathy, a transient dysfunction of the left ventricle, has been shown to be associated with both acute and former or chronic psychiatric diagnoses.[36] Up to 42.3% of Takotsubo patients had a psychiatric illness, and approximately half of these were affective disorders.[36]

BEHAVIORAL MECHANISMS

Depression

Depression is associated with cardiac risk factors such as smoking, obesity, and sedentary lifestyle.[7] Depression may also influence post-ACS outcomes through its effects on a patient's behaviors with regard to adherence to prescribed medications and primary or secondary prevention recommendations.[8,19] In addition, there may be disparities in the way the healthcare system behaves toward depressed patients, and these differences (e.g., the treatment they receive) may lead to worse outcomes. Although it is now widely accepted that post-ACS depression is associated with a poor medical prognosis, there remains a gap in our knowledge about which behavioral mechanisms underlie this association. See Fig. 26.6 for a schematic of the interplay between behavioral and biologic mechanisms underlying the association between depression and cardiovascular disease.

Adherence

Poor adherence to behaviors recommended for managing medical illnesses is well-established as an important factor in determining outcomes for a range of diseases. For example, treatment adherence accounted for 26% of the difference in outcomes among high adherers compared with low adherers in a meta-analysis.[19] Nonadherence to cardiovascular medications such as aspirin, statins, and β-blockers after ACS is clearly linked with poor medical outcomes, including cardiac outcomes, mortality, and composite endpoints with hazard ratios (HRs) between 3 and 3.8.[19]

Prior research shows that depression is associated with poor adherence among patients with a number of chronic medical illnesses, including ACS.[8] Patients with persistent depressive symptoms after ACS are less likely to adhere to secondary CHD prevention behaviors, such as exercising regularly and quitting smoking.[19] Although there are a number of potential behavioral mechanisms linking depression and post-ACS outcomes, poor medication adherence specifically represents the most promising and best-supported mechanism explaining this association. In an outpatient population of CHD patients, nearly 15% of those with MDD reported not taking their medication as prescribed, compared with 5% of those without depression.[19] In a post-ACS population, 42% of persistently depressed patients took their prescribed aspirin less than 75% of the time, whereas only approximately 11% of nondepressed patients demonstrated this level of nonadherence.[19]

Stigma

Finally, as a result of the cognitive, affective, and social characteristics of mental illnesses, patients with depression can be stigmatized by their illness, which may lead to lower rates of treatment for cardiac disease or poorer communication about secondary prevention behaviors.[19] For example, individuals with comorbid mental disorders are less likely to undergo coronary revascularization procedures than those without mental disorders. Additionally, patients with depression tend to have flat affect and be less engaging; therefore they may be most susceptible to such physician bias.

Anxiety

Much less is known about the association of anxiety with medication adherence or with adherence to secondary CHD prevention behaviors. Some studies indicate that anxious patients, in general, are more adherent, particularly when their anxiety takes the form of generalized anxiety disorder. However, other anxious patients with phobic or panic symptoms may be less likely to adhere. But, relatively little empiric evidence exists to strongly support any of these small-study findings and conjectures.

Stress

Stress may also be linked to poor CHD outcomes through behavioral mechanisms. For example, poor health behaviors that develop as a response to stress may result in obesity, hyperglycemia, and dyslipidemia — all of which are known cardiovascular risk factors.[29–31] Studies have attributed a portion of the effect of stress on CHD to the increased risk of metabolic syndrome among patients with high levels of perceived stress.[31]

TREATMENT OPTIONS

Depression

Treatment for depression may include psychotherapy, physical activity, or antidepressant drugs (Fig. 26.7).

Psychotherapy

Three types of psychotherapy have been shown to be effective in ameliorating depression.[37] Psychotherapy can be as effective as medication in treating depression and may be preferred in patients who cannot tolerate or do not want to take antidepressants.[8,14] Many depressed patients may respond better to a combination of antidepressants and

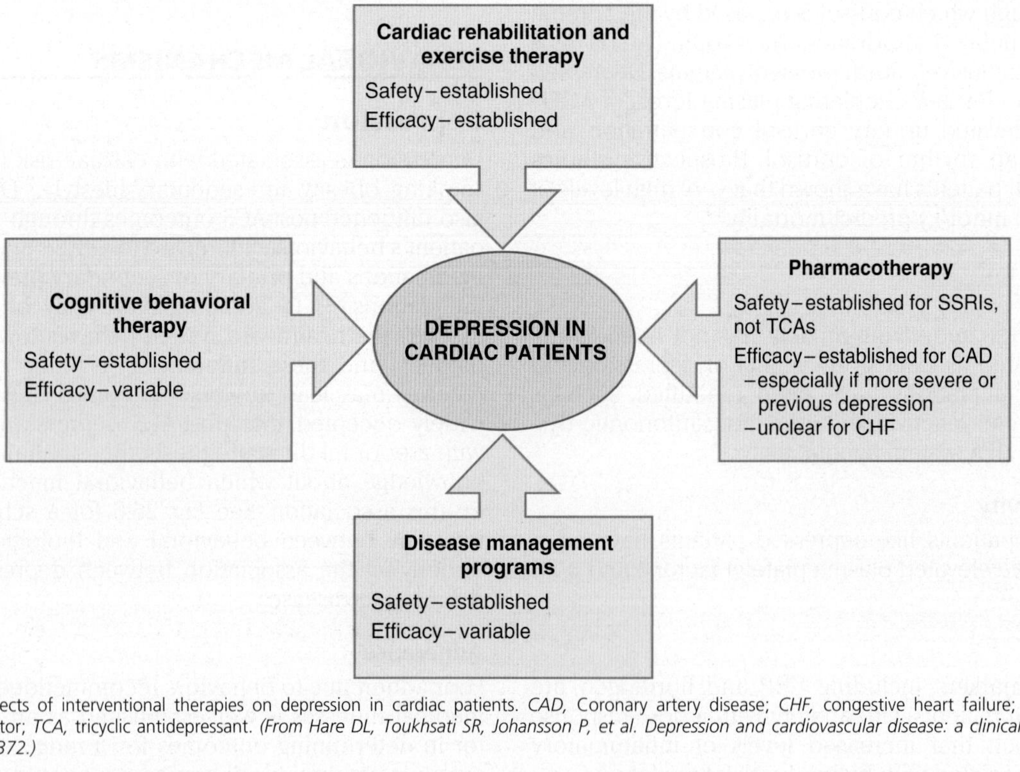

FIG. 26.7 The effects of interventional therapies on depression in cardiac patients. *CAD,* Coronary artery disease; *CHF,* congestive heart failure; *SSRI,* selective serotonin reuptake inhibitor; *TCA,* tricyclic antidepressant. *(From Hare DL, Toukhsati SR, Johansson P, et al. Depression and cardiovascular disease: a clinical review.* Eur Heart J. *2014;35(21):1365–1372.)*

psychotherapy, specifically cognitive behavioral therapy (CBT), than either treatment alone.

The most frequently used type of psychotherapy is CBT, which modifies thoughts and behaviors to decrease depressive symptoms. The second type of psychotherapy is interpersonal therapy, which focuses on interpersonal situations such as conflicts or role transitions.[38] These two therapies were found to have only modest improvements in depression in recent RCTs of CHD patients, although a recent trial of CABG patients showed good treatment effects for CBT.[39] Another study of CHD patients showed that 12 to 16 sessions of CBT over a period of 12 weeks helped achieve remission of depression.[39a]

Finally, problem-solving therapy teaches patients to improve their abilities to solve everyday problems,[40,41] and, when used in a patient preference design (in which patients are educated about the benefits and limitations of each therapy and then choose for themselves if they prefer problem-solving therapy and/or pharmacotherapy), improves depression in CHD patients.[42] Importantly, these psychotherapies can now be provided over the telephone, which is both cost effective and removes barriers to treatments for patients with mobility or transportation issues.[43]

Physical Activity

For patients with mild depressive symptoms, exercise can remediate depressive symptoms.[16] Exercise can improve both depressive symptoms and cardiovascular fitness.[8] The specific exercise regimen prescribed should be tailored to the cardiac condition and exercise capacity of each individual patient.[8]

Antidepressant Drugs

Depression can be treated with a variety of antidepressant drugs, including SSRIs, tricyclic antidepressants (TCAs), and monoamine oxidase inhibitors (MAOIs). Patients initiated on antidepressants should be closely monitored for the first 2 months of treatment and regularly thereafter to ensure adherence, detect adverse effects, and monitor suicidal risk.[8]

Tailored drug selection is critical among CHD patients, as antidepressants have been associated (but not tested in active comparator trials) with both increased and decreased cardiac risk.[8] Cardiologists should manage pharmacotherapy with careful consideration of each individual patient's cardiovascular disease and risk profile. Certain antidepressants may be associated with increased risk for arrhythmias, orthostatic hypotension, or hypertensive crisis, especially when combined with certain cardiovascular medications. Please see Tables 26.1, 26.2, and 26.3 for detailed information about antidepressant drug classes and individual drug cardiovascular side effects, potential interactions with cardiac medications, and pharmacokinetic interactions, respectively.

Selective Serotonin Reuptake Inhibitors

Treatment with an SSRI versus no antidepressant reduces death and recurrent MI among CHD patients who are depressed according to a nonrandomized, post hoc analysis.[8] Sertraline and citalopram are first-line antidepressant drugs for CHD patients as randomized clinical trials have shown them to be effective for the treatment of depression and safe for CHD patients without increasing the risk of cardiovascular adverse events.[7,8,14,44]

Tricyclic Antidepressants

TCAs are contraindicated for many CHD patients due to cardiotoxic effects and greater risk of cardiovascular adverse effects compared with SSRIs.[7] For example, they are likely proarrhythmic in post-MI patients due to sodium channel-blocking properties.[7]

Monoamine Oxidase Inhibitors

MAOIs are also contraindicated for many CHD patients due to cardiotoxic effects, such as orthostatic hypotension or hypertensive crisis. Given the evidence for blood pressure dysregulation, MAOIs have not been tested in trials of therapy for CHD patients.

Mood-Stabilizing Agents

The mood stabilizer lithium should be carefully managed in CAD patients. Lithium can be associated with arrhythmias, and its plasma levels can be increased by common cardiovascular medications such as thiazide, loop, and potassium-sparing diuretics, as well as angiotensin-converting enzyme (ACE) inhibitors (see Table 26.1).

Electroconvulsive Therapy

Depression that is refractive to antidepressant drugs may be treated with electroconvulsive therapy (ECT), which aims to incite secondary generalized tonic-clonic seizures while the patient is anesthetized. The APA has identified severe or unstable cardiovascular disease as associated with increased ECT-related risk.[45] There is also a risk associated with anesthesia administration. Moreover, during the tonic phase, patients experience a parasympathetic discharge, including heart block, bradycardia, and asystole, that can incite arrhythmias; during the clonic phase, patients experience a catecholamine surge that can incite tachycardia and hypertension. ECT may cause a reduction in left ventricular ejection fraction due to either global or regional wall motion abnormalities that tend to be transient.[46] Patients with cardiac disease have higher rates of cardiac complications from ECT, though most complications are transient and do not preclude completion of ECT.[47]

Anxiety

Anxiolytic Drugs

The first-line treatment for anxiety disorders—specifically, panic disorder, obsessive-compulsive disorder, and generalized anxiety disorder—is an SSRI. Benzodiazepines were first-line 2 decades ago, but they are now considered more appropriate for temporary use to bridge patients through the first 6 to 8 weeks of SSRI therapy, as the anxiolytic effects of SSRIs are delayed. This avoids long-term use of benzodiazepines and the accompanying risk of oversedation and physiologic or psychological dependence.[44]

Psychotherapy

Few studies have focused on the treatment of anxiety and stress in the context of CHD, thereby limiting the available evidence from which to draw inferences about the effectiveness of psychologic treatments for anxiety and stress in CHD.[48] Indeed, in most instances, psychologic conditions other than depression, such as anxiety and stress, were treated as secondary outcomes, and the size of the improvement for these conditions was not routinely reported.

TABLE 26.1 Cardiovascular Side Effects of Specific Antidepressant and Anxiolytic Medications

CLASS	CARDIOVASCULAR SIDE EFFECTS	LIKELY MECHANISM OF SIDE EFFECT	OTHER EFFECTS AND BENEFITS
Tricyclic and related cyclic antidepressants	Orthostatic hypotension	Postsynaptic α_1-receptor blockade	
Nortriptyline (Pamelor)			Lowest incidence of orthostatic hypotension with nortriptyline
Imipramine (Tofranil)			
Amitriptyline (Elavil)			
Desipramine (Norpramin)	Tachycardia	Secondary to hypotension	
Clomipramine (Anafranil)			
Doxepin (Sinequan)	Decreased heart rate variability	Postsynaptic cholinergic-receptor blockade	Urinary retention, dry mouth, constipation, confusion, exacerbation of narrow-angle glaucoma
Trimipramine (Surmontil)			
Protriptyline (Vivactil)	Slowing of intraventricular conduction	Quinidine-like effects	Avoid in patients with bifascicular block, left bundle branch block, QTc > 44 msec, or QRS > 11 msec
Monoamine oxidase inhibitors	Orthostatic hypotension	Inhibition of metabolism of serotonin and catecholamines	Fatal in overdose
Phenelzine (Nardil)	Hypertensive crisis		Requires adherence to tyramine-free diet and avoidance of other antidepressants and sympathomimetics
Tranylcypromine (Parnate)			
Isocarboxazid (Marplan)			
SSRIs		Postsynaptic serotonin-receptor blockade	Fatal in overdose Typical side effects: nausea, insomnia, sexual dysfunction, nervousness
Fluoxetine (Prozac)	Sinus bradycardia	Unknown	Requires 8 weeks for complete washout Inhibitor of CYP IID6 and CYP IIIA4 enzymes Also FDA approved for treatment of adult and pediatric OCD, bulimia, pediatric depression
Paroxetine (Paxil)	Clinically insignificant decreases in heart rate	Unknown	Inhibitor of CYP IID6 enzyme Also FDA indicated for treatment of social phobia, panic disorder, OCD, GAD
Sertraline (Zoloft)	None known		In high doses, inhibitor of CYP IID6 enzyme Also FDA indicated for treatment of panic disorder, adult and pediatric OCD, PTSD
Fluvoxamine (Luvox)	None known		Potent inhibitor of multiple CYP enzymes Also FDA approved for treatment of adult and pediatric OCD
Citalopram (Celexa)	None known		
Escitalopram (Lexapro)	None known		SSRI with most selective binding to serotonin transporter
Venlafaxine (Effexor)	Arrhythmia or cardiac block in overdose Decreased HRV Increased diastolic blood pressure in doses > 300 mg/day	Unknown Presynaptic inhibition of norepinephrine reuptake	No significant inhibition of CYP enzymes Also FDA indicated for treatment of GAD Side-effect profile similar to that of SSRIs

Presynaptic α_2-receptor antagonist			
Mirtazapine (Remeron)	None known	Postsynaptic histamine$_1$ receptor blockade	Very sedating in low doses Weight gain Minimal sexual side effects No significant inhibition of CYP enzymes
Dopamine and norepinephrine reuptake inhibitor			
Bupropion (Wellbutrin, Zyban)	Significant increases in blood pressure in patients with preexisting hypertension (rare)	Presynaptic inhibition of norepinephrine reuptake	No significant inhibition of CYP enzymes Minimal sexual side effects Not proven effective in the treatment of anxiety disorders FDA indicated for treatment of nicotine dependence
Atypical serotonergic agents			
Trazodone (Desyrel)	Orthostatic hypotension Cardiac arrhythmias rare	Postsynaptic α_1 receptor blockade Unknown	Sedation, confusion, dizziness Rare cases of priapism
Nefazodone (Serzone)	Sinus bradycardia	Unknown	Similar side-effect profile as trazodone (except without priapism) Minimal sexual side effects Potent inhibitor of multiple CYP enzymes Liver failure rare
Psychostimulants			
Dextroamphetamine (Dexedrine)	Rarely increases blood pressure or tachycardia in therapeutic doses	Release of dopamine and catecholamines	Avoid in patients with hyperthyroidism, severe hypertension, severe angina, tachyarrhythmias
Methylphenidate (Ritalin)			
Benzodiazepines		Allosteric alteration of $GABA_A$ receptors	Rapid relief of anxiety symptoms
Alprazolam (Xanax)			
Clonazepam (Klonopin)			
Lorazepam (Ativan)	Hypotension	Muscle relaxation of $GABA_A$ spinal cord receptors	Can cause fatigue, ataxia, drowsiness, amnesia, and behavioral dyscontrol
Oxazepam (Serax)			Relatively safe in overdose Physiologic and psychological dependence and withdrawal symptoms if dosage not gradually tapered
Partial 5-HT_{1A} receptor agonist			
Buspirone (BuSpar)	None known		FDA approved for treatment of GAD Nonaddictive
Omega$_1$ receptor agonist			
Zolpidem (Ambien)	None known	Potentiation of $GABA_A$ receptor	Sedating Nonaddictive
Zaleplon (Sonata)	None known		
Lithium	Sinus node dysfunction Sinoatrial block T-wave inversion or flattening, particularly in patients > 60 years Arrhythmias and sudden death in patients with cardiac disease	Unknown	Narrow therapeutic index (1.6–1.2 mmol/L) Many medications alter lithium plasma levels* Fatal in overdose Mood stabilizer for patients with bipolar disorder Yearly ECG in patients > 50 years

CYP, Cytochrome P450 enzyme; *ECG,* electrocardiogram; *FDA,* US Food and Drug Administration; *GABA,* gamma-aminobutyric acid; *GAD,* generalized anxiety disorder; *HRV,* heart rate variability; *OCD,* obsessive-compulsive disorder; *PTSD,* posttraumatic stress disorder; *SSRI,* selective serotonin reuptake inhibitor.

*Medications that increase lithium levels: nonsteroidal antiinflammatory drugs, diuretics (thiazides, ethacrynic acid, spironolactone, triamterene), angiotensin-converting enzyme inhibitors, metronidazole, tetracycline. Medications that decrease lithium levels: acetazolamide, theophylline, aminophylline, caffeine, osmotic diuretics. *(From Musselman DL, Evans DL, Nemeroff CB: The relationship of depression to cardiovascular disease: epidemiology, biology, and treatment,* Arch Gen Psychiatry *55(7):580–592, 1998.)*

TABLE 26.2 Interactions among Cardiovascular and Antidepressant Medications

CARDIOVASCULAR CONDITION	CARDIOVASCULAR DRUG/DRUG GROUP	RECOMMENDED ANTIDEPRESSANTS	ANTIDEPRESSANTS TO AVOID/USE WITH CAUTION		COMMENTS
Hypertension	β-adrenoceptor blocking drugs (e.g., propranolol, metoprolol, etc.)	Sertraline	**Avoid**	**Effect**	Paroxetine and fluoxetine may inhibit metabolism of doxasozin Mirtazapine and trazodone may antagonize effects of clonidine Duloxetine and venlafaxine are unstudied in CVD patients TCAs (amitriptyline, clomipramine, doxepin, imipramine, etc.) cause adverse cardiovascular events MAOIs (phenelzine, isocarboxazid, and tranylcypromine) cause adverse cardiovascular events
			TCAs	Increased risk of arrhythmia with sotalol	
			Venlafaxine	May worsen hypertension	
			Duloxetine	May worsen hypertension	
			Reboxetine	May worsen hypertension	
			Buproprion	May worsen hypertension	
			All MAOIs	Risk of hypertensive crisis	
			Caution	**Effect**	
			TCAs	Increased risk of postural hypotension; plasma levels increased by labetalol and propranolol	
			Citalopram/escitalopram	Increases plasma level of metoprolol	
			Paroxetine	May increase plasma levels of metoprolol	
			Fluvoxamine	Increases plasma levels of propranolol	
			Mirtazapine	Increased risk of postural hypotension	
			Trazodone	Increased risk of postural hypotension	
	Vasodilator drugs (e.g., diazoxide, hydralazine, prazosin, doxazosin)	Any alternative (e.g., SSRIs)	**Avoid**	**Effect**	
			Venlafaxine	May worsen hypertension	
			Duloxetine	May worsen hypertension	
			Reboxetine	May worsen hypertension	
			Buproprion	May worsen hypertension	
			All MAOIs	Risk of hypertensive crisis	
			Caution	**Effect**	
			TCAs	Increased risk of postural hypertension	
			Mirtazapine	Increased risk of postural hypertension	
	Centrally acting antihypertensives (e.g., methyldopa, clonidine, etc.)	Any alternative (e.g., SSRIs)	**Avoid**	**Effect**	
			TCAs	Antagonize effects of clonidine	
			Venlafaxine	May worsen hypertension	
			Duloxetine	May worsen hypertension	
			Reboxetine	May worsen hypertension	
			Bupropion	Hypertensive urgency when administered with clonidine	
			All MAOIs	Risk of hypertensive crisis	
			Caution	**Effect**	
			Mirtazapine	Increased risk of postural hypotension	
			Clonidine	Hypertensive urgency	
			Trazodone	Increased risk of postural hypotension	
	ACE inhibitors, angiotensin-II antagonists: renin inhibitors (e.g., captopril, enalapril, losartan, aliskiren)	Any alternative (e.g., SSRIs)	**Avoid**	**Effect**	
			MAOIs	May enhance hypotensive effects of ACE inhibitors and angiotensin antagonists	
			Venlafaxine	May worsen hypertension	
			Duloxetine	May worsen hypertension	
			Rexobetine	May worsen hypertension	
			Buproprion	May worsen hypertension	
			Lithium	Plasma levels increased by ACE inhibitors	
			Caution	**Effect**	
			TCAs	Increased risk of postural hypotension	
			Mirtazapine	Increased risk of postural hypotension	

Dyslipidemia	Bile acid sequestrants (e.g., colestipol, holestyramine)	Any	**Avoid** None specifically contraindicated **Caution** None specifically contraindicated		Omega-3 fatty acids may have antidepressant effects MAOIs (phenelzine, isocarboxazid, and tranylcypromine) cause adverse cardiovascular events
	Ezetimibe	Any	**Avoid** None specifically contraindicated **Caution** None specifically contraindicated		
	Fibrates (e.g., bezafibrate)	Any	**Avoid** MAOIs with bezafibrate	**Effect** Risk of hepatotoxicity	
	Statins (e.g., atorvastatin, simvastatin)	Any alternative (e.g., SSRIs, TCAs, others)	**Avoid** St. John's wort	**Effect** Reduces effect of simvastatin	
	Omega-3 fatty acids (e.g., MaxEPA, Omacor)	Any	**Avoid** None specifically contraindicated **Caution** None specifically contraindicated		
Angina	Nitrates (e.g., glyceryl trinitrate isosorbide, nononitrate)	Any alternative (e.g., SSRIs)	**Avoid** MAOIs **Caution** TCAs	**Effect** Increased hypotensive effects **Effect** Dry mouth may reduce absorption of sublingual tablets	Paroxetine has mild anticholinergic properties Tricyclics (amitriptyline, clomipramine, doxepin, imipramine, etc.) cause adverse cardiovascular events MAOIs (phenelzine, isocarboxazid, and tranylcypromine) cause adverse cardiovascular events
Heart failure	Cardiac glycosides (digoxin; digitoxin)	Any alternative (e.g., SSRIs, mirtazapine)	**Avoid** St. John's wort TCAs Venlafaxine Trazodone	**Effect** Reduces digoxin plasma levels Possibly proarrhythmic in cardiac disease Not recommended in those at risk of arrhythmia Increases digoxin plasma levels	May increase risk of antidepressant-associated hyponatremia Fluoxetine (SSRI) has a long half-life (3–4 weeks), which may be increased by heart failure Venlafaxine is unstudied in CVD patients Tricyclics (amitriptyline, clomipramine, doxepin, imipramine, etc.) cause adverse cardiovascular events MAOIs (phenelzine, isocarboxazid, and tranylcypromine) cause adverse cardiovascular events
	Thiazide diuretics (bendroflumethiazide, etc.)	Any alternative (e.g., SSRIs)	**Avoid** Reboxetine Lithium **Caution** MAOIs/tricyclics/mirtazapine	**Effect** Increased risk of hypokalemia Plasma levels increased by thiazides **Effect** Increased risk of postural hypotension	
	Loop diuretics (furosemide, bumetanide)	Any alternative (e.g., SSRIs, mirtazapine)	**Avoid** Reboxetine Lithium **Caution** MAOIs/TCAs	**Effect** Increased risk of hypocalcemia Plasma levels increased by loop diuretics **Effect** Increased risk of postural hypotension	
	Other diuretics (amiloride, eplerenone, etc.)	Any alternative (e.g., SSRIs)	**Avoid** St. John's wort	**Effect** Reduces eplerenone plasma levels	

Continued

TABLE 26.2 Interactions among Cardiovascular and Antidepressant Medications—cont'd

CARDIOVASCULAR CONDITION	CARDIOVASCULAR DRUG/DRUG GROUP	RECOMMENDED ANTIDEPRESSANTS	ANTIDEPRESSANTS TO AVOID/USE WITH CAUTION		COMMENTS
Cardiac arrhythmia	Antiarrhythmics (e.g., amiodarone, disopyramide, flecainide, lidocaine, propafenone, etc.)	Sertraline* Mirtazapine* Moclobemide* Mianserin* Citalopram† Escitalopram† Paroxetine Fluoxetine ****All recommended drugs should be used with caution*** *†QTc prolongation*	**Avoid** TCAs Citalopram/escitalopram Fluoxetine Paroxetine Duloxetine Venlafaxine **Caution** Trazodone Reboxetine	**Effect** Increased risk of arrhythmia Increases plasma levels of flecainide and propafenone Increases plasma levels of flecainide and propafenone Increases plasma levels of flecainide and propafenone Increases plasma levels of flecainide Possible increased risk of arrhythmia **Effect** Possibly increased risk of arrhythmia May cause hypokalemia	Venlafaxine is unstudied in CVD patients Tricyclics (amitriptyline, clomipramine, doxepin, imipramine, etc.) cause adverse cardiovascular events
Conditions requiring anticoagulation	Parenteral anticoagulates (e.g., heparin, LMW heparin)	Any alternative (e.g., trazodone, reboxetine, tricyclics)	**Avoid** SSRIs Venlafaxine Duloxetine	**Effect** Probable increased risk of bleeding Probable increased risk of bleeding Probable increased risk of bleeding	Venlafaxine is unstudied in CVD patients Tricyclics (amitriptyline, clomipramine, doxepin, imipramine, etc.) cause adverse cardiovascular events
	Oral anticoagulants (warfarin, phenindione)	Reboxetine Trazodone Mianserin ***All recommended drugs should be used with caution***	**Avoid** SSRIs TCAs Mirtazapine St. John's wort **Caution** Venlafaxine Duloxetine	**Effect** Enhanced anticoagulant effect Enhanced or reduced anticoagulant effect Enhanced anticoagulant effect Reduced warfarin plasma levels **Effect** Possibly enhanced anticoagulant effect Possibly enhanced anticoagulant effect	Fluvoxamine and fluoxetine inhibit warfarin metabolism Anticoagulant effects may be enhanced without change in INR Venlafaxine is unstudied in CVD patients

ACE, Angiotensin-converting enzyme; *CVD,* cardiovascular disease; *GTN,* glyceryl trinitrate; *INR,* International normalized ratio; *LMW,* low molecular weight; *MAOIs,* monoamine oxidase inhibitors; *SSRIs,* selective serotonin reuptake inhibitors; *TCA,* tricyclic antidepressant. *(Adapted from National Institute for Health and Clinical Excellence:* Depression in Adults with Chronic Physical Health Problems, *London, 2009, National Institute for Health and Clinical Excellence.* and *Bradley SM, Rumsfeld JS: Depression and cardiovascular disease,* Trends Cardiovasc Med *25(7):614–622, 2015.)*

TABLE 26.3 Pharmacokinetic Interactions of Antidepressant, Anxiolytic, and Cardiovascular Medications

CYP4501A2	CYP4502C9/19	CYP4502D6	CYP4503A4
Inhibited by:	**Inhibited by:**	**Inhibited by:**	**Inhibited by:**
Cimetidine	Cimetidine	Chlorpromazine	Amprenavir
Ciprofloxacin	Delavirdine	Duloxetine	Delavirdine
Erythromycin	Fluoxetine	Fluoxetine	Erythromycin
Fluvoxamine	Fluvoxamine	Fluphenazine	Fluoxetine
Paroxetine	Sertraline	Haloperidol Paroxetine Ritonavir Sertraline Tricyclics	Fluvoxamine Ketoconazole Nelfinavir Paroxetine Saquinavir Sertraline Tricyclics
Metabolizes:	**Metabolizes:**	**Metabolizes:**	**Metabolizes:**
Caffeine	Diazepam	Clozapine	Benzodiazepines
Clozapine	Omeprazole	Codeine	Calcium blockers
Duloxetine	Phenytoin	Donepezil	Carbamazepine
Tolbutamide	Flecainide	Cimetidine	Haloperidol
Mirtazapine	Tricyclics	Haloperidol	Clozapine
Warfarin	Metoprolol	Mirtazapine	Olanzapine
Propranolol		Phenothiazines	Donepezil
Theophylline		Pimozide	Erythromycin
Tricyclics		Propafenone Risperidone Tricyclics Tramadol Trazodone Venlafaxine	Galantamine Methadone Mirtazapine Reboxetine Risperidone Steroids Terfenadine Trazodone Tricyclics Valproate Venlafaxine Z-hypnotics

Medications indicated in red are psychiatric medications and those highlighted in yellow are cardiac medications. *(Adapted from National Institute for Health and Clinical Excellence:* Depression in Adults with Chronic Physical Health Problems, *London, 2009, National Institute for Health and Clinical Excellence.)*

Stress

Few interventions have been tested for stress, so this area is in dire need of further research. We could find no interventions that directly tested a pharmacologic intervention for stress, when stress was the primary complaint and was not comorbid with anxiety, depression, or other more commonly studied emotional dysregulations. Psychologic interventions for stress include CBT and muscle relaxation techniques.[30]

SHOULD PROFESSIONAL SOCIETY GUIDELINES/ADVISORIES/STATEMENTS BE FOLLOWED?

To recommend screening for a condition, the condition should be important, prevalent, not easily detected without screening, and treatable with treatment benefits that outweigh the risks as demonstrated in RCTs.[25] The AHA, AAFP, European societies, and NICE recommend screening for depression, anxiety, and stress in CHD patients. This is a large-scale healthcare policy and a potentially expensive practice, but it is not based on RCTs and, therefore, does not have rigorous evidence of effectiveness or benefit.

Evidence-based practice guidelines are often distinguished from consensus-based practice guidelines or advisories, as the former systematically review all available research on the specified topic and grade the level of evidence to make clinical recommendations. However, not all research designs are given equal weight. Standards of evidence for guidelines have evolved to place greater emphasis on RCTs because RCTs are the most replicable and have the fewest sources of bias. If all other variables are equal, RCTs have the greatest power to detect whether a screening practice or treatment results in a net benefit or harm.

It is important to examine the RCT evidence regarding screening and treating depression in CHD patients before changes in policy and practice are considered. Without RCTs, evidence-based guidelines cannot endorse screening, diagnosing, and treating depression, anxiety, or stress in CHD patients.

A recent systematic review and meta-analysis by Thombs et al.[25] found that there are no published RCTs investigating the effects of depression screening on either depression or cardiac outcomes in CAD patients. There are some RCTs showing that treating depression leads to modest improvements in depression symptoms among post-MI and stable CHD patients, as seen in Fig. 26.8,[25] but no RCTs show that treating depression improves cardiac outcomes.[25]

Depression

Treating Patients with Coronary Heart Disease for Depression: Randomized Controlled Trials

The establishment of depression as a risk marker in patients with CHD prompted the National Heart, Lung, and Blood Institute to fund the Enhancing Recovery in CHD Patients (ENRICHD) trial, which randomized almost 2500 patients to determine whether treating depression and social isolation after acute MI improves event-free survival.[49] There were no significant differences in all-cause mortality or nonfatal MI rates between the intervention and usual-care arms of ENRICHD, nor in underpowered trials such the Sertraline Antidepressant Heart-Attack Randomized Trial (SADHART)[50] and the Myocardial INfarction and Depression-Intervention Trial (MIND-IT).[51] ENRICHD and these first-generation phase II trials yielded only modest differences in depression between the treatment and control arms. Plausible reasons include: (1) the interventions were not efficacious, (2) the treatments were not well accepted, (3) the control conditions improved depression more than expected, and (4) the appropriate patient population was not studied. The ENRICHD investigators concluded that the next large, phase III trial should be postponed until more efficacious depression treatments are available and the subtypes of depression that are most responsible for increased medical morbidity and mortality have been identified. Progress since then includes the Sequenced Treatment Alternatives to Relieve Depression (STAR*D) trial,[52] which demonstrated that aggressive, algorithm-based delivery of existing therapies achieves better depression outcomes, several phase II clinical trials—described in the following section—that have demonstrated better depression outcomes in cardiac populations, and advances in our understanding of the characteristics of high-risk depression subtypes.

Freedland et al.[53] conducted an RCT involving 123 patients with major or minor depression who had recently

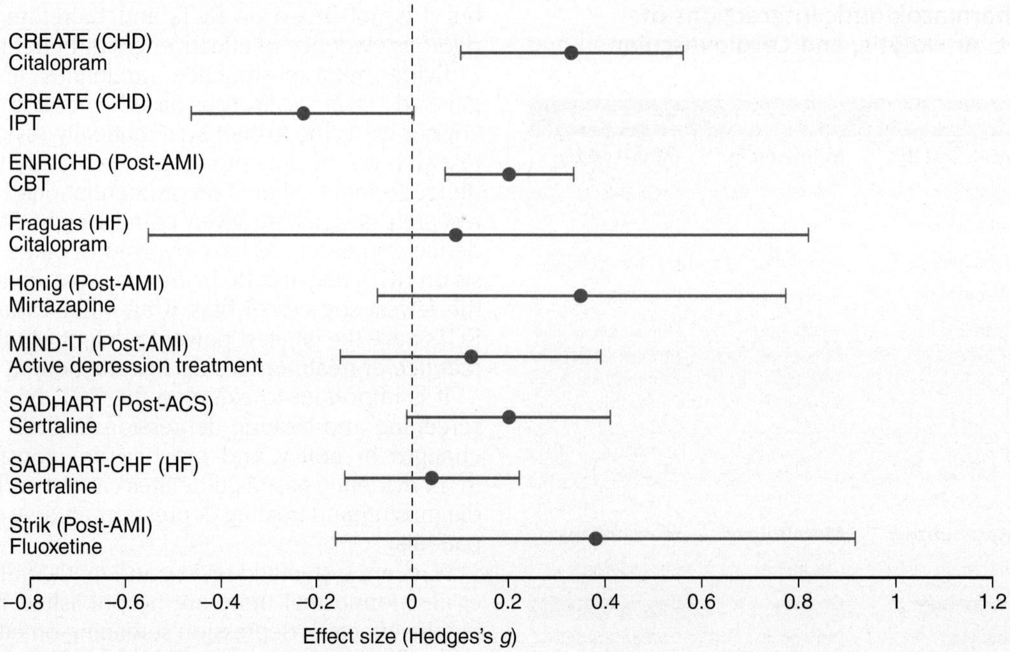

FIG. 26.8 Forest plot of effect sizes of depression treatment studies. *ACS,* Acute coronary syndrome; *AMI,* acute myocardial infarction; *CHD,* coronary heart disease; *HF,* heart failure. *(From Thombs BD, Roseman M, Coyne JC, et al. Does evidence support the American Heart Association's recommendation to screen patients for depression in cardiovascular care? An updated systematic review.* PLoS One. *2013;8(1):e52654.)*

undergone CABG surgery. The trial's primary purpose was to determine the efficacy of two behavioral treatments (CBT and supportive stress management) compared with usual care. The depression effect size for CBT at the end of 3 months yielded a Beck Depression Inventory (BDI) depression effect size of 0.85 (95% CI, 0.41–1.32). This effect was maintained 6 months after the end of the trial.

Huffman et al.[54] recently completed an RCT of 175 hospitalized depressed cardiac patients. They compared usual care with a low-intensity depression collaborative care treatment. The care was initiated in the hospital and continued by telephone. Depression was assessed by the PHQ-9 using the DSM-IV MDD criteria. All patients in the treatment arm received behavioral activation and, then, by patient preference and/or prior treatment history, received psychotherapy or pharmacotherapy. At 3 months (treatment end), treatment group patients had improved more than control patients, but this was not maintained at 6 months (when no treatment was offered).

The Coronary Psychosocial Evaluation Studies (COPES) II[42,55] post-ACS trial compared the acceptability and efficacy of 6-month stepped depression care, a patient preference-driven, stepped algorithm depression intervention, with referred depression care, in which depression screening was followed by physician notification and encouragement to initiate depression treatment. The protocol included 157 CHD patients with depressive symptoms, but was not limited to those who met DSM-IV criteria for MDD. This strategy targeted ACS patients who were at greatest mortality risk based on recent studies of depression and cardiac outcomes, namely those with postdischarge depressive symptoms. COPES II employed an aggressive, stepped-care, patient-preference, symptom-driven approach that increased the acceptability and efficacy of the depression intervention. Depression treatment acceptability was three times higher in the stepped depression care group than in the referred care group. The differential improvement in depression between groups was significantly larger in the stepped care arm (HR 0.59, 95% CI 0.18–1.00).

Whether the COPES intervention can be delivered as intended in multiple clinical centers was then addressed by Comparison of Depression Interventions after Acute Coronary Syndrome (CODIACS) I, a feasibility/vanguard study conducted at five US sites that showed significant improvement in depressive symptoms as measured by BDI scores with active treatment versus usual care.[56] In this vanguard, the COPES protocol was streamlined, case-finding made more efficient, and treatment delivery centralized and conducted by a web-based interface and then by telephone. Patients were randomized to 6 months of centralized depression care (patient preference for problem-solving treatment given via telephone or the Internet, pharmacotherapy, both, or neither), stepped every 6 to 8 weeks (active treatment group, $n = 73$) or to locally determined depression care after physician notification about the patient's depressive symptoms (usual care group, $n = 77$). The main outcomes were change in depressive symptoms during 6 months and total healthcare costs. The trial found that depressive symptoms were decreased significantly more in the active treatment group than in the usual care group (differential change between groups, –3.5 BDI points; 95% CI –6.1 to –0.7; $p = 0.01$). Although mental healthcare estimated costs were higher for active treatment than for usual care, overall healthcare estimated costs were not significantly different (difference adjusting for confounding, –\$325; 95% CI –\$2639 to \$1989; $p = 0.78$).[57]

The CODIACS trial concluded that for patients with post-ACS depression, active treatment had a substantial beneficial effect on depressive symptoms. Experts have concluded that it is time to conduct the next phase III depression trial in CHD patients.[58–61] To date, treating depression after ACS has not resulted in improved cardiovascular outcomes,[49,51] primarily because we do not have large RCTs that actually test this question.

Providing Patients with Coronary Heart Disease with the American Heart Association's Depression Screen and Treat Algorithm

There is a paucity of information from observational trials or RCTs on the costs and benefits of screening and treating depression in post-ACS patients. Only one randomized placebo-controlled trial of sertraline, SADHART[50] ($n = 369$), has been used to estimate costs, but this did not include cost-effectiveness and was not a depression screening RCT.[62] Many costs were not represented, as they were not collected.

A meta-analysis of RCTs testing depression screening with only notification of depression severity to primary care providers for primary care patients (*not* post-ACS patients) found that this strategy did not lead to increased detection or treatment of depression, and it showed no impact on health-related quality of life, depressive symptoms, or other patient outcomes, including cost-effectiveness.[63] An update of this Cochrane review found essentially the same disappointing results.[64] In a 2001 study examining the costs of screening for depression, the costs per QALY were unacceptable for screening annually, once a lifetime, or once every 5 years: the expected annual cost was $192,444/QALYs.[65] A nonstationary Markov model, using published literature, found that no depression screening was preferable over annual depression screening, and in the vast majority (99%) of scenarios, the cost per QALY was more than $50,000, with little expectation of patient benefit.[65] This low value of screening makes sense in a primary care setting in which the association of depression with clinical outcomes is less robust than in a post-ACS population and in which the prevalence of depression is lower. Thus, the evidence from RCTs in a primary care population is that screening and treating primary care patients for depression has minimal quality of life improvements and/or is cost ineffective.

The reasons for little positive effects of depression screening include high rates of false-positive results, small treatment effects, preexisting antidepressant use among CHD patients, and poor quality of routine mental healthcare.

Anxiety

Similar to the findings for the treatment of comorbid depression in CHD, pooled analyses of RCTs testing the effectiveness of psychologic interventions for anxiety (including cognitive techniques, relaxation training, and social support) indicate effect sizes for anxiety that are of equal magnitude to those observed for depression among patients with CHD (standardized mean differences = 0.25).[48] Although there are some small, single trials for stress reduction in patients with CHD, there are no systematic reviews of this evidence base.[66,67]

Stress

RCTs of stress interventions and cardiac outcomes have shown efficacy for treating "stress," even though definitions of stress have varied. A recent meta-analysis of 43 studies showed that psychological interventions targeted to stress reduction (including CBT, yoga, and muscle relaxation techniques) decreased 2-year mortality in men and event recurrence in all CHD patients by 27%.[68] No trials have yet examined the effects of stress reduction on CHD incidence.

PRACTICAL CONSIDERATIONS FOR TREATING COMORBID CORONARY HEART DISEASE AND DEPRESSION, ANXIETY, OR STRESS

Screening for Depression, Anxiety, or Stress

Staff-Assisted Depression Care Supports

Some patients who are screened for depression, anxiety, or stress will screen positive. Primary care providers or cardiovascular disease specialists who screen patients should be prepared to follow a practice-specific algorithm such as those executed by "staff-assisted depression care supports" for diagnosing, treating, and following-up patients identified as exhibiting symptoms of depression, anxiety, or stress.[69] According to the USPSTF (and formally recommended by the AAFP and American College of Physicians), such an algorithm should include referral for more complete interview and evaluation to confirm the diagnosis of depression according to DSM-IV.[69,36]

If a clinical practice does not have staff-assisted depression care supports, the net benefit of depression screening is likely minimal and is not recommended.[69,70] The AHA/ACC secondary prevention guidelines for CHD patients specifically recommend depression screening if patients have access to case management with collaborating primary care physicians and mental health specialists.[12]

Adverse Effects of Screening

Adverse effects of depression or anxiety screening include false-positive results, stigma of diagnosis, and management that leads to treatment of mild or transitory depression or anxiety with diversion of resources from patients who have more severe psychiatric conditions.

Further Evaluation of Depression, Anxiety, or Stress

Suicidality Screening

In one study of routine depression screening occurring over the course of 1 year among patients admitted with suspected CHD, 12% of patients reported suicidal ideation; all these patients underwent immediate psychiatric evaluation and upon formal assessment, 0.5% required hospitalization for imminent harm.[71] Depression screening in CHD patients should therefore be undertaken only if there is a system in place to treat or refer patients who are found be at risk of imminent harm.[22]

Screening for Manic Episodes

Depressive symptoms often occur as part of the clinical presentation of bipolar disorder.[22] Screening questions about current or previous manic or hypomanic episodes are needed to determine the appropriate psychiatric treatment course.

Assessment of Other Psychiatric Comorbidities

Subtle or overt psychotic processes, comorbid anxiety symptoms, personality disorders, dementia, illicit drug or alcohol dependence/abuse, and a number of other psychiatric comorbidities complicate the management of depression.[22] Clinicians should have a system in place for the immediate referral and follow-up with an appropriate mental health professional or setting, if any of these other comorbidities

BOX 26.3 Seven Key Challenges in Managing Depression

1. Make a diagnosis.
2. Educate and recruit the patient as a partner in treatment.
3. Start with the best possible treatment.
4. Use an adequate dose.
5. Treat long enough (patients often take 6 to 10 weeks to respond).
6. Follow outcomes and adjust treatment as needed. Consider consultation if patient is not improving.
7. Prevent relapse (50% risk after 1 episode, 70% after 2 episodes, and 90% after 3 episodes).

Adapted from Unützer J, Oishi S. *IMPACT Late-Life Depression Treatment Manual.* Los Angeles: UCLA NPI, Center for Health Services Research; 1999, 2004.

are discovered, as many of these conditions require close monitoring and follow-up.

Depression Caused by a General Medical Condition or Substance

When facing a positive depression screen result, clinicians should ensure that a coexisting medical condition or a current medication or substance is not causing the depressive symptoms. Examples of culprits include hypo- or hyperthyroidism, sleep apnea, vitamin B_{12} deficiency, vitamin D deficiency, and a variety of prescribed medications.[22] These conditions should be treated, after which depression should be reevaluated.

β-Blockers are a mainstay class of drugs for a variety of cardiac conditions, and there has been a historic concern that β-blocker use is associated with worse depressive symptoms. However, most studies supporting this concern had small sample sizes were not prospective in design, or did not use direct, validated measures of depression.[72] A recent prospective study of post-MI patients taking β-blockers compared with matched patients not taking β-blockers found that the groups did not significantly differ with regard to depressive symptoms as measured by the validated BDI after 1 year of follow-up.[72] A prospective study of patients undergoing implantable cardioverter-defibrillator placement did not find an association between β-blocker use and depressive symptoms.[73] Furthermore, a prospective study among post-cardiac catheterization patients found that β-blockers were associated with fewer depressive symptoms in a dose-response relationship.[74] Therefore, despite historic concerns, rigorously designed studies do not support that β-blockers are associated with depression.

Formal Evaluation

A mental health professional should confirm the diagnosis of depression or anxiety with a thorough evaluation based on standardized, semistructured interview or DSM criteria.

Managing Depression, Anxiety, or Stress

Patients diagnosed with depression, anxiety, or stress should be referred for management by a professional with the qualifications and experience to manage these conditions with psychotherapy and/or medical therapy.

Box 26.3 gives some key reminders of the best practices for managing depression.[75] If the patient does not meet the medical condition/risk rule-outs detailed previously and does not require immediate mental health/psychiatric attention, there are many evidence-based depression treatment options to consider. There is currently no preferred order or sequencing of treatments. Therefore, use of the modified IMPACT algorithm (Fig. 26.9) seems reasonable.[76] This algorithm was tested in an RCT of 157 post-ACS patients, and patients reported high satisfaction with depression care, a significant reduction in depressive symptoms, and a signal of decreased adverse cardiac events.[42] Patient preference for psychotherapy versus antidepressant medication may play a role in adherence to depression treatment regimen.[77] This suggests that if a patient reports a strong preference for either psychotherapy or antidepressant medication, the preference should be honored when possible.

Medical Management

Medical management offers benefits as well as adverse events to patients. Treating depression and anxiety with medical therapy risks both drug side effects and drug interactions that are detrimental to health, including cardiovascular health. Clinicians should be aware of these practical considerations, because the risks of treating depression or anxiety may outweigh any potential benefits.

Cardiovascular Side Effects of Psychotropic Drugs

Various antidepressants and anxiolytics are associated with increased cardiovascular side effects, ranging from elevated blood pressure to hypertensive crisis, bradycardia, tachycardia, and malignant arrhythmias (see Table 26.1).

Literature published over the past 15 years has suggested that SSRIs affect hemostasis by inhibiting serotonin uptake in platelets and thus weakly diminish platelet aggregation.[78] Gastrointestinal (GI) bleeding has been a frequently studied adverse effect of SSRIs, with a systematic literature review estimating that SSRI use is associated with an approximately two-fold increase in GI bleeds.[7] A systematic review showed that bleeding risk associated with SSRIs is increased with liver cirrhosis, portal hypertension, or liver failure.[79] Concomitant SSRI and nonsteroidal antiinflammatory drug or aspirin use, in particular, increases GI bleeding risk, according to systematic reviews.[78,80] Nearly all of the studies included in these reviews are observational, retrospective studies with matched control subjects that add rigor, though there were no RCTs.

SSRI use also increases general (not necessarily limited to GI) bleeding risk when combined with warfarin use among medicine and cardiac patients.[81] This phenomenon has been attributed to SSRIs' effect on the hepatic cytochrome P450 (CYP) isoenzyme system, resulting in inhibited warfarin metabolism. Fluvoxamine and fluoxetine seem most likely to enhance the anticoagulant effect of warfarin; paroxetine seems to have low-to-moderate risk; sertraline and citalopram appear to be least likely to interact with warfarin.[82] Patients initiating SSRI use when already using warfarin, or vice versa, should have their international normalized ratio levels carefully monitored.

The literature is more equivocal with regard to any increased risk of bleeding attributed to SSRI use among CHD patients. Kim et al.[83] found that CABG patients who received SSRIs did not have any increase in bleeding events compared with propensity-matched control subjects even when the SSRIs were used in combination with antiplatelet or anticoagulant drugs.[83] Labos et al.[84] found in a retrospective cohort study that acute MI patients who were taking an SSRI with aspirin or dual antiplatelet therapy were at increased

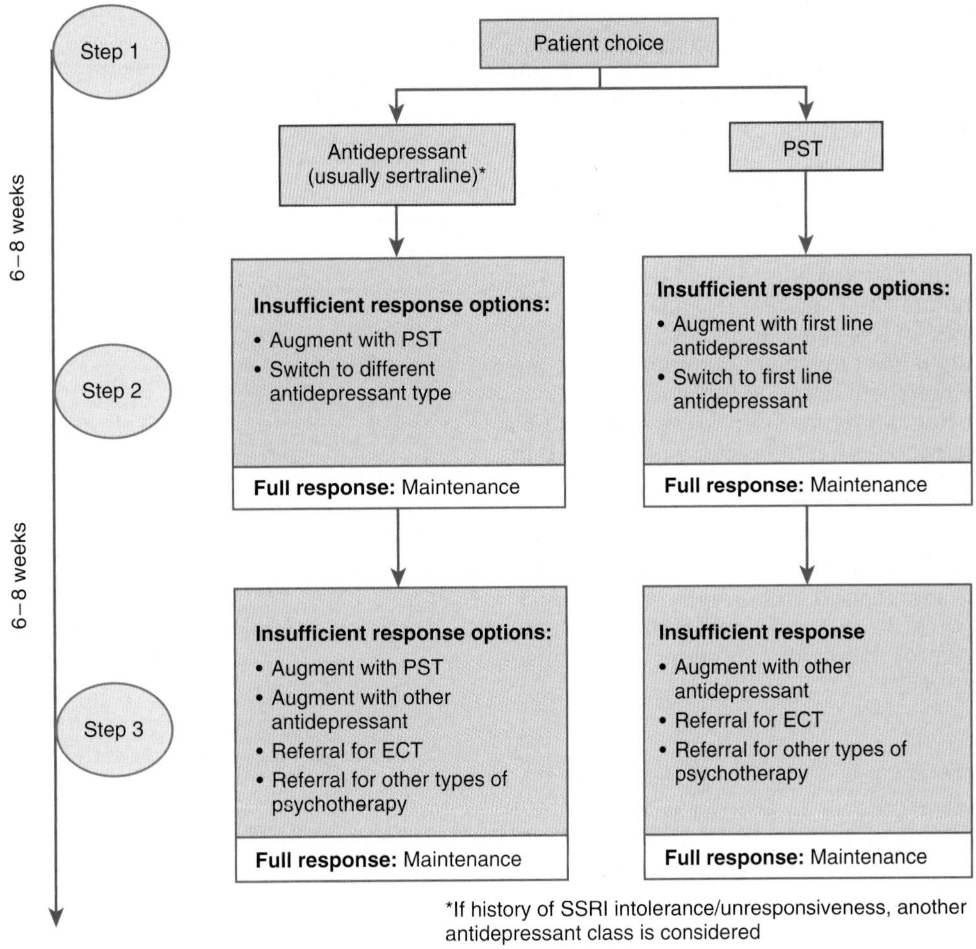

FIG. 26.9 Depression treatment algorithm to follow for depressed patients with coronary heart disease. *ECT*, Electroconvulsive therapy; *PST*, problem-solving therapy; *SSRI*, selective serotonin reuptake inhibitor. *(From Davidson KW. Depression and comorbid coronary heart disease.* Medscape Education Psychiatry and Mental Health. *2011.)*

risk of bleeding.[84] It is therefore prudent to be aware of this potential risk; SSRIs should be used thoughtfully and cautiously among cardiovascular patients requiring antiplatelet and/or anticoagulation agents who may already be at an increased bleeding risk.[7]

Drug Interactions

Depending on an individual patient's cardiovascular condition and medication regimen, specific psychotropic medications should be used with caution or avoided out of concern for side effects or drug-drug interactions. Table 26.2 details recommended antidepressants and those to be used with caution or avoided altogether according to cardiovascular conditions and cardiovascular medications.

Psychotropic drug pharmacokinetic interactions largely center on inhibition of hepatic CYP pathways, which can affect the metabolism of cardiovascular medications, as shown in Table 26.3. Most SSRIs inhibit CYP pathways in a dose-related fashion, leading to reduced metabolism of some cardiovascular medications and subsequent increased drug levels and side effects.[7,44]

The pharmacokinetic interaction concerns regarding lithium relate to its renal excretion. Cardiovascular medications such as ACE inhibitors or diuretics that alter renal function can reduce lithium excretion and lead to an increase in lithium levels as great as four-fold.[7] Renal function and lithium levels should be monitored regularly in such patients.[7]

The pharmacodynamic interactions of psychotropic medications are varied. SSRIs can increase the risk of hyponatremia, especially when diuretics that also reduce serum sodium are used.[7] TCAs antagonize α_1-adrenergic receptors and can, therefore, cause postural hypotension that can be additive with other α-blockers or antihypertensive agents.[7]

Other Considerations

When medical therapy is initiated for depression, there can be an initial increased risk of suicide. Patients and caregivers should be aware of this issue and be provided with a plan if suicidal ideation occurs or worsens.[22]

Psychotherapy

Most types of psychotherapy require professional training to be effective. Clinicians must take stock of the resources available for their patients and the system by which referrals would be made. Cost (lack of coverage by medical insurance plans) and waiting lists are barriers to the receipt of an effective treatment for depression.

Depression Is a Relapsing, Remitting Disorder

Relapse prevention and regular assessment should be planned at the end of a successful treatment course. There are three steps that can minimize depression relapses and partial remissions:[22]

1. Educate patients at the beginning of treatment, and particularly when depression is remitting, that relapses happen to everyone and that adherence to treatment and follow-up appointments is required to ensure continuing progress. Patients should also be taught at the start of treatment that treatment response is not immediate, that symptoms of depression may wax and wane, and that the clinician will work with them to augment or switch medication until remission has been achieved.
2. Maintain treatment. A systematic review has shown that those who continue their antidepressants have a 70% decreased chance of a depression relapse; therefore, 12 months of antidepressant treatment is commonly recommended, even when there is a good initial response.[85]
3. Reassess often. Regular depression assessment assures that early relapse and partial remission will be noted in the patient's progress, so that treatment can be tailored accordingly. A lack of initial response to treatment may be due to an incorrect diagnosis, insufficient psychotropic drug dose, insufficient duration of treatment, problems with medication adherence, and complicating factors such as comorbid psychiatric diseases, substance abuse, or medical conditions that cause depressive symptoms.

References

1. Thombs BD, Jewett LR, Knafo R, et al.: Learning from history: a commentary on the American Heart Association science advisory on depression screening, *Am Heart J* 158(4):503–505, 2009.
2. Smolderen KG, Spertus JA, Reid KJ, et al.: The association of cognitive and somatic depressive symptoms with depression recognition and outcomes after myocardial infarction, *Circ Cardiovasc Qual Outcomes* 2(4):328–337, 2009.
3. Smolderen KG, Buchanan DM, Amin AA, et al.: Real-world lessons from the implementation of a depression screening protocol in acute myocardial infarction patients: implications for the American Heart Association depression screening advisory, *Circ Cardiovasc Qual Outcomes* 4(3):283–292, 2011.
4. Thombs BD, de Jonge P, Ziegelstein RC: Depression screening in patients with heart disease–reply, *JAMA* 301(13):1338, 2009.
5. Hasnain M, Vieweg WVR, Lesnefsky EJ, et al.: Depression screening in patients with coronary heart disease: a critical evaluation of the AHA guidelines, *J Psychosom Res* 71(1):6–12, 2010.
6. Centers for Medicare and Medicaid Services: *2014 Clinical Quality Measures (CQMs) Adult Recommended Core Measures*, Baltimore, 2014, Centers for Medicare and Medicaid Services.
7. National Institute for Health and Clinical Excellence: *Depression in Adults with Chronic Physical Health Problems*, London, 2009, National Institute for Health and Clinical Excellence.
8. Lichtman JH, Bigger Jr JT, Blumenthal JA, et al.: Depression and coronary heart disease: recommendations for screening, referral, and treatment. A science advisory from the American Heart Association Prevention Committee of the Council on Cardiovascular Nursing, Council on Clinical Cardiology, Council on Epidemiology and Prevention, and Interdisciplinary Council on Quality of Care and Outcomes Research, *Circulation* 118(17):1768–1775, 2008.
9. Whooley MA, Avins AL, Miranda J, et al.: Case-finding instruments for depression. Two questions are as good as many, *J Gen Intern Med* 12(7):439–445, 1997.
10. Lichtman JH, Bigger Jr JT, Blumenthal JA, et al.: Depression and coronary heart disease: recommendations for screening, referral, and treatment: a science advisory from the American Heart Association Prevention Committee of the Council on Cardiovascular Nursing, Council on Clinical Cardiology, Council on Epidemiology and Prevention, and Interdisciplinary Council on Quality of Care and Outcomes Research: endorsed by the American Psychiatric Association, *Circulation* 118(17):1768–1775, 2008.
11. Mosca L, Banka CL, Benjamin EJ, et al.: Evidence-based guidelines for cardiovascular disease prevention in women: 2007 update, *J Am Coll Cardiol* 49(11):1230–1250, 2007.
12. Smith Jr SC, Benjamin EJ, Bonow RO, et al.: AHA/ACCF secondary prevention and risk reduction therapy for patients with coronary and other atherosclerotic vascular disease: 2011 update: a guideline from the American Heart Association and American College of Cardiology Foundation, *Circulation* 124(22):2458–2473, 2011.
13. Lichtman JH, Froelicher ES, Blumenthal JA, et al.: Depression as a risk factor for poor prognosis among patients with acute coronary syndrome: systematic review and recommendations: a scientific statement from the American Heart Association, *Circulation* 129(12):1350–1369, 2014.
14. Post-Myocardial Infarction Depression Clinical Practice Guideline Panel: AAFP guideline for the detection and management of post-myocardial infarction depression, *Ann Fam Med* 7(1):71–79, 2009.
15. Perk J, De Backer G, Gohlke H, et al.: European guidelines on cardiovascular disease prevention in clinical practice (version 2012): the fifth joint task force of the European Society of Cardiology and other societies on cardiovascular disease prevention in clinical practice (constituted by representatives of nine societies and by invited experts), *Int J Behav Med* 19(4):403–488, 2012.
16. *Depression in Adults with Chronic Physical Health Problems*, London, 2009, National Institute for Health and Clinical Excellence.
17. Arri SS, Ryan M, Redwood SR, et al.: Mental stress-induced myocardial ischaemia, *Heart* 102(6):472–480, 2016.
18. Tully PJ, Turnbull DA, Beltrame J, et al.: Panic disorder and incident coronary heart disease: a systematic review and meta-regression in 1,131,612 persons and 58,111 cardiac events, *Psychol Med* 45(14):2909–2920, 2015.
19. Davidson KW: Depression and coronary heart disease, *ISRN Cardiol* 2012, 2012:743813.
20. Bradley SM, Rumsfeld JS: Depression and cardiovascular disease, *Trends Cardiovasc Med* 25(7):614–622, 2015.
21. Seligman F, Nemeroff CB: The interface of depression and cardiovascular disease: therapeutic implications, *Ann N Y Acad Sci* 1345:25–35, 2015.
22. Davidson KW: Depression and comorbid coronary heart disease, *Medscape Education Psychiatry and Mental Health*, 2011.
23. Rozanski A, Blumenthal JA, Davidson KW, et al.: The epidemiology, pathophysiology, and management of psychosocial risk factors in cardiac practice: the emerging field of behavioral cardiology, *J Am Coll Cardiol* 45(5):637–651, 2005.
24. Whooley MA: Depression and cardiovascular disease: healing the broken-hearted, *JAMA* 295(24):2874–2881, 2006.
25. Thombs BD, Roseman M, Coyne JC, et al.: Does evidence support the American Heart Association's recommendation to screen patients for depression in cardiovascular care? An updated systematic review, *PLoS One* 8(1):e52654, 2013.
26. Hare DL, Toukhsati SR, Johansson P, et al.: Depression and cardiovascular disease: a clinical review, *Eur Heart J* 35(21):1365–1372, 2014.
27. Mujica-Mota RE, Roberts M, Abel G, et al.: Common patterns of morbidity and multi-morbidity and their impact on health-related quality of life: evidence from a national survey, *Qual Life Res* 24(4):909–918, 2015.
28. Cowles MK, Musselman DL, McDonald WM, et al.: Effects of mood and anxiety disorders on the cardiovascular system. In Fuster V, Walsh RA, Harrington RA, editors: *Hurst's The Heart*, ed 13, New York, 2011, McGraw-Hill, chapter 96.
29. Kershaw KN, Roux AVD, Bertoni A, et al.: Associations of chronic individual-level and neighbourhood-level stressors with incident coronary heart disease: the multi-ethnic study of atherosclerosis, *J Epidemiol Community Health* 69(2):136–141, 2015.
30. Richardson S, Shaffer JA, Falzon L, et al.: Meta-analysis of perceived stress and its association with incident coronary heart disease, *Am J Cardiol* 110(12):1711–1716, 2012.
31. Steptoe A, Kivimaki M: Stress and cardiovascular disease: an update on current knowledge, *Annu Rev Public Health* 34:337–354, 2013.
32. Nabi H, Kivimaki M, Batty GD, et al.: Increased risk of coronary heart disease among individuals reporting adverse impact of stress on their health: the Whitehall II prospective cohort study, *Eur Heart J* 34(34):2697–2705, 2013.
33. Georgiades A, Janszky I, Blom M, et al.: Financial strain predicts recurrent events among women with coronary artery disease, *Int J Cardiol* 135(2):175–183, 2009.
34. Laszlo KD, Ahnve S, Hallqvist J, et al.: Job strain predicts recurrent events after a first acute myocardial infarction: the Stockholm heart epidemiology program, *J Intern Med* 267(6):599–611, 2010.
35. Grippo AJ: Mechanisms underlying altered mood and cardiovascular dysfunction: the value of neurobiological and behavioral research with animal models, *Neurosci Biobehav Rev* 33(2): 171–180, 2009.
36. Maurer DM: Screening for depression, *Am Fam Physician* 85(2):139–144, 2012.
37. Cuijpers P, van Straten A, van Schaik A, et al.: Psychological treatment of depression in primary care: a meta-analysis, *Br J Gen Pract* 59(559):e51–e60, 2009.
38. Evans C: Review: interpersonal psychotherapy is slightly better and supportive therapy is worse than other therapies for depression, *Evid Based Med* 14(4):116, 2009.
39. Freedland KE, Skala JA, Carney RM, et al.: Treatment of depression after coronary artery bypass surgery: a randomized controlled trial, *Arch Gen Psychiatry* 66(4):387–396, 2009.
39a. Berkman LF, Blumenthal J, Burg M, et al.: Effects of treating depression and low perceived social support on clinical events after myocardial infarction: the Enhancing Recovery in Coronary Heart Disease Patients (ENRICHD) randomized trial, *JAMA* 289:3106–3116, 2003.
40. Unutzer J, Katon W, Callahan CM, et al.: Collaborative care management of late-life depression in the primary care setting: a randomized controlled trial, *JAMA* 288(22):2836–2845, 2002.
41. Burg MM, Lesperance F, Rieckmann N, et al.: Treating persistent depressive symptoms in post-ACS patients: the project COPES phase-I randomized controlled trial, *Contemp Clin Trials* 29(2): 231–240, 2008.
42. Davidson KW, Rieckmann N, Clemow L, et al.: Enhanced depression care for patients with acute coronary syndrome and persistent depressive symptoms: coronary psychosocial evaluation studies randomized controlled trial, *Arch Intern Med* 170(7):600–608, 2010.
43. Simon GE, Ludman EJ, Rutter CM: Incremental benefit and cost of telephone care management and telephone psychotherapy for depression in primary care, *Arch Gen Psychiatry* 66(10): 1081–1089, 2009.
44. Musselman DL, Evans DL, Nemeroff CB: The relationship of depression to cardiovascular disease: epidemiology, biology, and treatment, *Arch Gen Psychiatry* 55(7):580–592, 1998.
45. Committee on Electroconvulsive Therapy: *The Practice of Electroconvulsive Therapy: Recommendations for Treatment, Training, and Privileging: A Task Force Report of the American Psychiatric Association*. In Weiner RD, editor: ed 2, Washington, DC, 2001, American Psychiatric Association.
46. McCully RB, Karon BL, Rummans TA, et al.: Frequency of left ventricular dysfunction after electroconvulsive therapy, *Am J Cardiol* 91(9):1147–1150, 2003.
47. Zielinski RJ, Roose SP, Devanand DP, et al.: Cardiovascular complications of ECT in depressed patients with cardiac disease, *Am J Psychiatry* 150(6):904–909, 1993.
48. Whalley B, Thompson DR, Taylor RS: Psychological interventions for coronary heart disease: Cochrane systematic review and meta-analysis, *Int J Behav Med* 21(1):109–121, 2014.
49. Berkman LF, Blumenthal J, Burg M, et al.: Effects of treating depression and low perceived social support on clinical events after myocardial infarction: the Enhancing Recovery in Coronary Heart Disease Patients (ENRICHD) randomized trial, *JAMA* 289(23):3106–3116, 2003.
50. Glassman AH, O'Connor CM, Califf RM, et al.: Sertraline treatment of major depression in patients with acute MI or unstable angina, *JAMA* 288(6):701–709, 2002.
51. van Melle JP, de Jonge P, Honig A, et al.: Effects of antidepressant treatment following myocardial infarction, *Br J Psychiatry* 190:460–466, 2007.
52. Rush AJ, Trivedi MH, Wisniewski SR, et al.: Acute and longer-term outcomes in depressed outpatients requiring one or several treatment steps: a STAR*D report, *Am J Psychiatry* 163(11):1905–1917, 2006.
53. Freedland KE, Skala JA, Carney RM, et al.: Treatment of depression after coronary artery bypass surgery: a randomized controlled trial, *Arch Gen Psychiatry* 66(4):387–396, 2009.
54. Huffman JC, Mastromauro CA, Sowden G, et al.: Impact of a depression care management program for hospitalized cardiac patients, *Circ Cardiovasc Qual Outcomes* 4(2):198–205, 2011.
55. Burg MM, Lesperance F, Rieckmann N, et al.: Treating persistent depressive symptoms in post-ACS patients: the project COPES phase-I randomized controlled trial, *Contemp Clin Trials* 29(2): 231–240, 2007.
56. Whang W, Burg MM, Carney RM, et al.: Design and baseline data from the vanguard of the Comparison of Depression Interventions after Acute Coronary Syndrome (CODIACS) randomized controlled trial, *Contemp Clin Trials* 33(5):1003–1010, 2012.
57. Davidson KW, Bigger JT, Burg MM, et al.: Centralized, stepped, patient preference-based treatment for patients with post-acute coronary syndrome depression: CODIACS vanguard randomized controlled trial, *JAMA Intern Med* 173(11):997–1004, 2013.
58. Whang W, Davidson KW: Is it time to treat depression in patients with cardiovascular disease? *Circulation* 120(2):99–100, 2009.
59. Davidson KW, Kupfer DJ, Bigger JT, et al.: Assessment and treatment of depression in patients with cardiovascular disease: National Heart, Lung, and Blood Institute working group report, *Psychosom Med* 68(5):645–650, 2006.
60. Rumsfeld JS, Ho PM: Depression and cardiovascular disease: a call for recognition, *Circulation* 111(3):250–253, 2005.
61. Liu SS, Ziegelstein RC: Depression in patients with heart disease: the case for more trials, *Future Cardiol* 6(4):547–556, 2010.

62. Lattanzio F, Cherubini A, Furneri G, et al.: Sertraline treatment for depression associated with acute coronary syndromes: a cost analysis from the viewpoint of the Italian Healthcare System, *Aging Clin Exp Res* 20(1):76–80, 2008.
63. Gilbody S, House AO, Sheldon TA: Screening and case finding instruments for depression, *Cochrane Database Syst Rev*(4), 2005. CD002792.
64. Gilbody S, Sheldon T, House A: Screening and case-finding instruments for depression: a meta-analysis, *CMAJ* 178(8):997–1003, 2008.
65. Valenstein M, Vijan S, Zeber JE, et al.: The cost–utility of screening for depression in primary care, *Ann Intern Med* 134(5):345–360, 2001.
66. Gulliksson M, Burell G, Vessby B, et al.: Randomized controlled trial of cognitive behavioral therapy vs standard treatment to prevent recurrent cardiovascular events in patients with coronary heart disease: Secondary Prevention in Uppsala Primary Health Care Project (SUPRIM), *Arch Intern Med* 171(2):134–140, 2011.
67. Schneider RH, Grim CE, Rainforth MV, et al.: Stress reduction in the secondary prevention of cardiovascular disease: randomized, controlled trial of transcendental meditation and health education in blacks, *Circ Cardiovasc Qual Outcomes* 5(6):750–758, 2012.
68. Linden W, Phillips MJ, Leclerc J: Psychological treatment of cardiac patients: a meta-analysis, *Eur Heart J* 28(24):2972–2984, 2007.
69. Screening for depression in adults: U.S. preventive services task force recommendation statement, *Ann Intern Med* 151(11):784–792, 2009.
70. AAFP guideline for the detection and management of post-myocardial infarction depression, *Ann Fam Med* 7(1):71–79, 2009.
71. Shemesh E, Annunziato RA, Rubinstein D, et al.: Screening for depression and suicidality in patients with cardiovascular illnesses, *Am J Cardiol* 104(9):1194–1197, 2009.
72. van Melle JP, Verbeek DE, van den Berg MP, et al.: Beta-blockers and depression after myocardial infarction: a multicenter prospective study, *J Am Coll Cardiol* 48(11):2209–2214, 2006.
73. Hoogwegt MT, Kupper N, Theuns DAMJ, et al.: Beta-blocker therapy is not associated with symptoms of depression and anxiety in patients receiving an implantable cardioverter-defibrillator, *Europace* 14(1):74–80, 2012.
74. Battes LC, Pedersen SS, Oemrawsingh RM, et al.: Beta blocker therapy is associated with reduced depressive symptoms 12 months post percutaneous coronary intervention, *J Affect Disord* 136(3):751–757, 2011.
75. Unutzer J, Katon W, Callahan CM, et al.: Collaborative care management of late-life depression in the primary care setting: a randomized controlled trial, *JAMA* 288(22):2836–2845, 2002.
76. Davidson KW, Rieckmann N, Clemow L, et al.: Enhanced depression care for patients with acute coronary syndrome and persistent depressive symptoms: coronary psychosocial evaluation studies randomized controlled trial, *Arch Intern Med* 170(7):600–608, 2010.
77. Raue PJ, Schulberg HC, Heo M, et al.: Patients' depression treatment preferences and initiation, adherence, and outcome: a randomized primary care study, *Psychiatr Serv* 60(3):337–343, 2009.
78. Andrade C, Sandarsh S, Chethan KB, et al.: Serotonin reuptake inhibitor antidepressants and abnormal bleeding: a review for clinicians and a reconsideration of mechanisms, *J Clin Psychiatry* 71(12):1565–1575, 2010.
79. Weinrieb RM, Auriacombe M, Lynch KG, et al.: A critical review of selective serotonin reuptake inhibitor-associated bleeding: balancing the risk of treating hepatitis C-infected patients, *J Clin Psychiatry* 64(12):1502–1510, 2003.
80. Yuan Y, Tsoi K, Hunt RH: Selective serotonin reuptake inhibitors and risk of upper GI bleeding: confusion or confounding? *Am J Med* 119(9):719–727, 2006.
81. Hauta-Aho M, Tirkkonen T, Vahlberg T, et al.: The effect of drug interactions on bleeding risk associated with warfarin therapy in hospitalized patients, *Ann Med* 41(8):619–628, 2009.
82. Sansone RA, Sansone LA: Warfarin and antidepressants: happiness without hemorrhaging, *Psychiatry* 6(7):24–29, 2009.
83. Kim DH, Daskalakis C, Whellan DJ, et al.: Safety of selective serotonin reuptake inhibitor in adults undergoing coronary artery bypass grafting, *Am J Cardiol* 103(10):1391–1395, 2009.
84. Labos C, Dasgupta K, Nedjar H, et al.: Risk of bleeding associated with combined use of selective serotonin reuptake inhibitors and antiplatelet therapy following acute myocardial infarction, *CMAJ* 183(16):1835–1843, 2011.
85. Geddes JR, Carney SM, Davies C, et al.: Relapse prevention with antidepressant drug treatment in depressive disorders: a systematic review, *Lancet* 361(9358):653–661, 2003.

27 Refractory Angina

E. Marc Jolicoeur and Timothy D. Henry

INTRODUCTION

Angina is first and foremost a pain signal that originates from the heart to reach the brain. Typically, angina is triggered by myocardial ischemia. In addition to advanced coronary artery disease (CAD), microvascular dysfunction and vasospastic angina are well-described etiologies of myocardial ischemia resistant to medical therapy (Fig. 27.1). Angina is often simplified as the mere reflection of myocardial ischemia resulting from an imbalance between oxygen supply and demand (Fig. 27.2). However, the poor correlation between angina and the extent of coronary disease suggests that there is more than fixed epicardial coronary stenoses and oxygen deprivation to refractory angina. Angina becomes refractory when defective neurologic, psychogenic, or mitochondrial functions overlap with tissue ischemia to inappropriately maintain or enhance a persistent cardiac pain syndrome. Refractory anginas are therefore not a single disease but rather a mosaic of different systemic dysfunctions. Success in the treatment of refractory angina is unlikely to be achieved by addressing myocardial ischemia alone. Instead, the contemporary treatment of refractory angina also specifically addresses the neurogenic, psychogenic, and mitochondrial components of angina and cardiac pain (Fig. 27.3).

Angina can be considered refractory for several reasons. Refractory angina is a complex interaction between symptoms, myocardial perfusion, and coronary anatomy (Fig. 27.4). In some cases, patients with advanced CAD unsuitable for revascularization will experience persistent angina despite optimal doses of β-blockers, calcium-channel blockers (CCBs), and long-acting nitrates.[1] In other cases, angina caused by microvascular dysfunction or vasospasm can go unrecognized before a proper diagnosis is finally made and an adequate treatment is implemented. In North America alone, up to 500,000 Canadians and more than 1.8 million Americans are estimated to have refractory angina.[2] In Europe and the United States, it is estimated that between 5% and 15% of patients undergoing cardiac catheterization have refractory angina.[3,4] Whereas the annualized mortality rates among patients with refractory angina range between 2% and 4%,[5] the rates of ischemic endpoints (myocardial infarction [MI], stroke, cardiovascular rehospitalization, and revascularization) are approximately 50% in the 3 years following the diagnosis.[5a] The management of refractory angina is challenging, yet the condition is insufficiently studied and poorly covered by national practice guidelines. In this review, we discuss the pharmacologic, noninvasive, and interventional treatments of refractory angina in the context of past, present, and future innovations likely to influence how we treat refractory angina for the years to come.

DRUG THERAPY

The approach to refractory angina varies across different regions in the world, reflecting the local regulatory, organizational, and financial culture.[6] The choice of an add-on drug when symptoms persist despite β-blockers, CCBs, or long-acting nitrates can seem empirical, but some principles are available to help guide the selection of a new drug, such as the blood pressure (BP) and heart rate, the lack of tolerance to nitrates, and the presumptive defective system responsible for refractory angina. In a 2015 systematic review and meta-analysis, Belsey et al. studied the relative efficacy of adding ranolazine, trimetazidine, or ivabradine to patients with angina, despite treatment with β-blockers or CCBs (no comparative study was available for nicorandil)[6] (Fig. 27.5). The results suggest that the addition of ranolazine, trimetazidine, or ivabradine can delay the ischemic threshold and does improve the control of angina. The use of traditional therapies—β-blockers, nitrates, and CCBs—has been reviewed elegantly by Husted and Ohman[7] (see also Chapter 20). This section will focus on the evidence supporting the use of add-on antianginal drugs in patients with refractory angina.

Late Sodium Current Inhibitors

The tradition of treating angina with late sodium (Na) current inhibitors dates back to the 1960s when amiodarone was used in Europe.[8,9] Nowadays, amiodarone is anecdotally used for refractory angina.[10] Ranolazine, another late Na current inhibitor, has been extensively studied for stable angina with obstructive CAD and is considered in certain regions of the world to be on par with long-acting nitrates, ivabradine, or nicorandil as a second-line treatment after β-blockers or nondihydropyridine CCBs.[11] Ranolazine is

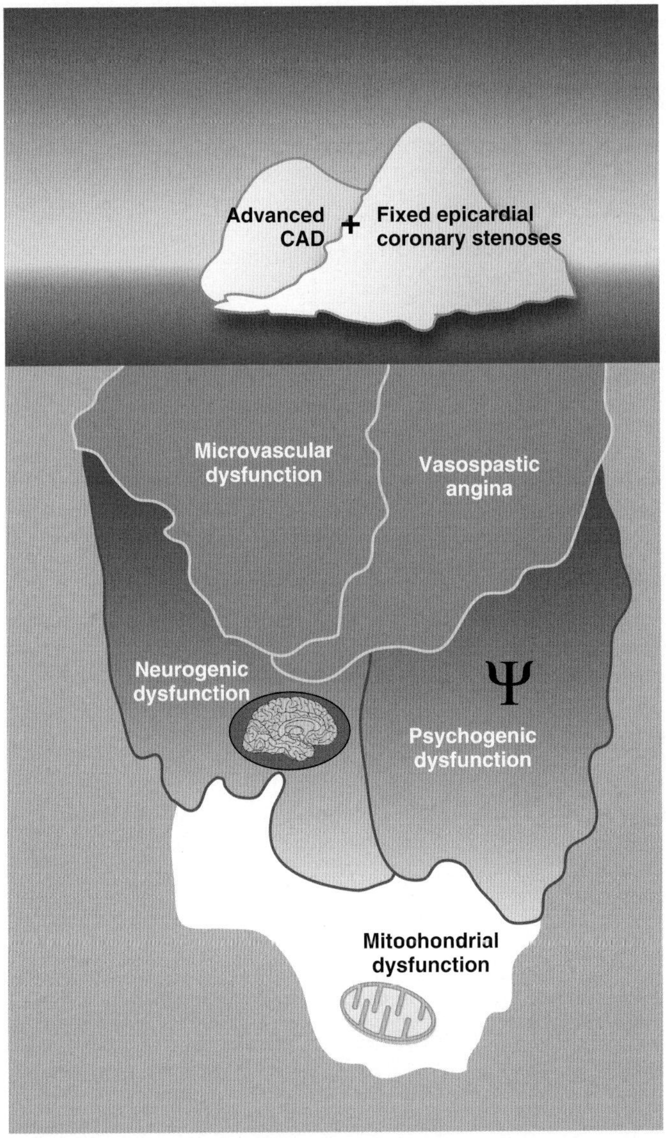

FIG. 27.1 The refractory anginas. Advanced coronary artery disease caused by fixed epicardial stenoses is the most frequently acknowledged etiology for refractory angina, but microvascular dysfunction and coronary vasospasm can also result in severe myocardial ischemia. Neurogenic, psychogenic, and mitochondrial dysfunctions can overlap with these ischemic substrates to trigger or enhance the cardiac pain signal seen in refractory angina. *CAD*, Coronary artery disease.

well suited for patients with persistent symptoms despite maximal tolerable doses of first-line antianginal agents, as its anti-ischemic effect is not related to heart rate or systemic BP lowering. The reason ranolazine is effective is debated, but likely involves an improved excitation-contraction coupling at the ventricular level and/or improved usage of oxygen at the mitochondrial level.[12] In the diseased heart, the exaggerated influx of Na^+ and calcium (Ca^{2+}) in the myocytes impairs relaxation, which increases diastolic stiffness and begets ischemia by preventing adequate ventricular perfusion. Ranolazine inhibits the late sodium current in cardiomyocytes and prevents the accumulation of Na^+ ions in the myocytes,[13] which in return prompts the sodium/calcium exchanger to expel calcium outside the myocytes to improve diastolic relaxation and coronary perfusion.[14] In experimental models, ranolazine also inhibits the β-oxidation of fatty acid in mitochondria.[12] This inhibition favors the oxidation of glucose, which requires less oxygen to yield similar amounts of adenosine triphosphate (ATP) production.[15]

Ranolazine improves total exercise duration and increases ischemic threshold in patients with chronic stable angina. In the Combination Assessment of Ranolazine In Stable Angina (CARISA) trial,[16] ranolazine (750 mg or 1000 mg for 12 weeks) compared to a placebo on top of amlodipine, atenolol, or diltiazem increased total exercise duration and times to angina and to ischemia (1 mm ST-segment depression). Ranolazine decreased angina (by approximately one episode per week) and reduced the use of nitroglycerin. Similar results were observed in the Efficacy of Ranolazine in Chronic Angina (ERICA) trial, where ranolazine (500 mg twice daily) or placebo for 1 week, followed by ranolazine (1000 mg twice daily) or placebo for 6 weeks, was added to amlodipine.[17] In the Type 2 Diabetes Evaluation of Ranolazine in Subjects with Chronic Stable Angina (TERISA) trial,[18] patients with type 2 diabetes mellitus and persistent angina despite one or two antianginal drugs experienced fewer angina episodes per week compared to placebo (3.8 vs. 4.3 episodes; $p < 0.01$) and consumed less sublingual nitroglycerin (1.7 vs. 2.1 doses; $p < 0.01$).

In a post hoc subgroup analysis of the Metabolic Efficiency with Ranolazine for Less Ischemia in Non–ST-Segment Elevation Acute Coronary Syndromes (MERLIN-TIMI 36) trial,[19] 3565 participants who had a history of chronic angina prior to their index acute coronary syndrome experienced a significant reduction of the primary endpoint (cardiovascular death, MI, and recurrent ischemia) with ranolazine compared to placebo (hazard ratio [HR], 0.86; 95% confidence interval [CI], 0.75–0.97; $p = 0.02$). This reduction was mostly driven by a drop in the number of recurrent ischemic episodes (HR, 0.78; 95% CI, 0.67–0.91; $p < 0.01$). Similar results were observed when the analysis was restricted to patients with a history of moderate-to-severe angina before enrollment (HR, 0.75; 95% CI, 0.63–0.91; $p < 0.01$), but ranolazine had no impact on the occurrence of cardiovascular death or MI. This antiischemic effect persisted in a 30-day landmark analysis, for up to a year (HR, 0.80; 95% CI, 0.67–0.96; $p = 0.02$). Of note, patients in this substudy were treated with 2.9 antianginal agents on average over the entire duration of the follow-up.

The favorable results seen in the MERLIN subgroup analysis fueled the enthusiasm for the Ranolazine in patients with incomplete revascularization after percutaneous coronary intervention (PCI) (RIVER-PCI) trial,[20] which assessed whether ranolazine 1000 mg twice daily was superior to placebo in 2651 participants with a history of chronic angina and incomplete revascularization post-PCI (residual lesions with diameter stenosis ≥ 50% in large coronary artery) at preventing the occurrence of ischemia-driven hospitalization with or without revascularization. Over a median follow-up of 643 days, the primary endpoint occurred in 345 participants (26%) assigned to ranolazine versus 364 participants (28%) assigned to placebo (HR, 0.95; 95% CI, 0.82–1.10; $p = 0.48$). Of note, the treatment effect of ranolazine for the primary endpoint remained the same in participants prescribed two to three anti-ischemic drugs, such as β-blockers, CCBs, or long-acting nitrates (HR, 1.04; 95% CI, 0.82–1.32; p interaction = 0.36). A safety subgroup analysis suggested that patients older than 75 years of age experienced higher rates of major adverse cardiovascular events (MACE) when given ranolazine compared to placebo. In this population, ranolazine provided no additional benefit to angina-related quality of life compared to placebo,[21] as quality of life improved

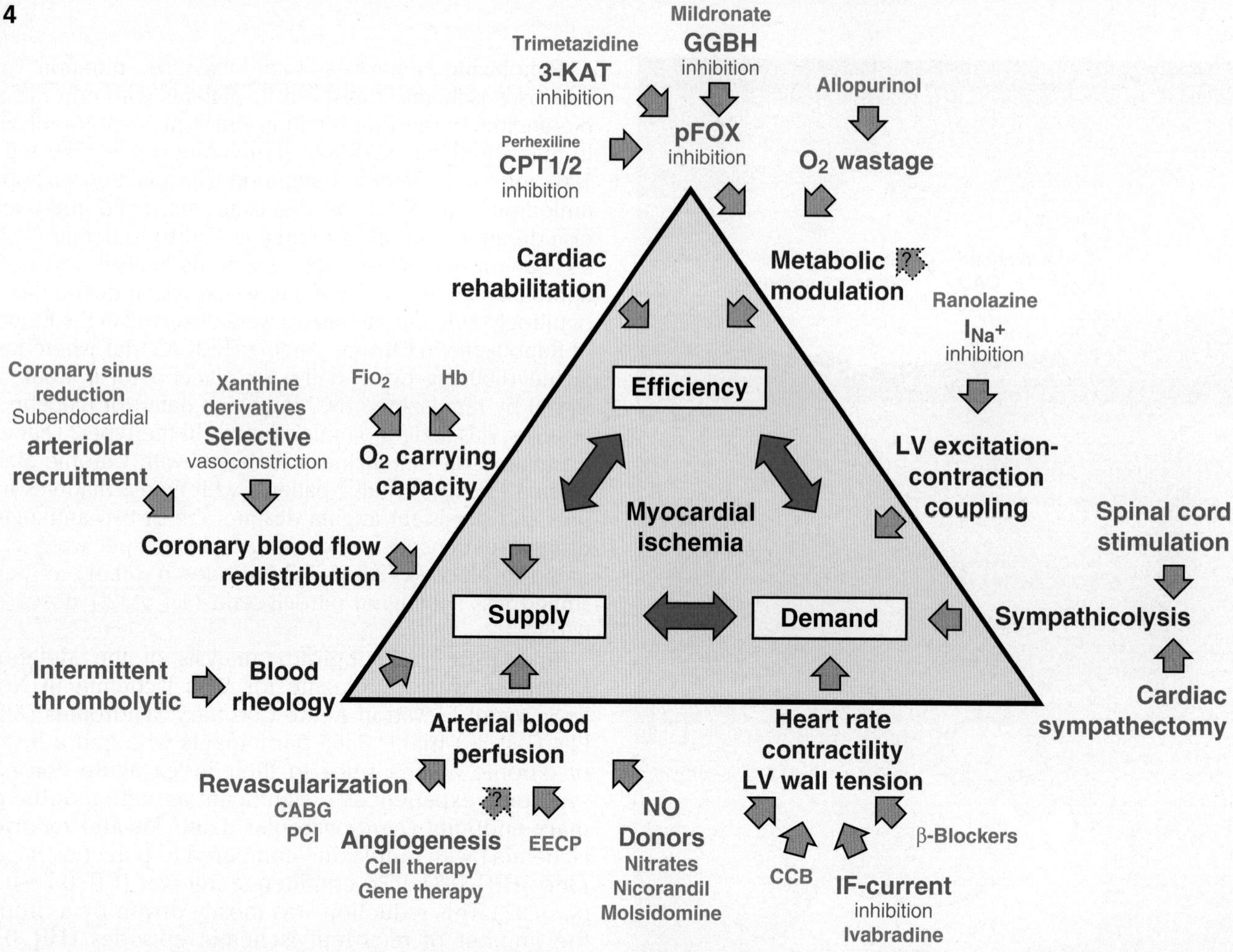

FIG. 27.2 Therapeutic principles of myocardial ischemia. Once described as a simple imbalance between oxygen supply and demand, myocardial ischemia is now also understood to result from an inefficient usage of oxygen and metabolites in the diseased myocardium. Therapeutic principles (represented in *red*) have been tested in refractory angina with varying success in the hope of increasing oxygen supply, reducing demand, and improving efficiency. Specific mechanisms of action and treatments are represented in *blue* and *green*, respectively. *CABG*, Coronary artery bypass graft; *CCB*, calcium-channel blocker; *CPT1/2*, carnitine *O*-palmitoyltransferase 1 and 2; *EECP*, enhanced external counterpulsation; *FiO₂*, fraction of inspired oxygen; *GGBH*, γ-butyrobetaine hydroxylase; *Hb*, hemoglobin; *3-KAT*, mitochondrial long-chain 3-ketoacyl-CoA thiolase; *LV*, left ventricle; *NO*, nitric oxide; *PCI*, percutaneous coronary intervention; *pFOX*, partial fatty acid oxidation.

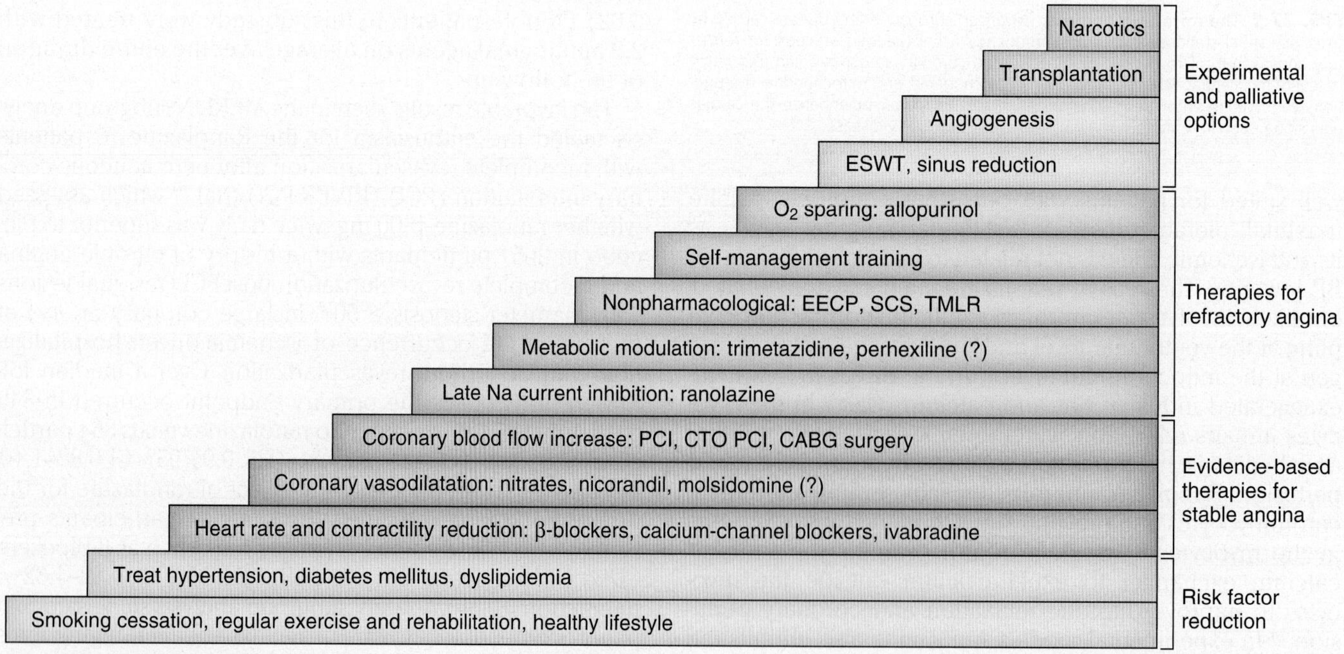

FIG. 27.3 Treatment options for refractory angina. The treatment of refractory angina starts with the management of risk factors (*yellow* steps) and the implementation of evidence-based therapy for chronic stable angina (*pink* steps). Available options for refractory angina include medical therapies and devices (*green* steps). The *blue* and *orange* steps display experimental and palliative options, which should be considered after lower options have been attempted. *CABG*, Coronary artery bypass graft; *CTO*, chronic total occlusion; *EECP*, enhanced external counterpulsation; *ESWT*; extracorporeal shock wave therapy; *PCI*, percutaneous coronary intervention; *SCS*, spinal cord stimulation; *TMLR*, transmyocardial laser revascularization. *(Reprinted from Henry TD, Satran D, Jolicoeur EM. Treatment of refractory angina in patients not suitable for revascularization.* Nat Rev Cardiol. *2014;11:78–95, courtesy of Nature Publishing Group.)*

drastically in both groups following the PCI. Overall, patients enrolled in RIVER-PCI had a low angina burden at baseline and follow-up, leaving little room for the quantification of an improvement, once the effect of the index PCI and the regression to the mean[22] were taken into account.

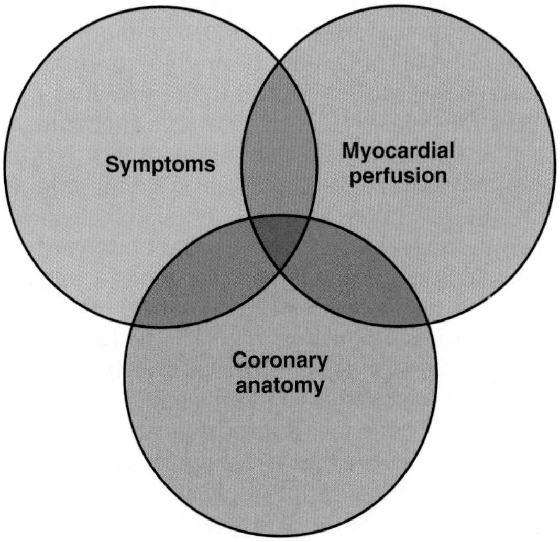

FIG. 27.4 **Refractory angina is a complex interaction between symptoms, myocardial perfusion, and coronary anatomy.**

Ranolazine has been associated with favorable outcomes in small pilot studies of microvascular angina,[23,24] and it was hypothesized that ranolazine could improve regional coronary in-flow in areas of myocardial ischemia.[25] Bairey Merz et al. (2016) reported the results of a trial in participants with microvascular dysfunction but without obstructive CAD who were randomized to either short-term oral ranolazine 500 to 1000 mg twice daily for 2 weeks or placebo, then crossed over to the alternate treatment arm.[26] The majority of patients were women treated with at least one antianginal drug, angiotensin converting enzyme inhibitors, and statins, and all participants had symptoms related to myocardial ischemia. Compared to placebo, ranolazine did not significantly improve the angina-related quality of life (measured by the Seattle Angina Questionnaire [SAQ]). In a mechanistic substudy, ranolazine failed to improve the myocardial perfusion reserve index (MPRI) measured by cardiac magnetic resonance imaging. One interesting finding was that the change in MPRI correlated with the change in SAQ score, suggesting that a modulation of microvascular dysfunction could lead to a new therapeutic avenue in patients with refractory angina. The suboptimal results in incompletely revascularized patients and those with microvascular disease might be a barrier to widespread use of ranolazine in this population.

ETT: Total time. Standardized mean difference. Random effects model

Study	*N* monotherapy	*N* dual therapy	SMD (95% CI)
Ranolazine added to BB or CCB			
Chaitman a	269	279	0.21 (0.20; 0.22)
Chaitman b	269	275	0.20 (0.18; 0.21)
Combined	**538**	**554**	**0.20 (0.19; 0.21)**
Test for heterogeneity: Q = 1.7; Chi² = 0.20; I2 = 39.9%			
Test for effect: SMD = 0.20; 95% CI = 0.19–0.21; *p* < 0.0001			
Trimetazidine added to BB or CCB			
Chazov	87	90	0.31 (0.26; 0.35)
Szwed	168	179	0.21 (0.19; 0.23)
Danchin a	653	654	0.07 (0.07; 0.08)
Danchin b	653	655	0.05 (0.05; 0.06)
Manchanda	32	32	−0.04 (−0.16; 0.08)
Sellier	106	117	−0.07 (−0.11; −0.04)
Levy	35	32	−0.31 (−0.43; 0.19)
Combined	**1734**	**1759**	**0.06 (0.02; 0.11)**
Test for heterogeneity: Q = 395; Chi² <0.0001; I2 = 98.5%			
Test for effect: SMD = 0.06; 95% CI = 0.02–0.11; *p* = 0.006			
Ivabradine added to BB			
Tardif	440	449	0.10 (0.09; 0.11)
Test effect: SMD = 0.10; 95% CI = 0.09–0.11; *p* < 0.0001			

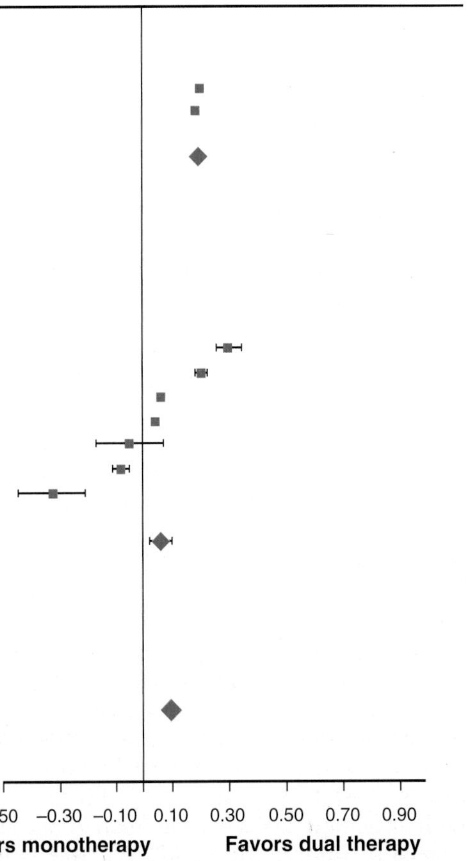

FIG. 27.5 **Relative efficacy of ranolazine, trimetazidine, and ivabradine as add-on therapy on total exercise duration in patients with stable angina.** Total exercise duration on exercise treadmill test. Data presented as standardized mean difference with a random effects model. *BB*, β-Blocker; *CCB*, calcium-channel blocker; *CI*, confidence interval; *ETT*, exercise treadmill test; *N*, number; *SMD*, standardized mean difference. *(Modified from Belsey J, Savelieva I, Mugelli A, Camm AJ. Relative efficacy of antianginal drugs used as add-on therapy in patients with stable angina: a systematic review and meta-analysis.* Eur J Prev Cardiol. *2015;22:837–848.)*

Due to pharmacologic interaction, ranolazine should not be used concomitantly with nondihydropyridine CCBs, ketoconazole, or macrolide antibiotics.

Partial Fatty Acid Oxidation Inhibitors

Trimetazidine

Trimetazidine (TMZ) is frequently presented as the archetype of partial fatty acid oxidation (pFOX) inhibitors. TMZ is proposed to modulate the mitochondrial metabolism by blocking the long-chain 3-ketoacyl-CoA thiolase (KAT), a key enzyme in the β-oxidation of fatty acids.[27] This blockade is thought to shift the mitochondrial substrate utilization toward glycolysis, which requires 10% to 15% less oxygen than the oxidation of fatty acid to yield the same energy. A partial inhibition of fatty acid oxidation has the potential to prevent the intracellular accumulation of lactate and protons, both of which are associated with impaired contraction–relaxation coupling in ischemic myocytes.[28] Although appealing, this presumptive mechanism of action is challenged by evidence suggesting that TMZ does not alter metabolic substrate oxidation in the human cardiac mitochondria but rather acts via an unidentified intracardiac mechanism,[29] possibly involving the adenosine monophosphate (AMP)-activated protein kinase (AMPK) and extracellular signal-related kinase (ERK) signaling pathway,[30] and the activation of p38 mitogen-activated protein kinase and Akt signaling.[31]

In the TRIMetazidine in POLand (TRIMPOL II) trial,[32] 426 participants with stable CAD and an abnormal treadmill stress test despite metoprolol 50 mg twice daily were randomized to either TMZ (20 mg three times daily over 12 weeks) or matching placebo. TMZ markedly improved the time to ST-segment depression compared to placebo (+ 86 s vs. + 24 s; $p < 0.01$). Likewise, TMZ reduced the weekly angina count (– 1.9 episodes vs. – 0.9 episode; $p < 0.01$).

In a recent meta-analysis of 1628 participants involved in 13 randomized trials from 1997 to 2013, TMZ in addition to antianginal medication was shown to be superior to antianginal medications at reducing the weekly angina count (weighted mean difference [WMD] = –0.95 episode; 95% CI, –1.30 episode to –0.61 episode; $p < 0.001$), the weekly nitroglycerin use (WMD = –0.98; 95% CI, –1.44 to –0.52; $p < 0.001$), and the time to 1-mm ST-segment depression (WMD = 0.30; 95% CI, 0.17 to 0.43; $p < 0.001$). Of note, only four of the trials included in the pooled analyses were appropriately blinded. These results contradict a previous meta-analysis that detected no benefit.[33] Importantly, TMZ has not been associated with a reduction in mortality or cardiovascular events.[33] TMZ is associated with adverse extrapyramidal reactions such as restless leg syndrome and parkinsonism.[34]

In summary, data supporting the use of TMZ are conflicting and further clinical trials are required. The European Medicines Agency (EMA) has restricted the use of TMZ as add-on therapy for patients who remain symptomatic or are intolerant to first-line antianginal treatments. The efficAcy and safety of Trimetazidine in Patients with angina pectoris having been treated by Percutaneous Coronary Intervention (ATPCI) trial (EudraCT Number: 2010-022134-89) is examining the efficacy of TMZ in patients with post-PCI angina. Results of this large trial are expected in 2017.

Perhexiline Maleate

Perhexiline is one of the oldest known antianginal drugs and was extensively studied in the 1970s before β-blockers and CCBs became mainstream therapies.[35,36] Despite its seeming efficacy, perhexiline was removed from the market in several countries due to cases of hepatotoxicity and neurotoxicity with chronic therapy,[37] predominantly explained by drug accumulation in slow CYP2D6 metabolizers.[38–41]

Perhexiline is a pFOX inhibitor that modulates mitochondrial metabolism by inhibiting the enzymes carnitine *O*-palmitoyltransferase (CPT) 1 and 2, which are responsible for the transfer of free fatty acids from the cytosol to the mitochondria.[42] These effects are systemic and not limited to the heart. Similar to TMZ, perhexiline is thought to shift the mitochondrial substrate utilization toward glucose oxidation, which is more energy efficient as it requires less oxygen to produce the same amount of ATP.[42] Based on stoichiometric models, an approximate 11% to 13% increase in oxygen efficiency would be expected by entirely blocking fatty acid metabolism in favor of an exclusive carbohydrate metabolism.[43] In practice, a predominant mitochondrial carbohydrate oxidation has been reported to be at least 30% to 40% more efficient than free fatty acid oxidation.[44] Animal metabolomic studies suggest that perhexiline may also favor lactate and amino acid uptake by the heart.[45] Perhexiline is also a weak L-type CCB,[46] a sodium channel blocker,[47] and a vasodilator, but these possible antianginal properties have never been fully delineated.[48]

In a systematic review counting 26 small, randomized, mostly cross-over, double-blind, controlled trials and 696 participants, perhexiline monotherapy was associated with a consistent reduction in the frequency of angina attacks and nitroglycerin consumption,[49] although there were concerns around the quality of reporting of the available trials. In a small, double-blind, controlled crossover trial ($n = 17$ participants), perhexiline was associated with a greater proportion (65%) of responders (measured by a reduction in angina as measured in a dedicated diary over 3 months) compared with placebo (18%, $p < 0.05$) in patients with refractory angina, despite the combination of β-blockers, nitrates, and CCBs. Likewise, all patients improved their performance on a treadmill stress test, compared with none when treated with placebo.[50] Five of 17 (29%) patients developed significant side effects despite plasma concentration monitoring, including four cases of transient ataxia. Similar findings were reported in patients treated with adequate β-blockade.[51] Of note, few trials have tested the efficacy of perhexiline at dosages deemed to be safe in most patients (100 to 200 mg/day). In a large 5-year retrospective series from two centers, perhexiline was associated with angina relief in most patients with otherwise refractory symptoms. However, the treatment was discontinued in 20% of patients due to side effects or out of safety concerns, despite careful therapeutic drug level monitoring.[52]

Therapeutic plasma monitoring opens the door to the personalized perhexiline administration in selected cases to avoid excessive drug accumulation. Short-term dizziness, nausea, vomiting, lethargy, and tremors are acute adverse effects observed with perhexiline. Perhexiline may be safely started at a dose of 100 mg twice daily and monitored at 1, 4, and 8 weeks to maintain plasma concentrations between 0.15 and 0.60 mg/L.[53] Perhexiline has been associated with occasional QT interval prolongation,[54] especially in patients with K^+-channel mutations (KCNQ1), and additional safety information will be required before it can be widely recommended in clinical practice. The genetic screening of allelic variants associated with slow cytochrome P450 2D6 hydroxylation may obviate the need for plasma monitoring in the future.[40] Mutations in CYP2D6 are present in 7% to 10% of Caucasians versus 2% of African Americans and less than 1% in Chinese and Japanese populations. Perhexiline is used for refractory angina in Australia and New Zealand.

Mildronate

Mildronate (better known as meldonium) has recently drawn a lot of attention after the suspension of a high-profile tennis player for doping.[55] Mildronate indirectly acts as a pFOX inhibitor by blocking the enzyme γ-butyrobetaine hydroxylase (GGBH), which catalyses the biosynthesis of carnitine.[56] Carnitine is essential for the transfer of long-chain fatty acids across the mitochondrial inner membrane for oxidation and ATP synthesis.[57] Mildronate also inhibits the activity of carnitine acetyltransferase (CAT), an enzyme that regulates the level of acetyl coenzyme A (acetyl-CoA) in the mitochondria, which plays a key role in several aspects of intermediary metabolism, including the oxidation of free fatty acids. In the phase II dose-finding MILSS (a dose-dependent improvement in exercise tolerance in patients with stable angina treated with mildronate) trial, 512 patients with chronic stable Canadian Cardiovascular Society (CCS) class II–III angina, despite β-blockers (> 94%), long-acting nitrates (> 70%), or CCB (35–50%), were blindly randomized to either mildronate (one of four doses: 100 mg, 300 mg, 1000 mg, or 3000 mg) or placebo for 12 weeks.[58] Mildronate resulted in a dose-related improvement in total exercise duration, as measured on a standard bicycle ergometer. Patients assigned to the 1000-mg dose (given as 500 mg twice daily) obtained the best effect compared to placebo (+35.2 s ± 53.3 s vs. −7.1 s ± 81.8 s, $p = 0.002$). No significant difference in the time to onset of angina was noted between the groups. Mildronate was developed in the former Soviet Union for the treatment of MI and stroke and has never been approved elsewhere. Mildronate is conceptually interesting for refractory angina, but insufficient evidence exists to support its use in clinical practice.

Nitric Oxide Donors

Nicorandil

Nicorandil is a coronary vasodilator with cardioprotective properties.[59] The nicotinamide-nitrate ester acts as an ATP-sensitive potassium channel (KATP) opener at the mitochondrial level to mimic ischemic preconditioning and prepare the myocytes against injury.[7] Similar to long-acting nitrates, nicorandil is a nitric oxide (NO) donor which directly vasodilates coronary arteries.[60] Unlike nitrates however, nicorandil does not impair endothelial function and is not associated with tachyphylaxis and tolerance.[61] Besides vasodilation, some evidence suggests that nicorandil may also have an intrinsic analgesic activity and may reduce the nociceptive response to angina.[62] Likewise, nicorandil may also improve the myocardial fatty acid metabolism.[63] For these reasons, nicorandil is conceptually appealing in patients with severe angina and advanced CAD, and in patients with vasospastic angina.

Nicorandil exerts effects similar to β-blockers,[64,65] long-acting nitrates,[66] and CCBs[67] in patients with stable CAD with no other background treatment. The Impact Of Nicorandil in Angina (IONA) trial compared nicorandil versus placebo in 5126 patients with chronic angina despite nitrates (87%), β-blockers (57%), or CCBs (55%). Nicorandil reduced the combined occurrence of cardiovascular death, nonfatal MI, or unplanned admissions to hospital for chest pain (13.1% vs. 15.5%; $p = 0.02$) and confirmed the cardioprotective effect of nicorandil in patients with CAD.[68] From this trial, no data were reported on the effect of nicorandil on angina symptoms or quality of life. At 6 months, 29.6% of patients assigned to nicorandil discontinued their study drug due to adverse effects, compared with 19.5% in patients assigned to placebo. No study has yet described the potential merit of nicorandil in patients with refractory angina despite classical antianginal drugs administered at maximal tolerable dose.[69]

The European Society of Cardiology (ESC) practice guidelines recommend nicorandil as a second-line treatment for the relief of angina/ischemia (class IIa indication), on par with long-acting nitrates, ivabradine, and ranolazine, according to heart rate, BP, and tolerance.[11] Surprisingly, no studies have been reported that describe the efficacy of nicorandil in an add-on role in angina.[6] Nicorandil is only available by special-access programs run by regulatory agencies in Canada and the United States. As is the case with all NO donors, nicorandil can cause headaches and hypotension. Not infrequently, nicorandil can induce oral, anal, or gastrointestinal ulceration, which typically subsides upon drug discontinuation.[70]

Molsidomine

Molsidomine is similar to long-acting nitrates, both in terms of mechanism of action and efficacy.[71,72] Molsidomine mediates its effect via NO and increases myocardial perfusion by vasodilating the coronary arterial system,[73] and reduces oxygen demand by increasing the peripheral venous capacitance, cardiac preload, and wall tension. Like long-acting nitrates, molsidomine could also be associated with tachyphylaxis and tolerance.[72]

Molsidomine has not been tested in refractory angina.[74] Two different formulations of molsidomine (8 mg twice daily vs. 16 mg daily) were compared to a placebo in a randomized trial of 533 patients with new onset angina pectoris where β-blockers, CCBs, and long-acting nitrates were prescribed.[75] Both formulations of molsidomine were better than placebo at reducing the weekly angina count (2.3 ± 3.2 episodes vs. 3.8 ± 3.7 episodes, $p < 0.001$) and reducing the use of short-acting nitrates, and resulted in a significantly improved total exercise duration. In the 2015 Effect of Molsidomine on the Endothelial Dysfunction in Patients with Angina Pectoris (MEDCORE) randomized controlled trial (RCT), molsidomine 16 mg once a day for 12 months as an add-on treatment to best of care medical therapy failed to improve endothelial dysfunction over placebo in patients who underwent a PCI for stable angina pectoris.[76] In real-world settings, molsidomine is well tolerated with only 9.1% of patients treated over the course of 1 year reporting drug-related adverse events (mostly headaches and hypotension).[77] Given the lack of evidence specific to refractory angina and the lack of safety data, molsidomine should probably be used cautiously in this population.

L-Arginine

The amino acid L-arginine is transformed by the NO synthases into NO, which mediates the endothelium-dependent vasodilatation.[78] Supplemental oral L-arginine (1 g TID) improves small-vessel coronary endothelial function in healthy individuals.[79] Whereas L-arginine has been shown to be better than a placebo at improving the total exercise duration on treadmill stress test in patients with stable CAD,[80] it has not been adequately investigated in refractory angina.[80] In a small factorial trial, Ruel et al. suggested that L-arginine (6 g per day) may potentiate the effect of vascular endothelial growth factor (VEGF)-165 plasmid DNA in patients with advanced CAD. Participants who received the combination of VEGF-165 plasmid DNA and L-arginine had improved anterior wall perfusion on positron emission tomography.[81]

I(*f*) Current Inhibitors

Ivabradine selectively inhibits the I(*f*) current which regulates the intrinsic chronotropic properties of the pacemaker cells in the sinoatrial node and lowers the heart rate. Ivabradine does not reduce BP nor does it exert a negative effect on the excitability of the heart and the conductive properties of the atrioventricular (AV) node.[82]

In the Efficacy and Safety of Ivabradine on Top of Atenolol in Stable Angina Pectoris (ASSOCIATE) trial, ivabradine up to 7.5 mg twice daily for 4 months was superior to placebo at improving the total exercise duration compared to placebo (+24.3 s ± 65.3 s vs. 7.7 s ± 63.8 s; $p < 0.001$) in patients with persistent angina despite atenolol 50 mg daily.[83] In small pilot trials performed in patients suffering microvascular angina, ivabradine (5 mg twice daily) has been superior to placebo at improving angina-related quality of life.[23,24] Ivabradine did not improve cardiovascular outcomes in patients with stable CAD and left ventricular systolic dysfunction.[84] However in the ivabradine for patients with stable coronary artery disease and left-ventricular systolic dysfunction (BEAUTIFUL) trial, the subgroup of participants who had limiting angina at baseline experienced a 24% reduction in cardiovascular death and hospitalization for MI or heart failure (HF). The majority of these patients were treated with β-blockers and long-acting nitrates.

In the Study assessInG the morbidity-mortality beNefits of the I(*f*) inhibitor ivabradine in patients with coronarY artery disease (SIGNIFY) trial,[85] a dose of ivabradine adjusted to reach a heart rate of 55 to 60 beats per minute (bpm) on top of guideline-directed medical therapy was not superior to placebo at improving the occurrence of cardiovascular death or MI in 19,102 patients with stable CAD and a heart rate of 70 bpm or greater (6.8% vs. 6.4%, respectively; HR, 1.08; 95% CI, 0.96–1.20; $p = 0.20$; median follow-up of 27.8 months). In the subgroup of patients with symptomatic angina (CCS class II or higher), a greater proportion of ivabradine-treated patients experienced an improvement in their CCS angina class (24.0% vs. 18.8%, $p = 0.01$). Despite these favorable findings, ivabradine was associated with a small yet significant increase in cardiovascular death and MI (HR, 1.18; 95% CI, 1.03–1.35; p interaction = 0.02) in this subgroup. Based on these results, caution has been advised regarding the prescription of ivabradine in patients with angina without HF.[86] Ivabradine might be considered in individuals with a heart rate of 70 bpm or greater who do not tolerate doses of β-blockers or when CCBs are contraindicated. Ivabradine has also been associated with new-onset atrial fibrillation, bradycardia, and blurred vision.[87]

Miscellaneous Pharmacologic Agents

Allopurinol

Allopurinol reduces oxygen wastage by inhibiting xanthine oxidase, an enzyme involved in the oxidative stress response.[88] Allopurinol may also improve endothelial function in patients with CAD.[89] In a small cross-over randomized trial, participants with stable CAD assigned to allopurinol (300 mg twice daily) did better than those assigned to placebo at improving their time to 1-mm ST-segment depression (+58 s; 95% CI, 45–77 s) and their time to chest pain (+43 s; 95% CI, 31–58 s) on exercise treadmill test.[90] The trial lacked power to detect a variation in angina burden, quality of life, or clinical outcomes. These findings are yet to be replicated independently. Allopurinol is cheap and could represent an interesting option in some regions of the world. At high dose (600 mg daily), toxic effects are possible and close monitoring is advised in patients with chronic renal failure.

Intermittent Thrombolytic

Intermittent thrombolytic is of historic importance as the case example of the principle of improved blood rheology to treat myocardial ischemia.[91] Poiseuille's law indicates that a reduced blood viscosity should translate into a superior flow in the coronary microcirculation. Because fibrinogen is a major determinant of plasma viscosity, its reduction by fibrinolysis should theoretically translate into reduced myocardial ischemia and angina. In a small randomized trial, a high dose of intermittent urokinase was better than a lower dose (500,000 IU vs. 50,000 IU IV, three times a week over 12 weeks) at improving the weekly angina count.[92]

Testosterone and Estrogen

Testosterone administration has been linked to an increased risk of adverse cardiovascular events.[93] However, it has been hypothesized that testosterone might improve the endothelium-dependent vasodilation of coronary arteries.[94] In small clinical studies, testosterone administration has been linked to improved angina threshold in men with chronic stable angina.[95–97] The recent US Food and Drug Administration (USFDA) restrictions on testosterone replacement therapy reinforce the notion that it should probably be avoided in high-risk patients until additional evidence becomes available. Similar to testosterone, estrogen has been investigated in patients with stable angina despite concern about increased cardiovascular risk in healthy postmenopausal US women.[98] Estrogen has been linked to improved endothelial function.[99] Estradiol-drospirenone hormone replacement therapy has been shown to improve myocardial perfusion reserve in postmenopausal women with angina pectoris.[100] In a small randomized double-blind trial, estradiol plus norethindrone acetate therapy for 16 weeks outperformed placebo at improving the total exercise duration (+32.7 s vs. 2.5 s, $p < 0.05$) and the time to 1-mm ST-segment depression (+99.1 s vs. 22.9 s, $p < 0.05$) compared to placebo in 74 Chinese postmenopausal women with established CAD.[101] Neither testosterone nor estrogen supplementation has been properly investigated in patients with advanced CAD and refractory angina.

Omapatrilat

The vasopeptidase inhibitor omapatrilat inhibits both the angiotensin-converting enzyme (ACE) and the neutral endopeptidase (NEP). NEP catalyses the breakdown of natriuretic peptides (atrial natriuretic peptide, brain-derived natriuretic peptide, and C-type natriuretic peptide) and of bradykinine.[102] The natriuretic peptides antagonize the sympathetic nervous system and the renin-angiotensin-aldosterone system, which might be beneficial in patients with significant myocardial ischemia. The concept of NEP inhibition in patients with chronic angina pectoris was tested in a proof-of-principle study where 348 participants with stable β-blocker monotherapy were blindly randomized to either omapatrilat (titrated up to 80 mg daily over 4 weeks) or matching placebo.[103] Participants assigned to omapatrilat significantly improved their total exercise duration in an exercise treadmill test compared to those assigned to placebo (76.6 s ± 84.2 s vs. 28.7 s ± 82.2 s, difference from baseline, $p < 0.001$). Likewise, omapatrilat also resulted in a significant improvement in the time to onset of 1-mm ST-segment depression (84 s ± 7 s vs. 34 s ± 7 s, $p < 0.001$). The anti-ischemic effect of omapatrilat was likely mediated by a blunting effect in systolic BP, as the rate–pressure product at peak exertion was lower in patients treated with the active drug compared to placebo (Δ – 609 ± –1254 to 36, $p = 0.06$). Omapatrilat was not approved by the USFDA due to concern over angioedema, possibly caused by an excessive bradykinin accumulation resulting from NEP inhibition. Sacubitril, a neprilysin neutral peptidase inhibitor combined with an angiotensin receptor antagonist to minimize angioedema, yielded favorable outcomes in patients with HF in the Prospective comparison of AR (angiotensin receptor) and NI (neprilysin inhibition) with ACE Inhibition to Determine Impact on Global Mortality and morbidity in Heart Failure (PARDIGM-HFT) trial.[104] The results are likely to revive the interest in the concept of broad vasopeptidase inhibition in angina.

Traditional Chinese Medicine

Traditional Chinese herbal medicines may be a valuable option to treat angina. Dantonic (T89) is a water extract of Danshen (Radix et Rhizoma Salviae Miltiorrhizae) and Sanqi (Radix et Rhizoma Notoginseng) combined with Bingpian (Borneol) to enhance absorption. Dantonic is currently being tested in a formal USFDA phase III placebo-controlled trial for efficacy in patients with CCS class II or III stable angina despite a β-blocker or a CCB and short-acting nitroglycerin. Enrollment ended in 2015 and results are expected in late 2016 (NCT01659580). Several mechanisms of action have been proposed to explain how dantonic may relieve angina, including improved blood rheology and antioxidant properties.[105–107] Other than Danshen and Sanqi, several traditional Chinese medicines have been tested in patients with angina, with inconsistent results. Other nontraditional methods such as herbal acupoint application[108] and acupuncture[109] have been advocated but have not been adequately tested.

INTERVENTIONAL THERAPIES

Chronic Total Occlusions

Chronic total occlusions (CTOs), once the last frontier of interventional cardiology, are now routinely recanalized in the hope of improving long-term outcomes and symptoms.[110] Current practice guidelines recommend that the percutaneous recanalization of CTOs should be considered in patients with symptoms or in the presence of objective evidence of viability/ischemia in the territory of the occluded artery.[111] The appropriate use criteria for coronary revascularization deem the recanalization of an isolated CTO appropriate if, despite maximal anti-ischemic medical therapy, moderate symptoms persist (angina CCS II or higher) and high-risk features are present on noninvasive testing, or severe symptoms persist (angina CCS III or more) with at least moderate risk features on noninvasive testing.[112] Pooled estimates from observational studies consistently report a lower mortality (odds ratio [OR], 0.52; 95% CI, 0.43–0.63), a lower risk of MACE (OR, 0.59; 95% CI, 0.44–0.79), and a lower need for subsequent coronary artery bypass graft (CABG) (OR, 0.18; 95% CI, 0.14–0.22)[113] in successfully recanalized CTO patients, compared to patients with failed recanalization. It is important to note that these observational comparisons of successful versus failed CTO PCIs are not sufficient to demonstrate the efficacy of this procedure on clinical outcomes.

The association between CTO PCIs and angina also remains controversial. In a recent meta-analysis with nine nonrandomized studies and 2536 patients covering 25 years, a successful CTO PCI was associated with a reduction in the risk of residual angina (OR, 0.38; 95% CI, 0.24–0.60) compared to a failed CTO PCI. Few of these observational studies used appropriate research tools to quantify post-PCI angina, and a sizable portion of the evidence originates from the pre-stent era. Olivari et al. reported a reduction in ischemic burden in patients with a successful CTO PCI, as they were more likely to have a normal exercise treadmill time at 12 months than were those with a failed CTO PCI (73% vs. 47%; $p < 0.001$).[114] Jolicoeur et al. failed to show an improvement in the rates of self-reported angina (20% vs. 24%; $p = 0.50$) and good-to-excellent quality of life (73% versus 68%; $p = 0.52$) 6 months after a successful and a failed CTO PCI, respectively.[115] Borgia et al. used the SAQ in 302 consecutive patients who underwent an attempt of CTO PCI at their center. Overall, a successful CTO PCI was associated with less limitation in physical activity and improved treatment satisfaction (53%), compared to 31% of patients with a failed CTO PCI.[116] Importantly, more than 75% of patients in the former group reported symptomatic improvement at late follow-up.

CTO PCIs are complex interventions with the potential for microvascular plugging and distal bed embolization.[117] In addition, patients with a CTO may have microvascular dysfunction[118] in addition to epicardial disease that can persist despite a successful recanalization. In a series of 120 consecutive patients with a successfully recanalized CTO, microvascular dysfunction quantified by coronary flow velocity reserve (CFVR) was measured immediately after the index PCI and repeated 5 months later.[119] On average, CFVR increased from 2.01 ± 0.58 at baseline to 2.50 ± 0.79 at follow-up ($p = 0.001$). Microvascular dysfunction, which in that study was defined as a CFVR < 2.0, was observed in 46% of patients after recanalization and persisted in 17% at follow-up. Diabetes mellitus was a major determinant of persistent microvascular dysfunction.

There are no reported RCTs comparing CTO PCI to medical therapy, but at least two large trials are under way that are expected to provide important new data to inform the field—the Drug-Eluting Stent Implantation Versus Optimal Medical Treatment in Patients with Chronic Total Occlusion (DECISION CTO) trial ($n = 1300$; NCT01078051) and the European Study on the Utilization of Revascularization Versus Optimal Medical Therapy for the Treatment of Chronic Total Coronary Occlusions (EURO-CTO) trial (NCT01760083).

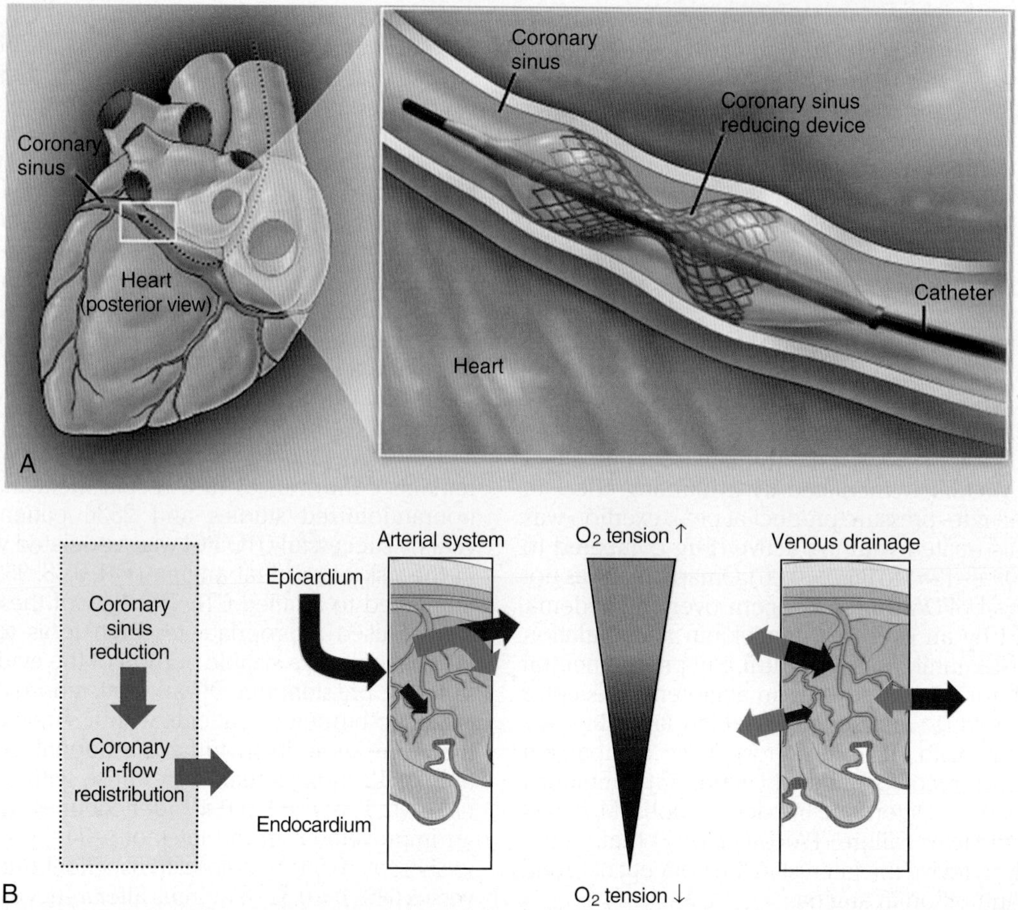

FIG. 27.6 (A) Coronary sinus reducer system. The complete system for the coronary sinus reducing device is comprised of a metal mesh device that is premounted on a balloon catheter and is shaped like an hourglass when expanded. After the device is implanted in the coronary sinus, local flow disruption and vascular reaction lead to a hyperplastic response in the vessel wall, with occlusion of the fenestrations in the metal mesh. The central orifice of the device remains patent and becomes the sole path for blood flow through the coronary sinus, leading to the development of an upstream pressure gradient that results in the redistribution of blood from the less ischemic epicardium to the ischemic endocardium. **(B) Coronary in-flow redistribution.** *([A] Courtesy of Verheye S, Jolicoeur EM, Behan MW, et al. Efficacy of a device to narrow the coronary sinus in refractory angina.* N Engl J Med. *2015;372:519–527. Copyright © 2015 Massachusetts Medical Society.)*

Reduction of the Coronary Sinus

Before CABGs were routinely performed to treat angina, Beck and Leighninger proposed in the mid-20th century a surgery to restrict the venous drainage of the heart.[120,121] The surgical narrowing of the coronary sinus (CS) was meant to favor a redistribution of the oxygenated blood into ischemic territories and was associated with a remarkable efficacy.[122] A contemporary exploitation of this concept is the percutaneous reduction of the CS in patients with refractory angina unsuitable for revascularization. The phase II Coronary Sinus Reducer for Treatment of Refractory Angina (COSIRA) trial tested a balloon-expandable stainless steel hourglass-shaped metal stent called Reducer in patients with severe refractory angina due to advanced CAD unsuitable for revascularization.[123] The device is implanted in the CS and creates a focal narrowing leading to an increase in CS pressures (Fig. 27.6A). In COSIRA, the Reducer was associated with a greater proportion of patients who improved by two CCS angina classes, compared to a blinded sham implantation (35% vs. 15%, $p = 0.02$).[130]

Other interventions that modulate the CS pressure have been investigated, including the pressure-controlled intermittent coronary sinus occlusion (PICSO) in diverse ischemic settings, including during CABG[124] and STEMI.[125] How exactly the modulation of the CS pressure can relieve angina is not clear. Experimental evidence supports the notion that pressure elevation in the CS favors the recruitment of collateral flow toward the ischemic myocardium.[126] A reduction of the coronary sinus is thought to apply a backward pressure to the venules and capillaries,[127,128] which is thought to recruit arterioles and preferentially reduce the resistance to flow in the ischemic subendocardium[129] (see Fig. 27.6B).

In the healthy heart, the subendocardium is preferentially perfused during stress due to a physiologic vasoconstriction in the subepicardial layers. In the diseased heart, this compensatory mechanism is impaired, leading to a relative hypoperfusion of the subendocardium (see Fig. 27.6B, *red arrows*) and a proportional reduction in venous drainage (see Fig. 27.6B, *purple arrows*). In addition, any increase in the left ventricular (LV) end-diastolic pressure (LVEDP) further compromises the flow in the subendocardial capillaries. In response to a narrowing of the CS, the backward pressure applied to the venules and capillaries (see Fig. 27.6B, *green arrows*) is thought to recruit arterioles and preferentially reduce the resistance to flow in the ischemic subendocardium,[129] which improves perfusion, contractility, and reduces LVEDP and breaks the vicious cycle of ischemia.[130]

Myocardial infarction

Study or subgroup	Stem cell Events	Stem cell Total	Control Events	Control Total	Weight	Odds ratio M-H, fixed, 95% CI	Year
Losordo 2007	0	6	0	18		Not estimable	2007
PROTECT-CAD 2007	0	19	1	9	12.9%	0.15 (0.01, 3.94)	2007
Wang 2010	0	56	0	56		Not estimable	2010
ACT34-CMI (High) 2011	3	56	7	56	43.8%	0.40 (0.10, 1.62)	2011
ACT34-CMI (Low) 2011	3	55	7	56	43.3%	0.40 (0.10, 1.65)	2011
Total (95% CI)		**192**		**195**	**100.0%**	**0.37 (0.14, 0.95)**	
Total events	**6**		**15**				

Heterogeneity: Chi2 = 0.33, df = 2 (*p* = 0.85); F = 0%
Test for overall effect Z = 2.07 (*p* = 0.04)

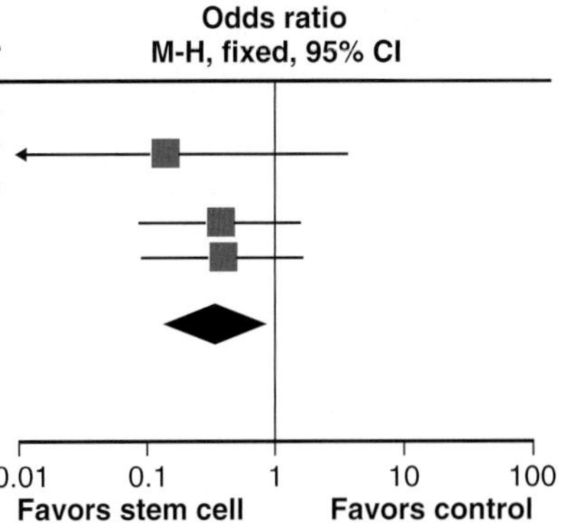

A

Death

Study or subgroup	Stem cell Events	Stem cell Total	Control Events	Control Total	Weight	Odds ratio M-H, fixed, 95% CI	Year
Losordo 2007	0	6	0	18		Not estimable	2007
PROTECT-CAD 2007	0	9	0	19		Not estimable	2007
Ramshorst 2009	1	25	0	25	6.4%	3.12 (0.12, 80.39)	2009
Wang 2010	0	56	0	56		Not estimable	2010
ACT34-CMI (High) 2011	0	58	3	56	47.0%	0.14 (0.01, 2.68)	2011
ACT34-CMI (Low) 2011	0	55	3	56	46.6%	0.14 (0.01, 2.73)	2011
Total (95% CI)		**207**		**230**	**100.0%**	**0.33 (0.08, 1.39)**	
Total events	**1**		**6**				

Heterogeneity: Chi2 = 2.51, df = 2 (*p* = 0.28); F = 20%
Test for overall effect Z = 1.51 (*p* = 0.13)

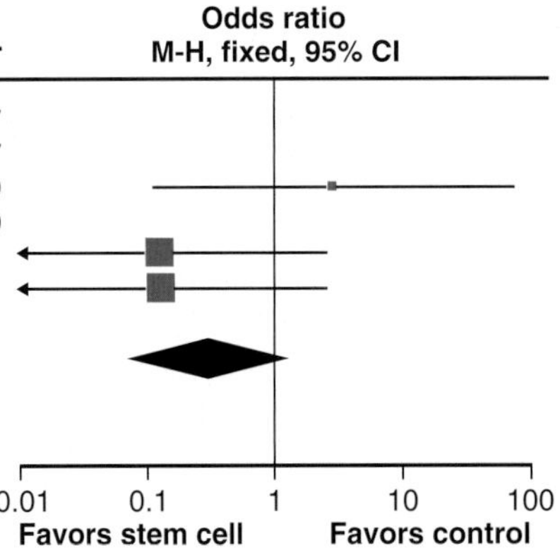

B

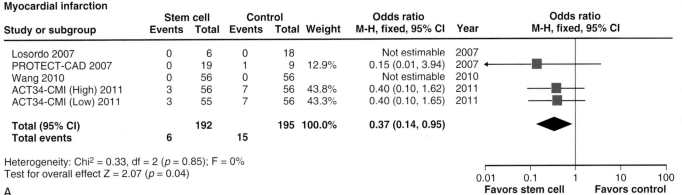

FIG. 27.7 Cell therapy is associated with improved clinical outcomes in patients with refractory angina. Forest plot of odds ratio for myocardial infarction **(A)** and death **(B)** in the stem cell group compared with the control group. *ACT34-CMI (High)*, High-dose CD34+ cell group; *ACT34-CMI (Low)*, low-dose CD34+ cell group; *CI*, confidence interval; *df*, degree of freedom; *M-H*, Mantel-Haenszel; *PROTECT-CAD*, Prospective Randomized Trial of Direct Endomyocardial Implantation of Bone Marrow Cells for Treatment of Severe Coronary Artery Diseases. *(Courtesy of Li N, Yang YJ, Zhang Q, et al. Stem cell therapy is a promising tool for refractory angina: a meta-analysis of randomized controlled trials.* Can J Cardiol. *2013;29:908–914.)*

Therapeutic Angiogenesis

Protein and Gene Therapy

Recombinant growth factors and gene therapy have been tested in the hope of enhancing the natural angiogenesis process in patients with advanced CAD. The intracoronary delivery of angiogenic proteins VEGF and fibroblast growth factor (FGF) both failed to meet their primary endpoint (total exercise duration) in large, randomized, placebo-controlled trials, although there were positive secondary endpoints.[131,132] To address the lack of efficacy of short half-life protein therapy, cardiac gene therapy has been developed in the hope of allowing a sustained expression of angiogenic factors in ischemic territories. The efficacy signal observed with the intracoronary (IC) delivery of an adenovirus encoding FGF5 (Ad5FGF) in the early-phase Angiogenic Gene Therapy (AGENT) and AGENT-II trials[133,134] prompted the phase III trials AGENT-III and AGENT-IV, which compared different doses of Ad5FGF-4 (up to 1×10^{10} viral particles) to placebo. A pooled analysis of both trials (n = 532 participants) revealed no significant change in total exercise duration 12 weeks after therapy with Ad5FGF-4 compared to placebo.[135] Post-hoc analyses suggested a substantial exercise benefit in high-risk patients (aged > 55 years, angina class III or higher, and baseline exercise duration inferior to 300 s). Likewise, a significant beneficial effect was observed in women, who improved their total exercise duration and functional class. These findings await prospective validation in a dedicated trial. The direct intramyocardial injection of VEGF-165 gene therapy in patients with advanced CAD failed to improve the perfusion of ischemic myocardium in two distinct placebo-controlled trials.[136,137] Other smaller, open-label trials have reached discordant results.[138,139] The ongoing KAT301 trial testing endocardial VEGF-D gene therapy in patients with advanced CAD is likely to bring additional information to the discussion (NCT01002430). The future of gene-based therapeutic angiogenesis may lie in the use of multiple growth factor therapies embedded in biologic scaffolds.

Cell Therapy

Besides the potential direct dependent of collaterals, cell therapy is hypothesized to locally release proangiogenic cytokines that promote angiogenesis and improve blood supply to the ischemic myocardium. Cell therapy is also thought to favorably alter myocardial function, reduce apoptosis, and recruit both resident and circulating stem cells.[140] Some evidence links cell therapy to reduced mortality and improved functionality in the long term in patients with ischemic heart disease[141] (Fig. 27.7). At this time, fewer than 10 randomized placebo-controlled trials have been conducted to assess cell therapy specifically in patients with intractable or refractory angina.[142–148] A pooled analysis of 331 participants enrolled in five phase I/II trials has suggested that cell therapy (either autologous CD34+ cells or bone marrow mononuclear cells) may be better than a placebo delivery at decreasing the weekly angina count (by seven episodes per week; 95% CI, 1–13; $p = 0.02$), at increasing the total exercise duration on a stress test (by 61 s; 95% CI, 18–104 s; $p = 0.005$), and at reducing the odds of experiencing an MI (OR = 0.37; 95% CI, 0.14–0.95; $p = 0.04$).[149]

Autologous CD34+ cells are endothelial progenitors isolated from granulocyte colony-stimulating factor (G-CSF)-mobilized peripheral blood, which may be partially effective. Wang et al. assessed the efficacy of autologous CD34+ cells (mean dose of 5.6×10^7 cells) compared to a placebo transfused in the coronary arteries of 112 patients with refractory angina. At 6 months, the weekly angina count was significantly reduced in patients treated with autologous CD34+ cells (−15.6 ± 4.0 episodes) compared with placebo (−3.0 ± 1.2 episodes; $p < 0.01$).[145] Likewise, Lee et al. found that the intracoronary transfusion of CD34+ cells was superior to a sham delivery at improving left ventricular ejection fraction (LVEF), possibly via an improved neovascularization. However, exercise tolerance and symptoms remained similar in both groups.[150] The largest experience is with intramyocardial CD34+ cell therapy that included phase I/IIa,[143] IIb,[142] and III[147] trials. In the phase IIb ACT34+ trial, intramyocardial CD34+ cells (1×10^5 cells per kg) improved weekly angina count compared to a sham placebo intervention (−6.8 ± 1.1 episodes vs. −10.9 ± 1.2 episodes; $p = 0.02$). Similar results were found for total exercise duration in a treadmill stress test (139 s ± 115 s versus 69 s ± 122 s; $p = 0.01$).[142] CD34+ cell therapy was associated with a persistent improvement in angina at 2 years.[151] These favorable results prompted the phase III Efficacy and Safety of Targeted Intramyocardial Delivery of Auto CD34+ Stem Cells for Improving Exercise Capacity in Subjects with Refractory Angina (RENEW) trial,[147] which stopped after 112 participants (of the 444 initially planned) had been randomized due to a financial decision by the sponsors. Although underpowered, the results seen in RENEW were consistent with those observed in the phase II trial.[152]

In an uncontrolled study, autologous mesenchymal stromal cells (MSCs) injected directly into the ischemic myocardium of patients with advanced CAD have been associated with improved total exercise duration and angina class up to 3 years.[153] In a phase I/II RCT, CD133 cells injected directly into the myocardium reduced significantly the monthly angina count (−8.5 episodes; 95% CI, −15.0 episodes to −4.0 episodes) and the angina functional class compared to no cell therapy.[148] Mechanistic studies even suggest that repeating the intramyocardial injection of bone marrow mononuclear cells in previous responders can further improve ischemia and relieve angina.[154] Although the results are promising, cell therapy is an investigational product and its use should remain confined to formal clinical investigations.

Neuromodulation

The heart muscle does not ache.[155] The genesis of angina is a complex neurogenic phenomenon that involves both the receptors of the sympathetic and vagal afferent pathways. How ischemia triggers a pain signal is still unclear and likely results from a multitude of substances such as lactates, adenosine, bradykinin, and potassium that irritates the chemosensitive endings of unmyelinated (C) fibers and of myelinated (Aδ) fibers embedded in the myocardium. Sympathetic fibers coalesce toward the cardiac sympathetic afferent nerve and reach the paravertebral sympathetic ganglia, which form the sympathetic cervical chain, including the stellate ganglia. Excitation of the sympathetic afferent fibers at the myocardial level stimulates the spinothalamic tract cells in the cervico-thoracic spinal segments and mediates the angina located in the chest and arm. Excitation of the vagal afferent fibers mediates the angina located in the neck and jaw.[156]

The nervous system has several points of convergence where specific information transits (such as the cardiac pain impulse). In the peripheral nervous system, some of these points are readily accessible for targeted interventions, such as the stellate ganglia or the spinal tract. However, because of the duplicity of the afferent pathways involved in the transmission of noxious cardiac signals, it is unlikely that single interventions—however targeted they may be—may entirely suppress angina. The cardiac nociceptive signal is also processed centrally by the thalamus, which plays the role of a gate,[157] and the cortex. The latter seems to be amenable to modulation by interventions such as self-management training or selective serotonin-reuptake inhibitor (SSRI).

Cardiac neuromodulation involves the deception or the interruption of a nociceptive signal using chemical, electrical, or mechanical means that can be applied at any level in the transmission pathway from the heart to the central nervous system. Conceptually, neuromodulation is appealing for the relief of cardiac pain with a prominent neurogenic component, as is the case with inappropriate cardiac pain perception. Because neuromodulation can potentially alter any cardiac pain signal, regardless of the pathophysiology, neuromodulation may be useful in patients with refractory angina. Neuromodulation may also favorably alter the sympathetic afference responsible for coronary artery vasoconstriction. The evidence available to support the various possible declinations of neuromodulation is still suboptimal.

Spinal Cord Stimulation

Spinal cord stimulation (SCS) achieves electroanalgesia after a multipolar electrode is positioned in the epidural space near the dorsal column between the C7 and T4 vertebrae where the cardiac afferent sympathetic fibers synapse with second-order sensory neurons in the dorsal horns. The electrodes stimulate the dorsal horn and blur the transmission of the nociceptive impulse en route toward the spinothalamic tract. The main effect of SCS is to replace the unpleasant experience of angina with more tolerable precordial paresthesias.[158] How SCS mediates its effect is not entirely elucidated, but it has been hypothesized to change the dorsal horn chemistry by promoting the release of γ-aminobutyric acid (GABA) and of β-endorphins, which antagonizes the descending inhibitory pathways, otherwise known to favor the transmission of nociceptive impulses.[159] In addition to an analgesic effect, SCS may have an anti-ischemic effect by downmodulating the autonomic nervous system through a partial sympatholysis[160] with ensuing vasodilation and improved flow in the coronary microcirculation.[161,162] Although appealing, this association has not been consistent in the literature.[163]

SCS has been tested in several small clinical trials against various comparators, such as optimal medical therapy, transmyocardial laser, and even CABG. The available trials were frequently interrupted prematurely due to poor enrollment, and were unblinded due to the obvious paresthesia caused by SCS once activated. A meta-analysis with seven RCTs and 270 patients suggested that SCS significantly improved the total exercise duration (standardized mean difference [SMD] 0.76; 95% CI 0.07–1.46; $p = 0.03$) and health-related quality of life (SMD 0.83; 95% CI, 0.32–1.34; $p = 0.001$).[164] SCS in patients with advanced CAD has also been associated with an improvement in LVEF.[165] The potential benefits of SCS are now being explored in patients with chronic HF, but the efficacy is uncertain.[166] Small studies have suggested that SCS plus medical therapy is cost-effective despite the higher costs at the initiation of therapy.[167,168] Randomized trials from 2015[169] and real-life observational studies[170] support these findings.

An interesting variation to SCS is subcutaneous electrical nerve stimulation (SENS) where two multipolar electrodes are subcutaneously implanted in each side of the sternum at the level where the retrosternal pain radiates during an angina episode. SENS targets subcutaneous nerve endings and has been associated with improved angina and reduced sublingual nitrate consumption in a small study.[171]

Based on moderate-quality evidence, most cardiology practice guidelines weakly recommend SCS, suggesting it may be considered to improve exercise capacity[172] and quality of life[11] in patients with refractory angina. When considered, SCS requires a multidisciplinary approach including a discussion regarding the safety and timing of stopping oral anticoagulants and antiplatelet agents to avoid epidural bleeding. SCS is generally performed as a minor surgical procedure under local anesthesia. SCS elevates the angina threshold, but breakthrough angina episodes are still possible despite active stimulation, such as when the signal is particularly intense. The concerns around silencing life-threatening ischemic episodes are therefore unsubstantiated.[169] Interactions between SCS pulse generators and implantable defibrillators are possible and warrant proper surveillance.[173]

Cardiac Sympathectomy

In addition to allowing the retropropagation of cardiac nociceptive impulses to the brain, the sympathetic nervous system can cause myocardial ischemia directly by favoring vasoconstriction and indirectly by favoring systemic humoral activation leading to higher catecholamine concentrations. It therefore appears logical that interventions that specifically downmodulate the sympathetic system would effectively relieve angina. However, due to the lack of appropriate studies, cardiac sympathectomy is not regularly performed in cardiology and its use remains largely empirical.

Stellate Ganglion Blockade

The left stellate (cervicothoracic) sympathetic ganglion is a point of convergence for sympathetic fibers before they synapse to the intermediolateral gray column in the thoracic spinal cord. Neuroanatomy provides compelling arguments in favor of stellate ganglion blockades to relieve angina, yet the evidence to support this practice is lacking.[11,172]

The left stellate ganglion is typically located between the carotid artery and the cricoid cartilage at the level of C6, although anatomic variants and right-sided duplicity are possible. The left stellate ganglion can be safely accessed under ultrasound guidance and injected with various anesthetic substances to temporarily block (in theory) the transmission of nociceptive afference signals to the brain.[174] In a case series of 59 consecutive patients, the mean period for angina relief was 3.5 weeks with stellate ganglion blockades with 15 mL of 0.5% bupivacaine, compared to 2.80 weeks for paravertebral blockades. These procedures could be performed serially with complication rates of approximately 3% (mostly reversible episodes of vertigo and hypotension, but also hematoma).[175] The Horner syndrome is also another complication described as a result of the intervention. Permanent effects have been described with the direct ablation of the stellate ganglion using radiofrequency for angina,[176] and other complex regional pain syndromes.[177]

High Thoracic Epidural Analgesia

In a case series of 152 consecutive patients with refractory angina, serial epidural analgesia with bupivacaine through a permanent epidural catheter inserted at thoracic level 2 to 5 was associated with improved angina symptoms and quality of life for up to 6 years.[178] Whereas there were no central nervous system infections, some patients developed cutaneous infection, a temporary drop in BP, and Horner syndrome.

Surgical Thoracic Sympathectomy

Surgical thoracic sympathectomy is a historic intervention that has been anecdotally used in refractory angina with varying success rates despite permanent sequelae.[179] If considered, surgical thoracic sympathectomy should be preceded by temporary sympathetic blockade to establish the suspected contribution of sympathetic mediation to the cardiac pain.

Imipramine

Imipramine is a tricyclic antidepressant that has been tested in a small, randomized, cross-over, placebo-controlled trial in patients (predominantly female) with normal coronary angiogram, negative ergonovine provocation test, and prominent cardiac pain, despite previous attempt of β-blockers, CCBs, or long-acting nitrates. Unlike any other medications given to treat angina related to myocardial ischemia, imipramine was shown to reduce the sensitivity to cardiac pain triggered by either right ventricle (RV) pacing or IC adenosine (2.2 mg/min for 2 min). Patients treated with imipramine (50 mg nightly for 3 weeks) not only experienced a reduction in their angina count compared to placebo (−52% ± 25% vs. −1% ± 86%, $p = 0.03$) but were also more likely to report an improvement of their repeated RV pacing/IC adenosine cardiac pain sensitivity tests (60% vs. 12.5%, $p = 0.01$).[180] These findings were confirmed by a group of independent investigators, who also reported a lack of efficacy on quality of life, likely due to the high incidence of side effects (mostly anticholinergic) associated with imipramine.[181] Despite its unique effect on cardiac sensitivity, imipramine remains inadequately studied in patients with advanced CAD and refractory angina. The drug should probably be reserved for patients with a prominent neurogenic component to their angina, such as patients with sensitive heart syndrome.

MENTAL STRESS–INDUCED MYOCARDIAL ISCHEMIA

Mental stress–induced myocardial ischemia (MSIMI) describes the objective evidence of myocardial ischemia during a mental stress task. Mental stress tests are rarely performed in clinical practice but typically include elements such as mental arithmetic, mirror trace, and public speaking with anger recall. During a mental stress test, subjects are monitored for the occurrence of ischemic markers such as ST-segment depression on electrocardiogram (ECG), any development of regional wall motion, or a drop in LVEF on echocardiogram.

The available evidence suggests that MSIMI may be associated with a twofold increase in the risk of death and cardiac events.[182] The underlying pathophysiology of MSIMI is unknown but is likely to be multifactorial. Microvascular dysfunction,[183] cardiac autonomic nervous system imbalance, and even enhanced platelet aggregation[184] have all been suggested as possible contributory factors. Mental stress is an effective inducer of coronary vasospasm,[185] and MSIMI has been classified by some groups as a subtype of vasospastic angina.[186] Besides ischemia, angina is a nociceptive signal and its perception can be centrally modulated by affects.[187] MSIMI is typically evoked in patients without epicardial coronary disease (see Chapter 25) but is thought to be much more prevalent among patients with established CAD.[183]

In the Responses of Mental Stress Induced Myocardial Ischemia to Escitalopram Treatment (REMIT) trial, more patients with MSIMI treated with escitalopram (5 mg daily) were free of the disease after 6 weeks of treatment compared to placebo (34.2% vs. 17.5%; OR, 2.62; p = 0.04).[188] Escitalopram was not associated with a significant change in scores of symptoms of depression, trait anxiety, or perceived stress compared to placebo, nor did it alter exercise capacity. SSRIs may modulate the hypothalamic-pituitary-adrenal axis and its ensuing effect on coronary microvascular function. Escitalopram should not to be confused with citalopram, which can prolong the QT interval. Escitalopram should be administered under the guidance of psychiatrists in patients with major depression, as its use has been associated with suicidal hazard.

Other nonpharmacologic approaches, such as patient self-management training, can help to mitigate the impact that emotions and stress may have on symptom perception and quality of life[189] (see also Chapter 26).

REFRACTORY VASOSPASTIC ANGINA

Recurrent chest pain with normal coronary angiogram is a common reason for consultation in specialized refractory angina clinics. Vasospastic angina is often referred to as *atypical* when compared to the angina resulting from fixed atherosclerotic lesions, but still presents with its own typical pattern: angina occurs at rest, particularly between the night and the early morning, and is associated with a considerable variation of exercise capacity during the day, especially pronounced in the morning. In addition, episodes can be provoked by hyperventilation.[186] Vasospastic angina is often overlooked because of the lack of demonstrable ischemia with most standard noninvasive diagnostic approaches, in the presence of seemingly normal coronary arteries. The Prinzmetal variant angina is a subtype of acute/unstable vasospastic angina that associates nitrate-responsive rest angina with transient ST-segment elevation on the ECG.[190] The Coronary Vasomotion Disorders International Study Group (COVADIS) defines vasospastic angina as the combined occurrence of nitrate-responsive episodes of angina with either transient ischemic ECG changes (such as 1-mV ST-segment depression or elevation, or new negative U waves) or coronary artery spasms (transient total or subtotal [90%] coronary artery occlusion)[191] in response to IC acetylcholine or ergonovine. The definition of vasospastic angina has been refined to include the notion of microvascular spasm that combines angina with transient ischemic ECG changes but no or incomplete coronary spasms (less than 70% luminal occlusion).[192,193] Nosologists are yet to clarify the overlap that may exist between microvascular spasms and endothelium-dependent microvascular dysfunction[194,195] (see Fig. 27.2). Both diagnoses can also coexist with advanced CAD.[196]

Invasive provocative coronary artery spasm testing should be performed whenever the diagnosis is suspected, especially in high-risk patients or those who are severely symptomatic.[186] Acknowledgment of the diagnosis is important and is a necessary step in the differentiation from other conditions such as sensitive heart syndrome or microvascular dysfunction, which may actually respond to the appropriate treatments. Most cases of vasospastic angina will respond to short- and long-acting nitrates, CCBs,[197] and to the avoidance of noxious stimuli (e.g., smoking, alcohol, β-blockers, ergot derivatives, cocaine, and other sympathomimetics), but it is estimated that 10% to 20% of patients are poor responders to first-line therapies.[198,199] In addition to a poor quality of life due to recurrent angina, these patients are at increased risk of sudden cardiac death, syncope, and MI with sequelae.

The lack of immediate response to nitrates strongly suggests that the diagnosis of vasospastic angina is unlikely.[186] However, nitrate tolerance following chronic administration remains a possibility,[61] although some patients will not tolerate nitrates due to side effects (e.g., headaches, hypotension). As per the Guidelines for Diagnosis and Treatment of Patients with Vasospastic Angina by the Japanese Circulation Society, nicorandil receives a class IIa recommendation for the treatment of vasospastic angina.[186] Nicorandil exerts a strong vasodilatory effect on coronary arteries[60] and has been successfully used in small case series of patients with persistent rest angina despite the combination of CCBs and nitrates.[200]

The field of refractory vasospastic angina has not been studied with large, adequately powered clinical trials. Instead, the best available evidence often stems from small case series and uncontrolled trials. In refractory cases, high doses of CCBs can be attempted (such as verapamil or diltiazem 960 mg/day; nifedipine 100 mg/day). Both nondihydropyridine and dihydropyridine CCBs can be combined to maximize the vasodilatory effects.[201] β-Blockers are proscribed as theoretically they might exacerbate spasms by leaving α-mediated vasoconstriction unopposed by β-mediated vasodilatation.

Fasudil is an IV/IC Rho-kinase inhibitor, which possibly decreases the calcium sensitization of vascular smooth muscle to prevent vasospasm.[202] Fasudil has a limited availability outside Japan and is of limited utility for patients requiring long-term oral therapy.[203] Oral Rho-kinase inhibitors with better bioavailability may eventually become useful to treat this indication.

Cilostazol is a selective inhibitor of phosphodiesterase III (PDE III) with pleiotropic properties, including vasodilation and platelet inhibition. Cilostazol is thought to mediate vasodilation via a reduction in cytosolic calcium concentration in vascular smooth muscle cells.[204] Cilostazol has been used with relative success in patients with symptomatic peripheral arterial disease. In the Study to evaluaTe the Efficacy and safety of Pletal (ciLostazoL) in subjects with vasospastic Angina (STELLA) randomized, double-blind trial, 50 patients with newly diagnosed vasospastic angina who had at least one angina episode per week despite amlodipine therapy (5 mg/day) were randomly assigned to either cilostazol (50 mg twice daily for 2 weeks, then 100 mg twice daily for 2 weeks) or placebo for 4 weeks. Patients assigned to cilostazol experienced a greater drop in their weekly angina count (−3.7 ± 0.5 episodes vs. −1.9 ± 0.6 episodes, respectively, $p = 0.03$).[205] Headache was the most common adverse event.

In a small nonrandomized study ($n = 73$), the peroxisome proliferator-activated receptor gamma (PPAR-γ) activator pioglitazone (15–30 mg/day) added to CCBs was associated with a better suppression of acetylcholine-induced coronary spasm compared to CCBs alone (50% vs. 21.6%, $p < 0.001$).[206] Cardiac rehabilitation performed with aerobic interval exercise training in the afternoon (when vasospastic episodes are less likely) may also help to improve symptoms.[207]

Anecdotal successes have been reported with estradiol (in postmenopausal women),[208] left stellate ganglion blockade,[209] thoracic sympathectomy,[210] vitamin C,[211] glutathione[212] (antioxidant), guanethidine (antiadrenergic drug that reduces the release of norepinephrine in the sympathetic nerve) with clonidine,[213] and corticosteroids.[214] Magnesium sulfate (IV infusion of 0.27 mM/kg)[215,216] and complete cardiac denervation by autotransplantion[217,218] have been used historically but yielded questionable results.

Optical coherence tomography (OCT) studies indicate that intimal erosion, fibrous cap disruption, and lumen irregularity are more frequently found at the site of focal spasm.[219] If true, this observation opens the door to selective PCI in spasmodic coronary segments, which has been historically performed in highly symptomatic individuals.[220,221]

REFRACTORY ANGINA IN PATIENTS WITH CORONARY MICROVASCULAR DYSFUNCTION

Beyond the readily visible epicardial coronary stenoses, coronary microvascular dysfunction is likely an attendant break to blood flow in most patients with advanced CAD. Whereas diagnostic algorithms[222,223] have been proposed for coronary microvascular dysfunction in the absence of obstructive CAD, the documentation of abnormal coronary reactivity, vasospasm, or myocardial perfusion index in patients with advanced CAD can be challenging (see Fig. 27.3). Patients with chest pain and nonobstructive CAD have a high prevalence of coronary microvascular abnormalities.[224] Recognizing that angina, ischemia, and cardiac pain are all possible with nonocclusive coronary arteries is an important step in the treatment of a large contingent of patients with persistent chest pain. Microvascular dysfunction may not result in detectable myocardial ischemia when standard scintigraphic diagnostic methods are used, because of the scattered distribution of perfusion defects in the microvasculature, and may not result in measurable contractile dysfunction because of the preserved contractile function of the surrounding nonischemic myocardial tissue.

Xanthine Derivatives

Therapeutic options for microvascular dysfunction are reviewed in detail in Chapters 5 and 25. Regarding patients with refractory symptoms, xanthine derivatives offer a conceptually appealing treatment option, as they antagonize the effect of adenosine, which theoretically favors the redistribution of coronary blood flow toward areas of microvascular dysfunction.[225] Adenosine achieves maximal vasodilation independently from the endothelium. In response to adenosine, dysfunctional microvascular segments fail to vasodilate, while healthy microvascular segments do. Adenosine antagonists are thought to selectively constrict nondysfunctional coronary microcirculation and to prevent norepinephrine reuptake in sympathetic nerve endings.[226] Adenosine antagonists may also have an analgesic effect by preventing the sensitizing effect of adenosine on the nociceptors involved in cardiac pain.[227] Pentoxifylline,[228] bamiphylline,[229] and amoniphylline[230,231] have been tested in patients with syndrome X, with varying success. In a small double-blind cross-over trial, 13 patients were randomized to either oral aminophylline (225–350 mg twice daily) or placebo for 3 weeks. Aminophylline resulted in a better total exercise duration compared to placebo (632 s ± 202 s vs. 522 s ± 264 s) but failed to improve angina episode.[230] Insufficient evidence exists to support the use of xanthine derivatives in refractory angina. Xanthine derivatives have been given a class IIb (level of evidence B) by the ESC for the treatment of patients with microvascular angina.[11]

Endothelin-1 Receptor Blockade

Endothelin (ET) is a peptide that mediates vasoconstriction. Endothelin-1 (ET-1) receptor blockade has been tested in patients with acute MI under the premise that it would improve microvascular function.[232] Experimental evidence suggests that ET-1 is essential to mediate coronary vasospasm and that ET-1 receptor blockage may indeed prevent vasospasm[233] and improve microvascular function.[234] Selective ET-1 receptor blockade is a promising strategy but has not been properly tested in patients with angina due to microvascular dysfunction.[235]

NONINVASIVE THERAPIES

Extracorporeal Shock Wave Therapy

Extracorporeal shock wave therapy (ESWT) employs brief, low-energy, high-amplitude acoustic pressure pulses delivered focally in ischemic cardiac segments. In response to the acoustic field, the naturally occurring microbubbles inside and outside the myocytes oscillate and collapse to exert a focal shear stress that favors the in situ release of proangiogenic cytokines, such as stromal cell-derived factor 1 and VEGF,[236,237] and the recruitment of progenitor cells.[238,239] As observed in other conditions, such as orthopedic and soft tissue diseases, ESWT may exert an early vasodilatory effect in the ischemic heart that may explain the early onset of angina relief associated with ESWT in refractory angina.[240]

ESWT is applied during diastole via electrocardiographic R-wave gating to avoid theoretical malignant ventricular arrhythmias and is delivered noninvasively under echographic guidance to target the border zone between the ischemic and the healthy myocardium in the hope of promoting angiogenesis. Although protocols vary, ESWT is typically administered over nine sessions lasting approximately 20 minutes each, over 3 months, divided in three clusters of three sessions per week followed by a treatment-free interval of 3 weeks (to allow the neovascularization effect to take place). During each session, up to 10 focal spots are repeatedly pulsed (up to 200 times) with low-energy shock waves (0.09 mJ/mm^2, which is approximately one-tenth of the energy delivered for renal lithotripsy).[241] The treatment is generally well tolerated with no evidence of discomfort, side effects, or myocardial injury.[240–242] Patients with a poor acoustic window are equally poor candidates for ESWT. ESWT is considered safe even at a high-energy level (as is the case for renal lithotripsy) as it exerts a differential effect on resilient and calcified tissues.

In nonrandomized studies, ESWT has been associated with an improvement in symptoms and hospitalization rates in patients with advanced CAD. Whether or not ESWT improves myocardial perfusion is still controversial.[240,242,243] Shock wave therapy has been inadequately studied in refractory angina. A 2015 meta-analysis summarized the clinical experience in ischemic heart disease and included six randomized trials (total n = 307 participants) and eight nonrandomized studies (total n = 209 patients). In this analysis, shock wave therapy was associated with an improvement in CCS angina class (–0.86; 95% CI, –1.2 to –0.65; $p < 0.001$), a reduced weekly nitrate intake (–0.71; 95% CI –1.08 to –0.33; $p < 0.01$), and an improved angina-related quality of life (measured with the SAQ; 5.64, 95% CI, 3.12–8.15; $p < 0.001$), compared to a sham intervention or standard medical therapy.[244] Only one trial used proper random sequence generation and blinding.[245] In their trial, Wang et al. compared two ESWT protocols (accelerated over 1 month vs. standard over 3 months) to a sham intervention in 55 patients with refractory angina unsuitable for revascularization. Both the accelerated and the standard ESWT protocols improved the mean 6-min walking test distance at 12 months compared to the sham intervention (329 m ± 134 m to 452 m ± 117 m vs. 344 m ± 106 m to 478 m ± 105 m vs. 364 m ± 151 m to 348 m ± 132 m, respectively; $p = 0.02$). ESWT was also associated with a significant improvement in CCS angina class. Additional evidence is required before this treatment can be widely adopted in clinical practice.

Enhanced External Counterpulsation

Enhanced external counterpulsation (EECP) uses three sets of pneumatic cuffs around the lower extremities, which mimics externally what an intra-aortic balloon pump does internally.[246] The prompt inflation of cuffs at the onset of diastole augments coronary blood flow, while the deflation immediately before systole decreases afterload and increases venous return.[247] The augmented diastolic coronary perfusion is thought to recruit coronary collaterals[248] and favor the release of proangiogenic cytokines.[249,250] EECP has been associated with improved endothelial function and peripheral training effect.[251] EECP also improves systolic BP in patients with refractory angina.[5a]

In refractory angina, EECP has been tested in a single randomized trial, Multicenter Study of Enhanced External Counterpulsation (MUST-EECP), which compared standard EECP (with cuff inflation up to 350 mm Hg) to an inactive counterpulsation (cuff inflation lower than 75 mm Hg) in 139 patients with advanced CAD and refractory angina. Treatments were administered as 35 sessions of 1 h each over 4 to 7 weeks. The inactive counterpulsation was meant as a control to preserve the appearance and feel of a real counterpulsation without augmenting the diastolic BP and increasing the coronary perfusion. Objectively, EECP improved the time to 1-mm ST-segment depression compared to the sham intervention (+37 s ± 11 s vs. –4 s ± 12 s; $p = 0.01$) but did not significantly improve the total exercise duration.[253] The variation in daily angina count was numerically but not statistically improved in patients treated with EECP (–0.11 ± 0.21 episodes vs. 0.13 ± 0.22 episodes; $p = 0.09$), whereas the daily use of short-acting nitrates showed no significant difference. A meta-analysis that included 18 nonrandomized prospective studies and 1768 patients suggested that angina class improved by at least one CCS class in 85% of patients treated with EECP (95% CI, 0.81–0.88).[254] EECP has also been associated with improved quality of life,[255] myocardial perfusion,[256] and persistent reduction of MACEs.[254] Because EECP relies on ECG gating, it may be challenging to use in patients with rapid atrial fibrillation or with frequent ventricular ectopy. EECP is contraindicated in patients with abdominal aortic aneurysm, aortic insufficiency, and decompensated HF. Patients with severe peripheral arterial disease may derive less benefit from EECP given the reduced augmentation transmitted to the heart. EECP has been given a class IIb indication in the United States and Canada and a class IIa in Europe for the management of CCS class III and IV refractory angina. In the future, endovascular counterpulsation devices may help amplify coronary flow in patients with advanced CAD.[257]

Cardiac Rehabilitation

The idea of exercising patients with CCS class III/IV angina appears counterintuitive to most clinicians due to the fear of triggering ischemia-related malignant arrhythmias or acute coronary syndromes. However, rehabilitation has been shown to improve the quality of life of several populations with ischemic heart disease. At the present time, practice guidelines do not address the concept of cardiac rehabilitation in patients with refractory angina.[172,258] Most patients with refractory angina are reasonably stable and not at immediate risk of an adverse event.[5,259]

In a small study, 42 patients with refractory angina were randomized to an 8-week outpatient cardiac rehabilitation exercise program or no exercise at all.[260] The program involved supervised aerobic conditioning sessions in a dedicated center combined with home exercises and was aimed at improving functional capacity and muscular strength. During exercise, patients were asked to exercise at 60% to 75% of their age-predicted heart rate reserve (when LVEF was preserved), or 40% to 60% (when LVEF was less than 40%). Participants randomized to cardiac rehabilitation experienced no deterioration of their angina frequency and severity and were able to increase their walked distance by approximately 50 m. No difference was seen however in the severity or frequency of angina between groups, possibly due to an ischemic threshold adaptation in patients assigned to rehabilitation.[261] A validation of the safety of cardiac rehabilitation in an appropriately powered trial should be performed before it can be widely recommended in patients with refractory angina.

In a related trial, aerobic interval exercise training in the afternoon reduced the number of angina episodes in 26 patients with documented vasospastic angina.[207] The authors hypothesized that exercise reduced the coronary spastic angina by improving endothelial function and reducing oxidative stress.

HOW TO APPROACH PATIENTS WITH REFRACTORY ANGINA

The concept of refractory angina has evolved from a concept of advanced CAD that cannot be controlled by a

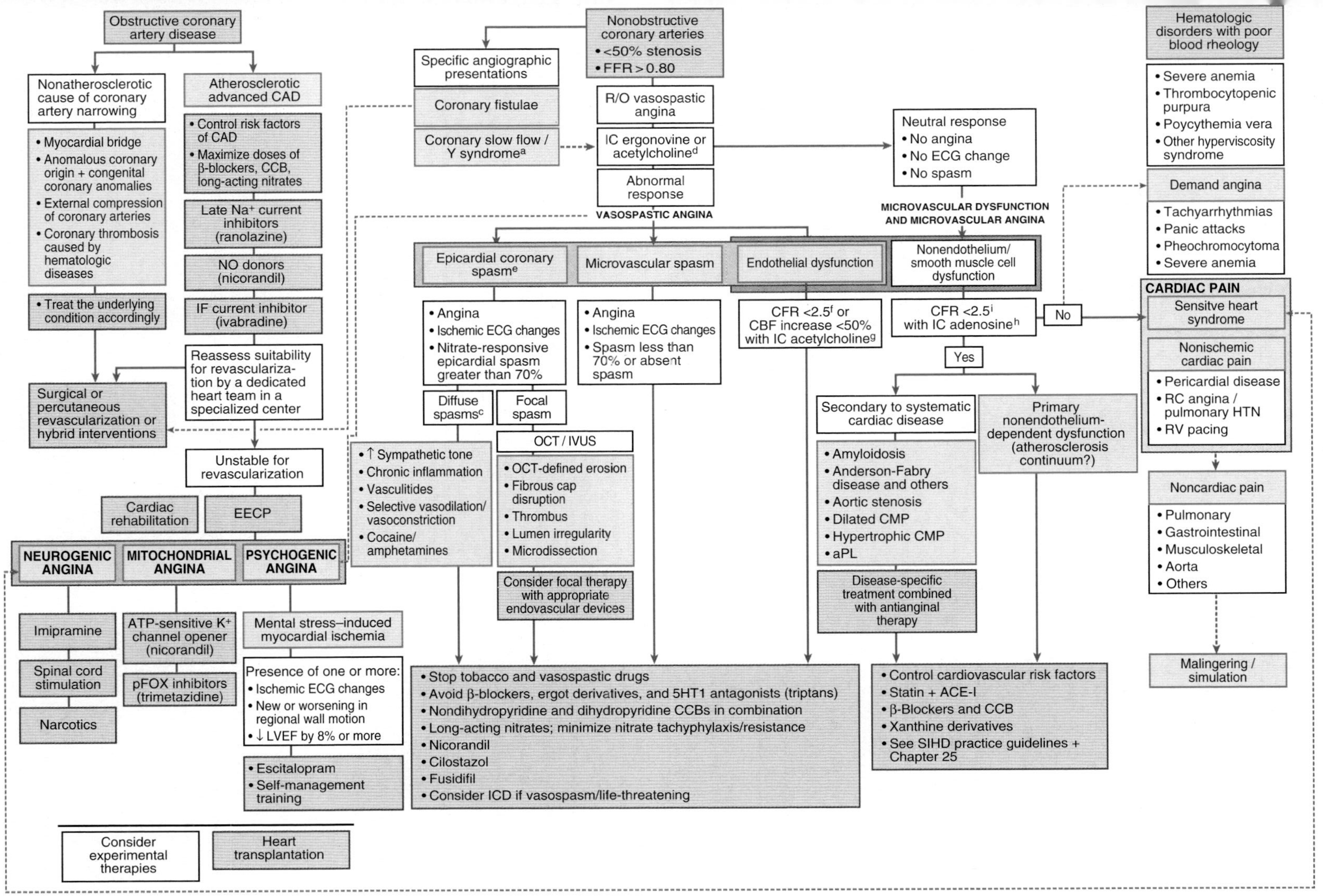

FIG. 27.8 Refractory anginas united. Box color scheme: *Blue*, presenting condition; *white*, diagnostic algorithm; *green*, diagnoses; *pink*, specific treatments.

a, Y syndrome is a disputed clinical entity defined as the presence of angina with nonobstructive coronary arteries and a marked delayed opacification of the distal vasculature.[263]

b, Ischemic electrocardiogram (ECG) changes recorded in at least two contiguous leads on the 12-lead ECG and defined as a transient ST-segment elevation of 0.1 mV or more, an ST depression of 0.1 mV or more, or new negative U waves.

c, Defined as occurring in more than one Collaborative Study in Coronary Artery Surgery coronary segment, or in more than one coronary artery.

d, Long-acting nitrates and calcium-channel blockers (CCBs) should be withheld for 48 h or longer. Invasive intracoronary ergonovine or acetylcholine should be reserved for high-risk or for highly symptomatic patients. Hyperventilation testing has been proposed as an alternative test in patients suspected of having vasospastic angina with low frequency of episodes.[186]

e, Catheter-induced spasm is not considered diagnostic for vasospastic angina.

f, Various diagnostic coronary flow reserve (CFR) cut-offs have been proposed in the literature, with 2.5 and lower being more sensitive and 2.0 and lower being more specific. Invasive CFR measurements (intracoronary Doppler, thermodilution) are considered the gold standard, but invasive myocardial perfusion reserve has also been proposed, notably with the use of positron emission tomography scan and by cardiac magnetic resonance imaging. Noninvasive imaging does not allow the discrimination of epicardial and microvascular disease and correlates poorly with invasive quantification methods.[224] Likewise, noninvasive tests relying on contractility (such as echocardiography) may not be adequate to detect microvascular perfusion defects because of the sparse nature of ischemia combined with the preserved contractile function of the surrounding nonischemic myocardial tissue.

g, Cold pressor test has been proposed as an alternative to acetylcholine to assess endothelium-dependent microvascular dysfunction. However, a cold pressor test is generally not recommended for the detection of epicardial spasm.[186]

h, Epicardial spasm, or the lack of an increased coronary blood flow of at least 50% in response to intracoronary nitrate, is also suggestive of macrovascular nonendothelial dysfunction.

ACE-I, Angiotensin-converting enzyme inhibitor; *aPL*, antiphospholipid syndrome; *ATP*, adenosine triphosphate; *CABG*, coronary artery bypass graft; *CAD*, coronary artery disease; *CBF*, coronary blood flow; *CCB*, calcium-channel blockers; *CFR*, coronary flow reserve; *CIHD*, chronic ischemic heart disease; *CMP*, cardiomyopathy; *CTO*, chronic total occlusion; *ECG*, electrocardiogram; *EECP*, enhanced external counterpulsation; *FFR*, fractional flow reserve; *5HT1*, 5-hydroxytryptamine receptor; *HTN*, hypertension; *IC*, intracoronary; *ICD*, implantable cardioverter defibrillator; *IVUS*, intravascular ultrasound; *LVEF*, left ventricular ejection fraction; *MI*, myocardial infarction; *Na+*, sodium; *NO*, nitric oxide; *OCT*, optical coherence tomography; *PCI*, percutaneous coronary intervention; *pFOX*, partial fatty acid oxidation; *R/O*, rule out; *RV*; right ventricle; *SIHD*, stable ischemic heart disease.

combination of medical therapy, angioplasty, and coronary bypass surgery[3] to a concept of cardiac pain caused by ischemia secondary to advanced CAD, microvascular dysfunction, or spasm and perpetuated because of a neurogenic, psychological, or mitochondrial dysfunction. Fig. 27.8 proposes an algorithmic approach to a wide range of presentations for refractory angina. When obstructive CAD is considered the main explanation for myocardial ischemia, second-line antianginal medications such as ranolazine, nicorandil, or ivabradine should be added to maximal tolerable doses of β-blockers, long-acting nitrates, and CCBs. The unsuitability of further revascularization is a dynamic decision that may change in time in response to patient-specific characteristics and available medical expertise. PCI or bypass surgery should be withheld when they cannot be reasonably attempted or are not expected to improve perfusion, as determined by a consensus decision by a heart team with interest in the field of refractory angina.[196] If needed, the coronary angiogram should be repeated periodically, even in patients previously deemed unsuitable for revascularization, as the disease may have progressed in new coronary segments now amenable to revascularization. This is frequently seen in patients who experience an abrupt deterioration of their angina. When revascularization is not possible, EECP and supervised rehabilitation can be considered. When symptoms persist despite multiple anti-ischemic therapies, the neurogenic component of the cardiac pain can be mitigated with imipramine, SCS, and ultimately narcotics.

One key message of Fig. 27.8 is that refractory angina is possible in patients with seemingly normal coronary arteries. When no significant obstructive coronary arteries are present, vasospastic angina and microvascular dysfunction should be formally ruled out. The noninvasive diagnosis of vasospastic angina is difficult as most modalities will not discriminate between epicardial and microvascular disease and will not document the dynamic nature of the coronary blood flow. Intracoronary ergonovine and acetylcholine provocation tests can be attempted in patients with seemingly normal coronary arteries to document the presence of epicardial or microvascular spasm. Depending on the response observed (focal vs. diffuse), different therapies have been proposed. In all instances, tobacco should be discouraged and vasospastic drugs discontinued. CCBs and nitrates are the mainstay in treatment of vasospastic angina, but nicorandil and cilostazol have been successfully used in selected cases. In the presence of life-threatening vasospastic angina, an implantable cardioverter defibrillator (ICD) should be considered.[262]

In the absence of vasospastic angina and endothelial dysfunction, nonendothelial-dependent microvascular dysfunction can be diagnosed by measuring the variation in coronary flow reserve in response to IC adenosine. Whenever an invasive assessment is not possible or is not desired, the noninvasive quantification of myocardial perfusion reserve (MPR) by positron emission tomography (PET) scan and by cardiac magnetic resonance (CMR) imaging can be considered. When detected, microvascular dysfunction should be approached as a primary disorder except when a systemic heart disease is concomitantly diagnosed, as is the case with various storage diseases or with hypertrophic cardiomyopathy.

Finally, when neither epicardial disease nor microvascular dysfunction can be objectified, consideration should be given to disorders of inappropriate cardiac pain perception and to nonischemic cardiac pain. In such instances, psychiatric disease, substance abuse, and drug-seeking behavior should all be considered as alternate diagnoses. Dealing with these various complex presentations often requires interdisciplinary, specialized clinics with advanced clinical care and the implementation of psychological and self-management approaches.[189]

References

1. Jolicoeur EM, Granger CB, Henry TD, et al.: Clinical and research issues regarding chronic advanced coronary artery disease: part I: contemporary and emerging therapies, *Am Heart J* 155:418–434, 2008.
2. McGillion M, L'Allier PL, Arthur H, et al.: Recommendations for advancing the care of Canadians living with refractory angina pectoris: a Canadian Cardiovascular Society position statement, *Can J Cardiol* 25:399–401, 2009.
3. Mannheimer C, Camici P, Chester MR, et al.: The problem of chronic refractory angina; report from the ESC Joint Study Group on the Treatment of Refractory Angina, *Eur Heart J* 23: 355–370, 2002.
4. Williams B, Menon M, Satran D, et al.: Patients with coronary artery disease not amenable to traditional revascularization: prevalence and 3-year mortality, *Catheter Cardiovasc Interv* 75: 886–891, 2010.
5. Henry TD, Satran D, Hodges JS, et al.: Long-term survival in patients with refractory angina, *Eur Heart J* 34:2683–2688, 2013.

5a. Campbell AR, Satran D, Zenovich AG, et al.: Enhanced external counterpulsation improves systolic blood pressure in patients with refractory angina, *Am Heart J* 156:1217–1222, 2008.

6. Belsey J, Savelieva I, Mugelli A, Camm AJ: Relative efficacy of antianginal drugs used as add-on therapy in patients with stable angina: a systematic review and meta-analysis, *Eur J Prev Cardiol* 22:837–848, 2015.
7. Husted SE, Ohman EM: Pharmacological and emerging therapies in the treatment of chronic angina, *Lancet* 386:691–701, 2015.
8. Charlier R, Deltour G, Tondeur R, Binon F: Studies in the benzofuran series. VII. Preliminary pharmacological study of 2-butyl-3-(3,5-diiodo-4-beta-N-diethylaminoethoxybenzoyl)-benzofuran, *Arch Int Pharmacodyn Ther* 139:255–264, 1962.
9. Singh BN, Vaughan Williams EM: The effect of amiodarone, a new anti-anginal drug, on cardiac muscle, *Br J Pharmacol* 39:657–667, 1970.
10. Meyer BJ, Amann FW: Additional antianginal efficacy of amiodarone in patients with limiting angina pectoris, *Am Heart J* 125:996–1001, 1993.
11. Montalescot G, Sechtem U, Achenbach S, et al.: 2013 ESC guidelines on the management of stable coronary artery disease: the Task Force on the management of stable coronary artery disease of the European Society of Cardiology, *Eur Heart J* 34:2949–3003, 2013.
12. McCormack JG, Barr RL, Wolff AA, Lopaschuk GD: Ranolazine stimulates glucose oxidation in normoxic, ischemic, and reperfused ischemic rat hearts, *Circulation* 93:135–142, 1996.
13. Antzelevitch C, Belardinelli L, Zygmunt AC, et al.: Electrophysiological effects of ranolazine, a novel antianginal agent with antiarrhythmic properties, *Circulation* 110:904–910, 2004.
14. Belardinelli L, Shryock JC, Fraser H: Inhibition of the late sodium current as a potential cardioprotective principle: effects of the late sodium current inhibitor ranolazine, *Heart* 92(Suppl 4):iv6–iv14, 2006.
15. Stanley WC, Recchia FA, Lopaschuk GD: Myocardial substrate metabolism in the normal and failing heart, *Physiol Rev* 85:1093–1129, 2005.
16. Chaitman BR, Pepine CJ, Parker JO, et al.: Effects of ranolazine with atenolol, amlodipine, or diltiazem on exercise tolerance and angina frequency in patients with severe chronic angina: a randomized controlled trial, *JAMA* 291:309–316, 2004.
17. Stone PH, Gratsiansky NA, Blokhin A, Huang IZ, Meng L: Antianginal efficacy of ranolazine when added to treatment with amlodipine: the ERICA (Efficacy of Ranolazine in Chronic Angina) trial, *J Am Coll Cardiol* 48:566–575, 2006.
18. Kosiborod M, Arnold SV, Spertus JA, et al.: Evaluation of ranolazine in patients with type 2 diabetes mellitus and chronic stable angina: results from the TERISA randomized clinical trial (Type 2 Diabetes Evaluation of Ranolazine in Subjects with Chronic Stable Angina), *J Am Coll Cardiol* 61:2038–2045, 2013.
19. Wilson SR, Scirica BM, Braunwald E, et al.: Efficacy of ranolazine in patients with chronic angina observations from the randomized, double-blind, placebo-controlled MERLIN-TIMI (Metabolic Efficiency with Ranolazine for Less Ischemia in Non-ST-Segment Elevation Acute Coronary Syndromes) 36 Trial, *J Am Coll Cardiol* 53:1510–1516, 2009.
20. Weisz G, Genereux P, Iniguez A, et al.: Ranolazine in patients with incomplete revascularisation after percutaneous coronary intervention (RIVER-PCI): a multicentre, randomised, double-blind, placebo-controlled trial, *Lancet* 387:136–145, 2016.
21. Alexander KP, Weisz G, Prather K, et al.: Effects of ranolazine on angina and quality of life after percutaneous coronary intervention with incomplete revascularization: results from the Ranolazine for Incomplete Vessel Revascularization (RIVER-PCI) Trial, *Circulation* 133: 39–47, 2016.
22. Jolicoeur EM, Ohman EM, Temple R, et al.: Clinical and research issues regarding chronic advanced coronary artery disease part II: trial design, outcomes, and regulatory issues, *Am Heart J* 155:435–444, 2008.
23. Villano A, Di FA, Nerla R, et al.: Effects of ivabradine and ranolazine in patients with microvascular angina pectoris, *Am J Cardiol* 112:8–13, 2013.
24. Mehta PK, Goykhman P, Thomson LE, et al.: Ranolazine improves angina in women with evidence of myocardial ischemia but no obstructive coronary artery disease, *JACC Cardiovasc Imaging* 4:514–522, 2011.
25. Stone PH, Chaitman BR, Stocke K, et al.: The anti-ischemic mechanism of action of ranolazine in stable ischemic heart disease, *J Am Coll Cardiol* 56:934–942, 2010.
26. Bairey Merz CN, Handberg EM, Shufelt CL, et al.: A randomized, placebo-controlled trial of late Na current inhibition (ranolazine) in coronary microvascular dysfunction (CMD): impact on angina and myocardial perfusion reserve, *Eur Heart J* 37:1504–1513, 2016.
27. Kantor PF, Lucien A, Kozak R, Lopaschuk GD: The antianginal drug trimetazidine shifts cardiac energy metabolism from fatty acid oxidation to glucose oxidation by inhibiting mitochondrial long-chain 3-ketoacyl coenzyme A thiolase, *Circ Res* 86:580–588, 2000.
28. Henry TD, Satran D, Jolicoeur EM: Treatment of refractory angina in patients not suitable for revascularization, *Nat Rev Cardiol* 11:78–95, 2014.
29. Cavar M, Ljubkovic M, Bulat C, et al.: Trimetazidine does not alter metabolic substrate oxidation in cardiac mitochondria of target patient population, *Br J Pharmacol* 173:1529–1540, 2016.
30. Liu Z, Chen JM, Huang H, et al.: The protective effect of trimetazidine on myocardial ischemia/reperfusion injury through activating AMPK and ERK signaling pathway, *Metabolism* 65:122–130, 2016.

31. Khan M, Meduru S, Mostafa M, et al.: Trimetazidine, administered at the onset of reperfusion, ameliorates myocardial dysfunction and injury by activation of p38 mitogen-activated protein kinase and Akt signaling, *Journal Pharmacol Exp Ther* 333:421–429, 2010.
32. Szwed H, Sadowski Z, Elikowski W, et al.: Combination treatment in stable effort angina using trimetazidine and metoprolol: results of a randomized, double-blind, multicentre study (TRIMPOL II). TRIMetazidine in POLand, *Eur Heart J* 22:2267–2274, 2001.
33. Ciapponi A, Pizarro R, Harrison J: Trimetazidine for stable angina, *Cochrane Database Syst Rev* CD003614, 2005.
34. Masmoudi K, Masson H, Gras V, Andrejak M: Extrapyramidal adverse drug reactions associated with trimetazidine: a series of 21 cases, *Fundam Clin Pharmacol* 26:198–203, 2012.
35. Lyon LJ, Nevins MA, Risch S, Henry S: Perhexilene maleate in treatment of angina pectoris, *Lancet* 1:1272–1274, 1971.
36. Burns-Cox CJ, Chandrasekhar KP, Ikram H, et al.: Clinical evaluation of perhexiline maleate in patients with angina pectoris, *Br Med J* 4:586–588, 1971.
37. Fraser DM, Campbell IW, Miller HC: Peripheral and autonomic neuropathy after treatment with perhexiline maleate, *Br Med J* 2:675–676, 1977.
38. Singlas E, Goujet MA, Simon P: Pharmacokinetics of perhexiline maleate in anginal patients with and without peripheral neuropathy, *Eur J Clin Pharmacol* 14:195–201, 1978.
39. Singlas E, Goujet MA, Simon P: Perhexilline maleate: relationship between side-effects, plasma concentrations and rate of metabolism (author's transl), *Nouv Presse Med* 7:1631–1632, 1978.
40. Barclay ML, Sawyers SM, Begg EJ, et al.: Correlation of CYP2D6 genotype with perhexiline phenotypic metabolizer status, *Pharmacogenetics* 13:627–632, 2003.
41. Chong CR, Drury NE, Licari G, et al.: Stereoselective handling of perhexiline: implications regarding accumulation within the human myocardium, *Eur J Clin Pharmacol* 71:1485–1491, 2015.
42. Kennedy JA, Kiosoglous AJ, Murphy GA, Pelle MA, Horowitz JD: Effect of perhexiline and oxfenicine on myocardial function and metabolism during low-flow ischemia/reperfusion in the isolated rat heart, *J Cardiovasc Pharmacol* 36:794–801, 2000.
43. Opie LH, Lopaschuck GD: Fuels, aerobic and anaerobic metabolism. In Opie LH, editor: *Heart Physiology, From Cell to Circulation*, ed 4, Philadelphia, 2004, Lippincott, Williams, Wilkins, pp 306–354.
44. Ashrafian H, Horowitz JD, Frenneaux MP: Perhexiline, *Cardiovasc Drug Rev* 25:76–97, 2007.
45. Yin X, Dwyer J, Langley SR, et al.: Effects of perhexiline-induced fuel switch on the cardiac proteome and metabolome, *J Mol Cell Cardiol* 55:27–30, 2013.
46. Barry WH, Horowitz JD, Smith TW: Comparison of negative inotropic potency, reversibility, and effects on calcium influx of six calcium channel antagonists in cultured myocardial cells, *Br J Pharmacol* 85:51–59, 1985.
47. Grima M, Velly J, Decker N, Marciniak G, Schwartz J: Inhibitory effects of some cyclohexylaralkylamines related to perhexiline on sodium influx, binding of [3H]batrachotoxinin A 20-alpha-benzoate and [3H]nitrendipine and on guinea pig left atria contractions, *Eur J Pharmacol* 147:173–185, 1988.
48. Ono H, Kimura M: Effect of Ca^{2+}-antagonistic vasodilators, diltiazem, nifedipine, perhexiline and verapamil, on platelet aggregation in vitro, *Arzneimittelforschung* 31:1131–1134, 1981.
49. Killalea SM, Krum H: Systematic review of the efficacy and safety of perhexiline in the treatment of ischemic heart disease, *Am J Cardiovasc Drugs* 1:193–204, 2001.
50. Cole PL, Beamer AD, McGowan N, et al.: Efficacy and safety of perhexiline maleate in refractory angina. A double-blind placebo-controlled clinical trial of a novel antianginal agent, *Circulation* 81:1260–1270, 1990.
51. White HD, Lowe JB: Antianginal efficacy of perhexiline maleate in patients refractory to beta-adrenoreceptor blockade, *Int J Cardiol* 3:145–155, 1983.
52. Phan TT, Shivu GN, Choudhury A, et al.: Multi-centre experience on the use of perhexiline in chronic heart failure and refractory angina: old drug, new hope, *Eur J Heart Fail* 11:881–886, 2009.
53. Gupta AK, Winchester D, Pepine CJ: Antagonist molecules in the treatment of angina, *Expert Opin Pharmacother* 14:2323–2342, 2013.
54. Drake FT, Haring O, Singer DH, Dirnberger G: Proceedings: evaluation of anti-arrhythmic efficacy of perhexiline maleate in ambulatory patients by Holter monitoring, *Postgrad Med J* 49(Suppl 3):52–63, 1973.
55. Arduini A, Zammit VA: A tennis lesson: sharp practice in the science behind the Sharapova case, *Postgrad Med J* 92:429–430, 2016.
56. Simkhovich BZ, Shutenko ZV, Meirena DV, et al.: 3-(2,2,2-Trimethylhydrazinium)propionate (THP)–a novel gamma-butyrobetaine hydroxylase inhibitor with cardioprotective properties, *Biochem Pharmacol* 37:195–202, 1988.
57. Zammit VA, Ramsay RR, Bonomini M, Arduini A: Carnitine, mitochondrial function and therapy, *Adv Drug Deliv Rev* 61:1353–1362, 2009.
58. Dzerve V: A dose-dependent improvement in exercise tolerance in patients with stable angina treated with mildronate: a clinical trial "MILSS I," *Medicina (Kaunas)* 47:544–551, 2011.
59. Treese N, Erbel R, Meyer J: Acute hemodynamic effects of nicorandil in coronary artery disease, *J Cardiovasc Pharmacol* 20(Suppl 3):S52–S56, 1992.
60. Aizawa T, Ogasawara K, Nakamura F, et al.: Effect of nicorandil on coronary spasm, *Am J Cardiol* 63:75j–79j, 1989.
61. Munzel T, Daiber A, Gori T: Nitrate therapy: new aspects concerning molecular action and tolerance, *Circulation* 123:2132–2144, 2011.
62. Dutra MM, Nascimento Junior EB, Godin AM, et al.: Opioid pathways activation mediates the activity of nicorandil in experimental models of nociceptive and inflammatory pain, *Eur J Pharmacol* 768:160–164, 2015.
63. Nishimura M, Okamoto Y, Takatani T, et al.: Improvement of myocardial fatty acid metabolism by oral nicorandil in hemodialysis patients without coronary artery disease, *J Nephrol* 28:227–234, 2015.
64. Di SS, Liguori V, Petitto M, et al.: A double-blind comparison of nicorandil and metoprolol in stable effort angina pectoris, *Cardiovasc Drugs Ther* 7:119–123, 1993.
65. Hughes LO, Rose EL, Lahiri A, Raftery EB: Comparison of nicorandil and atenolol in stable angina pectoris, *Am J Cardiol* 66:679–682, 1990.
66. Doring G: Antianginal and anti-ischemic efficacy of nicorandil in comparison with isosorbide-5-mononitrate and isosorbide dinitrate: results from two multicenter, double-blind, randomized studies with stable coronary heart disease patients, *J Cardiovasc Pharmacol* 20(Suppl 3):S74–S81, 1992.
67. Guermonprez JL, Blin P, Peterlongo F: A double-blind comparison of the long-term efficacy of a potassium channel opener and a calcium antagonist in stable angina pectoris, *Eur Heart J* 14(Suppl B):30–34, 1993.
68. Effect of nicorandil on coronary events in patients with stable angina: the Impact Of Nicorandil in Angina (IONA) randomised trial, *Lancet* 359:1269–1275, 2002.
69. Belsey J, Savelieva I, Mugelli A, Camm AJ: Relative efficacy of antianginal drugs used as add-on therapy in patients with stable angina: a systematic review and meta-analysis, *Eur J Prev Cardiol* 22:837–848, 2015.
70. Toquero L, Briggs CD, Bassuini MM, Rochester JR: Anal ulceration associated with nicorandil: case series and review of the literature, *Colorectal Dis* 8:717–720, 2006.
71. Wagner F, Gohlke-Barwolf C, Trenk D, Jahnchen E, Roskamm H: Differences in the antiischaemic effects of molsidomine and isosorbide dinitrate (ISDN) during acute and short-term administration in stable angina pectoris, *Eur Heart J* 12:994–999, 1991.
72. Schartl M, Dougherty C, Rutsch W, Schmutzler H: Hemodynamic effects of molsidomine, isosorbide dinitrate, and nifedipine at rest and during exercise, *Am Heart J* 109:649–653, 1985.
73. Belhassen L, Carville C, Pelle G, et al.: Molsidomine improves flow-dependent vasodilation in brachial arteries of patients with coronary artery disease, *J Cardiovasc Pharmacol* 35:560–563, 2000.
74. Messin R, Boxho G, De Smedt J, Buntinx IM: Acute and chronic effect of molsidomine extended release on exercise capacity in patients with stable angina, a double blind cross-over clinical trial versus placebo, *J Cardiovasc Pharmacol* 25:558–563, 1995.
75. Messin R, Opolski G, Fenyvesi T, et al.: Efficacy and safety of molsidomine once-a-day in patients with stable angina pectoris, *Int J Cardiol* 98:79–89, 2005.
76. Barbato E, Herman A, Benit E, et al.: Long-term effect of molsidomine, a direct nitric oxide donor, as an add-on treatment, on endothelial dysfunction in patients with stable angina pectoris undergoing percutaneous coronary intervention: results of the MEDCOR trial, *Atherosclerosis* 240:351–354, 2015.
77. Messin R, Bruhwyler J, Dubois C, Famaey JP, Geczy J: Tolerability to 1-year treatment with once-daily molsidomine in patients with stable angina, *Adv Ther* 23:601–614, 2006.
78. Moncada S, Higgs A: The L-arginine-nitric oxide pathway, *N Engl J Med* 329:2002–2012, 1993.
79. Lerman A, Burnett Jr JC, Higano ST, McKinley LJ, Holmes Jr DR: Long-term L-arginine supplementation improves small-vessel coronary endothelial function in humans, *Circulation* 97:2123–2128, 1998.
80. Ceremuzynski L, Chamiec T, Herbaczynska-Cedro K: Effect of supplemental oral L-arginine on exercise capacity in patients with stable angina pectoris, *Am J Cardiol* 80:331–333, 1997.
81. Ruel M, Beanlands RS, Lortie M, et al.: Concomitant treatment with oral L-arginine improves the efficacy of surgical angiogenesis in patients with severe diffuse coronary artery disease: the Endothelial Modulation in Angiogenic Therapy randomized controlled trial, *J Thorac Cardiovasc Surg* 135:762–770, 2008. 770.e1.
82. Tardif JC, Ford I, Tendera M, Bourassa MG, Fox K: Efficacy of ivabradine, a new selective I(f) inhibitor, compared with atenolol in patients with chronic stable angina, *Eur Heart J* 26:2529–2536, 2005.
83. Tardif JC, Ponikowski P, Kahan T: Efficacy of the I(f) current inhibitor ivabradine in patients with chronic stable angina receiving beta-blocker therapy: a 4-month, randomized, placebo-controlled trial, *Eur Heart J* 30:540–548, 2009.
84. Fox K, Ford I, Steg PG, Tendera M, Ferrari R: Ivabradine for patients with stable coronary artery disease and left-ventricular systolic dysfunction (BEAUTIFUL): a randomised, double-blind, placebo-controlled trial, *Lancet* 372:807–816, 2008.
85. Fox K, Ford I, Steg PG, et al.: Ivabradine in stable coronary artery disease without clinical heart failure, *N Engl J Med* 371:1091–1099, 2014.
86. Ambrosio G, Komajda M, Mugelli A, et al.: Management of stable angina: a commentary on the European Society of Cardiology guidelines, *Eur J Prev Cardiol*, 23(13):1401–1412, 2016 sep.
87. Cammarano C, Silva M, Comee M, Donovan JL, Malloy MJ: Meta-analysis of ivabradine in patients with stable coronary artery disease with and without left ventricular dysfunction, *Clin Ther* 38:387–395, 2016.
88. Rajendra NS, Ireland S, George J, et al.: Mechanistic insights into the therapeutic use of high-dose allopurinol in angina pectoris, *J Am Coll Cardiol* 58:820–828, 2011.
89. George J, Carr E, Davies J, Belch JJ, Struthers A: High-dose allopurinol improves endothelial function by profoundly reducing vascular oxidative stress and not by lowering uric acid, *Circulation* 114:2508–2516, 2006.
90. Noman A, Ang DS, Ogston S, et al.: Effect of high-dose allopurinol on exercise in patients with chronic stable angina: a randomised, placebo controlled crossover trial, *Lancet* 375:2161–2167, 2010.
91. Leschke M: Rheology and coronary heart disease, *Dtsch Med Wochenschr* 133(Suppl 8):S270–S273, 2008.
92. Leschke M, Schoebel FC, Mecklenbeck WG, et al.: Long-term intermittent urokinase therapy in patients with end-stage coronary artery disease and refractory angina pectoris: a randomized dose-response trial, *J Am Coll Cardiol* 27:575–584, 1996.
93. Basaria S, Coviello AD, Travison TG, et al.: Adverse events associated with testosterone administration, *N Engl J Med* 363:109–122, 2010.
94. Kloner RA, Carson 3rd C, Dobs A, Kopecky S, Mohler 3rd ER: Testosterone and cardiovascular disease, *J Am Coll Cardiol* 67:545–557, 2016.
95. English KM, Steeds RP, Jones TH, Diver MJ, Channer KS: Low-dose transdermal testosterone therapy improves angina threshold in men with chronic stable angina: a randomized, double-blind, placebo-controlled study, *Circulation* 102:1906–1911, 2000.
96. Mathur A, Malkin C, Saeed B, et al.: Long-term benefits of testosterone replacement therapy on angina threshold and atheroma in men, *Eur J Endocrinol* 161:443–449, 2009.
97. Rosano GM, Leonardo F, Pagnotta P, et al.: Acute anti-ischemic effect of testosterone in men with coronary artery disease, *Circulation* 99:1666–1670, 1999.
98. Rossouw JE, Anderson GL, Prentice RL, et al.: Risks and benefits of estrogen plus progestin in healthy postmenopausal women: principal results from the Women's Health Initiative randomized controlled trial, *JAMA* 288:321–333, 2002.
99. Chandrasekar B, Nattel S, Tanguay JF: Coronary artery endothelial protection after local delivery of 17beta-estradiol during balloon angioplasty in a porcine model: a potential new pharmacologic approach to improve endothelial function, *J Am Coll Cardiol* 38:1570–1576, 2001.
100. Knuuti J, Kalliokoski R, Janatuinen T, et al.: Effect of estradiol-drospirenone hormone treatment on myocardial perfusion reserve in postmenopausal women with angina pectoris, *Am J Cardiol* 99:1648–1652, 2007.
101. Sanderson JE, Haines CJ, Yeung L, et al.: Anti-ischemic action of estrogen-progestogen continuous combined hormone replacement therapy in postmenopausal women with established angina pectoris: a randomized, placebo-controlled, double-blind, parallel-group trial, *J Cardiovasc Pharmacol* 38:372–883, 2001.
102. Trippodo NC, Fox M, Natarajan V, et al.: Combined inhibition of neutral endopeptidase and angiotensin converting enzyme in cardiomyopathic hamsters with compensated heart failure, *J Pharmacol Exp Ther* 267:108–116, 1993.
103. Chaitman BR, Ivleva AY, Ujda M, et al.: Antianginal efficacy of omapatrilat in patients with chronic angina pectoris, *Am J Cardiol* 95:1283–1289, 2005.
104. McMurray JJV, Packer M, Desai AS, et al.: Angiotensin–neprilysin inhibition versus enalapril in heart failure, *N Engl J Med* 371:993–1004, 2014.
105. Yao Y, Feng Y, Lin W: Systematic review and meta-analysis of randomized controlled trials comparing compound danshen dripping pills and isosorbide dinitrate in treating angina pectoris, *Int J Cardiol* 182:46–47, 2015.
106. Jia Y, Huang F, Zhang S, Leung SW: Is danshen (*Salvia miltiorrhiza*) dripping pill more effective than isosorbide dinitrate in treating angina pectoris? A systematic review of randomized controlled trials, *Int J Cardiol* 157:330–340, 2012.
107. Wang G, Wang L, Xiong ZY, Mao B, Li TQ: Compound salvia pellet, a traditional Chinese medicine, for the treatment of chronic stable angina pectoris compared with nitrates: a meta-analysis, *Med Sci Monit* 12:Sr1–7, 2006.
108. Ren Y, Li D, Zheng H, et al.: Acupoint application in patients with chronic stable angina pectoris: study protocol of a randomized, double-blind, controlled trial, *Evid Based Complement Alternat Med* 2014:619706, 2014. http://dx.doi.org/10.1155/2014/619706.
109. Li D, Yang M, Zhao L, et al.: Acupuncture for chronic, stable angina pectoris and an investigation of the characteristics of acupoint specificity: study protocol for a multicenter randomized controlled trial, *Trials* 15:50, 2014.
110. Azzalini L, Vo M, Dens J, Agostoni P: Myths to debunk to improve management, referral, and outcomes in patients with chronic total occlusion of an epicardial coronary artery, *Am J Cardiol* 116:1774–1780, 2015.

111. Windecker S, Kolh P, Alfonso F, et al.: 2014 ESC/EACTS guidelines on myocardial revascularization: the Task Force on Myocardial Revascularization of the European Society of Cardiology (ESC) and the European Association for Cardio-Thoracic Surgery (EACTS) Developed with the special contribution of the European Association of Percutaneous Cardiovascular Interventions (EAPCI), *Eur Heart J* 35:2541–2619, 2014.
112. Patel MR, Dehmer GJ, Hirshfeld JW, Smith PK, Spertus JA: ACCF/SCAI/STS/AATS/AHA/ASNC/HFSA/SCCT 2012 appropriate use criteria for coronary revascularization focused update: a report of the American College of Cardiology Foundation Appropriate Use Criteria Task Force, Society for Cardiovascular Angiography and Interventions, Society of Thoracic Surgeons, American Association for Thoracic Surgery, American Heart Association, American Society of Nuclear Cardiology, and the Society of Cardiovascular Computed Tomography, *J Am Coll Cardiol* 59:857–881, 2012.
113. Christakopoulos GE, Christopoulos G, Carlino M, et al.: Meta-analysis of clinical outcomes of patients who underwent percutaneous coronary interventions for chronic total occlusions, *Am J Cardiol* 115:1367–1375, 2015.
114. Olivari Z, Rubartelli P, Piscione F, et al.: Immediate results and one-year clinical outcome after percutaneous coronary interventions in chronic total occlusions: data from a multicenter, prospective, observational study (TOAST-GISE), *J Am Coll Cardiol* 41:1672–1678, 2003.
115. Jolicoeur EM, Sketch MJ, Wojdyla DM, et al.: Percutaneous coronary interventions and cardiovascular outcomes for patients with chronic total occlusions, *Catheter Cardiovasc Interv* 79:603–612, 2012.
116. Borgia FF, Viceconte NF, Ali OF, et al.: Improved cardiac survival, freedom from MACE and angina-related quality of life after successful percutaneous recanalization of coronary artery chronic total occlusions, *Int J Cardiol* 161:31–38, 2012.
117. Jaffe R, Charron T, Puley G, Dick A, Strauss BH: Microvascular obstruction and the no-reflow phenomenon after percutaneous coronary intervention, *Circulation* 117:3152–3156, 2008.
118. Ladwiniec A, Cunnington MS, Rossington J, et al.: Microvascular dysfunction in the immediate aftermath of chronic total coronary occlusion recanalization, *Catheter Cardiovasc Interv* 87:1071–1079, 2016.
119. Werner GS, Emig U, Bahrmann P, Ferrari M, Figulla HR: Recovery of impaired microvascular function in collateral dependent myocardium after recanalisation of a chronic total coronary occlusion, *Heart* 90:1303–1309, 2004.
120. Beck CS, Leighninger DS: Operations for coronary artery disease, *J Am Med Assoc* 156:1226–1233, 1954.
121. Beck CS, Leighninger DS: Scientific basis for the surgical treatment of coronary artery disease, *J Am Med Assoc* 159:1264–1271, 1955.
122. Wising PJ: The Beck-I operation for angina pectoris: medical aspects, *Acta Med Scand* 174:93–98, 1963.
123. Jolicoeur EM, Banai S, Henry TD, et al.: A phase II, sham-controlled, double-blinded study testing the safety and efficacy of the coronary sinus reducer in patients with refractory angina: study protocol for a randomized controlled trial, *Trials* 14:46, 2013.
124. Mohl W, Simon P, Neumann F, Schreiner W, Punzengruber C: Clinical evaluation of pressure-controlled intermittent coronary sinus occlusion: randomized trial during coronary artery surgery, *Ann Thorac Surg* 46:192–201, 1988.
125. van de Hoef TP, Nijveldt R, van der Ent M, et al.: Pressure-controlled intermittent coronary sinus occlusion (PICSO) in acute ST-segment elevation myocardial infarction: results of the Prepare RAMSES safety and feasibility study, *EuroIntervention* 11:37–44, 2015.
126. Mohl W, Kajgana I, Bergmeister H, Rattay F: Intermittent pressure elevation of the coronary venous system as a method to protect ischemic myocardium, *Interact Cardiovasc Thorac Surg* 4:66–69, 2005.
127. Ido A, Hasebe N, Matsuhashi H, Kikuchi K: Coronary sinus occlusion enhances coronary collateral flow and reduces subendocardial ischemia, *Am J Physiol Heart Circ Physiol* 280:H1361–H1367, 2001.
128. Beyar R, Guerci AD, Halperin HR, Tsitlik JE, Weisfeldt ML: Intermittent coronary sinus occlusion after coronary arterial ligation results in venous retroperfusion, *Circ Res* 65:695–707, 1989.
129. Konigstein M, Verheye S, Jolicoeur EM, Banai S: Narrowing of the coronary sinus: a device-based therapy for persistent angina pectoris, *Cardiology in Review* 24:238–243, 2016.
130. Verheye S, Jolicoeur EM, Behan MW, et al.: Efficacy of a device to narrow the coronary sinus in refractory angina, *N Engl J Med* 372:519–527, 2015.
131. Henry TD, Annex BH, McKendall GR, et al.: The VIVA trial: vascular endothelial growth factor in Ischemia for Vascular Angiogenesis, *Circulation* 107:1359–1365, 2003.
132. Simons M, Annex BH, Laham RJ, et al.: Pharmacological treatment of coronary artery disease with recombinant fibroblast growth factor-2: double-blind, randomized, controlled clinical trial, *Circulation* 105:788–793, 2002.
133. Grines CL, Watkins MW, Helmer G, et al.: Angiogenic Gene Therapy (AGENT) trial in patients with stable angina pectoris, *Circulation* 105:1291–1297, 2002.
134. Grines CL, Watkins MW, Mahmarian JJ, et al.: A randomized, double-blind, placebo-controlled trial of Ad5FGF-4 gene therapy and its effect on myocardial perfusion in patients with stable angina, *J Am Coll Cardiol* 42:1339–1347, 2003.
135. Henry TD, Grines CL, Watkins MW, et al.: Effects of Ad5FGF-4 in patients with angina: an analysis of pooled data from the AGENT-3 and AGENT-4 trials, *J Am Coll Cardiol* 50:1038–1046, 2007.
136. Kastrup J, Jorgensen E, Ruck A, et al.: Direct intramyocardial plasmid vascular endothelial growth factor-A165 gene therapy in patients with stable severe angina pectoris A randomized double-blind placebo-controlled study: the Euroinject One trial, *J Am Coll Cardiol* 45:982–988, 2005.
137. Stewart DJ, Kutryk MJ, Fitchett D, et al.: VEGF gene therapy fails to improve perfusion of ischemic myocardium in patients with advanced coronary disease: results of the NORTHERN trial, *Mol Ther* 17:1109–1115, 2009.
138. Giusti II, Rodrigues CG, Salles FB, et al.: High doses of vascular endothelial growth factor 165 safely, but transiently, improve myocardial perfusion in no-option ischemic disease, *Hum Gene Ther Methods* 24:298–306, 2013.
139. Favaloro L, Diez M, Mendiz O, et al.: High-dose plasmid-mediated VEGF gene transfer is safe in patients with severe ischemic heart disease (Genesis-I). A phase I, open-label, two-year follow-up trial, *Catheterization Cardiovasc Interv* 82:899–906, 2013.
140. Losordo DW, Dimmeler S: Therapeutic angiogenesis and vasculogenesis for ischemic disease. Part I: angiogenic cytokines, *Circulation* 109:2487–2491, 2004.
141. Fisher SA, Brunskill SJ, Doree C, et al.: Stem cell therapy for chronic ischaemic heart disease and congestive heart failure, *Cochrane Database Syst Rev* Cd007888, 2014. http://dx.doi.org/10.1002/14651858.CD007888.pub2.
142. Losordo DW, Henry TD, Davidson C, et al.: Intramyocardial, autologous CD34+ cell therapy for refractory angina, *Circ Res* 109:428–436, 2011.
143. Losordo DW, Schatz RA, White CJ, et al.: Intramyocardial transplantation of autologous CD34+ stem cells for intractable angina: a phase I/IIa double-blind, randomized controlled trial, *Circulation* 115:3165–3172, 2007.
144. van Ramshorst J, Bax JJ, Beeres SLMA, et al.: Intramyocardial bone marrow cell injection for chronic myocardial ischemia: a randomized controlled trial, *JAMA* 301:1997–2004, 2009.
145. Wang S, Cui J, Peng W, Lu M: Intracoronary autologous CD34+ stem cell therapy for intractable angina, *Cardiology* 117:140–147, 2010.
146. Tse HF, Thambar S, Kwong YL, et al.: Prospective randomized trial of direct endomyocardial implantation of bone marrow cells for treatment of severe coronary artery diseases (PROTECT-CAD trial), *Eur Heart J* 28:2998–3005, 2007.
147. Povsic TJ, Junge C, Nada A, et al.: A phase 3, randomized, double-blinded, active-controlled, unblinded standard of care study assessing the efficacy and safety of intramyocardial autologous CD34+ cell administration in patients with refractory angina: design of the RENEW study, *Am Heart J* 165:854–861.e2, 2013.
148. Jimenez-Quevedo P, Gonzalez-Ferrer JJ, Sabate M, et al.: Selected CD133(+) progenitor cells to promote angiogenesis in patients with refractory angina: final results of the PROGENITOR randomized trial, *Circ Res* 115:950–960, 2014.
149. Li N, Yang YJ, Zhang Q, et al.: Stem cell therapy is a promising tool for refractory angina: a meta-analysis of randomized controlled trials, *Can J Cardiol* 29:908–914, 2013.
150. Lee FY, Chen YL, Sung PH, et al.: Intracoronary transfusion of circulation-derived CD34+ cells improves left ventricular function in patients with end-stage diffuse coronary artery disease unsuitable for coronary intervention, *Crit Care Med* 43:2117–2132, 2015.
151. Henry TD, Schaer GL, Traverse JH, et al.: Autologous CD34+ Cell Therapy for Refractory Angina: 2-year Outcomes from the ACT34-CMI Study, *Cell Transplant* 25 :1701–1711, 2016.
152. Povsic TJ, Henry TD, Traverse JH, et al.: The RENEW Trial: efficacy and safety of intramyocardial autologous CD34+ cell administration in patients with refractory angina, *JACC Cardiovasc Interv* 9:1576–1585, 2016.
153. Mathiasen AB, Haack-Sorensen M, Jorgensen E, Kastrup J: Autotransplantation of mesenchymal stromal cells from bone-marrow to heart in patients with severe stable coronary artery disease and refractory angina—final 3-year follow-up, *Int J Cardiol* 170:246–251, 2013.
154. Mann I, Rodrigo SF, van Ramshorst J, et al.: Repeated intramyocardial bone marrow cell injection in previously responding patients with refractory angina again improves myocardial perfusion, anginal complaints, and quality of life, *Circ Cardiovasc Interv* 8, 2015. http://dx.doi.org/10.1161/CIRCINTERVENTIONS.115.002740.
155. San Mauro MP, Patronelli F, Spinelli E, et al.: Nerves of the heart: a comprehensive review with a clinical point of view, *Neuroanatomy* 8:26–31, 2009.
156. Foreman RD: Mechanisms of cardiac pain, *Annu Rev Physiol* 61:143–167, 1999.
157. Rosen SD: From heart to brain: the genesis and processing of cardiac pain, *Can J Cardiol* 28:S7–S19, 2012.
158. Deer TR, Mekhail N, Provenzano D, et al.: The appropriate use of neurostimulation of the spinal cord and peripheral nervous system for the treatment of chronic pain and ischemic diseases: the Neuromodulation Appropriateness Consensus Committee, *Neuromodulation* 17:515–550, 2014. discussion 550.
159. Prager JP: What does the mechanism of spinal cord stimulation tell us about complex regional pain syndrome? *Pain Med* 11:1278–1283, 2010.
160. Latif OA, Nedeljkovic SS, Stevenson LW: Spinal cord stimulation for chronic intractable angina pectoris: a unified theory on its mechanism, *Clin Cardiol* 24:533–541, 2001.
161. Hautvast RW, Blanksma PK, DeJongste MJ, et al.: Effect of spinal cord stimulation on myocardial blood flow assessed by positron emission tomography in patients with refractory angina pectoris, *Am J Cardiol* 77:462–467, 1996.
162. de Jongste MJ, Haaksma J, Hautvast RW, et al.: Effects of spinal cord stimulation on myocardial ischaemia during daily life in patients with severe coronary artery disease. A prospective ambulatory electrocardiographic study, *Br Heart J* 71:413–418, 1994.
163. Kingma Jr JG, Linderoth B, Ardell JL, et al.: Neuromodulation therapy does not influence blood flow distribution or left-ventricular dynamics during acute myocardial ischemia, *Auton Neurosci* 91:47–54, 2001.
164. Taylor RS, De VJ, Buchser E, DeJongste MJ: Spinal cord stimulation in the treatment of refractory angina: systematic review and meta-analysis of randomised controlled trials, *BMC Cardiovasc Disord* 9:13, 2009.
165. Kujacic V, Eliasson T, Mannheimer C, et al.: Assessment of the influence of spinal cord stimulation on left ventricular function in patients with severe angina pectoris: an echocardiographic study, *Eur Heart J* 14:1238–1244, 1993.
166. Zipes DP, Neuzil P, Theres H, et al.: Determining the Feasibility of Spinal Cord Neuromodulation for the Treatment of Chronic Systolic Heart Failure: the DEFEAT-HF Study, *JACC Heart Fail* 4:129–136, 2016.
167. Levy RM: Spinal cord stimulation for medically refractory angina pectoris: can the therapy be resuscitated? *Neuromodulation* 14:1–5, 2011.
168. Kumar K, Rizvi S: Cost-effectiveness of spinal cord stimulation therapy in management of chronic pain, *Pain Med* 14:1631–1649, 2013.
169. Tsigaridas N, Naka K, Tsapogas P, Pelechas E, Damigos D: Spinal cord stimulation in refractory angina. A systematic review of randomized controlled trials, *Acta Cardiol* 70:233–243, 2015.
170. Andrell P, Yu W, Gersbach P, et al.: Long-term effects of spinal cord stimulation on angina symptoms and quality of life in patients with refractory angina pectoris—results from the European Angina Registry Link Study (EARL), *Heart* 96:1132–1136, 2010.
171. Buiten MS, DeJongste MJ, Beese U: Subcutaneous electrical nerve stimulation: a feasible and new method for the treatment of patients with refractory angina, *Neuromodulation* 14:258–265, 2011.
172. McGillion M, Arthur HM, Cook A, et al.: Management of patients with refractory angina: Canadian Cardiovascular Society/Canadian Pain Society joint guidelines, *Can J Cardiol* 28(Suppl A):S20–S41, 2012.
173. Guinand A, Noble S, Frei A, et al.: Extra-cardiac stimulators: what do cardiologists need to know? *Europace* 18(9):1299–1307, 2016.
174. Dobias M, Michalek P, Neuzil P, Stritesky M, Johnston P: Interventional treatment of pain in refractory angina. A review, *Biomed Pap Med Fac Univ Palacky Olomouc Czech Repub* 158:518–527, 2014.
175. Moore R, Groves D, Hammond C, Leach A, Chester MR: Temporary sympathectomy in the treatment of chronic refractory angina, *J Pain Symptom Manage* 30:183–191, 2005.
176. Forouzanfar T, van Kleef M, Weber WE: Radiofrequency lesions of the stellate ganglion in chronic pain syndromes: retrospective analysis of clinical efficacy in 86 patients, *Clin J Pain* 16:164–168, 2000.
177. Roy C, Chatterjee N: Radiofrequency ablation of stellate ganglion in a patient with complex regional pain syndrome, *Saudi J Anaesth* 8:408–411, 2014.
178. Richter A, Cederholm I, Fredrikson M, et al.: Effect of long-term thoracic epidural analgesia on refractory angina pectoris: a 10-year experience, *J Cardiothorac Vasc Anesth* 26:822–828, 2012.
179. Gramling-Babb P, Miller MJ, Reeves ST, Roy RC, Zile MR: Treatment of medically and surgically refractory angina pectoris with high thoracic epidural analgesia: initial clinical experience, *Am Heart J* 133:648–655, 1997.
180. Cannon III RO, Quyyumi AA, Mincemoyer R, et al.: Imipramine in patients with chest pain despite normal coronary angiograms, *N Engl J Med* 330:1411–1417, 1994.
181. Cox ID, Hann CM, Kaski JC: Low dose imipramine improves chest pain but not quality of life in patients with angina and normal coronary angiograms, *Eur Heart J* 19:250–254, 1998.
182. Wei J, Rooks C, Ramadan R, et al.: Meta-analysis of mental stress-induced myocardial ischemia and subsequent cardiac events in patients with coronary artery disease, *Am J Cardiol* 114:187–192, 2014.
183. Ma H, Guo L, Huang D, et al.: The role of the myocardial microvasculature in mental stress-induced myocardial ischemia, *Clin Cardiol* 39:234–239, 2016.
184. Jiang W, Boyle SH, Ortel TL, et al.: Platelet aggregation and mental stress induced myocardial ischemia: results from the Responses of Myocardial Ischemia to Escitalopram Treatment (REMIT) study, *Am Heart J* 169:496–507.e1, 2015.

185. Yoshida K, Utsunomiya T, Morooka T, et al.: Mental stress test is an effective inducer of vasospastic angina pectoris: comparison with cold pressor, hyperventilation and master two-step exercise test, *Int J Cardiol* 70:155–163, 1999.
186. Guidelines for diagnosis and treatment of patients with vasospastic angina (coronary spastic angina) (JCS 2013), *Circ J* 78:2779–2801, 2014.
187. Dimsdale JE: Psychological stress and cardiovascular disease, *J Am Coll Cardiol* 51:1237–1246, 2008.
188. Jiang W, Velazquez EJ, Kuchibhatla M, et al.: Effect of escitalopram on mental stress-induced myocardial ischemia: results of the REMIT trial, *JAMA* 309:2139–2149, 2013.
189. McGillion M, Arthur H, Victor JC, Watt-Watson J, Cosman T: Effectiveness of psychoeducational interventions for improving symptoms, health-related quality of life, and psychological well being in patients with stable angina, *Curr Cardiol Rev* 4:1–11, 2008.
190. Prinzmetal M, Kennamer R, Merliss R, Wada T, Bor N: Angina pectoris. I. A variant form of angina pectoris; preliminary report, *Am J Med* 27:375–388, 1959.
191. Beltrame JF, Crea F, Kaski JC, et al.: International standardization of diagnostic criteria for vasospastic angina, *Eur Heart J*, 2015. http://dx.doi.org/10.1093/eurheartj/ehv351" 10.1093/eurheartj/ehv351.
192. Sun H, Mohri M, Shimokawa H, et al.: Coronary microvascular spasm causes myocardial ischemia in patients with vasospastic angina, *J Am Coll Cardiol* 39:847–851, 2002.
193. Mohri M, Koyanagi M, Egashira K, et al.: Angina pectoris caused by coronary microvascular spasm, *Lancet* 351:1165–1169, 1998.
194. Ong P, Athanasiadis A, Borgulya G, et al.: Clinical usefulness, angiographic characteristics, and safety evaluation of intracoronary acetylcholine provocation testing among 921 consecutive white patients with unobstructed coronary arteries, *Circulation* 129:1723–1730, 2014.
195. Pepine CJ, Kerensky RA, Lambert CR, et al.: Some thoughts on the vasculopathy of women with ischemic heart disease, *J Am Coll Cardiol* 47:S30–S35, 2006.
196. Jolicoeur EM, Cartier R, Henry TD, et al.: Patients with coronary artery disease unsuitable for revascularization: definition, general principles, and a classification, *Can J Cardiol* 28(Suppl A):S50–S59, 2012.
197. Yasue H, Takizawa A, Nagao M, et al.: Long-term prognosis for patients with variant angina and influential factors, *Circulation* 78:1–9, 1988.
198. Taylor SH: Usefulness of amlodipine for angina pectoris, *Am J Cardiol* 73:28a–33a, 1994.
199. Beltrame JF, Crea F, Kaski JC, et al.: The who, what, why, when, how and where of vasospastic angina, *Circ J* 80:289–298, 2016.
200. Araki H, Hayata N, Matsuguchi T, Nakamura M: Effects of nicorandil on rest and effort angina unresponsive to combination therapy with a calcium antagonist and oral nitrate, *Clin Ther* 9:174–182, 1987.
201. Phaneuf DC, Waters DD, Dauwe F, et al.: Refractory variant angina controlled with combined drug therapy in a patient with a single coronary artery, *Cathet Cardiovasc Diagn* 6:413–421, 1980.
202. Mohri M, Shimokawa H, Hirakawa Y, Masumoto A, Takeshita A: Rho-kinase inhibition with intracoronary fasudil prevents myocardial ischemia in patients with coronary microvascular spasm, *J Am Coll Cardiol* 41:15–19, 2003.
203. Masumoto A, Mohri M, Shimokawa H, et al.: Suppression of coronary artery spasm by the Rho-kinase inhibitor fasudil in patients with vasospastic angina, *Circulation* 105:1545–1547, 2002.
204. Shiraishi Y, Kanmura Y, Itoh T: Effect of cilostazol, a phosphodiesterase type III inhibitor, on histamine-induced increase in $[Ca^{2+}]i$ and force in middle cerebral artery of the rabbit, *Br J Pharmacol* 123:869–878, 1998.
205. Shin ES, Lee JH, Yoo SY, et al.: A randomised, multicentre, double blind, placebo controlled trial to evaluate the efficacy and safety of cilostazol in patients with vasospastic angina, *Heart* 100:1531–1536, 2014.
206. Morita S, Mizuno Y, Harada E, et al.: Pioglitazone, a peroxisome proliferator-activated receptor gamma activator, suppresses coronary spasm, *Coron Artery Dis* 25:671–677, 2014.
207. Morikawa Y, Mizuno Y, Harada E, et al.: Aerobic interval exercise training in the afternoon reduces attacks of coronary spastic angina in conjunction with improvement in endothelial function, oxidative stress, and inflammation, *Coron Artery Dis* 24:177–182, 2013.
208. Kawano H, Motoyama T, Hirai N, et al.: Estradiol supplementation suppresses hyperventilation-induced attacks in postmenopausal women with variant angina, *J Am Coll Cardiol* 37:735–740, 2001.
209. Abbate A, Hamza M, Cassano AD, et al.: Sympathectomy as a treatment for refractory coronary artery spasm, *Int J Cardiol* 161:e7–e9, 2012.
210. Cardona-Guarache R, Pozen J, Jahangiri A, et al.: Thoracic sympathectomy for severe refractory multivessel coronary artery spasm, *Am J Cardiol* 117:159–161, 2016.
211. Kugiyama K, Motoyama T, Hirashima O, et al.: Vitamin C attenuates abnormal vasomotor reactivity in spasm coronary arteries in patients with coronary spastic angina, *J Am Coll Cardiol* 32:103–109, 1998.
212. Kugiyama K, Miyao Y, Sakamoto T, et al.: Glutathione attenuates coronary constriction to acetylcholine in patients with coronary spastic angina, *Am J Physiol Heart Circ Physiol* 280:H264–H271, 2001.
213. Frenneaux M, Kaski JC, Brown M, Maseri A: Refractory variant angina relieved by guanethidine and clonidine, *Am J Cardiol* 62:832–833, 1988.
214. Dominguez Franco AJ, Gomez Doblas JJ, Garcia Pinilla JM, et al.: Treatment of refractory vasospastic angina with corticosteroids. A case report, *Int J Cardiol* 118:e51–e53, 2007.
215. Miyagi H, Yasue H, Okumura K, et al.: Effect of magnesium on anginal attack induced by hyperventilation in patients with variant angina, *Circulation* 79:597–602, 1989.
216. Sueda S, Saeki H, Otani T, et al.: Limited efficacy of magnesium for the treatment of variant angina, *J Cardiol* 34:139–147, 1999.
217. Clark DA, Quint RA, Mitchell RL, Angell WW: Coronary artery spasm. Medical management, surgical denervation, and autotransplantation, *J Thorac Cardiovasc Surg* 73:332–339, 1977.
218. Bertrand ME, Lablanche JM, Tilmant PY, et al.: Treatment of a severe coronary artery spasm, refractory to complete denervation of the heart (autotransplantation), *Arch Mal Coeur Vaiss* 75:717–723, 1982.
219. Shin ES, Ann SH, Singh GB, et al.: OCT-defined morphological characteristics of coronary artery spasm sites in vasospastic angina, *JACC Cardiovasc Imaging* 8:1059–1067, 2015.
220. Gaspardone A, Tomai F, Versaci F, et al.: Coronary artery stent placement in patients with variant angina refractory to medical treatment, *Am J Cardiol* 84:96–98, 1999. A8.
221. Chu G, Zhang G, Zhang Z, et al.: Clinical outcome of coronary stenting in patients with variant angina refractory to medical treatment: a consecutive single-center analysis, *Med Princ Pract* 22:583–587, 2013.
222. Radico F, Cicchitti V, Zimarino M, De Caterina R: Angina pectoris and myocardial ischemia in the absence of obstructive coronary artery disease: practical considerations for diagnostic tests, *JACC Cardiovasc Interv* 7:453–463, 2014.
223. Zaya M, Mehta PK, Merz CN: Provocative testing for coronary reactivity and spasm, *J Am Coll Cardiol* 63:103–109, 2014.
224. Sara JD, Widmer RJ, Matsuzawa Y, et al.: Prevalence of coronary microvascular dysfunction among patients with chest pain and nonobstructive coronary artery disease, *JACC Cardiovasc Interv* 8:1445–1453, 2015.
225. Lanza GA, Parrinello R, Figliozzi S: Management of microvascular angina pectoris, *Am J Cardiovasc Drugs* 14:31–40, 2014.
226. Minamino T, Kitakaze M, Morioka T, et al.: Bidirectional effects of aminophylline on myocardial ischemia, *Circulation* 92:1254–1260, 1995.
227. Gaspardone A, Crea F, Tomai F, et al.: Substance P potentiates the algogenic effects of intraarterial infusion of adenosine, *J Am Coll Cardiol* 24:477–482, 1994.
228. Insel J, Halle AA, Mirvis DM: Efficacy of pentoxifylline in patients with stable angina pectoris, *Angiology* 39:514–519, 1988.
229. Lanza GA, Gaspardone A, Pasceri V, et al.: Effects of bamiphylline on exercise testing in patients with syndrome X, *G Ital Cardiol* 27:50–54, 1997.
230. Elliott PM, Krzyzowska-Dickinson K, Calvino R, Hann C, Kaski JC: Effect of oral aminophylline in patients with angina and normal coronary arteriograms (cardiac syndrome X), *Heart* 77:523–526, 1997.
231. Radice M, Giudici V, Pusineri E, et al.: Different effects of acute administration of aminophylline and nitroglycerin on exercise capacity in patients with syndrome X, *Am J Cardiol* 78:88–92, 1996.
232. Adlbrecht C, Andreas M, Redwan B, et al.: Systemic endothelin receptor blockade in ST-segment elevation acute coronary syndrome protects the microvasculature: a randomised pilot study, *EuroIntervention* 7:1386–1395, 2012.
233. Osugi T, Saitoh S, Matumoto K, et al.: Preventive effect of chronic endothelin type A receptor antagonist on coronary microvascular spasm induced by repeated epicardial coronary artery endothelial denudation in pigs, *J Atheroscler Thromb* 17:54–63, 2010.
234. Saitoh S, Matsumoto K, Kamioka M, et al.: Novel pathway of endothelin-1 and reactive oxygen species in coronary vasospasm with endothelial dysfunction, *Coron Artery Dis* 20:400–408, 2009.
235. Kothawade K, Bairey Merz CN: Microvascular coronary dysfunction in women: pathophysiology, diagnosis, and management, *Curr Probl Cardiol* 36:291–318, 2011.
236. Nishida T, Shimokawa H, Oi K, et al.: Extracorporeal cardiac shock wave therapy markedly ameliorates ischemia-induced myocardial dysfunction in pigs in vivo, *Circulation* 110:3055–3061, 2004.
237. Aicher A, Heeschen C, Sasaki K, et al.: Low-energy shock wave for enhancing recruitment of endothelial progenitor cells: a new modality to increase efficacy of cell therapy in chronic hind limb ischemia, *Circulation* 114:2823–2830, 2006.
238. Chavakis E, Koyanagi M, Dimmeler S: Enhancing the outcome of cell therapy for cardiac repair: progress from bench to bedside and back, *Circulation* 121:325–335, 2010.
239. Assmus B, Walter DH, Seeger FH, et al.: Effect of shock wave-facilitated intracoronary cell therapy on LVEF in patients with chronic heart failure: the CELLWAVE randomized clinical trial, *JAMA* 309:1622–1631, 2013.
240. Alunni G, Marra S, Meynet I, et al.: The beneficial effect of extracorporeal shockwave myocardial revascularization in patients with refractory angina, *Cardiovasc Revasc Med* 16:6–11, 2015.
241. Schmid JP, Capoferri M, Wahl A, Eshtehardi P, Hess OM: Cardiac shock wave therapy for chronic refractory angina pectoris. A prospective placebo-controlled randomized trial, *Cardiovasc Ther* 31:e1–e6, 2013.
242. Prasad M, Wan Ahmad WA, Sukmawan R, et al.: Extracorporeal shockwave myocardial therapy is efficacious in improving symptoms in patients with refractory angina pectoris—a multicenter study, *Coron Artery Dis* 26:194–200, 2015.
243. Slikkerveer J, de Boer K, Robbers LF, van Rossum AC, Kamp O: Evaluation of extracorporeal shock wave therapy for refractory angina pectoris with quantitative analysis using cardiac magnetic resonance imaging: a short communication, *Neth Heart J* 24:319–325, 2016.
244. Wang J, Zhou C, Liu L, Pan X, Guo T: Clinical effect of cardiac shock wave therapy on patients with ischaemic heart disease: a systematic review and meta-analysis, *Eur J Clin Invest* 45:1270–1285, 2015.
245. Wang Y, Guo T, Ma TK, et al.: A modified regimen of extracorporeal cardiac shock wave therapy for treatment of coronary artery disease, *Cardiovasc Ultrasound* 10:35, 2012.
246. Michaels AD, McCullough PA, Soran OZ, et al.: Primer: practical approach to the selection of patients for and application of EECP, *Nat Clin Pract Cardiovasc Med* 3:623–632, 2006.
247. Sinvhal RM, Gowda RM, Khan IA: Enhanced external counterpulsation for refractory angina pectoris, *Heart* 89:830–833, 2003.
248. Michaels AD, Raisinghani A, Soran O, et al.: The effects of enhanced external counterpulsation on myocardial perfusion in patients with stable angina: a multicenter radionuclide study, *Am Heart J* 150:1066–1073, 2005.
249. Masuda D, Nohara R, Hirai T, et al.: Enhanced external counterpulsation improved myocardial perfusion and coronary flow reserve in patients with chronic stable angina; evaluation by ^{13}N-ammonia positron emission tomography, *Eur Heart J* 22:1451–1458, 2001.
250. Kiernan TJ, Boilson BA, Tesmer L, et al.: Effect of enhanced external counterpulsation on circulating CD34+ progenitor cell subsets, *Int J Cardiol* 153:202–206, 2011.
251. Bonetti PO, Holmes Jr DR, Lerman A, Barsness GW: Enhanced external counterpulsation for ischemic heart disease: what's behind the curtain? *J Am Coll Cardiol* 41:1918–1925, 2003.
252. Deleted in proofs.
253. Arora RR, Chou TM, Jain D, et al.: The multicenter study of enhanced external counterpulsation (MUST-EECP): effect of EECP on exercise-induced myocardial ischemia and anginal episodes, *J Am Coll Cardiol* 33:1833–1840, 1999.
254. Zhang C, Liu X, Wang X, et al.: Efficacy of enhanced external counterpulsation in patients with chronic refractory angina on Canadian Cardiovascular Society (CCS) angina class: an updated meta-analysis, *Medicine* 94:e2002, 2015.
255. Shah SA, Shapiro RJ, Mehta R, Snyder JA: Impact of enhanced external counterpulsation on Canadian Cardiovascular Society angina class in patients with chronic stable angina: a meta-analysis, *Pharmacotherapy* 30:639–645, 2010.
256. Urano H, Ikeda H, Ueno T, et al.: Enhanced external counterpulsation improves exercise tolerance, reduces exercise-induced myocardial ischemia and improves left ventricular diastolic filling in patients with coronary artery disease, *J Am Coll Cardiol* 37:93–99, 2001.
257. Nussinovitch U, Shtenberg G, Roguin A, Feld Y: A novel intra-aortic device designed for coronary blood flow amplification in unrevascularizable patients, *J Cardiovasc Transl Res* 9:315–320, 2016.
258. National Clinical Guidelines Centre: National Institute for Health and Clinical Excellence: Guidance. Stable Angina: Methods, Evidence & Guidance, London, 2011, Royal College of Physicians (UK) National Clinical Guidelines Centre.
259. Povsic TJ, Broderick S, Anstrom KJ, et al.: Predictors of long-term clinical endpoints in patients with refractory angina, *J Am Heart Assoc* 4, 2015. http://dx.doi.org/10.1161/JAHA.114.001287.
260. Asbury EA, Webb CM, Probert H, et al.: Cardiac rehabilitation to improve physical functioning in refractory angina: a pilot study, *Cardiology* 122:170–177, 2012.
261. Goldman L, Cook EF, Mitchell N, et al.: Pitfalls in the serial assessment of cardiac functional status. How a reduction in "ordinary" activity may reduce the apparent degree of cardiac compromise and give a misleading impression of improvement, *J Chronic Dis* 35:763–771, 1982.
262. Eschalier R, Souteyrand G, Jean F, et al.: Should an implanted defibrillator be considered in patients with vasospastic angina? *Arch Cardiovasc Dis* 107:42–47, 2014.
263. Beltrame JF, Limaye SB, Wuttke RD, Horowitz JD: Coronary hemodynamic and metabolic studies of the coronary slow flow phenomenon, *Am Heart J* 146:84–90, 2003.

SECTION V

PREVENTION

28 Primary Prevention of Atherosclerotic Cardiovascular Disease

Jennifer G. Robinson

The atherosclerotic process begins in childhood and manifests clinically in adulthood as an acute atherothrombotic event (acute coronary syndrome or stroke) or as symptomatic obstructive disease (angina or claudication) (Fig.28.1).[1] The major risk factors for atherosclerotic cardiovascular disease (ASCVD) are well characterized in populations around the world (advancing age, male sex, increased total and low-density lipoprotein cholesterol [LDL-C], low high-density lipoprotein cholesterol [HDL-C], smoking, elevated blood pressure, and diabetes mellitus) and are largely driven by unhealthy lifestyle habits over the life course.[2–4]

Adherence to healthy lifestyle habits should be encouraged for all children and adults. Avoidance of smoking, a Mediterranean-type diet, regular physical activity, and avoidance of obesity are all associated with a lower risk of ASCVD events.[4] Drug treatment is recommended to reduce an increased risk of ASCVD events in many higher-risk individuals with advancing age and in those with familial or genetic hypercholesterolemia.[5] After age 75, trajectories of comorbidity begin to widely differ among individuals, and preventive efforts may be of less importance for some patients. Thus, the priorities for clinical intervention shift throughout the lifespan (Table 28.1).

This chapter will focus on the primary prevention of ASCVD in adults of 20 years of age or older. Recommendations from the 2013 prevention guidelines from the American College of Cardiology (ACC)/American Heart Association (AHA) are the focus because they were based on a rigorous systematic evidence review performed under the direction of the National Heart, Lung, and Blood Institute (NHLBI).[5–9] A similar approach to statin initiation is recommended by current cholesterol treatment guidelines from the American Diabetes Association and the United Kingdom National Institute for Health and Care Excellence.[10,11] The 2013 ACC/AHA recommendations are contrasted with the 2016 European Society of Cardiology (ESC)/ European Atherosclerosis Society (EAS), which are similar to the previous 2012 ESC/EAS prevention guidelines. Additional recommendations from other groups are also discussed, including recent guidelines from the Centers for Disease Control and Prevention (CDC) and the US Preventive Services Task Force.

Those interested in ASCVD prevention in children and adolescents are referred to the NHLBI pediatric guidelines.[12] However, clinicians should be aware that if a parent has an LDL-C of 190 mg/dL or higher, the offspring, as well as other first-degree relatives, should be screened for familial hypercholesterolemia.

ENCOURAGE LONG-TERM ADHERENCE

As part of an ongoing therapeutic relationship with the patient, adherence to lifestyle and drug therapy should be reinforced at each visit.[5] Blood pressure and body mass index (BMI) should be assessed regularly.[9,13] A fasting lipid

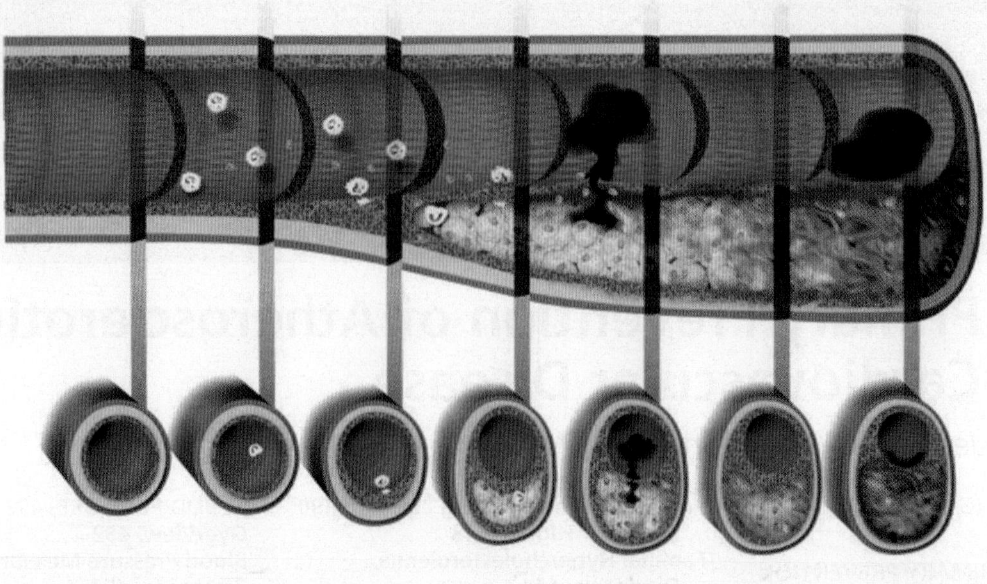

FIG. 28.1 Progression of atherosclerosis throughout the lifespan, which can manifest clinically as acute or chronic cardiovascular events. *(From Libby P.* Circulation. *2001;104:365–372. FIG. 1.)*

TABLE 28.1 Lifestyle and Drug Therapy Recommendations for Prevention. The Strongest Randomized Trial Evidence for Drug Therapy Is Highlighted in Bold

20–49 YEARS	50–75 YEARS	> 75 YEARS
	HEALTHY LIFESTYLE HABITS *Avoid smoking – Healthy diet – Regular physical activity – Control obesity* *Moderate sodium intake – Alcohol in moderation*	
Statins – LDL-C ≥ 190 mg/dL – Diabetes 40–79 years – Consider in selected other high-risk patients	**Statins** **– LDL-C ≥ 190 mg/dL** **– Diabetes age 50–75 years** **– ≥ 7.5% 10-year ASCVD risk** **– Consider 5–< 7.5% 10-year ASCVD risk in selected lower-risk patients**	Statins – Consider in selected primary prevention patients
Antihypertensive drugs – Consider in selected patients with BP ≥ 140/or ≥ 90 mm Hg	**Antihypertensive drugs** **– Goal BP < 140/90 mm Hg** **– Consider SBP goal < 120 mm Hg in selected patients**	**Antihypertensive drugs** **– Goal < 150/90 mm Hg unless frail or orthostatic** **– Goal SBP < 140 mm Hg is reasonable** **– Consider goal SBP < 120 mm Hg in selected patients**
	Aspirin **50–59 years: Low-dose aspirin if ≥ 10-year ASCVD risk at low risk for bleeding** **60–69 years: Consider in selected patients with ≥ 10 year ASCVD risk at low risk for bleeding**	
	EMPHASIZE ADHERENCE TO LIFESTYLE AND DRUG THERAPY	

ASCVD, Atherosclerotic cardiovascular disease; *BP*, blood pressure; *LDL-C*, low-density lipoprotein cholesterol; *SBP*, systolic blood pressure.

panel should be performed at the initial visit, every 4–6 years as part of ASCVD risk assessment in patients who are not receiving statins, and annually in those receiving statins, or more frequently as needed.[5]

Barriers to adherence should be addressed. Adverse effects during drug therapy often occur and should be addressed in a systematic fashion as outlined in Box 28.1.

OVERVIEW OF PRIMARY PREVENTION PRIORITIES BY AGE GROUP

Lifestyle and drug treatment priorities may be different in those 20–49 years, 50–75 years, and over age 75 years (see Table 28.1). Therefore, the main recommendations from the US and European guidelines are summarized by age. Guideline recommendations and randomized trial evidence are discussed in more detail in the respective sections on cholesterol, blood pressure, and aspirin therapy. ASCVD risk prediction is discussed in more detail in the cholesterol section, and links to online resources are provided.

Before Age 50

Lifestyle

Adherence to healthy lifestyle habits should be strongly encouraged as the foundation for ASCVD prevention. Changes in lifestyle habits have been shown to slow progression of atherosclerosis in this age group.[14] Smoking cessation is a necessity and should be addressed at every visit.

BOX 28.1 Management of Symptoms During Statin Therapy (2013 ACC/AHA Cholesterol Guideline)

Choice of statin and dose

To maximize the safety of statins, selection of the appropriate statin and dose in men and nonpregnant/nonnursing women should be based on patient characteristics, level of ASCVD* risk, and potential for adverse effects. Moderate-intensity statin therapy should be used in individuals in whom high-intensity statin therapy would otherwise be recommended when characteristics predisposing them to statin-associated adverse effects are present.

Characteristics predisposing individuals to statin adverse effects include but are not limited to:

- Multiple or serious comorbidities, including impaired renal or hepatic function.
- History of previous statin intolerance or muscle disorders.
- Unexplained ALT elevations ≥3 times ULN.
- Patient characteristics or concomitant use of drugs affecting statin metabolism.
- Age >75 years.

Additional characteristics that could modify the decision to use higher statin intensities might include but are not limited to:

- History of hemorrhagic stroke.
- Asian ancestry

Management of symptoms

The large majority of patients with symptoms during statin therapy can be successfully rechallenged with statin therapy. It is reasonable to evaluate and treat muscle symptoms, including pain, tenderness, stiffness, cramping, weakness, or fatigue, in statin-treated patients according to the following management algorithm:

- To avoid unnecessary discontinuation of statins, obtain a history of prior or current muscle symptoms to establish a baseline before initiation of statin therapy.
- If unexplained severe muscle symptoms or fatigue develop during statin therapy, promptly discontinue the statin and address the possibility of rhabdomyolysis by evaluating CK and creatinine and performing urinalysis for myoglobinuria.
- If mild to moderate muscle symptoms develop during statin therapy:
    - Discontinue the statin until the symptoms can be evaluated.
    - Evaluate the patient for other conditions that might increase the risk for muscle symptoms (e.g., hypothyroidism, reduced renal or hepatic function, rheumatologic disorders such as polymyalgia rheumatica, steroid myopathy, vitamin D deficiency, or primary muscle diseases).
    - If muscle symptoms resolve, and if no contraindication exists, give the patient the original or a lower dose of the same statin to establish a causal relationship between the muscle symptoms and statin therapy.
    - If a causal relationship exists, discontinue the original statin. Once muscle symptoms resolve, use a low dose of a different statin.
    - Once a low dose of a statin is tolerated, gradually increase the dose as tolerated.
    - If, after 2 months without statin treatment, muscle symptoms or elevated CK levels do not resolve completely, consider other causes of muscle symptoms listed above.
    - If persistent muscle symptoms are determined to arise from a condition unrelated to statin therapy, or if the predisposing condition has been treated, resume statin therapy at the original dose.

Other symptoms are very unlikely to be due to statin therapy and can be managed using a similar strategy of discontinuation and rechallenge.

Monitoring

- Creatine kinase

Do not routinely measure creatine kinase levels (although baseline levels may be helpful in patients with a history of statin intolerance, or if muscle symptoms develop)

- Hepatic transaminases

Do not routinely measure hepatic transaminases (unless baseline alanine aminotransferase (ALT) is elevated or symptoms of hepatoxoicity develop)

- Glucose and hemoglobin A1c

Do not routinely monitor glycemic parameters. Patients should be monitored as recommended by expert guidelines.

From *Stone NJ, Robinson JG, Lichtenstein AH, et al. 2013 ACC/AHA Guideline on the Treatment of Blood Cholesterol to Reduce Atherosclerotic Cardiovascular Risk in Adults: A Report of the American College of Cardiology/American Heart Association Task Force on Practice Guidelines.* J Am Coll Cardiol. *2014;63:2889-2934.*

Cholesterol

Statin therapy is recommended for primary prevention in high-risk patients older than 50 years if they have:[5,15]

- Familial or other genetic hypercholesterolemia (cut-off in the United States, LDL-C ≥ 190 mg/dL; in Europe, total cholesterol > 8 mmol/L or 310 mg/dL).
- Diabetes (in the United States, age ≥ 40 years; in Europe, depends on LDL-C level).
- Multiple or severe risk factor elevations (in Europe, this includes moderate chronic kidney disease).

For lower-risk primary prevention patients, 10-year cardiovascular risk should be estimated using calculators appropriate to the population under treatment. In the United States, the 2013 ACC/AHA Pooled Cohort Equations should be used as the starting point for estimating 10-year ASCVD risk for those aged 40–75 years if LDL-C is greater than 190 mg/dL.[5,7] Statin therapy should be considered for those with a 7.5% or higher 10-year ASCVD risk and may be reasonable for those with a 5% to < 7.5% 10-year ASCVD risk. Selected lower-risk patients may also benefit from statin therapy.

In Europe, the Systematic Coronary Risk Estimation (SCORE) equations should be the starting point for estimating 10-year risk of fatal ASCVD in Caucasians who are not otherwise characterized as high risk.[15] The calculated SCORE 10-year fatal ASCVD risk can then characterize patient risk in individuals aged 40–65 years and be used to identify an LDL-C treatment goal: very high risk (≥ 10%; LDL-C goal < 1.8 mmol/L or 70 mg/dL), high risk (5 to < 10%; LDL-C goal < 2.6 mmol/L or 100 mg/dL), moderate (≥ 1% to < 5%; LDL-C goal < 3.0 mmol/L or 115 mg/dL), or low (< 1%; LDL-C goal < 3.0 mmol/L or 115 mg/dL).

Race/ethnic-specific equations (QRISK2) for major cardiovascular disease have been developed for the United Kingdom.[16,17]

Blood Pressure

Elevated blood pressure should first be addressed through lifestyle modification, including weight loss, increasing regular physical activity, and reducing sodium intake. Although there is little clinical trial evidence in individuals under 50 years of age, antihypertensive drug therapy can be considered if systolic blood pressure remains greater than 140 mm Hg or diastolic blood pressure remains higher than 90 mm Hg on multiple occasions both in and outside the office, especially if other risk factors are present.[6,15]

Aspirin

There is no indication for aspirin therapy in individuals under 50 years of age.[18]

Age 50-75 Years

Lifestyle

Smoking avoidance and healthy lifestyle habits should continue to be encouraged. However, the primary clinical focus should turn to consideration of preventive drug therapies. The largest body of evidence for preventive drug therapy comes from randomized trials in those aged 50–75 years.

In this age group, atherosclerosis is usually well advanced (see Fig. 28.1), with extensive fibrocalcific plaque development in most individuals.[1] The risk of clinical events is significantly increased, and more aggressive risk factor reduction is needed. The randomized trials of drug therapy were all performed on a background of advice to maintain a healthy diet and regular physical activity.[5] However, the modest changes in risk factor levels associated with these lifestyle interventions have not been shown to reduce ASCVD events in this age group.[19,20]

Cholesterol

Statin therapy is strongly recommended for individuals aged 50–75 years with:[5,15]

- Familial or other genetic hypercholesterolemia (cut-off in the United States, LDL-C ≥ 190 mg/dL; in Europe, total cholesterol > 8 mmol/L or 310 mg/dL).
- Diabetes (in the United States, age ≥ 40 years; in Europe, depends on LDL-C level).
- Multiple or severe risk factor elevations (in Europe, this includes moderate chronic kidney disease).
- Increased ASCVD risk based on risk prediction equations.

In the United States, statins should be considered in individuals up to age 75 years with a 7.5% or greater 10-year ASCVD risk and may be reasonable in those with 5% to < 7.5% 10-year ASCVD risk.[5] Lower-risk patients in the 50–75-year age group may also benefit from statin therapy.

In Europe, SCORE charts can be used for estimating 10-year risk of fatal ASCVD in Caucasians aged 40–65 years who are not otherwise characterized as high risk.[15] The calculated SCORE 10-year fatal ASCVD risk can then characterize patient risk in individuals aged 40–65 years and be used to identify an LDL-C treatment goal: very high risk (≥ 10%; LDL-C goal < 1.8 mmol/L or 70 mg/dL), high risk (5 to < 10%; LDL-C goal < 2.6 mmol/L or 100 mg/dL), moderate (≥ 1% to < 5%; LDL-C goal < 3.0 mmol/L or 115 mg/dL), or low (< 1%; LDL-C goal < 3.0 mmol/L or 115 mg/dL).

Blood Pressure

Antihypertensive drug therapy is recommended in those aged 50 or older if systolic blood pressure remains at 140 mm Hg or higher or diastolic blood pressure remains at 90 mm Hg or higher on multiple occasions both in and outside the office.[6,15] Greater absolute risk reduction occurs from antihypertensive therapy in higher-risk individuals, and there are little data for those without cardiovascular risk factors less than 80 years of age. In selected high-risk individuals tolerating the current drug regimen, another antihypertensive drug could be considered if systolic blood pressure remains greater than 120 mm Hg.[22]

Aspirin

Aspirin therapy can be considered for those aged 50–59 years at low risk of bleeding and is reasonable to consider in those 60–69 years, with a 10-year or greater ASCVD risk at low risk of bleeding.[18]

Age over 75 Years

Lifestyle

Smoking avoidance and healthy lifestyle habits should continue to be encouraged. Observational evidence suggests health benefits occur from smoking cessation at any age.[23] Regular physical activity, although not shown to reduce ASCVD events or mortality, may be beneficial for improving quality of life.[24]

Cholesterol

Persons in good to excellent health at age 75 are likely to live at least another 10–15 years and so may benefit from preventive drug therapy.[25] Less evidence for primary prevention with statins is available for individuals greater than 75 years, and the randomized trials that are available have conflicting results.[5] The absolute risk of ASCVD events is highest after age 75, but high rates of competing causes of mortality and morbidity may alter the potential net benefit from statin therapy.

In the United States, after age 75 years, there are no strong recommendations for primary prevention statin therapy.[5] Patient preferences for prevention, and concerns about safety, should contribute to the decision to initiate (or continue) statin therapy.

In Europe, age over 75 years is not mentioned as a factor in the decision to initiate statin therapy. The SCORE charts do not estimate 10-year fatal ASCVD risk after age 65 years.[15]

Blood Pressure

Numerous randomized trials have evaluated the effect of antihypertensive therapy on ASCVD outcomes, heart failure, and mortality in generally healthy persons over 75 years. The strongest evidence for those over 75 years supports treating blood pressure greater than 150/or greater than 90 mm Hg, but recent evidence suggests a benefit from treating to blood pressure levels less than 140/<90 mm Hg in persons 75 years of age or older.[6,22]

Aspirin

Few randomized trial data are available for aspirin in persons over 75 years of age, and aspirin therapy is generally not recommended for primary prevention in this age group due to the excess risk of bleeding in older individuals.[18]

LIFESTYLE RECOMMENDATIONS

A healthy lifestyle is the foundation of health promotion and disease prevention efforts and should be addressed at every visit (Table 28.2).[5,8,15] Regular counseling to improve diet or increase physical activity changes health behaviors and is associated with small improvements in adiposity, blood pressure, and lipid levels.[27] Smoking cessation is discussed in Chapter 18.

Lifestyle Interventions

Diet

The 2013 ACC/AHA lifestyle guideline, ESC/EAS prevention guidelines, and other guidelines recommend a dietary pattern rich in fruits, vegetables, and whole grains that includes low-fat dairy products, poultry, fish, legumes, nuts, and

TABLE 28.2 Recommendations to Reduce LDL-C, Non–HDL-C, and Blood Pressure and General Physical Activity Recommendations from the 2013 ACC/AHA Lifestyle Guideline, Centers for Disease Control, and ESC/EAS Prevention Guideline

DIET	CLASS/LOE
1. Consume a dietary pattern that: • Emphasizes intake of vegetables, fruits, and whole grains • Includes low-fat dairy products, poultry, fish, legumes, non-tropical vegetable oils, and nuts • Limits intake of sweets, sugar-sweetened beverages, and red meats • Adapts appropriate calorie requirements, personal and cultural food preferences, and nutrition therapy for other medical conditions (including diabetes mellitus) • Follows plans such as the DASH dietary pattern, the USDA Food Pattern, or the AHA Diet	I A
2. Aim for a dietary pattern that achieves 5% to 6% of calories from saturated fat	I A
3. Reduce percent calories from saturated fat	I A
4. Reduce percent calories from *trans* fat	I A
5. For those who would benefit from blood pressure lowering, reduce sodium intake	I A
Sodium intake ≤ 2400 mg daily is advised Sodium intake ≤ 1500 mg daily can result in greater blood pressure reduction Reducing sodium by at least 1000 mg daily can lower blood pressure	IIa B
Physical Activity	
1. For important health benefits, adults should: • Engage in at least 150 minutes' moderate aerobic activity (e.g., brisk walking) each week • Alternatively, engage in 75 minutes of vigorous-intensity aerobic activity (e.g., jogging or running) each week • Aerobic activity sessions should be at least 10 minutes in duration • For even greater health benefits, increase moderate intensity physical activity to 300 minutes per week or vigorous intensity physical activity for 150 minutes per week • Engage in muscle strengthening activities at least twice a week that engage all major muscle groups	CDC
2. In general, advise adults to engage in aerobic physical activity to reduce LDL-C, non–HDL-C, and blood pressure • 3–4 sessions a week • Lasting on average 40 minutes per session • Involving moderate to vigorous physical activity	IIa A

LOE, Level of evidence; *CDC*, Centers for Disease Control and Prevention.
Modified from Eckel RH, Jakicic JM, Ard JD, et al. 2013 AHA/ACC guideline on lifestyle management to reduce cardiovascular risk: a report of the American College of Cardiology/American Heart Association Task Force on practice guidelines. J Am Coll Cardiol. *2014;63:2960–2984; Physical Activity Guidelines Advisory Committee.* Physical Activity Guidelines Advisory Committee Report, 2008. *Washington, DC: US Department of Health and Human Services. 2008; Piepoli MF, Hoes AW, Agewall S, et al. 2016 European guidelines on cardiovascular disease prevention in clinical practice:* Eur Heart J. *2016;37(29):2315–2381. pii: ehw106.*

non-tropical vegetable oils (see Table 28.2).[8,15,28] Intake of sweets, sugar-sweetened beverages, and red meats should be limited. Saturated fat intake should be limited to 5% to 6% of calories and *trans* fats should be avoided. The caloric content of the diet should be based on the need of the patient to lose, maintain, or gain weight. Alcohol consumption should be limited to two glasses per day (20 g/day of alcohol) for men and one glass per day for women (10 g/day).[15] This dietary pattern can be achieved by following plans such as the Dietary Approaches to Stop Hypertension (DASH) dietary pattern, the United States Department of Agriculture (USDA) Food Pattern, or the American Heart Association Diet.

Randomized trials of the DASH dietary pattern have been shown to reduce blood pressure, and the effect of this diet is enhanced by reducing sodium intake.[8] Restricting sodium to no more than 2400 mg daily is advised for those who would benefit from lowering blood pressure, and greater restriction may be beneficial for some patients.

Physical Activity

For important health benefits, the CDC and the ESC/EAS prevention guidelines recommend at least 150 minutes of moderate-intensity physical activity (e.g., walking) every week, along with muscle strengthening activities on two or more days a week that work all major muscle groups (legs, back, abdomen, chest, shoulders, and arms) (see Table 28.2).[15,24] Alternatively, more vigorous activity (such as jogging or running) can be performed for 75 minutes each week. Activity can be performed throughout the day, as long as moderate to intense effort occurs for at least 10 minutes. Even greater health benefits accrue by increasing moderate-intensity physical activity to 300 minutes per week or vigorous-intensity physical activity to 150 minutes per week.

The 2013 ACC/AHA lifestyle guideline recommends that adults in general should be advised to engage in regular aerobic physical activity to reduce LDL-C, non–HDL-C, and blood pressure.[8] The systematic review of randomized trials performed by the guideline panel found that three to four sessions of moderate-to vigorous-intensity physical activity lasting on average 40 minutes significantly reduced all three risk factors. Reducing sedentary activity, independent of physical activity levels, also appears to have benefits for cardiovascular health.[15,29]

Obesity Prevention and Control

Maintenance of a healthy weight is recommended by all primary prevention guidelines.[5,9,15] Obese or overweight individuals may aim to reduce weight in order to lower blood pressure, improve lipid levels, and reduce the risk of developing type 2 diabetes mellitus.[15] Recommendations from the 2013 AHA/ACC/The Obesity Society (TOS) obesity guideline are summarized in Table 28.3.[9]

BMI (weight in kilograms divided by height in meters squared) should be assessed annually. A BMI of 25.0–29.9 kg/m^2 is considered overweight and a BMI of 30 kg/m^2 or greater is considered obese. The higher the BMI above 25 kg/m^2, the greater the risk of ASCVD, diabetes, other morbidities, and mortality from all causes. However, cut-points for BMI may not apply to nonwhite racial groups. BMI cut-points that

TABLE 28.3 2013 ACC/AHA/TOS Obesity Guideline Recommendations

OBESITY	CLASS/LOE
1. Identifying those who need to lose weight	
1a. Measure height and weight and calculate BMI at annual visits or more frequently	I C
1b. Use categories for BMI to identify individuals at increased risk • Overweight 25.0–29.9 kg/m² – at increased CVD risk • Obesity ≥ 30 kg/m² – at increased of all-cause mortality risk	I B
1c. Advise overweight and obese individuals that the greater the BMI, the greater the risk of CVD, type 2 diabetes, and all-cause mortality	I B
1d. Measure the waist circumference at annual visits or more frequently in overweight and obese adults • Advise adults that the greater the waist circumference, the greater the risk of CVD, type 2 diabetes, and all-cause mortality. Use the NIH/NHLBI or WHO/IDF cut-points for now.	IIa B
2. Matching the treatment benefits with risk profiles	
Counsel overweight and obese adults with CVD risk factors that lifestyle changes that produce modest, sustained weight loss of 3–5% produce meaningful health benefits, and greater weight loss causes greater benefits • Reductions in blood glucose, hemoglobin A1c, triglycerides • Reduced risk of diabetes • > 5% weight loss – reductions in blood pressure & antihypertensive medications, LDL-C, increases in HDL-C, and further reductions in blood glucose and triglycerides	I A
3. Diets for weight loss	
3a. Prescribe a diet to achieve reduced calorie intake for overweight or obese individuals who would benefit from weight loss, as part of a comprehensive lifestyle intervention. Any of the following methods can be used: • 1200–1500 kcal/day for women; 1500–1800 kcal/day for men • 500–750 kcal/day energy deficit • Evidence-based diet that restricts certain food types (such as high carbohydrate foods, low fiber foods, or high fat foods) to create a calorie deficit	I A
3b. Base prescription on patient preferences and health status, preferably referring to a nutrition professional for counseling	I A
4. Lifestyle intervention and counseling	
4a. Advise overweight and obese individuals who would benefit from weight loss to participate for ≥ 6 months in a *comprehensive lifestyle program* that assists participants in adhering to a lower calorie diet and increasing physical activity	I A
4b. Prescribe on-site, high-intensity (i.e., ≥ 14 sessions in 6 months) comprehensive weight loss interventions provided in individual or group sessions by a trained interventionist	I A
4c. Electronically delivered weight loss programs (including by telephone) that include personalized feedback from a trained interventionist (although may be less effective than in-person interventions)	IIa A
4d. Some commercial programs that provide comprehensive lifestyle interventions that have peer-reviewed published evidence of their efficacy and safety are an option	IIa A
4e. Avoid very low calorie (< 800 kcal/day) diets, except in limited circumstances and administered by a trained practitioner in a medical setting	IIa A
4f. Advise overweight and obese individuals who have lost weight to participate in a long-term (≥ 1 year) weight loss maintenance program	I A
4g. For weight loss maintenance, face-to-face or telephone-delivered programs with monthly or more frequent contact with a trained interventionist who helps participants engage in high levels of physical activity (i.e., 200–300 min/week), monitor body weight weekly or more frequently, and consume a reduced calorie diet to maintain body weight	I A
5. Selecting patients for bariatric surgical treatment for obesity	
5a. Advise adults with BMI ≥ 40 kg/m² with obesity-related comorbid conditions, who are motivated to lose weight, and who have not responded to behavioral treatment with or without pharmacotherapy with sufficient weight loss to achieve targeted health outcomes, that bariatric surgery may be an appropriate option to improve health • Offer referral to an experienced bariatric surgeon for consultation and evaluation	IIa A
5b. For individuals with BMI < 35 kg/m², there is insufficient evidence to recommend for or against bariatric surgical procedures	--
5c. Advise patients that choice of a bariatric surgical procedure may be affected by patient factors, including age, severity of obesity, obesity-related comorbid conditions, other operative risk factors, risk of short- and long-term complications, behavioral and psychosocial factors, and patient tolerance for risk, as well as provide factors (surgeon and facility)	IIb C

ACC, American College of Cardiology; *AHA*, American Heart Association; *BMI*, body mass index; *CVD*, cardiovascular disease; *IDF*, International Diabetes Federation; *LDL-C*, low-density lipoprotein cholesterol; *HDL-C*, high-density lipoprotein cholesterol; *NHLBI*, National Heart, Lung, and Blood Institute; *NIH*, National Institutes of Health; *TOS*, The Obesity Society; *WHO*, World Health Organization. *From Jensen MD, Ryan DH, Apovian CM, et al. 2013 AHA/ACC/TOS guideline for the management of overweight and obesity in adults: a report of the American College of Cardiology/American Heart Association Task Force on Practice Guidelines and The Obesity Society.* J Am Coll Cardiol. *2014;63:2985–3023.*

confer increased ASCVD risk may be higher for individuals of African ancestry due to greater muscle mass, and lower in individuals of Asian, Pacific Islander, or Native American ancestry.[30]

Increasing waist circumference and waist/hip ratio also confers an increased risk of ASCVD.[9] These indices may be a better measure for identifying at-risk individuals (see Table 28.3). Waist circumference cut-points may differ for various racial/ethnic groups.[30]

Overweight and obese adults with cardiovascular risk factors should be advised to lose and sustain a 3% to 5% reduction in body weight.[9] The systematic review of randomized trials performed by the 2013 AHA/ACC/TOS guideline panel found numerous randomized trials demonstrating that this amount of weight loss reduces blood glucose, hemoglobin A1c, and triglycerides, and reduces the risk of developing type 2 diabetes mellitus. A greater than 5% weight loss results in further reductions in blood pressure, down-titration of antihypertensive medications, further reductions in blood glucose and triglycerides, and increases in HDL-C.

Once it has been determined that a patient may benefit from weight loss, a comprehensive lifestyle program should be advised.[9] Participation in structured weight loss programs, whether provided though healthcare systems or community, commercial, or internet or phone-based programs, has been shown to be helpful. Once the patient achieves the desired weight loss, participation in weight maintenance programs should be encouraged.

Compared with nonsurgical treatment of obesity, bariatric surgery leads to greater body weight loss and higher remission rates of type 2 diabetes and metabolic syndrome, although long-term follow-up data are sparse.[31,32] Based on this evidence, the 2013 ACC/AHA obesity guideline recommended consideration of bariatric surgery for patients with BMI of 40 kg/m^2 or greater and obesity-related comorbid conditions who have not responded to behavioral treatment with or without pharmacotherapy with sufficient weight loss to achieve targeted health outcomes, who are motivated to lose weight.[9] They considered there to be insufficient evidence to support bariatric surgery in those with BMI less than 40 kg/m^2. In 2016, however, the American Diabetes Association recommended consideration of bariatric surgery in adults with type 2 diabetes whose BMI is greater than 35 kg/m^2, especially if their diabetes is difficult to control or associated comorbidities are difficult to control with lifestyle and pharmacologic therapy.[10] Bariatric surgery and its complications are costly, and outcomes vary depending on the procedure and experience of the surgeon. Long-term disadvantages may include weight regain, dumping syndrome, and vitamin and mineral deficiencies.

CHOLESTEROL MANAGEMENT

Overview

Total cholesterol and LDL-C levels are associated with an increased risk of ASCVD events across the adult lifespan.[33] Family and genetic epidemiology studies show that individuals with high LDL-C levels are at high risk of premature ASCVD and, conversely, those with low LDL-C are at low lifetime ASCVD risk.[34–37] Support for a causal role for LDL-C in ASCVD comes from Mendelian randomization studies that have shown that elevated LDL-C levels due to genetic polymorphisms are associated with increased ASCVD risk.[34,38] Long-term epidemiologic studies have shown that individuals whose non–HDL-C level remains below 130 mg/dL during young adulthood through middle age are at minimal risk of developing advanced atherosclerosis.[39] This correlates with an LDL-C below 100 mg/dL.

The causal role of LDL-C is now conclusively established through the numerous cardiovascular outcomes trials of statin therapy and in a cardiovascular outcomes trial with ezetimibe.[40,41] Although statins have non–LDL-C effects (often called *pleiotropic*), these effects are not associated with cardiovascular risk reduction beyond that expected from the magnitude of LDL-C lowering.[42,43] LDL-C lowering with statin therapy is the most effective method of reducing cardiovascular risk over a period of 2 to 5 years.[5] However, it is critical to consider the potential for a net benefit from statin or nonstatin therapy when deciding whom to treat. The magnitude of ASCVD risk reduction, adverse effects, cost, and patient preferences all need to be considered before initiating drug therapy to reduce ASCVD risk.

Limited controversy still exists regarding the use of statins for primary prevention. However, recent analyses overwhelmingly support the use of statins for cardiovascular prevention even in low-risk adults, who experience an even greater reduction in the relative risk of cardiovascular events than do higher-risk patients.[44,45] Statins also reduce total mortality in both high-risk and low-risk individuals.

Although muscle and other symptoms are common in statin-treated patients, the rates of muscle, hepatic, and other adverse effects were similar in placebo and statin-treated patients in randomized trials. Notably, double-blind placebo-controlled trials have found that the large majority of patients intolerant to two or more statins are able to tolerate a moderate-intensity statin on rechallenge.[46,47] An approach to the management of symptoms on statins is outlined hereafter.

Screening

Systematic cardiovascular risk assessment, including a lipid panel, is recommended in the United States starting at age 21, and in Europe after age 40 in men and age 50 in women.[5,7,15] Screening should be repeated every 4 to 6 years thereafter. Although a fasting lipid panel is preferred, a nonfasting lipid panel will identify those with total cholesterol over 200 mg/dL who should then undergo further assessment with a fasting lipid panel.[48]

In the United States, screening for familial hypercholesterolemia should begin in childhood (universal screening at age 9–11 years and again at age 17–20 years; targeted screening at age 2 if a family history of premature ASCVD or familial hypercholesterolemia).[12,49] Once an individual with suspected familial hypercholesterolemia, or an LDL-C of 190 mg/dL or greater, is identified, cascade screening of family members is recommended by familial hypercholesterolemia experts around the world.[49–51]

Overview of the 2013 ACC/AHA Cholesterol Guideline

The 2013 ACC/AHA guideline on the treatment of blood cholesterol to reduce atherosclerotic cardiovascular disease risk in adults was based on a rigorous systematic review of randomized drug therapy trials with cardiovascular outcomes.[5] Recommendations were based on the strength of evidence for a net ASCVD risk-reduction benefit from a drug therapy. Consequently, statins were recommended for four groups of patients: those with (1) clinical ASCVD, (2) untreated LDL-C of 190 mg/dL or greater, (3) diabetes and aged between 40 and 75 years, and (4) a 7.5% or greater 10-year ASCVD risk (Fig. 28.2). Moderate evidence supports the use of statins in those with a 5% to < 7.5% 10-year ASCVD risk.

The focus on the reduction in nonfatal and fatal ASCVD risk is an important advance over previous guidelines that

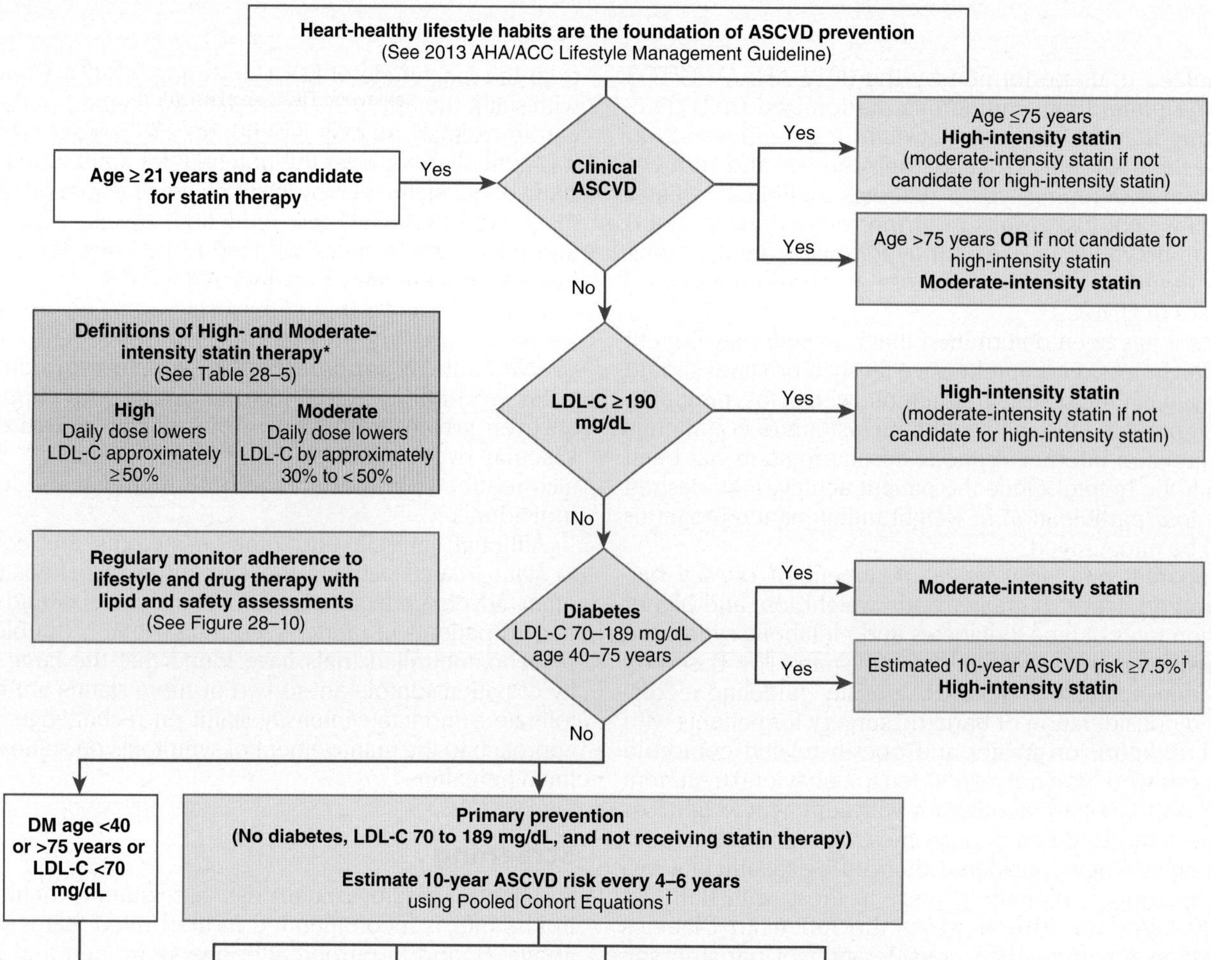

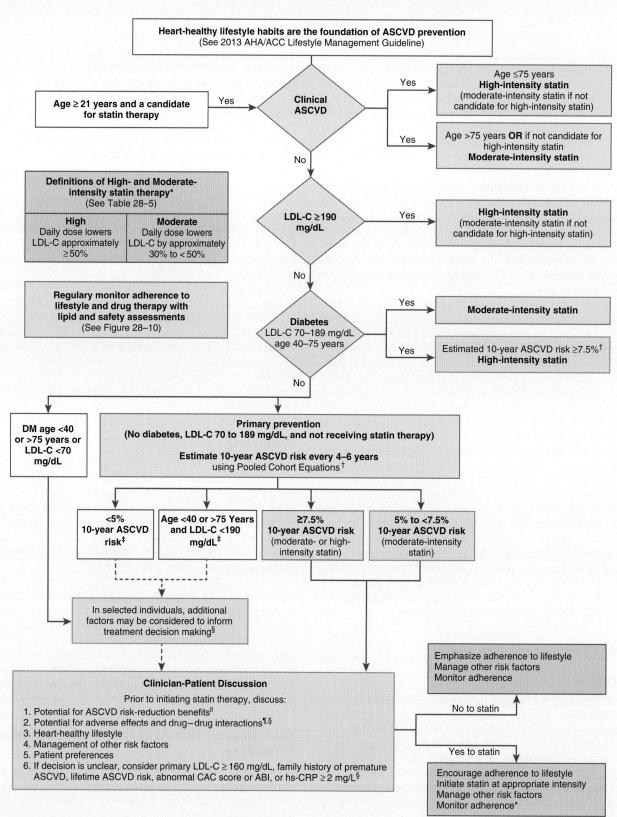

FIG. 28.2 2013 ACC/AHA cholesterol guideline recommendations for initiation of statin therapy. Colors correspond to the Classes of Recommendation (*I*, green, *IIa*, yellow, *IIb*, orange). *Percent reduction in LDL-C can be used as an indication of response and adherence to therapy, but is not in itself a treatment goal. †The Pooled Cohort Equations can be used to estimate 10-year ASCVD risk in individuals with and without diabetes. The estimator within this application should be used to inform decision-making in primary prevention patients not on a statin. ‡Consider moderate-intensity statin as more appropriate in low-risk individuals. §For those in whom a risk assessment is uncertain, consider factors such as primary LDL-C ≥ 160 mg/dL or other evidence of genetic hyperlipidemias, family history of premature ASCVD with onset < 55 years of age in a first-degree male relative or < 65 years of age in a first-degree female relative, hs-CRP ≥ 2 mg/L, CAC score ≥ 300 Agatston units, or ≥ 75th percentile for age, sex, and ethnicity (for additional information, see http://www.mesa-nhlbi.org/CACReference.aspx), ABI < 0.9, or lifetime risk of ASCVD. Additional factors that may aid in individual risk assessment may be identified in the future. ‖Potential ASCVD risk-reduction benefits. The absolute reduction in ASCVD events from moderate- or high-intensity statin therapy can be approximated by multiplying the estimated 10-year ASCVD risk by the anticipated relative risk reduction from the intensity of statin initiated (~30% for moderate-intensity statin or ~45% for high-intensity statin therapy). The net ASCVD risk-reduction benefit is estimated from the number of potential ASCVD events prevented with a statin, compared to the number of potential excess adverse effects. ¶Potential adverse effects. The excess risk of diabetes is the main consideration in ~0.1 excess cases per 100 individuals treated with a moderate-intensity statin for 1 year and ~0.3 excess cases per 100 individuals treated with a high-intensity statin for 1 year. In RCTs, both statin-treated and placebo-treated participants experienced the same rate of muscle symptoms. The actual rate of statin-related muscle symptoms in the clinical population is unclear. Muscle symptoms attributed to statin therapy should be evaluated (see Table 8, Safety Recommendation 8 in the 2013 ACC/AHA cholesterol guideline report). *ABI*, Ankle-brachial index; *ASCVD*, atherosclerotic cardiovascular disease; *CAC*, coronary artery calcium; *hs-CRP*, high-sensitivity C-reactive protein; *LDL-C*, low-density lipoprotein cholesterol; *MI*, myocardial infarction; *RCT*, randomized controlled trial. *(Reprinted with permission of the authors of Stone NJ, Robinson JG, Lichtenstein AH, et al. 2013 ACC/AHA guideline on the treatment of blood cholesterol to reduce atherosclerotic cardiovascular risk in adults: a report of the American College of Cardiology/American Heart Association Task Force on Practice Guidelines.* J Am Coll Cardiol. *2014;63(25, Part B):2889–2934).*

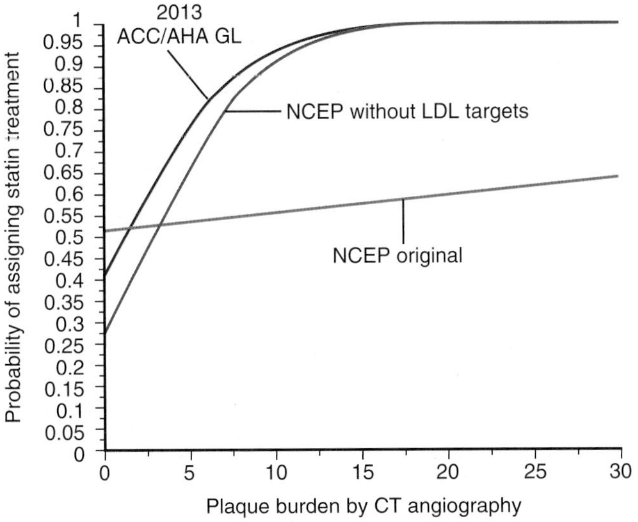

FIG. 28.3 Probability of assigning statin therapy versus plaque burden: 2013 ACC/AHA cholesterol guideline (GL) versus the National Cholesterol Education Program (NCEP) Adult Treatment Panel 3 guideline. *ACC,* American College of Cardiology; *AHA,* American Heart Association; *CT,* computed tomography; *LDL,* low-density lipoprotein. *(Adapted from Johnson KM et al.* JACC *2014;64:910–919.)*

addressed only coronary heart disease risk.[48] The risk of stroke increases with advancing age, especially in white women and African-American women and men.[53,54] In addition to reducing coronary events, statins also reduce the risk of ischemic and total stroke, as well as peripheral arterial disease events.[40]

The 2013 ACC/AHA cholesterol guideline was a major paradigm shift from previous guidelines, as well as the recent 2016 ESC/EAS guidelines, which focus on achieving specific cholesterol targets. Multiple analyses have confirmed that the 2013 ACC/AHA cholesterol guideline approach, when compared to the National Cholesterol Education Program Adult Treatment Panel III (NCEP ATP III) guidelines and the 2012 ESC/EAS guidelines, better identifies individuals at high ASCVD risk for the appropriate intensity of statin therapy and avoids statin treatment in lower-risk patients.[54,56–60] Comparisons with the 2016 ESC/EAS guideline have not yet been performed.

An important consequence of the LDL-C goal approach used in previous guidelines is that these goals may turn into LDL-C thresholds for treatment. Thus, higher-risk patients who are "at goal" are unlikely to be treated, despite evidence of benefit from additional LDL-C lowering from randomized cardiovascular outcomes trials (Fig. 28.3).

There appears to be additional ASCVD risk-reduction benefit when LDL-C levels below the previously recommended targets (<30, <100, or <70 mg/dL) are achieved with statin therapy (Figs. 28.4 and 28.5).[61,62] Thus, it is not clear what the optimal target should be. Nor is there sufficient data to determine the potential for net benefit (e.g., benefits – adverse effects) from adding nonstatin therapies to maximal statin therapy to achieve a specific cholesterol goal. Additional rationales supporting the move away from LDL-C goals are provided in Box 28.2.

For primary prevention in individuals aged between 40 and 75 years with LDL-C below 190 mg/dL, assessment of 10-year ASCVD risk is recommended to inform the decision to initiate statin therapy. The 2013 ACC/AHA risk assessment guideline recommends the use of the Pooled Cohort Equations for white and African-American men and women.[7] Other factors such as premature family history of ASCVD, lifetime ASCVD risk, coronary artery calcification,

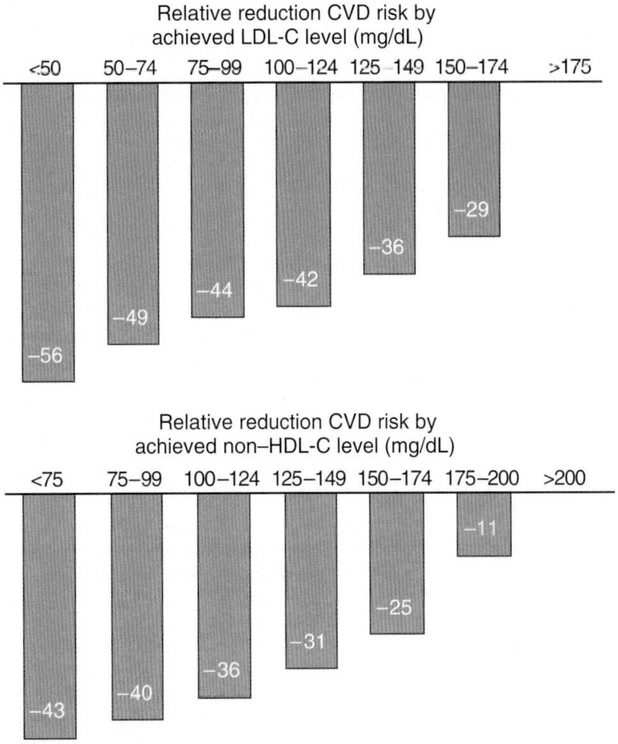

FIG. 28.4 Relative risk reduction cardiovascular events by achieved LDL-C level—meta-analysis of eight statin trials evaluating high- and moderate-intensity statins. *CDV,* Cardiovascular disease; *LDL-C,* low-density lipoprotein cholesterol. *(Adapted from Boekholdt SM, Hovingh GK, Mora S, et al.* JACC *2014;64:485–494.)*

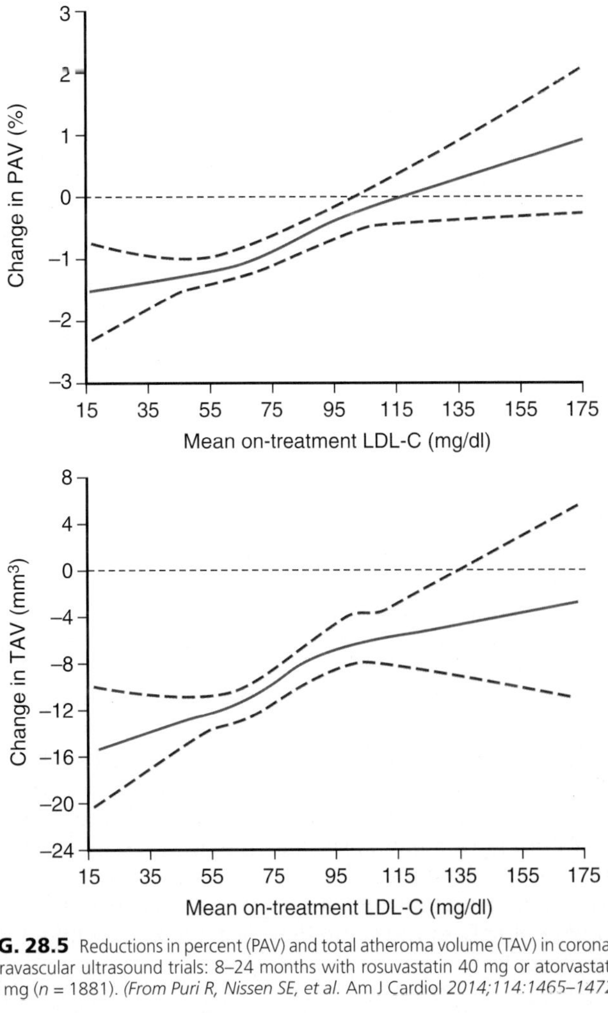

FIG. 28.5 Reductions in percent (PAV) and total atheroma volume (TAV) in coronary intravascular ultrasound trials: 8–24 months with rosuvastatin 40 mg or atorvastatin 80 mg (n = 1881). *(From Puri R, Nissen SE, et al.* Am J Cardiol *2014;114:1465–1472.)*

BOX 28.2 2013 ACC/AHA Cholesterol Guideline: A New Perspective on LDL-C and/or Non–HDL-C Goals

1. The difficulty of giving up the treat-to-goal paradigm was deliberated extensively over a 3-year period. Many clinicians use targets such as LDL-C < 70 mg/dL and LDL-C < 100 mg/dL for secondary and primary ASCVD prevention (non–HDL-C targets are 30 mg/dL higher). However, the RCT evidence clearly shows that ASCVD events are reduced by using the maximum-tolerated statin intensity in those groups shown to benefit. After a comprehensive review, no RCTs were identified that titrated drug therapy to specific LDL-C or non–HDL-C goals to improve ASCVD outcomes. However, one RCT was identified that showed no additional ASCVD event reduction from the addition of nonstatin therapy to further treat non–HDL-C levels once an LDL-C goal was reached. In AIM-HIGH,[68b] the additional reduction in non–HDL-C levels (as well as additional reductions in Apo B, Lp(a), and triglycerides in addition to HDL-C increases) with niacin therapy **DID NOT** further reduce ASCVD risk in individuals treated to LDL-C levels of 40–80 mg/dL.
2. Use of LDL-C targets may result in under treatment with evidence-based statin therapy or overtreatment with nonstatin drugs that have not been shown to reduce ASCVD events in RCTs (even though the drug may additionally lower LDL-C and/or non–HDL-C). Implications of treating to an LDL-C goal may mean that a suboptimal intensity of statin is used because the goal has been achieved, or that adding a nonstatin therapy to achieve a specific target results in down-titration of the evidence-based intensity of statin for safety reasons. However, when RCT evidence is available that a nonstatin therapy further reduces ASCVD events when added to statin therapy, the nonstatin therapy may be considered.
3. Modest physiologic or laboratory measurement variations in LDL-C and non–HDL-C with little impact on the pathophysiology of atherosclerosis may result in excursions above or below goal, resulting in therapeutic changes that may provide little or no additional net ASCVD risk reduction benefit to the patient.
4. Some examples comparing a strategy based on the four statin benefit groups to a strategy using LDL-C/non–HDL-C targets:
   A. Secondary prevention – evidence supports high-intensity statin therapy for this group to maximally lower LDL-C. It does not support the use of an LDL-C target. For example, if a secondary-prevention patient achieves an LDL-C of 78 mg/dL on a dose of 80 mg of atorvastatin, the patient is receiving evidence-based therapy. As of yet, there are no data to show that adding nonstatin drug(s) to high-intensity statin therapy will provide incremental ASCVD risk-reduction benefit with an acceptable margin of safety. Indeed, AIM-HIGH[68b] demonstrated the futility of adding niacin in individuals with low HDL-C and high triglycerides, and ACCORD[126] demonstrated the futility of adding fenofibrate in persons with diabetes. Although an ACCORD subgroup analysis of those with high triglycerides and low HDL-C levels suggested that fenofibrate may reduce ASCVD events in patients with diabetes, this is hypothesis generating and needs further testing in comparison to the evidence-based use of a high-intensity statin. In addition, not having a goal of < 70 mg/dL for LDL-C means that the patient who is adhering to optimal lifestyle management and receiving a high-intensity statin avoids additional, non–evidence-based therapy just because his/her LDL-C is higher than an arbitrary cut-point. Indeed, the LDL-C goal approach can make this patient unnecessarily feel like a failure.
   B. Familial hypercholesterolemia with LDL-C ≥ 190 mg/dL – In many cases, individuals with familial hypercholesterolemia are unable to achieve an LDL-C goal < 100 mg/dL. For example, an individual with familial hypercholesterolemia may achieve an LDL-C of only 120 mg/dL despite use of three cholesterol-lowering drugs. Although this individual may have fallen short of the 100 mg/dL goal, he/she has decreased his/her LDL-C by > 50% (starting from an untreated LDL-C level of ~325–400 mg/dL). These patients are not treatment failures, as observational data has shown significant reductions in ASCVD events without achieving specific LDL-C targets. This is an area where observational data supports the recommended approach.
   C. Type 2 diabetes – For those 40–75 years of age with risk factors, the potential benefits of LDL-C lowering with a high-intensity statin are substantial. Because those with diabetes often have lower LDL-C levels than those without diabetes, "goal"-directed therapy often encourages use of a lower statin dose than is supported by the RCTs, and nonstatin drugs may be added to address low HDL-C or high triglycerides, for which RCT evidence of an ASCVD event reduction is lacking. Giving a maximally tolerated statin intensity should receive primary emphasis because it most accurately reflects the data that statins reduce the relative risk of ASCVD events similarly in individuals with and without diabetes, and in primary and secondary prevention in those with diabetes, along with evidence that high-intensity statins reduce ASCVD events more than moderate-intensity statins.
   D. Estimated 10-year ASCVD risk ≥ 7.5% – data have shown that statins used for primary prevention have substantial ASCVD risk-reduction benefits across the range of LDL-C levels of 70–189 mg/dL. Moreover, the Cochrane meta-analysis,[15] as well as a meta-analysis by the Cholesterol Treatment Trialists confirms that primary prevention with statins reduces total mortality as well as nonfatal ASCVD events.[44]

ACC, American College of Cardiology; *ACCORD,* Action to Control Cardiovascular Risk in Diabetes; *AHA,* American Heart Association; *AIM-HIGH,* Atherothrombosis Intervention in Metabolic Syndrome with Low HDL/High Triglycerides: Impact on Global Health Outcomes; *ASCVD,* atherosclerotic cardiovascular disease; *HDL-C,* high-density lipoprotein cholesterol; *LDL-C,* low-density lipoprotein cholesterol; *RCT,* randomized controlled trial. From Stone N, Robinson J, Lichtenstein A, et al. 2013 ACC/AHA guideline on the treatment of blood cholesterol to reduce atherosclerotic cardiovascular risk in adults. *Circulation.* 2014;129[suppl 2]:S1–S45. Reprinted with permission of the author JG Robinson.

reduced ankle-brachial index, and elevated C-reactive protein, race, and ethnicity may be considered for informing risk assessment.

The potential for an ASCVD risk-reduction benefit from adding a nonstatin to further lower LDL-C is of particular importance in lower-risk primary prevention in patients with LDL-C below 190 mg/dL, where the margin of ASCVD risk-reduction benefit may be smaller, yet the burden of additional therapy, costs, and risk of adverse effects is unchanged.[5] Ezetimibe is the preferred nonstatin due to clear demonstration that it reduces ASCVD events when added to background statin therapy with an excellent margin of safety.

Overview of the 2016 ESC/EAS Cholesterol Guideline

The 2016 ESC/EAS prevention guideline continues to use the risk stratification and LDL-C goal paradigm of previous ESC/EAS guidelines (Box 28.3).[15,63] Patients are stratified into four groups: (1) very high risk (documented cardiovascular disease), diabetes with target organ damage or a major cardiovascular risk factor, severe chronic kidney disease, or a calculated SCORE greater than or equal to 10%; (2) high risk (marked elevation of single risk factors, in particular total cholesterol > 8 mmol/L or > 310 mg/dL), other people with diabetes mellitus, moderate chronic kidney

BOX 28.3 2016 ESC/EAS Prevention Guideline (Clinical Indications for Out-of-Office Blood Pressure Measurements)

Suspicion of white-coat or masked hypertension
- High office BP in individuals without organ damage and at low total CV risk.
- Normal office BP in individuals with organ damage or at high total CV risk.
- Considerable variability of office BP over the same or different visits.
- Autonomic, postural, postprandial, siesta- and drug-induced hypotension.
- Elevated office BP or suspected pre-eclampsia in pregnant women.
- Identification of true and false resistant hypertension.

Specific indications for ABPM
- Marked discordance between office BP and home BP.
- Assessment of dipping status.
- Suspicion of nocturnal hypertension or absence of dipping, such as in patients with sleep apnea, CKD, or DM.
- Assessment of BP variability.

ABPM, Ambulatory blood pressure monitoring; *BP*, blood pressure; *CKD*, chronic kidney disease; *CV*, cardiovascular; *DM*, diabetes mellitus.
From Piepoli MF, Hoes AW, Agewall S, et al. 2016 European guidelines on cardiovascular disease prevention in clinical practice. *Eur Heart J*. 2016;37(29):2315–2381. pii: ehw106.

disease, or a calculated SCORE of 5% to less than 10%; (3) moderate risk (SCORE ≥ 1% and < 5%); and (4) low risk (SCORE < 1%) (see Table 28.4). Premature family history of ASCVD, psychosocial factors, coronary artery calcium, carotid plaque, ankle-brachial index, and the presence of autoimmune disease can also be considered as part of the risk assessment.

The level of patient risk identifies LDL-C treatment goal: very high risk (≥ 10%; LDL-C goal < 1.8 mmol/L or 70 mg/dL); high risk (5 to < 10%; LDL-C goal < 2.6 mmol/L or 100 mg/dL); moderate risk (≥ 1% to < 5%; LDL-C goal < 3.0 mmol/L or 115 mg/dL); or low risk (< 1%; LDL-C goal < 3.0 mmol/L or 115 mg/dL) (see Table 28.4).

Statins are recommended as the first choice in patients with hypercholesterolemia or combined hyperlipidemia. Nonstatins are recommended as combination therapy with statins in selected patients when a specific goal is not reached with the maximal tolerated dose of statin. Ezetimibe may be preferred based on IMProved Reduction of Outcomes: Vytorin Efficacy International Trial (IMPROVE-IT). Niacin and bile acid sequestrants are not recommended. Fenofibrate may be useful in some patients with hypertriglyceridemia, with the excess risk of myopathy clearly communicated.

Non–HDL-C is considered a reasonable alternative treatment goal, although it has not been an endpoint in cardiovascular outcomes trials. Non–HDL-C is calculated by subtracting HDL-C from total cholesterol, thus reflecting all the circulating apolipoprotein B–containing atherogenic lipoproteins, including LDL-C. Non–HDL-C is particularly helpful in hypertriglyceridemic patients and can be calculated when triglycerides are above 400 mg/dL (unlike calculated LDL-C). Non–HDL-C does not require fasting and is approximately 0.8 mmol/L (30 mg/dL) higher than the LDL-C level. Non–HDL-C treatment goals are: very high risk less than 2.6 mmol/L (< 100 mg/dL), high risk less than 3.3 mmol/L (< 130 mg/dL), and in moderate–low risk less than 3.8 mmol/L (< 145 mg/dL).

The remainder of this section will focus on the 2013 ACC/AHA cholesterol guideline recommendations, with additional information from the shorter cholesterol treatment section of the 2016 ESC/AHA prevention guideline provided as needed.

Statin Intensity

The 2013 ACC/AHA cholesterol guideline recommends moderate- or high-intensity statin therapy based on the strength of evidence and likelihood of a net ASCVD risk-reduction benefit. Statin intensity is defined in Table 28.5.[5] High-risk patients up to age 75 years should receive a high-intensity statin, unless safety concerns are present. Three trials have demonstrated high-intensity statins reduce ASCVD events more than moderate-intensity statins and are well tolerated in high-risk patient populations aged 75 years or older.[64–66] In lower-risk patients (< 7.5%), and in those over 75 years, moderate-intensity statins are preferred. In those unable to tolerate high- or moderate-intensity statins, the maximally tolerated statin dose should be used.

Primary Prevention with LDL-C of 190 mg/dL or Higher

When a patient is first identified with an LDL-C of 190 mg/dL or higher (or triglycerides ≥ 500 mg/dL), secondary causes of hypercholesterolemia should be ruled out (Table 28.6).[5] Management of hypertriglyceridemia is discussed briefly later in this section. Readers are referred to the AHA triglyceride statement for a more detailed discussion.[67]

Individuals of any age with a primary elevation of LDL-C of 190 mg/dL or higher have a strong genetic contribution to their hypercholesterolemia and are at increased risk of premature ASCVD.[5] Healthy lifestyle habits, avoidance of smoking, and control of blood pressure are all very important. However, substantial LDL-C reduction in LDL-C levels is required to significantly reduce the premature risk of ASCVD in these patients.

The 2013 ACC/AHA cholesterol guideline recommends that all individuals with primary LDL-C of 190 mg/dL or higher be treated with a high-intensity statin. LDL-C should be reduced by at least 50%. Because high-intensity statins reduce LDL-C more than moderate-intensity statins,[64–66] a high-intensity statin should be initiated unless safety considerations are present.[5] Many patients with untreated LDL-C levels of 190 mg/dL or higher will require the addition of a nonstatin to further lower LDL-C to desirable levels.

Although no evidence is available for nonstatins added to statin therapy in patients with genetic hypercholesterolemia, the 2013 ACC/AHA cholesterol guideline panel considered the potential benefit of additional LDL-C reduction in these patients to be significant based on extrapolation of the Cholesterol Treatment Trialists meta-analysis of statin therapy, where each 1 mmol/L (39 mg/dL) reduction in LDL-C was associated with a 21% reduction in major cardiovascular events (Fig. 28.6).[68a] Therefore, an expert recommendation was made to add nonstatin therapy to achieve the desired level of LDL-C, preferably a nonstatin(s) shown to reduce ASCVD events.[51] The recommended treatment strategy is outlined in Fig. 28.7.

The 2016 ESC/EAS guideline recommends an LDL-C goal below 100 mg/dL for high-risk primary prevention patients with total cholesterol greater than 8 mmol/L

TABLE 28.4 2016 ESC/EAS Prevention Guidelines: Patient Risk Categories and Lipid Treatment Recommendations

RISK LEVEL	CHARACTERISTICS	RECOMMENDATION	CLASS	LEVEL
Very high risk	• Documented CVD, clinical or unequivocal on imaging. Documented clinical CVD includes previous AMI, ACS, coronary revascularization and other arterial revascularization procedures, stroke and TIA, aortic aneurysm and PAD. Unequivocally documented CVD on imaging includes significant plaque on coronary angiography or carotid ultrasound. It does NOT include some increase in continuous imaging parameters such as intima-media thickness of the carotid artery • DM with target organ damage such as proteinuria or with a major risk factor such as smoking or marked hypercholesterolemia or marked hypertension • Severe CKD (GFR < 30 mL/min per 1.73 m^2) • A calculated SCORE ≥ 10%	An LDL-C goal < 1.8 mmol/L (< 70 mg/dL), or a reduction of at least 50% if the baseline is between 1.8 and 3.5 mmol/L (70 and 135 mg/dL) is recommended	I	B
High risk	• Markedly elevated single risk factors, in particular cholesterol > 8 mmol/L (> 310 mg/dL) (e.g., in familial hypercholesterolemia) or BP ≥ 180/110 mm Hg • Most other people with DM (with the exception of young people with type 1 DM and without major risk factors that may be at low or moderate risk) • Moderate CKD (GFR 30–59 mL/min per 1.73 m^2) • A calculated SCORE ≥ 5% and < 10%	LDL-C goal < 2.6 mmol/L (< 100 mg/dL), or a reduction of at least 50% if the baseline is between 2.6 and 5.1 mmol/L (100 and 200 mg/dL) is recommended	I	B
Moderate risk	SCORE is ≥ 1% and < 5% at 10 years. Many middle-aged subjects belong to this category	In the remaining patients on LDL-C lowering treatment, an LDL-C goal < 3.0 mmol/L (< 115 mg/dL) should be considered	IIa	C
Low risk	SCORE < 1%.			

AMI, Acute myocardial infarction; *ACS*, acute coronary syndrome; *BP*, blood pressure; *CKD*, chronic kidney disease; *CVD*, cardiovascular disease; *DM*, diabetes mellitus; GFR, glomerular filtration rate; *LDL-C*, low-density lipoprotein cholesterol; *PAD*, peripheral artery disease; *TIA*, transient ischemic attack. *From Piepoli MF, Hoes AW, Agewall S, et al. 2016 European Guidelines on cardiovascular disease prevention in clinical practice.* Eur Heart J. *2016;37(29):2315–2381.*

TABLE 28.5 High-, Moderate-, and Low-Intensity Statin Therapy*

	DAILY DOSE		
STATIN THERAPY	**High Intensity ↓LDL-C ≥ 50%**	**Moderate Intensity ↓LDL-C 30-< 50%**	**Low Intensity ↓LDL-C < 30%**
Atorvastatin	(40)–80 mg‖	10 *(20)* mg	
Rosuvastatin	20 *(40)* mg	*(5)* 10 mg	
Simvastatin		20–40 mg¶	*10 mg*
Pravastatin		40 *(80)* mg	10–20 mg
Lovastatin		40 mg	20 mg
Fluvastatin		*80 mg (Fluvastatin XL)*	*20–40 mg*
Fluvastatin		40 mg**	
Pitavastatin		*2–4 mg*	*1 mg*

*Individual responses to statin therapy varied in randomized, controlled trials and vary in clinical practice. A less-than-average response may have a biologic basis. Statins and dosages in bold were reduced in major cardiovascular events in randomized, controlled trials. Statins and doses in italics were approved by the FDA but were not tested in randomized, controlled trials.
‖Evidence from one randomized, controlled trial only; down-titration if patient is unable to tolerate atorvastatin, 80 mg.
¶Although simvastatin 80 mg was evaluated in randomized, controlled trials, the FDA recommends against initiation of or titration to 80 mg of simvastatin because of increased risk for myopathy and rhabdomyolysis.
**Twice daily.
FDA, US Food and Drug Administration; *LDL-C*, low-density lipoprotein cholesterol; *XL*, extended-release.
From Stone NJ, Robinson JG, Lichtenstein AH, et al. 2013 ACC/AHA guideline on the treatment of blood cholesterol to reduce atherosclerotic cardiovascular risk in adults: a report of the American College of Cardiology/American Heart Association Task Force on Practice Guidelines. J Am Coll Cardiol. *2014;63(25, Part B):2889–2934. Reprinted with permission of the author JG Robinson.*

(> 310 mg/dL).[15] The National Lipid Association has recommended achieving an LDL-C below 100 mg/dL for these patients.

Familial Hypercholesterolemia Diagnosis

Individuals with familial hypercholesterolemia are at particularly high risk of premature ASCVD due to exposure to high LDL-C levels from birth.[35,51] In adulthood, familial hypercholesterolemia can be diagnosed as an untreated LDL-C of 190 mg/dL or higher and a family history of familial hypercholesterolemia or premature-onset ASCVD in a first-degree relative (before age 55 years in men; before age 65 years in women).[35] The presence of an LDL-C–raising gene defect (LDL receptor, apolipoprotein B, or PCSK9) is also diagnostic, although not present in all cases of familial hypercholesterolemia. Once a patient with familial hypercholesterolemia is diagnosed, cascade screening of relatives should be performed, including in children age 2 or older. Early treatment with statins markedly reduces the premature risk of ASCVD in patients with genetic hypercholesterolemia.[50]

TABLE 28.6 Secondary Causes of Hyperlipidemia

SECONDARY CAUSE	ELEVATED LDL-C OR NON–HDL-C	ELEVATED TRIGLYCERIDES
Diet	**Saturated or *trans* fats, large weight gain**, anorexia	**Large weight gain**, high fat intake, **high refined carbohydrate intake, excessive alcohol intake**, very low fat diets if high in refined carbohydrates
Drugs	**Glucocorticoids**, cyclosporine, anticonvulsants, oral contraceptives, anabolic steroids, diuretics, sirolimus, amiodarone	**Glucocorticoids**, oral estrogens, anabolic steroids, bile acid sequestrants, highly active retroviral therapy, retinoic acid (isotretinoin), sirolimus, tacrolimus, raloxifene, tamoxifen, β-blockers (not carvedilol), thiazides, cyclophosphamide, L-asparaginase, second-generation antipsychotics (clozapine and olanzapine)
Diseases	Biliary obstruction, nephrotic syndrome, gammaglobulinopathy	**Proteinuria**, nephrotic syndrome, chronic renal failure, glomerulonephritis, Cushing syndrome, HIV, lipodystrophies, gammaglobulinopathy, systemic lupus erythematosus, automimmune chylomicronemia, chronic idiopathic urticaria
Disorders and altered states of metabolism	**Obesity**, hypothyroidism, pregnancy*	**Diabetes (poorly controlled), obesity**, lipodystrophy, hypothyroidism, pregnancy,* polycystic ovarian syndrome

Common causes of secondary hyperlipidemia (most common causes in **bold**; leading causes underlined).
*Cholesterol and triglycerides rise progressively throughout pregnancy.

Secondary causes of hyperlipidemia should be evaluated in patients with:
- Newly identified LDL-C ≥ 160 mg/dL or non–HDL-C ≥ 190 mg/dL.
- Newly identified triglycerides ≥ 500 mg/dL.
- Worsening LDL-C, non–HDL-C, or triglyceride levels despite adherences to lifestyle and drug therapy.

Initial laboratory tests should include:
- Fasting glucose or hemoglobin A1C (HbA1C).
- Thyroid-stimulating hormone (TSH).
- Alkaline phosphatase, bilirubin, and alanine aminotransferase (ALT).
- Creatinine/glomerular filtration rate (GFR).
- Urinary albumin.

Additional tests include:
- Total protein
- Women of childbearing age – beta human chorionic gonadotropin (β-hCG).

Used with permission of Robinson JG. Clinical Lipid Management. Professional Communications Inc, West Islip, NY, 2015.

Primary Prevention in Patients with Diabetes

Individuals with type 1 or 2 diabetes are also at very high lifetime risk of ASCVD events.[5] These patients often have dyslipidemia characterized by lower LDL-C and HDL-C and higher triglyceride and non–HDL-C levels than patients without diabetes.[69] However, for ASCVD risk reduction, the focus remains on LDL-C lowering with statin therapy, which reduces risk across the spectrum of other lipid abnormalities and patient characteristics in patients with diabetes (Fig. 28.8).[68] Primary prevention patients with diabetes experience the same relative reduction in cardiovascular risk as those with clinical ASCVD.

Based on a strong body of evidence from multiple clinical trials, the 2013 ACC/AHA cholesterol guideline recommends statin therapy for all patients with diabetes aged between 40 and 75 years.[5] Only moderate-intensity statins have been evaluated in primary prevention populations of patients with diabetes. However, as in other patient groups, the reduction in cardiovascular risk is proportional to the magnitude of LDL-C reduction.[68] Therefore, the 2013 ACC/AHA cholesterol guideline recommends consideration of high-intensity statin therapy in patients with diabetes who have a 7.5% or higher 10-year ASCVD risk. Ten-year and lifetime ASCVD risk can be estimated using the ACC/AHA risk calculator Pooled Cohort Equations.[7]

Statin therapy for primary prevention can also be considered in patients with diabetes younger than age 40 or older than age 75. The American Diabetes Association recommends statin therapy in individuals under 40 years who have cardiovascular risk factors (defined as LDL-C ≥ 100 mg/dL, high blood pressure, smoking, or overweight/obesity).[10] Statin therapy is also recommended for patients with diabetes over age 75: moderate intensity if no risk factors and moderate or high intensity if cardiovascular risk factors are present.

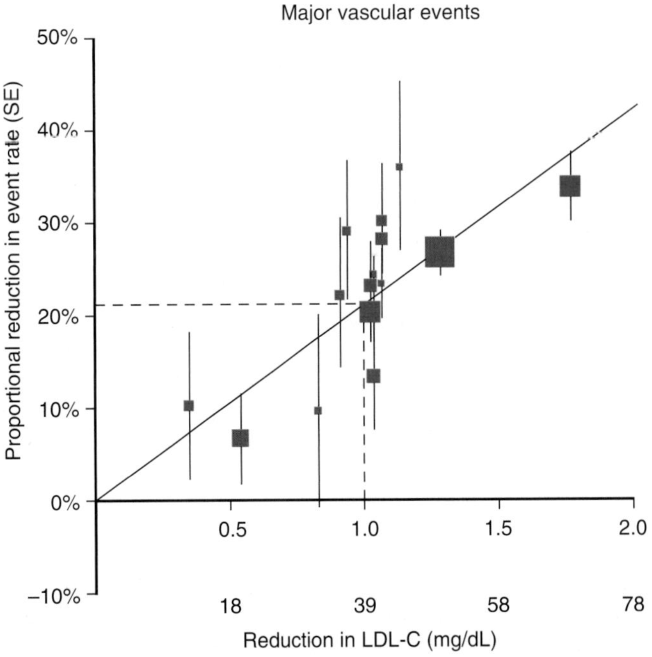

FIG. 28.6 Relationship between the reduction in LDL-C and relative reduction in ASCVD events and the relative risk reduction in ASCVD events observed by year. *(Cholesterol Treatment Trialists, C. Efficacy and safety of cholesterol-lowering treatment: prospective meta-analysis of data from 90,056 patients in 14 randomized trials of statins.* Lancet *2005;366:1267–1278.)*

Primary Prevention among Individuals Without Diabetes and with LDL-C Less Than 190 mg/dL

Whether the first clinical manifestation of ASCVD occurs prematurely or in advanced old age largely depends on genetic susceptibility and the risk factor burden over the

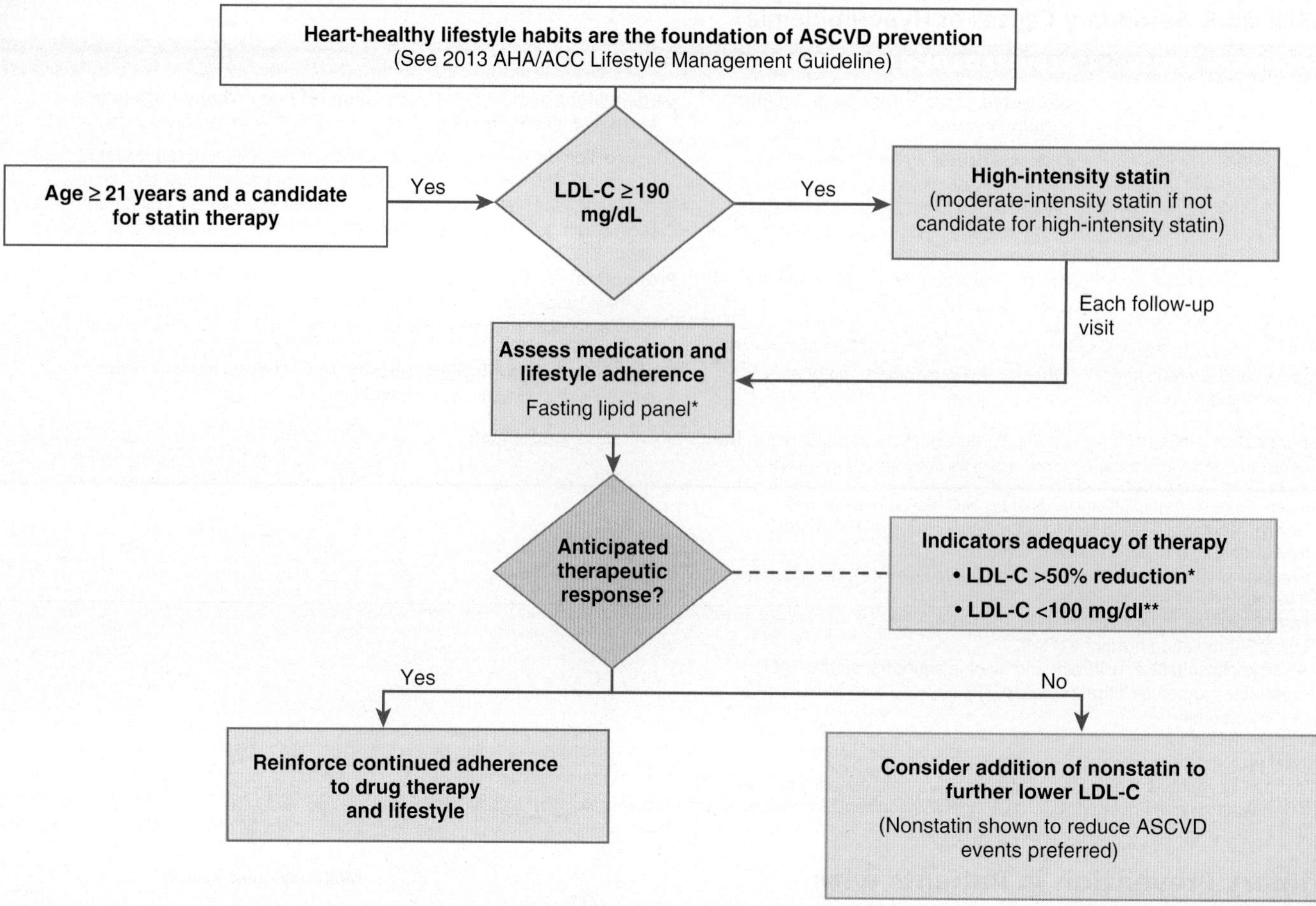

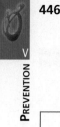

FIG. 28.7 Treatment strategy genetic hypercholesterolemia when LDL-C ≥190 mg/dl. [Green Class 1 recommendation – "should do"; Yellow Class II a recommendation – "reasonable to do"] *Adapted with permission of author from Stone NJ, Robinson JG, Lichtenstein AH, et al. 2013 ACC/AHA Guideline on the Treatment of Blood Cholesterol to Reduce Atherosclerotic Cardiovascular Risk in Adults: A Report of the American College of Cardiology/American Heart Association Task Force on Practice Guidelines. J Am Coll Cardiol. 2014;63(25, Part B):2889-2934).* *For patients with familial combined hyperlipidemia (FCH) and non–HDL-C≥ 220 mg/dL and/or severe hypertriglyceridemia, a 50% reduction in non–HDL-C and non–HDL-C<130 mg/dL may be used as indicators of adequacy of therapy. ** Per the National Lipid Association Familial Hypercholesterolemia statement. *(Goldberg AC, Hopkins PN, Toth PP, et al. Familial hypercholesterolemia: screening, diagnosis and management of pediatric and adult patients: clinical guidance from the National Lipid Association Expert Panel on Familial Hypercholesterolemia.* J Clin Lipidol *2011;5:S1–S8.)*
(From Cholesterol Treatment Trialists. Efficacy and safety of cholesterol-lowering treatment: prospective meta-analysis of data from 90,056 patients in 14 randomized trials of statins. Lancet *2005;366:1267–1278.)*

lifetime.[70,71] Unfortunately, currently available tools cannot accurately predict risk for an individual patient but must rely on probabilistic estimates derived from epidemiologic population data. With this framework in mind, the clinical approach to statins for primary prevention relies heavily on shared decision-making with patients without diabetes who have an LDL-C below 190 mg/dL.

Clinical Trial Evidence

The 2013 ACC/AHA cholesterol guideline developed primary prevention recommendations based on evidence from three purely primary prevention cardiovascular outcomes trials.[72–74] Strong evidence supports a net ASCVD risk-reduction benefit in individuals aged between 40 and 75 years with a 7.5% or higher 10-year ASCVD risk for moderate- or high-intensity statins. Moderate evidence supports the use of moderate-intensity statins in individuals aged between 40 and 75 years with 5% to less than 7.5% 10-year ASCVD risk.[74]

The clinical trial evidence for those aged under 40 years and over 75 years is insufficient. No primary prevention trials enrolled individuals under 40 years. The evidence for primary prevention statin therapy in individuals over 75 years is equivocal. One trial found a cardiovascular risk-reduction benefit with high-intensity statin therapy, but another trial found no benefit with moderate-intensity statin therapy.[75,76] Therefore the decision to initiate statin therapy in these age groups must be individualized with particular consideration of patient preferences.

Statin Safety

When compared with higher-risk secondary prevention patients, safety considerations more strongly influence the decision to initiate statins for lower-risk primary prevention patients, where the margin of ASCVD risk-reduction benefit may be smaller. The most serious adverse effects of serious myopathy and hemorrhagic stroke are rare.[40]

Although muscle symptoms are commonly reported by statin-treated patients, they occurred no more commonly in the moderate- and high-intensity statin-treated groups than in the placebo group in the cardiovascular outcomes trials (management of symptoms in statin-treated patients is discussed hereafter).[5] Of course, these trials excluded patients with serious comorbidities or conditions requiring complex drug regimens that could influence safety (such as HIV or organ transplantation). It should be noted, however, that moderate-intensity statins had a rate of adverse events comparable to placebo in two trials of in patients with Class II–IV heart failure and in two trials of patients receiving maintenance hemodialysis.[78–81]

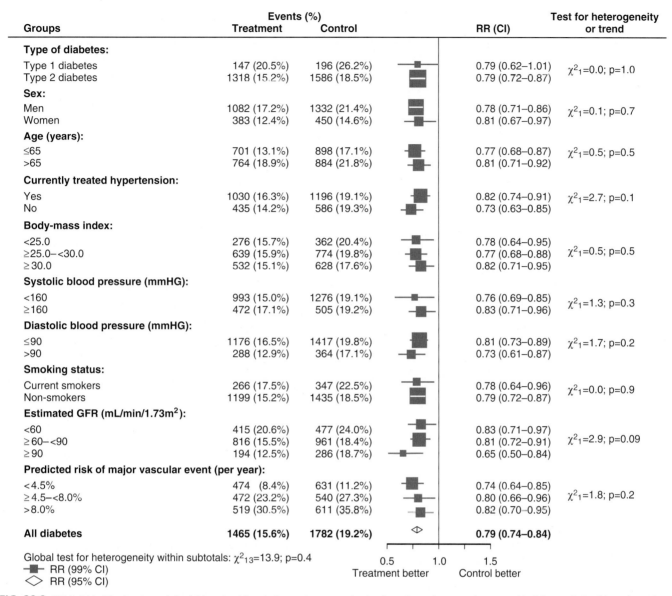

Groups	Events (%) Treatment	Control	RR (CI)	Test for heterogeneity or trend
Type of diabetes:				
Type 1 diabetes	147 (20.5%)	196 (26.2%)	0.79 (0.62–1.01)	χ^2_1=0.0; p=1.0
Type 2 diabetes	1318 (15.2%)	1586 (18.5%)	0.79 (0.72–0.87)	
Sex:				
Men	1082 (17.2%)	1332 (21.4%)	0.78 (0.71–0.86)	χ^2_1=0.1; p=0.7
Women	383 (12.4%)	450 (14.6%)	0.81 (0.67–0.97)	
Age (years):				
≤65	701 (13.1%)	898 (17.1%)	0.77 (0.68–0.87)	χ^2_1=0.5; p=0.5
>65	764 (18.9%)	884 (21.8%)	0.81 (0.71–0.92)	
Currently treated hypertension:				
Yes	1030 (16.3%)	1196 (19.1%)	0.82 (0.74–0.91)	χ^2_1=2.7; p=0.1
No	435 (14.2%)	586 (19.3%)	0.73 (0.63–0.85)	
Body-mass index:				
<25.0	276 (15.7%)	362 (20.4%)	0.78 (0.64–0.95)	
≥25.0–<30.0	639 (15.9%)	774 (19.8%)	0.77 (0.68–0.88)	χ^2_1=0.5; p=0.5
≥30.0	532 (15.1%)	628 (17.6%)	0.82 (0.71–0.95)	
Systolic blood pressure (mmHG):				
<160	993 (15.0%)	1276 (19.1%)	0.76 (0.69–0.85)	χ^2_1=1.3; p=0.3
≥160	472 (17.1%)	505 (19.2%)	0.83 (0.71–0.96)	
Diastolic blood pressure (mmHG):				
≤90	1176 (16.5%)	1417 (19.8%)	0.81 (0.73–0.89)	χ^2_1=1.7; p=0.2
>90	288 (12.9%)	364 (17.1%)	0.73 (0.61–0.87)	
Smoking status:				
Current smokers	266 (17.5%)	347 (22.5%)	0.78 (0.64–0.96)	χ^2_1=0.0; p=0.9
Non-smokers	1199 (15.2%)	1435 (18.5%)	0.79 (0.72–0.87)	
Estimated GFR (mL/min/1.73m²):				
<60	415 (20.6%)	477 (24.0%)	0.83 (0.71–0.97)	
≥60–<90	816 (15.5%)	961 (18.4%)	0.81 (0.72–0.91)	χ^2_1=2.9; p=0.09
≥90	194 (12.5%)	286 (18.7%)	0.65 (0.50–0.84)	
Predicted risk of major vascular event (per year):				
<4.5%	474 (8.4%)	631 (11.2%)	0.74 (0.64–0.85)	
≥4.5–<8.0%	472 (23.2%)	540 (27.3%)	0.80 (0.66–0.96)	χ^2_1=1.8; p=0.2
>8.0%	519 (30.5%)	611 (35.8%)	0.82 (0.70–0.95)	
All diabetes	**1465 (15.6%)**	**1782 (19.2%)**	**0.79 (0.74–0.84)**	

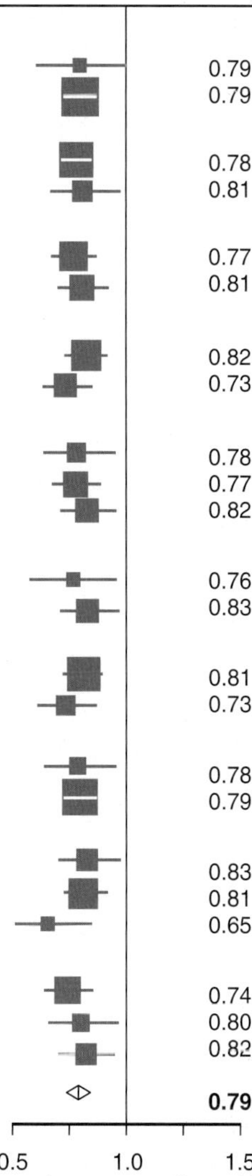

Global test for heterogeneity within subtotals: χ^2_{13}=13.9; p=0.4
RR (99% CI)
RR (95% CI)

FIG. 28.8 CTT individual level meta-analysis of 14 statin trials—cardiovascular event reduction for various subgroups of persons with diabetes. *CI*, Confidence interval; *RR*, relative risk. *(From Cholesterol Treatment Trialists Collaborators CTT, Kearney P, Blackwell L, et al. Efficacy of cholesterol-lowering therapy in 18,686 people with diabetes in 14 randomised trials of statins.* Lancet *2008;371:117–125.)*

A modest excess of statin-associated diabetes has been observed in cardiovascular outcomes trials of moderate-intensity statins, with somewhat higher rates observed with high-intensity statins.[82,83] However, this observation is likely to be of little clinical significance because only patients with diabetes risk factors experienced the excess risk of statin-associated diabetes, and the statin-treated patients were diagnosed with diabetes only 2 to 4 months earlier than patients in the placebo groups.[84]

The 2013 ACC/AHA cholesterol guideline evaluated the number needed to treat to prevent an ASCVD event (NNT) and the number needed to treat to cause one adverse event (harm; NNH) across the range of 10-year ASCVD risk.[85] Considering the risk of serious myopathy, hemorrhagic stroke, and the excess of statin-associated diabetes combined, the NNT exceeded the NNH for moderate-intensity statins even for very low-risk patients (Fig. 28.9). The margin of benefit for high-intensity statins was narrower. However, if the excess risk of diabetes is excluded from the calculation of harm, the NNH of 1000 is well below the NNT for moderate- and high-intensity statins.[84] This suggests there may be additional benefit (with no significant excess of harm) from using high-intensity statins for primary prevention.

Statin Initiation—Age 40 to 75 Years

In patients between 40 and 75 years without diabetes, the 2013 ACC/AHA cholesterol guideline recommends a multi-step process of shared decision-making (see Fig. 28.2):[5]

1. Start by estimating 10-year ASCVD risk in those who are not on a statin and have an LDL-C below 190 mg/dL. Use the ACC/AHA risk calculator. Download from http://my.americanheart.org/professional/StatementsGuidelines/Prevention-Guidelines_UCM_457698_SubHomePage.jsp or http://tools.acc.org/ASCVD-Risk-Estimator.
2. Determine whether the patient has the potential to experience a net ASCVD risk-reduction benefit. Strong evidence: ≥7.5% 10-year ASCVD risk, moderate evidence: 5% to <7.5% 10-year ASCVD risk. In patients with <5% risk, statin therapy can still be considered in selected patients.
3. Consider other characteristics that may influence safety, including drug–drug interactions.

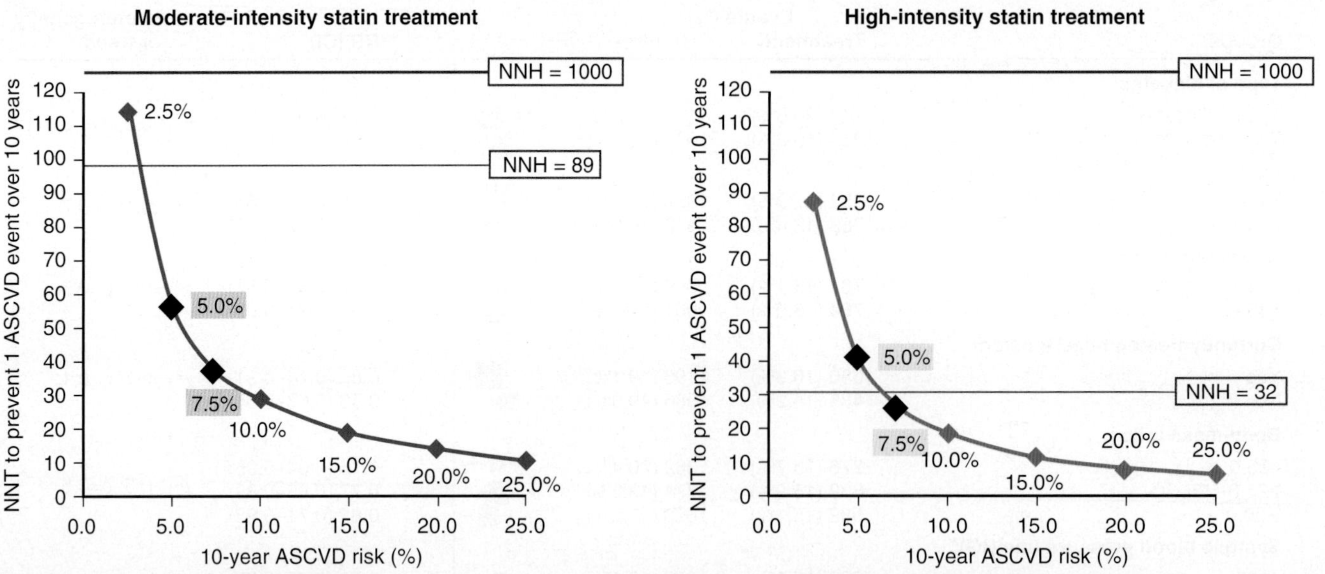

FIG. 28.9 Comparison of the number needed to treat to prevent one ASCVD event (NNH) and the number needed to treat to cause one adverse event (harm; NNH) across the range of 10-year ASCVD risk for moderate- and high-intensity statin therapy. If the excess risk of diabetes is excluded, the NNH is 1000 based on the excess risk of serious myopathy and hemorrhagic stroke. Moderate-intensity statin treatment assumes a 35% relative risk reduction in ASCVD from moderate-intensity statin treatment NNT to prevent one ASCVD event varies by baseline estimated 10-year ASCVD risk. NNH based on one excess case of incident diabetes per 100 individuals* treated with statins for 10 years. High-intensity statin treatment assumes a 45% relative risk reduction in ASCVD from high- intensity statin treatment NNT to prevent one ASCVD event varies by baseline estimated 10-year ASCVD risk NNH based on three excess cases of incident diabetes* per 100 individuals treated with statins for 10 years. *A conservative estimate of adverse events includes excess cases of incident diabetes, myopathy, and hemorrhagic stroke. The NNH is dominated by excess cases of diabetes, with minimal contribution by myopathy (approximately 0.01 excess case per 100) and hemorrhagic stroke (approximately 0.01 excess case per 100 for hemorrhagic stroke). *ASCVD*, Atherosclerotic cardiovascular disease. *(Adapted from Stone N, Robinson J, Lichtenstein A, et al. 2013 ACC/AHA guideline on the treatment of blood cholesterol to reduce atherosclerotic cardiovascular risk in adults.* Circulation. *2014;129[suppl 2]:S1-S45. Full Report online supplement.)*

4. Elicit the preferences of the informed patient.
5. If the decision is unclear, other factors can be considered to refine the risk estimate (see following).

Initial Risk Assessment

The ACC/AHA risk calculator Pooled Cohort Equations should only be used in patients who do not have ASCVD and whose LDL-C is below 190 mg/dL.[5,7] The 10-year ASCVD risk can be estimated in individuals between 40 and 79 years.

The ACC/AHA risk calculator also estimates lifetime risk in individuals aged between 20 and 59 years. After age 60 years, 10-year and lifetime risk converge. Lifetime risk may inform the clinician–patient discussion. In younger patients with risk factors, 10-year ASCVD risk may be low, but lifetime risk may be very high.[7] These patients should address lifestyle and risk factor control and may wish to initiate statin therapy to decrease the lifetime ASCVD risk.

In the United States, estimation of 10-year ASCVD risk should start with the Pooled Cohort Equations, developed as part of the 2013 ACC/AHA risk assessment guideline.[7] The Pooled Cohort Equations were developed from five epidemiologic cohorts supported by the National Heart, Lung, and Blood Institute. These cohorts include non-Hispanic white and African Americans from young adulthood to old age. The Pooled Cohort Equations predict nonfatal and fatal myocardial infarction and stroke. By including stroke, these race- and sex-specific equations perform better in white women and African-American women and men than does the Framingham Score used in earlier cholesterol guidelines, which was derived from a white population and predicted only coronary heart disease.[54]

According to the 2016 ESC/EAS guideline, in Europe, the SCORE equations for low- and high-risk countries should be used to estimate the 10-year risk of fatal ASCVD in primary prevention individuals aged over 40 years who are not otherwise categorized as high or very high risk (e.g., clinical ASCVD, diabetes, chronic kidney disease, or highly elevated single risk factor) (http://www.escardio.org/Guidelines-&-Education/Practice-tools/CVD-prevention-toolbox/SCORE-Risk-Charts).[15] The performance of these equations in non-Caucasians has not been evaluated. However, race/ethnic specific equations have been developed for the United Kingdom (QRISK2) (http://www.qrisk.org/).[16,17]

Revising the Risk Assessment

The 2013 ACC/AHA risk assessment guideline also recommends starting with the Pooled Cohort Equations, and then considering revising the risk estimate downward in individuals from populations known to be at lower ASCVD risk (East Asians and Mexican Americans).[7] Upward revision of risk should also be considered for individuals from populations known to be at higher ASCVD risk (south Asians from India, Pakistan, Bangladesh, Pacific Islanders, some Hispanics of Puerto Rican origin, and Native Americans).

Not surprisingly, the Pooled Cohort Equations have been shown to over-predict ASCVD risk in low-risk populations such as health professionals who volunteered for a clinical trial, Chinese or Hispanic Americans, individuals whose risk factors were well-treated after entry into the study, individuals enrolled in a health maintenance organization in Northern California, or people from low-risk European countries.[86–89] When applied to the general US population of African-American and white men and women who might be considered candidates for statin therapy, the Pooled Cohort Equations perform quite well.[90] Thus, it appears that information on socioeconomic status and race/ethnicity may be informative when revising the risk estimate.

The 2013 ACC/AHA risk assessment guideline also evaluated other biomarkers and patient characteristics to determine if they added sufficient new information to revise the initial risk assessment based on risk factor levels.[7] They identified a number of characteristics that could be considered when the decision to initiate statin therapy for primary prevention is uncertain. A family history of premature ASCVD, elevated coronary artery calcium, a C-reactive protein greater than or equal to 2 mg/L, and low ankle-brachial index were all found to add risk prediction information. Lifetime risk may also be a consideration deciding to initiate statin therapy. LDL-C of 160 mg/dL or higher was added by the 2013 ACC/AHA cholesterol guideline as a characteristic that may indicate increased net benefit from statin therapy due to the greater magnitude of LDL-C reduction as well as likelihood of long-term exposure to genetically high LDL-C levels.[91]

Emerging evidence suggests elevated lipoprotein(a) (Lp[a]) levels may improve risk prediction, especially if there is a family history of premature ASCVD.[92–94] An Lp(a) of 50 mg/dL or higher for non-Hispanic white and an Lp(a) of 30 mg/dL or higher in African Americans may indicate increased ASCVD risk.[95] Some evidence suggests a coronary artery calcium score of zero may modestly downclassify coronary heart disease and ASCVD risk in white men in the 55–65-year age group.[96] However, there is insufficient evidence to determine if this is true for white women, nonwhite adults, and individuals under 55 years.

Characteristics that may be considered when a treatment decision is uncertain are summarized in Box 28.4.

BOX 28.4 Characteristics That May Be Considered to Refine ASCVD Risk Estimation

Recommended indicators of increased ASCVD risk—2013 ACC/AHA risk assessment guideline

1. Family history of premature cardiovascular disease (first-degree relative: male < 55 years or female < 65 years).
2. High sensitivity C-reactive protein ≥ 2.0 mg/L.
3. Coronary artery calcium score ≥ 300 Agatston units or 75th percentile for age/sex/ethnicity.
4. Ankle-brachial index < 0.9.

Other factors to consider—2013 ACC/AHA risk assessment guideline

1. May be at increased ASCVD risk—South Asian ancestry (e.g., India, Pakistan, Bangladesh), some Hispanic groups (e.g., Puerto Rican), Pacific Islander ancestry, Native American ancestry.
2. May be at lower ASCVD risk—East Asian ancestry (China, Japan, etc.), some Hispanic groups (Mexican Americans).

Other factors to consider—2013 ACC/AHA cholesterol guideline

1. LDL-C ≥ 160 mg/dL.
2. Lifetime ASCVD risk.

Other factors that could be considered

1. Lower risk if health professional, high socioeconomic status or educational level.
2. Higher risk of Lp(a) ≥ 50 mg/dL in white or ≥ 30 mg/dL in African Americans.
3. Citizen of a European country with low cardiovascular risk.

ACC, American College of Cardiology; *AHA,* American Heart Association; *ASCVD,* atherosclerotic cardiovascular disease.

Statin Initiation—Age under 40 Years

Healthy lifestyle habits and avoidance of smoking should be the primary emphasis in patients under 40 years. Although no randomized trial evidence is available to guide the decision to initiate statin therapy in patients under 40 years, statin therapy may still be considered in selected patients at increased ASCVD risk.[5] Characteristics that might influence the decision to initiate statin therapy for the primary prevention of ASCVD before age 40 years:

1. An LDL-C ≥ 160 mg before age 40 years indicates a high genetic burden contributing to increased ASCVD risk.
2. The ACC/AHA risk calculator can be used to estimate lifetime ASCVD risk in individuals aged 20–59 years.
3. The 10-year ASCVD risk estimator could also be used to demonstrate the risk at age 40 if risk factors remain unchanged.
4. Family history of premature ASCVD (onset before age 55 years in a first-degree male relative or before age 65 years in a first-degree female relative).

Lipoprotein(a) may be helpful, as previously summarized, especially if a family history of premature ASCVD is present.[92] Coronary artery calcium is unhelpful in this age group, and a score of zero may give a false reassurance regarding ASCVD risk, especially if there is a family history of premature ASCVD.[97] There are few data regarding C-reactive protein or ankle-brachial index and ASCVD risk prediction in this age group.

Statin Initiation—Age over 75 Years

Although the absolute risk of ASCVD events and death is highest after age 75, the decision to initiate statins for primary prevention is less clear.[5] Aging trajectories begin to diverge after age 75 years, and prevention may be less of a clinical or patient priority.[98,99] Nonetheless, even patients in average health at age 75 years are likely to live at least 10 more years, a time frame over which statins might be expected to provide an ASCVD risk-reduction benefit.[25] However, the randomized trial data are equivocal for primary prevention patients over 75 years and no clear evidence-based recommendation can be made.

The ACC/AHA risk calculator can be used to estimate risk up to age 79 years. After age 60 years, 10-year risk estimates converge with lifetime ASCVD risk estimates, so lifetime risk is not calculated.[7] Noninvasive assessment of atherosclerosis may be helpful in those over 75 years, in that a zero or very low coronary artery calcium score may reflect a low 10-year coronary heart disease risk (albeit not zero risk).[100] Stroke risk may still be increased, however, because coronary artery calcium is a weaker predictor of stroke than coronary artery disease.[96,100] An ankle-brachial index greater than 0.90 indicates an individual at high ASCVD risk.[101] A C-reactive protein greater than 2 mg/L may also be helpful because this was an eligibility criterion for the primary prevention Justification for the Use of Statins in Prevention: an Intervention Trial Evaluating Rosuvastatin (JUPITER) trial, where high-intensity statin therapy (rosuvastatin 20 mg) was shown to reduce ASCVD risk in those aged 70 years or older with similar adverse events rate as placebo.[75]

Women

Statins are pregnancy category X and should not be used during pregnancy or by nursing mothers.[5] Nonstatin lipid-lowering agents other than bile acid sequestrants should also be avoided in these women. This consideration primarily affects women with untreated LDL-C of 190 mg/dL or higher and women with diabetes. A woman with genetic hypercholesterolemia should begin statin therapy no later than age 21, so she can experience the maximum potential impact on atherosclerosis progression earlier in the course of the disease, and discontinue therapy during the reproductive period with minimal concern.[35]

The best approach is to counsel the woman and her partner on the potential for harm to the fetus and baby and to confirm that effective contraceptive measures will be undertaken.[102] Statin and nonstatin therapy should be discontinued 2 to 3 months before conception efforts begin. Drug therapy can be resumed after nursing is completed.

White women without diabetes who have LDL-C less than 190 mg/dL are at relatively lower ASCVD risk before age 75 compared to white men and African-American women and men.[4] Fewer women have been enrolled in primary prevention cardiovascular outcomes trials, but the available evidence suggests that women experience similar relative risk reduction to that experienced by men.[103] The Pooled Cohort Equations work particularly well for predicting ASCVD risk in both white and African-American women.[7,54]

Special Clinical Populations

Patients with heart failure and end-stage renal failure are at high risk of cardiovascular events and death. However, statins have not been shown to reduce ASCVD events in patients with Class II–IV heart failure of ischemic or non-ischemic origin,[78,79] nor do statins reduce ASCVD events in patients receiving maintenance hemodialysis.[80,81] The decision to initiate statin therapy in these patients needs to be considered on an individual basis. Notably, moderate-intensity statins were well-tolerated in these trials.

The lack of benefit from statin therapy in these two high-risk groups of patients with serious comorbidities, and the potential for drug–drug interactions, has brought into question the potential for a net ASCVD risk reduction from statins used for primary prevention in other groups of patients with serious comorbidities. Patients with HIV infection, chronic inflammatory or rheumatologic conditions, organ transplantation, and cancer survivors may all be at increased ASCVD risk.[85,104] Statins can certainly be considered for primary prevention, but the statin and dose should be carefully considered to enhance safety.

Monitoring

The success of primary prevention efforts can be enhanced through an ongoing therapeutic relationship between clinicians, patients, and their families. Adherence to lifestyle and medications needs to be assessed regularly. The 2013 ACC/AHA cholesterol guideline recommends regular follow-up visits to assess response to therapy, adverse effects, and adherence (Fig. 28.10).[5] The panel noted that the reduction in cardiovascular events and excellent safety record of statins in the cardiovascular outcomes trials occurred within the context of regular clinical visits.

Although the 2013 ACC/AHA cholesterol guideline moved away from the treat-to-target approach, it did provide some benchmarks for assessing therapeutic efficacy.[5] On average, a 50% or greater reduction in LDL-C will occur with a high-intensity statin, and a 30% to less than 50% reduction will occur with a moderate-intensity statin. When the baseline LDL-C is unknown, it was noted that an LDL-C below 100 mg/dL was observed in the high-intensity statin trials. If, after several visits, it is determined that the patient might benefit from additional LDL-C reduction, the statin dose can be intensified or the addition of a nonstatin can be considered.

Nonstatin Therapy

Nonstatins such as niacin, bile acid sequestrants, and fibrates were shown to reduce ASCVD events in trials performed in highly select high-risk populations in the prestatin era.[5] However, until recently, there was little evidence that nonstatins further reduced ASCVD events when added to background statin therapy.

The 2013 ACC/AHA cholesterol guideline recommended consideration of the addition of a nonstatin in selected high-risk patients who might benefit from additional LDL-C lowering, such as those with LDL-C of 190 mg/dL or higher, those with clinical ASCVD, those with diabetes aged between 40 and 75 years who were unable to tolerate a high-intensity statin, or those who had a less than 50% reduction in LDL-C.[5] Nonstatins shown to reduce ASCVD events were preferred. Ezetimibe would be the preferred nonstatin on the basis of cardiovascular outcomes trial data, although this will likely change as ongoing cardiovascular outcomes trials are completed. The 2016 ESC/EAS guideline recommends the consideration of added nonstatin therapy to achieve risk-based LDL-C or non–HDL-C targets (see Table 28.4).[15]

Ezetimibe

Ezetimibe lowers LDL-C by 15% to 25% when added to background statin therapy.[105,106] The IMPROVE-IT trial for the first time provided clear evidence that adding a nonstatin, ezetimibe, further reduced ASCVD events in statin-treated patients.[41] This trial provides support for the addition of ezetimibe for further lowering LDL-C to reduce ASCVD risk in very high-risk patients such as those with acute coronary syndromes and an additional high-risk characteristic such as diabetes. For lower-risk primary prevention, the addition of ezetimbe is unlikely to have the potential for a meaningful reduction in ASCVD risk unless LDL-C levels are very high, as in patients with familial hypercholesterolemia or high-risk statin-intolerant patients.[107]

One approach that has been suggested for the lower-risk primary prevention setting is to reserve nonstatins for patients most likely to benefit.[108,110-111] This might include those with familial or other genetic hypercholesterolemia whose LDL-C remains above 100 mg/dL on maximally tolerated statin therapy.[51] Patients with a 10-year ASCVD risk of 15% to 20% or greater (with or without diabetes) may benefit from the addition of a nonstatin to further lower LDL-C if LDL-C remains at 130 mg/dL or higher on maximally tolerated statin therapy. The margin of benefit is likely narrower if the LDL-C level is below 130 mg/dL.

PCSK9 Inhibitors

Several cardiovascular outcomes trials are ongoing for proprotein convertase subtilisin-like/kexin type 9 (PCSK9) monoclonal antibodies.[112–114] These drugs lower LDL-C by 45% to 70% and lipoprotein(a) by approximately 25%, with minimal effects of triglycerides and HDL-C.[115,116] Preliminary

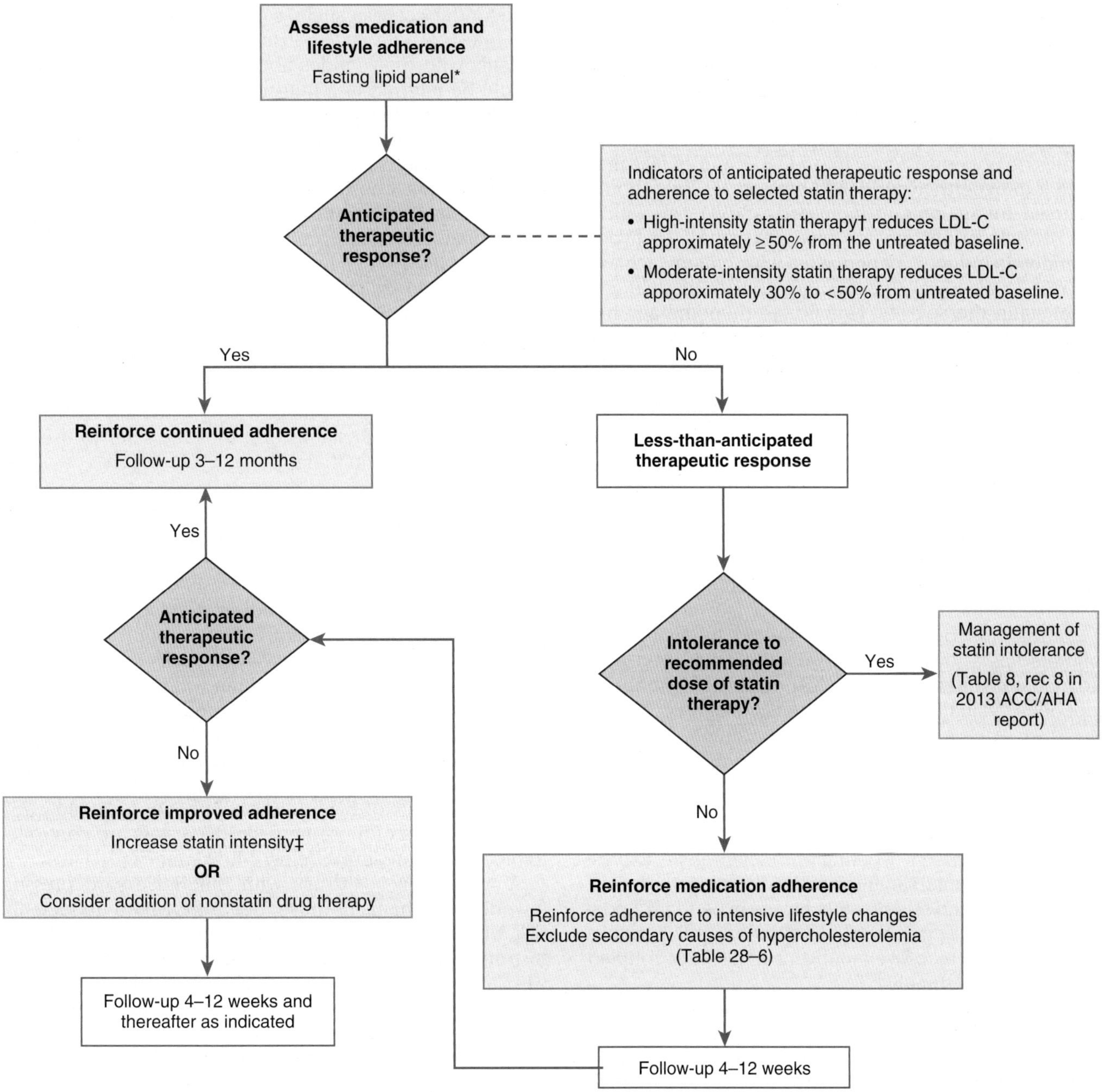

FIG. 28.10 Monitoring therapeutic response and adherence. Colors correspond to the Classes of Recommendation (I = green, IIa = yellow, IIb = orange). *Fasting lipid panel preferred. In a nonfasting individual, a nonfasting non–HDL-C level > 220 mg/dL may indicate genetic hypercholesterolemia that requires further evaluation or a secondary etiology. If nonfasting triglycerides are > 500 mg/dL, a fasting lipid panel is required. †In those already on a statin, in whom baseline LDL-C is unknown, an LDL-C < 100 mg/dL was observed in most individuals receiving high-intensity statin therapy in RCTs. ‡See Section 6.3.1 of 2013 ACC/AHA cholesterol guideline report. *(Reprinted with permission of the authors–Stone NJ, Robinson JG, Lichtenstein AH, et al. 2013 ACC/AHA guideline on the treatment of blood cholesterol to reduce atherosclerotic cardiovascular risk in adults: a report of the American College of Cardiology/American Heart Association Task Force on Practice Guidelines.* J Am Coll Cardiol. *2014;63(25, Part B):2889–2934).*

data from 11–18-month efficacy/safety trials suggest that PCSK9 mAbs may further reduce ASCVD events and mortality in patients receiving background statin therapy.[115,116] However, the magnitude of risk reduction and long-term safety of these has yet to be determined.

In 2015, the PCSK9 monoclonal antibodies alirocumab and evolocumab received Food and Drug Administration (FDA) approval for patients with heterozygous familial hypercholesterolemia and for patients with clinical ASCVD, who are receiving maximally tolerated statin therapy and require additional LDL-C lowering.[117,118] Evolocumab was also approved for use in patients with homozygous familial hypercholesterolemia. These expensive drugs are not considered cost-effective at current wholesale pricing, which has limited patient access.[119]

Other Lipid-Modifying Nonstatins

Other LDL-C lowering drugs include niacin and bile acid sequestrants. Both niacin and bile acid sequestrants used as monotherapy have been shown to reduce ASCVD events in hypercholesterolemic male patients with and without coronary heart disease, respectively.[120,121] Niacin should be avoided in primary prevention. Niacin has not demonstrated added ASCVD event reduction efficacy when added to background statin therapy in patients with ASCVD and has a number of serious adverse effects limiting its use.[68b,122] Niacin should not be used in patients with diabetes and increases the risk of diabetes even in normoglycemic individuals.

No cardiovascular outcomes trials have evaluated bile acid sequestrants added to statin therapy. Bile acid sequestrants should not be used when triglycerides are 300 mg/dL or higher and have numerous drug interactions.[5]

Fibrates do not consistently lower LDL-C and, in fact, may increase it in hypertriglyceridemia patients.[123] They should be reserved for patients at increased ASCVD risk with a history of triglycerides greater than 1000 mg/dL or hypertriglyceridemia-induced pancreatitis, who cannot achieve triglyceride levels lower than 500 mg/dL with lifestyle and maximal statin therapy.[67,124] Fenofibrate monotherapy has been shown to reduce ASCVD events in primary prevention patients with diabetes, but not when added to background statin therapy.[125,126] Subgroup analysis in the Action to Control Cardiovascular Risk in Diabetes (ACCORD) trial suggests fenofibrate may have reduced ASCVD events in patients with low HDL-C and high triglycerides but also showed it increased ASCVD events in women.[126] Gemfibrozil monotherapy has been shown to reduce ASCVD events in primary prevention hypercholesterolemic men and in men with coronary heart disease and low LDL-C, HDL-C, and high triglycerides.[127,128] However, gemfibrozil dramatically increases the risk of serious myopathy when used with statins, and concomitant use should be avoided.[129] Fenofibrate has a lower risk of myopathy when used with low-to moderate-intensity statins.[126] The safety of fenofibrate has not been evaluated with high-intensity statins.

Hypertriglyceridemia

Mild to moderate hypertriglcyeridemia (150–499 mg/dL; 1.7–5.6 mmol/L) is common. Hypertriglyceridemia results from the interaction between hypertriglyceridemic gene expression and environmental stimuli from the diet, excess adiposity, physical inactivity, and other factors. Severe hypertriglyceridemia of 1000 mg/dL or greater (> ≈10 mmol/L) usually results from an autosomal recessive monogenetic disorder coupled with environmental stimuli.[130]

Triglyceride levels above 150 mg/dL are associated with increased ASCVD risk in univariate analyses.[67] But in the majority of studies, hypertriglyceridemia does not appear to be independently associated with increased ASCVD risk once adjusted for other risk factors, including low HDL-C levels.

Drug therapy to lower triglycerides per se has not been shown to reduce ASCVD risk.[132] Hypertriglyceridemic patients with triglyceride levels below 500 mg/dL are managed with the appropriate intensity of statin therapy to reduce their ASCVD risk.[5] High-intensity statin therapy may reduce triglycerides by up to 30%. Patients with triglycerides of 500 mg/dL or higher (5.6 mmol/L) are often treated to reduce their risk of pancreatitis, although pancreatitis is more likely once triglycerides are above 1000 mg/dL (> ≈ 10 mmol/L).[15,131] No cardiovascular outcomes trials or pancreatitis prevention trials have been performed in this population.

Regardless of the genetic etiology, the treatment approach is the same. Lifestyle habits and secondary causes are the major contributors and should be the primary focus of treatment. Although randomized outcomes trials are lacking, triglyceride-lowering therapy is often considered reasonable by experts if triglycerides remain above 500 mg/dL (5.6 mmol/L) despite maximal lifestyle efforts and control of secondary causes, such as diabetes or excessive alcohol or refined carbohydrate consumption (see Table 28.6).[67] All patients with triglycerides above 500 mg/dL (5.6 mmol/L) should be referred to a nutritional therapist for counseling for a low-fat (< 15% total fat), low refined carbohydrate diet and counseled to lose weight and engage in regular, aerobic physical activity.

Fibrates are considered first-line therapy for reducing triglycerides to prevent pancreatitis.[15,67,131] Fenofibrate and gemfibrozil lower triglycerides by 20% to 50%, with variable effects on other lipids depending on the lipid disorder.[111] Gemfibrozil should not be used with statin therapy due to myotoxicity concerns. Marine omega-3 fatty acids, eicosapentaenoic acid (EPA) and docosahexaenoic acid (DHA), reduce triglycerides in a dose-dependent fashion. A 3.5-g to 4-g dose of EPA + DHA will lower triglycerides by approximately 25%.[133] Omega-3 fatty acids appear to have no interactions with statins and thus are safer to use with higher-intensity statin therapy.

BLOOD PRESSURE

Overview

High blood pressure is a leading risk factor for chronic disease burden and premature death around the world.[134] Hypertension affects 30% to 45% of adults.[4,134] After age 65 years, over 65% of men and women will have hypertension. Systolic and diastolic blood pressure levels are associated with an increased risk of ASCVD events, as well as heart failure, chronic renal failure, atrial fibrillation, and eye disease. In the United States, despite high levels of patient awareness of the diagnosis of hypertension, only approximately 75% are treated, and of those treated, 50% or less are controlled to blood pressure levels below 140/90 mm Hg.[4]

A wide range of drugs with differing blood pressure lowering mechanisms have been shown to reduce the risk of stroke, coronary heart disease, and heart failure in primary and secondary prevention and in individuals with and without diabetes or chronic renal disease (Fig. 28.11).[6,15,135–137] For primary prevention patients, diuretics, angiotensin-converting enzyme inhibitors/angiotensin receptor blockers, and calcium-channel blockers appear to be more effective overall than β- or α-blocking agents.[138] The benefits of treatment are mainly driven by the magnitude of blood pressure reduction, not by type of drug.[15]

Blood Pressure Measurement

Office blood pressure measurement can be performed manually or with an automated sphygmomanometer. The proper protocol is to use the mean of two blood pressure measurements taken while the patient is seated, allowing for 5 minutes or more between entry into the office and blood pressure measurement.[139] An appropriate-sized arm cuff should be used, with the patient's arm at the level of the right atrium. Ambulatory and home blood pressure monitoring can be used to confirm a diagnosis of hypertension, or exclude "white coat" hypertension, after the initial screening.

Screening

The United States Preventive Services Task Force (USPTF) recommends screening for high blood pressure in adults

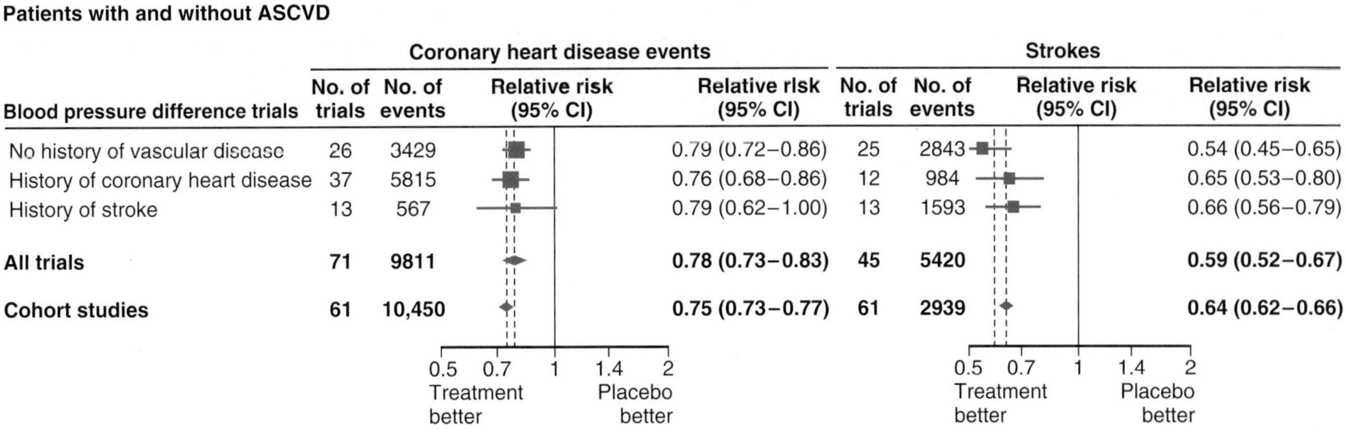

Patients with and without ASCVD
Coronary heart disease events
Strokes
Blood pressure difference trials
No. of trials
No. of events
Relative risk (95% CI)
No history of vascular disease 26 3429 0.79 (0.72–0.86) 25 2843 0.54 (0.45–0.65)
History of coronary heart disease 37 5815 0.76 (0.68–0.86) 12 984 0.65 (0.53–0.80)
History of stroke 13 567 0.79 (0.62–1.00) 13 1593 0.66 (0.56–0.79)
All trials 71 9811 0.78 (0.73–0.83) 45 5420 0.59 (0.52–0.67)
Cohort studies 61 10,450 0.75 (0.73–0.77) 61 2939 0.64 (0.62–0.66)
0.5 0.7 1 1.4 2
Treatment better
Placebo better

FIG. 28.11 Association of each 10-mm Hg reduction in systolic blood pressure and reduction in events from meta-analyses of antihypertensive drug trials. *(From Law M, Morris J, Wald N. Use of blood pressure lowering drugs in the prevention of cardiovascular disease: meta-analysis of 147 randomised trials in the context of expectations from prospective epidemiological studies.* BMJ *2009;338:b1665.)*

aged 18 or older.[139] Adults aged 40 years or older and persons at increased risk for hypertension (including those with systolic blood pressure ≥130 mm Hg or diastolic blood pressure ≥85 mm Hg) should be screened annually. Others should be rescreened every 3 to 5 years. Multiple measurements over time are better than a single measurement. Blood pressure measurements outside the clinical setting may be needed for diagnostic confirmation, including ambulatory and home blood pressure monitoring.

The 2016 ESC/EAS guideline recommends office blood pressure for screening and diagnosis of hypertension, with at least two blood pressure measurements per visit and at least two visits.[15] Repeated measures over several months are needed to identify the patient's "usual" blood pressure and determine treatment. See Box 28.3 for clinical indications for out-of-office blood pressure measurements.

Hypertension Diagnosis

The ESC/EAS and previous Joint National Commission (JNC) 7 guidelines use the same definitions and classification of blood pressure levels, with hypertension defined as a systolic blood pressure of 140 mm Hg or higher and/or a diastolic blood pressure of 90 mm Hg or higher (Table 28.7). The 2016 ESC/EAS guideline identifies different blood pressure thresholds for hypertension diagnosis based on out-of-office measurements (Table 28.8).

Randomized trial evidence now supports a treatment threshold below 140 mm Hg in moderate-risk primary prevention patients. Recent data from the Heart Outcomes Prevention Evaluation (HOPE)-3 trial supports the treatment of systolic blood pressure between 140 and 160 mm Hg in moderate-risk persons.[140] HOPE-3 enrolled an international population of men aged 55 years or over and women aged 65 years or over with at least one additional risk factor (elevated waist-hip ratio, low HDL-C, smoking, dysglycemia without diabetes, premature family history of coronary heart disease, or mild renal dysfunction). However, antihypertensive treatment was of no benefit and caused an excess of adverse events in those with systolic blood pressure below 140 mm Hg at baseline.

Hypertension Treatment

The 2016 ESC/EAS prevention guideline recommendations for the treatment of hypertension are listed in Table 28.9. Although a blood pressure goal below 140/90 mm Hg can be considered for all patients under 60 years old if lifestyle measures fail to reduce blood pressure, the strongest recommendations are for initiation of drug therapy in those aged 60 years or older or with severe hypertension (≥ 180/and or ≥110 mm Hg). In patients 60 years of age or older, with systolic blood pressure of 160 mm Hg or higher, reducing systolic blood pressure to between 140 and 150 mm Hg is recommended, unless the patient is frail or there are concerns about safety.

TABLE 28.7 Definitions and Classification of ESC/EAS Prevention and JNC 7 Hypertension Guidelines

CATEGORY	SYSTOLIC BP (mm Hg)		DIASTOLIC BP (mm Hg)
Optimal	< 120	and	< 80
Normal	120–129	and/or	80–84
High-normal	130–139	and/or	85–89
Grade 1 hypertension	140–159	and/or	90–99
Grade 2 hypertension	160–179	and/or	100–109
Grade 3 hypertension	≥ 180	and/or	≥ 110
Isolated systolic hypertension	≥ 140	and	< 90

Modified from Piepoli MF, Hoes AW, Agewall S, et al. 2016 European guidelines on cardiovascular disease prevention in clinical practice. Eur Heart J. *2016;37(29):2315–2381; Chobanian AV, et al. The Seventh Report of the Joint National Committee on Prevention, Detection, Evaluation, and Treatment of High Blood Pressure: The JNC 7 Report.* JAMA. *2003;289:2560–2571.*

TABLE 28.8 2016 ESC/EAS Prevention Guideline (Blood Pressure Thresholds for Defining Hypertension with Different Types of Blood Pressure Measurement)

	SBP (mm Hg)	DBP (mm Hg)
Office or clinic	140	90
24-hour	125–130	80
Day	130–135	85
Night	120	70
Home	130–135	85

DBP, diastolic blood pressure; *SBP,* systolic blood pressure.
From Piepoli MF, Hoes AW, Agewall S, et al. 2016 European Guidelines on cardiovascular disease prevention in clinical practice: Eur Heart J. 2016;37(29):2315–2381. pii: ehw106.

TABLE 28.9 2016 ESC/EAS Prevention Guideline (Recommendations for the Management of Hypertension)

RECOMMENDATIONS	CLASS[a]	LEVEL[b]
Lifestyle measures (weight control, increased physical activity, alcohol moderation, sodium restriction, and increased consumption of fruits, vegetables, and low-fat dairy products) are recommended in all patients with hypertension and in individuals with high normal BP	I	A
All major BP-lowering drug classes (i.e., diuretics, ACE-I, calcium antagonists, ARBs, and β-blockers) do not differ significantly in their BP-lowering efficacy and thus are recommended as BP-lowering treatment	I	A
In asymptomatic subjects with hypertension but free of CVD, CKD, and DM, total CV risk stratification using the SCORE model is recommended	I	B
Drug treatment is recommended in patients with grade 3 hypertension irrespective of CV risk, as well as in patients with grade 1 or 2 hypertension who are at very high CV risk	I	B
Drug treatment should be considered in patients with grade 1 or 2 hypertension who are at high CV risk	IIa	B
In patients at low to moderate total CV risk and with grade 1 or 2 hypertension, lifestyle measures are recommended	I	B
In patients at low to moderate total CV risk and with grade 1 or 2 hypertension, if lifestyle measures fail to reduce BP, drug treatment may be considered	IIb	B
SBP < 140 mm Hg and DBP < 90 mm Hg are recommended in all treated hypertensive patients < 60 years old	I	B
In patients > 60 years old with SBP ≥ 160 mm Hg, it is recommended to reduce SBP to between 150 and 140 mm Hg	I	B
In fit patients < 80 years old, a target SBP < 140 mm Hg may be considered if treatment is well tolerated. In some of these patients a target SBP < 120 mm Hg may be considered if at (very) high risk and tolerate multiple BP-lowering drugs	IIb	B
In individuals < 80 years and with initial SBP ≥ 160 mm Hg, it is recommended to reduce SBP to between 150 and 140 mm Hg, provided they are in good physical and mental condition	I	B
In frail elderly patients, a careful treatment intensity (e.g., number of BP-lowering drugs) and BP targets should be considered, and clinical effects of treatment should be carefully monitored	IIa	B
Initiation if BP-lowering therapy with a two-drug combination may be considered in patients with markedly elevated baseline BP or at high CV risk. Combination of two drugs at fixed doses in a single pill may be considered because of improved adherence	IIb	C
β-blockers and thiazide diuretics are not recommended in hypertensive patients with multiple metabolic risk factors,[c] due to the increased risk of DM.	III	B

[a]Class of recommendation. [b]Level of evidence. [c]Overweight, obesity, dyslipidemia, impaired glucose tolerance.
ACE-I, Angiotensin-converting enzyme inhibitor; *ARBs,* angiotensin receptor blockers; *BP,* blood pressure; *CKD,* chronic kidney disease; *CV,* cardiovascular; *CVD,* cardiovascular disease; *DBP,* diastolic blood pressure; *SBP,* systolic blood pressure; *SCORE,* Systematic Coronary Risk Estimation.
From Piepoli MF, Hoes AW, Agewall S, et al. 2016 European guidelines on cardiovascular disease prevention in clinical practice: Eur Heart J. *2016;37(29):2315–2381. pii: ehw106.*

Updated US hypertension guidelines were in development at the time this chapter was prepared. The JNC 8 hypertension guideline panel was convened at the same time as the updated previously mentioned cholesterol guideline.[6] The JNC 8 panel performed a similarly rigorous systematic review of randomized cardiovascular outcomes trials. Based on the trials available at the time, they did not find sufficient evidence to treat everyone to blood pressure levels below 140/90 mm Hg, as recommended in the earlier JNC 7 guideline, although an expert recommendation was made to treat blood pressure to below 140/90 mm Hg.[141]

Interpreting SPRINT

After the JNC 8 recommendations were completed, important data from the Systolic Blood Pressure Intervention Trial (SPRINT) has become available.[22] SPRINT randomized primary and secondary prevention US patients at increased cardiovascular risk (age ≥ 50 years without diabetes and at least one of the following: clinical or subclinical cardiovascular disease other than stroke, chronic kidney disease with glomerular filtration rate [GFR] 20–60 mL/min per1.73 m^2 of body surface area, 10-year cardiovascular risk ≥ 15 on the basis of the Framingham Score, or age 75 years or older) and with a systolic blood pressure 130–180 mm Hg to a systolic BP below 120 mm Hg treatment target, compared to those randomized to a systolic BP below 140 mm Hg. SPRINT ended early due a mortality benefit emerging in those after 3.26 years of treatment (hazard ratio 0.73, 95% confidence interval [CI] 0.60–0.90, $p = 0.003$). The mean blood pressure in the less than 140 mm Hg arm was 136 mm Hg, and in the less than 120 mm Hg arm was 121 mm Hg. This means approximately half of the participants randomized to the less than 120 mm Hg goal group had systolic blood pressure greater than 120 mm Hg during the trial. The mean number of antihypertensive drugs was two drugs in the less than 140 mm Hg group and three drugs in the less than 120 mm Hg group. An excess of serious adverse events was observed in the less than 120 mm Hg treatment group: hypotension, syncope, electrolyte abnormalities, and acute kidney failure or injury. Injurious falls were similar in both groups.

A straightforward interpretation of SPRINT[22] and the HOPE-3 trial,[140] described previously, may support:

1. Initiation of drug therapy when blood pressure levels are ≥ 140/or ≥ 90 mm Hg in patients ≥ 50 years with one or more risk factors.
2. Consideration of adding another antihypertensive drug if systolic blood pressure is closer to 140 mm Hg than to 120 mm Hg in those who are tolerating current antihypertensive drug therapy. This is because less than half of the participants in the intensive treatment arm achieved a systolic BP less than 120 mm Hg, and adverse events were higher in the greater than 120 mm Hg group.

Age over 75 Years

The European hypertension guidelines address hypertension treatment after age 75 in a thoughtful evidence-based

TABLE 28.10 ESH/ASC Guidelines for the Management of Arterial Hypertension in the Elderly

RECOMMENDATIONS	CLASS[a]	LEVEL[b]
In elderly hypertensives with SBP ≥ 160 mm Hg there is solid evidence to recommend reducing SBP to between 150 and 140 mm Hg	I	A
In fit elderly patients < 80 years old antihypertensive treatment may be considered at SBP values ≥ 140 mm Hg with a target SBP < 140 mm Hg if treatment is well tolerated	IIb	C
In individuals older than 80 years with an initial SBP ≥ 160 mm Hg it is recommended to reduce SBP to between 150 and 140 mm Hg, provided they are in good physical and mental condition	I	B
In frail elderly patients, it is recommended to leave decisions on antihypertensive therapy to the treating physician, and based on monitoring of the clinical effects of treatment	I	C
Continuation of well-tolerated antihypertensive treatment should be considered when a treated individual becomes an octogenarian	IIa	C
All hypertensive agents are recommended and can be used in the elderly, although diuretics and calcium antagonists may be preferred in isolated systolic hypertension	I	A

[a]Class of recommendation. [b]Level of evidence. *SBP*, Systolic blood pressure.
From Mancia G, et al. Eur Heart J. *2013;31:1281–1357.*

set of recommendations that incorporate consideration of differences in aging trajectories after age 75 (Table 28.10).[142] As in the JNC 8 guideline, strong evidence supports treating systolic blood pressure of 160 mm Hg or higher to between 140 and 150 mm Hg in elderly patients, with the further provision that the patient should be in good physical and mental condition. SPRINT suggests treating to a systolic blood pressure below 140 mm Hg may be reasonable in these patients.[26] However, treatment of hypertension in frail elderly patients needs to be individualized, with careful monitoring for adverse effects, including orthostatic hypertension.[142]

Lifestyle

Lifestyle measures are recommended for all individuals with hypertension (systolic blood pressure ≥ 140 mm Hg or diastolic blood pressure ≥ 90 mm Hg) or high normal blood pressure (systolic blood pressure 130–139 mm Hg or diastolic blood pressure 85–89 mm Hg).[8,15] Diet and physical activity recommendations are listed in Table 28.4. This pattern can be achieved by plans such as the DASH dietary pattern, the American Heart Association Diet, or the US Department of Agriculture (USDA) Food Pattern. Along with weight control and regular physical activity, these lifestyle changes may be sufficient to control modest blood pressure elevations.[15] Reducing sodium intake to 2400 mg/day, or a 1000 mg/day reduction, is recommended, and further reduction in sodium to 1500 mg/day can be considered.[8]

Choice of Antihypertensive Drug Therapy

The JNC 8, USPTF, and ESC/EAS guidelines all recommend initial treatment with a thiazide diuretic, calcium-channel blocker, angiotensin-converting enzyme inhibitor, or angiotensin receptor blocker for non–African-American patients.[6,15,139] For African-American patients, initial treatment is a thiazide or a calcium-channel blocker. For patients with chronic kidney disease, either an angiotensin-converting enzyme inhibitor or angiotensin receptor blocker (but not both) should be initial or add-on treatment.

Antihypertensive therapy can be continued into advanced age as long as it is well tolerated.[6,139,142] Diuretics and calcium antagonists may be preferred in isolated systolic hypertension, although all agents can be used in the elderly.

Monitoring

Generally, antihypertensive therapy should be maintained indefinitely. JNC 8 recommended a clinic follow-up visit within 1 month, with intensification of therapy if needed.[6] In SPRINT, medications were up-titrated to the randomized goal on a monthly basis based on an average of three automated blood pressure measurements taken at the office visit after the patient had been sitting quietly for 5 minutes. On this basis, the 2016 Canadian hypertension guideline recommends the use of automated office blood pressure measurements to guide intensification of drug therapy.[143] Once the desired blood pressure level is achieved, a visit interval of every 3 to 6 months is reasonable.[15] With proper patient instruction and device calibration, home-based blood pressure monitoring may improve blood pressure control.[15]

ASPIRIN

ASCVD remains the leading cause of death in the United States, and colorectal cancer is the third most common cancer.[4,144] The effects of aspirin for reducing the risk of myocardial infarction and stroke are considered primarily due to aspirin's antiplatelet effects, as is the increased risk of bleeding.[145]

The clinical trial evidence for aspirin in primary prevention is much weaker and more inconsistent than the data supporting statins for primary prevention. In a meta-analysis performed to support the 2016 USPTF aspirin recommendations, aspirin modestly reduced the relative risk of nonfatal myocardial infarction by 22% and all-cause mortality by 6%.[146] Only aspirin in doses of 100 mg/day or less reduced the risk of nonfatal stroke (–14%); however, all-cause mortality was not reduced at these doses. In addition, a 2014 trial in a Japanese population found no benefits from aspirin and only an excess of bleeding.[147] Aspirin had no effect on colorectal cancer incidence in the first 10 years of treatment, but reduced colorectal cancer by 40% after 10 years of continuous treatment.[148] Across all primary prevention trials, aspirin increases the risk of major gastrointestinal bleeding by 58% and hemorrhagic stroke by 27%.[149] Estimated excess risk of a major bleeding event was 0.02% per year for a community-based sample taking aspirin.

The ESC/EAS prevention does not recommend aspirin for primary prevention due to the increased risk of major bleeding.[15]

Based on the systematic review of the evidence of cardiovascular benefits and bleeding harms previously described, the USPTF considered aspirin of moderate benefit for reducing the risk of nonfatal myocardial infarction and stroke in adults aged between 50 and 69 years with a 10% or greater 10-year ASCVD risk.[18] Aspirin was also found to reduce the incidence of colorectal cancer after 10 years of use. Counterbalancing the potential benefits of aspirin are the risk of gastrointestinal bleeding and hemorrhagic stroke. These risk are small before age 60 years and small to moderate in those aged 60 to 69 years. There was insufficient evidence to support aspirin for primary prevention in those under 50 years or those 70 years or older. The USPTF risk-benefit analysis used the 2013 ACC/AHA risk assessment guideline's Pooled Cohort Equations, previously described.[7]

Among US adults without cardiovascular disease, 47% take aspirin for primary prevention.[150] Clinicians may consider counseling primary prevention patients who are already on aspirin about the potential benefits and harms of continued aspirin use.

Age 50 to 59 Years

The USPTF made a moderate recommendation for low-dose aspirin for the primary prevention of ASCVD and colorectal cancer in adults aged 50 to 59 years who have a 10% or greater 10-year ASCVD risk provided they have a life expectancy of at least 10 years and are willing to take low-dose aspirin daily for at least 10 years.

Age 60 to 69 Years

The USPTF recommends consideration of low-dose aspirin on an individual basis in persons aged 60 to 69 years with a 10% or greater 10-year ASCVD risk who have a life expectancy of at least 10 years, are at low risk of bleeding, and are willing to take low-dose aspirin daily for at least 10 years. Patient preferences for the potential to benefit versus the potential for harm play an important role due to the narrow margin of benefit versus harm from bleeding.

Age Under 50 or Age 70 Years or Older

Aspirin is not recommended for primary prevention in individuals under 50 years or over 70 years due to insufficient evidence to assess the balance of benefits and harms. The ongoing ASPirin in Reducing Events in the Elderly (ASPREE) trial is evaluating the potential benefits and harms of enteric-coated aspirin (100 mg) for primary prevention in individuals over 65 years of age.[151]

Aspirin Dosage

The optimal aspirin dose is unknown.[18] Primary prevention trials have demonstrated benefits with doses of 75 and 100 mg/day, and 100 and 325 mg every other day. The 75-mg dose seems to be as effective as higher doses but may have a lower risk of bleeding. A pragmatic approach is to use 81 mg/day in the United States and 75 mg in countries outside the United States, as these are the most widely available low- dose preparations.

Bleeding Risk Factors

The USPTF identified numerous risk factors for gastrointestinal bleeding with low-dose aspirin: aspirin dose, history of gastrointestinal ulcers or upper gastrointestinal pain, bleeding disorders, renal failure, severe liver disease, and thrombocytopenia.[18] A meta-analysis of trials that included patients with chronic kidney disease found no reduction in cardiovascular risk but an excess of harm with aspirin treatment.[152] Risk factors for intracranial bleeding include concurrent anticoagulation or nonsteroidal antiinflammatory drug (NSAID) therapy, uncontrolled hypertension, male sex, and older age.

CONCLUSIONS

Healthy lifestyle habits are the foundation of cardiovascular prevention. An extensive body of evidence supports statins and antihypertensive drug therapy for the primary prevention of ASCVD in adults between 50 and 75 years of age. Younger individuals with severe risk factor elevations also benefit from risk factor control. With advancing age, patient preferences and comorbidities may influence preventive therapy.

References

1. Libby P: Current concepts of the pathogenesis of the acute coronary syndromes, *Circulation* 104(3):365–372, 2001.
2. Yusuf S, Rangarajan S, Teo K, et al.: Cardiovascular risk and events in 17 low-, middle-, and high-income countries, *N Engl J Med* 371(9):818–827, 2014.
3. Pencina MJ, D'Agostino Sr RB, Larson MG, et al.: Predicting the 30-year risk of cardiovascular disease: the Framingham Heart Study, *Circulation* 119:3078–3084, 2009.
4. Mozaffarian D, Benjamin EJ, Go AS, et al.: Heart disease and stroke statistics—2015 update: a report from the American Heart Association, *Circulation* 131(4):e29–e322, 2015.
5. Stone NJ, Robinson JG, Lichtenstein AH, et al.: 2013 ACC/AHA guideline on the treatment of blood cholesterol to reduce atherosclerotic cardiovascular risk in adults: a report of the American College of Cardiology/American Heart Association Task Force on Practice Guidelines, *J Am Coll Cardiol* 63(25, Part B):2889–2934, 2014.
6. James PA, Oparil S, Carter BL, et al.: 2014 evidence-based guideline for the management of high blood pressure in adults: report from the panel members appointed to the Eighth Joint National Committee (JNC 8), *JAMA* 311(5):507–520, 2014.
7. Goff Jr DC, Lloyd-Jones DM, Bennett G, et al.: 2013 ACC/AHA guideline on the assessment of cardiovascular risk: a report of the American College of Cardiology/American Heart Association Task Force on Practice Guidelines, *J Am Coll Cardiol* 63(25, Part B):2935–2959, 2014.
8. Eckel RH, Jakicic JM, Ard JD, et al.: 2013 AHA/ACC guideline on lifestyle management to reduce cardiovascular risk: a report of the American College of Cardiology/American Heart Association Task Force on Practice Guidelines, *J Am Coll Cardiol* 63(25, Part B):2960–2984, 2014.
9. Jensen MD, Ryan DH, Apovian CM, et al.: 2013 AHA/ACC/TOS guideline for the management of overweight and obesity in adults: a report of the American College of Cardiology/American Heart Association Task Force on Practice Guidelines and The Obesity Society, *J Am Coll Cardiol* 63(25, Part B):2985–3023, 2014.
10. American Diabetes Association: Standards of care—2016, *Diab Care* 39(Suppl 1):S1–S116, 2016.
11. National Institute for Health and Care Excellence: Lipid modification: cardiovascular risk assessment and the modification of blood lipids for the primary and secondary prevention of cardiovascular disease (Clinical guideline 181), 2014. Available from: http://www.nice.org.uk/guidance/CG181.
12. Expert Panel on Integrated Guidelines for Cardiovascular Health and Risk Reduction in Children and Adolescents: Expert Panel on Integrated Guidelines for Cardiovascular Health and Risk Reduction in Children and Adolescents: summary report, *Pediatrics* 128(Supplement 5):S213–S56, 2011.
13. Siu AL, S: Preventive Services Task Force. Screening for high blood pressure in adults: U.S. Preventive Services Task Force Recommendation Statement, *Ann Intern Med* 163(10):778–786, 2015.
14. Spring B, Moller AC, Colangelo LA, et al.: Healthy lifestyle change and subclinical atherosclerosis in young adults: Coronary Artery Risk Development in Young Adults (CARDIA) study, *Circulation* 130(1):10–17, 2014.
15. Piepoli MF, Hoes AW, Agewall S, et al.: 2016 European guidelines on cardiovascular disease prevention in clinical practice, *Eur Heart J* 37(29):2315–2381, 2016. pii: ehw106.
16. Rabar S, Harker M, O'Flynn N, et al.: Lipid modification and cardiovascular risk assessment for the primary and secondary prevention of cardiovascular disease: summary of updated NICE guidance, 2014.
17. Board J: Joint British Societies' consensus recommendations for the prevention of cardiovascular disease (JBS3), *Heart* 100(Suppl 2):ii1–ii67, 2014.
18. U.S. Preventive Services Task Force: Draft Recommendation Statement: aspirin to prevent cardiovascular disease and cancer, September 2015.
19. Howard BV, Van Horn L, Hsia J, et al.: Low-fat dietary pattern and risk of cardiovascular disease: the Women's Health Initiative randomized controlled dietary modification trial, *JAMA* 295:655–666, 2006.
20. The Look AHEAD Research Group. Cardiovascular effects of intensive lifestyle intervention in type 2 diabetes, *N Engl J Med* 369:145–154, 2013.
21. Deleted in proofs.
22. The SPRINT Investigators: A randomized trial of intensive versus standard blood-pressure control, *N Engl J Med* 373(22):2103–2116, 2015.

23. Mons U, Müezzinler A, Gellert C, et al.: Impact of smoking and smoking cessation on cardiovascular events and mortality among older adults: meta-analysis of individual participant data from prospective cohort studies of the CHANCES consortium, *BMJ* 350, 2015.
24. Physical Activity Guidelines Advisory Committee: *Physical Activity Guidelines Advisory Committee Report, 2008*, Washington, DC, 2008, US Department of Health and Human Services.
25. Holmes HM, Hayley DC, Alexander GC, et al.: Reconsidering medication appropriateness for patients late in life, *Arch Intern Med* 166:605–609, 2006.
26. Deleted in proofs.
27. Lin JS, O'Connor E, Whitlock EP, et al.: Behavioral counseling to promote physical activity and a healthful diet to prevent cardiovascular disease in adults: a systematic review for the U.S. Preventive Services Task Force, *Ann Intern Med* 153(11):736–750, 2010.
28. U.S. Department of Agriculture, Services USDoHaH: Dietary Guidelines for Americans, 2010. Available from: http://health.gov/dietaryguidelines/dga2010/dietaryguidelines2010.pdf.
29. Thorp AA, Owen N, Neuhaus M, et al.: Sedentary behaviors and subsequent health outcomes in adults: a systematic review of longitudinal studies, 1996–2011, *Am J Prev Med* 41(2):207–215, 2011.
30. Rao G, Powell-Wiley TM, Ancheta I, et al.: Identification of obesity and cardiovascular risk in ethnically and racially diverse populations: a scientific statement from the American Heart Association, *Circulation* 132(5):457–472, 2015.
31. Gloy VL, Briel M, Bhatt DL, et al.: Bariatric surgery versus non-surgical treatment for obesity: a systematic review and meta-analysis of randomised controlled trials, *BMJ* 347, 2013.
32. Puzziferri N, Roshek TB, Iii, et al.: Long-term follow-up after bariatric surgery: a systematic review, *JAMA* 312(9):934–942, 2014.
33. Prospective Studies Collaboration: Blood cholesterol and vascular mortality by age, sex, and blood pressure: a meta-analysis of individual data from 61 prospective studies with 55,000 vascular deaths, *Lancet* 370:1829–1839, 2007.
34. Ference BA, Yoo W, Alesh I, et al.: Effect of long-term exposure to lower low-density lipoprotein cholesterol beginning early in life on the risk of coronary heart disease: a Mendelian randomization analysis, *J Am Coll Cardiol* 60:2631–2639, 2012.
35. Gidding SS, Ann Champagne M, de Ferranti SD, et al.: The agenda for familial hypercholesterolemia: a scientific statement from the American Heart Association, *Circulation* 132(22):2167–2192, 2015.
36. Khera AV, Won H-H, Peloso GM, et al.: Diagnostic yield and clinical utility of sequencing familial hypercholesterolemia genes in patients with severe hypercholesterolemia, *J Am Coll Cardiol* 67(22):2578–2589, 2016.
37. Cohen JC, Boerwinkle E, Mosley Jr TH, et al.: Sequence variations in PCSK9, low LDL, and protection against coronary heart disease, *N Engl J Med* 354:1264–1272, 2006.
38. Voight BF, Peloso GM, Orho-Melander M, et al.: Plasma HDL cholesterol and risk of myocardial infarction: a Mendelian randomisation study, *Lancet* 380(9841):572–580, 2012.
39. Navar-Boggan AM, Peterson ED, D'Agostino RB, et al.: Hyperlipidemia in early adulthood increases long-term risk of coronary heart disease, *Circulation* 131(5):451–458, 2015.
40. Cholesterol Treatment Trialists Collaboration: Efficacy and safety of more intensive lowering of LDL cholesterol: a meta-analysis of data from 170,000 participants in 26 randomised trials, *Lancet* 376:1670–1681, 2010.
41. Cannon CP, Blazing MA, Giugliano RP, et al.: Ezetimibe added to statin therapy after acute coronary syndromes, *N Engl J Med* 372(25):2387–2397, 2015.
42. Robinson JG, Smith B, Maheshwari N, et al.: Pleiotropic effects of statins: benefit beyond cholesterol reduction? A meta-regression analysis, *J Am Coll Cardiol* 46:1855–1862, 2005.
43. Robinson JG: Models for describing relations among the various statin drugs, low-density lipoprotein cholesterol lowering, pleiotropic effects, and cardiovascular risk, *Am J Cardiol* 101:1009–1015, 2008.
44. Cholesterol Treatment Trialists Collaborators: The effects of lowering LDL cholesterol with statin therapy in people at low risk of vascular disease: meta-analysis of individual data from 27 randomised trials, *Lancet* 380:581–590, 2012.
45. Taylor F, Huffman M, Macedo A, et al.: Statins for the primary prevention of cardiovascular disease, *Cochrane Database Syst Rev* CD004816, 2013.
46. Moriarty PM, Jacobson TA, Bruckert E, et al.: Efficacy and safety of alirocumab, a monoclonal antibody to PCSK9, in statin-intolerant patients: design and rationale of ODYSSEY ALTERNATIVE, a randomized phase 3 trial, *J Clin Lipidol* 8(6):554–561, 2014.
47. Nissen SE, Stroes E, Dent-Acosta RE, et al.: Efficacy and tolerability of evolocumab vs ezetimibe in patients with muscle-related statin intolerance: the GAUSS-3 Randomized Clinical Trial, *JAMA* 315(15):1580–1590, 2016.
48. National Cholesterol Education Panel: Third Report of the National Cholesterol Education Program (NCEP) Expert Panel on Detection, Evaluation, and Treatment of High Blood Cholesterol in Adults (Adult Treatment Panel III) Final Report, *Circulation* 106:3143–3421, 2002.
49. Gidding SS, Ann Champagne M, de Ferranti SD, et al.: The agenda for familial hypercholesterolemia: a scientific statement from the American Heart Association, *Circulation* 132(22):2167–2192, 2015.
50. Wiegman A, Gidding SS, Watts GF, et al.: Familial hypercholesterolaemia in children and adolescents: gaining decades of life by optimizing detection and treatment, *Eur Heart J* 36(36):2425–2437, 2015.
51. Goldberg AC, Hopkins PN, Toth PP, et al.: Familial hypercholesterolemia: screening, diagnosis and management of pediatric and adult patients: clinical guidance from the National Lipid Association Expert Panel on Familial Hypercholesterolemia, *J Clin Lipidol* 5(3, Suppl 1):S1–S8, 2011.
52. Deleted in proofs.
53. Mozaffarian D, Benjamin EJ, Go AS, et al.: Heart Disease and Stroke Statistics—2016 Update: a report from the American Heart Association, *Circulation* 133(4):e38–e360, 2016.
54. Karmali KN, Goff Jr DC, Ning H, et al.: A systematic examination of the 2013 ACC/AHA pooled cohort risk assessment tool for atherosclerotic cardiovascular disease, *J Am Coll Cardiol* 64:959–968, 2014.
55. Deleted in proofs.
56. Paixao ARM, Ayers CR, Berry JD, et al.: Atherosclerotic cardiovascular prevention: a comparison between the Third Adult Treatment Panel and the New 2013 Treatment of Blood Cholesterol Guidelines, *Circulation Qual Cardiovasc Outcomes* 7:778–779, 2014.
57. Pencina MJ, Navar-Boggan AM, D'Agostino RB, et al.: Application of new cholesterol guidelines to a population-based sample, *N Engl J Med* 370:1422–1431, 2014.
58. Johnson KM, Dowe DA: Accuracy of statin assignment using the 2013 AHA/ACC Cholesterol Guideline versus the 2001 NCEP ATP III Guideline: correlation with atherosclerotic plaque imaging, *J Am Coll Cardiol* 64:910–919, 2014.
59. Pursnani A, Massaro JM, D'Agostino RB, et al.: Guideline-based statin eligibility, coronary artery calcification, and cardiovascular events, *JAMA* 314(2):134–141, 2015.
60. Mortensen M, Nordestgaard BG, Afzal S, et al.: ACC/AHA guidelines superior to ESC/EAS guidelines for primary prevention with statins in nondiabetic Europeans: the Copenhagen General Population Study, *Eur Heart J*, 2016. in press.
61. Puri R, Nissen SE, Shao M, et al.: Impact of baseline lipoprotein and C-reactive protein levels on coronary atheroma regression following high-intensity statin therapy, *Am J Cardiol* 114:1465–1472, 2014.
62. Boekholdt SM, Hovingh GK, Mora S, et al.: Very low levels of atherogenic lipoproteins and the risk for cardiovascular events: a meta-analysis of statin trials, *J Am Coll Cardiol* 64:485–494, 2014.
63. Perk J, De B, Gohlke H, et al.: European guidelines on cardiovascular disease prevention in clinical practice (version 2012). The Fifth Joint Task Force of the European Society of Cardiology and Other Societies on Cardiovascular Disease Prevention in Clinical Practice (constituted by representatives of nine societies and by invited experts). Developed with the special contribution of the European Association for Cardiovascular Prevention & Rehabilitation (EACPR), *Eur Heart J* 33(13):1635–1701, 2012.
64. LaRosa JC, Grundy SM, Waters DD, et al.: Intensive lipid lowering with atorvastatin in patients with stable coronary disease, *N Engl J Med* 352:1425–1435, 2005.
65. Pedersen TR, Faergeman O, Kastelein JJP, et al.: High-dose atorvastatin vs usual-dose simvastatin for secondary prevention after myocardial infarction: the IDEAL Study: a randomized controlled trial, *JAMA* 294:2437–2445, 2005.
66. Cannon C, Braunwald E, McCabe C, et al.: Intensive versus moderate lipid lowering with statins after acute coronary syndromes, *N Engl J Med* 350:1495–1504, 2004.
67. Miller M, Stone NJ, Ballantyne C, et al.: Triglycerides and cardiovascular disease: a scientific statement from the American Heart Association, *Circulation*, 2011.
68. Cholesterol Treatment Trialists Collaborators: Efficacy of cholesterol-lowering therapy in 18,686 people with diabetes in 14 randomised trials of statins: a meta-analysis, *Lancet* 371:117–125, 2008.
68a. Cholesterol Treatment Trialists' (CTT) Collaborators, Efficacy and safety of cholesterol-lowering treatment: prospective meta-analysis of data from 90,056 participants in 14 randomised trials of statins, *Lancet* 366:p. 1267–1278, 2005.
68b. The AIM-HIGH Investigators, Niacin in Patients with Low HDL Cholesterol Levels Receiving Intensive Statin Therapy, *N Engl J Med* 365:p. 2255–2267, 2011.
69. Taskinen M-R, Borén J: New insights into the pathophysiology of dyslipidemia in type 2 diabetes, *Atherosclerosis* 239(2):483–495, 2015.
70. Lloyd-Jones DM, Hong Y, Labarthe D, et al.: Defining and setting national goals for cardiovascular health promotion and disease reduction: the American Heart Association's strategic impact goal through 2020 and beyond, *Circulation* 121:586–613, 2010.
71. Salfati E, Nandkeolyar S, Fortmann SP, et al.: Susceptibility loci for clinical CAD and subclinical coronary atherosclerosis throughout the life-course, *Circ Cardiovasc Genet* 8(6):803–811, 2015.
72. Ridker P, Danielson E, Fonseca F, et al.: Rosuvastatin to prevent vascular events in men and women with elevated C-reactive protein, *N Engl J Med* 359:2195–2207, 2008.
73. Downs J, Clearfield M, Weis S, et al.: Primary prevention of acute coronary events with lovastatin in men and women with average cholesterol levels. Results of AFCAPS/TexCAPS, *JAMA* 279:1615–1622, 1998.
74. Nakamura H, Arakawa K, Itakura H, et al.: Primary prevention of cardiovascular disease with pravastatin in Japan (MEGA Study): a prospective randomised controlled trial, *Lancet* 368:1155–1163, 2006.
75. Glynn RJ, Koenig W, Nordestgaard BrG, et al.: Rosuvastatin for primary prevention in older persons with elevated C-reactive protein and low to average low-density lipoprotein cholesterol levels: exploratory analysis of a randomized trial, *Ann Intern Med* 152(8):488–496, 2010.
76. Shepherd J, Blauw G, Murphy M, et al.: Pravastatin in elderly individuals at risk of vascular disease (PROSPER): a randomised controlled trial, *Lancet* 360:1623–1630, 2002.
77. Deleted in proofs.
78. Kjekshus J, Apetrei E, Barrios V, et al.: Rosuvastatin in older patients with systolic heart failure, *N Engl J Med* 357:2248–2261, 2007.
79. Gissi-HF Investigators: Effect of rosuvastatin in patients with chronic heart failure (the GISSI-HF trial): a randomised, double-blind, placebo-controlled trial, *Lancet* 372:1231–1239, 2008.
80. Wanner C, Krane V, Marz W, et al.: Atorvastatin in patients with type 2 diabetes mellitus undergoing hemodialysis, *N Engl J Med* 353:238–248, 2005.
81. Fellstrom B, Jardine A, Schmieder M, et al.: Rosuvastatin and cardiovascular events in patients undergoing hemodialysis, *N Engl J Med* 360:1395–1407, 2009.
82. Ridker PM, Pradhan A, MacFadyen JG, et al.: Cardiovascular benefits and diabetes risks of statin therapy in primary prevention: an analysis from the JUPITER trial, *Lancet* 380:565–571, 2012.
83. Sattar N, Preiss D, Murray H, et al.: Statins and risk of incident diabetes: a collaborative meta-analysis of randomized statin trials, *Lancet* 375:735–742, 2010.
84. Robinson J: Statins and diabetes risk: how real is it and what are the mechanisms? *Curr Opin Lipidol* 26:228–235, 2015.
85. Stone N, Robinson J, Lichtenstein A, et al.: 2013 ACC/AHA guideline on the treatment of blood cholesterol to reduce atherosclerotic cardiovascular risk in adults, *Circulation* 129(Suppl 2):S1–S45, 2014.
86. Ridker PM, Cook NR: Statins: new American guidelines for prevention of cardiovascular disease, *Lancet* 382:1762–1765, 2013.
87. DeFilippis AP, Young R, Carrubba CJ, et al.: An analysis of calibration and discrimination among multiple cardiovascular risk scores in a modern multiethnic cohort, *Ann Intern Med* 162(4):266–275, 2015.
88. Kavousi M, Leening MG, Nanchen D, et al.: Comparison of application of the ACC/AHA guidelines, Adult Treatment Panel III guidelines, and European Society of Cardiology guidelines for cardiovascular disease prevention in a European cohort, *JAMA* 311(14):1416–1423, 2014.
89. Rana JS, Tabada GH, Solomon MD, et al.: Accuracy of the atherosclerotic cardiovascular risk equation in a large contemporary, multiethnic population, *J Am Coll Cardiol* 67(18):2118–2130, 2016.
90. Muntner P, Colantonio LD, Cushman M, et al.: Validation of the atherosclerotic cardiovascular disease pooled cohort risk equations, *JAMA* 311(14):1406–1415, 2014.
91. Soran H, Schofield JD, Durrington PN: Cholesterol, not just cardiovascular risk, is important in deciding who should receive statin treatment, *Eur Heart J* 36(43):2975–2983, 2015.
92. Nordestgaard BG, Chapman MJ, Ray K, et al.: Lipoprotein(a) as a cardiovascular risk factor: current status, *Eur Heart J* 31(23):2844–2853, 2010.
93. Kamstrup PR, Tybjærg-Hansen A, Nordestgaard BG: Extreme lipoprotein(a) levels and improved cardiovascular risk prediction, *J Am Coll Cardiol* 61(11):1146–1156, 2013.
94. Willeit P, Kiechl S, Kronenberg F, et al.: Discrimination and net reclassification of cardiovascular risk with lipoprotein(a): prospective 15-year outcomes in the Bruneck study, *J Am Coll Cardiol* 64:851–860, 2014.
95. Guan W, Cao J, Steffen BT, et al.: Race is a key variable in assigning lipoprotein(a) cutoff values for coronary heart disease risk assessment: the Multi-Ethnic Study of Atherosclerosis, *Arterioscler Thromb Vasc Biol* 35(4):996–1001, 2015.
96. Nasir K, Bittencourt MS, Blaha MJ, et al.: Implications of coronary artery calcium testing among statin candidates according to American College of Cardiology/American Heart Association Cholesterol Management Guidelines: MESA (Multi-Ethnic Study of Atherosclerosis), *J Am Coll Cardiol* 66(15):1657–1668, 2015.
97. Patel J, Al Rifai M, Blaha MJ, et al.: Coronary artery calcium improves risk assessment in adults with a family history of premature coronary heart disease: results from Multiethnic Study of Atherosclerosis, *Circ Cardiovass Imaging* 8(6):e003186, 2015.
98. Cho H, Klabunde CN, Yabroff KR, et al.: Comorbidity-adjusted life expectancy: a new tool to inform recommendations for optimal screening strategies, *Ann Intern Med* 159(10):667–676, 2013.
99. American Geriatrics Society: Patient-centered care for older adults with multiple chronic conditions: a stepwise approach from the American Geriatrics Society, *J Am Geriatr Soc*, 2012. http://dx.doi.org/10.1111/j.532–5415.2012.04187.x.

100. McClelland RL, Jorgensen NW, Budoff M, et al.: 10-Year coronary heart disease risk prediction using coronary artery calcium and traditional risk factors: derivation in the MESA (Multi-Ethnic Study of Atherosclerosis) with validation in the HNR (Heinz Nixdorf Recall) Study and the DHS (Dallas Heart Study), *J Am Coll Cardiol* 66(15):1643–1653, 2015.
101. Diehm C, Allenberg JR, Pittrow D, et al.: Mortality and vascular morbidity in older adults with asymptomatic versus symptomatic peripheral artery disease, *Circulation* 120(21):2053–2061, 2009.
102. Ito MK, McGowan MP, Moriarty PM: Management of familial hypercholesterolemias in adult patients: recommendations from the National Lipid Association Expert Panel on Familial Hypercholesterolemia, *J Clin Lipidol* 5(3, Suppl 1):S38–S45, 2011.
103. Cholesterol Treatment Trialists Collaborators: Efficacy and safety of LDL-lowering therapy among men and women: meta-analysis of individual data from 174,000 participants in 27 randomized trials, *Lancet*, 2015. http://dx.doi.org/10.1016/S0140-6736(14)61368-4.
104. Feinstein MJ, Achenbach CJ, Stone NJ, et al.: A systematic review of the usefulness of statin therapy in HIV-infected patients, *Am J Cardiol* 115(12):1760–1766, 2015.
105. Robinson J, Davidson M: Combination therapy with ezetimibe and simvastatin to acheive aggressive LDL reduction, *Expert Rev Cardiovasc Ther* 4:461–476, 2006.
106. Cannon CP, Blazing MA, Giugliano RP, et al.: Ezetimibe added to statin therapy after acute coronary syndromes, *N Engl J Med* 372(25):2387–2397, 2015.
107. Robinson JG, Ray K: Counterpoint: low-density cholesterol targets are not needed in lipid treatment guidelines, *Arterioscler Thromb Vasc Biol* 36(4):586–590, 2016.
108. Robinson JG, Stone NJ: The 2013 ACC/AHA guideline on the treatment of blood cholesterol to reduce atherosclerotic cardiovascular disease risk: a new paradigm supported by more evidence, 2015.
109. Deleted in proofs.
110. Lloyd-Jones DM, Morris PB, Ballantyne CM, et al.: 2016 ACC expert consensus decision pathway on the role of non-statin therapies for LDL-cholesterol lowering in the management of atherosclerotic cardiovascular disease risk. A report of the American College of Cardiology Task Force on Clinical Expert Consensus Documents, *J Am Coll Cardiol* 68(1):92–125, 2016.
111. Robinson JG: *Clinical Lipid Management*, ed 1, West Islip, NY, 2016, Professional Communications, Inc.
112. Amgen: Further cardiovascular outcomes research with PCSK9 inhibition in subjects with elevated risk (FOURIER), ClinicalTrials.gov. Identifier: NCT01764633, 2014. Available from: https://clinicaltrials.gov/ct2/show/NCT01764633?term=fourier+amgen&rank=1.
113. Sanofi/Regeneron: ODYSSEY Outcomes: evaluation of cardiovascular outcomes after an acute coronary syndrome during treatment with alirocumab SAR236553 (REGN727), ClinicalTrials.gov. Identifier: NCT01663402, 2015. Available from: https://clinicaltrials.gov/ct2/show/NCT01663402?term=odyssey+outcomes&rank=1.
114. Pfizer: The evaluation of bococizumab (PF-04950615; RN316) in reducing the occurrence of major cardiovascular events in high risk subjects (SPIRE-2b), ClinicalTrials.gov. Identifier: NCT01975389, 2015. Available from: https://clinicaltrials.gov/ct2/show/NCT01975389?term=pfizer+SPIRE&rank=3.
115. Sabatine MS, Giugliano RP, Wiviott SD, et al.: Efficacy and safety of evolocumab in reducing lipids and cardiovascular events, *N Engl J Med* 372(16):1500–1509, 2015.
116. Robinson JG, Farnier M, Krempf M, et al.: Efficacy and safety of alirocumab in reducing lipids and cardiovascular events, *N Engl J Med* 372(16):1489–1499, 2015.
117. Sanofi Aventis, Regeneron Pharmaceuticals Inc: Praluent (alirocumab injection) manufacturer's prescribing information. Available from: http://products.sanofi.us/praluent/praluent.pdf, 2015.
118. Amgen: Repatha (evolocumab) injection prescribing information. Available from: http://pi.amgen.com/united_states/repatha/repatha_pi_hcp_english.pdf, 2015.
119. Tice JA, Kazi DS, Pearson SD: Proprotein convertase subtilisin/kexin type 9 (PCSK9) inhibitors for treatment of high cholesterol levels: effectiveness and value, *JAMA Intern Med* 176(1):107–108, 2016.
120. Lipid Research Clinics Program: The Lipid Research Clinics Coronary Primary Prevention Trial results. I. Reduction in incidence of coronary heart disease, *JAMA* 251:351–364, 1984.
121. Coronary Drug Project: Clofibrate and niacin in coronary heart disease, *JAMA* 231:360–380, 1975.
122. The HPS2-THRIVE Collaborative Group. Effects of extended-release niacin with laropiprant in high-risk patients, *N Engl J Med* 371:203–2012, 2014.
123. Abourbih S, Filion KB, Joseph L, et al.: Effect of fibrates on lipid profiles and cardiovascular outcomes: a systematic review, *Am J Med* 122(10):962, 2009. e1-e8.
124. Berglund L, Brunzell JD, Goldberg AC, et al.: Evaluation and treatment of hypertriglyceridemia: an Endocrine Society clinical practice guideline, *J Clin Endocrinol Metab* 97(9):2969–2989, 2012.
125. The FIELD Study Investigators: Effects of long-term fenofibrate therapy on cardiovascular events in 9795 people with type 2 diabetes mellitus (the FIELD study): randomised controlled trial, *Lancet* 366:1849–1861, 2005.
126. The ACCORD Study Group: Effects of combination lipid therapy in type 2 diabetes mellitus, *N Engl J Med* 362:1563–1574, 2010.
127. Rubins H, Robins S, Collins D, et al.: Gemfibrozil for the secondary prevention of coronary heart disease in men with low levels of high-density lipoprotein cholesterol. Veterans Affairs High-Density Lipoprotein Cholesterol Intervention Trial Study Group, *N Engl J Med* 341:410–418, 1999.
128. Manninen V, Elo MO, Frick MH, et al.: Lipid alterations and decline in the incidence of coronary heart disease in the Helsinki Heart Study, *JAMA* 260:641–651, 1988.
129. Davidson MH, Armani A, McKenney JM, et al.: Safety considerations with fibrate therapy, *Am J Cardiol* 99(6, Suppl 1):S3–S18, 2007.
130. Hegele RA, Ginsberg H, Chapman J, et al.: The polygenic nature of hypertriglcyeridaemia: implications for definition, diagnosis, and management, *Lancet Diab Endocrinol* 655–666, 2014.
131. Miller M, Stone NJ, Ballantyne C, et al.: Triglycerides and cardiovascular disease: a scientific statement from the American Heart Association, *Circulation* 123(20):2292–2333, 2011.
132. Briel M, Ferreira-Gonzalez I, You JJ, et al.: Association between change in high density lipoprotein cholesterol and cardiovascular disease morbidity and mortality: systematic review and meta-regression analysis, *BMJ* 338:b92, 2009.
133. Deleted in proofs.
134. Tzoulaki I, Elliott P, Kontis V, et al.: Worldwide exposures to cardiovascular risk factors and associated health effects: current knowledge and data gaps, *Circulation* 133(23):2314–2333, 2016.
135. Emdin CA, Anderson SG, Callender T, et al.: Usual blood pressure, peripheral arterial disease, and vascular risk: cohort study of 4.2 million adults, *BMJ* 351, 2015.
136. Blood Pressure Lowering Treatment Trialists' Collaboration: Blood pressure lowering and major cardiovascular events in people with and without chronic kidney disease: meta-analysis of randomised controlled trials, *BMJ* 347, 2013.
137. Law M, Morris J, Wald N: Use of blood pressure lowering drugs in the prevention of cardiovascular disease: meta-analysis of 147 randomised trials in the context of expectations from prospective epidemiological studies, *BMJ* 338: b1665, 2009.
138. Fretheim A, Odgaard-Jensen J, Brors O, et al.: Comparative effectiveness of antihypertensive medication for primary prevention of cardiovascular disease: systematic review and multiple treatments meta-analysis, *BMC Med* 10(1):33, 2012.
139. Siu AL: Screening for high blood pressure in adults: U.S. Preventive Services Task Force Recommendation Statement, *Ann Intern Med* 163(10):778–786, 2015.
140. Lonn EM, Bosch J, López-Jaramillo P, et al.: Blood-pressure lowering in intermediate-risk persons without cardiovascular disease, *N Engl J Med* 374(21):2009–2020, 2016.
141. Chobanian AV, Bakris GL, Black HR, et al.: The Seventh Report of the Joint National Committee on Prevention, Detection, Evaluation, and Treatment of High Blood Pressure: the JNC 7 Report, *JAMA* 289:2560–2571, 2003.
142. Mancia G, Fagard R, Narkiewicz K, et al.: 2013 ESH/ESC guidelines for the management of arterial hypertension: the Task Force for the Management of Arterial Hypertension of the European Society of Hypertension (ESH) and of the European Society of Cardiology (ESC), *Eur Heart J* 34(28):2159–2219, 2013.
143. Padwal R, Rabi DM, Schiffrin EL: Recommendations for intensive blood pressure lowering in high-risk patients, the canadian viewpoint, *Hypertension* 68(1):3–5, 2016.
144. Siegel R, Ma J, Zou Z, et al.: Cancer statistics, 2014 *Cancer J Clin*64:9–29, 2014.
145. Patrono C: The multifaceted clinical readouts of platelet inhibition by low-dose aspirin, *J Am Coll Cardiol* 66(1):74–85, 2015.
146. Gauirguis-Blake J, Evans C, Senger A, et al.: *Aspirin for the primary prevention of cardiovascular events: a systematic evidence review for the US Preventive Services Task Force. Evidence Synthesis No 131*, Rockville (MD), 2015, Agency for Healthcare Research and Quality (US). http://www.ncbi.nlm.nih.gov/books/NBK321623/.
147. Ikeda Y, Shimada K, Teramoto T, et al.: Low-dose aspirin for primary prevention of cardiovascular events in Japanese patients 60 years and older with atherosclerotic risk factors: a randomized clinical trial, *JAMA* 312:2510–2520, 2014.
148. Chubak J, Kamineni A, Buist D, et al.: *Aspirin use for the prevention of colorectal cancer: an updated systematic evidence review for the U.S. Preventive Services Task Force*, Rockville (MD), 2015, Agency for Healthcare Research and Quality (US): U.S. Preventive Services Task Force Evidence Syntheses, formerly Systematic Evidence Reviews. http://www.ncbi.nlm.nih.gov/pubmedhealth/PMH0079342/.
149. Whitlock EP, Burda BU, Williams SB, et al.: Bleeding risks with aspirin use for primary prevention in adults: a systematic review for the U.S. Preventive Services Task Force, *Ann Intern Med* 164(12):826–835, 2016.
150. Williams CD, Chan AT, Elman MR, et al.: Aspirin use among adults in the U.S.: results of a national survey, *Am J Prev Med* 48(5):501–508, 2015.
151. Minneapolis Medical Research Foundation: Aspirin Reducing Events in the Elderly (ASPREE). ClinicalTrials.gov. Identifier: NCT01038583. Available from: http://clinicaltrials.gov/ct2/show/NCT01038583?term=aspree&rank=1.
152. Major RW, Oozeerally I, Dawson S, et al. Aspirin and cardiovascular primary prevention in non-endstage chronic kidney disease: a meta-analysis. Atherosclerosis. 251:177–182, 2016.

29 Screening for Atherosclerotic Cardiovascular Disease in Asymptomatic Individuals

Erin D. Michos, Michael J. Blaha, Seth S. Martin, and Roger S. Blumenthal

INTRODUCTION

Despite a 31% decline in the death rate from atherosclerotic cardiovascular disease (ASCVD) (i.e., coronary heart disease [CHD] or stroke) between 2001 and 2011, ASCVD remains the cause of approximately one of three deaths in the United States.[1] More than a third of deaths attributed to ASCVD occur among individuals aged less than 75 years, which is younger than the current life expectancy of 79 years.[1] ASCVD exists on a spectrum, with many high-risk primary prevention patients having ASCVD event rates similar to lower-risk secondary prevention patients (those who have had a prior ASCVD event).

As over half of major ASCVD events occur in previously asymptomatic people, it is critical to identify "at-risk" individuals for early implementation of preventive strategies and treatments. The long incubation period of atherosclerosis allows for such intervention. Indeed, intensive risk factor modification via both lifestyle improvements and pharmacologic treatments of cholesterol, blood pressure, and glycemic control has been shown to modestly regress and stabilize existing atherosclerotic plaques and ultimately reduce ASCVD events.[2]

Unfortunately, unhealthy lifestyle habits and suboptimal risk factor control remain unacceptably high in most populations. Some of the most effective interventions for ASCVD risk reduction are lifestyle modifications. Emphasis must be placed on both preventing ASCVD risk factor development (primordial prevention) and treating existing risk factors (primary prevention).

In 1985, Geoffrey Rose wrote a seminal article entitled "Sick individuals and sick populations." It conveyed the key message that, despite the fact that high-risk individuals gain the most from preventive measures, the greatest number of deaths from ASCVD occur among individuals at the low- or medium-risk end of the risk distribution, simply because many more people fall into these categories.[3] This became known as the classic *Rose paradox* and highlights that both "high-risk" and "population-based" preventive strategies are needed and are in fact complementary.[4] It is therefore imperative to employ both population-based and individualized approaches for comprehensive ASCVD prevention (Fig. 29.1). The purpose of individualized risk assessment is to identify persons at a stage when interventions could effectively alter the course of the disease and reduce ASCVD morbidity and/or mortality.

In this chapter, we discuss various tests that can be potentially used for "screening" the asymptomatic individual for the detection of ASCVD. We will distinguish between the roles of traditional population-based screening and individualized risk assessment as strategies for reducing ASCVD risk and optimizing cardiovascular health. There are other tests more commonly used for diagnostic purposes in the evaluation and management of patients with CHD or symptoms suggestive of CHD (e.g., echocardiography, pharmacologic stress testing, coronary computed tomography angiography, cardiac magnetic resonance imaging, and coronary angiography). They are not discussed here in much detail as we will focus on assessment of the asymptomatic individual. Table 29.1 outlines our conceptual distinction between true *screening*, individualized *risk assessment*, and *diagnostic testing*.

Distinction Between Traditional Screening and Individualized Risk Assessment

Traditional screening is defined as the routine evaluation of a general population with the goal of *detection* of disease among people without signs or symptoms of the disease, not *exclusion* of disease.[5] In 1968, Wilson and Jungner outlined 10 criteria for a valid screening program for the World Health Organization (WHO) (Box 29.1)[5] that still hold true today. Briefly, a screening program should be targeted at a disease that is an important health problem, a disease that has a long latent phase where early detection is possible, where treating in an early stage is more beneficial than treating at a later stage, and where potential benefits of screening outweigh the costs.

Thus, screening for ASCVD meets all of these WHO criteria and has great appeal due to the long disease latency, emerging technologies for early detection, and existence of

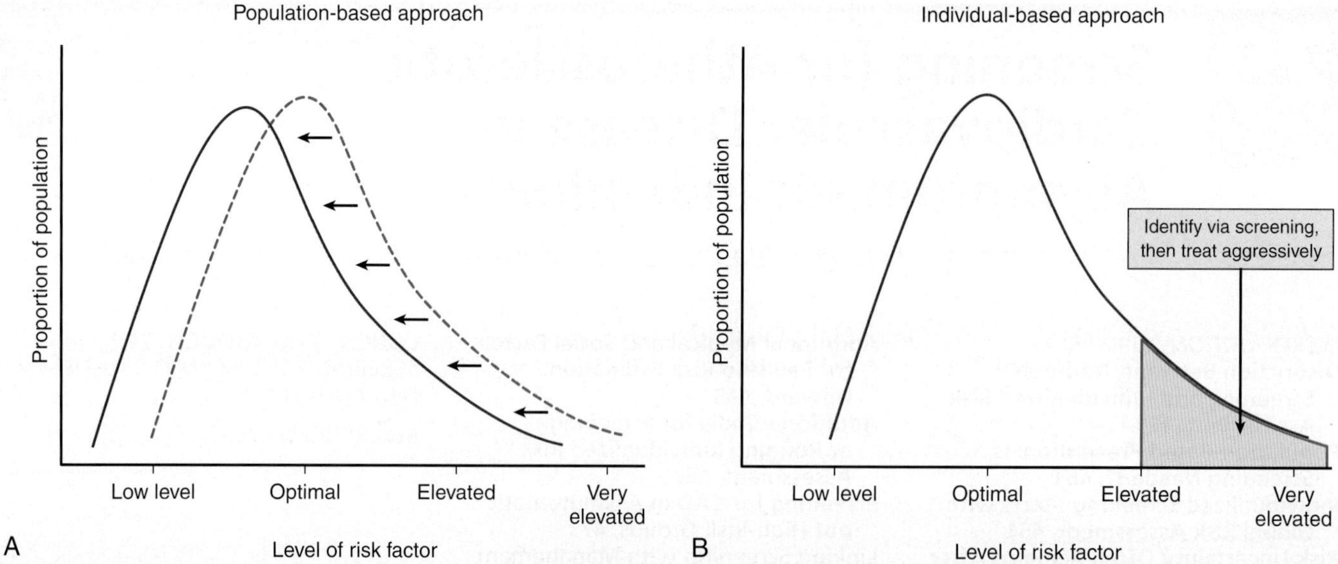

FIG. 29.1 (A) Population-based approach to control of risk factors. **(B)** Individual-based approach to control of risk factors. *(From Blaha MJ, Gluckman T, Blumenthal RS. Chapter 1 – Preventive cardiology: past, present, and future. In: Blumenthal RS, Wong N, Foody D, editors. Preventive Cardiology: A Companion to Braunwald's Heart Disease. 2011: Chapter 1.)*

TABLE 29.1 Interpretations of the Term *Screening* for Atherosclerotic Cardiovascular Disease

	GOAL	TARGET POPULATION	SCREENING OUTCOMES	PARAMETERS OF EFFICACY	EXAMPLE OF POTENTIALLY EFFECTIVE STRATEGY	GUIDELINES
Traditional screening	Early detection of unheralded disease	Healthy people General asymptomatic population	Identify high-risk cases	Sensitivity Specificity PPV NPV	Population-based screening for total cholesterol and blood pressure	USPSTF
Individual risk assessment	Individualize risk to inform clinical decision-making	Individual patients "Intermediate" risk Those in whom "treatment decisions uncertain"	Identify lower than expected risk ("derisk") AND Identify higher than expected risk	C-statistic NRI NNT NNH	Global risk scoring Coronary artery calcium scoring	ACC/AHA ESC/EAS
Diagnostic testing	Confirm clinical suspicion, make diagnosis	Symptomatic patients	Make clinical diagnosis	Sensitivity Specificity Negative and positive likelihood ratios	Stress echocardiography	ACC/AHA

ACC, American College of Cardiology; *AHA,* American Heart Association; *EAS,* European Atherosclerosis Society; *ESC,* European Society of Cardiology; *NNH,* number need to harm; *NNT,* number needed to treat; *NPV,* negative predictive value; *NRI,* net reclassification index; *PPV,* positive predictive value; *USPSTF,* US Preventive Services Task Force.

BOX 29.1 The Wilson–Jungner Criteria for a Screening Program

1. The condition being screened for should be an important health problem.
2. The natural history of the condition should be adequately understood.
3. There should be a latent stage of disease where early detection is possible.
4. Treatment at an early stage should be of more benefit than at a later stage.
5. A suitable test should be devised for the early stage.
6. The test should be acceptable to the population.
7. Intervals for repeating the test should be determined.
8. Adequate health service provision should be made for the extra clinical workload resulting from screening.
9. The risks, both physical and psychological, should be less than the benefits.
10. The costs should be balanced against the benefits.

From Wilson JMG, Jungner G. *Principles and Practice of Screening for Disease.* Geneva: World Health Organization; 1968.

proven therapies that slow its natural history. Nonetheless, various experts have pointed to potential problems with ASCVD screening due to false-positive test results, inappropriate downstream testing, and creation of "pseudodisease."[6] Pseudodisease means that some individuals with subclinical atherosclerosis may not be destined to have an ASCVD event and there is a risk of overtreatment with medications.

One of the WHO criteria is that costs should be balanced against potential benefits. For ASCVD screening, costs include not only the direct cost of the screening test itself but downstream costs from additional testing, specialty referrals, and treatments; sometimes screening can even lead to more invasive procedures such as coronary angiography and revascularization, which have their own associated risks and expense.[7] In addition, there might be psychological harm from anxiety or being labeled as "diseased" because of subclinical atherosclerosis or mild left ventricular dysfunction.

Several organizations have issued guidelines on ASCVD screening, including the United States Preventive Service Task

Force (USPSTF), the American College of Cardiology (ACC)/American Heart Association (AHA), and the European Society of Cardiology (ESC)/European Atherosclerosis Society (EAS). Interestingly, these guidelines often reach different conclusions, owing in large part to different interpretations of the role of screening in routine clinical care. Table 29.2 outlines potential screening or risk assessment tools and the recommendations for or against their use in asymptomatic individuals by these major guideline bodies.

The USPSTF has consistently advised against *routine* screening for ASCVD beyond measurement of traditional ASCVD risk factors such as total cholesterol and blood pressure.[8] The recommendations from the USPSTF are best understood in the context of our definition of traditional screening. Because most current tests for the diagnosis of CHD are limited by a low positive predictive value for future CHD events (thus, there is concern for false-positive tests and overtreatment), these tests fail as broad-based population-wide screening tests per the USPSTF criteria.

The ACC/AHA guidelines[9,10] and the ESC guidelines[11] take a different approach to screening, targeting their recommendations at the individual patient rather than the larger population. This approach is commonly referred to as *clinical risk assessment*. The goal of individual risk assessment is to inform therapy decisions, particularly in intermediate-risk patients or in patients in whom treatment decisions are otherwise uncertain. As opposed to traditional screening, which focuses exclusively on disease detection, when conducting individual risk assessment, the identification of low ASCVD risk (and, therefore, persons not in need of the aggressive pharmacologic prevention treatment) is equally important. The hallmark of individual risk assessment is that patients may move both up and down the risk spectrum after testing (i.e., risk reclassification). Clinical risk assessment offers the opportunity to rule out high-risk states (and the potential to reduce the intensity of preventive interventions and avoid or withdraw pharmacologic therapy) in a patient who would otherwise have qualified for aggressive treatment based purely on risk factor–based ASCVD screening.

Population-Based Prevention: Is Screening Needed?

Several strategies for ASCVD prevention do not require any type of screening. Foremost among these are purely population-based strategies, which seek to modify risk for everyone across an entire population and are a primary tool for primordial ASCVD prevention. Examples of successful population-based prevention strategies include public smoking bans, trans-fat bans, and salt reduction in packaged and prepared foods.

Some experts have advocated for dismissal of formal screening and adoption of a simple "treat-all" approach to ASCVD prevention. For example, some cost-effectiveness analyses have suggested that treating all adults aged 55 years and over with a low-cost statin may be more cost-effective than any currently available screening strategy.[12] A related strategy adapted to populations with less healthcare resources is the polypill, where all older patients are treated with a combination pill including a statin, aspirin, angiotensin-converting enzyme inhibitor or angiotensin receptor blocker, and thiazide diuretic.[13] Interestingly, the 2013 ACC/AHA Cholesterol Guidelines,[14] which lowered the threshold for recommending statin therapy, have inched closer toward a modified age-based treat-all approach with statin therapy for men over the age of 60 and women over the age of 65. As a general rule, when treatment thresholds are lowered, the importance of traditional population-based screening decreases (because most people will already have qualified for pharmacologic treatment) and the importance of individual risk assessment increases (to determine which individuals might avoid pharmacologic treatment at that point in time and for the next few years).

As a result, in most industrialized countries with greater healthcare budgets, there is an increasing push for greater personalization of preventive therapy. A fundamental goal of individual risk assessment is to limit overtreatment by matching the intensity of preventive therapy to the absolute risk of the patient, thereby maximizing potential benefit while minimizing the potential for harm (Fig. 29.2).

Individualized Screening Starts with Global Risk Assessment

The typical initial approach to screening is ascertainment of traditional ASCVD risk factors, and for specific age-groups (generally excluding the young and the elderly), to estimate one's 10-year global risk for ASCVD. Multiple risk prediction models have been developed (Table 29.3). Most models include age, sex, smoking status, systolic blood pressure (as well as antihypertensive treatment), total cholesterol, high-density lipoprotein cholesterol, and diabetes mellitus. Some additionally consider family history of ASCVD (Reynolds risk score,[15,16] QRISK,[17] ASSIGN,[18] PROCAM[19]) or markers of inflammation (Reynolds risk score), and some of the European risk scoring models (QRISK, ASSIGN) are unique by including measures of social deprivation.

The ESC/EAS guidelines recommend using the SCORE[20] system, which estimates 10-year risk of fatal ASCVD, with separate risk estimations for high- and low-risk regions in Europe.[21] In the ESC/EAS guidelines, recommendations for drug treatment of dyslipidemia (vs lifestyle alone) are based on both one's estimated 10-year risk of fatal ASCVD using SCORE (with < 1% being low risk, 1–4% moderate risk, 5–10% high risk, and ≥ 10% very high risk) and one's low-density lipoprotein cholesterol (LDL-C) level.[21] In general, individuals at higher predicted fatal ASCVD risk are recommended for drug treatment at much lower LDL-C levels.

In the United States, the 2013 ACC/AHA guideline on the assessment of cardiovascular risk[10] endorses risk factor screening every 4 to 6 years for those aged 20 to 79 years and application of the pooled cohort equations in asymptomatic adults aged 40 to 79 years to estimate 10-year risk for a first "hard" ASCVD event (myocardial infarction [MI] or stroke). The ACC/AHA risk estimator was not designed to be used in those already on statin therapy. In contrast to previous cardiovascular risk scores, there are now separate models by race (e.g., non-Hispanic whites and blacks) and by sex for more refined risk prediction. These guidelines are linked to the ACC/AHA cholesterol guidelines,[14] which state that higher-risk individuals (10-year predicted risk of ASCVD ≥ 7.5%) are recommended for statin treatment, after a clinician-patient discussion.[22] Moreover, those persons with a 5% to 7.4% risk over the next decade can also be considered for moderate-intensity statin therapy after a clinician-patient discussion. In addition, the ACC/AHA guidelines support estimating a 30-year or lifetime ASCVD risk based on traditional risk factors for adults aged 20 to 59 who are not at high short-term (i.e., 10-year) risk.

TABLE 29.2 Potential Atherosclerotic Cardiovascular Disease (ASCVD) Screening or Risk Assessment Tools and Their Recommended Use by the USPSTF, ACC/AHA, and ESC/EAS Guidelines

	USPSTF	ACC/AHA	ACC/AHA	ESC/EAS
Grading of recommendations	*Grade A:* Recommend. High certainty of significant benefit. *Grade B:* Recommend. High certainty of moderate benefit or moderate certainty of moderate to significant benefit. *Grade C:* May be considered in select patients. For most, only small benefit likely. *Grade D:* Not recommended. Moderate to high certainty that there is no benefit or harms outweigh benefits. *Grade I:* No recommendation. Insufficient evidence to balance benefits and harms.	*Class I:* Recommend. Benefits much greater than risk. *Class IIa:* Reasonable. Benefit generally greater than risk. *Class IIb:* May be considered. Usefulness less well established. *Class III:* No benefit or harm. Not recommended.	*Class I:* Recommend. Benefits much greater than risk. *Class IIa:* Reasonable. Benefit generally greater than risk. *Class IIb:* May be considered. Usefulness less well established. *Class III:* No benefit or harm. Not recommended.	*Class I:* Recommend. Benefits much greater than risk. *Class IIa:* Reasonable. Benefit generally greater than risk. *Class IIb:* May be considered. Usefulness less well established. *Class III:* No benefit or harm. Not recommended.
	USPSTF	**ACC/AHA 2010 Risk Assessment[9]**	**ACC/AHA 2013 Risk Assessment[10]**	**ESC/EAS**
Global risk assessment	2009[8] Clinicians should use the Framingham risk model to assess CHD risk and to guide risk-based therapy until further evidence is obtained.	2010 Global risk scores (such as FRS) should be performed in all asymptomatic adults without known CHD (*class I*).	2013 Apply race-/sex-specific pooled cohort equations to predict 10-year risk of ASCVD events among non-Hispanic blacks and whites, age 40 to 79 years old (*class I*) and consider using for other race/ethnic populations (*class IIb*). Measure ASCVD risk factors every 4 to 6 years in adults aged 20 to 79 years and estimate 10-year ASCVD risk every 4 to 6 years in adults aged 40 to 79 without known ASCVD (*IIa*). Assess 30-year or lifetime risk in adults aged 20 to 59 without ASCVD who are not at high short-term risk (*IIb*).	2011[21] Lipid screening is recommended in those with established ASCVD, diabetes, hypertension, smoking, obesity, family history of ASCVD, family history of dyslipidemias, chronic inflammatory diseases, and chronic kidney disease (*class I*) and in men over age 40 and women over age 50 (*class IIb*). 2012[11] Global risk estimation using multiple risk factors such as the SCORE estimator is recommended for asymptomatic adults without evidence of ASCVD (*class I, level of evidence [LOE] C*).
Electrocardiogram (ECG) at rest	2012[83] Recommend against use of a resting ECG for screening asymptomatic adults at *low* risk for CHD events (*grade D*). Insufficient evidence for the use of a resting ECG for screening asymptomatic adults at *intermediate to high* risk for CHD events (*grade I*).	2010 May be reasonable in asymptomatic adults with hypertension and diabetes (*IIa*) or among those without hypertension/diabetes (*IIb*).	2013 Not addressed.	
Treadmill stress ECG	2012[83] Recommend against the use of an exercise ECG for screening asymptomatic adults at low risk for CHD events (*grade D*). Insufficient evidence for the use of an exercise ECG for screening asymptomatic adults at *intermediate to high* risk for CHD events (*grade I*).	2010 May be reasonable for risk assessment of intermediate-risk asymptomatic adults, especially if non-ECG factors are considered as exercise capacity (*IIb*).	2013 No recommendation for or against measuring cardiorespiratory fitness.	2012[11] Exercise ECG may be considered for ASCVD risk assessment in moderate-risk asymptomatic adults (including sedentary adults considering starting a vigorous exercise program), particularly when attention is paid to non-ECG markers, e.g., cardiorespiratory fitness (*class IIB, LOE B*).

Coronary artery calcium (CAC)	2009[8] Insufficient evidence for using CAC screening among intermediate-risk adults (*grade I*).	2010 May be reasonable for risk assessment among intermediate-risk adults (10% to 20% ATP III FRS) (*IIa*) or could be considered for low to intermediate risk (6% to 10%) (*IIb*).	2013 If risk-based treatment decision is uncertain, CAC ≥ 300 or ≥ 75th age/gender/race percentile may prompt consideration of revising risk assessment upward (*IIb*).	2012[11] Measurement of CAC should be considered for ASCVD risk assessment in asymptomatic adults at moderate risk (*class IIa, LOE B*).
Carotid intima-media thickness (cIMT)	2014[155] Do not screen for carotid stenosis in general population (*grade D*). 2009[8] Insufficient evidence for using cIMT for risk assessment of intermediate-risk adults (*grade I*).	2010 May be reasonable for risk assessment among intermediate-risk adults (*IIa*).	2013 Not recommended (*class III*).	2012[11] Measurement of cIMT and/or screening for carotid plaques should be considered for ASCVD risk assessment in asymptomatic adults at moderate risk (*class IIa, LOE B*).
Ankle-brachial index (ABI)	2013[164] Insufficient evidence to recommend for or against screening in general population (*grade I*); if any benefit, it would be among those at increased risk for peripheral artery disease who are not already receiving interventions for ASCVD risk reduction. 2009[8] Insufficient evidence for using ABI for risk assessment of intermediate-risk adults (*grade I*).	2010 May be reasonable for intermediate risk (*IIa*).	2013 If risk-based treatment decision is uncertain, ABI < 0.9 may promote consideration of revising risk assessment upward (*IIb*).	2012[11] Measurement of ABI should be considered for ASCVD risk assessment in the asymptomatic adult at moderate risk (*class IIa, LOE B*).
High-sensitivity C-reactive protein (hs-CRP)	2009[8] Insufficient evidence for using for risk stratification among intermediate-risk adults (*grade I*).	2010 Among men ≥ 50 or women ≥ 60 years of age with LDL-C < 130 mg/dL not already on statins (i.e., JUPITER eligibility criteria), may be useful for selecting statin therapy (*IIa*). Among intermediate-risk asymptomatic men < 50 and women < 60 years of age, may be reasonable for risk assessment (*IIb*). Not recommended for high-risk or low-risk adults (men < 50, women < 60 years) (*class III*).	2013 If risk-based treatment decision is uncertain, hs-CRP ≥ 2 mg/L may promote consideration of revising risk assessment upward (*IIb*).	2012[11] hs-CRP may be considered to refine risk assessment in patients with unusual or moderate ASCVD risk profile (*class IIb, LOE B*). hs-CRP should not be measured in asymptomatic low-risk individuals and high-risk individuals to assess 10-year ASCVD risk (*class III, LOE B*).
Coronary CT angiography (CTA)		2010 Not recommended for risk assessment among asymptomatic adults (*class III*).	2013 Not addressed.	2013[190] Not recommended as a screening test in asymptomatic individuals without a clinical suspicion of CHD (class I).

ACC, American College of Cardiology; *AHA*, American Heart Association; *CHD*, coronary heart disease; *CT*, computed tomography; *EAS*, European Atherosclerosis Society; *ESC*, European Society of Cardiology; *FRS*, Framingham risk score; *LDL-C*, low-density lipoprotein cholesterol; *USPSTF*, US Preventive Services Task Force.

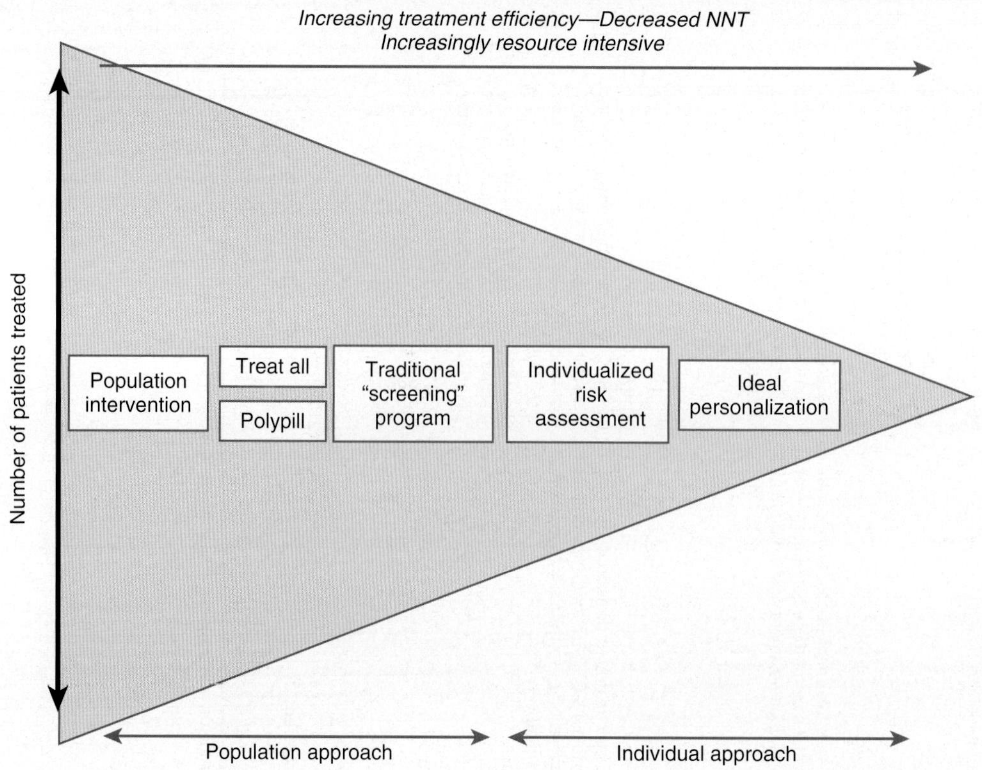

FIG. 29.2 Population-based versus individual-based approaches to preventive therapy: selection of target groups. The number needed to treat (NNT) decreases and resource utilization increases as the treatment spectrum narrows from population-based to individual-based approaches.

TABLE 29.3 Comparison of Global Cardiovascular Risk Prediction Estimators

	REGION	VARIABLES INCLUDED	OUTCOMES PREDICTED	NOTES ON SUBGROUP
SCORE[20] (2003)	Europe	Age, sex, smoking, SBP, and total cholesterol	10-year risk of fatal* total ASCVD (MI, stroke, occlusive arterial disease, sudden cardiac death)	Separate equations for low- and high-risk regions of Europe Diabetics already considered high risk
Framingham CHD[191] (1998)	Framingham, MA, USA	Age, sex, total cholesterol or LDL-C, HDL-C, SBP, diabetes, smoking	10-year risk for total CHD (angina, unstable angina, MI, CHD death)	
Framingham global CVD[192] (2008)	Framingham, MA, USA	Age, sex, total cholesterol, HDL-C, SBP, BP treatment, diabetes, smoking	10-year risk of hard ASCVD plus cardiac failure (MI, CHD death, stroke, stroke death, heart failure)	
ATP III[193] (2001)	Framingham, MA, USA	Age, sex, total cholesterol, HDL-C, SBP, BP treatment, smoking	10-year risk of hard CHD (MI or CHD death)	Diabetics already considered high risk
Reynolds risk score (2008, men;[16] 2007, women[15])	USA	Men: age, total cholesterol, HDL-C, hs-CRP, SBP, smoking, family history of premature CHD Women: age, total cholesterol, HDL-C, hs-CRP, SBP, hemoglobin A_{1c}, family history of premature CHD	Total CHD including revascularizations (MI, CHD death, stroke, stroke death, coronary revascularizations)	Separate equations for men and women, and for non-Hispanic whites and non-Hispanic blacks
QRisk[17] (2007)	United Kingdom	Age, sex, smoking, SBP, BP treatment, ratio of total cholesterol to HDL-C, body mass index, family history of premature CVD, social deprivation	10-year risk of total CHD including revascularizations (angina, unstable angina, revascularizations, MI, CHD death, stroke, stroke death, TIA)	
ACC/AHA pooled cohort equations[10] (2013)	USA	Age, sex, race, total cholesterol, HDL-C, SBP, BP treatment, smoking, diabetes	10-year risk of hard ASCVD (MI, CHD death, stroke, stroke death)	Races other than white and black should use equation for white race/ethnicity
PROCAM[19] (2002)	Germany	Age, LDL-C, HDL-C, SBP, diabetes, smoking, family history of CVD	10-year risk of hard CHD (MI and CHD death)	Equation for men only
ASSIGN[18] (2007)	Scotland	Age, sex, postal code (geography), social deprivation, smoking status and cigarette dosing, family history of CVD, total cholesterol, HDL-C, SBP, diabetes	10-year ASCVD (CHD, cerebrovascular disease, ASCVD death, revascularization)	

*To estimate risk for nonfatal + fatal ASCVD, multiply by 3 in men, by 4 in women, and slightly less for older adults.

ASCVD, Atherosclerotic cardiovascular disease; *CHD*, coronary heart disease; *HDL-C*, high-density lipoprotein cholesterol; *hs-CRP*, high sensitivity C-reactive protein; *LDL-C*, low-density lipoprotein cholesterol; *MI*, myocardial infarction; *SBP*, systolic blood pressure; *TIA*, transient ischemic attack.

The USPSTF also recently posed draft recommendations on statin use for the primary prevention of ASCVD in adults on its website.[23] They recommended that the people who benefit most from statin use are 40 to 75 years of age with at least one other risk factor for ASCVD and have a 10-year ASCVD risk estimate of 10% or greater (grade B recommendation). They advise that those with a 7.5% to 10% estimated 10-year risk are less likely to benefit and should talk to their doctor (grade C recommendation).

Risk Uncertainty Often Remains After Global Risk Assessment

In contrast to the ASCVD risk estimation tools developed for the United States and Europe, there are many areas of the world such as the BRICS countries (Brazil, Russia, India, China, and South Africa) where accurate tools have not been developed; yet these countries have a large burden of cardiovascular disease.[24] Current risk estimation calculators may over- or underestimate risk in these populations. Caution should be used when applying the ACC/AHA pooled cohort equations to groups outside the United States and to groups that are neither white nor black within the United States. This may result in overestimation of ASCVD risk among those of Chinese/East Asian descent and underestimation in American Indians and those of South Asian descent.

In addition, in the context of epidemiologic trends pointing toward continually decreasing ASCVD rates in the United States[25] and in many developed countries, there remains a concern that risk scores such as the ACC/AHA pooled cohort equations that are based on historic data may systematically overestimate ASCVD risk in modern populations.[26,27]

Furthermore, with all risk calculators, applying the results from population-based estimators to clinical decision-making at the individual level can be problematic. Specifically, these calculators estimate the average risk in a group of individuals who have similar risk factor profiles; however, a given risk score is far more accurate for this group than it is for any individual within the group. Indeed, with respect to the individual, each estimate has a theoretical confidence interval that is unknown and that may overlap personalized treatment thresholds.[28]

A critical feature of the 2013 ACC/AHA guidelines is the acknowledgment that in many cases after initial 10-year risk estimation, the treatment decision about statin therapy will still remain uncertain to either the patient or the clinician. The guidelines allow for revising one's risk status *upward* if one of the following is present: elevated lifetime risk, family history of premature ASCVD, high-sensitivity C-reactive protein (hs-CRP) ≥ 2.0 mg/L, LDL-C ≥ 160 mg/dL, abnormal coronary artery calcium (CAC) score (Agatston score ≥ 300 or ≥ 75th percentile for one's age and sex), or ankle-brachial index (ABI) < 0.9.[10,29]

The ESC/EAS guidelines, which endorsed the SCORE estimator as a starting point, also acknowledged uncertainty by including many important "qualifiers" in their document where risk estimation may need to be adjusted upward or downward based on an individual's pretest probability.[21] These guidelines state that (1) risk will be overestimated in countries with falling ASCVD mortality rates and underestimated in countries where mortality is increasing; (2) at a given age, women will have a lower predicted 10-year ASCVD risk than men, but this may be misleading because eventually similar numbers of women will die of ASCVD compared to men; (3) risk will be higher in individuals with social deprivation; (4) risk will be higher among those who are sedentary and have central obesity; (5) risk will be higher among those with low high-density lipoprotein (HDL)-C, increased triglycerides, increased apolipoprotein B, or increased hs-CRP; (6) risk will be higher among asymptomatic individuals with evidence of subclinical atherosclerosis; (7) risk will be higher among those with impaired renal function; (8) risk will be higher among those with a family history of premature ASCVD; and (9) risk will be lower among those with high HDL-C or a family history of longevity.

Despite these limitations, global risk estimation tools are helpful in initiating a risk-based discussion of preventive pharmacologic therapy, and we strongly endorse their routine use as a starting point. But, given these caveats of risk underestimation among certain patient subgroups (i.e., potential for undertreatment) alongside concerns for risk overestimation in other populations combined with much lower treatment thresholds (i.e., potential for overtreatment), the need for further individualized risk assessment has become increasingly important.

With their extensive safety data and the availability of low-cost generic statins, combined with much lower treatment thresholds, many more patients are now eligible for statin therapy under the 2013 ACC/AHA guidelines.[30] The group previously recommended for risk reclassification (the "intermediate-risk" group) has become much more narrow and with lower absolute risk;[31] however, uncertainty of risk often remains among a broad range of estimated risk scores (5–15% 10-year risk). We discuss later in this chapter how selective use of additional tools may help refine personalization of risk assessment. Select tests are discussed in detail hereafter, with a particular emphasis on exercise stress testing (to assess cardiorespiratory fitness or exercise capacity) and noncontrast cardiac computed tomography (CT) (to measure the presence of or the amount of CAC), which appear to be the best predictors of long-term survival.[32]

Additional Medical and Social Factors for Revising Risk Estimation Upward

Before one considers ordering additional testing to refine risk, there are additional elements that can be obtained from a detailed medical and social history that help guide risk assessment. For example, there are many risk factors for ASCVD that are not included in the pooled cohort equations including a family history of premature or later-onset ASCVD, former cigarette smoking, secondhand exposure to smoke, history of erectile dysfunction (ED), history of adverse pregnancy outcomes (i.e., preeclampsia or gestational diabetes), insulin resistance/prediabetes/metabolic syndrome, sedentary behavior, autoimmune disease, human immunodeficiency virus infection, chronic kidney disease, obstructive sleep apnea, and hepatosteatosis. Several of these are discussed herafter.

It would be cumbersome and impractical to add these and other unique risk factors to a universal risk prediction model. However, physicians require further direction on how best to categorize individuals with unique risk factors. It is especially in this setting that further risk stratification with tests that inherently individualize risk, such as measuring subclinical atherosclerosis, may better delineate those who would most likely benefit from preventive therapies.

Family History of Premature Coronary Heart Disease

Screening for ASCVD in the asymptomatic individual should incorporate a detailed family history. A history of premature

CHD among first-degree relatives has been shown in multiple epidemiologic studies to be strongly associated with incident ASCVD including MI, coronary death, and stroke.[33–38] Studies have demonstrated a 2- to 7-fold increase in risk of CHD associated with a positive family history, with men younger than 60 years of age being the most affected.[39]

Family history, which is asked by virtually every clinician conducting clinical risk assessments, was considered for inclusion in the 2013 ACC/AHA risk models. However, it was not included as part of the ACC/AHA pooled cohort equations because it did not adequately improve model performance, likely because it was not distinguished from a family history of *premature* CHD—a well-established predictor of subsequent ASCVD events.[37] On the other hand, other risk score calculators (Reynolds risk score, QRISK, ASSIGN, PROCAM) do include family history of premature ASCVD in risk assessment.

However, the ACC/AHA risk assessment guidelines do state that the presence of a family history of premature CHD (described as occurring in male first-degree relatives before age 55 and female first-degree relatives before age 65) could be used to revise one's risk estimation upward (IIb recommendation, level of evidence B).[10] A family history of premature CHD is similarly endorsed as a significant risk factor by experts in the 2011 AHA effectiveness-based guidelines for the prevention of cardiovascular disease in women.[40] Additionally, the Canadian Cardiovascular Society guidelines recommended that a person's estimated risk be doubled with a family history of premature ASCVD.[41] A family history of premature CHD in a subject's parents is one of the factors included in the Reynolds risk score for ASCVD prediction.[15,16] A history of ASCVD in a sibling is an even stronger risk factor than a parental history.[38]

However, not everyone with a positive family history of premature CHD is destined to have an ASCVD event, and thus upgrading the risk category (and potential eligibility for statins) for everyone with a family history may be inappropriate. Moreover, many individuals with a family history of premature CHD have few or no other risk factors, and it may be difficult to accurately determine their risk. When risk is uncertain, selective use of subclinical atherosclerosis imaging tools such as CAC may help guide the risk discussion.[36]

Autoimmune Diseases

Autoimmune diseases, such as systemic lupus erythematous, scleroderma, psoriatic arthritis, and rheumatoid arthritis, affect approximately 8% of the population, 78% of whom are women.[42] Inflammation underlies the development of atherosclerosis, and autoimmune rheumatic diseases are associated with higher rates of cardiovascular morbidity and mortality due to accelerated atherosclerosis. Multiple studies have demonstrated the association between rheumatoid arthritis or systemic lupus erythematous and increased risk for ASCVD.[43–45] Thus, patients with autoimmune diseases may warrant more intensive preventive therapies or may be candidates for additional second-tier risk assessment tools such as CAC, if risk is uncertain. Additionally, treatment with biologic agents, such as antitumor necrosis factor agents, has been shown to decrease the risk for cardiovascular events in rheumatoid arthritis patients.[46]

Adverse Pregnancy Outcomes

Pregnancy complications, such as gestational diabetes and preeclampsia, give insight into a mother's long-term ASCVD risk.[47] Thus women (even years past their child-bearing days) should be asked about their prior pregnancy outcomes as part of an office-based ASCVD risk assessment.

Gestational diabetes is associated with long-term adverse maternal ASCVD risks, such as type 2 diabetes mellitus, hypertension, and metabolic syndrome.[48–50] Nearly half of women with a history of gestational diabetes mellitus will develop type 2 diabetes mellitus within 10 years.[51] However, gestational diabetes is also a risk factor for the development of ASCVD independent of conventional risk factors, especially among women with elevated body mass index.[52]

Preeclampsia is a multisystem disease that occurs after 20 weeks of gestation, mediated by abnormalities in the placental vasculature leading to both short- and long-term endothelial dysfunction and inappropriate vasoconstriction in multiple vascular beds.[53] It presents with hypertension and proteinuria and complicates approximately 2% to 8% of pregnancies.[54] Some risk factors such as diabetes and obesity may predispose women both to preeclampsia during child-bearing age and also to increased ASCVD risk later in life (i.e., the pregnancy "unmasks" underlying predisposition to atherosclerotic vascular disease). Alternatively, preeclampsia may directly have a causal effect on the vasculature that contributes to ASCVD later in life.

Preeclampsia is independently associated with an increased risk for ASCVD events.[55] Women with a history of preeclampsia have nearly double the risk of CHD and stroke approximately 10 to12 years later and a nearly 50% increased risk of all-cause mortality at an average of 15 years' follow-up.[56] Thus, the 2011 AHA women's prevention guidelines consider these adverse pregnancy outcomes to be significant risk factors for ASCVD[40]—on par with traditional risk factors such as smoking and hypertension.

Erectile Dysfunction

ED is very common, affecting 40% of men older than 40 and 70% of those over 70 years of age.[57] Up to 80% of ED is from vascular etiologies. Data from the National Health and Nutrition Examination Survey (NHANES) found that almost 90% of men with ED had at least one major ASCVD risk factor (hypertension, hypercholesterolemia, current smoking, or diabetes).[57] A 2013 Australian study of 95,000 men with no known heart problems found that those with severe ED had a 60% higher risk of developing heart disease and nearly twice the risk of dying, compared with those without ED.[58] Other studies have reaffirmed these findings.

ED may be a marker of generalized endothelial dysfunction. Because ED symptoms can precede ASCVD, screening for ED can be used as an early marker to identify men at higher risk of ASCVD who might benefit from intensive treatment of risk factors and a detailed cardiovascular assessment.[59] More than 40% of men with ED and risk factors for ASCVD are unaware of their risk.[60] The ESC guidelines state that all men with ED should undergo ASCVD risk estimation and risk management (class IIa recommendation).[11]

A 2015 study determined that screening men with ED for ASCVD risk would be a cost-effective strategy that would not only help avert ASCVD events but also potentially save more than $21 billion dollars in healthcare expenses over 20 years in the United States alone.[60] When ASCVD risk is uncertain, the use of personalized prognostic tools, such as the CAC score, may aid in cardiovascular risk stratification and management of men with vascular ED.[61]

Assessment of Physical Inactivity and Sedentary Behavior

The AHA recommends that assessment of physical activity levels should be a vital health measure that is screened for at regular intervals similar to all other major modifiable ASCVD risk factors (i.e., diabetes mellitus, hypertension, hyperlipidemia, obesity, smoking) and tracked over time.[62] More than half of the American population perform less than the recommended levels of physical activity,[63] and annually approximately 250,000 deaths in the United States can be attributed to the consequences of physical inactivity.[64] Furthermore, from a global perspective it is estimated that 31% of the world's population are not getting recommended levels of physical activity, and physical inactivity has been cited as the fourth leading cause of death worldwide.[65]

The AHA has released a document establishing goals to improve the cardiovascular health of all Americans by 20%, while reducing deaths from ASCVD by 20% before 2020. In this statement, ideal cardiovascular health is defined by seven factors, one of which is performing recommended levels of physical activity.[66] Similarly, WHO and other global advocacy groups have listed physical activity as a public health priority.[65]

Recent data have highlighted the importance of sedentary behavior as a distinct risk factor.[67] Whereas physical inactivity is the failure to meet the recommended moderate to vigorous physical activity threshold, sedentary behavior refers to the time spent in behaviors that result in ≤ 1.5 metabolic equivalents of task (METs).[68] This commonly includes any seated or reclined posture at a desk, in a car or bus, using a computer, or watching television and generally excludes time sleeping. Therefore, even individuals who exercise on a treadmill each morning can have prolonged sedentary time if much of their day is spent working at a desk, driving in a car, and relaxing at home in the evening. Biswas et al. showed that prolonged sedentary time is independently associated with ASCVD events, cardiovascular mortality, all-cause mortality, and other adverse health outcomes.[69]

The study of Biswas et al. and much of the physical inactivity and sedentary behavior research literature have a limitation in that they rely on self-report and use of surrogate measures such as time spent watching television. Lack of access to more objective data on behavior is also a challenge in medical practice. One option to consider using is the standard pedometer in conjunction with a step count diary. In addition, new mobile health (mHealth) technologies, namely built-in smartphone activity trackers and wearable connected health devices, equipped with triaxial accelerometry, are increasing in popularity and appear accurate.[70,71] These devices may facilitate even easier access to longitudinal information on step counts, the time spent in various forms of activity, and the pattern of activity. They likely will enhance the quality of future research in this field, and, when data are integrated with the electronic medical record, this could facilitate implementation of physical activity/sedentary behavior as a vital sign in clinic. Moreover, a digital data stream could enable automated interventions providing real-time coaching to increase physical activity and reduce sedentary behavior.[72]

Chronic Kidney Disease

Chronic kidney disease (CKD) is an independent risk factor for ASCVD, and the risk of ASCVD among CKD patients is not fully captured by traditional risk factor models such as the Framingham risk score or the 2013 ACC/AHA pooled cohort equations.[73] More than 50% of deaths in CKD patients are attributed to ASCVD, and CKD patients are more likely to die from ASCVD than to progress to end-stage renal disease.[74] Patients with CKD should be assessed for ASCVD risk, and they may benefit from more intensive preventive therapies similar to those for patients with established CHD. The 2011 AHA women's prevention guidelines consider CKD a high-risk condition, similar to clinically manifest ASCVD and diabetes.[40] The ESC guidelines also give a class I recommendation that patients with CKD should have risk factors managed in a similar way as individuals with very high ASCVD risk.[11] In the REasons for Geographic and Racial Differences in Stroke (REGARDS) study (a natural history study), only approximately 8% of patients with CKD in the 50 to 79 years age range did not meet 2013 ACC/AHA cholesterol guideline criteria for initiating a statin regimen.[75]

Metabolic Syndrome

The metabolic syndrome, a constellation of three or more of abdominal obesity, prehypertension, prediabetes, low HDL-C, and high triglycerides, is an important marker of risk for ASCVD and new-onset type 2 diabetes, largely due to the influence of abdominal obesity and insulin resistance. Although not itself a risk-scoring tool, the metabolic syndrome clinical construct is meant to draw attention to the clustering of cardiometabolic risk factors in certain predisposed individuals.[76,77] A clinical diagnosis of metabolic syndrome can help facilitate communication with patients and other providers about the core causative factors of a patients ASCVD risk, the risk of developing diabetes, and importance of lifestyle modification.

There are several ancillary hallmarks of metabolic syndrome that can be important for identifying ASCVD risk. For example, the most common liver function abnormality in the United States is asymptomatic fatty liver disease (hepatosteatosis), which is a core component of the pathophysiology of atherogenic dyslipidemia in metabolic syndrome. Obstructive sleep apnea is also commonly seen among patients with the metabolic syndrome and is associated with ASCVD risk beyond what would be predicted by traditional risk factors alone. The ESC guidelines state that all individuals with obstructive sleep apnea should undergo ASCVD risk assessment and risk factor management.[11]

Predisposition to metabolic syndrome is also one of the reasons why patients of South Asian ancestry appear to have elevated ASCVD risk beyond what would be predicted by traditional risk factors alone. Other patients predisposed to metabolic syndrome include patients with human immunodeficiency virus, patients with depression, patients treated with antipsychotics, treated cancer survivors, and patients with prior organ transplants.

Additional Tools for Screening or Refining Individualized Risk Assessment

Resting Electrocardiogram

One of the simplest potential screening tests for ASCVD is a resting electrocardiogram (ECG); this is a low-cost test, with essentially no direct risk from the test itself, and it is readily available in most clinical practices. Major ECG abnormalities include Q waves suggestive of silent MI, evidence of left ventricular hypertrophy (LVH), complete bundle branch block, atrial fibrillation or flutter, or major ST-T wave changes. Minor ECG abnormalities include minor ST-T changes.

In several population-based studies of asymptomatic adults, ECG abnormalities predicted incident CHD events and mortality.[78–80] In a population based study of older adults (aged 70 to 79 years), both major and minor ECG abnormalities were associated with increased risk of CHD events when added to a model with traditional risk factors (although not when added to the Framingham risk score); the largest reclassification was seen for the intermediate-risk group (14% reclassified).[81] Of note, the main contribution to the net reclassification improvement in this study came from reclassifying patients to lower, not higher, risk, which actually would result in fewer patients receiving preventive pharmacologic treatment;[82] if this downward reclassification was not appropriate, this could adversely lead to fewer ASCVD events prevented. A resting ECG is not a sensitive enough tool to exclude the presence of moderate or advanced coronary artery disease (CAD).

Although not endorsed in the 2013 ACC/AHA risk assessment guidelines, the 2010 ACC/AHA guideline for the assessment of cardiovascular risk in asymptomatic adults stated that an ECG at rest may be reasonable in asymptomatic adults with hypertension or diabetes (class IIa recommendation). They also gave a weaker but still generally supportive recommendation even among those without hypertension or diabetes (class IIb).[9]

In contrast, based on a systematic review, the USPSTF did not recommend screening asymptomatic adults at low CHD risk with a resting or exercise ECG for the prediction of CHD events (grade D recommendation).[83] Similarly, this same sentiment was also endorsed in a 2015 statement by the American College of Physicians, which stated that clinicians should not screen asymptomatic low-risk adults with a resting or exercise ECG for the detection of cardiac disease given low pretest probability and low likelihood that positive results will affect treatment decisions and clinical outcomes, plus the potential harms of false-positives leading to unnecessary tests and procedures.[7]

Resting Echocardiogram

A resting transthoracic echocardiogram is widely used to assess patients with suspected cardiac symptoms or structural heart disease, both for diagnostic purposes and management. However, it is not recommended for routine use for screening of asymptomatic individuals.[84]

The majority of echocardiograms are ordered by primary care physicians, rather than cardiologists.[85] Population-based studies of asymptomatic individuals screened by echocardiography have found that incidental findings such as asymptomatic left ventricular (LV) dysfunction and LVH can predict cardiovascular and all-cause mortality independent of blood pressure and other risk factors.[86,87] The 2010 ACC/AHA guidelines for assessment of cardiovascular risk in asymptomatic adults provide weak support for selective use of echocardiography screening to detect LVH and LV dysfunction for asymptomatic adults with hypertension (class IIb recommendation) but a class III (no benefit) for those without hypertension.[9]

Of note, the population-based Tromsø study in Norway evaluated outcomes among asymptomatic participants who were randomly assigned to a screening echocardiogram or to a control group.[88] Participants with abnormal findings on echocardiogram newly detected by screening (including myxoma, LV dysfunction, wall motion abnormality, or valvular disease) were referred to a cardiologist for further evaluation (approximately 9% of participants). However, despite cardiology referral for these diagnoses, ASCVD events and all-cause mortality during 15 years of follow-up were unchanged between the screened and nonscreened groups.

In response to the growing use of echocardiography (~8% annual increase[85]), in 2011 the American Society of Echocardiography (ASE) updated its appropriate use criteria consensus statement in conjunction with the ACC and AHA.[89] This document reaffirmed that echocardiography should not be used for routine screening in an unselected general population, including patients with asymptomatic hypertension. The consensus statement also does not endorse screening asymptomatic family members of individuals with ASCVD with echocardiography unless there is a first-degree relative with inherited cardiomyopathy or suspected connective tissue disease.[89]

Although echocardiography does not use any ionizing radiation, a normal resting echocardiogram does not exclude risk for significant CAD. Therefore, patients with a "normal" appearing echocardiogram may be falsely reassured and not follow through with other recommended screening or preventive measures. Mild abnormalities or questionable test results may lead to additional testing associated with expense and potential for harm.

Exercise Treadmill Testing

Some patients and providers may equate screening for CHD with exercise treadmill testing (ETT). However, ETT can generally only detect obstructive CHD, whereas the majority of MIs occur from acute plaque rupture from thin-capped fibroatheromas producing < 50% diameter stenosis.[90] Whereas ETT is commonly used to evaluate symptoms suggestive of possible CHD for diagnostic purposes, current guidelines do not support routine ETT in the vast majority of asymptomatic individuals.

For certain subgroups of asymptomatic patients, however, ETT may be useful.[91] The previous 2010 ACC/AHA guidelines gave a modest class IIb recommendation that ETT may be considered for ASCVD risk stratification for the intermediate-risk individual, particularly when non-ECG parameters such as exercise capacity (i.e., METS achieved) are considered.[9] Other older ACC/AHA guidelines felt it was reasonable (class IIa recommendation) to screen asymptomatic diabetic individuals who plan to start vigorous exercise but gave a weak endorsement (class IIb) for older nondiabetic individuals before vigorous exercise.[92] Similarly the ESC stated in their guidelines that exercise ECG may be considered for ASCVD risk assessment in moderate-risk asymptomatic adults (including sedentary adults considering starting a vigorous exercise program), particularly when attention is paid to non-ECG markers like cardiorespiratory fitness (class IIb).[11]

However, in contrast to the older ACC/AHA and ESC guidelines, given the low prevalence of significant obstructive CAD among asymptomatic individuals screened, the USPSTF determined there was insufficient evidence for routine stress testing before exercise training and did not endorse screening.[93]

Unfortunately, no randomized controlled trials (RCTs) have addressed the utility of ETT in asymptomatic individuals, even those pursuing a vigorous exercise program or competition. Further discussion regarding screening of competitive athletes is found in the "special populations" section of this chapter.

The role of ETT screening for high-risk occupations like commercial and military pilots and competitive athletes also remains highly controversial, but current evidence does not support the role of routine screening among these individuals either. A study analyzing the use of ETT screening of asymptomatic US Air Force pilots found a very low positive predictive value of CAD of only 16%, and thus screening ETT was not felt to be efficacious.[94]

An abnormal ETT is associated with an increased risk of MI and sudden cardiac death, though the positive predictive value is low. Many parameters obtained by ETT individually have prognostic value, and they include ST-segment changes, assessment of exercise capacity, heart rate recovery, arrhythmias, and blood pressure response. Reduced exercise capacity (METs) and poor heart rate recovery are strongly predictive of ASCVD death even independent of traditional ASCVD risk factors.[95] Conversely, those with excellent exercise capacity generally have a favorable long-term prognosis.[96]

Exercise capacity/physical fitness is one of the strongest overall predictors of survival. The Henry Ford Exercise Testing Project (FIT) evaluated over 58,000 patients without known CHD who underwent a clinically indicated ETT and then were followed for an average of 10 years for mortality and CHD outcomes. After age and sex, the factors most predictive of survival were METs achieved and percentage of maximal predicted heart rate achieved.[97] This FIT treadmill score, using standard parameters obtained from ETT, as well as age and sex, can be used to estimate one's 10-year mortality risk and potentially refine ASCVD risk prediction. This score is defined as percentage of maximum predicted heart rate + 12 (METs) − 4 (age) + 43 if female. For prognostic purposes, the FIT treadmill score, which runs from −200 to 200, can be considered to be included in all ETT reports for patients who have no existing ASCVD and have a negative ECG portion on their stress test.

In addition to being inversely associated with CHD events and mortality, greater fitness (assessed by METs) is also associated with decreased risk of other important outcomes such as atrial fibrillation,[98] incident diabetes,[99] incident hypertension,[100] and heart failure.[101] Importantly, high fitness/exercise capacity achieved antecedent of a first heart attack is perhaps the best predictor of heart attack survival.[102] The good news is that only moderate fitness levels are required to significantly improve the coronary risk factor profile.[103]

As previously discussed, greater levels of physical activity are strongly associated with reduced ASCVD risk. Because most asymptomatic patients do not undergo an ETT for risk stratification, asking about physical activity is frequently used as a surrogate for fitness in clinical practice. However self-reported physical activity is only modestly correlated with directly measured fitness and when discordant, measured fitness is a better marker of cardiometabolic risk.[104]

Despite the strong prognostic value of fitness measures for identifying individuals at increased risk for ASCVD outcomes, it remains unclear how to use the ETT risk-stratification results to alter the management of patients compared to current guideline recommendations. Achievement of a high MET level (generally > stage 4 on the Bruce protocol) and high FIT score confer excellent prognostic information; such individuals may generally be reassured and recommended to continue following a healthy active lifestyle. However, less favorable findings from an ETT could lead toward more targeted and intensified efforts at promoting improved physical activity and risk factor control for at-risk individuals (i.e., aggressive lipid-lowering therapy[105]).

Coronary Artery Calcium

ASCVD risk prediction models are heavily weighted toward chronologic age, yet "arterial" or "biologic age" is frequently discordant with chronologic age. Assessment of CAC is a useful surrogate measure of total coronary atherosclerotic burden and therefore arterial age.[106]

CAC is performed using noncontrast cardiac-gated CT scanning. CAC scans can be performed on any modern CT equipment and thus can be performed similarly around the world. The entire procedure takes about 10 minutes, with most of the time spent placing electrodes and positioning the patient on the table. With modern scanners, scans are acquired in under a second using approximately 0.5 to 2 mSv of radiation (approximately equivalent to 2 bilateral mammograms or 10 chest x-rays). In most metropolitan centers in the United States, CAC scans cost between $75 and $150.

CAC scanning leverages the fact that calcified deposits in the coronary arteries strongly attenuate x-rays and are thus visible on unenhanced images. Contiguous voxels approximately 130 Hounsfield units are considered to be calcium. CAC scans are generally scored using the Agatston score, which is a summed score of all calcified lesions in the coronary arteries through the complete z-axis of the heart, weighted for the density (x-ray attenuation) of the calcium. Agatston scoring uses a 120-kV electron, variable mA based on patient body weight, acquiring up to 40 slices at a fixed 2.5-mm to 3-mm slice increment. The ideal way to score a CAC scan remains controversial, with potential benefit in differently accounting for the density of calcium and regional distribution of calcium, as well as extracoronary calcification.[107] Future advancements will likely increase the sensitivity to minute calcium deposits and will likely further reduce the associated radiation.[107]

CAC scoring does not identify isolated noncalcified plaque, although its prevalence is less common when calcium is not present anywhere in the coronary tree. Current evidence does not support a strong incremental predictive value for the detection of isolated noncalcified plaque in the asymptomatic primary prevention patient.[108,109]

When added to traditional risk factor models, CAC improves risk discrimination more than any other available test. In the community-based Multi-Ethnic Study of Atherosclerosis (MESA), the area under the receiver operating characteristic (ROC) curve for the prediction of CHD events was significantly improved when a CAC-based model was compared to a model with only traditional risk factors.[110] Individuals without risk factors but elevated CAC have substantially higher event rates than those who have multiple risk factors but no CAC.[111,112] In MESA, individuals with no risk factors and CAC greater than 300 had an event rate 3.5 times higher than individuals with 3 or more risk factors and CAC of 0.[112] Even minimal CAC (scores 1 to 10) is associated with 3-fold increased CHD risk compared to those with a CAC of 0.[113] Additionally, there appears to be no upper threshold of risk with increasing CAC scores.[114]

In addition to its role in "upgrading" or elevating predicted risk in younger patients when significant CAC is present,[29] perhaps the most important potential role of CAC testing in the modern era using currently available risk scores may be for downgrading or "derisking" an older adult with a CAC score of 0 who might otherwise be recommended

TABLE 29.4 Potential Use of CAC = 0 for Derisking: Data from the Multi-Ethnic Study of Atherosclerosis (MESA)

STUDY (REF. NUMBER)	POPULATION SIMULATED IN MESA	THERAPY	WITH CAC = 0	EVENT RATES PER 1000 PERSON-YEARS	ESTIMATED NNT_5 FOR CAC = 0	CONCLUSION
Blaha[116]	JUPITER trial-eligible patients	Rosuvastatin	47%	**CHD** CAC = 0: 0.8 CAC 1–100: 4.8 CAC > 100: 20.2	549 (CHD)	Unfavorable NNT when treating CAC = 0 with rosuvastatin
Bittencourt[118]	Eligible for polypill trials	Primary prevention polypill	TIPS: 59% Poly-IRAN: 55% Wald: 39% PILL: 41%	**CHD** CAC = 0: 1.2–1.9 CAC 1–100: 4.6– 5.5 CAC > 100: 11.6–13.3	170–269 (CHD)	Unfavorable risk:benefit ratio treating CAC = 0 with primary prevention polypill
Martin[117]	Dyslipidemic patients without known atherosclerotic cardiovascular disease (ASCVD) and not on statins at baseline	Moderate-intensity generic statin	By number of lipid abnormalities (LAs): 0 LAs: 58% 1 LA: 55% 2 LAs: 45% 3 LAs: 50%	**ASCVD** CAC = 0: 2.4–6.2 CAC 1–100: 7.6–17.2 CAC > 100: 22.2–29.2	154–267 (ASCVD)	Unfavorable NNT treating CAC = 0 with generic statin
Miedema[119]	Candidates for aspirin therapy	Low-dose aspirin	56%	**CHD** CAC = 0: 1.3 CAC 1–100: 4.1 CAC > 100: 11.6	808–2036 (CHD)	Unfavorable risk:benefit treating CAC = 0 with aspirin
Nasir[120]	Statin use *recommended* by the 2013 ACC/AHA cholesterol guidelines Statin use *considered* by the 2013 ACC/AHA cholesterol guidelines	Statin therapy (assumes 30% risk reduction)	44%	**ASCVD** CAC = 0: 5.2 CAC 1–100: 8.8 CAC > 100: 15.4 **ASCVD** CAC = 0: 1.5 CAC 1–100: 7.8 CAC > 100: 6.3	64 38 33 223 43	Heterogeneity of event rates among statin eligible groups. NNT less favorable when CAC = 0

ASCVD, Atherosclerotic cardiovascular disease; *CAC,* coronary artery calcium; *CHD,* coronary heart disease; *NNT,* number needed to treat.

for pharmacologic therapy based on models that are dominated by chronologic age.[115] We have previously found that the number needed to treat to prevent one ASCVD event would generally be unfavorable using a high- or moderate-intensity statin,[116,117] a polypill,[118] or aspirin[119] for primary prevention when CAC = 0 (Table 29.4).

A recent analysis from MESA showed that there is substantial heterogeneity among groups of asymptomatic adults recommended for statin therapy under the 2013 ACC/AHA guidelines.[120] Of the MESA participants who would be recommended or considered for statins under the guidelines, nearly half (44%) had CAC = 0 at baseline and their observed 10-year ASCVD event rate was overall low (4.2 events/1000 person-years). Of note, approximately half of these events are strokes, and a good number of them are not atherosclerotic in nature but are secondary to hypertension and/or atrial fibrillation, and it is unclear if statin therapy would be helpful in these conditions. In contrast, the respective ASCVD event rates for those with any CAC greater than 0 was 11.2/1000 person-years.

With specific relevance to individuals reluctant to take preventive medicines, recent cost-effectiveness analyses suggest that CAC is broadly cost-effective for steering treatment toward those with measurable CAC when the mild disutility of taking daily prevention medication is factored into decision-making.[12,121] Importantly, a score of CAC = 0 is associated with an excellent long-term prognosis with annual mortality of less than 1% up to 15 years in asymptomatic adults.[122,123] When compared to other "negative" risk markers (carotid intimal medial thickness < 25th percentile, absence of carotid plaque, ABI > 0.9 and < 1.3, hs-CRP < 2 mg/L, homocysteine < 10 μmol/L, N-terminal pro-brain natriuretic peptide <100 pg/mL, no microalbuminuria, no family history of CHD, absence of metabolic syndrome, and healthy lifestyle), the absence of CAC conferred the greatest downward shift in ASCVD risk.[124]

Clinicians now have a tool for incorporating CAC scores into estimates of 10-year risk. The MESA CHD risk score,[125] available online at http://www.mesa-nhlbi.org/MESACHDRisk/MesaRiskScore/RiskScore.aspx, allows entry of age, sex, race/ethnicity, traditional Framingham risk factors, family history of CHD, and CAC score with resultant 10-year risks of CHD (distinct from the ASCVD endpoint used in the 2013 guidelines) before and after incorporation of CAC data. We believe that a MESA CHD risk score greater than 5% is a reasonable threshold for consideration of initiating more aggressive preventive therapy, i.e., a statin and possibly aspirin.

The Early Identification of Subclinical Atherosclerosis by Noninvasive Imaging Research (EISNER) study[126] found that randomization to CAC scanning versus no scanning did not increase overall downstream medical testing; rather randomization to CAC scanning was associated with modestly improved risk factor control. Findings from a population-based cohort showed that identification of severe CAC (> 400) was associated with higher rates of initiation and continuation of important preventive medications including lipid-lowering agents, blood pressure-lowering agents, and aspirin.[127]

Limitations of CAC scoring include the modest amount of radiation exposure (as discussed earlier) and the detection of incidental findings (most commonly, noncalcified lung nodules) in approximately 4% to 8% of persons,[128] who may need follow-up CT scans to document stability. Also, it is imperative that clinicians are advised how to use CAC scores in their management practices (i.e., initiating aspirin and high-intensity statin when scores are high); misunderstanding of how to use CAC could lead to unnecessary referrals for coronary angiography in asymptomatic individuals (and the potential complications and expense stemming from that procedure).

Additionally, of concern to some, is the lack of definitive clinical trial evidence demonstrating that CAC-based treatment decision-making is superior to traditional global risk assessment in reducing ASCVD outcomes in a cost-effective manner. It is important to note that we do not have any RCTs for ASCVD risk estimators either. Due to the low risk and low cost of a CAC scan and the cost involved for a large RCT, it seems unlikely in the near future that a CAC-based clinical trial (or any clinical trials comparing CHD risk assessment modalities among asymptomatic individuals) will be funded in the United States. However, the ROBINSCA clinical trial of CAC screening versus risk factor screening is ongoing in the Netherlands and may offer future insights.[129] In the meantime, approaches to ASCVD risk assessment must rely on the best evidence from observational studies.[130]

Most guidelines suggest that men starting at age 40 and women at age 45 with at least one additional risk factor such as a family history of premature atherosclerotic vascular disease or an ASCVD 10-year risk estimate of at least 5% could be considered for a CAC scan. The 2013 ACC/AHA prevention guidelines state that an Agatston score of 300 units or more, or a score on or above the 75th percentile for age, sex, and ethnicity, is a factor that indicates that the person is likely at a higher risk level and would warrant strong consideration of statin therapy and intensified lifestyle changes. Other data from MESA indicates that an Agatston score of at least 100 units portends a "CHD-equivalent level" of risk.[116] Prior data suggest that the absolute CAC score is a better indicator of near-term risk than age/sex/race percentiles, although percentiles may have more value for communicating lifetime risk.[131]

Whereas CAC progression is strongly predictive of outcomes,[132] there is no need to rescan a person who has a higher CAC score (e.g., > 100) because clinical decision-making will likely not change. It is reasonable to rescan a patient with a CACs of 0 approximately 4 to 5 years later.[133] However, in a smoker[134] or a person with diabetes,[135] a CAC score of 0 provides less reassurance for a very low ASCVD event rate; in these patients, this low-risk finding should be supported by other clinical information and rescanning should be considered after a shorter interval.

Finally, appropriate use criteria and some guidelines have stated that it is reasonable to do an ETT or stress myocardial perfusion imaging (MPI) in asymptomatic persons with high CAC scores (> 400) if they are planning to engage in vigorous physical activity; this can help to rule out high-grade obstructive disease. Prior AHA guidelines have also stated that asymptomatic diabetics with a CAC score greater than 400 may be considered for stress MPI for more advanced cardiovascular risk assessment (IIb recommendation).[9] However, all patients with advanced subclinical coronary atherosclerosis should undergo aggressive lifestyle and pharmacologic management of their risk factors.

Coronary Computed Tomography Angiography

One limitation of CAC scoring (obtained by noncontrast CT) is that it cannot identify noncalcified plaques or coronary stenoses. It can only identify the vulnerable *patient*, not the vulnerable *lesion*, although the value of such a plaque-based approach remains debatable. Thus, coronary CTA (performed with intravenous [IV] contrast) may initially appear to be an attractive screening tool given that it can assess coronary atherosclerosis and anatomy with reasonable accuracy,[136] characterize features of high-risk plaque lesions,[137] and add prognostic information to both traditional risk factors and CAC scoring, at least for symptomatic patients.[138] However, at this time, the role of coronary CTA is best served to evaluate symptomatic patients with known or suspected CHD as the additive value beyond CAC in asymptomatic patients has not been demonstrated. In a large registry of over 7500 individuals without chest pain or known CHD who underwent coronary CTA, there was very little incremental prognostic value added by coronary CTA over prediction models that incorporated CAC and Framingham risk factors; the incremental improvements of C-statistic and net reclassification index conferred by coronary CTA of 0.03 and 0.09, respectively, were small.[108]

Although the prevalence of occult coronary atherosclerosis in asymptomatic individuals is not uncommon (22% in one study had atherosclerotic plaques, with 5% having significant stenoses), short-term prognosis for these patients is still reasonably good.[139,140] A prior study that evaluated coronary CTA screening of asymptomatic patients in South Korea compared with a matched control group who did not have screening found that abnormal test findings were predictive of increased use of preventive medications like aspirin and statins but also led to increased use of invasive tests, with no difference in ASCVD event rates at 18 months.[141]

Concerns regarding risks of ionizing radiation (although this is decreasing over time with modern protocols), risks of IV contrast exposure, greater incidental findings versus noncontrast CT for CAC scoring, and costs (both direct and downstream) limit its use as a screening tool at this time. The 2010 ACC/AHA guidelines did not recommend coronary CTA for screening of the asymptomatic individual (class III).[9]

Carotid Intima-Media Thickness

Carotid intima-media thickness (cIMT) assessed by B-mode ultrasound is another surrogate measure of atherosclerotic burden.[142] It has many attractive features for a screening tool compared with CAC, including lack of radiation, ability to detect noncalcified plaques, and ability to detect atherosclerosis even in younger adults.[143] However, a prior analysis from MESA found CAC to be a substantially better predictor of ASCVD events than cIMT.[144]

One important issue limiting assessment of cIMT is that across studies there is substantial variation of how cIMT is reported, including the number and location of carotid segments assessed (i.e., common carotid artery, internal carotid artery, or carotid bulb), which measurements were reported (i.e., mean or maximal thickness, mean of the mean, or mean of the maximum), and whether plaque was included in cIMT assessment. Measuring the far wall of the common carotid artery appears to be the most reliable method for assessing cIMT.[145] In 2008, the ASE expert task force set forth guidelines on how cIMT should be measured.[142]

Although some studies found cIMT was a predictor of future CHD events,[146,147] many others failed to show that cIMT added prognostic information over and above traditional risk factor assessment using tools such as the Framingham risk score.[148,149] A prior systematic review and meta-analysis concluded that the addition of cIMT did little to improve the performance of traditional ASCVD risk prediction models.[150] Thus, because of lack of compelling incremental predictive value beyond traditional risk factor models, the 2013 ACC/AHA guidelines did not recommend routine use of cIMT for the screening of asymptomatic adults for ASCVD risk assessment.

There are some caveats to this recommendation. Measuring cIMT from the internal carotid artery may be more predictive than the common carotid artery, but it is harder to perform accurately.[151] Importantly, assessing carotid plaque at the time of ultrasound adds to prognostic yield, particularly for the prediction of stroke.[152,153] Plaque is more likely to represent definite areas of atherosclerosis versus medial hypertrophy alone. Thus, relative to cIMT, carotid plaque has a stronger association with ASCVD, and it is not recommended to measure cIMT alone without also considering plaque.[154] Whereas CAC has been shown to be superior to carotid plaque for prediction of total ASCVD events, CAC and carotid plaque performed similarly for prediction of strokes and transient ischemic attacks.[153]

In contrast to the 2013 AHA/ACC guidelines, the 2012 ESC guidelines were more favorable regarding the use of cIMT along with carotid plaque for risk stratification of the asymptomatic adult at moderate ASCVD risk (class IIa recommendation).[11] However, the population-based MESA study found that both assessment of low cIMT and absence of carotid plaque were inferior to CAC for "derisking" (i.e., shifting ASCVD risk downward).[124]

Regarding carotid ultrasound for the detection of obstructive carotid artery disease (i.e., stenosis), the USPSTF also recommended against screening for asymptomatic carotid stenosis in the general population without a history of transient ischemic attack, stroke, or neurologic symptoms.[155]

High-Sensitivity C-Reactive Protein

CRP is a marker of inflammation and is associated with the metabolic syndrome. In a cohort of apparently healthy women, hs-CRP was a better predictor of risk for ASCVD events than LDL-C and added prognostic information to models based on traditional risk factors.[156] Results from the Justification for the Use of Statins in Primary Prevention: An Intervention Trial Evaluating Rosuvastatin (JUPITER) clinical trial support the use of statins in older adults with elevated hs-CRP of greater than or equal to 2 mg/L and LDL-C of less than 130 mg/dL.[157] The 2013 ACC/AHA risk assessment guidelines do state that a hs-CRP value of greater than or equal to 2 mg/L could be used to revise risk estimation upward, when risk is uncertain.[10] On the other hand, the ESC guidelines gave only a weak endorsement for hs-CRP (class IIb recommendation) for further risk assessment among asymptomatic adults at moderate ASCVD risk and recommended against measurement of hs-CRP in low- and high-risk adults to assess 10-year ASCVD risk (class III recommendation).[11]

Several issues limit our enthusiasm for routine risk assessment with hs-CRP. It is an inferior risk predictor compared with CAC,[116,148] is closely linked with other metabolic syndrome traits, and suffers from the same lack of RCT evidence as all other tests. As JUPITER did not enroll participants with normal hs-CRP levels,[158] this trial does not provide evidence to support measurement of hs-CRP for screening. Low hs-CRP does not offer the same value in derisking as that achieved with a CAC of 0.[116,124] Thus, in contrast to risk assessment with CAC scanning, screening with hs-CRP leads to more overall treatment and less accurate matching of treatment with risk.

Ankle-Brachial Index

Asymptomatic peripheral arterial disease (PAD) is highly prevalent in older adults. Based on NHANES data from 1999–2004, it is estimated that more than 12% of adults over the age of 60 and 23% of adults over the age of 70 have an ABI of less than 0.9.[159] A low ABI is not just a measure of PAD but a marker of generalized atherosclerosis.[160]

Compared with those without PAD, asymptomatic individuals with PAD have higher rates of all-cause and vascular mortality,[161] rates similar to those with symptomatic PAD.[162] Approximately 1 in 5 PAD patients has an MI, stroke, hospitalization for ASCVD event, or ASCVD death each year. Thus, patients with asymptomatic PAD are a high-risk group that warrant aggressive preventive intervention.

Prior meta-analyses showed that the addition of ABI to the Framingham risk score could improve cardiovascular risk prediction, resulting in reclassification of risk categories and modification of treatment recommendation in approximately 19% of men and 36% of women.[163] The 2013 ACC/AHA risk guidelines advise that the presence of an ABI of less than 0.9 could also be used to revise the risk estimate into a higher category.[10] Yet, similar to hs-CRP, ABI also compares unfavorably with CAC, with inferior discrimination and risk reclassification[148] and does not offer the same potential for derisking.[124] Moreover, abnormal ABI is rare in an asymptomatic patient without a history of diabetes and/or cigarette smoking.[148] In their systematic review, the USPSTF concluded that there was insufficient current evidence regarding the balance of benefits and harms of screening for PAD with the ABI for ASCVD risk assessment among unselected populations.[164]

High-Sensitivity Troponin

Cardiac troponins T and I are well-established biomarkers of myocardial injury and are used clinically to guide diagnosis and management of patients suspected of having acute coronary syndromes. However, elevated levels may be due to cardiac damage associated with chronic structural heart disease rather than from acute ischemia, especially when levels remain generally consistent over the short term.[165] New high-sensitivity assays have expanded the role of cardiac troponin as a prognostic marker even among asymptomatic individuals without suspected acute coronary syndrome.

High-sensitivity cardiac troponin elevations, even among those without known clinical ASCVD, are associated with increased risk for incident CHD and heart failure events.[166] A recent systematic review of 21 prospective community-based cohort studies involving nearly 65,000 patients found that an elevated cardiac troponin level was associated with a near tripling of risk for all-cause and ASCVD mortality among asymptomatic individuals.[167] Thus, although it is currently not measured routinely in clinical practice in the asymptomatic individual, it also has the potential as a screening tool for refining risk prediction.

However, further work is needed to determine whether the excess risk associated with elevated cardiac troponin is modifiable with intensification of preventive therapies.[167] In the JUPITER primary prevention RCT, although high-sensitivity troponin I was associated with increased risk of vascular events and mortality, the benefits of rosuvastatin for ASCVD event reduction were similar across all baseline categories of high-sensitivity troponin; thus, those with higher troponin levels did not benefit more from statin therapy than those with lower troponin levels.[168] Furthermore in the Bypass Angioplasty Revascularization Investigation 2 Diabetes (BARI-2D) RCT of patients with stable CHD and diabetes, whereas again an elevated high-sensitivity troponin was associated with greater risk of ASCVD events, it did not identify a group of patients who benefited more from early coronary revascularization compared with medical therapy alone.[169] Therefore, how to manage patients differently on the basis of the identification of an elevated high-sensitivity troponin is uncertain and thus limits this biomarker's utility as a screening tool at this time. The 2013 ACC/AHA risk assessment guidelines did not give any endorsement for or against high-sensitivity cardiac troponin as a marker to guide risk assessment.

Screening for CAD in Asymptomatic but High-Risk Groups

The 2013 ACC/AHA risk assessment guidelines did not provide any recommendations regarding utility of imaging in high-risk subpopulations.[10] This is in contrast to the 2010 ACC/AHA guidelines for assessment of cardiovascular risk in asymptomatic adults, which gave a class IIb recommendation for stress MPI for asymptomatic adults with diabetes or family history of CHD.[9]

Diabetes

Risk in diabetes is heterogeneous, and diabetes is no longer considered a CHD risk equivalent as was the case in prior lipid-lowering guidelines. Risk in diabetes varies according to age of onset, duration, severity, and presence or absence of accompanying metabolic risk factors.[170]

The Detection of Ischemia in Asymptomatic Diabetics (DIAD) was a randomized multicenter study that assessed whether screening asymptomatic patients with diabetes with nuclear stress testing affected outcomes;[171] 1123 participants with type 2 diabetes and no symptoms of CAD were randomly assigned to adenosine-stress radionuclide MPI or no MPI. No detailed advice regarding the need for more aggressive risk factor modification was provided for how to manage abnormal stress MPI results. Overall, cardiac event rates were low and perhaps this group of diabetics was healthier than a general diabetic population. Event rates were not significantly reduced by MPI screening for myocardial ischemia over 4.8 years.

Similar to ETT, stress MPI generally only identifies flow-limiting stenoses and approximately two-thirds of acute coronary syndrome events stem from non–flow-limiting lesions. It is possible, however, that any stress-induced myocardial ischemia may be related to disease of the coronary microcirculation and coronary artery vasoconstriction due to endothelial dysfunction.[172,173] Any screening strategy needs to be coupled with an effective preventive strategy directed at managing abnormal test results; such a strategy should involve more aggressive risk factor management through appropriate use of medications to optimize lipid and blood pressure, as well as dietary and exercise habits.

Whereas stress MPI provides a functional assessment of ischemia, coronary CTA, as previously described, can identify coronary anatomy, including the presence of non–flow-limiting stenosis due to calcified, noncalcified, and mixed atherosclerotic plaques. The FACTOR-64 study was an RCT involving 45 clinics of a single health system (Intermountain Healthcare, UT) that enrolled 900 patients with either type 1 or type 2 diabetes of at least 3 to 5 years' duration and without symptoms of CAD.[174] Participants were randomized to CHD screening with coronary CTA versus standard diabetes care based on national guidelines. Standard versus aggressive risk factor reduction targets were recommended based on the coronary CTA findings.

The use of coronary CTA to screen for CHD did not significantly reduce the composite primary endpoint of all-cause mortality, nonfatal MI, or unstable angina requiring hospitalization at 4 years among this population of asymptomatic diabetic patients, though the actual event rate was much lower than had been anticipated. Whereas the point estimate for the primary endpoint was consistent with a 20% lower risk in the coronary CTA group, the trial was not sufficiently powered to determine whether this was due to chance or the use of CTA to guide management decisions.

Although coronary CTA can provide information on both calcified and noncalcified plaque and determine the extent of stenosis, a simple noncontrast CAC score might suffice for risk-stratification of diabetic patients. All-cause mortality risk in diabetics rises in proportion to severity of CAC score; diabetics with a CAC score of 0 (up to 40% of asymptomatic individuals with diabetes) have a low short-term risk for death, similar to nondiabetics with a 0 CAC.[175] Prior 2010 AHA guidelines had stated that in asymptomatic adults with diabetes 40 years of age or over, measurement of CAC is reasonable for ASCVD risk assessment (class IIa recommendation).

In summary, the available evidence does not support screening with MPI or coronary CTA in asymptomatic diabetic patients. Of note, both DIAD and FACTOR-64 included lower-risk diabetics, and thus the role of screening in higher-risk diabetics is still uncertain. Regardless of such testing, the 2013 cholesterol guidelines identify diabetics as a group that generally warrants treatment with a moderate- to high-intensity statin along with intensive lifestyle modification.[14] As MESA showed that among individuals with CAC = 0, having diabetes did not increase the risk of adverse events in the short-term, CAC could be helpful in refining risk in diabetics who are hesitant to start aggressive pharmacologic measures such as aspirin and statin therapy or who are contemplating dual lipid-lowering therapy to treat mixed hyperlipidemia. However, as also mentioned, the warranty period and level of reassurance for a CAC = 0 is less among diabetic than nondiabetic patients.[135] Patients with diabetes may be considered for a rescan within a shorter interval if uncertainty still remains regarding their ASCVD risk.

Family History of Premature Coronary Heart Disease

As previously described, a family history of premature CHD could potentially be used, according to the 2013 ACC/AHA risk assessment guidelines, to revise the risk category upward. But do individuals with a family history of premature CHD benefit from stress imaging? A study evaluated 1287 asymptomatic siblings of patients who had premature CHD at less than 60 years of age who underwent risk factor screening and treadmill exercise stress testing with MPI and were followed for CHD events for up to 25 years.[176] The study found that, whereas inducible ischemia by stress MPI was associated with a worse prognosis, male siblings with negative tests still had a relatively high risk of ASCVD, suggesting that male siblings over 40 years of age should be considered for aggressive primary prevention pharmacotherapy regardless of stress MPI results. For women, the presence of inducible ischemia was also associated with risk, but the prevalence of ischemia was low enough that routine stress MPI did not appear to be warranted.

Data from the MESA study found that CAC in asymptomatic patients with a family history of premature CHD was a strong predictor of both absolute and relative increased risk of ASCVD, whereas cIMT was not.[36] Nearly half of individuals with a family history of premature CHD had a CAC of 0, with a low absolute event rate, and thus might have considerably less net benefit from aspirin and statin therapy. These data suggest that not everyone with a family history of premature CHD needs to be elevated to a higher-risk category. Confidence in the reporting of family history should be considered, and the use of CAC is also likely to be helpful to refine risk in this population, although perhaps this risk restratification with CAC works better for a middle-aged or older patient than a younger patient.[177]

Competitive Athletes

After the introduction of a preparticipation athletic screening program in Italy (first with physical examination and ECG, and then echocardiography if needed), the incidence of sudden cardiac death in athletes declined.[178] The diseases being screened for in these young adult athletes are generally not ASCVD but rather inherited cardiomyopathies such as hypertrophic cardiomyopathy or arrhythmogenic right ventricular cardiomyopathy, or occasionally anomalous coronary artery origins.

The ESC has formally endorsed screening initiatives of competitive athletes with ECGs.[179] In contrast, in the United States, the AHA does not endorse mandatory routine screening with ECG among competitive athletes with a normal cardiovascular exam and no cardiac symptoms.[180] Concerns cited were the risk of false-positive findings that could lead to additional testing and unnecessary anxiety and/or disqualification, the cost of implementing such a mass screening program, and the low prevalence of disease in this population. Similarly, the ASE does not endorse routine echocardiography screening for athletes participating in competitive sports who have normal findings on cardiovascular exam.[89] The role for cardiovascular screening of presumably healthy athletes remains highly controversial, given generally low rates of sudden cardiac death in this population.

Linking Screening with Management Decisions

Screening tests, by themselves, cannot improve the prognosis of patients. To improve patient care, they must be linked to more accurate risk-based therapy decisions. Therefore, none of the above risk assessment tools should be performed if management decisions will not be altered by the test results.

The ABCs of ASCVD Risk Management

All healthcare providers should participate in creating a more heart-healthy environment for sustained population-wide primordial prevention. Incorporating the recommendations from the many ACC/AHA, Canadian, and European guideline documents is quite challenging for clinicians. Use of an "ABCDE" approach (Table 29.5)[181] can integrate the most recent cardiovascular guidelines,[10] assist clinician adherence to guideline-based care, and promote participation in the Million Hearts Initiative,[182] the AHA 2020 goal,[66] and the 25 × 25 target; each of these programs are aimed at reducing strokes and heart attacks and promoting health over the next decade.

In the preceding sections of this chapter, we have discussed in the detail the first "A"—Assessment of risk. This begins with a global risk assessment, with selective use of additional risk stratification tools to refine risk when risk is uncertain. Quantification of subclinical atherosclerosis can provide the clinician and patient with an integrated view of risk factor exposure. At this time though, CAC is likely the only marker of risk that significantly improves discrimination and calibration and substantially reclassifies risk beyond traditional risk estimation.[148]

We outline Antiplatelet therapy and Cholesterol management hereafter, as using aspirin and high-intensity statins are generally recommended when CAC scores are high. We address Blood pressure management, Cigarettes, Diet, Diabetes, and Exercise in Table 29.5.

Antiplatelet Therapy

Aspirin Use in Primary Prevention

Aspirin can reduce the risk of atherothrombotic events in high-risk patients, but it comes at the cost of increased risk of bleeding. The data regarding the use of aspirin in primary prevention are equivocal. In the Antithrombotic Trialists' Collaboration, an analysis was done of 95,456 subjects in 6 clinical trials. Treatment with aspirin was associated with a small reduction in serious vascular events (0.51% vs 0.57% per year; $p = 0.0001$), but this was accompanied by a slight increase in the rate of major extracranial and gastrointestinal bleeding (0.10% vs 0.07% per year; $p < 0.0001$).[183] Since this 2009 publication, other studies have called into question the value of aspirin in primary prevention.[184,185]

Finding an appropriate balance between an increased bleeding risk with aspirin and prevention of ASCVD events is an area of active research. Prior aspirin guidelines recommended aspirin if the 10-year risk of an MI/CHD death was at least 10% and the potential benefit outweighed the bleeding risk. However, the 2013 prevention guidelines no longer recommend the use of the ATP III modified Framingham risk score that was used to estimate risk of MI/CHD death; instead, the algorithm that clinicians are encouraged to use now is the same one for statin eligibility (the pooled cohort equations), which estimates the risk of an MI or stroke.

It remains to be seen if upcoming ACC/AHA recommendations endorse a threshold of a 10% risk of MI/CVA for aspirin eligibility or not. Of note, a 2015 draft recommendation by the USPSTF did generally recommend (with a grade B recommendation) aspirin therapy for primary prevention of ASCVD and colorectal cancer for adults aged 50 to 59 with a 10% or greater 10-year ASCVD risk who are not at increased risk of bleeding using the pooled cohort equations.[186] The USPSTF also endorsed, although with a slightly weaker grade C recommendation, aspirin use for primary prevention for adults aged 60 to 69 years with a 10% or greater 10-year ASCVD risk who are not at increased risk for bleeding.

An interesting analysis by Miedema et al. looked at the potential of CAC scoring to guide aspirin use in primary prevention.[119] They studied 4220 subjects who were free of diabetes and calculated number needed to treat by applying an 18% relative CHD reduction to the observed event rates and compared those estimates with a 5-year number needed to harm based on risk of major bleeding reported in a large aspirin meta-analysis. They concluded that participants with a CAC of 100 or higher had favorable risk/benefit estimations for aspirin use whereas participants with no CAC would likely receive net harm from aspirin.

TABLE 29.5 ABCDEs for Primary Atherosclerotic Cardiovascular Disease (ASCVD) Prevention*

	ABCDE COMPONENT	RECOMMENDATION
A	Assess risk	Assess for ASCVD risk factors at least every 4 to 6 years beginning at age 20 Apply the pooled cohort equations (or similar global risk estimator) in asymptomatic adults aged 40 to 79 years old (not already on statins) to estimate 10-year risk for a first hard ASCVD event Consider selective use of CAC when risk-based treatment decisions are uncertain
A	Antiplatelet therapy	Consider aspirin 81 mg/day if 50 to 69 years old and 10-year ASCVD risk ≥ 10% if potential benefit outweighs risk of bleeding after clinician-patient risk discussion; no role for dual antiplatelet therapy
B	Blood pressure	Lifestyle interventions (i.e., weight management, exercise, sodium restriction) Pharmacotherapy as needed to reach blood pressure targets BP goal: <150/90 mm Hg among older adults (≥ 60 years); <140/90 mm Hg for those < 60 years, with diabetes, and/or with chronic kidney disease (Recent clinical trial data indicates that a person over age 50 with a cardiac risk factor should likely strive for an SBP < 130 mm Hg)
C	Cholesterol	Lifestyle changes are the major emphasis Statins recommended if within 1 of 4 statin benefit groups (per 2013 ACC/AHA lipid guidelines)[14] after clinician/patient discussion Among those not in one of the statin benefit groups or for whom a risk decision is still uncertain, statin use may be considered in the presence of one or more additional factors such as LDL-C ≥ 160 mg/dL, family history of premature ASCVD, high lifetime risk (among younger patients where short-term ASCVD risk is low), abnormal CAC score, ABI < 0.9, and hs-CRP ≥ 2.0 mg/L
C	Cigarette/tobacco cessation	Education Assessment, counseling, pharmacotherapy 5As: Ask, Advise, Assess, Assist, Arrange
D	Diet and weight management	Endorse diet that is low in trans-fats, saturated fats, and sodium; emphasizes fruits, vegetables, whole grains, lean protein, and nuts; minimizes sweets and sweetened beverages Goal body mass index: 18.5 to 24.9 kg/m^2; waist circumference: < 40 inches (men), < 35 inches (women) If weight loss needed: (1) lose 3% to 5% of body weight; (2) low-calorie diet: 1200 to 1500 kcal/day (women); 1500 to 1800 kcal/day (men); (3) energy deficit via decreased calorie intake and increased physical activity; (4) comprehensive lifestyle program; (5) weight loss maintenance
D	Diabetes prevention and treatment	Prevention: lifestyle interventions; goal: normal fasting blood glucose and hemoglobin A_{1c} < 5.7% Treatment: lifestyle interventions, metformin, oral hypoglycemic, insulin; goal: hemoglobin A_{1c} < 7% if obtained without significant hypoglycemia
E	Exercise	Regular aerobic physical activity; goal: 3 to 4 sessions a week, lasting on average 40 min/session involving moderate- to vigorous-intensity physical activity Education in sitting/sedentary time; goal: aim for 10,000 steps/day of walking

*High-risk: follow secondary prevention guidelines.
ABI, Ankle-brachial index; *BP,* blood pressure; *CAC,* coronary artery calcium; *hs-CRP,* high-sensitivity C-reactive protein, *LDL-C,* low-density lipoprotein cholesterol; *SBP,* systolic blood pressure.

In summary, the decision to use aspirin for the primary prevention of ASCVD requires an individualized approach that involves a clinician-patient risk discussion. This may involve further risk stratification using modalities such as CAC or biomarkers such as hs-CRP while incorporating risk of bleeding to make the decision about whether aspirin therapy should be recommended.

Cholesterol

Statin therapy undisputedly reduces morbidity and mortality among secondary prevention and moderate- to high-risk primary prevention individuals.[187] The 2013 ACC/AHA cholesterol guidelines formally endorse the absolute risk model, whereby the intensity of cholesterol treatment is directly linked to the estimated absolute ASCVD risk.[14] Four groups of patients who would benefit from statin therapy were identified; those with clinical ASCVD; those aged 40 to 75 years with diabetes mellitus and LDL-C 70 to 189 mg/dL; those with LDL-C of 190 mg/dL or greater; and those aged 40 to 75 years old with LDL-C of 70 to 189 mg/dL with an estimated 10-year risk of 7.5% or higher (with moderate evidence also supporting consideration of a moderate-intensity statin for those at 5% to < 7.5% 10-year risk). The guidelines recommend, particularly in this last group, that a clinician-patient risk discussion be conducted before statin initiation.[14] Statins have an excellent safety profile, but RCTs and meta-analyses have suggested an increased risk of diabetes with statins, particularly with high-intensity statins among individuals with prediabetes and metabolic syndrome.[188] Thus, this risk discussion between patients and their clinicians should address potential for ASCVD risk reduction, potential for adverse effects, and patient preferences, and encourage heart-healthy lifestyle and management of other risk factors.

Statins should be the first-line lipid-modifying agents used for primary prevention of ASCVD. However, some high-risk patients remain intolerant of statins even after a rechallenge; in these cases, a second-line agent with proven outcome and safety data (such as ezetimibe or the PCSK9 inhibitors) could be considered. Furthermore, there may be certain very-high-risk groups such as those with familial hyperlipidemia, a very strong family history of premature ASCVD, and/or advanced subclinical atherosclerosis that would benefit from combination lipid-lowering therapy (i.e., the addition of a second lipid-modifying agent on top of a maximal statin). These decisions should be made in the context of a clinician-patient risk discussion.

CONCLUDING THOUGHTS ON SCREENING THE ASYMPTOMATIC INDIVIDUAL

Critical to an informed clinician-patient discussion is communication of the most accurate and personalized risk information. Among individuals not in the above-mentioned statin-benefit groups or among those in whom treatment decisions are uncertain (i.e., the statin-reluctant patient or patients with unique risk factors such as ED or autoimmune diseases), additional factors can guide decision-making. These include an abnormal CAC score or ABI, family history of premature ASCVD, high hs-CRP, LDL-C level of 160 mg/dL or higher, or elevated lifetime risk. Additional factors that may aid in individual risk assessment may be identified in the future.

However, many clinicians and patients may still find that these guidelines lead to more aggressive treatment than they are comfortable with, especially in patients with an LDL-C of less than 100 mg/dL. All pharmacotherapy is associated with cost, as well as some disutility, such as burden of taking a daily drug and potential side effects. Rather than moving closer to an age-based treat-nearly-all strategy, individualized risk assessment may allow the opportunity to engage in a more sophisticated patient-centered risk discussion where patient preferences, competing medical risks, polypharmacy, and the disutility of taking medications can also be considered. Many questions remain, however, including how best and when to incorporate individualized risk assessment measures, how best to incorporate lifetime risk assessments, and whether making treatment decisions (i.e., initiation or titration of statins) based on these measures can improve outcomes.

In our clinical practice, we recommend the ABCDE approach as a way to provide a consistent and comprehensive organizational method for writing template-based notes and managing cardiovascular risk personalized for the individual patient. It is appropriate that the very first step of our approach is "A: Assessment of risk." As a starting point, we endorse screening with traditional ASCVD risk factors and applying the pooled cohort equations (in asymptomatic adults aged 40 to 79, not already on a statin), and embrace the concept of the clinician-patient risk discussion. When risk-based treatment decisions remain uncertain, which is common in those with an estimated ASCVD risk of 5% to 15%, other tools can be considered to help refine individual risk assessment. We feel that the current evidence supports the selective use of CAC as the best tool for further risk stratification. Again, there is no role in screening if the selected test does not change management strategies. Further patient discussions regarding "A: Antiplatelet therapy," "B: Blood pressure management," "C: Cholesterol management," "C: Cigarette smoking cessation," "D: Diet," "D: Diabetes prevention or management," and "E: Exercise" directly stem from the guideline recommendations and personalized risk assessment.[181]

Involving the patient in a risk discussion recognizes the importance of patient autonomy and value of shared decision-making in patient-centered care. Potential benefits from proper attention to clinician-patient risk discussions include a stronger clinician-patient relationship, increased patient engagement, and greater adherence to the treatment plan.

References

1. Mozaffarian D, Benjamin EJ, Go AS, et al.: Heart disease and stroke statistics–2015 update: a report from the American Heart Association, *Circulation* 131:e29–e322, 2015.
2. Robinson JG, Gidding SS: Curing atherosclerosis should be the next major cardiovascular prevention goal, *J Am Coll Cardiol* 63:2779–2785, 2014.
3. Rose G: Sick individuals and sick populations, *Int J Epidemiol* 14:32–38, 1985.
4. Cooney MT, Dudina A, Whincup P, et al.: Re-evaluating the Rose approach: comparative benefits of the population and high-risk preventive strategies, *Eur J Cardiovasc Prev Rehabil* 16:541–549, 2009.
5. Wilson JMG, Jungner G: *Principles and Practice of Screening for Disease*, Geneva, 1968, World Health Organization.
6. Lauer MS: Pseudodisease, the next great epidemic in coronary atherosclerosis? Comment on "Impact of coronary computed tomographic angiography results on patient and physician behavior in a low-risk population," *Arch Intern Med* 171:1268–1269, 2011.
7. Chou R: High Value Care Task Force of the American College of Physicians. Cardiac screening with electrocardiography, stress echocardiography, or myocardial perfusion imaging: advice for high-value care from the American College of Physicians, *Ann Intern Med* 162:438–447, 2015.
8. US Preventive Services Task Force: Using nontraditional risk factors in coronary heart disease risk assessment: U.S. Preventive Services Task Force recommendation statement, *Ann Intern Med* 151:474–482, 2009.
9. Greenland P, Alpert JS, Beller GA, et al.: 2010 ACCF/AHA guideline for assessment of cardiovascular risk in asymptomatic adults: a report of the American College of Cardiology Foundation/American Heart Association Task Force on Practice Guidelines, *J Am Coll Cardiol* 56:e50–e103, 2010.
10. Goff Jr DC, Lloyd-Jones DM, Bennett G, et al.: 2013 ACC/AHA guideline on the assessment of cardiovascular risk: a report of the American College of Cardiology/American Heart Association Task Force on Practice Guidelines, *Circulation* 129:S49–S73, 2014.
11. Perk J, De Backer G, Gohlke H, et al.: European guidelines on cardiovascular disease prevention in clinical practice (version 2012). The Fifth Joint Task Force of the European Society of Cardiology and Other Societies on Cardiovascular Disease Prevention in Clinical Practice (constituted by representatives of nine societies and by invited experts), *Eur Heart J* 33:1635–1701, 2012.
12. Pletcher MJ, Pignone M, Earnshaw S, et al.: Using the coronary artery calcium score to guide statin therapy: a cost-effectiveness analysis, *Circ Cardiovasc Qual Outcomes* 7:276–284, 2014.
13. Castellano JM, Sanz G, Penalvo JL, et al.: A polypill strategy to improve adherence: results from the FOCUS project, *J Am Coll Cardiol* 64:2071–2082, 2014.
14. Stone NJ, Robinson JG, Lichtenstein AH, et al.: 2013 ACC/AHA guideline on the treatment of blood cholesterol to reduce atherosclerotic cardiovascular risk in adults: a report of the American College of Cardiology/American Heart Association Task Force on Practice Guidelines, *Circulation* 129:S1–S45, 2014.
15. Ridker PM, Buring JE, Rifai N, et al.: Development and validation of improved algorithms for the assessment of global cardiovascular risk in women: the Reynolds risk score, *JAMA* 297:61120619, 2007.
16. Ridker PM, Paynter NP, Rifai N, et al.: C-reactive protein and parental history improve global cardiovascular risk prediction: the Reynolds risk score for men, *Circulation* 118:2243–2251, 2008.
17. Hippisley-Cox J, Coupland C, Vinogradova Y, et al.: Derivation and validation of QRISK, a new cardiovascular disease risk score for the United Kingdom: prospective open cohort study, *BMJ* 335:136, 2007.
18. Woodward M, Brindle P, Tunstall-Pedoe H, et al.: Adding social deprivation and family history to cardiovascular risk assessment: the ASSIGN score from the Scottish Heart Health Extended Cohort (SHHEC), *Heart* 93:172–176, 2007.
19. Assmann G, Cullen P, Schulte H: Simple scoring scheme for calculating the risk of acute coronary events based on the 10-year follow-up of the prospective cardiovascular Munster (PROCAM) study, *Circulation* 105:310–315, 2002.
20. Conroy RM, Pyorala K, Fitzgerald AP, et al.: Estimation of ten-year risk of fatal cardiovascular disease in Europe: the SCORE project, *Eur Heart J* 24:987–1003, 2003.
21. European Association for Cardiovascular Preventation and Rehabilitation, Reiner Z, Catapano AL, et al.: ESC/EAS Guidelines for the management of dyslipidaemias: the task force for the management of dyslipidaemias of the European Society of Cardiology (ESC) and the European Atherosclerosis Society (EAS), *Eur Heart J* 32:1769–1818, 2011.
22. Martin SS, Sperling LS, Blaha MJ, et al.: Clinician-patient risk discussion for atherosclerotic cardiovascular disease prevention: importance to implementation of the 2013 ACC/AHA Guidelines, *J Am Coll Cardiol* 65:1361–1368, 2015.
23. http://www.uspreventiveservicestaskforce.org/Page/Document/draft-recommendation-statement175/statin-use-in-adults-preventive-medication1.
24. Araujo F, Gouvinhas C, Fontes F, et al.: Trends in cardiovascular diseases and cancer mortality in 45 countries from five continents (1980–2010), *Eur J Prev Cardiol* 21:1004–1017, 2014.
25. Krumholz HM, Normand SL, Wang Y: Trends in hospitalizations and outcomes for acute cardiovascular disease and stroke, 1999–2011, *Circulation* 130:966–975, 2014.
26. Cook NR, Ridker PM: Further insight into the cardiovascular risk calculator: the roles of statins, revascularizations, and underascertainment in the Women's Health Study, *JAMA Intern Med* 174:1964–1971, 2014.
27. DeFilippis AP, Young R, Carrubba CJ, et al.: An analysis of calibration and discrimination among multiple cardiovascular risk scores in a modern multiethnic cohort, *Ann Intern Med* 162:266–275, 2015.
28. McEvoy JW, Diamond GA, Detrano RC, et al.: Risk and the physics of clinical prediction, *Am J Cardiol* 113:1429–1435, 2014.
29. Yeboah J, Polonsky TS, Young R, et al.: Utility of nontraditional risk markers in individuals ineligible for statin therapy according to the 2013 American College of Cardiology/American Heart Association cholesterol guidelines, *Circulation* 132:916–922, 2015.
30. Pencina MJ, Navar-Boggan AM, D'Agostino Sr RB, et al.: Application of new cholesterol guidelines to a population-based sample, *N Engl J Med* 370:1422–1431, 2014.
31. Blaha MJ, Dardari ZA, Blumenthal RS, et al.: The new "intermediate risk" group: a comparative analysis of the new 2013 ACC/AHA risk assessment guidelines versus prior guidelines in men, *Atherosclerosis* 237:1–4, 2014.
32. Blaha MJ, Feldman DI, Nasir K: Coronary artery calcium and physical fitness—the two best predictors of long-term survival, *Atherosclerosis* 234:93–94, 2014.
33. Myers RH, Kiely DK, Cupples LA, et al.: Parental history is an independent risk factor for coronary artery disease: the Framingham Study, *Am Heart J* 120:963–969, 1990.
34. Sesso HD, Lee IM, Gaziano JM, et al.: Maternal and paternal history of myocardial infarction and risk of cardiovascular disease in men and women, *Circulation* 104:393–398, 2001.
35. Kardia SL, Modell SM, Peyser PA: Family-centered approaches to understanding and preventing coronary heart disease, *Am J Prev Med* 24:143–151, 2003.
36. Patel J, Al Rifai M, Blaha MJ, et al.: Coronary artery calcium improves risk assessment in adults with a family history of premature coronary heart disease: results from multiethnic study of atherosclerosis, *Circ Cardiovasc Imaging* 8:e003186, 2015.
37. Lloyd-Jones DM, Nam BH, D'Agostino RB, et al.: Parental cardiovascular disease as a risk factor for cardiovascular disease in middle-aged adults: a prospective study of parents and offspring, *JAMA* 291:2204–2211, 2004.
38. Murabito JM, Pencina MJ, Nam BH, et al.: Sibling cardiovascular disease as a risk factor for cardiovascular disease in middle-aged adults, *JAMA* 294:3117–3123, 2005.
39. Jorde LB, Williams RR: Relation between family history of coronary artery disease and coronary risk variables, *Am J Cardiol* 62:708–713, 1988.
40. Mosca L, Benjamin EJ, Berra K, et al.: Effectiveness-based guidelines for the prevention of cardiovascular disease in women 2011 update: a guideline from the American Heart Association, *Circulation* 123:1243–1262, 2011.
41. Anderson TJ, Gregoire J, Hegele RA, et al.: 2012 update of the Canadian Cardiovascular Society guidelines for the diagnosis and treatment of dyslipidemia for the prevention of cardiovascular disease in the adult, *Can J Cardiol* 29:151–167, 2013.
42. Fairweather D, Frisancho-Kiss S, Rose NR: Sex differences in autoimmune disease from a pathological perspective, *Am J Pathol* 173:600–609, 2008.

43. del Rincon ID, Williams K, Stern MP, et al.: High incidence of cardiovascular events in a rheumatoid arthritis cohort not explained by traditional cardiac risk factors, *Arthritis Rheum* 44:2737–2745, 2001.
44. Manzi S, Meilahn EN, Rairie JE, et al.: Age-specific incidence rates of myocardial infarction and angina in women with systemic lupus erythematosus: comparison with the Framingham Study, *Am J Epidemiol* 145:408–415, 1997.
45. Salmon JE, Roman MJ. Subclinical atherosclerosis in rheumatoid arthritis and systemic lupus erythematosus, *Am J Med* 121:S3–S8, 2008.
46. Nurmohamed M, Bao Y, Signorovitch J, et al.: Longer durations of antitumour necrosis factor treatment are associated with reduced risk of cardiovascular events in patients with rheumatoid arthritis, *RMD Open* 1:e000080, 2015.
47. Rich-Edwards JW: The predictive pregnancy: what complicated pregnancies tell us about mother's future cardiovascular risk, *Circulation* 125:1336–1338, 2012.
48. Bellamy L, Casas JP, Hingorani AD, et al.: Type 2 diabetes mellitus after gestational diabetes: a systematic review and meta-analysis, *Lancet* 373:1773–1779, 2009.
49. Lauenborg J, Mathiesen E, Hansen T, et al.: The prevalence of the metabolic syndrome in a Danish population of women with previous gestational diabetes mellitus is three-fold higher than in the general population, *J Clin Endocrinol Metab* 90:4004–4010, 2005.
50. Pirkola J, Pouta A, Bloigu A, et al.: Prepregnancy overweight and gestational diabetes as determinants of subsequent diabetes and hypertension after 20-year follow-up, *J Clin Endocrinol Metab* 95:772–778, 2010.
51. Metzger BE, Buchanan TA, Coustan DR, et al.: Summary and recommendations of the Fifth International Workshop-Conference on Gestational Diabetes Mellitus, *Diabetes Care* 30(Suppl 2): S251–S260, 2007.
52. Fadl H, Magnuson A, Ostlund I, et al.: Gestational diabetes mellitus and later cardiovascular disease: a Swedish population based case-control study, *BJOG* 121:1530–1536, 2014.
53. Evans CS, Gooch L, Flotta D, et al.: Cardiovascular system during the postpartum state in women with a history of preeclampsia, *Hypertension* 58:57–62, 2011.
54. Ahmed R, Dunford J, Mehran R, et al.: Pre-eclampsia and future cardiovascular risk among women: a review, *J Am Coll Cardiol* 63:1815–1822, 2014.
55. Ray JG, Vermeulen MJ, Schull MJ, et al.: Cardiovascular health after maternal placental syndromes (CHAMPS): population-based retrospective cohort study, *Lancet* 366:1797–1803, 2005.
56. Bellamy L, Casas JP, Hingorani AD, et al.: Pre-eclampsia and risk of cardiovascular disease and cancer in later life: systematic review and meta-analysis, *BMJ* 335:974, 2007.
57. Selvin E, Burnett AL, Platz EA: Prevalence and risk factors for erectile dysfunction in the US, *Am J Med* 120:151–157, 2007.
58. Banks E, Joshy G, Abhayaratna WP, et al.: Erectile dysfunction severity as a risk marker for cardiovascular disease hospitalisation and all-cause mortality: a prospective cohort study, *PLoS Med* 10:e1001372, 2013.
59. Gandaglia G, Briganti A, Jackson G, et al.: A systematic review of the association between erectile dysfunction and cardiovascular disease, *Eur Urol* 65:968–978, 2014.
60. Pastuszak AW, Hyman DA, Yadav N, et al.: Erectile dysfunction as a marker for cardiovascular disease diagnosis and intervention: a cost analysis, *J Sex Med* 12:975–984, 2015.
61. Shah NP, Cainzos-Achirica M, Feldman DI, et al.: Cardiovascular disease prevention in men with vascular erectile dysfunction: the view of the preventive cardiologist, *Am J Med* 129(3):251–259, 2015.
62. Strath SJ, Kaminsky LA, Ainsworth BE, et al.: Guide to the assessment of physical activity: clinical and research applications: a scientific statement from the American Heart Association, *Circulation* 128:2259–2279, 2013.
63. Centers for Disease Control and Prevention: Adult participation in recommended levels of physical activity–United States, 2001 and 2003, *MMWR Morb Mortal Wkly Rep* 54:1208–1212, 2005.
64. Booth FW, Gordon SE, Carlson CJ, et al.: Waging war on modern chronic diseases: primary prevention through exercise biology, *J Appl Physiol (1985)* 88:774–787, 2000.
65. Kohl III HW, Craig CL, Lambert EV, et al.: The pandemic of physical inactivity: global action for public health, *Lancet* 380:294–305, 2012.
66. Lloyd-Jones DM, Hong Y, Labarthe D, et al.: Defining and setting national goals for cardiovascular health promotion and disease reduction: the American Heart Association's strategic impact goal through 2020 and beyond, *Circulation* 121:586–613, 2010.
67. Same RV, Feldman DI, Shah N, et al.: Relationship between sedentary behavior and cardiovascular risk, *Curr Cardiol Rep* 18:6, 2016.
68. Owen N, Sparling PB, Healy GN, et al.: Sedentary behavior: emerging evidence for a new health risk, *Mayo Clin Proc* 85:1138–1141, 2010.
69. Biswas A, Oh PI, Faulkner GE, et al.: Sedentary time and its association with risk for disease incidence, mortality, and hospitalization in adults: a systematic review and meta-analysis, *Ann Intern Med* 162:123–132, 2015.
70. Burke LE, Ma J, Azar KM, Bennett GG, et al.: Current science on consumer use of mobile health for cardiovascular disease prevention: a scientific statement from the American Heart Association, *Circulation* 132:1157–1213, 2015.
71. Case MA, Burwick HA, Volpp KG, et al.: Accuracy of smartphone applications and wearable devices for tracking physical activity data, *JAMA* 313:625–626, 2015.
72. Martin SS, Feldman DI, Blumenthal RS, et al.: A randomized clinical trial of an automated mhealth intervention for physical activity promotion, *J Am Heart Assoc* 4, 2015.
73. Sarnak MJ, Levey AS, Schoolwerth AC, et al.: Kidney disease as a risk factor for development of cardiovascular disease: a statement from the American Heart Association Councils on Kidney in Cardiovascular Disease, High Blood Pressure Research, Clinical Cardiology, and Epidemiology and Prevention, *Hypertension* 42:1050–1065, 2003.
74. Briasoulis A, Bakris GL: Chronic kidney disease as a coronary artery disease risk equivalent, *Curr Cardiol Rep* 15:340, 2013.
75. Colantonio LD, Baber U, Banach M, et al.: Contrasting cholesterol management guidelines for adults with CKD, *J Am Soc Nephrol* 26:1173–1180, 2015.
76. Blaha MJ, Elasy TA: Clinical definitions of the metabolic syndrome: why the confusion? *Clinical Diabetes* 24:125–131, 2006.
77. Blaha MJ, Tota-Maharaj R. Metabolic Syndrome: From Risk Factors to Treatment. SEEd publishers, Italy. Handbook. 192 pages. May 31, 2012. ISBN-13: 978-8897419198 (Two Editions: English and Italian).
78. Kannel WB, Anderson K, McGee DL, et al.: Nonspecific electrocardiographic abnormality as a predictor of coronary heart disease: the Framingham Study, *Am Heart J* 113:370–376, 1987.
79. Menotti A, Seccareccia F: Electrocardiographic Minnesota code findings predicting short-term mortality in asymptomatic subjects. The Italian RIFLE Pooling Project (risk factors and life expectancy), *G Ital Cardiol* 27:40–49, 1997.
80. De Bacquer D, De Backer G, Kornitzer M, et al.: Prognostic value of ECG findings for total, cardiovascular disease, and coronary heart disease death in men and women, *Heart* 80:570–577, 1998.
81. Auer R, Bauer DC, Marques-Vidal P, et al.: Association of major and minor ECG abnormalities with coronary heart disease events, *JAMA* 307:1497–1505, 2012.
82. Greenland P: Should the resting electrocardiogram be ordered as a routine risk assessment test in healthy asymptomatic adults? *JAMA* 307:1530–1531, 2012.
83. Moyer VA: U.S. Preventive Services Task Force. Screening for coronary heart disease with electrocardiography: U.S. Preventive Services Task Force recommendation statement, *Ann Intern Med* 157:512–518, 2012.
84. Michos ED, Abraham TP: Echoing the appropriate use criteria: the role of echocardiography for cardiovascular risk assessment of the asymptomatic individual, *JAMA Intern Med* 173:1598–1599, 2013.
85. Pearlman AS, Ryan T, Picard MH, et al.: Evolving trends in the use of echocardiography: a study of Medicare beneficiaries, *J Am Coll Cardiol* 49:2283–2291, 2007.
86. Sundstrom J, Lind L, Arnlov J, et al.: Echocardiographic and electrocardiographic diagnoses of left ventricular hypertrophy predict mortality independently of each other in a population of elderly men, *Circulation* 103:2346–2351, 2001.
87. Wang TJ, Evans JC, Benjamin EJ, et al.: Natural history of asymptomatic left ventricular systolic dysfunction in the community, *Circulation* 108:977–982, 2003.
88. Lindekleiv H, Lochen ML, Mathiesen EB, et al.: Echocardiographic screening of the general population and long-term survival: a randomized clinical study, *JAMA Intern Med* 173:1592–1598, 2013.
89. ACCF/ASE/AHA/ASNC/HFSA/HRS/SCAI/SCCM/SCCT/SCMR 2011 Appropriate Use Criteria for Echocardiography. A Report of the American College of Cardiology Foundation Appropriate Use Criteria Task Force, American Society of Echocardiography, American Heart Association, American Society of Nuclear Cardiology, Heart Failure Society of America, Heart Rhythm Society, Society for Cardiovascular Angiography and Interventions, Society of Critical Care Medicine, Society of Cardiovascular Computed Tomography, and Society for Cardiovascular Magnetic Resonance Endorsed by the American College of Chest Physicians, *J Am Coll Cardiol* 57:1126–1166, 2011.
90. Yeghiazarians Y, Braunstein JB, Askari A, et al.: Unstable angina pectoris, *N Engl J Med* 342: 101–114, 2000.
91. Balady GJ, Arena R, Sietsema K, et al.: Clinician's guide to cardiopulmonary exercise testing in adults: a scientific statement from the American Heart Association, *Circulation* 122:191–225, 2010.
92. Gibbons RJ, Balady GJ, Bricker JT, et al.: ACC/AHA 2002 guideline update for exercise testing: summary article. A report of the American College of Cardiology/American Heart Association Task Force on Practice Guidelines (committee to update the 1997 exercise testing guidelines), *J Am Coll Cardiol* 40:1531–1540, 2002.
93. Fowler-Brown A, Pignone M, Pletcher M, et al.: Exercise tolerance testing to screen for coronary heart disease: a systematic review for the technical support for the U.S. Preventive Services Task Force, *Ann Intern Med* 140:W9–W24, 2004.
94. Davenport E, Palileo E, Kruyer W, et al.: Screening with echocardiography or stress testing in asymptomatic USAF aviators—not efficacious, *J Am Coll Cardiol* 65, 2015.
95. Mora S, Redberg RF, Cui Y, et al.: Ability of exercise testing to predict cardiovascular and all-cause death in asymptomatic women: a 20-year follow-up of the Lipid Research Clinics Prevalence Study, *JAMA* 290:1600–1607, 2003.
96. Kodama S, Saito K, Tanaka S, et al.: Cardiorespiratory fitness as a quantitative predictor of all-cause mortality and cardiovascular events in healthy men and women: a meta-analysis, *JAMA* 301:2024–2035, 2009.
97. Ahmed HM, Al-Mallah MH, McEvoy JW, et al.: Maximal exercise testing variables and 10-year survival: fitness risk score derivation from the FIT Project, *Mayo Clin Proc* 90:346–355, 2015.
98. Qureshi WT, Alirhayim Z, Blaha MJ, et al.: Cardiorespiratory fitness and risk of incident atrial fibrillation: results from the Henry Ford exercise testing (FIT) project, *Circulation* 131:1827–1834, 2015.
99. Juraschek SP, Blaha MJ, Blumenthal RS, et al.: Cardiorespiratory fitness and incident diabetes: the FIT (Henry Ford ExercIse Testing) project, *Diabetes Care* 38:1075–1081, 2015.
100. Aladin AI, Al Rifai M, Rasool SH, et al.: The association of resting heart rate and incident hypertension: the Henry Ford Hospital exercise testing (FIT) project, *Am J Hypertens* 29(2):251–257, 2015.
101. Echouffo-Tcheugui JB, Butler J, Yancy CW, et al.: Association of physical activity or fitness with incident heart failure: a systematic review and meta-analysis, *Circ Heart Fail* 8:853–861, 2015.
102. Shaya GE, Al-Mallah MH, Hung RK, et al.: High exercise capacity attenuates risk of early mortality after first myocardial infarction: the Henry Ford exercise testing (FIT) project, *Mayo Clin Proc* 91(2):129–139, 2016.
103. Kokkinos PF, Holland JC, Pittaras AE, et al.: Cardiorespiratory fitness and coronary heart disease risk factor association in women, *J Am Coll Cardiol* 26:358–364, 1995.
104. Minder CM, Shaya GE, Michos ED, et al.: Relation between self-reported physical activity level, fitness, and cardiometabolic risk, *Am J Cardiol* 113:637–643, 2014.
105. Hung RK, Al-Mallah MH, Qadi MA, et al.: Cardiorespiratory fitness attenuates risk for major adverse cardiac events in hyperlipidemic men and women independent of statin therapy: the Henry Ford exercise testing project, *Am Heart J* 170:390–399, 2015.
106. McClelland RL, Nasir K, Budoff M, et al.: Arterial age as a function of coronary artery calcium (from the Multi-Ethnic Study of Atherosclerosis [MESA]), *Am J Cardiol* 103:59–63, 2009.
107. Alluri K, Joshi PH, Henry TS, et al.: Scoring of coronary artery calcium scans: history, assumptions, current limitations, and future directions, *Atherosclerosis* 239:109–117, 2015.
108. Cho I, Chang HJ, Sung JM, et al.: Coronary computed tomographic angiography and risk of all-cause mortality and nonfatal myocardial infarction in subjects without chest pain syndrome from the CONFIRM Registry (coronary CT angiography evaluation for clinical outcomes: an international multicenter registry), *Circulation* 126:304–313, 2012.
109. Joshi PH, Blaha MJ, Blumenthal RS, et al.: What is the role of calcium scoring in the age of coronary computed tomographic angiography? *J Nucl Cardiol* 19:1226–1235, 2012.
110. Polonsky TS, McClelland RL, Jorgensen NW, et al.: Coronary artery calcium score and risk classification for coronary heart disease prediction, *JAMA* 303:1610–1616, 2010.
111. Nasir K, Rubin J, Blaha MJ, et al.: Interplay of coronary artery calcification and traditional risk factors for the prediction of all-cause mortality in asymptomatic individuals, *Circ Cardiovasc Imaging* 5:467–473, 2012.
112. Silverman MG, Blaha MJ, Krumholz HM, et al.: Impact of coronary artery calcium on coronary heart disease events in individuals at the extremes of traditional risk factor burden: the Multi-Ethnic Study of Atherosclerosis, *Eur Heart J* 35:2232–2241, 2014.
113. Budoff MJ, McClelland RL, Nasir K, et al.: Cardiovascular events with absent or minimal coronary calcification: the Multi-Ethnic Study of Atherosclerosis (MESA), *Am Heart J* 158:554–561, 2009.
114. Patel J, Blaha MJ, McEvoy JW, et al.: All-cause mortality in asymptomatic persons with extensive Agatston scores above 1000, *J Cardiovasc Comput Tomogr* 8:26–32, 2014.
115. Blaha MJ, Blumenthal RS, Budoff MJ, et al.: Understanding the utility of zero coronary calcium as a prognostic test: a Bayesian approach, *Circ Cardiovasc Qual Outcomes* 4:253–256, 2011.
116. Blaha MJ, Budoff MJ, DeFilippis AP, et al.: Associations between C-reactive protein, coronary artery calcium, and cardiovascular events: implications for the JUPITER population from MESA, a population-based cohort study, *Lancet* 378:684–692, 2011.
117. Martin SS, Blaha MJ, Blankstein R, et al.: Dyslipidemia, coronary artery calcium, and incident atherosclerotic cardiovascular disease: implications for statin therapy from the Multi-Ethnic Study of Atherosclerosis, *Circulation* 129:77–86, 2014.
118. Bittencourt MS, Blaha MJ, Blankstein R, et al.: Polypill therapy, subclinical atherosclerosis, and cardiovascular events—implications for the use of preventive pharmacotherapy: MESA (Multi-Ethnic Study of Atherosclerosis), *J Am Coll Cardiol* 63:434–443, 2014.
119. Miedema MD, Duprez DA, Misialek JR, et al.: Use of coronary artery calcium testing to guide aspirin utilization for primary prevention: estimates from the Multi-Ethnic Study of Atherosclerosis, *Circ Cardiovasc Qual Outcomes* 7:453–460, 2014.
120. Nasir K, Bittencourt MS, Blaha MJ, et al.: Implications of coronary artery calcium testing among statin candidates according to American College of Cardiology/American Heart Association Cholesterol Management Guidelines: MESA (Multi-Ethnic Study of Atherosclerosis), *J Am Coll Cardiol* 66:1657–1668, 2015.

121. Roberts ET, Horne A, Martin SS, et al.: Cost-effectiveness of coronary artery calcium testing for coronary heart and cardiovascular disease risk prediction to guide statin allocation: the Multi-Ethnic Study of Atherosclerosis (MESA), *PLoS One* 10:e0116377, 2015.
122. Valenti V, Ó Hartaigh B, Heo R, et al.: A 15-year warranty period for asymptomatic individuals without coronary artery calcium: a prospective follow-up of 9,715 individuals, *JACC Cardiovasc Imaging* 8:900–909, 2015.
123. Shaw LJ, Giambrone AE, Blaha MJ, et al.: Long-term prognosis after coronary artery calcification testing in asymptomatic patients: a cohort study, *Ann Intern Med* 163:14–21, 2015.
124. Blaha MJ, Cainzos-Achirica M, Greenland P, et al.: Role of coronary artery calcium score of zero and other negative risk markers for cardiovascular disease: the Multi-Ethnic Study of Atherosclerosis (MESA), *Circulation* 133:849–858, 2016.
125. McClelland RL, Jorgensen NW, Budoff M, et al.: 10-year coronary heart disease risk prediction using coronary artery calcium and traditional risk factors: derivation in the MESA (Multi-Ethnic Study of Atherosclerosis) with validation in the HNR (Heinz Nixdorf Recall) study and the DHS (Dallas Heart Study), *J Am Coll Cardiol* 66:1643–1653, 2015.
126. Rozanski A, Gransar H, Shaw LJ, et al.: Impact of coronary artery calcium scanning on coronary risk factors and downstream testing the EISNER (Early Identification of Subclinical Atherosclerosis by Noninvasive Imaging Research) prospective randomized trial, *J Am Coll Cardiol* 57:1622–1632, 2011.
127. Nasir K, McClelland RL, Blumenthal RS, et al.: Coronary artery calcium in relation to initiation and continuation of cardiovascular preventive medications: the Multi-Ethnic Study of Atherosclerosis (MESA), *Circ Cardiovasc Qual Outcomes* 3:228–235, 2010.
128. Horton KM, Post WS, Blumenthal RS, et al.: Prevalence of significant noncardiac findings on electron-beam computed tomography coronary artery calcium screening examinations, *Circulation* 106:532–534, 2002.
129. http://www.robinsca.nl/wp-content/uploads/2014/10/82355-ErasmusMC-Robinsca-Informatiebrochure-deelnemer-Engels-def.pdf.
130. McEvoy JW, Blaha MJ: Coronary artery calcium testing: exploring the need for a randomized trial, *Circ Cardiovasc Imaging* 7:578–580, 2014.
131. Budoff MJ, Nasir K, McClelland RL, et al.: Coronary calcium predicts events better with absolute calcium scores than age-sex-race/ethnicity percentiles: MESA (Multi-Ethnic Study of Atherosclerosis), *J Am Coll Cardiol* 53:345–352, 2009.
132. Budoff MJ, Young R, Lopez VA, et al.: Progression of coronary calcium and incident coronary heart disease events: MESA (Multi-Ethnic Study of Atherosclerosis), *J Am Coll Cardiol* 61:1231–1239, 2013.
133. Min JK, Lin FY, Gidseg DS, et al.: Determinants of coronary calcium conversion among patients with a normal coronary calcium scan: what is the "warranty period" for remaining normal? *J Am Coll Cardiol* 55:1110–1117, 2010.
134. McEvoy JW, Blaha MJ, Rivera JJ, et al.: Mortality rates in smokers and nonsmokers in the presence or absence of coronary artery calcification, *JACC Cardiovasc Imaging* 5:1037–1045, 2012.
135. Valenti V, ÓHartaigh B, Cho I, et al.: Absence of coronary artery calcium identifies asymptomatic diabetic individuals at low near-term but not long-term risk of mortality: a 15-year follow-up study of 9715 patients, *Circ Cardiovasc Imaging* 9:e003528, 2016.
136. Arbab-Zadeh A, Di Carli MF, Cerci R, et al.: Accuracy of computed tomographic angiography and single-photon emission computed tomography-acquired myocardial perfusion imaging for the diagnosis of coronary artery disease, *Circ Cardiovasc Imaging* 8:e003533, 2015.
137. Braunwald E: Progress in the noninvasive detection of high-risk coronary plaques, *J Am Coll Cardiol* 66:347–349, 2015.
138. Hou ZH, Lu B, Gao Y, et al.: Prognostic value of coronary CT angiography and calcium score for major adverse cardiac events in outpatients, *JACC Cardiovasc Imaging* 5:990–999, 2012.
139. Choi EK, Choi SI, Rivera JJ, et al.: Coronary computed tomography angiography as a screening tool for the detection of occult coronary artery disease in asymptomatic individuals, *J Am Coll Cardiol* 52:357–365, 2008.
140. Hulten E, Bittencourt MS, Ghoshhajra B, et al.: Incremental prognostic value of coronary artery calcium score versus CT angiography among symptomatic patients without known coronary artery disease, *Atherosclerosis* 233:190–195, 2014.
141. McEvoy JW, Blaha MJ, Nasir K, et al.: Impact of coronary computed tomographic angiography results on patient and physician behavior in a low-risk population, *Arch Intern Med* 171:1260–1268, 2011.
142. Stein JH, Korcarz CE, Hurst RT, et al.: Use of carotid ultrasound to identify subclinical vascular disease and evaluate cardiovascular disease risk: a consensus statement from the American Society of Echocardiography Carotid Intima-Media Thickness Task Force. Endorsed by the Society for Vascular Medicine, *J Am Soc Echocardiogr* 21:93–111, 2008. quiz 189–190.
143. Johnson HM, Douglas PS, Srinivasan SR, et al.: Predictors of carotid intima-media thickness progression in young adults: the Bogalusa Heart Study, *Stroke* 38:900–905, 2007.
144. Folsom AR, Kronmal RA, Detrano RC, et al.: Coronary artery calcification compared with carotid intima-media thickness in the prediction of cardiovascular disease incidence: the Multi-Ethnic Study of Atherosclerosis (MESA), *Arch Intern Med* 168:1333–1339, 2008.
145. Naqvi TZ, Lee MS: Carotid intima-media thickness and plaque in cardiovascular risk assessment, *JACC Cardiovasc Imaging* 7:1025–1038, 2014.
146. Chambless LE, Heiss G, Folsom AR, et al.: Association of coronary heart disease incidence with carotid arterial wall thickness and major risk factors: the Atherosclerosis Risk in Communities (ARIC) study, 1987–1993, *Am J Epidemiol* 146:483–494, 1997.
147. Bots ML, Hoes AW, Koudstaal PJ, et al.: Common carotid intima-media thickness and risk of stroke and myocardial infarction: the Rotterdam Study, *Circulation* 96:1432–1437, 1997.
148. Yeboah J, McClelland RL, Polonsky TS, et al.: Comparison of novel risk markers for improvement in cardiovascular risk assessment in intermediate-risk individuals, *JAMA* 308:788–795, 2012.
149. Simon A, Megnien JL, Chironi G: The value of carotid intima-media thickness for predicting cardiovascular risk, *Arterioscler Thromb Vasc Biol* 30:182–185, 2010.
150. van den Oord SC, Sijbrands EJ, ten Kate GL, et al.: Carotid intima-media thickness for cardiovascular risk assessment: systematic review and meta-analysis, *Atherosclerosis* 228:1–11, 2013.
151. Polak JF, Pencina MJ, Pencina KM, et al.: Carotid-wall intima-media thickness and cardiovascular events, *N Engl J Med* 365:213–221, 2011.
152. Nambi V, Chambless L, He M, et al.: Common carotid artery intima-media thickness is as good as carotid intima-media thickness of all carotid artery segments in improving prediction of coronary heart disease risk in the Atherosclerosis Risk in Communities (ARIC) study, *Eur Heart J* 33:183–190, 2012.
153. Gepner AD, Young R, Delaney JA, et al.: Comparison of coronary artery calcium presence, carotid plaque presence, and carotid intima-media thickness for cardiovascular disease prediction in the Multi-Ethnic Study of Atherosclerosis, *Circ Cardiovasc Imaging* 8, 2015.
154. Nambi V, Brunner G, Ballantyne CM: Ultrasound in cardiovascular risk prediction: don't forget the plaque! *J Am Heart Assoc* 2:e000180, 2013.
155. LeFevre ML: U.S. Preventive Services Task Force. Screening for asymptomatic carotid artery stenosis: U.S. Preventive Services Task Force recommendation statement, *Ann Intern Med* 161:356–362, 2014.
156. Ridker PM, Rifai N, Rose L, et al.: Comparison of C-reactive protein and low-density lipoprotein cholesterol levels in the prediction of first cardiovascular events, *N Engl J Med* 347:1557–1565, 2002.
157. Ridker PM, Danielson E, Fonseca FA, et al.: Rosuvastatin to prevent vascular events in men and women with elevated C-reactive protein, *N Engl J Med* 359:2195–2207, 2008.
158. Kim J, McEvoy JW, Nasir K, et al.: Critical review of high-sensitivity C-reactive protein and coronary artery calcium for the guidance of statin allocation: head-to-head comparison of the JUPITER and St. Francis Heart Trials, *Circ Cardiovasc Qual Outcomes* 7:315–322, 2014.
159. Ostchega Y, Paulose-Ram R, Dillon CF, et al.: Prevalence of peripheral arterial disease and risk factors in persons aged 60 and older: data from the National Health and Nutrition Examination Survey 1999–2004, *J Am Geriatr Soc* 55:583–589, 2007.
160. Newman AB, Siscovick DS, Manolio TA, et al.: Ankle-arm index as a marker of atherosclerosis in the Cardiovascular Health Study. Cardiovascular Heart Study (CHS) collaborative research group, *Circulation* 88:837–845, 1993.
161. Hooi JD, Kester AD, Stoffers HE, et al.: Asymptomatic peripheral arterial occlusive disease predicted cardiovascular morbidity and mortality in a 7-year follow-up study, *J Clin Epidemiol* 57:294–300, 2004.
162. Diehm C, Allenberg JR, Pittrow D, et al.: Mortality and vascular morbidity in older adults with asymptomatic versus symptomatic peripheral artery disease, *Circulation* 120:2053–2061, 2009.
163. Ankle Brachial Index Collaboration, Fowkes FG, Murray GD, et al.: Ankle brachial index combined with Framingham risk score to predict cardiovascular events and mortality: a meta-analysis, *JAMA* 300:197–208, 2008.
164. Moyer VA: U.S. Preventive Services Task Force. Screening for peripheral artery disease and cardiovascular disease risk assessment with the ankle-brachial index in adults: U.S. Preventive Services Task Force recommendation statement, *Ann Intern Med* 159:342–348, 2013.
165. Jaffe AS: Chasing troponin: how low can you go if you can see the rise? *J Am Coll Cardiol* 48:1763–1764, 2006.
166. Saunders JT, Nambi V, de Lemos JA, et al.: Cardiac troponin T measured by a highly sensitive assay predicts coronary heart disease, heart failure, and mortality in the Atherosclerosis Risk in Communities Study, *Circulation* 123:1367–1376, 2011.
167. Sze J, Mooney J, Barzi F, et al.: Cardiac troponin and its relationship to cardiovascular outcomes in community populations—a systematic review and meta-analysis, *Heart Lung Circ* 25(3): 217–228, 2015.
168. Everett BM, Zeller T, Glynn RJ, et al.: High-sensitivity cardiac troponin I and B-type natriuretic peptide as predictors of vascular events in primary prevention: impact of statin therapy, *Circulation* 131:1851–1860, 2015.
169. Everett BM, Brooks MM, Vlachos HE, et al.: Troponin and cardiac events in stable ischemic heart disease and diabetes, *N Engl J Med* 373:610–620, 2015.
170. Wannamethee SG, Shaper AG, Whincup PH, et al.: Impact of diabetes on cardiovascular disease risk and all-cause mortality in older men: influence of age at onset, diabetes duration, and established and novel risk factors, *Arch Intern Med* 171:404–410, 2011.
171. Young LH, Wackers FJ, Chyun DA, et al.: Cardiac outcomes after screening for asymptomatic coronary artery disease in patients with type 2 diabetes: the DIAD study: a randomized controlled trial, *JAMA* 301:1547–1555, 2009.
172. Blumenthal RS, Becker DM, Yanek LR, et al.: Detecting occult coronary disease in a high-risk asymptomatic population, *Circulation* 107:702–707, 2003.
173. Blumenthal RS, Becker DM, Yanek LR, et al.: Comparison of coronary calcium and stress myocardial perfusion imaging in apparently healthy siblings of individuals with premature coronary artery disease, *Am J Cardiol* 97:328–333, 2006.
174. Muhlestein JB, Lappe DL, Lima JA, et al.: Effect of screening for coronary artery disease using CT angiography on mortality and cardiac events in high-risk patients with diabetes: the FACTOR-64 randomized clinical trial, *JAMA* 312:2234–2243, 2014.
175. Raggi P, Shaw LJ, Berman DS, et al.: Prognostic value of coronary artery calcium screening in subjects with and without diabetes, *J Am Coll Cardiol* 43:1663–1669, 2004.
176. Kral BG, Becker LC, Vaidya D, et al.: Silent myocardial ischaemia and long-term coronary artery disease outcomes in apparently healthy people from families with early-onset ischaemic heart disease, *Eur Heart J* 32:2766–2772, 2011.
177. Knapper JT, Khosa F, Blaha MJ, et al.: Coronary calcium scoring for long-term mortality prediction in patients with and without a family history of coronary disease, *Heart*, 2015.
178. Corrado D, Basso C, Pavei A, et al.: Trends in sudden cardiovascular death in young competitive athletes after implementation of a preparticipation screening program, *JAMA* 296:1593–1601, 2006.
179. Corrado D, Pelliccia A, Bjornstad HH, et al.: Cardiovascular pre-participation screening of young competitive athletes for prevention of sudden death: proposal for a common European protocol. Consensus Statement of the Study Group of Sport Cardiology of the Working Group of Cardiac Rehabilitation and Exercise Physiology and the Working Group of Myocardial and Pericardial Diseases of the European Society of Cardiology, *Eur Heart J* 26:516–524, 2005.
180. Maron BJ, Levine BD, Washington RL, et al.: Eligibility and disqualification recommendations for competitive athletes with cardiovascular abnormalities: Task Force 2: preparticipation screening for cardiovascular disease in competitive athletes: a scientific statement from the American Heart Association and American College of Cardiology, *Circulation* 132:e267–e272, 2015.
181. Kohli P, Whelton SP, Hsu S, et al.: Clinician's guide to the updated ABCs of cardiovascular disease prevention, *J Am Heart Assoc* 3:e001098, 2014.
182. Frieden TR, Berwick DM: The "million hearts" initiative—preventing heart attacks and strokes, *N Engl J Med* 365:e27, 2011.
183. Antithrombotic Trialists' (ATT) Collaboration, Baigent C, Blackwell L, et al.: Aspirin in the primary and secondary prevention of vascular disease: collaborative meta-analysis of individual participant data from randomised trials, *Lancet* 373:1849–1860, 2009.
184. Ogawa H, Nakayama M, Morimoto T, et al.: Low-dose aspirin for primary prevention of atherosclerotic events in patients with type 2 diabetes: a randomized controlled trial, *JAMA* 300: 2134–2141, 2008.
185. Fowkes FG, Price JF, Stewart MC, et al.: Aspirin for prevention of cardiovascular events in a general population screened for a low ankle brachial index: a randomized controlled trial, *JAMA* 303:841–848, 2010.
186. http://www.uspreventiveservicestaskforce.org/Page/Document/draft-recommendation-statement/aspirin-to-prevent-cardiovascular-disease-and-cancer.
187. Cholesterol Treatment Trialists Collaborative, Mihaylova B, Emberson J, et al.: The effects of lowering LDL cholesterol with statin therapy in people at low risk of vascular disease: meta-analysis of individual data from 27 randomised trials, *Lancet* 380:581–590, 2012.
188. Desai CS, Martin SS, Blumenthal RS: Non-cardiovascular effects associated with statins, *BMJ* 349: g3743, 2014.
189. Blaha MJ, Gluckman T, Blumenthal RS: Chapter 1–Preventive cardiology: past, present, and future. In: Blumenthal RS, Wong N, Foody D, editors. Preventive Cardiology: A Companion to Braunwald's Heart Disease. 2011: [Chapter 1].
190. Task Force Members, Montalescot G, Sechtem U, et al.: 2013 ESC guidelines on the management of stable coronary artery disease: the Task Force on the management of stable coronary artery disease of the European Society of Cardiology, *Eur Heart J* 34:2949–3003, 2013.
191. Wilson PW, D'Agostino RB, Levy D, et al.: Prediction of coronary heart disease using risk factor categories, *Circulation* 97:1837–1847, 1998.
192. D'Agostino Sr RB, Vasan RS, Pencina MJ, et al.: General cardiovascular risk profile for use in primary care: the Framingham Heart Study, *Circulation* 117:743–753, 2008.
193. Expert Panel on Detection and Treatment of High Blood Cholesterol in Adults: Executive summary of the third report of the National Cholesterol Education Program (NCEP) expert panel on detection, evaluation, and treatment of high blood cholesterol in adults (Adult Treatment Panel).

30 Secondary Prevention of Coronary Artery Disease

Karol E. Watson, Yuanlin Guo, and Sheila Sahni

INTRODUCTION

Great strides have been made in reducing morbidity and mortality from heart disease in recent decades. Despite this, coronary artery disease (CAD) rates remain unacceptably high. CAD is the single largest cause of mortality in the United States[1] and preventing morbidity and mortality from chronic CAD remains a top priority. The objective of primary prevention of CAD is to prevent cardiac events from occurring in asymptomatic individuals. The subject of this chapter is secondary prevention, the goals of which are to prevent progression of CAD and to prevent recurrent coronary events. Individuals with a prior cardiac event have an increased risk of having a future event of more than 20-fold compared to individuals without prior cardiovascular disease (CVD).[2] In secondary prevention clinical trials, more than 80% of the mortality occurs due to cardiovascular causes.[3] Therefore, with secondary prevention, many fewer patients need to be treated in order to save one life or prevent one clinical event compared with primary prevention strategies. Goals of secondary prevention can broadly be placed into one of two categories: (1) to prevent morbidity and mortality from cardiovascular events, and (2) to improve quality of life and well-being. Effective secondary prevention involves: (1) risk factor management, (2) optimal pharmacologic therapy, and (3) appropriate preventive strategies (Fig. 30.1). This chapter will review current medications and strategies for secondary prevention. With each recommendation, the strength of the evidence base behind the recommendation will be given as a "level of evidence (LOE)." The LOEs include:

- LOE A, indicating several high-quality studies with consistent results or one large, high-quality multicenter trial;
- LOE B, indicating one high-quality study or several studies of moderate quality;
- LOE C, indicating expert opinion.

RISK FACTOR MANAGEMENT

The same risk factors that contribute to the initial development of atherosclerosis also contribute to its progression. There is impressive evidence that risk factor modification (Box 30.1) is effective in preventing recurrent cardiac events.[4] An analysis by Capewell et al. was undertaken to determine how much of the decline in mortality from CAD during the period 1980–2000 could be explained by improvements in interventions and how much could be explained by changes in cardiovascular risk factors.[5] The study estimated that approximately 47% of this decline in mortality was attributable to improved interventions and medical therapies, whereas approximately 44% was attributable to improvements in major risk factors. These data highlight the important role played by risk factor modification in preventing cardiovascular events.

However, despite clear evidence of benefit from risk factor modification for secondary prevention, the level of risk factor control in clinical practice has been disappointing.[6–9] The risk factors that appear to have the largest impact on secondary prevention of CAD are diabetes mellitus, hypertension, dyslipidemia, and smoking.

Diabetes Mellitus

It is widely acknowledged that diabetes is a significant cardiovascular risk factor, being associated with accelerated and more severe CAD (see Chapter 24). Although type 1 and type 2 diabetes mellitus have many differences in pathogenesis, age of onset, and strategies for glucose-lowering, both types are associated with greatly increased cardiovascular event rates.[10–12]

Because one of the hallmarks of diabetes is elevated glucose levels, and because prior epidemiologic studies showed an association between lower glucose levels and reduced cardiovascular events,[13] intensive glucose lowering was postulated to have a beneficial effect on secondary prevention of CAD. Despite the epidemiologic evidence, however, randomized controlled clinical trials evaluating intensive glucose lowering in patients with diabetes to reduce cardiovascular events have not been convincing. The Action to Control Cardiovascular Risk in Diabetes (ACCORD) trial[14] showed that a strategy of intensive glucose control (glycated hemoglobin [HbA1c] < 6% versus a goal of between 7% and 7.9%) did not reduce the primary endpoint, which was a composite of fatal and nonfatal cardiovascular events. Additionally, medications for intensive glucose control have often been associated with increased cardiovascular events, particularly heart failure events. In a meta-analysis including

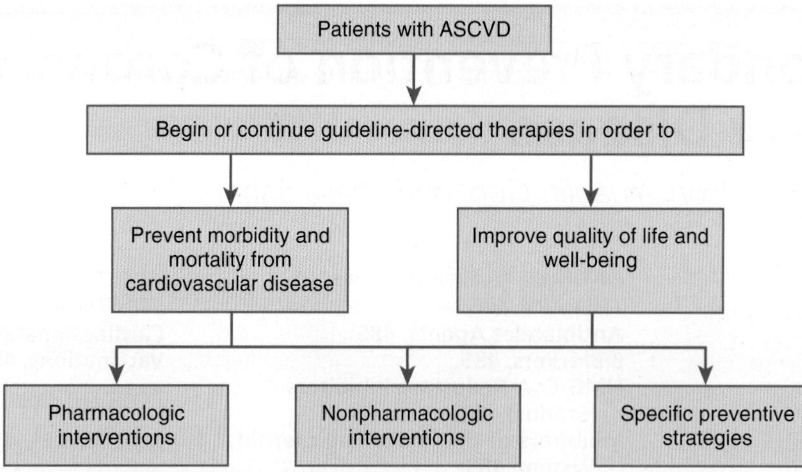

FIG. 30.1 **Effective secondary prevention involves pharmacologic interventions, nonpharmacologic interventions, and specific preventive strategies.** *ASCVD*, Atherosclerotic cardiovascular disease.

BOX 30.1 Secondary Prevention Strategies

PHARMACOLOGIC STRATEGIES	NONPHARMACOLOGIC STRATEGIES
• Antiplatelet agents • β-Blockers • HMG Co-A reductase inhibitors (statins) • ACE-I or ARBs	• Smoking cessation (with assistance) • Weight management • Mediterranean diet • Completion of cardiac rehab program • Physical activity

ACE-I, Angiotensin-converting enzyme inhibitors; *ARBs*, angiotensin receptor blockers; *HMG Co-A reductase inhibitors*, 3-hydroxy-3-methylglutaryl coenzyme A reductase inhibitors (statins).

data from 14 trials and 95,502 patients,[15] glucose-lowering drugs or strategies were associated with a 1.7-kg weight gain and an increased risk of heart failure compared with standard care (relative risk [RR] 1.14, 95% confidence interval [CI] 1.01–1.30; $p = 0.041$).

Of the currently available oral glucose lowering medications, metformin is perhaps the most studied. In the United Kingdom Prospective Diabetes Study (UKPDS), overweight patients with newly diagnosed type 2 diabetes mellitus were randomized to an intensive glucose control strategy that included metformin versus usual care.[16] Whereas lowering blood glucose had no significant effect on cardiovascular complications in the overall trial, there was a 16% reduction (which was not statistically significant, $p = 0.052$) in the risk of combined fatal or nonfatal myocardial infarction (MI) and sudden death in the metformin arm. The current recommendation from the 2012 American College of Cardiology Foundation (ACCF)/American Heart Association (AHA) Guideline for the Diagnosis and Management of Patients With Stable Ischemic Heart Disease (SIHD) recommends that patients with ischemic heart disease (IHD) and diabetes mellitus be treated to a HbA1c goal of less than 7% (LOE: B).[17] These guidelines further specifically state that the drug rosiglitazone should not be initiated in patients with SIHD (LOE: C).

A potentially promising new class of oral hypoglycemic agents is the sodium/glucose cotransporter 2 (SGLT2) inhibitor class. In normal physiologic states, glucose is filtered from the blood by the kidney but is then "reclaimed" into the bloodstream via renal reabsorption of glucose (which has been postulated to be an evolutionary adaptation aimed at preserving calories). Renal SGLT2 is expressed in the proximal tubule and responsible for the majority (>90%) of glucose reabsorption through active transport of glucose (against a concentration gradient) by coupling it to the downhill transport of sodium (Na^+). When SGLT2 is inhibited, less glucose is reclaimed and more Na^+ is excreted.[18] For hypertensive patients with diabetes, these agents have demonstrated an additional benefit of blood pressure (BP) reduction compared with placebo through renal sodium loss.[19]

The 2015 EMPA Reg trial[20] showed beneficial results with the SGLT2 inhibitor empagliflozin. The EMPA Reg trial involved 7020 patients with type 2 diabetes and high cardiovascular risk who, in addition to receiving standard care, were randomized to receive empagliflozin or placebo. The individuals randomized to empagliflozin had a lower rate of the primary composite cardiovascular outcome and of death from any cause than did patients randomized to placebo.

Hypertension

Multiple randomized controlled trials have demonstrated that treating hypertension reduces cardiovascular events in patients both with and without known IHD, even in very-elderly hypertensive individuals.[21–24] This has not been controversial. What has been controversial, however, is the optimal blood pressure goal to achieve this benefit. Whereas it is widely accepted that elevated blood pressure is a significant risk factor, excessively low blood pressure is also of concern, especially in patients with known CAD. According to the J-curve phenomenon, an excessive lowering of diastolic BP might impair coronary perfusion, leading to adverse cardiovascular events.[25–27] In order to find the relationship between on-treatment BP and cardiovascular outcomes in patients with CAD, the J-curve revisited study evaluated 10, 001 patients with CAD in the Treating to New Targets Trial. The investigators found a nonlinear relationship between BP and CVD events, with a higher risk of CVD at lower BPs (110–120/60–70 mm Hg). The adverse events which were higher with lower BP were all-cause mortality, cardiovascular mortality, nonfatal MI, and angina. Conversely, stroke outcomes were reduced with the lower BPs.[28] In another recent post hoc analysis of data of 22,576 patients with hypertension and CAD studied in the International Verapamil-Trandolapril Study (INVEST), the relationship between BP and the primary outcome of all-cause mortality and total MI was found to be J-shaped, particularly for diastolic BP, with a nadir at 119/84 mm Hg. For the outcome of stroke, the investigators did not find a J-curve.[29] However, other investigators note that there is no evidence of harm in treating BP down to a level of 115/75 mm Hg.[30] The 2012 American College of Cardiology (ACC)/AHA SIHD guidelines recommend a BP goal of below 140/90 mm Hg (LOE: A).[17]

Nonetheless, since these guidelines were released, a new study suggests that a lower BP goal will provide even better outcomes for high cardiovascular–risk patients.[31] The Systolic Blood Pressure Intervention Trial (SPRINT) randomized 9361 patients at high cardiovascular risk (61% with a Framingham 10-year CVD risk score ≥ 15%, 20% with CVD, 28% with chronic kidney disease, and 28% older than 75 years) to either a standard BP treatment arm or an intensive BP treatment arm. A total of 4678 patients were assigned to the intensive arm with a goal systolic BP of less than 120 mm Hg, and 4683 were assigned to the standard treatment arm with a goal systolic BP of less than 140 mm Hg. The participants were followed for an average of 3.2 years before the trial was prematurely terminated due to benefit. The investigators found a 25% reduction in the primary outcome (a composite of MI, heart failure, stroke, and total mortality) and a 27% reduction in all-cause mortality among participants who were randomized to the more intensive systolic BP goal of less than 120 mm Hg, compared to participants assigned to the standard treatment arm with a goal of less than 140 mm Hg.

Of note, there were more side effects associated with tighter BP control in SPRINT. Rates of serious adverse events of hypotension, syncope, electrolyte abnormalities, and acute kidney injury were higher in the intensive-treatment group than in the standard-treatment group. An important caveat is that SPRINT was an open-label study, i.e., was not blinded. In addition, patients with diabetes or prior stroke were excluded from this trial, so these results may not be generalizable to these populations. Finally, the elevated risk profile seen in SPRINT was largely driven by advancing age and chronic kidney disease. Notwithstanding these caveats, current evidence suggests that, in patients with CAD, a systolic BP goal of less than 120 mm Hg may improve outcomes. Consistent with these findings, a 2015 meta-analysis by Ettehad et al. analyzed 123 studies with 613,815 participants and came to similar conclusions.[32] These investigators found that for every 10 mm Hg reduction in systolic BP there was a significant reduction in the risk of major cardiovascular disease events (RR 0.80, 95% CI 0.77–0.83), coronary heart disease (0.83, 0.78–0.88), stroke (0.73, 0.68–0.77), and heart failure (0.72, 0.67–0.78), and a significant 13% reduction in all-cause mortality (0.87, 0.84–0.91). The investigators concluded that there is "strong support for lowering blood pressure to systolic blood pressures less than 130 mm Hg."[32]

In patients with hypertension and chronic CAD, most will require a combination of medications, including a thiazide-type diuretic, to achieve optimal BP control. Angiotensin-converting enzyme inhibitors (ACE-I) may also improve outcomes in patients with CAD, especially in those with a history of MI, left ventricular (LV) dysfunction, chronic kidney disease (CKD) or diabetes mellitus. Angiotensin receptor blockers (ARBs) may improve outcomes in the same groups of patients but should be avoided in combination with ACE-I due to an increase in serious adverse events with this combination. β-Blockers improve outcomes in specific populations such as patients with angina pectoris, a history of MI, or LV dysfunction. Aldosterone antagonists improve outcomes in patients with LV dysfunction and heart failure, and calcium antagonists may be useful in the treatment of angina.

Dyslipidemia

Dyslipidemia is a powerful risk factor for atherosclerotic cardiovascular disease (ASCVD). In 2013, the ACC and AHA published guideline recommendations on managing blood cholesterol to reduce ASCVD risk.[33] As with prior cholesterol guidelines, these new recommendations were written with the goal of reducing the risk of atherosclerotic disease, but unlike prior recommendations these guidelines were written using only the highest quality evidence base (randomized controlled trials, or high quality systematic reviews, and meta-analyses). This evidence base was used to specifically define which lipid-modulating strategies were most effective at reducing hard cardiovascular outcomes such as MI, stroke, and cardiovascular death and concluded that the most powerful strategy, with the greatest evidence base, was statin therapy. This is distinct from prior guidelines, which offered several options for pharmacotherapies to reduce cholesterol. These guidelines also stressed that the appropriate intensity of statin therapy should be used with the recommended intensity being defined by an individual's cardiovascular risk rather than the absolute low-density lipoprotein cholesterol (LDL-C) level. These guidelines further define which patients are expected to benefit from statin therapy, and these are known as the *statin benefit* groups. The four statin benefit groups are:

1. adults with clinical established ASCVD,
2. adults with LDL-C > 190 mg/dL,
3. adults (40–75 years of age) with either type 1 or type 2 diabetes with LDL-C of 70–189 mg/dL,
4. adults (40–75 years of age) with > 7.5% 10-year ASCVD risk with LDL-C of 70–189 mg/dL.

At the time of writing of the 2013 cholesterol guidelines, no other lipid-altering medications had been shown in randomized controlled clinical trials to provide additional cardiovascular risk reduction above and beyond statin therapy for secondary prevention and some therapies had demonstrated potential harms.

The Atherothrombosis Intervention in Metabolic Syndrome With Low HDL/High Triglycerides: Impact on Global Health Outcomes (AIM-HIGH) trial tested a strategy of adding niacin-based therapy to statin therapy and found that there was no clinical benefit from the addition of niacin to simvastatin.[34] More recently, the Heart Protection Study 2–Treatment of HDL to Reduce the Incidence of Vascular Events (HPS2-THRIVE) trial confirmed similar findings with the use of extended-release niacin–laropiprant added to the background of simvastatin 40 mg. In this trial there was a significant increase in serious adverse events such as an increased incidence of diabetes and gastrointestinal and musculoskeletal side effects with the addition of the niacin-based therapy to statin therapy.[35] Similarly, the Action to Control Cardiovascular Risk in Diabetes (ACCORD) trial demonstrated no additional benefit of adding fenofibrate to statin therapy in patients with diabetes.[36]

Since these guidelines were released, however, the results of the Improved Reduction of Outcomes: Vytorin Efficacy International Trial (IMPROVE-IT) were released.[37] IMPROVE-IT showed that the combination of simvastatin and ezetimibe compared to simvastatin alone had a 2% absolute risk reduction in the primary composite cardiovascular outcome in patients with recent acute coronary syndrome (ACS). Subgroup analysis showed that the benefits were greatest in the subgroup of patients with diabetes. Given that this trial took approximately 7 years to complete, the results also showed the excellent safety of this combination therapy in patients with prior ACS.

The 2013 ACC/AHA guidelines for management of blood cholesterol in the United States departed from a prior paradigm focused on lipid levels, toward a new paradigm focused primarily on cardiovascular risk. By contrast, the current European guidelines for the management of hyperlipidemia rely on a combination of lipid levels and CVD risk to identify adults in need of statin therapy. In 2011, the European Society of Cardiology (ESC) and European Atherosclerosis Society (EAS) released guidelines for the management of dyslipidemias.[38] These EAS/ESC dyslipidemia guidelines recommend a "treat to risk group" approach and categorize patients into four risk levels: very high risk, high risk, moderate risk, and low risk. Very-high-risk patients include any of the following: (1) documented CVD by invasive or noninvasive testing; (2) previous MI, ACS, percutaneous coronary intervention (PCI), coronary artery bypass graft (CABG), ischemic stroke, or peripheral arterial disease; (3) diabetes mellitus type 2 or type 1 with target organ damage; (4) moderate to severe chronic kidney disease (defined as glomerular filtration rate < 60 mL/min per 1.73m^2); or (5) a calculated 10-year risk SCORE (Systematic Coronary Risk Estimation) of greater than or equal to 10%. Table 30.1 displays the ESC and ACC/AHA guidelines for secondary prevention.

Another promising class of cholesterol-lowering agents for CAD secondary prevention is the proprotein convertase subtilisin/kexin type 9 (PCSK9) inhibitor monoclonal antibodies. The two currently Food and Drug Administration (FDA)-approved PCSK9 inhibitors are alirocumab[39] and evolocumab,[40] which have been shown to produce LDL-C reductions of up to 73%.[40,41] While we await outcomes studies with these two agents, there is currently no specific place for routine use of these agents in secondary prevention, but these agents may ultimately have a role in: (1) ASCVD patients on maximally tolerated statin therapy with inadequate LDL-C reduction, (2) ASCVD patients with recurrent cardiovascular (CV) events while on maximally tolerated statin therapy, and (3) patients with statin intolerance.[42] The guidelines also emphasize the importance of long-term therapeutic lifestyle changes in addition to pharmacologic therapy.

Smoking Cessation

Tobacco use greatly increases the risk of a first or a recurrent cardiac event. Patients with CAD who continue to smoke are more likely to have postinfarction angina[43] and are twice as likely to suffer a subsequent MI as those who quit.[44] Observational studies suggest that smoking cessation will reduce the risk of cardiovascular mortality by up to 50% over the ensuing years;[45] thus smoking cessation remains one of the most effective secondary prevention interventions available. A 2004 systematic review from the Cochrane database[46] reviewed twenty studies that evaluated the effect of smoking cessation on subsequent cardiac events. This analysis found that there was a 36% reduction in the RR of mortality for patients who quit smoking compared with those who continued smoking (RR 0.64, 95% CI 0.58–0.71). There was also a significant reduction in nonfatal MIs (RR 0.68, 95% CI 0.57–0.82). The authors concluded that smoking cessation is associated with a substantial reduction in all-cause mortality among patients with CHD and that this 36% risk reduction compares favorably with other secondary preventive strategies.

In addition to cessation of active smoking, avoidance of exposure to second-hand smoke (SHS) is also important as a secondary preventive measure. Several reports, including two recent separate meta-analyses of 17 and 18 individual studies, assessed the association of SHS with heart disease.[47–50] Both estimated that nonsmoking spouses of smoking partners experience an increased risk of heart disease of approximately 25% (95% CI 17%–32%).[49,50] A review of six studies examining the association between workplace SHS and CVD found a positive association in five of the six studies and a significant dose (exposure)–response relationship between the intensity of exposure to SHS (number of cigarettes smoked by coworkers) and

TABLE 30.1 American College of Cardiology/American Heart Association and European Society of Cardiology/European Atherosclerosis Society Dyslipidemia Management Guidelines for Secondary Prevention

ACC/AHA GUIDELINES			ESC/EAS GUIDELINES		
	Recommendation	Class of Evidence, LOE		Recommendation	Class of Evidence, LOE
Age < 75 years with clinical ASCVD without contraindications to statin therapy, drug-drug interactions, or statin intolerance	High-intensity statin therapy	I, A	Very-high CV risk patients (Calculated SCORE > 10%)	Lifestyle changes and consider drug therapy irrespective of LDL-C. Specifically, in patients with MI statin therapy is recommended irrespective of LDL-C level.	IIa, A
Age > 75 years or safety concerns	Moderate-intensity statin therapy	IIa, B			

ACC, American College of Cardiology; *AHA*, American Heart Association; *ASCVD*, atherosclerotic cardiovascular disease; *CV*, cardiovascular; *EAS*, European Atherosclerosis Society; *ESC*, European Society of Cardiology; *LDL-C*, low-density lipoprotein cholesterol; *LOE*, level of evidence.

From Stone NJ, Robinson JG, Lichtenstein AH, et al., members of the American College of Cardiology/American Heart Association Task Force on Practice Guidelines. 2013 ACC/AHA guideline on the treatment of blood cholesterol to reduce atherosclerotic cardiovascular risk in adults: a report of the American College of Cardiology/American Heart Association Task Force on Practice Guidelines. J Am Coll Cardiol. *2014;63:2889–2934; European Association for Cardiovascular Prevention & Rehabilitation, Reiner Z, Catapano AL, et al. ESC/EAS Guidelines for the management of dyslipidaemias: the Task Force for the management of dyslipidaemias of the European Society of Cardiology (ESC) and the European Atherosclerosis Society (EAS).* Eur Heart J. *2011;32:1769–1818.*

coronary risk.[51] Finally, studies in which coronary event rates were assessed in municipalities that have instituted complete outdoor smoking bans, before and after the bans took place, have revealed impressive reductions in MIs within months of initiation of the smoking bans.[52–54] These data strongly suggest that avoidance of all environmental smoke is prudent as a secondary prevention measure (LOE: B).[55–58]

Lifestyle Risk Factors

All patients with chronic CAD should be counseled about the need for lifestyle modification including smoking cessation, weight control, increased physical activity, alcohol moderation, and sodium reduction, along with emphasis on increased consumption of fresh fruits, vegetables, and low-fat dairy products (LOE: B).

Weight Management

Obesity is associated with increased CAD morbidity and mortality (see Chapter 19).[59] Obesity is typically classified by body mass index (BMI), which is reported as kg/m^2.[60] BMI under 18.5 kg/m^2 is considered to be in the underweight category, BMI of 18.5 to 24.9 kg/m^2 is the normal weight category, BMI of 25.0 to 29.9 kg/m^2 is in the overweight category, and a BMI of 30.0 kg/m^2 or higher is in the obese category.[60] For patients with CAD, weight loss is indicated for those classified as overweight or obese. The AHA recommends measuring BMI at each office visit, then providing objective feedback and consistent counseling on weight loss strategies (LOE: B).[61] Long-term weight maintenance is best achieved by balancing energy expenditure (basal metabolic rate plus physical activity) and energy intake (calories from food).[61] Whereas the recommendation is to maintain BMI within the normal category, improvements in cardiac risk factors are commonly observed with even modest weight loss (10% of baseline weight).[62] Whereas weight loss has been shown to improve cardiovascular risk factors, insufficient evidence exists to determine whether weight reduction decreases cardiovascular events. Nonetheless, achievement of optimal BMI (18.5–24.9 kg/m^2) and waist circumference of less than 40 inches (102 cm) in men and less than 35 (88 cm) inches in women is appropriate.

Diet Modifications

Several trials have examined the effect of dietary modifications (see Chapter 18) on weight loss and cardiovascular risk factors, but fewer studies have examined the effects of specific diets on CAD morbidity and mortality. Currently recommended diets typically fall into one of three categories: (1) low-carbohydrate, (2) low-fat, or (3) Mediterranean-type diets.[63–68]

Low-carbohydrate diets have been shown to lead to weight loss and improvement in some cardiovascular risk factors, however cardiovascular outcome studies are lacking. A recent randomized controlled trial of 311 premenopausal women showed greater mean weight loss at 1 year in participants following the Atkins very-low-carbohydrate diet (4.7 kg mean weight loss) compared with dieters using the Zone moderate carbohydrate–restriction diet (1.6 kg mean weight loss), the Ornish very-low-fat diet (2.2 kg mean weight loss), or the LEARN (Lifestyle, Exercise, Attitudes, Relationships, and Nutrition) carbohydrate-restricted diet (2.6 kg mean weight loss).[67] No studies have determined differences in morbidity, mortality, or cardiovascular outcomes with low-carbohydrate diets, and in fact a recent analysis of a Swedish female cohort showed an increase in overall mortality rates among women with increased protein and decreased carbohydrate intake.[68]

Low-fat diets typically limit dietary fat intake to achieve weight loss. Low-fat diets have also been evaluated as strategies to prevent CAD. One low-fat diet plan that has been shown to improve CAD is the Ornish diet.[69] This diet incorporates a vegetarian diet with very-low-fat intake (approximately 10% of total calories). This plan also integrates exercise, meditation, stress management, and smoking cessation.[70] In a 5-year study of the Ornish program, 48 men who were diagnosed with CAD were enrolled in the Lifestyle Heart Trial. In this study, the Ornish diet lowered low-density lipoprotein (LDL) levels by approximately 20%, whereas triglyceride and high-density lipoprotein (HDL) levels did not change. Those on the Ornish diet also lost an average of 5.8 kg compared with no change in the control group. At 5 years, subjects in the intervention arm had a 72% decrease in anginal symptoms whereas the control group had a 36% increase in anginal symptoms.[71] Myocardial perfusion also improved in the intervention group, as did atherosclerosis severity by quantitative coronary angiography with an average 8% improvement compared to a 27% progression in the control group.[72]

Another diet with a strong evidence base is the Mediterranean diet. The Mediterranean diet has many different interpretations, but it is generally defined as a diet plan that is characteristic of the traditional diets of southern Mediterranean countries.[73] These diets consist of several principal components including high consumption of fruits, vegetables, legumes, grains, and unrefined cereals; generous use of olive oil; moderate to high consumption of fish; moderate consumption of dairy products (cheese and yogurt); moderate consumption of wine; and low consumption of other meat products, especially red meat.[73] Studies of the Mediterranean diet have shown associated improvements in LDL-C, high-density lipoprotein cholesterol (HDL-C), C-reactive protein, and insulin levels.[74,75] The Mediterranean diet has also been evaluated for its role in the reduction and prevention of cardiac events. The Lyon Diet Heart Study[76] was the first trial to demonstrate cardiovascular event reduction with the Mediterranean diet. This study was a prospective randomized controlled trial of 605 patients below 70 years of age who had an MI within the prior 6 months. Patients were randomly assigned to either a control group that received only usual dietary advice, or a group that followed the Mediterranean dietary guidelines. Specifically, the latter group were to consume more bread, root vegetables, and green vegetables; to consume at least one serving of fruit every day; to eat more fish and less red meat (replaced by poultry); and to replace butter and cream with a canola oil spread (which was supplied by the study and was high in the omega-3 fatty acid, alpha linolenic acid). After 27 months, the Mediterranean diet group had a 73% RR reduction in the composite endpoint of fatal plus nonfatal MIs. There was also a 70% RR reduction in total mortality. The endpoints of angina, stroke, heart failure, pulmonary embolism, and deep venous thrombosis were also significantly reduced. These findings were independent of cholesterol levels, systolic BP, sex, or aspirin use. Importantly, it was also discovered that these benefits persisted. A follow-up study of the original trial was published 5 years later and

BOX 30.2 Dietary Recommendations for Coronary Artery Disease Secondary Prevention

1. Saturated fatty acids to account for < 10% of total energy intake, through replacement by polyunsaturated fatty acids
2. Trans unsaturated fatty acids < 1% of total energy intake
3. < 5 g of salt per day
4. 30–45 g fiber per day, from wholegrain products, fruits and vegetables
   200 g of fruit per day (2–3 servings)
   200 g of vegetables per day (2–3 servings)
5. Fish at least twice a week, one being oily fish
   Consumption of alcoholic beverages should be limited to 2 glasses per day (20 g/day of alcohol) for men and 1 glass per day (10 g/day of alcohol) for non-pregnant women

From Task Force Members, Montalescot G, Sechtem U, et al. 2013 ESC guidelines on the management of stable coronary artery disease: the Task Force on the management of stable coronary artery disease of the European Society of Cardiology. *Eur Heart J*. 2013;34(38):2949–3003; Table 25.

found that the benefits originally seen persisted.[77] Box 30.2 and Table 30.2 list recommended dietary guidelines and the three evidence-based diets.

Exercise

Multiple controlled clinical trials have examined the benefits of aerobic exercise (see Chapter 18) in patients with SIHD. A 2004 systematic review and meta-analysis examined 48 randomized controlled trials of exercise-based rehabilitation programs in 8940 patients with IHD.[78] This study revealed that exercise training resulted in a 20% reduction in all-cause mortality and a 26% reduction in cardiac mortality. There were also trends toward a reduction in nonfatal MI and need for coronary revascularization procedures. The reduction in mortality with exercise might be explained by improvements in traditional cardiovascular risk factors, but this has not been proven. In addition to aerobic exercise, the value of resistance exercise has been shown to improve functional capacity and quality of life in patients with SIHD.[79] The 2012 ACC/AHA SIHD guidelines[17] recommend that all patients with SIHD perform 30 to 60 min of moderate-intensity aerobic activity, such as brisk walking, at least 5 days and preferably 7 days per week (LOE: B). This document also recommends that patients increase their daily lifestyle activities like walking, gardening, or household work, and further recommends that for all patients, risk assessment with a physical activity history and/or an exercise test should be used to guide prognosis and exercise prescription (LOE: B). Not all guidelines mandate cardiac testing before recommending exercise to a patient with SIHD, but clinicians should individually evaluate the safety of patients to enter into exercise programs and perform additional cardiac testing if there are any questions or concerns about cardiac safety.

Alcohol

Numerous epidemiologic studies have consistently shown an inverse relationship between alcohol consumption and CAD incidence. Moderate alcohol intake (one to two drinks per day, or 10–30 g/d) is associated with reduced risk of CAD events in both primary prevention and secondary prevention populations.[80] To date, no randomized controlled clinical trials have been performed to verify the cardioprotective benefits of alcohol. Thus, in the absence of data from

TABLE 30.2 Evidence-Based Diets for Cardiovascular Risk Reduction

DASH	FOOD GROUP	SERVING SIZE (PER DAY UNLESS OTHERWISE NOTED)
	Grains and grain products	6–8
	Vegetables	4–5
	Fruit	4–5
	Low-fat or fat-free dairy	2–3
	Lean meat, fish, poultry	2 or less
	Nuts, seeds, dry beans	4–5 per week
	Fats and oils	2–3
	Sweets	5 or less per week
	Sodium	1500–2300 mg
MEDITERRANEAN	**FOOD GROUP**	**SERVING SIZE (PER DAY UNLESS OTHERWISE NOTED)**
	Olive oil	≥ 4 tablespoons
	Tree nuts and peanuts	≥ 3 per week
	Fruits	≥ 3
	Vegetables	≥ 2
	Legumes	≥ 3 per week
	Seafood/fish (particularly fatty fish)	≥ 3 per week
	White meat	Replace red meat
	Optional: wine with meals (only for habitual drinkers)	≥ 7 glasses per week
ORNISH	**NUTRITIONAL CONTENT**	
	Fat	10% of total calories per day
	Cholesterol	10 mg or less per day
	Simple/refined carbohydrates	In moderation
	Animal products	None except egg whites and non-fat milk products
	Calories	Unrestricted unless for weight management
	Sodium	In moderation
	Caffeine	Green tea only—maximum of 2 cups
	Full-fat soy	1 serving full-fat soy product per day (naturally occurring fat from soy typically > 3 g fat per serving)
	Required nutritional supplement	1. Multivitamin 100% daily value with minerals with a 2.4 μg vitamin B_{12} and no iron 2. Cholesterol-free omega-3 fatty acid, approx. 600 mg EPA and 400 mg DHA daily for women and men

DASH, Dietary Approaches to Stop Hypertension; *DHA*, docosahexaenoic acid; *EPA*, eicosapentaenoic acid.
From Moore TJ, Conlin PR, Ard J, Svetkey LP. DASH (Dietary Approaches to Stop Hypertension) diet is effective treatment for stage 1 isolated systolic hypertension. Hypertension. *2001;38:155–158; Estruch R, Ros E, Salas-Salvadó J, et al. Primary prevention of cardiovascular disease with a Mediterranean diet.* N Engl J Med. *2013;368:1279–1290; Ornish, D. Nutrition: Spectrum Guidelines. http://ornishspectrum.com/proven-program/nutrition/.*

randomized controlled clinical trials, no firm recommendations regarding alcohol consumption as a secondary preventive measure can be made. A meta-analysis by Costanzo et al. found J-shaped curves for alcohol consumption and mortality, with a significant maximal protection against cardiovascular mortality with consumption of approximately 26 g/d and maximal protection against mortality from any cause with consumption in the range of 5–10 g/d.[82] The pattern and amount of alcohol intake appears to be more important than the type.

Psychological Factors

Multiple observational studies have demonstrated an association between depression and cardiovascular events (see Chapter 26).[83] Approximately 20% of patients with angiographic evidence of CAD, and a similar percentage of those recovering from acute myocardial infarction (AMI), have comorbid depression. For this reason, the 2012 SIHD guidelines state that it is reasonable to consider screening SIHD patients for depression and to refer or treat when indicated (LOE: B). However, it is important to note that despite the documented association between depression and adverse cardiovascular outcomes, no clinical trials have established a reduction in cardiovascular risk with either counseling or antidepressant therapy.

OPTIMAL PHARMACOLOGIC THERAPY (BOX 30.1)

Antiplatelet Agents

Numerous randomized clinical trials have reported beneficial effects of antiplatelet agents (see Chapter 21) in patients with known CAD.[84] The benefits are impressive in secondary prevention with an approximate 31% reduction in nonfatal re-infarction, a 42% reduction in nonfatal stroke, and a 13% reduction in cardiovascular mortality. The most well-studied antiplatelet agent is the cyclo-oxygenase-1-inhibitor aspirin (acetylsalicylic acid). Thus, current recommendations state that aspirin should be used in all secondary prevention patients. The doses studied in the various clinical trials range from 50 mg to 500 mg daily. A dose of 75 mg/d appears to be equally as effective as higher doses in prevention of CAD events with lower bleeding rates; thus guidelines recommend that treatment with aspirin 75 to 162 mg/d should be continued indefinitely in the absence of contraindications in patients with SIHD (LOE: A).[17] Another important class of antiplatelet agents is the adenosine diphosphate (ADP)-dependent $P2Y_{12}$ inhibitor class, which includes clopidogrel, ticagrelor, and prasugrel.[85] Current guidelines recommend 12 months of dual antiplatelet therapy with aspirin and a $P2Y_{12}$ inhibitor for patients who are post-MI or post stent placement. Longer-term dual antiplatelet therapy beyond 1 year may be considered in selected patients with chronic CAD (see Chapter 21); however the balance between reduction in ischemic events versus the increase in bleeding events must always be considered when dual antiplatelet therapy is employed.

β-Blockers

β-Blockers have been extensively studied in secondary prevention and have been found to reduce the risk of re-infarction by approximately 25%, the risk of sudden death by 32%, and the risk of dying by 23% post-MI.[86] It is not completely understood how β-blockers exert their protective mechanisms, but reduction in heart rate is believed to play a role. Current guidelines[17] recommend that β-blocker therapy should be started and continued for 3 years in all patients with normal LV function post ACS (LOE: B). The guidelines also recommend that β-blocker therapy should be used in all patients with LV systolic dysfunction (ejection fraction [EF] < 40%) with heart failure or prior MI, unless contraindicated (LOE: A). Carvedilol, metoprolol succinate, or bisoprolol are recommended, because these agents have been shown in large-scale trials to improve outcomes[87–89] (LOE: A). These guidelines also state that β-blockers may be considered as chronic therapy for all other patients with coronary or other vascular disease (LOE: C). However, it is not clear that β-blockers improve outcomes among patients with stable CAD without recent MI or left ventricular systolic dysfunction. A recent longitudinal, observational study using propensity score matched analysis analyzed 44,708 patients with a median follow-up of 44 months. The results showed the event rates were not significantly different in patients on β-blocker therapy compared to those who were not on β-blocker therapy, even in those with a prior MI. Only in patients with a recent MI (within 1 year) was β-blocker use associated with a lower incidence of CVD.[90]

HMG-CoA Reductase Inhibitors (Statins)

As previously noted, statins are the cholesterol-lowering medications with the greatest clinical trial evidence demonstrating a reduction in coronary events. Therefore, high-intensity statin therapy should be offered to all adults under the age of 75 years with clinically established ASCVD (LOE: A). Moderate-intensity statin therapy may be used in patients who cannot tolerate higher-dose statins or in patients over the age of 75 years (LOE: B).

Inhibitors of the Renin-Angiotensin System

Multiple clinical trials have demonstrated that ACE-I reduce the risk of ischemic events and mortality[91–95] both in patients with and without known CAD. Clinical studies have demonstrated benefits in patients after MI and in patients with and without LV dysfunction. ARBs have been shown to have similar benefits.[96,97] Both classes of agents reduce BP, but there appear to be both BP-dependent and BP-independent effects. In a meta-analysis of 26 trials including patients with both hypertension and cardiovascular disease,[98] the effects of ACE-I and ARBs on major vascular events were compared. In this study, there were no significant differences between the effects of ACE-I–based regimens or ARB-based regimens on the risk of stroke, ischemic heart disease, or heart failure for equivalent BP reduction. In studies without BP reduction, however, there appeared to be greater benefits for ACE-I–based regimens compared to ARB-based regimens. In one study, ACE-I were associated with a 9% reduced risk for ischemic heart disease compared to ARBs ($p = 0.004$), whereas no differences were observed in the risk of stroke or heart failure. The 2012 guidelines[17] recommend that ARBs be substituted for ACE-I in patients with SIHD and hypertension who are intolerant of ACE-I (LOE: A). They also recommend that ACE-I be prescribed in all patients with SIHD who also have hypertension, diabetes mellitus, left ventricular ejection fraction

(LVEF) 40% or less, or CKD, unless contraindicated (LOE: A). These guidelines recommend that ARBs be prescribed in patients with SIHD who have hypertension, diabetes mellitus, LV systolic dysfunction, or CKD, and have indications for, but are intolerant of, ACE-I (LOE: A).

ADDITIONAL PREVENTIVE STRATEGIES (BOX 30.1)

Cardiac Rehabilitation

Studies of cardiac rehabilitation (see Chapter 18) following MI have demonstrated reduced mortality. As previously noted, a meta-analysis incorporating data from 8940 patients revealed that exercise training resulted in a 20% reduction in all-cause mortality and a 26% reduction in cardiac mortality.[78] A meta-analysis of 10 randomized trials demonstrated a 24% reduction in total mortality and a 25% reduction in cardiovascular mortality in the exercise group.[99] Another meta-analysis of 22 randomized trials of cardiac rehabilitation post-MI found similar results with a 20% reduction in total mortality and a 22% reduction in cardiovascular mortality after 3 years.[100] Because of these strong, consistent results, current guidelines recommend medically supervised programs (cardiac rehabilitation) and physician-directed, home-based programs for at-risk patients with SIHD at the time of first diagnosis (LOE: A).[17] Unfortunately, whereas many patients are eligible to attend cardiac rehabilitation, many patients are never referred. There are opportunities through continued research, cost-effective analysis, and performance improvement measures to help close the gap in cardiac referral rates for secondary prevention of CAD.[101]

Vaccinations

A 2015 Cochrane systematic review[102] that included eight clinical trials and 12,029 participants compared clinical outcomes in patients who had received influenza vaccination with those who received either placebo or no vaccination. Cardiovascular mortality was significantly reduced by influenza vaccination (RR of 0.45, 95% CI 0.26–0.76; $p = 0.003$), and the authors concluded that in patients with cardiovascular disease, influenza vaccination may reduce cardiovascular mortality and combined cardiovascular events. The 2012 guidelines[17] recommend that patients with SIHD receive an annual influenza vaccination (LOE: B). The Centers for Disease Control recommend the use of pneumococcal polysaccharide vaccine (Pneumovax) in patients with chronic heart failure or cardiomyopathy. Pneumococcal pneumonia has been associated with acute cardiac events such as arrhythmia, MI, and acute heart failure.[103]

CONCLUSIONS

Once cardiovascular disease is manifest in patients, they remain at elevated risk for a recurrent cardiac event. Application of guideline-directed medical therapy has been shown to decrease future cardiac events, thus it is imperative that secondary prevention efforts are applied to all patients at risk. In one study using the Duke Databank for Cardiovascular Disease,[104] consistent use of guideline-directed medical therapies (GDMT) was analyzed in relation to cardiovascular outcomes. In this study, consistent use of GDMT was associated with lower adjusted mortality as follows: consistent aspirin use (hazard ratio [HR] 0.58, 95% CI 0.54–0.62); consistent β-blocker use (HR 0.63, 95% CI 0.59–0.67); consistent lipid-lowering therapy (HR 0.52, 95% CI 0.42–0.65); and consistent use of all three (HR 0.67, 95% CI 0.59–0.77).

It is important to remember that the approach to secondary prevention requires partnerships among the healthcare team, the patient, his or her family, and his or her community. The goal of these partnerships is to assure an effective exchange of information, sharing of concerns, and an improved understanding of treatments, with the aim of improving quality of life and health outcomes. If appropriate strategies and medications are employed, clinical trials have proven that patient outcomes will be significantly improved.

References

1. Mozaffarian D, Benjamin EJ, Go AS, et al. on behalf of the American Heart Association Statistics Committee and Stroke Statistics Subcommittee. Heart Disease and Stroke Statistics—2016 Update. http://circ.ahajournals.org/content/early/2015/12/16/CIR.0000000000000350.
2. Pekkanen J, Linn S, Heiss G, et al.: Ten-year mortality from cardiovascular disease in relation to cholesterol level among men with and without preexisting cardiovascular disease, *New Engl J Med* 322:1700, 1990.
3. Rossouw JE, Lewis B, Rifkind BM: The value of lowering cholesterol after myocardial infarction, *New Engl J Med* 323:1112, 1990.
4. Haskell WL, Alderman EL, Fair JM, et al.: Effects of intensive multiple risk-factor reduction on coronary atherosclerosis and clinical cardiac events in men and women with coronary artery disease, The Stanford Coronary Risk Intervention Project (SCRIP), *Circulation* 89:975, 1994.
5. Ford ES, Ajani UA, Croft JB, et al.: Explaining the decrease in U.S. deaths from coronary disease, 1980-2000, *N Engl J Med* 356:2388, 2007.
6. Wood D, De Bacquer D, De Backer G, et al.: on behalf of the EUROASPIRE Study Group. A European Society of Cardiology survey of secondary prevention of coronary heart disease: principal results, *Eur Heart J* 18:1569–1582, 1997.
7. Bhatt DL, Steg PG, Ohman EM, et al.: for the REACH Registry Investigators. International prevalence, recognition, and treatment of cardiovascular risk factors in outpatients with atherothrombosis, *JAMA* 295:180–189, 2006.
8. Farkouh ME, Boden WE, Bittner V, et al.: Risk factor control for coronary artery disease secondary prevention in large randomized trials, *J Am Coll Cardiol* 61:1607–1615, 2013.
9. Mehta RH, Bhatt DL, Steg PG, et al.: on behalf of the REACH Registry Investigators. Modifiable risk factors control and its relationship with 1 year outcomes after coronary artery bypass surgery: insights from the REACH registry, *Eur Heart J* 29:3052–3060, 2008.
10. Seshasai SR, Kaptoge S, Thompson A, et al.: on behalf of the Emerging Risk Factors Collaboration. Diabetes mellitus, fasting glucose, and risk of cause-specific death, *N Engl J Med* 364:829–841, 2011.
11. Haffner SM, Lehto S, Rönnemaa T, et al.: Mortality from coronary heart disease in subjects with type 2 diabetes and in nondiabetic subjects with and without prior myocardial infarction, *N Engl J Med* 339:229, 1998.
12. Schramm TK, Gislason GH, Køber L, et al.: Diabetes patients requiring glucose-lowering therapy and nondiabetics with a prior myocardial infarction carry the same cardiovascular risk: a population study of 3.3 million people, *Circulation* 117:1945, 2008.
13. Selvin E, Steffes MW, Zhu H, et al.: Glycated hemoglobin, diabetes, and cardiovascular risk in nondiabetic adults, *N Engl J Med* 362:800, 2010.
14. Gerstein HC, Miller ME, Byington RP, et al.: on behalf of the Action to Control Cardiovascular Risk in Diabetes Study Group. Effects of intensive glucose lowering in type 2 diabetes, *N Engl J Med* 358:2545–2559, 2008.
15. Udell JA, Cavender MA, Bhatt DL, et al.: Glucose-lowering drugs or strategies and cardiovascular outcomes in patients with or at risk for type 2 diabetes: a meta-analysis of randomised controlled trials, *Lancet Diabetes Endocrinol* 3:356–366, 2015.
16. Holman RR, Paul SK, Bethel A, et al.: 10-year follow-up of intensive glucose control in type 2 diabetes, *N Engl J Med* 359:1577–1589, 2008.
17. Fihn SD, Gardin JM, Abrams J, et al.: American College of Cardiology Foundation/American Heart Association Task Force: 2012 ACCF/AHA/ACP/AATS/PCNA/SCAI/STS guideline for the diagnosis and management of patients with stable ischemic heart disease, *Circulation* 126:e354–e471, 2012.
18. Chao EC, Henry RR: SGLT2 inhibition—a novel strategy for diabetes treatment, *Nat Rev Drug Discov* 9:551–559, 2010.
19. Weir MR, Januszewicz A, Gilbert RE, et al.: Effect of canagliflozin on blood pressure and adverse events related to osmotic diuresis and reduced intravascular volume in patients with type 2 diabetes mellitus, *Clin Hypertens (Greenwich)* 16:875, 2014.
20. Zinman B, Wanner C, Lachin JM, et al.: Empagliflozin, cardiovascular outcomes, and mortality in type 2 diabetes, *N Engl J Med* 373:2117, 2015.
21. Blood Pressure Lowering Treatment Trialists' Collaboration, Sundström J, Arima H, et al.: Blood pressure-lowering treatment based on cardiovascular risk: a meta-analysis of individual patient data, *Lancet* 384:591–598, 2014.
22. Lewington S, Clarke R, Qizilbash N, et al.: Age-specific relevance of usual blood pressure to vascular mortality: a meta-analysis of individual data for one million adults in 61 prospective studies, *Lancet* 360:1903, 2002.
23. Law MR, Morris JK, Wald NJ. Use of blood pressure lowering drugs in the prevention of cardiovascular disease: meta-analysis of 147 randomised trials in the context of expectations from prospective epidemiological studies, *BMJ* 338:B1665, 2009. http://dx.doi.org/10.1136/bmj.b1665.
24. Beckett NS, Peters R, Fletcher AE, et al.: HYVET Study Group. Treatment of hypertension in patients 80 years of age or older, *N Engl J Med* 358:1887, 2008.
25. Verdecchia P, Angeli F, Cavallini C, et al.: The optimal blood pressure target for patients with coronary artery disease, *Curr Cardiol Rep* 12:302, 2010.
26. Rabkin SW, Waheed A, Poulter RS, et al.: Myocardial perfusion pressure in patients with hypertension and coronary artery disease: implications for DBP targets in hypertension management, *J Hypertens* 31:975, 2013.

27. Bangalore S, Kumar S, Volodarskiy A, et al.: Blood pressure targets in patients with coronary artery disease: observations from traditional and Bayesian random effects meta-analysis of randomised trials, *Heart* 99:601, 2013.
28. Bangalore S, Messerli FH, Wun CC, et al.: J-curve revisited: an analysis of blood pressure and cardiovascular events in the Treating to New Targets (TNT) Trial, *Eur Heart J* 31:2897, 2010.
29. Messerli FH, Mancia G, Conti CR, et al.: Dogma disputed: can aggressively lowering blood pressure in hypertensive patients with coronary artery disease be dangerous? *Ann Intern Med* 144:884, 2006.
30. Fuchs FD, Fuchs SC: Blood pressure targets in the treatment of high blood pressure: a reappraisal of the J-shaped phenomenon, *J Hum Hypertens* 28:80, 2014.
31. SPRINT Research Group, Wright Jr JT, Williamson JD, et al.: A randomized trial of intensive versus standard blood pressure control, *N Engl J Med* 373:2103–2116, 2015.
32. Ettehad D, Emdin CA, Kiran A, et al.: Blood pressure lowering for prevention of cardiovascular disease and death: a systematic review and meta-analysis, *Lancet* 387:957–967, 2016.
33. Stone NJ, Robinson JG, Lichtenstein AH, et al, members of the American College of Cardiology/American Heart Association Task Force on Practice Guidelines. 2013 ACC/AHA guideline on the treatment of blood cholesterol to reduce atherosclerotic cardiovascular risk in adults: a report of the American College of Cardiology/American Heart Association Task Force on Practice Guidelines, *J Am Coll Cardiol* 63:2889–2934, 2014.
34. AIM-HIGH Investigators: The role of niacin in raising high-density lipoprotein cholesterol to reduce cardiovascular events in patients with atherosclerotic cardiovascular disease and optimally treated low-density lipoprotein cholesterol: baseline characteristics of study participants. The Atherothrombosis Intervention in Metabolic syndrome with low HDL/high triglycerides: Impact on Global Health outcomes (AIM-HIGH) trial, *Am Heart J* 161: 538–534, 2011.
35. HPS2-THRIVE Collaborative Group, Landray MJ, Haynes R, et al.: Effects of extended-release niacin with laropiprant in high-risk patients, *N Engl J Med* 371:203, 2014.
36. Margolis KL, O'Connor PJ, Morgan TM, et al.: Outcomes of combined cardiovascular risk factor management strategies in type 2 diabetes: the ACCORD randomized trial, *Diabetes Care* 37:1721, 2014.
37. Cannon CP, Blazing MA, Giugliano RP, et al.: Ezetimibe added to statin therapy after acute coronary syndromes, *New Engl J Med* 372:2387, 2015.
38. European Association for Cardiovascular Prevention & Rehabilitation, Reiner Z, Catapano AL, et al.: ESC/EAS Guidelines for the management of dyslipidaemias: the Task Force for the management of dyslipidaemias of the European Society of Cardiology (ESC) and the European Atherosclerosis Society (EAS), *Eur Heart J* 32:1769–1818, 2011.
39. Schwartz GG, Bessac L, Berdan LG, et al.: Effect of alirocumab, a monoclonal antibody to PCSK9, on long-term cardiovascular outcomes following acute coronary syndromes: rationale and design of the ODYSSEY outcomes trial, *Am Heart J* 168:682, 2014.
40. Stein EA, Honarpour N, Wasserman SM, et al.: Effect of the PCSK9 monoclonal antibody, AMG 145, in homozygous familial hypercholesterolemia, *Circulation* 128:2113, 2013.
41. Raal F, Scott R, Somaratne R, et al.: Low-density lipoprotein cholesterol-lowering effects of AMG 145, a monoclonal antibody to proprotein convertase subtilisin/kexin type 9 serine protease in patients with heterozygous familial hypercholesterolemia: the Reduction of LDL-C with PCSK9 Inhibition in Heterozygous Familial Hypercholesterolemia Disorder (RUTHERFORD) randomized trial, *Circulation* 126:2408, 2012.
42. Navarese EP, Kolodziejczak M, Schulze V, et al.: Effects of proprotein convertase subtilisin/kexin type 9 antibodies in adults with hypercholesterolemia: a systematic review and meta-analysis, *Ann Intern Med* 163:40–51, 2015.
43. Daly LE, Graham IM, Hickey N, Mulcahy R: Does stopping smoking delay onset of angina after infarction? *Br Med J (Clin Res Ed)* 291:935–937, 1985.
44. Hubert HB, Holford TR, Kannel WB: Clinical characteristics and cigarette smoking in relation to prognosis of angina pectoris in Framingham, *Am J Epidemiol* 115:231, 1982.
45. Wilhelmsson C, Vedin JA, Elmfeldt D, et al.: Smoking and myocardial infarction, *Lancet* 1:415, 1975.
46. Critchley J, Capewell S: Smoking cessation for the secondary prevention of coronary heart disease, *Cochrane Database Syst Rev* 1:CD003041, 2004.
47. Glantz SA, Parmley WW: Passive smoking and heart disease: mechanisms and risk, *JAMA* 273:1047, 1995.
48. Wells AJ: Heart disease from passive smoking in the workplace, *J Am Coll Cardiol* 31:1, 1998.
49. Thun M, Henley J, Apicella L: Epidemiologic studies of fatal and nonfatal cardiovascular disease and ETS from spousal smoking, *Environ Health Perspect* 107:841, 1999.
50. He J, Vupputuri S, Allen K, et al.: Passive smoking and the risk of coronary heart disease: a meta-analysis of epidemiologic studies, *N Engl J Med* 340:920, 1999.
51. Kawachi I, Colditz GA: Workplace exposure to passive smoking and risk of cardiovascular disease: summary of epidemiologic studies, *Environ Health Perspect* 107:847, 1999.
52. Bar CD, Diez DM, Wang Y, et al.: Comprehensive smoking bans and acute myocardial infarction among Medicare enrollees in 387 US counties: 1999–2008, *Am J Epidemiol* 176:642–648, 2012.
53. Jones MR, Barnova J, Stranges S, et al.: Cardiovascular events following smoke-free legislations: an updated systematic review and meta-analysis, *Curr Environ Health Rep* 1:239, 2014.
54. Tan CE, Glantz SA: Association between smoke-free legislation and hospitalizations for cardiac, cerebrovascular, and respiratory diseases: a meta-analysis, *Circulation* 126:2177, 2012.
55. Hubbard R, Lewis S, Smith C, et al.: Use of nicotine replacement therapy and the risk of acute myocardial infarction, stroke, and death, *Tob Control* 14:416, 2005.
56. Tonstad S, Farsang C, Klaene G, et al.: Bupropion SR for smoking cessation in smokers with cardiovascular disease: a multicentre, randomised study, *Eur Heart J* 24:946, 2003.
57. Rigotti NA, Pipe AL, Benowitz NL, et al.: Efficacy and safety of varenicline for smoking cessation in patients with cardiovascular disease. A randomized trial, *Circulation* 121:221, 2010.
58. Pipe AL, Papadakis S, Reid RD: The role of smoking cessation in the prevention of coronary artery disease, *Curr Atheroscler Rep* 12:145, 2010.
59. National Institutes of Health (NIH), National Heart, Lung, and Blood Institute (NHLBI): *The Practical Guide: Identification, Evaluation, and Treatment of Overweight and Obesity in Adults*, Bethesda, National Institutes of Health, NIH publication 00-4084; 2000.
60. Smith Jr SC, Allen J, Blair SN, et al.: AHA/ACC guidelines for secondary prevention for patients with coronary and other atherosclerotic vascular disease: 2006 update: endorsed by the National Heart, Lung, and Blood Institute, *Circulation* 113:2363, 2006.
61. Yancy Jr WS, Olsen MK, Guyton JR, et al.: A low-carbohydrate, ketogenic diet versus a low-fat diet to treat obesity and hyperlipidemia: a randomized, controlled trial, *Ann Intern Med* 140:769, 2004.
62. Klein S, Burke LE, Bray GA, et al.: Clinical implications of obesity with specific focus on cardiovascular disease: a statement for professionals from the American Heart Association Council on Nutrition, Physical Activity, and Metabolism: endorsed by the American College of Cardiology Foundation, *Circulation* 110:2952, 2004.
63. Foster GD, Wyatt HR, Hill JO, et al.: A randomized trial of a low-carbohydrate diet for obesity, *N Engl J Med* 348:2082, 2003.
64. Sondike SB, Copperman N, Jacobson MS: Effects of a low-carbohydrate diet on weight loss and cardiovascular risk factor in overweight adolescents, *J Pediatr* 142:253, 2003.
65. Samaha FF, Iqbal N, Seshadri P, et al.: A low-carbohydrate as compared with a low-fat diet in severe obesity, *N Engl J Med* 348:2074, 2003.
66. Gardner CD, Kiazand A, Alhassan S, et al.: Comparison of the Atkins, Zone, Ornish, and LEARN diets for change in weight and related risk factors among overweight premenopausal women: the A to Z Weight Loss Study: a randomized trial, *JAMA* 297:969–977, 2007.
67. Dansinger ML, Gleason JA, Griffith JL, et al.: Comparison of the Atkins, Ornish, Weight Watchers, and Zone diets for weight loss and heart disease risk reduction: a randomized trial, *JAMA* 293:43, 2005.
68. Lagiou P, Sandin S, Weiderpass E, et al.: Low carbohydrate-high protein diet and mortality in a cohort of Swedish women, *J Intern Med* 261:366, 2007.
69. Ornish D: Very-low fat diets, *Circulation* 100:1013, 1999.
70. Ornish D, Scherwitz LW, Doody R, et al.: Effects of stress management training and dietary changes in treating ischemic heart disease, *JAMA* 249:54, 1983.
71. Ornish D, Scherwitz LW, Billings JH, et al.: Intensive lifestyle changes for reversal of coronary heart disease, *JAMA* 280:2001, 1998.
72. Gould KL, Ornish D, Scherwitz L, et al.: Changes in myocardial perfusion abnormalities by positron emission tomography after long-term, intense risk factor modification, *JAMA* 274:894, 1995.
73. Ferro-Luzzi A, Sette S: The Mediterranean diet: an attempt to define its present and past composition, *Eur J Clin Nutr* 43(Suppl 2):13, 1989.
74. Esposito K, Marfella R, Ciotola M, et al.: Effect of a Mediterranean-style diet on endothelial dysfunction and markers of vascular inflammation in the metabolic syndrome: a randomized trial, *JAMA* 292:1440, 2004.
75. Chrysohoou C, Panagiotakos DB, Pitsavos C, et al.: Adherence to the Mediterranean diet attenuates inflammation and coagulation process in healthy adults: the ATTICA Study, *J Am Coll Cardiol* 44:152, 2004.
76. de Lorgeril M, Salen P, Martin JL, et al.: Mediterranean diet, traditional risk factors, and the rate of cardiovascular complications after myocardial infarction: final report of the Lyon Diet Heart Study, *Circulation* 99:779, 1999.
77. de Lorgeril M, Salen P, Martin J-L, et al.: Mediterranean diet, traditional risk factors, and the rate of cardiovascular complications after myocardial infarction: final report of the Lyon Diet Heart Study, *Circulation* 99:779, 1999.
78. Taylor RS, Brown A, Ebrahim S, et al.: Exercise-based rehabilitation for patients with coronary heart disease: systematic review and meta-analysis of randomized controlled trials, *Am J Med* 116:682, 2004.
79. McCartney N, McKelvie RS, Haslam DR, et al.: Usefulness of weightlifting training in improving strength and maximal power output in coronary artery disease, *Am J Cardiol* 67:939, 1991.
80. Mukamal KJ, Maclure M, Muller JE, et al.: Prior alcohol consumption and mortality following acute myocardial infarction, *JAMA* 285:1965, 2001.
81. Deleted in proofs.
82. Di Castelnuovo A, Costanzo S, Bagnardi V, et al.: Alcohol dosing and total mortality in men and women: an updated meta-analysis of 34 prospective studies, *Arch Intern Med* 166:2437, 2006.
83. Poole L, Dickens C, Steptoe A: The puzzle of depression and acute coronary syndrome: reviewing the role of acute inflammation, *J Psychosom Res* 71:61, 2011.
84. Antiplatelet Trialists Collaboration: Collaborative overview of randomised trials of antiplatelet therapy—I: prevention of death, myocardial infarction, and stroke by prolonged antiplatelet therapy in various categories of patients, *BMJ* 308:81–106, 1994.
85. Cattaneo M: New P2Y12 Inhibitors, *Circulation* 121:171–179, 2010.
86. Freemantle N, Cleland J, Young P, et al.: Beta blockade after myocardial infarction: systematic review and meta regression analysis, *BMJ* 318:1730–1737, 1999.
87. Packer M, Bristow MR, Cohn JN, et al.: The effect of carvedilol on morbidity and mortality in patients with chronic heart failure. U.S. Carvedilol Heart Failure Study Group, *N Engl J Med* 334:1349, 1996.
88. Leizorovicz A, Lechat P, Cucherat M, et al.: Bisoprolol for the treatment of chronic heart failure: a meta-analysis on individual data of two placebo-controlled studies—CIBIS and CIBIS II. Cardiac Insufficiency Bisoprolol Study, *Am Heart J* 143:301, 2002.
89. Poole-Wilson PA, Swedberg K, Cleland JG, et al.: Comparison of carvedilol and metoprolol on clinical outcomes in patients with chronic heart failure in the Carvedilol Or Metoprolol European Trial (COMET): randomised controlled trial, *Lancet* 362:7, 2003.
90. Bangalore S, Steg G, Deedwania P, et al.: β-Blocker use and clinical outcomes in stable outpatients with and without coronary artery disease, *JAMA* 308:1340, 2012.
91. Lonn EM, Yusuf S, Jha P, et al.: Emerging role of angiotensin converting enzyme inhibitors in cardiac and vascular protection, *Circulation* 90:2056, 1994.
92. Pfeffer MA, Braunwald E, Moye LA, et al.: Effect of captopril on mortality and morbidity in patients with left ventricular dysfunction after myocardial infarction. Results of the survival and ventricular enlargement trial. The SAVE Investigators, *N Engl J Med* 327:669, 1992.
93. Al-Mallah MH, Tleyjeh IM, bdel-Latif AA, et al.: Angiotensin converting enzyme inhibitors in coronary artery disease and preserved left ventricular systolic function: a systematic review and meta-analysis of randomized controlled trials, *J Am Coll Cardiol* 47:1576, 2006.
94. Pitt B, O'Neill B, Feldman R, et al.: The QUinapril Ischemic Event Trial (QUIET): evaluation of chronic ACE inhibitor therapy in patients with ischemic heart disease and preserved left ventricular function, *Am J Cardiol* 87:1058, 2001.
95. Heart Outcomes Prevention Evaluation Study Investigators: Effects of ramipril on cardiovascular and microvascular outcomes in people with diabetes mellitus: results of the HOPE study and MICRO-HOPE substudy, *Lancet* 355:253–259, 2000.
96. ONTARGET Investigators, Yusuf S, Teo KK, Pogue J, et al.: Telmisartan, ramipril, or both in patients at high risk for vascular events, *N Engl J Med* 358:1547–1559, 2008.
97. Munger MA: Use of angiotensin receptor blockers in cardiovascular protection: current evidence and future directions, *P T* 36:22–40, 2011.
98. Turnbull F, Neal B, Pfeffer M, et al.: Blood pressure-dependent and independent effects of agents that inhibit the renin-angiotensin system, *J Hypertens* 25:951, 2007.
99. Oldridge NB, Guyatt GH, Fischer ME, Rimm AA: Cardiac rehabilitation after myocardial infarction. Combined experience of randomized clinical trials, *JAMA* 260:945, 1988.
100. O'Connor GT, Buring JE, Yusuf S, et al.: An overview of randomized trials of rehabilitation with exercise after myocardial infarction, *Circulation* 80:234, 1989.
101. Arena R, Williams M, Forman DE, et al.: Increasing referral and participation rates to outpatient cardiac rehabilitation: the valuable role of healthcare professionals in the inpatient and home health settings: a science advisory from the American Heart Association, *Circulation* 125: 1321–1329, 2012.
102. Clar C, Oseni Z, Flowers N, et al.: Influenza vaccines for preventing cardiovascular disease, *Cochrane Database Syst Rev* 5:CD005050, 2015. http://dx.doi.org/10.1002/14651858.CD005050.pub3.
103. Musher DM, Rueda AM, Kaka AS, Mapara SM: The association between pneumococcal pneumonia and acute cardiac events, *Clin Infect Dis* 45:158, 2007.
104. Newby LK, LaPointe NM, Chen AY, et al.: Long-term adherence to evidence-based secondary prevention therapies in coronary artery disease, *Circulation* 113:203, 2006.

Index

Note: Page numbers followed by "*b*", "*t*", and "*f*" refer to boxes, tables, and figures respectively.